Arterial Treatment of Neurological Diseases

Shailendra Joshi
Editor

Arterial Treatment of Neurological Diseases

Current Status and Future Directions

Springer

Editor
Shailendra Joshi, MBBS,MD Anesthesiology,FFARCS(I)
Associate Professor
Department of Anesthesiology
Columbia University Irving Medical Center
New York, NY, USA

ISBN 978-3-031-80172-3 ISBN 978-3-031-80173-0 (eBook)
https://doi.org/10.1007/978-3-031-80173-0

This Springer imprint is published by the registered company Springer Nature Switzerland AG
The registered company address is: Gewerbestrasse 11, 6330 Cham, Switzerland

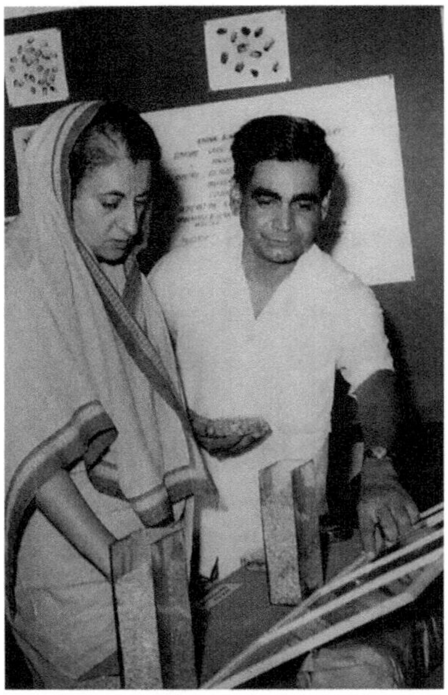

This book is dedicated to my late parents, Jaya and Lalit Mohan Joshi. My father, Lalit Mohan, seen here with the Indian Prime Minister, Mrs. Indira Gandhi, played an essential role in increasing India's wheat production. Known for his stubborn honesty, he was called a "Scientist's scientist." He cautioned me that there were no shortcuts on the road to excellence. My mother, Jaya, warned me that a single letter tarnishes a whole page of excellent handwriting. These two early childhood lessons have been challenging and inspiring throughout my life.

Foreword: Arterial Drug Delivery—The Neurosurgical Perspective

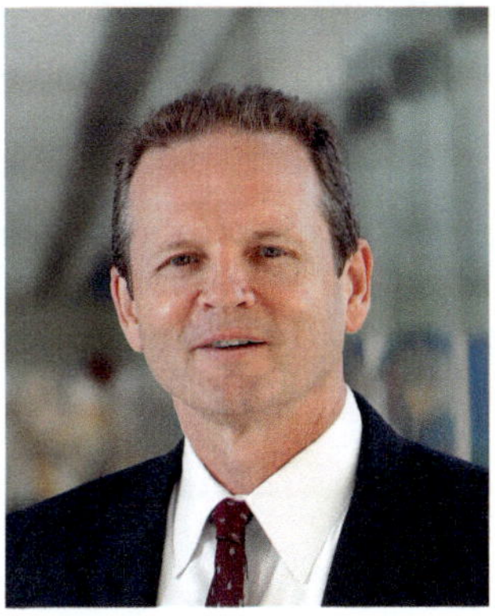

Drug delivery has remained a significant hurdle to the treatment of brain tumors. The first attempt to treat brain tumors with arterial injections began in the 1950s. The idea of selectively delivering drugs by arterial injections to brain tumors will soon celebrate its 75th anniversary. Yet, the failure to demonstrate increased survival of patients in randomized clinical trials has resulted in waning interest in this approach. Very few groups have persisted with this mode of drug delivery. In fairness, other modes of drug delivery have also struggled to impact patient survival, particularly for those with glioblastoma multiforme.

This book provides a timely review of arterial drug delivery technology for treating neurological diseases. As interest in arterial brain tumors has waned over the last two decades, endovascular technology has dramatically advanced. Modern endovascular approaches using stenting devices and embolic materials have provided novel approaches to treating cerebrovascular diseases. However, the field of endovascular pharmacology has not advanced. From the neurosurgical perspective, arterial drug treatments fall into three broad groups: (a) Those widely accepted and considered safe and effective, including Wada testing for mapping brain functions; (b) those clinically used in extremis with inconsistent benefits, such as intraarterial vasodilator treatment of cerebral vasospasm or thrombolysis for acute ischemic stroke; and (c) experimental or sporadic applications, such as for treating brain tumors.

This book, *Arterial Treatment of Neurological Diseases*, presents the current status and future applications of arterial drug delivery technology in the context of brain diseases. Arterial drug delivery is a deceptively simple concept. The primary challenge in arterial delivery is to maximize the drug uptake during its initial pass through the cerebral circulation safely and, if possible, without disrupting the blood–brain barrier. Optimizing first-pass drug uptake is a complex pharmacological and bioengineering problem. Since this transit occurs in 1–5 s, it is difficult to investigate by conventional tissue sampling means. Yet, arterial drug delivery promises substantial rewards. The ideal goal of arterial drug delivery is to provide simpler, safer, and more efficacious treatments with substantially reduced drug doses and without local or systemic complications. Thus, a wide-angle review of the field is merited. This book covers the history, models, and methods to investigate drug delivery, current applications of arterial drugs, catheters, tools for arterial delivery, and pathways to arterial drug development. It covers arterial gene and stem cell therapy and the application of robotics and artificial intelligence for advancing arterial pharmacology.

I have followed Dr. Joshi's research for many years. His laboratory developed optical methods to assess drug delivery by tracking the delivery of drugs and dyes. These ultrafast measurements helped him to identify carriers for drug delivery. He was able to significantly improve drug delivery and circumvent the need to disrupt the blood–brain barrier. These studies should be followed up. Beyond reviewing its current applications, this book documents the techniques developed in his laboratory and presents a vision for the future applications of arterial drugs.

In summation, this is perhaps the first book on arterial drug delivery for treating neurological diseases. It is relevant to a broad audience, from clinicians and basic science researchers involved in the care of neurosurgical patients to pharmacologists and optical engineers who could further advance such research. I commend Dr. Joshi for his efforts.

Jeffrey N. Bruce, M.D., F.A.C.S.
Edgar N. Housepian Professor of Neurological Surgery
Department of Neurological Surgery
Columbia University Irving Medical Center
New York, NY, USA
jnb2@cumc.columbia.edu

Foreword: Arterial Drug Delivery—The Interventional Radiology Perspective

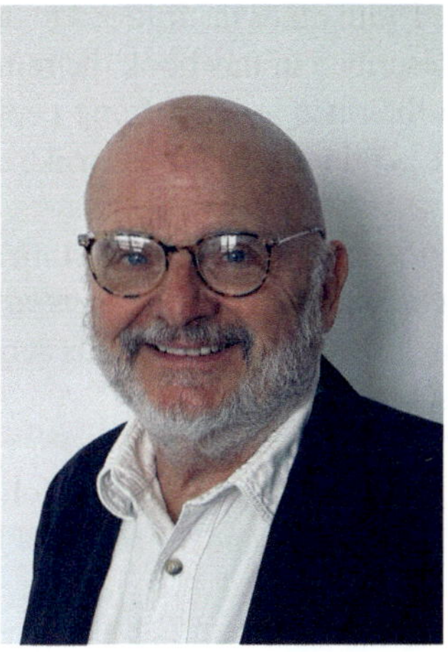

Late Charles Dotter, the father of interventional radiology, regarded the catheter as a surgical instrument. When Dotter died in 1985, the field of interventional radiology was still in its infancy. Since then, and especially in the last two decades, catheter-based endovascular technology has advanced immensely, leading to novel treatments of neurological diseases deemed challenging even a decade ago. Novel clot-aspirating techniques, stents, coils, embolic materials, and vascular-closing devices have greatly augmented the reach and safety of neuroradiological interventions. Advances in imaging technologies, with faster imaging, less radiation exposure, greater resolution, and sophisticated post-image processing, have greatly helped in the planning, execution, and assessment of such procedures. With steady advances in material sciences, hardware engineering, computational capabilities, and informatics, it is easily foreseeable that this progress will continue well into the future.

Yet, despite all these advances in treating neurological diseases, there remains a startling deficiency. While mechanical endovascular devices have advanced, endovascular pharmacology has remained stranded in the late 1990s. Intraarterial drug injections are currently used for Wada testing, treating cerebral vasospasm, and disrupting the blood–brain barrier. However, other applications are less well accepted. Mechanical clot extraction has largely supplanted intraarterial fibrinolytic use in acute ischemic stroke. In brain tumor treatments, arterial chemotherapy remains an experimental intervention. Attempts to deliver stem cells and gene vectors have also faced technical hurdles. The logistics and cost of isotope handling have dissuaded investigators from using ^{133}Xe isotope-based CSF measurements, foundational to cerebrovascular research for decades. Thus, while diagnostic angiography and mechanical interventions are gaining popularity, endovascular pharmacology seems to be in retreat.

Against this declining trend, this book litigates the value of arterial drug delivery. Taking an over-the-horizon approach to challenges in arterial pharmacology, it points out some of the current limitations and offers novel solutions. This book emphasizes the need to extract drugs in their initial pass through the cerebral circulation, develop optical tools to monitor the first-pass delivery, develop carrier systems that are safe and effective for this purpose, assess the outcome with multimodal imaging tools, and interpret the results recognizing the immense complexity of neurological diseases. It also looks at two widely accepted clinical applications of arterial drugs for treating liver cancers and retinoblastoma to glean what could be applied to neurological diseases.

It is not surprising to me that Dr. Joshi embarked on an effort to collect such diverse sources of information under a single title. I have known Dr. Joshi ever since he joined our research group at Columbia University under the mentorship of my friend and colleague, the late William L. Young. Under Bill's guidance, Dr. Joshi learned the basics of arterial drug delivery. After Bill's departure to UCSF, he established a cerebral vascular laboratory focused on arterial drug delivery and collaborated with other institutions to develop novel techniques to investigate arterial drug kinetics. As described in this book, he relied on optical methods to identify suitable carriers. Culminating in their use in identifying peptides for treating brain tumors in preclinical models. Some of those peptides could treat stroke and other neurological diseases in the future.

I am enthusiastic about recommending this book to clinical and translational neuroscience researchers because it provides a broad review of an essential route of drug delivery. The ubiquitous applications of arterial drugs and delivery methods across organs make this book potentially relevant beyond the neuroscience audience.

John Pile-Spellman, M.D., F.A.C.R.
Founder and Chief Scientist, Hibernia Medical LLC
Uniondale, NY, USA

Professor, Department of Radiology
Nassau University Medical Center of Stony Brook University
East Meadow, NY, USA

Former Vice-Chairman (Research), Department of Radiology
Columbia University Irving Medical Center
New York, NY, USA
johnpilespellman@gmail.com

Preface

I am only a child playing on the beach while the vast oceans of truth lie undiscovered before me.

Sir Issac Newton (1643–1727), Mathematician, Physicist, Astronomer, Alchemist, and Theologian

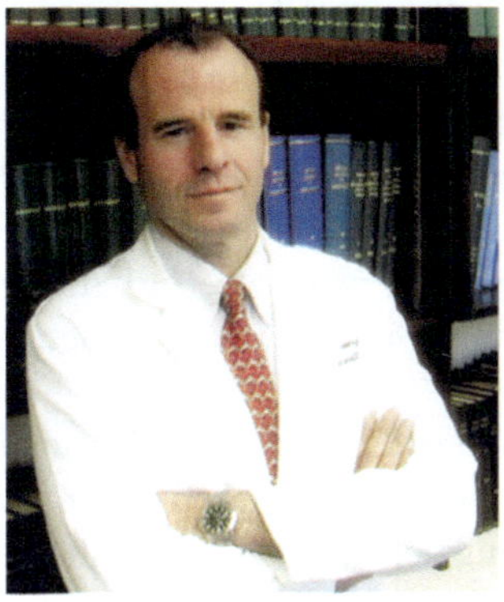

William Lawrence Young, MD (1954-2013)

Around 2003, I sat across the table from my late mentor, William Lawrence Young [1, 2], at our annual American Society of Anesthesiologists meeting. I told him I wanted to focus on arterial drug delivery. Bill was blunt and said, "Avoid it!" He was very skeptical that I would succeed. He wanted me to focus on elucidating the mechanisms that regulate human cerebral blood flow using arterial drug injections, the problem I had worked on for the previous 7 years. Little did he realize that there was a catch. How could one do mechanistic research when one could not reproduce tissue drug concentrations after such injections? Going against a highly respected mentor's advice was not easy. Much of the arterial drug delivery research was done at the National Institute of Health (NIH) in the 1980s–1990s. So, I emailed a set of questions to one of NIH's lead researchers, Dr. Robert L. Dedrick [3]. Bob was also skeptical of arterial drug delivery, although he did not directly answer my questions.

Over the seven preceding years, while working with Bill, I had measured cerebral blood flow several hundred times with arterial ^{133}Xe injections in human subjects and non-human primates. The technique was safe and reproducible. So why was arterial drug delivery ineffective? It was clear to me, having observed hundreds of ^{133}Xe washout curves, that arterial drug delivery is unlikely to have a significant clinical impact unless the drug is trapped in the tissues during its first pass through the regional circulation. *Maximizing the first-pass uptake and retention of the drugs was the central requirement of arterial drug delivery.* Solving this problem was not going to be easy. Although, at the time, there was extensive brain uptake indices data, it did not provide a complete pharmacokinetic picture. Rare positron emission tomographic (PET) studies provided some pharmacokinetic insights. However, these scans were often done at 10-min intervals. Arterial drugs transit through the human cerebral circulation in 5–7 s and far more quickly in laboratory animals, so a few PET studies would not crack the problem.

Understanding the first-pass kinetics of arterial drug injection requires continuous or sub-second assessment of tissue drug concentrations, preferably without invading the tissue. While isotopic studies can permit such measurement, radiolabeling drugs and carriers is expensive and raises safety concerns. In contrast, if the skull is removed or thinned, optical methods such as diffuse reflectance spectroscopy (DRS) can determine the tissue concentration of certain drugs and carrier dye conjugates. DRS provides ultrafast tissue concentration measurements. Joining forces with Irving J. Bigio, Professor of Biomedical Engineering at Boston University, who pioneered the DRS or the optical pharmacokinetic (OP) technique, was an immense help [4, 5]. Using optical methods, we could rapidly screen carriers suitable for arterial drug delivery that had significant tissue uptake and sustained retention for hours after a single injection. What we could do within a few hours using a single animal by optical means would take hundreds of animals and months of effort by conventional tissue sampling method.

We had no problems securing NIH funds when developing techniques to identify carriers or improve delivery methods. However, as we ventured into the treatment of brain tumors and stroke, our luck ran out. It was clear our grant applications were being dismissed without any serious review. The reviewers cited past failures of arterial drug delivery. Others conflated intravenous and intraarterial studies. Some were even bothered by the investigator's academic rank! Despite the best efforts of Dr. Houston Baker, the Program Official at the National Cancer Institute, our project was mothballed. The lab's closure in the spring of 2021 was a bitter disappointment. It came at a time when our carriers were working. Brain tumor models revealed that our treatment approach was safe, our results suggested at least a two-fold improvement in survival. The improvement could be achieved with 1/4 to 1/8 the dose of the chemotherapeutic drug.

This book aims to showcase the potential for arterial treatment of brain diseases. That past failures are not emblematic of what such delivery has to offer. The book provides a history of technologies related to arterial drug delivery, the conceptual rationale for making such delivery the most effective, the use of optical methods to study arterial delivery, the identification of suitable carriers, the current clinical application of arterial drugs, and lessons from treating liver cancers and retinoblastomas or the complications of accidental arterial injections that could be applied to arterial drug development. The book envisions the future of arterial drug delivery, given advances in angiographic techniques, nanoparticle technologies, blood-brain barrier disruption, pharmacological advances, stem cell and gene therapy research, artificial intelligence, robotics, and complex problem-solving.

I am sure many other investigators have faced the same skepticism in seeking funding for arterial drug delivery research. Reviewers often believe that past failures of arterial treatment do not justify any future investment. They overlook that arterial drug delivery can access all regions of the body with the same core angiographic techniques. The technology uses image guidance and will require rudimentary robotic controls for automation. It can be a force multiplier for other tissue-targeting drug delivery technologies. It can offer novel treatment with multiple drug interventions for tissue ablation, repair, and functional recovery. Arterial drug delivery is not a footnote of history but a prologue of the future. The principal goal of this book is to create a vision for grant reviewers so they do not have to dwell on past failures while rejecting novel approaches. Arterial drug delivery has a vast untapped potential that deserves a fair peer review unencumbered by past failures.

I am immensely grateful for the help and encouragement from Dr. Irving J. Bigio at Boston University, Dr. Robert Straubinger at Buffalo University, and Dr. Houston Baker at the National Cancer Institute's Imaging Program. On a personal note, I want to thank my family for their constant support and encouragement throughout my research and this book project.

New York, NY, USA

Shailendra Joshi, MBBS,MD
Anesthesiology,FFARCS(I)
sj121@cumc.columbia.edu

References

1. Mohr J, Kim H, Pawlikowska L, Su H. In memoriam: William L. Young, MD. Stroke. 2014;45:2–3.
2. Warner DS, Lanier WL. Mr. Piano Man: reflections on the life of physician, scientist, and humanitarian, William L. Young, MD (1954–2013). J Neurosurg Anesthesiol. 2014;26(1):1–3.
3. Dedrick RL. Arterial drug infusion: pharmacokinetic problems and pitfalls. J Natl Cancer Inst. 1988;80(2):84–9.
4. Mourant JR, Bigio IJ, Boyer J, Conn RL, Johnson T, Shimada T. Spectroscopic diagnosis of bladder cancer with elastic light scattering. Lasers Surg Med. 1995;17(4):350–7.
5. Mourant JR, Bigio IJ, Boyer JD, Johnson TM, Lacey J, Bohorfoush Iii AG, et al. Elastic scattering spectroscopy as a diagnostic tool for differentiating pathologies in the gastrointestinal tract: preliminary testing. J Biomed Opt. 1996;1(2):192–9.

Contents

About the Author

Shailendra Joshi, MBBS,MD Anesthesiology,FFARCS(I) After his medical graduation from the University of Delhi, Dr. Joshi trained in anesthesiology in India and England and later specialized in neuroanesthesiology in the United States. He joined Columbia University in 1995 for a post-doctoral fellowship under Professor William L. Young. At the time, Professor Young and Professor John Pile-Spellman were conducting studies on mechanisms of blood flow regulation in the human cerebral circulation. A part of that project was investing in the effects of intraarterial vasodilators. Dr. Joshi focused on developing the basic science side of the project, which involved non-human primates and other animal models. Realizing the need for ultrafast measurements to investigate arterial drug kinetics, his lab focused on using an optical approach to evaluate arterial delivery. Starting with video microscopy and the spectroscopic method developed by Dr. Irving Bigio at Boston University, his laboratory expanded the use of optical devices to track tracer-tagged carrier delivery to the brain in whole animal experiments. This book summarizes his experience with arterial drug delivery and those of other investigators.

Dr. Joshi is an Associate Professor of Anesthesiology at Columbia University. He has over 50 peer-reviewed scientific publications, most focused on arterial drug delivery. He has contributed to prestigious neuroanesthesiology texts, and is a long-standing editorial board member of the *Journal of Neurosurgical Anesthesiology*. His textbook, *Neuroanesthesiology Case Companion*, was published in 2023. He holds several design and utility patents.

1 The Evolution of Arterial Drug Delivery: The Underlying Concepts and Technology

Samrat Worah and Shailendra Joshi

Study the past if you want to define the future.
Confucius (551–479 BCE), Chinese Philosopher

Introduction

History often garners contempt that belies its real value. It is humbling to note that many scientific advances are frequently rediscoveries of past achievements. Therefore, knowing history, analyzing its failures, and applying new concepts and technologies to solve persistent problems can provide rich grounds for future technological advances. Scientific breakthroughs need four elements to come together, which can be abbreviated in an acronym: "NIFE." *The first* component is the "Need." There has to be a pressing need to solve a problem. Need helps direct resources to the problem or get the needed attention. *The second* component, though the least important component, is the "Individual"—a person with sufficient capacity and tenacity to solve the problem. The *third* is "Feasibility." The available technology should be able to solve the problem. *Fourth* is the "Environment." Scientific discoveries often need an environment that fosters the solution. Many scientific advances have been hindered because of hostility to novel concepts. The scientific community rejected many classical medical advances, such as handwashing before surgery, the germ theory of disease, and the use of anesthesia in surgery, as they did not fit the accepted views of their time. The NIFE approach could be used retrospectively and perhaps prospectively to assess the successes and failures of many research efforts. Therefore, knowing, analyzing, and addressing past events can provide a road map for future progress. Figure 1.1 shows the drivers of arterial drug delivery, conceptual and technological, that can address unmet oncologic and non-oncologic needs. It shows many converging pathways of technological development, suggesting that now is the time to investigate and develop arterial drug delivery and treatments. This chapter describes the development of intraarterial (IA) drugs while focusing on IA chemotherapy. It traces the evolution of various threads of knowledge that helped us understand IA drug delivery from antiquity to the present.

S. Worah · S. Joshi (✉)
Department of Anesthesiology, Columbia University Irving Medical Center, New York, NY, USA
e-mail: sw3909@cumc.columbia.edu; sj121@cumc.columbia.edu

S. Joshi (ed.), *Arterial Treatment of Neurological Diseases*, https://doi.org/10.1007/978-3-031-80173-0_1

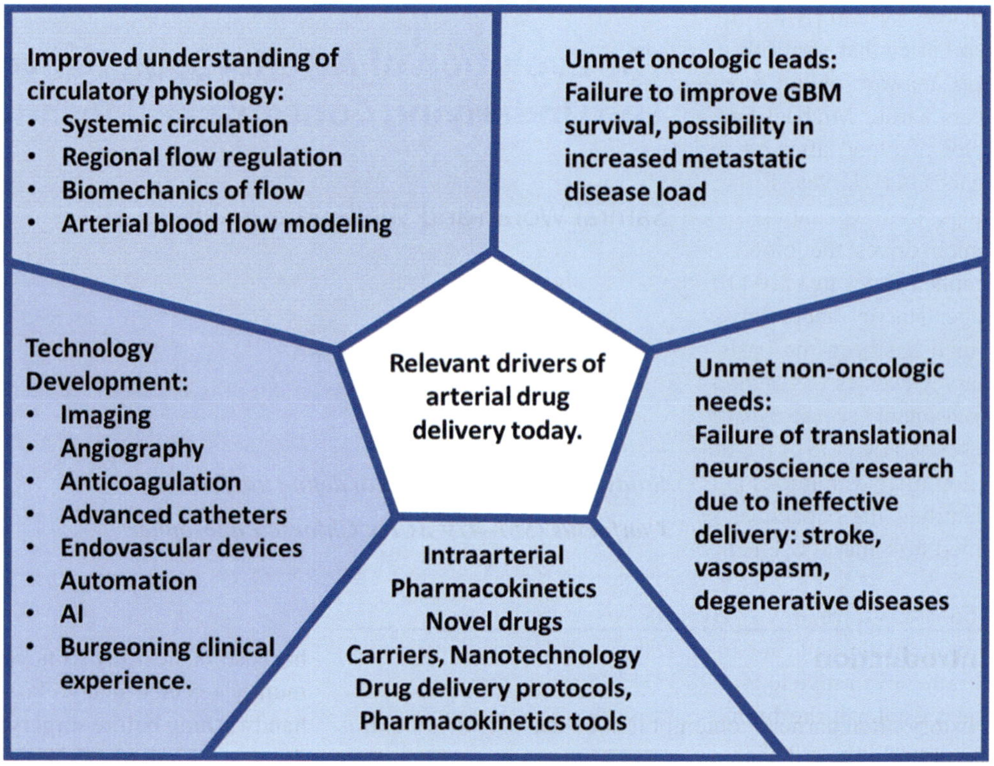

Fig. 1.1 An overview of drivers of intraarterial drug delivery in the early twenty-first century

The Dawn of Circulatory Physiology

Arteries and veins were known to the anatomists of antiquity, but their physiological role was a mystery. Understanding cardiovascular physiology based on dissections of rotting corpses was fundamentally flawed. Such errors are best reflected in the erroneous anatomical diagrams of the human torso by Leonardo da Vinci. Despite Leonardo's solid command of mechanical principles, his anatomical drawings reflect a lack of understanding of circulatory physiology. The erroneous interpretation of the circulatory system was further complicated by its assumed anatomical and functional relationship with the lungs and the gut, partly due to rationalizing the concept of disease based on the inhalation of foul air.

Over the last twenty-five hundred years, the concept of the circulatory system passed through four conceptual stages, as was recently reviewed by Aird [1]:

- *Erasistratus, around 250 BC,* described the open-ended circulatory system. He described the heart as a pump and distinguished between arteries and veins. While veins delivered blood to different regions of the body, Erasistratus believed that the arteries contained air and distributed pneuma or the animal spirit.
- *Galen of Pergamon, around 129 AD*, described veins and arteries as containing blood. Venous blood could transfer through perforations in the heart to the arterial side, and arterial and venous blood perfused the organs independently.
- *Realdo Colombo*, 1515–1559, discovered that the valves in the heart permitted blood flow in one direction. He concluded that venous blood goes from the heart to the lungs and blood returns to the heart to be dispersed by the arteries to the rest of the body.
- *William Harvey, in 1628,* laid the foundation of modern circulatory physiology. Harvey described pulmonary and systemic circulation as closed loops where the blood circulates constantly. He deduced this by the valves' direction, indicating the blood flow pattern. He estimated that over 24 h, a dog's heart ejected 245 kg of blood. It would be impossible to synthesize or absorb such a large volume of blood. Therefore, the only rational explanation was that blood was constantly being recirculated. Using graded pressure, Harvey demonstrated higher pressure in the arteries, enabling blood flow into the veins. He postulated the existence of pores that permit blood to flow from the arterial to the venous side.

Interestingly, Harvey studied astronomy while he was a student in Padua. At that time, Galileo was a Professor of Astronomy at the university, advancing the idea of heliocentric planetary orbits. A debatable resonance exists between the planetary circulation around the sun and the blood circulation centered on the heart. On return to England, Harvey correctly elaborated on the functional organization of the circulatory system [2–4]. However, Harvey was unaware of the capillaries that were observed only after his death. He was also unaware of the function of the lungs, although a 100 years earlier Michael Servetus had noted the change in the color of blood after passing through the lungs [5–8]. Fifty years after Harvey, Robert Boyle identified the role of the lungs in oxygenating blood [9]. Arterial blood pressure, which drives the blood flow, was first measured by Rev. Stephen Hales in 1710 [10, 11]. Despite such gaps in knowledge, Harvey accurately described the circulatory system, which has been the basis of cardiac physiology ever since. Harvey even assessed the cardiac output as 4 L/min, which is a reasonably accurate estimate. Giovanni Alfonso Borelli first described the role of the heart as a piston pump driving circulation in a posthumous publication in 1680 [12]. Borelli also identified the capacitive nature of arteries in smoothening blood flow that is cyclically ejected from the heart [13, 14].

The Measurement of Arterial Blood Pressure Once the overall picture of the circulatory system had evolved, it became imperative to establish physiological parameters that could establish the biomechanics of blood circulation. The critical parameter needed to advance cardiovascular physiology was determining arterial blood pressure. In 1730, *Rev Steven Hales* cannulated the carotid artery of a mare; he found that the column of blood extended to almost 9 ft, corresponding to a pressure of about 200 mmHg. However, when he slowly bled out the animal, the pressure decreased. The column height was 2 ft or 40 mmHg when the animal died. Encouraged by Sir Isaac Newton, he published his findings in a series of books on blood pressure measurements. Hales also poured wax into the animal's left ventricle and determined its volume to be 160 mL. Given a heart rate of 36 beats per minute, he estimated the animal's cardiac output to be 6 L. Hales also determined that the systole was one-third of the cardiac cycle [15]. Furthermore, he showed that the distal arteries were the principal site of flow resistance. Stephen Hales and Euler have been called the fathers of hemodynamics. Stephen Hale is credited with the first arterial blood pressure measurement. However, invasive blood pressure measurement methods that led to the animal's death had little clinical relevance. Table 1.1 lists the significant landmarks in measuring arterial blood pressure noninvasively, which are critical towards understanding arterial and cerebral blood flow [16].

Measurement of systemic blood pressure only provides a global parameter for assessing cerebral perfusion. However, modeling cerebral circulation, assessing pathology, and controlling regional perfusion to optimize drug delivery require invasively measuring local arterial blood pressure [28]. Although IA blood pressure could be measured directly using a manometer, transducers were required for its reliable quantification [29–31]. Since 1990, invasive arterial blood pressure monitoring has become routine in critical care, whether in the operating room or elsewhere. Intravascular pressure measurements use microcatheters and transducer systems to assess stenosis; however, sensor technology is rapidly evolving. In recent years, intravascular pressure transducers that have a 50 nm sensor on the tip of a wire 0.014 inches (0.36 mm) in diameter have been developed. These technological innovations have generated new insight into cardiovascular physiology and disease treatment [32, 33].

Table 1.1 History of arterial blood pressure measurement

Year	Investigator	Significance	Reference
1628	William Harvey	Described the circulation of blood	[17]
1733	Stephen Hales	Direct measurement of arterial blood pressure in animals	[10]
1826	Jean Poiseuille	First U tube mercury manometer and measured ABP in mmHg	[18]
1847	Carl Ludwig	First mercury manometer to record ABP	[19]
1856	Jean Faivre	Recorded ABP using a kymograph during lower limb amputation	[20]
1855	Karl Vierordt	Attempted noninvasive measurement of ABP with arterial occlusion with a cuff placed around the arm. The measurements were unreliable	[21]
1860	Etienne-Jules Marey	Used a sphygmograph to measure heart rate accurately, but noninvasive blood pressure measurement remained unreliable	[22]
1882	Robert Ellis Dudgeon	The first widely used portable sphygmograph	[23]
1881	Samuel Ritter von Basch	Sphygmomanometer using balloon occlusion of the artery	[24]
1889	Pierre-Carl Potain	Introduced pneumatic compression cuff to occlude the artery	[25]
1896	Scipione Riva-Rocci	Used an inflatable pneumatic cuff and mercury manometer	[26]
1905	Nikolai Korotkoff	Described method to detect systolic and diastolic blood pressure	[26]
1973	Penaz, J	Development of noninvasive continuous BP monitor	[27]
1974	Panasonic Inc.	Automated blood pressure	[26]

Understanding Arterial Blood Flow

Besides encouraging Stephen Hales, Sir Isaac Newton played a significant role in advancing the understanding of blood flow through arteries. Newton's law of viscosity was described in the *Principia Mathematica*, published in 1684. Newton described shear stress (τ) = Force (F)/Area (A) parallel to the direction of applied force. The law states that shear stress is the product of viscosity multiplied by spatial velocity gradient. In Newton's model flow model, viscosity plays a critical role [16].

Daniel Bernoulli, in 1738, applied the law of energy conservation in flowing fluids. Bernoulli showed that the sum of the potential, kinetic, and pressure energy during fluid flow is constant. For example, when a tube is narrowed, flow velocity in the narrowed region increases, thereby conserving its kinetic energy. However, to solve his equations, Bernoulli had to ignore viscosity's effect, which has a profound and detrimental impact on flow by dissipating energy. Thus, the energy conservation described by Bernoulli applies only to perfect fluids with zero viscosity but fails to represent blood flow accurately [34].

While Newtonian fluid mechanics is relatively easy to apply to uniform rigid tubes, applying them to elastic blood vessels poses enormous complexity. In addition, the pulsatile nature of arterial pressure, nonuniform diameter, and branching of blood vessels make arterial blood flow modeling very challenging. *Leonhard Euler* undertook the one-dimensional modeling of fluid flow through rigid and elastic tubes with a piston pump (1742, printed and dated 1775). While the flow model worked for the rigid tubes, it failed to describe flow through elastic tubes. However, Euler's approach has successfully been modeled with advances in computational capabilities. The mathematical equations and the fundamental construction of Euler's circulatory model are still valid two centuries later. The one-dimensional Euler model is still used to describe blood flow; however, it can also be applied to compressible gases and flow in shallow water channels. The physical concept of elasticity that Euler described preceded its formal description by Thomas Young by almost 80 years [35].

Claude-Louis Navier in 1817 and George Gabriel Strokes in 1845 independently addressed the Bernoulli model's limitation of ignoring viscosity [36, 37]. Navier-Strokes equations form a complete set of three-dimensional differential equations that accurately describe viscous fluid flow in vessels with simplified geometries and flow conditions [38].

Around 1840, *Jean Leonard Marie Poiseuille* demonstrated that for fluid flow in a cylindrical tube, the pressure drop was proportional to the viscosity, length, and flow divided by the fourth power of the radius. The "Poiseuille law" could be applied to vessels of different sizes. It showed that the resistance to flow significantly increased as their diameter decreased [39]. In 1828, Poiseuille invented the mercury manometer and found that the pressure in the aorta was approximately the same as in the smaller arteries [40]. The lack of pressure decrease in the large arteries compared to the heart was consistent with Stephen Hale's observations a century earlier. Twenty years later, Gotthilf Hagenbach successfully applied the Navier-Strokes equation to steady-state flow in straight, circular tubes consistent with the Poiseuille law and Newton's law of viscosity. The Poiseuille-Hagenbach equation, Fig. 1.2, has remained the foundational equation for describing regional blood flow [16].

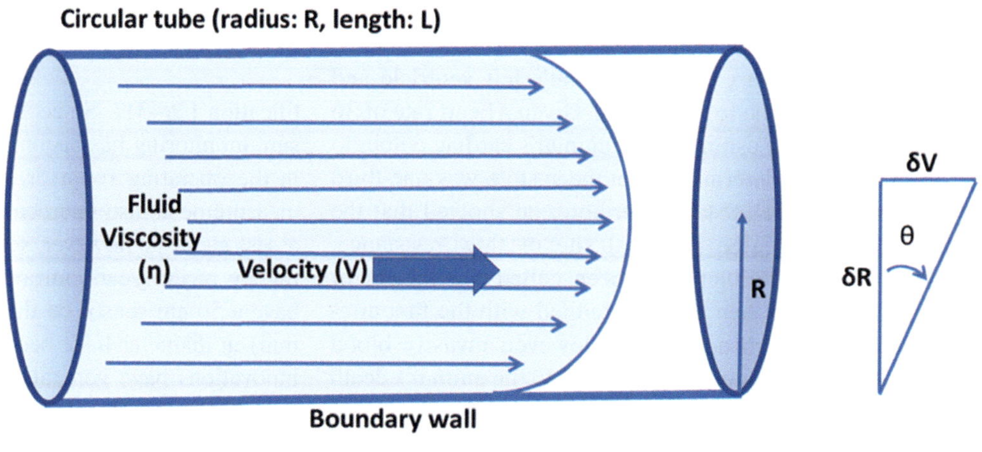

Newton's Law of Viscosity (1684):
Shear stress = Viscosity (η) X velocity gradient
velocity gradient =(δV/ δR)

$$\text{Flow (Q)} = \frac{\pi\ X\ Pressure\ X\ radius^{4}}{8\ X\ \eta\ X\ Length}$$

Poiseuille Law (1840) verified by Hagenbach (1860)

Fig. 1.2 Key concepts in arterial blood flow

Over time, though, the concept of resistance was replaced with impedance to model the pulsatile nature of the flow. In addition, the assumption that flow would be laminar with a parabolic flow velocity was challenged by clinical observations of bruits that *Laennec* had described in the 1820s. Bruits indicated turbulence in flow and usually occurred in the region of significant arterial narrowing [41, 42]. In 1883, *Osborne Reynolds* described the dimensionless Reynolds' number. Below this number, the flow is laminar, and above it, it becomes turbulent. Reynolds' number for circular tubes resulted from the diameter and velocity divided by viscosity [43]. Thus, the number would double if the diameter was reduced by half and there was a fourfold increase resulting in flow velocity. The creation of turbulence results in energy loss and complicates the mathematical models.

Anatomical factors (such as a change in diameter or branching) and physiological factors (such as pulsatile flow, turbulence, and elasticity of the vessel walls) were the foremost hurdles to arterial blood flow modeling until the twentieth century. However, in the later part of the twentieth century, those challenges were further compounded by advances in cell biology. Advances in cell biology revealed that vascular endothelium played a dynamic role in modulating blood flow. Thus, despite the advances in mathematics and computational capabilities, understanding blood flow in arteries is still undergoing considerable refinement. The early twenty-first-century blood flow models can describe the delivery of drugs and nanoparticles for general hypothesis development and testing and, recently, for patient-specific arterial networks (Chap. 3) [16].

Development of Angiography

The three components needed for an angiographic procedure include the X-ray imager, the radiocontrast, and the development of catheters for contrast and drug delivery.

The Advances in X-Ray Generation

The mysterious nature of waves on the electromagnetic spectrum between the ultraviolet and the gamma rays led to their designation as X-rays. Although the X-rays were officially discovered in 1895, these rays had been under investigation for a long time earlier (Table 1.2). The landmark image of his wife's hand by Wilhelm Conrad Röntgen on December 22, 1895, provided indisputable evidence of potential medical applications of X-rays [44]. Röntgen did not seek a patent for his discovery. The lack of a patent significantly accelerated X-ray research. Almost half of the Nobel Prizes in the first quarter of the twentieth century were X-ray-related. By 1916, Marie Curie and her daughter used mobile X-ray units in field hospitals during the First World War [45].

Table 1.2 Historical landmarks in X-ray discovery

Year	Development	References
1857	Heinrich Geissler produced a colorful light with partially evacuated vacuum tubes	[46, 47]
1875	William Crookes achieved a greater vacuum for the electrons to reach the anode and the glass wall to cause fluorescence	[48, 49]
1876	Eugen Goldstein described the cathode rays	[50]
1881	Ivan Puluj experimented with cold light and observed the degradation of photographic plates	[51]
1894	Nikola Tesla investigated X-rays, but his laboratory burned down	[52, 53]
1895	On November 8, Röntgen observed that X-rays from a Crookes tube penetrated cardboard; on December 28, Röntgen first reported using X-rays for imaging	[54]
1896	Puluj and Tesla also report the discovery of the X-rays	[51, 53]

Immediately after Röntgen discovered X-rays, efforts were underway to improve the Crookes tube by enhancing the X-ray flux and beam's focus. These improvements were initially achieved in the Coolidge (1913) tube by heating the cathode, introducing a focusing shield, and improving the vacuum in the tube [55]. In these tubes, the flux of the electrons and the X-rays could be controlled by changing the voltage and the current. Focusing the beam remained a concern. Earlier efforts to focus the X-ray beam relied on shaping the anode. Over time, the electron beam became more powerful and narrowly focused on the target [56]. The focal point in the sealed tubes is about 10 μm in diameter, which results in heating and degradation of the target site on the anode. In the 1930s, rotating anodes were introduced [57]. These offered a constantly changing target for the electron beam, thereby minimizing the risk of heating and degradation of the anode. Target burnout remains a problem with sealed tubes, thus limiting the X-rays they can generate [58]. Figure 1.3 describes the key aspects of advances in X-ray generation.

In the 1940s, the availability of better vacuum pumps led to the development of open X-ray tubes. The open X-ray tubes permit easy replacement of the cathode and the anodes and could, therefore, be operated at higher energies, producing better focusing and X-ray flux. These methods have greatly expanded the application of X-ray for electron microscopy, materials sciences, and industrial applications. Since then, other sources of X-rays have developed. These include the evolution of powerful, focused X-ray beans for nonmedical applications. The synchrotron and lanthanum hexa-borate as electron sources. At the same time, develop-

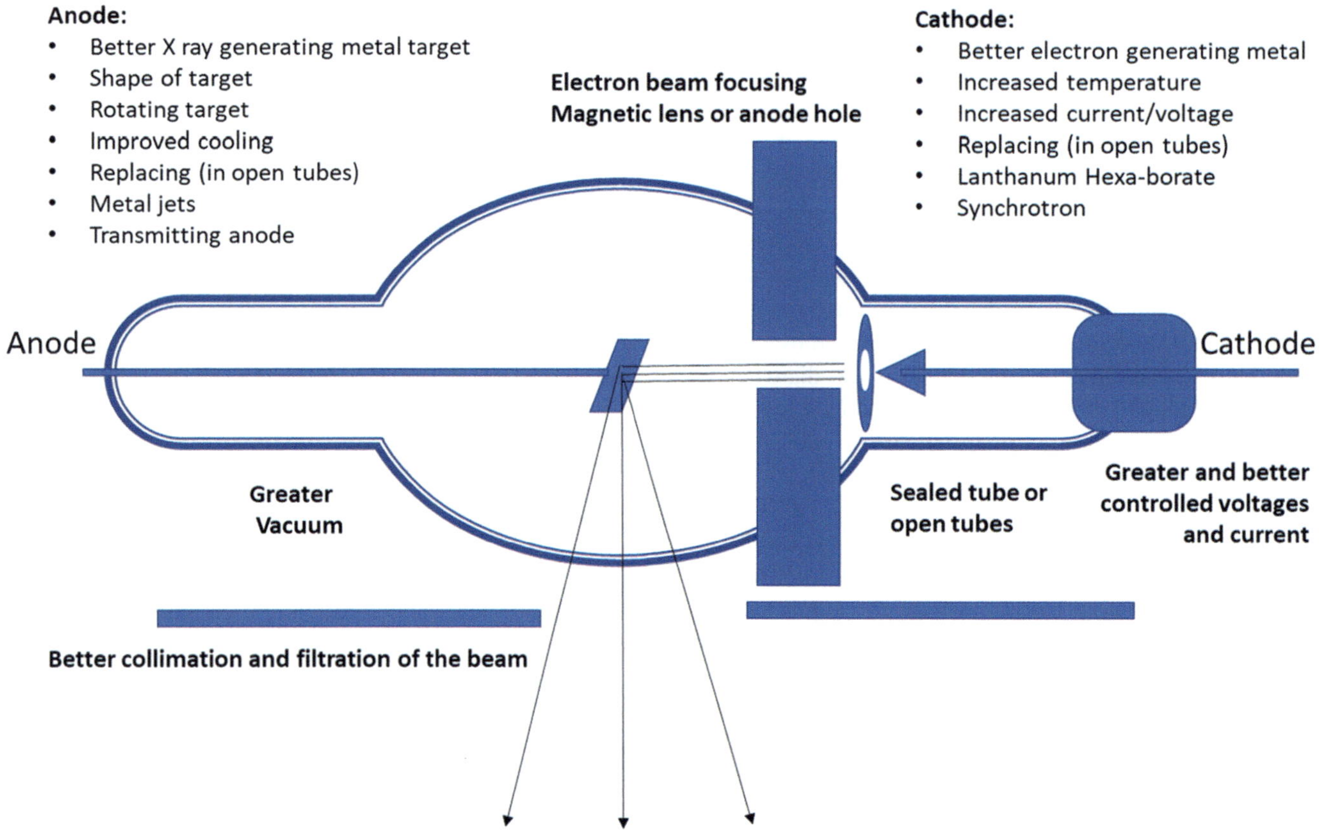

Fig. 1.3 Some of the technological advances in X-ray generation since Röntgen

ing a liquid metal jet anode provided a constantly changing target for the electron beam to generate focused high-powered X-rays without the risk of heating and wearing out [59, 60].

Advances in X-Ray Imaging

Broadly, the advances in X-ray imaging can be described in three phases: chemical image processing, digital imaging, and post-digital image manipulation [61].

- *Acquisition of images on plates and films by chemical means*: Photographic glass plates were initially used to capture X-ray images. However, these glass plates were inefficient, heavy, and fragile. Flexible cellulose nitrate-containing films that evolved around 1910 were unsatisfactory due to their high inflammability. The emergence of cellulose triacetate polyester films in the 1920s decreased the chances of flammability. The X-rays led to image formation in these films by interacting directly with silver halide. However, the effect of X-ray fluorescence can be significantly boosted by interposing a layer of scintillators. The scintillators convert the X-ray to UV light. Thus, the invention of X-ray plates and fluorescence screens with a scintillating layer decreased the X-rays needed to generate the image. Initially, a calcium tungstate class of scintillators for high-energy X-rays was developed. These were replaced with rare earth scintillators that were more suitable for clinical use for low-energy X-rays. However, chemical film processing was needed after exposure to the X-ray. This wet process was automated in the 1950s [62].
- *Digital X-ray image acquisition*: X-rays excite a phosphor layer during digital imaging. The excited phosphor layer activates the electroconductive layer that traps electrons and spatially retains the information. The latent image can be read by laser light stimulation that produces luminescence or recorded by charged-coupled devices. The digital data is processed to reduce noise, increase the signal-noise ratio, increase or decrease contrast, and improve image resolution [63].
- *Improvement in digital image processing*: The ability to manipulate digitized data with advanced computational capabilities has created a positive feedback loop in advancing X-ray hardware and increasingly faster and more sophisticated X-ray imaging. These advances are best reflected in the development of CT scanners. While the first-generation CT scanners needed 30 min, the latest CT scanners can complete scans in 1–2 s. The radiation dose can also be decreased by 70%. The quality of images

has been dramatically improved. Using dual-energy or multi-energy CT scanning that can be undertaken simultaneously can help differentiate bone and iodinated contrast and is useful for angiography [64–66].

- *Angiographic flow assessment*: Processing digital images rapidly and accurately to determine the time needed for contrast to transit cerebral circulation is essential for arterial drug delivery. Hitherto, contrast transit time has provided a semiquantitative assessment of cerebral blood flow, but technology is rapidly evolving. Reliable evaluation of cerebral blood flow can optimize arterial drug delivery. It can also assess neuropathology, the safety of embolization, and the effectiveness of treatments [67–70].
- *Role of magnetic resonance imaging (MRI) as an alternative to X-ray angiography*: The increasing availability of MRI, primarily driven by the urgency of stroke treatments, creates novel opportunities to use arterial drug delivery in such an environment. MR can provide detailed images of vascular morphology, assess blood flow and blood-brain barrier integrity, and guide arterial delivery [71–75].
- *Role of intravascular ultrasonic imaging*: Attempts to image vessels from within with ultrasound began in the early 1960s [76]. However, the rapid development of angiography stymied their progress. In recent years, though, flow piezo crystal-tipped 0.014-in-sized guide wires have been used to assess blood flow. Ultrasound-guided drug infusion protocols have been developed for coronary diseases that could have potential implications for cerebral arterial drug delivery [77].

Development of Contrast Agents

Immediately after Röntgen published his report, the limitation of X-rays in detecting subtle differences in the translucency of the soft tissue was evident. It was known that elements with greater atomic weights absorb X-rays. In January 1896, less than a month after the first X-ray report, the first cadaveric angiogram was reported in an amputated hand using chalk, mercury sulfide, and Vaseline to generate a detailed image of the arterial network of the hand [78]. By 1920, the search for contrast agents had begun earnestly [79]. At that time, iodinated compounds were used to treat syphilis. Binz and Rath, in the early 1920s, synthesized several safe iodopyridine compounds that could be used for syphilis treatment. It was observed that intravenous sodium iodide used to treat syphilis produced opaque urine to X-rays. Moses Swick demonstrated that iodopyridine compounds could delineate the kidneys and the urinary tract. By 1930, Binz and Rath patented mono- and di-iodinated derivatives of iodopyridine as clinically used contrast agents. Iodine is the only element that can be safely given in concentrations for tissue imaging purposes [80]. In the late 1920s, Thorotrast, a 25% solution of thorium iodide, was introduced but was found to be carcinogenic, leading to the formation of thorotrastomas [81].

The credit for doing the first arterial cerebral angiogram in vivo goes to Egas Moniz in 1927 [82, 83] Due to the radiolucency of brain tissue, plain X-rays of the skull were of limited value in diagnosing brain pathologies. In 1916, in the USA, Walter Dandy pioneered air injection in the ventricles to delineate brain tumors [84, 85]. Jean Sicard, in 1921, in Paris, demonstrated the compression of the medulla by using lipiodol [86, 87]. He also injected the compound in the femoral vein of dogs and observed the blood vessels. IV lipiodol delineated the inferior vena cava and the heart. It resulted in pulmonary emboli, which were evident in the chest X-ray. Joseph Berberich and Hirsch (1923) used strontium bromide in an occluded antecubital vein to perform the first retrograde angiography. They later injected the femoral artery to get the first femoral angiogram [78, 88].

Moniz started his experiments with cerebral angiography, first in cadavers and dogs. Moniz required the compound to be radiopaque, harmless, and nonfatty to avoid embolic stroke during cerebral angiography. He experimented with lithium bromide, strontium bromide, sodium bromide, and sodium iodide. Lithium injections caused considerable pain and were abandoned. His first four angiographic attempts with percutaneous strontium bromide injections failed. In two patients, the injections were extravascular; one had hemorrhage, while the fourth had poor-quality images. In his second attempt, he used surgical exposure of the carotid artery. He obtained good images with strontium bromide, but one of the patients died of a massive stroke 8 h later. Therefore, he recommended using 5–6 cc of 25% sodium iodide for the procedure. He took precautions to avoid accidental air injection or letting the blood enter the needle to prevent clot formation and embolization. Cerebral angiography opened new avenues for the diagnosis and treatment of neurological diseases. Moniz was nominated for the Nobel Prize thrice and eventually won it in 1949. However, it was not for cerebral angiography that is widely used today but for prefrontal leucotomy, which has long been abandoned [78]!

The Development of Catheters

Catheters have been used to drain urine since antiquity. According to the Edwin Smith papyri (dated 1500 BC or earlier), they were made from rolled leaves, reeds, straws, or bronze tubes almost 3000 years ago [89]. The arterial and venous catheterization procedures were initially performed using quills soon after Harvey discovered blood circulation. Stephen Hales used brass cannulae connected to glass tubes. Claude Bernard perhaps did the first left and right heart cardiac catheterization in a dog using glass tubes. It is claimed that the first cardiac catheterization was done in the early 1900s by Fritz Bleichroder, Ernst Unger, and William Loeb in dogs. Later, Bleichroder volunteered to undergo catheterization on himself. While undergoing a third procedure, he had severe chest pain, and the catheter had to be withdrawn before its location could be documented. Although it could have been the first cardiac catheterization, as has been claimed, it was not adequately documented [90].

The credit for the first cardiac catheterization in human subjects goes to Werner Forssmann in 1929. He passed a well-lubricated "ureteric" catheter through the antecubital vein into his heart and then X-rayed its position. Although a report mentions it was a plastic catheter, it could be in error because most catheters at the time were made of rubber. Plastic catheters were unavailable until the second half of the twentieth century. Before vulcanization, rubber catheters could disintegrate during use. Thus, rubber was not an ideal material for catheter construction. The details of Werner's device are not mentioned in most reports [91, 92].

Andre Cournand pioneered cardiac catheterization in the United States and used a ureteric catheter. The catheter was made of silk with a smooth lacquered surface and a rounded tip to prevent vascular injury. It was constantly flushed with 15 drops per minute of normal saline during the procedure to minimize clot formation. The Cournand technique minimized the two principal risks of angiography: thrombus formation and vascular injury [93–95].

Modern angiographic catheters are constructed from polyamides, polyurethane Teflon, and silicone. These materials provide flexibility, tensile strength, and smooth, minimally thrombogenic surfaces. They can also be molded into desired shapes and are flexible enough to be wire-guided into millimeter-scale vessels. They can also be manufactured with pressure-tolerant balloons for vascular dilation. Super selective and balloon-occluding catheters can permit selective drug delivery while occluding blood flow. However, modern catheters do not allow long-term cannulation without the risk of thrombus formation. They need angiographic verification before use due to the possibility of migration after placement.

The Oncologic Applications of Arterial Drug Delivery

Discovery of Chemotherapy

The dawn of modern chemotherapy is often attributed to the bombing of the Italian port city of Bari during the Second World War. Nestled on the eastern side of southern Italy, the port was considered a safe harbor that was out of reach of the German Air Force. When USS John Harvey arrived at the port of Bari in late November 1943, the need to unload its top-secret cargo could not be publicly disclosed. The port of Bari was the transit point for ammunition needed to liberate Italy. It was unprotected [97].

On the afternoon of December 2, 1943, a Luftwaffe reconnaissance pilot observed intense activities at the port. In addition, the port city was lit at night to unload the cargo. It was an easy target for a nighttime raid. USS John Harvey was still waiting at the harbor when 105 German bombers attacked the port that night. Harvey was among the 28 ships destroyed that night, while 12 others were damaged. It had sustained a direct hit and caught fire. All its crew perished, alongwith a thousand other men who died within 90 min. Noone could account for the mysterious garlic odor emanating from the burning ship. The attack on Bari is a relatively unknown maritime disaster called the "Little Pearl Harbor." It took over a year for the port to recover. The destruction of Bari was shrouded in secrecy and a long time afterward for an excellent reason [97].

Unknown to the port operators and the public, John Harvey was carrying a deadly cargo of some 12,000 M47A1 bombs, each containing 60–70 pounds of sulfur mustard. Mustard gas as a chemical weapon has been used since the First World War. Its toxic blistering effects were well known at the time. However, there was a general understanding not to use chemical weapons during the Second World War. President Dwight Eisenhower personally approved the deadly cargo onboard John Harvey. Any public report of an American warship carrying chemical ammunition could trigger a retaliatory chemical attack. However, the contamination of the port city by sulfur mustard dispersed by the toxic plume of the fire and in the water by the ship's sinking was hard to conceal. Within a day, some 600 military personnel reported unexplained blindness and chemical burns. Many civilian complaints soon followed. Lt. Col. Stewart Francis Alexander was tasked to investigate these symptoms. As an expert in chemical warfare, Col. Alexander mapped the distribution of the cases. He sourced the origin to John Harvey and, in the wreckage, found the fragment of the M47A1 bomb. His report was censored and withheld from the public. The injuries were attributed to physical burns and conventional war injuries. However, Col. Alexander attributed the symptoms to nitrogen mustard. Due to the sinking of the ships, fuel was released into the water along with the sulfur mustard. The fuel served as a solvent for the nitrogen mustards to penetrate the skin. Although the military command insisted on its denial, Col. Alexander instituted treatment for mustard gas poisoning. Some 83 of the 638 hospitalized military personnel died within a month after the raid. Col. Alexander documented the decreased white cell count due to the suppression of the bone marrow in these patients, and he preserved tissue samples for further investigations [97].

The Use of Nitrogen Mustard: The First Chemotherapy Drug

The lethality of mustard gas has been well-known since the First World War. Fritz Haber synthesized several chemical compounds for warfare during the First World War. The toxic effects of the mustard gas were most evident in the battle of Ypres when some 10,000 troops died in 1917. Only 2 years earlier, in 1915, Haber had developed the method to mass-produce ammonia, which accounts for 50% of the world's food production today. Haber won the Nobel Prize for Chemistry in 1918. Haber's wife—herself a chemist—opposed the development of chemicals for use in war and committed suicide when he decided to supervise gas warfare [98, 99].

After the First World War, the race for chemical weapons began, as did the desire to protect against their effects. Milton Winternitz, the Dean of Yale 1920–1935, wrote in 1920 about the need to investigate these compounds. At some point, he initiated research into the effects of chemical warfare agents at the university, which must have antedated the attack on Bari. At the university, Louis Goodman and Alfred Gilman undertook systematic investigations into the bone marrow suppressive effects of nitrogen mustard. In animal models, they demonstrated the effectiveness of this compound in treating lymphomas [100]. Subsequently, they treated an advanced non-Hodgkin's lymphoma, probably a lymphosarcoma. The patient had sizeable axillary lymph nodes that restricted the movements of his arm. His jaw tumor prevented him from eating food. The tumors were also causing respiratory distress. He received the first dose (0.1 mg/kg) of "synthetic lymphocidal chemical" on August 27, 1942. After five daily treatments, there was a dramatic improvement in this clinical condition with softening and regressing of his tumors. The biopsy after the tenth treatment reported no tumor tissue. He continued to improve but developed bleeding and petechial hemorrhages, requiring blood transfusions. The disease relapsed, and he needed two more courses of treatment. He died 94 days later [100, 101].

The Dawn of Intraarterial Drug Delivery

The first use of IA drugs was probably in Spain in 1909 when Jose Goyanes Capdevila produced regional anesthesia with an IA injection of local anesthetic [102–104]. Goyanes also demonstrated the safety of arterial puncture and had tested his technique in animals a year earlier with IA cocaine. Goyanes tested several local anesthetic drugs: cocaine, procaine, and eucaine [105]. He showed that IA anesthetics effectively blocked the nerve endings by applying two tourniquets [104]. Goyanes reported the successful use of IA novocaine for limb surgery in 70 patients with only 2 failures [104]. In 1914, Fiolle in France [106] and Heddaus in Germany [107] experimented with IA drug delivery. Glasser, in 1945, used IA penicillin for limb infections [108]. Donovan used IA heparin for treating thromboembolism [109]. Kappert treated peripheral vascular insufficiency with intravenous and IA delivery of ergot alkaloid [110].

While these were examples of intravenous drugs being injected into arteries, cerebral angiography represented the first IA compounds developed specifically for IA delivery. In many ways, the development of radiocontrast agents revealed potential hazards for IA delivery unrelated to the drugs, such as bleeding, vascular dissections, perforation, and hematomas [78–80]. The early contrast agents were hyperosmotic, painful, and tissue-toxic [111–114]. Accidental air injection and the crude construction of the catheters further aggravated the risks associated with its use.

Beginning in early 1940, along with the introduction of intravenous anesthetic drugs, namely, pentothal, a slew of reports started to emerge regarding accidental IA injection of drugs. Pentothal was introduced to clinical practice in the 1930s [115, 116]. However, the doses and concentrations of the drug were not standardized. It was available in concentrations of 2.5%, 5%, and 10%. Poor dosing protocols had disastrous consequences when a standard dose of 0.5 g was administered to survivors of the Pearl Harbor bombing on December 7, 1941. Pentothal was initially blamed for 1000 deaths, and a surgeon described it as a tool for euthanasia [117]. As a result, it was less popular in the United States than in Europe and elsewhere. Several reports of accidental IA drug injections soon appeared in the literature [116, 118]. Since then, similar complications have been reported with arterial injections of several other drugs. The clinical symptoms are listed in Table 1.3. The underlying mechanisms are unclear and may not be independent of each other. These include crystal embolization, lipid-soluble drugs, vasospasm, inflammation, arterial and venous thrombosis, direct cytotoxicity, osmotic stress, and endothelial injury [119, 120]. These injections were often made in patients who were in shock, in whom detection of acci-

Table 1.3 Evolution of vascular injuries after accidental arterial injections

Time	Symptoms
On injection	Pain, redness, numbness, weakness
0–30 min	Pallor, poor capillary refill
<24 h	Swelling, pain, mottled cyanosis, cramps, paresthesia, and motor weakness
<48 h	Skin: cyanosis, bullae, vesicles, Muscles: compartment syndrome with swelling, muscle pain, and tenderness with painful movements Sensations: numbness, tingling, or burning
<1 week	Muscle necrosis, contracture
>1 week	Necrosis, contractures, gangrene, amputation

dental arterial cannulation might have been difficult due to hypotension.

Ironically, while complications of accidental arterial injections were reported in the 1940s, highly viscous radiocontrast agents were developed for injection into the arteries during angiography. In 1949, Juhn Atsushi Wada, a Japanese neurologist and neurosurgeon, reported using an IA anesthetic drug to locate speech function before surgery. Wada first used IA amytal to suppress seizures in a patient with protracted seizures despite intensive medical treatment. He observed that although intracarotid amytal aborted the seizures, it resulted in transient hemiplegia and aphasia. In 1949, Wada published his report on IA amytal injection for localization of speech function. In 1954, Wada introduced his test to Wilder Penfield at the Montreal Neurological Institute [121].

Between 1948 and 1954, Wada conducted 80 such tests with no complications. Typically, 50–300 mg of 10% sodium amytal was used. Furthermore, in nonhuman primate experiments, Wada revealed that 20× the human equivalent dose of IA amytal was safely tolerated. Most clinical reports reveal the Wada test is exceedingly safe, with complications ranging from 0.3% to 11% [122]. The latter publication is an extreme case in which most complications were attributed to encephalopathy, yet only 2% of the patients needed any intervention. Routine cerebral angiography is associated with a 1–3% complication rate without IA drug injection. Seizures, transient neurological complications, occasional TIA, and sporadic strokes are expected due to patient population, surgical intervention, and preoperative withholding of anti-epileptic drugs for testing purposes. Using any test for 70 years is a compelling testament to the procedure's safety [121, 123].

The Development of Intraarterial Chemotherapy

Concerns regarding the safety of IA drug delivery cannot be rhetorically dismissed. Any IA injection carries small but potentially significant risks due to the procedure itself independent of drug delivery. Therefore, the real question is not the absolute risks involved but the risk relative to the benefits of the treatment. In this light, Calvin Klopp considered complications of IA injection of nitrogen mustard to be an acceptable risk. However, the accidental IA injection did cause erythema, blistering, and ulceration of the arm [124].

Klopp observed that the arm recovered after such an injury. Klopp then proceeded to test IA delivery in rabbits and dogs. There was evidence of tissue injury that was related to the dose. He also observed necrosis of implanted tumors in rabbits. However, due to spontaneous necrosis, it wasn't easy to discern the effect of the treatment. He observed that kidneys perfused with nitrogen mustard were undamaged, while all implanted tumors showed necrosis. Therefore, it was likely that the treatment was safe enough to treat tumors if the dose was fractionated to enhance tumor selectivity, similar to radiation treatments. Klopp proceeded to test IA nitrosourea on ten human subjects. The media picked up his report, which was presented in April 1949. TIME© magazine a fortnight later reported Klopp expected a tenfold reduction in drug dosing with IA injections [124–126].

Although seven of the ten patients had died, they all showed temporary improvement. One of the patients who was rendered blind by his brain tumor could even read again. Of the ten patients Klopp investigated, seven had head and neck tumors, two had malignant brain tumors, and one had fibrosarcoma of the thigh. Understandably, Klopp's results were reasonably encouraging and triggered several investigations into IA treatment of cancers in various organs (Table 1.4). In April 1950, H. R. Bierman, who also pioneered IA delivery of nitrogen mustards, published his results supporting the work done by Klopp's findings [124, 127].

Development of Pumps for Arterial Chemotherapy

The prime example of the benefits of long-term arterial drug infusion in clinical practice has been in the treatment of liver cancer. It was shown in the 1960s that prolonged chemotherapy infusion directly into the artery can improve survival. However, such treatment benefits were limited by complications due to drug delivery. Due to catheter migration, there was non-target site delivery of potent chemotherapeutic drugs into the stomach and elsewhere. Surgical isolation of the hepatic artery could decrease those complications. However, the quality of life was poor, with the patient requiring prolonged hospitalization to enable drug delivery. Perry Lynnfield Blackshear Jr. at the University of Minnesota developed the first implantable pump in 1980. The pump was initially designed to deliver heparin to prevent the clotting of catheters; however, it was soon adapted to deliver chemotherapy. The development of the implantable pump greatly impacted the quality of the patient's life as it permitted outdoor activities, including swimming, and enabled treatment on an outpatient basis. Subsequently, the availability of silicone catheters further decreased the risk of thromboembolism and increased the safety of prolonged arterial drug delivery. Continuous hepatic artery infusion with implantable pumps provides a template for safe and effective prolonged arterial chemotherapy development [96].

Table 1.4 Reports of oncologic applications of arterial chemotherapy

Year	Type of cancer	Drug	Author	Reference
1952	Brain cancer	Nitrogen mustard	French J	[128]
1952	Vaginal and cervical cancer	Nitrogen mustard	Cromer J	[130]
1954	Retinoblastoma	Triethylenemelamine (TEM)	Reese AB	[129]
1959	Head and neck	Methotrexate	Sullivan RD	[131]
1961	Breast cancer	Nitrogen mustard	Byron RL	[132]
1961	Liver cancer	Nitrogen mustard	Byron RL	[133]
1975	Penile cancer	Methotrexate	Tarquini	[134]
1998	Pancreatic cancer	Mitomycin C, Cisplatin, 5FU	Aigner KD	[135]

Table 1.5 Early reports of non-oncologic applications of arterial drugs

Year	Application	Drug	Author	Reference
1908	Regional analgesia	Cocaine, novocaine, eucaine	Goyenes	[103]
1927	Angiography	Sodium iodide	Monize	[83]
1944	Local infection	Penicillin	Glesser	[108]
1954	Regional thromboembolism	Heparin	Lefebvre	[136]
1947	Regional ischemia	Ergot alkaloids	Kappert	[110]
1949	Location of the speech center	Amytal	Wada	[121]
1971	Cerebrovascular insufficiency	Papaverine	Olesen	[137]
1979	Myocardial infarction	Nitroglycerin and streptokinase	Rentrop	[138]
1980	Blood-brain barrier disruption	Mannitol	Neuwelt	[139, 140]
1992	Cerebral vasospasm after SAH	Papaverine	Kaku	[141]
1996	Peripheral vascular insufficiency	Plasmid phVEGF165	Isner	[142]
2007	Stroke	Stem cells	Correa	[143]

The Non-oncologic Applications of Arterial Drug Delivery

IA regional anesthesia pioneered by Goyanes was the first non-oncologic application of IA drug delivery. As Glasser referenced in his 1945 paper, in 1914, Jean Folies in France and Heddaus in Germany also used IA drugs [108]. It is not easy to ascertain the purpose and results of their injections. Glasser introduced IA injection of penicillin, which was a subject of intense investigation in the 1950s, primarily due to the drug's scarcity. Some of the other non-oncologic uses of IA drugs are listed in Table 1.5.

Development of Pharmacokinetic Models

The intuitive appeal of IA drug delivery to achieve high concentrations at the target site betrays the complexity of the underlying pharmacokinetics. Many researchers determine the arterial concentrations by dividing the delivered dose by blood flow. This approach, for example, ignores the biomechanics of injection, the mixing of drugs with blood, and the extent of drug binding.

Ekman described an early pharmacokinetic model revealing the benefits of arterial delivery in 1974 [144]. The model showed how increased cardiac output and systemic clearance adversely affected arterial drug delivery and revealed the importance of the fraction extracted by the target site [145]. The rate of uptake and efflux from the target site determined local drug concentration. Target site concentrations were determined by increased local extraction, prolonged half-life, and decreased systemic uptake.

Simpler two-compartment pharmacokinetic models was later developed by Dedrick in 1986 and 1988 (Fig. 1.4) [145, 146]. This model revealed that IA drug delivery is effective when there is greater regional extraction, low regional blood flow, and high systemic clearance. Though these models provided a theoretical construct to develop a hypothesis, none accurately reflected experimental observations. The Deidrick model was recently updated to show the enormous impact of tissue avidity/retention on arterial drug delivery [147].

A significant problem in arterial pharmacokinetics models is *streaming*. Steaming is the uneven distribution of the drug in arterial branches downstream of the point of injection due to preferential flow in some of those arteries [148–150]. The uniformity of drug concentration depends on the site of injection, underlying blood flow, phase of cardiac cycle, and the rate and volume of drug injection [148]. Only in this century have arterial models emerged in the context of nanoparticle delivery that account for the flow conditions. Some of the enormous complexities in modeling arterial blood flow were discussed earlier [151]. Modeling arterial drug delivery is far more complex given the anatomic com-

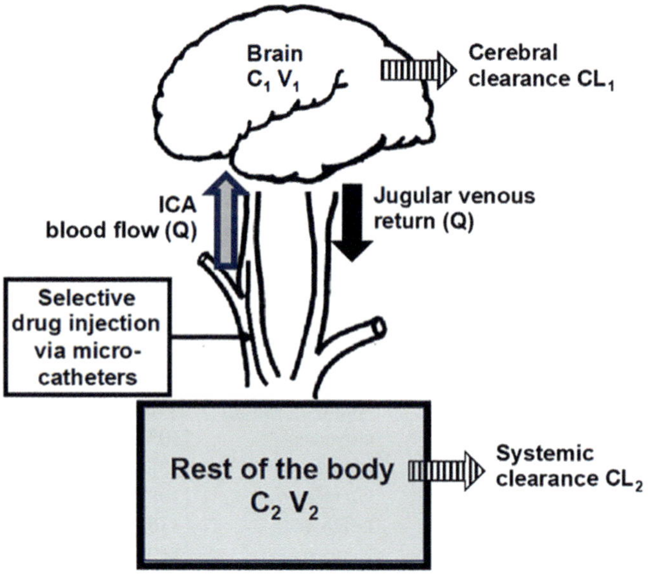

Fig. 1.4 The Dedrick (1988) model as applied to intracarotid drug delivery, C_1 C_2 and V_1 V_2 are concentrations and volumes in the brain (1) and the remainder of the body (2), respectively. Q is the regional blood flow, and CL_1 and CL_2 are cerebral and remaining body clearances

plexities of the arterial networks, biomechanics of the arterial wall, changing flow conditions, streaming, systemic hemodynamic factors, and biological responsiveness of the system. Although MRI-based patient-specific drug delivery models have been described, these models are still in the preliminary stages of development [151].

Development of Drug Infusion Protocols

Klopp et al. (1950) noted in the preliminary animal studies that bolus injection of the total dose of nitrogen mustard resulted in serious tissue injury [124]. The situation was analogous to the severe side effects observed if a total radiation dose was given in a single setting. Klopp, therefore, recommended that the total dose be fractionated and given in smaller amounts to minimize side effects. Other investigators used a continuous infusion of multiple drugs through an indwelling catheter over several days [152]. However, low-volume infusion rates could increase the likelihood of streaming and result in unpredictable tissue concentrations [150]. To minimize streaming, it was recommended that drug injections were delivered as pulses during diastole [148]. Cloughesy et al. recommended that the drug dose delivered via pulsatile delivery be proportional to the regional blood flow [153]. An innovative approach developed was the use of thiosulfate to neutralize the recirculating drug to minimize systemic toxicity [154]. Oldfield used a physical hemoperfusion approach to increase systemic clearance during arterial chemotherapy [155, 156].

Aigner, in 1998, recommended that drug uptake would be better if the arterial blood flow was reduced or even stopped during drug infusion [157]. Around the time, Pile-Spellman et al. demonstrated the feasibility of adenosine-induced flow arrest to assist the delivery of embolic materials to treat high-flow arteriovenous malformation [158]. Flow arrest drug delivery offered many advantages, including:

- Better localizing the drug at the target site.
- Minimizing and avoiding contact with blood to achieve high arterial blood concentrations.
- Avoiding binding to cells and proteins in the arterial blood.
- Increasing the transit time of the drug to traverse the capillary circulation.
- Decreasing shear force on nanoparticles to enhance endothelial attachment and uptake.
- Avoiding streaming-related variability in arterial drug concentrations.

Joshi et al. revealed that the tissue concentrations of carmustine were 6× greater when the injections were made during flow arrest compared to conventional arterial infusions [159]. Using video microscopy, they showed that during transient flow arrest, the drug completely displaces blood from the vascular network and avoids any contact with blood, thereby fundamentally changing the pharmacokinetic profile of arterial injections. Rinna et al. (2010) demonstrated the technical feasibility of highly targeted arterial drug delivery using super-selective arterial catheterization and flow arrest using a balloon occluding catheter [160].

Development of Drugs for Intraarterial Delivery

The modified Dedrick model shows that IA drugs should be rapidly absorbed and avidly bound to the target tissue [147]. To that end, the term extraction is somewhat misleading, as the drug should be extracted and retained or avidly bound to the tissue for a sufficient duration to have the desired effect. The drug's tissue concentration has to be maintained for a sufficient duration to have the desired pharmacodynamic effect [146]. Much of the emphasis on drug and drug conjugate development has been on the uptake by the target site. An overlooked strategy for arterial drug development is to develop rapidly metabolized drugs. Due to rapid metabolism, limiting the drug's regional effects to arterial irrigation might be possible. Adenosine is a drug prototype with a half-life of 0.6–10 s [161]. Hence, large doses of adenosine can be infused arterially without systemic side effects to augment blood flow [162].

Hitherto, the development of drugs specifically for therapeutic arterial delivery has primarily evolved around the treatment of liver cancers. The success of hepatic artery chemotherapy is due to several unique characteristics of the liver, including dual sources of tissue perfusion, selective perfusion of tumors by the hepatic artery, the inherent ability of the liver to clear drugs such as 5FU from the circulating blood, and the ability to regenerate if injured [163]. The liver can be safely embolized with embolic materials loaded with sustained-release chemotherapy or locally irradiative isotopes. Unsurprisingly, between 1964 and 2022, almost 60% of publications on IA treatments dealt with liver cancer, an area of intense innovation (Fig. 1.5).

However, the challenges in developing drugs for treating neurological diseases are significantly different from those for the liver. In contrast to hepatocytes, neurons are exquisitely vulnerable to ischemia and have no regenerative capacity. The blood-brain barrier also protects the brain, which can restrict drug delivery. Since 1970, IA drug delivery has usually focused on disruption or delivery across the blood-brain barrier [164–166]. However, small molecular weight lipid-soluble drugs, such as temozolomide, that are not restricted by the barrier have not been helpful for IA treatments. High regional concentrations of the drug and increased lipid solubility could trap the drug in the white matter and predispose it to injury [139, 167, 168]. Disrupting the blood-brain barrier with hyperosmotic agents can be highly variable [169]. Osmotic BBB disruption is effective in treating certain brain tumors [170, 171]. Improving blood-brain barrier penetration might be more relevant to large molecular weight compounds such as peptides and monoclonal antibodies, especially when the disruption is super selective and limited in scale [172, 173].

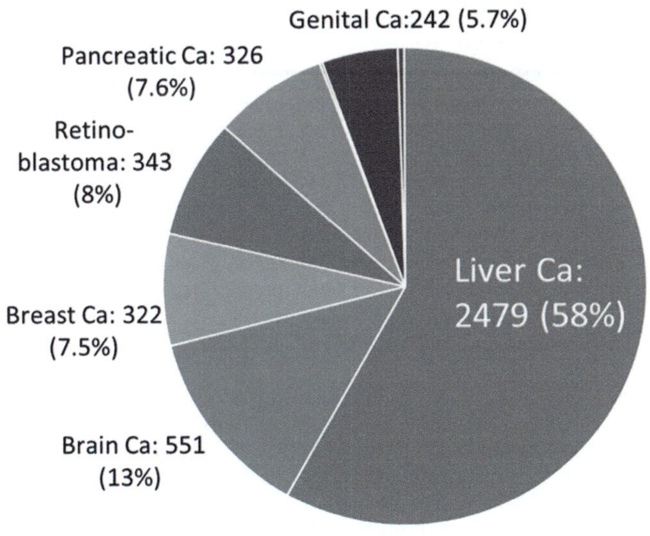

Fig. 1.5 Number of publications on Pub med with Intraarterial treatment of various cancers between 1964 and 2022

Due to its high resting cerebral blood flow, any drug crossing the blood-brain barrier will rapidly diffuse back, promptly cleared once the arterial infusion ceases. During the 1980s, the increased lipid solubility of chemotherapeutic drugs led to the development of chlorambucil tertiary butyl ester [174]. However, drug delivery to the brain did not significantly improve. Other investigators relied on carrier-conjugated drugs, which exploited the transporter systems across the blood-brain barrier using transferrin antibodies [175]. These have been clinically assessed. One problem in identifying suitable drug formulations for arterial drug delivery is determining tissue concentrations in the sub-second time frame needed to track arterial drug delivery. Although positron emission tomography is available, it is not practical for high-volume studies needed to optimize drug development [176]. The duration of electrocerebral silence after arterial anesthetic injections was used as a surrogate of drug concentrations to investigate the relationship between blood flow and arterial drug effects [177–179]. Using the optical pharmacokinetic method developed by Bigio and Mourant [180–182], Joshi et al. were able to investigate cationic micelles [183, 184], liposomes [185–189], and peptides [189] that were avidly retained by rodent brain tumors. These compounds are yet to be thoroughly evaluated in larger models.

Synthesis and Future Directions

The persistent belief that injecting the drugs arterially leads to increased local drug delivery with resulting therapeutic benefits has stymied the neurological applications of this method of drug delivery. As this historical review shows, the technology for improving arterial drug delivery is still improving. These include better catheters, imaging devices, and drug formulations. However, there is a paucity of robust models of first-pass uptake of arterial drugs that can be used for developing drug delivery protocols. Most drug delivery protocols ignore the underlying flow conditions. The critical role of background blood flow in determining the efficacy and side effects of arterial treatments is typically not recognized. Klopp, for example, observed that renal arterial injections of drugs were safe, while limb injections caused cutaneous injury. Renal arterial blood flow is estimated to be 160–190 mL/100 g/min, while the skin blood flow is 1–3 mL/100 g/min. Thus, even in the earliest studies, there was evidence of the critical role blood flow plays in determining the net effects of arterial drug injection. Still, blood flow modulation was ignored in many studies [124].

While arterial drug delivery has been proven safe and effective during Wada testing, it has yet to find a place in treating malignant brain tumors and other neurological diseases. In defense of arterial delivery, it is the observation that most other treatments for malignant brain tumors have also not proven to be very successful. However, treatment failure is not an excuse for abandoning arterial drug delivery research. Arterial drug delivery has three conceptual components: (a) a complex set of bioengineering factors determining arterial blood drug concentrations, (b) the first pass uptake and elimination from the target site determining the site-specific drug concentrations, and (c) the systemic pharmacokinetics of the effluent drug determining the recirculating drug concentrations. Arterial drug delivery is as much a fluid engineering problem as a pharmacokinetic one. Unless the drug delivery problem is addressed holistically, the conventional piecemeal approach will likely fail. This chapter provided a historical perspective on underlying tools and concepts of arterial delivery. Other chapters in this book describe specific successes and failures of such treatments. The optical pharmacokinetic method to understand arterial drug delivery, development of novel carriers, and delivery protocol could further advance brain cancer treatment. The goal of arterial chemotherapy for malignant brain tumors should be a dramatic reduction of drug dosing to enable novel treatment of brain tumors and other neurological diseases.

Conclusions

The first drug to be injected intravenously to enable surgery was the tincture of opium, which was tested on dogs. Three hundred and seventy years later, intravenous drug infusion protocols are still developing, a testament to the slow evolution of medical technologies. Ironically, the first IA drug injected was also an anesthetic to enable surgery on dogs a century ago. Although arterial drug delivery has come a long way, the technology is still in its infancy. Much of the technology is still developing; there is a need for better imaging that can map drug distribution while quantifying blood flow. Better computational models to understand and improve delivery; catheters that are super selective, non-thrombogenic, and capable of modulating the blood flow; better delivery protocols with drug formulations that are optimized for arterial delivery; and selection of appropriate drug cargos that are effective within the time constraints placed by the delivery method are some examples of advancements in technology that would enhance IA drug delivery. If all these advances come into play, they will reveal the vast oncologic and non-oncologic potential of arterial drug delivery. This review shows how the individual components of arterial drug delivery have evolved over the last century. It also reveals how advances in pharmacology, materials sciences, biomedical imaging, and computational capabilities can usher in novel arterial treatments of neurological diseases hitherto unachievable by conventional means.

References

1. Aird WC. Discovery of the cardiovascular system: from Galen to William Harvey. J Thromb Haemost. 2011;9(Suppl 1):118–29.
2. Bolli R. William Harvey and the discovery of the circulation of the blood. Circ Res. 2019;124(10):1428–9.
3. Bolli R. William Harvey and the discovery of the circulation of the blood. Circ Res. 2019;124(9):1300–2.
4. Bolli R. William Harvey and the discovery of the circulation of the blood. Circ Res. 2019;124(8):1169–71.
5. Bosmia A, Watanabe K, Shoja MM, Loukas M, Tubbs RS. Michael Servetus (1511–1553): physician and heretic who described the pulmonary circulation. Int J Cardiol. 2013;167(2):318–21.
6. Canale DJ. Michael Servetus, theologian, physician and heretic: a reappraisal of his contribution to physiology and medicine. J Med Biogr. 2001;9(3):137–42.
7. Cattermole GN. Michael Servetus: physician, Socinian and victim. J R Soc Med. 1997;90(11):640–4.
8. West JB. History of respiratory gas exchange. Compr Physiol. 2011;1(3):1509–23.
9. Fitting JW. From breathing to respiration. Respiration. 2015;89(1):82–7.
10. Lewis O. Stephen Hales and the measurement of blood pressure. J Hum Hypertens. 1994;8(12):865–71.
11. Macklem PT. Stephen Hales, an unrecognized giant of medicine. Osler Libr Newsl. 2010;114:1–4.
12. Maquet P. Borelli: De Motu Animalium. A first treatise on biomechanics. Acta Orthop Belg. 1989;55(4):541–6.
13. Castel-Branco N. Physico-mathematics and the life sciences: experiencing the mechanism of venous return, 1650s–1680s. Ann Sci. 2022;79(4):442–67.
14. Des Chene D. Mechanisms of life in the seventeenth century: Borelli, Perrault, Regis. Stud Hist Phil Biol Biomed Sci. 2005;36(2):245–60.
15. Smith IB. The impact of Stephen Hales on medicine. J R Soc Med. 1993;86(6):349–52.
16. Archie JP Jr. Presidential address: A brief history of arterial blood flow—from Harvey and Newton to computational analysis. J Vasc Surg. 2001;34(3):398–404.
17. Steinke H. William Harvey revisited. Ther Umsch. 2015;72(7):421–7.
18. Karamanou M, Papaioannou TG, Tsoucalas G, Tousoulis D, Stefanadis C, Androutsos G. Blood pressure measurement: lessons learned from our ancestors. Curr Pharm Des. 2015;21(6):700–4.
19. Ding XR, Zhao N, Yang GZ, Pettigrew RI, Lo B, Miao F, et al. Continuous blood pressure measurement from invasive to unobtrusive: celebration of 200th birth anniversary of Carl Ludwig. IEEE J Biomed Health Inform. 2016;20(6):1455–65.
20. Tsyrlin VA, Kuzmenko N, Pliss M. The history of blood pressure measurement: from Hales to our days. Arterial'naya Gipertenziya (Arterial Hypertens). 2016;22(2):144–52.
21. Major RH. Karl Vierordt. Ann Med Hist. 1938;10(6):463–73.
22. Booth J. A short history of blood pressure measurement. Proc R Soc Med. 1977;70(11):793–9.
23. Anonymous. Obituary: Dr. Robert Ellis Dudgeon. BMJ. 1904;2:954.
24. Soto-Perez-de-Celis E. Karl Samuel Ritter Von Basch: the sphygmomanometer and the Empire. J Hypertens. 2007;25(7):1507–9.
25. Anonymous. South Australian Medical Heritage Society Inc. https://www.samhs.org.au/Virtual%20Museum/Medicine/Blood_pressure/Blood_pressure.html.
26. Diegel U. A short history of blood pressure. 2018. https://www.bloodpressurehistory.com/blood-pressure-history.

27. Penaz J. Photoelectric measurement of blood pressure, volume, and flow in the finger. In: Digest of the 10th International Conference on Medical and Biological Engineering; 1973.
28. Duong DH, Young WL, Vang MC, Sciacca RR, Mast H, Koennecke HC, et al. Feeding artery pressure and venous drainage pattern are primary determinants of hemorrhage from cerebral arteriovenous malformations. Stroke. 1998;29(6):1167–76.
29. Lam S, Liu H, Jian Z, Settels J, Bohringer C. Intraoperative invasive blood pressure monitoring and the potential pitfalls of invasively measured systolic blood pressure. Cureus. 2021;13(8):e17610.
30. Parker KH. A brief history of arterial wave mechanics. Med Biol Eng Comput. 2009;47(2):111–8.
31. Ball C, Westhorpe RN. Direct blood pressure monitoring. Anaesth Intensive Care. 2009;37(4):515.
32. Cerrato E, Tomassini F, Salinas P, Pavani M, Conrotto F, Echavarria-Pinto M, et al. Simplified hybrid algorithms for pressure wire interrogation exploiting advantages of a baseline and contrast Pd/Pa ratio indexes to predict stenosis significance: insight from the SPARE multicenter prospective study. Catheter Cardiovasc Interv. 2018;92(6):1090–6.
33. Echavarria-Pinto M, Collet C, Escaned J, Piek JJ, Serruys PW. State of the art: pressure wire and coronary functional assessment. EuroIntervention. 2017;13(6):666–79.
34. O'Connor JJ, Robertson EF. Daniel Bernoulli School of Mathematics. Scotland: University of St. Andrews; 1998. https://mathshistory.st-andrews.ac.uk/Biographies/Bernoulli_Daniel/.
35. Bistafa SR. Euler, father of hemodynamics. Adv Histor Stud. 2018;7:97–111.
36. O'Connor JJ, Robertson EF. Claude Louis Marie Henri Navier. 2000. https://mathshistory.st-andrews.ac.uk/Biographies/Navier/.
37. O'Connor JJ, Robertson EF. George Gabriel Strokes. 2003. https://mathshistory.st-andrews.ac.uk/Biographies/Stokes/.
38. Anonymous. Navier-Strokes Equations: 3 dimensional unsteady NASA Glenn Research Center. 2021. https://www.grc.nasa.gov/www/k-12/airplane/nseqs.html.
39. Sutera SP, Skalak R. The history of Poiseuille's law. Annu Rev Fluid Mech. 1993;25:1–19.
40. Poiseuille and the mercury manometer—1828. JAMA J Am Med Assoc. 1928;91(1):31–2.
41. Gurdjian ES, Gurdjian ES. History of occlusive cerebrovascular disease I. From Wepfer to Moniz. Arch Neurol. 1979;36(6):340–3.
42. Gurdjian ES, Gurdjian ES. History of occlusive cerebrovascular disease. II. After Moniz, with special reference to surgical treatment. Arch Neurol. 1979;36(7):427–32.
43. Nachtigall W. On the significance of Reynold's number and the fluid mechanical phenomena connected to it in swimming physiology and flight biophysics (author's transl). Fortschr Zool. 1977;24(2–3):13–56.
44. Mishra NL. 125th year of the discovery of X-rays. Sci Report. 2021;58:44–6.
45. Dunn PM. Wilhelm Conrad Roentgen (1845–1923), the discovery of x rays and perinatal diagnosis. Arch Dis Child Fetal Neonatal Ed. 2001;84(2):F138–9.
46. Mayr A. Prof. Heinrich Geissler. Berl Munch Tierarztl Wochenschr. 1979;92(13):249–50.
47. Dorfel G. The master and his school—on the biography and action of instrument developer Heinrich Geissler. Sudhoffs Arch. 2014;98(1):91–108.
48. Baskervilie C. Sir William Crookes. Science. 1910;31(786):100–3.
49. Parsons JH. Specimens of experimental glasses prepared by Sir William Crookes, O.M., P.R.S. Proc R Soc Med. 1914;7(Sect Ophthalmol):48–50.
50. Editors. Eugen Goldstein. Encyclopedia Britannica. 2023.
51. Pai-Dhungat J. Ivan Puluj—forgotten man of X-rays. J Assoc Physicians India. 2021;69(6):11–2.
52. Babic RR, Stankovic Babic G, Babic SR, Babic NR. 120 Years since the discovery of X-rays. Med Pregl. 2016;69(9–10):323–30.
53. Vucevic D, Dordevic D, Radosavljevic T. Nikola Tesla and medicine: 160th anniversary of the birth of the genius who gave light to the world—Part I. Med Pregl. 2016;69(9–10):313–22.
54. James T. The centenary of the discovery of X-rays by Röntgen—8 November 1895. Adler Mus Bull. 1995;21(1):11–5.
55. Kanikovskii VB. Increasing the anode characteristics of sharp-focused Coolidge X-ray tubes by changing from a high to a low vacuum. Med Tekh. 2002;5:9–13.
56. Aronowitz JN. Transformative technologies: the Crookes, Coolidge, and Cascade tubes. Int J Radiat Oncol Biol Phys. 2016;96(5):931–3.
57. Fradin M. Why use rotating anodes? J Radiol Electrol Arch Electr Medicale. 1950;31(1–2):104–5.
58. Konoplev EE, Stoliarov VN, Stoliarov IN. New structural materials for rotating anodes of diagnostic X-ray tubes. Med Tekh. 2011;5:6–10.
59. Prellwitz F. History of medical x-ray tubes. 1. Rontgenpraxis. 1974;27(2):38–47.
60. Prellwitz F. History of medical x-ray tubes. Rontgenpraxis. 1974;27(1):17–22 contd.
61. Ou X, Chen X, Xu X, Xie L, Chen X, Hong Z, et al. Recent development in X-ray imaging technology: future and challenges. Research (Wash D C). 2021;2021:9892152.
62. Howell JD. Early clinical use of the X-ray. Trans Am Clin Climatol Assoc. 2016;127:341–9.
63. Oborska-Kumaszynska D, Wisniewska-Kubka S. Analog and digital systems of imaging in roentgenodiagnostics. Pol J Radiol. 2010;75(2):73–81.
64. Gomez LP, Mejuto J, Vidal JJ. A low-cost system for digital image processing of moving images in real time: application to X-ray fluoroscopy. Comput Methods Prog Biomed. 1992;39(1–2):43–9.
65. Mairgunther RH. Film-less digital x-ray image processing—new prospects with the RadioVisioGraphy equipment. Schweiz Monatsschr Zahnmed. 1994;104(1):31–4.
66. Rowlands JA. The physics of computed radiography. Phys Med Biol. 2002;47(23):R123–66.
67. Asai K, Nakamura H, Watabe T, Nishida T, Sakaguchi M, Hatazawa J, et al. X-ray angiography perfusion imaging with an intra-arterial injection: comparative study with (15)O-gas/water positron emission tomography. J Neurointerv Surg. 2018;10(8):780–3.
68. Brunozzi D, Shakur SF, Ismail R, Linninger A, Hsu CY, Charbel FT, et al. Correlation between contrast time-density time on digital subtraction angiography and flow: an in vitro study. World Neurosurg. 2018;110:e315–e20.
69. Donaldson C, O'Neill AH, Slater LA, Chong W, Lai LT, Chandra RV. Feasibility of real-time angiographic perfusion imaging in the treatment of cerebral vasospasm. Interv Neurol. 2017;6(3–4):163–9.
70. Wakhloo AK, Lieber BB, Rudin S, Fronckowiak MD, Mericle RA, Hopkins LN. A novel approach to flow quantification in brain arteriovenous malformations prior to enbucrilate embolization: use of insoluble contrast (Ethiodol droplet) angiography. J Neurosurg. 1998;89(3):395–404.
71. Asaduddin M, Roh HG, Kim HJ, Kim EY, Park SH. Perfusion maps acquired from dynamic angiography MRI using deep learning approaches. J Magn Reson Imaging. 2023;57(2):456–69.
72. Larsson HBW, Vestergaard MB, Lindberg U, Iversen HK, Cramer SP. Brain capillary transit time heterogeneity in healthy volunteers measured by dynamic contrast-enhanced T(1)-weighted perfusion MRI. J Magn Reson Imaging. 2017;45(6):1809–20.
73. Agus O, Ozkan M, Aydin K, Sahinbas M, Sencer S. Evaluation of hemodynamic perfusion MR images. Conf Proc IEEE Eng Med Biol Soc. 2005;2005:5794–7.

74. Martinez P, Nault G, Steiner J, Wempe MF, Pierce A, Brunt B, et al. MRI-guided focused ultrasound blood-brain barrier opening increases drug delivery and efficacy in a diffuse midline glioma mouse model. Neurooncol Adv. 2023;5(1):vdad111.
75. Malysz-Cymborska I, Golubczyk D, Kalkowski L, Kwiatkowska J, Zawadzki M, Glodek J, et al. Intra-arterial transplantation of stem cells in large animals as a minimally-invasive strategy for the treatment of disseminated neurodegeneration. Sci Rep. 2021;11(1):6581.
76. Fraser AG, Monaghan MJ, van der Steen AFW, Sutherland GR. A concise history of echocardiography: timeline, pioneers, and landmark publications. Eur Heart J Cardiovasc Imaging. 2022;23(9):1130–43.
77. Newby DE, Fox KA. Invasive assessment of the coronary circulation: intravascular ultrasound and Doppler. Br J Clin Pharmacol. 2002;53(6):561–75.
78. Van Tiggelen R. The rise of contrast-enhanced Roentgenology: an illustrated and chronological overview. J Belg Soc Radiol. 2016;100(1):102.
79. Smolik ED, Nash FP. Cerebral angiography. A brief outline of its history and experiences with Conray, a new contrast medium. Vasc Dis. 1964;1:21–8.
80. Mohammed AQ, Sawmiller CJ, Sumpio BE. Radio contrast agents: history and evolution. In: Chang JB, editor. Textbook of angiology. New York: Springer; 2000.
81. Tauber WB. Clinical consequences of Thorotrast in a long-term survivor. Health Phys. 1992;63(1):13–9.
82. Rangappa P. Egaz Moniz. J Assoc Physicians India. 2015;63(3):95–6.
83. [Egaz Moniz]. Rev Neurol (Paris). 1957;96(1):49–50.
84. Kilgore EJ, Elster AD. Walter Dandy and the history of ventriculography. Radiology. 1995;194(3):657–60.
85. Horwitz NH. Walter Edward Dandy (1886–1946). Neurosurgery. 1997;40(1):211–5.
86. Steimle RH, Jean A. Sicard (1872–1929). His pioneer work in nervous diseases. Neuroradiology. 1990;32(1):1–3.
87. Steimle R, Jean A. Sicard (1872–1929). J Neurol. 2013;260(7):1946–7.
88. Wake R, Yoshiyama M. Chapter 4: History of coronary angiography. In: Kirac S, editor. Advances in the diagnosis of coronary atherosclerosis. InTech; 2011. p. 69–80.
89. Anonymous. Brief history of urinary catheters. UroToday. 2023. https://www.urotoday.com/urinary-catheters-home/history-of-urinary-catheters.html.
90. Berry D. Pioneers in cardiology. Eur Heart J. 2009;30:1296–7.
91. Forssmann-Falck R. Werner Forssmann: a pioneer of cardiology. Am J Cardiol. 1997;79(5):651–60.
92. Afshar A, Steensma DP, Kyle RA. Werner Forssmann: a Pioneer of interventional cardiology and auto-experimentation. Mayo Clin Proc. 2018;93(9):e97–e8.
93. Riley RL. Andre Cournand. Bull Eur Physiopathol Respir. 1979;15(5):695–7.
94. Lequime J. In memoriam Andre Cournand (1895–1988). His role in the development of modern cardiology. Acta Cardiol. 1988;43(4):437–42.
95. Franch RH, Andre F. Cournand: father of clinical cardiopulmonary physiology. Clin Cardiol. 1986;9(2):82–6.
96. Anteby R, Kemeny NE, Kingham TP, D'Angelica MI, Wei AC, Balachandran VP, et al. Getting chemotherapy directly to the liver: the historical evolution of hepatic artery chemotherapy. J Am Coll Surg. 2021;232(3):332–8.
97. Infield GB. Disaster at Bari. New English Library; 1976.
98. Dunikowska M, Turko L. Fritz Haber: the damned scientist. Angew Chem Int Ed Engl. 2011;50(43):10050–62.
99. Stern F. Fritz Haber: flawed greatness of person and country. Angew Chem Int Ed Engl. 2012;51(1):50–6.
100. Christakis P. The birth of chemotherapy at Yale. Bicentennial lecture series: surgery grand round. Yale J Biol Med. 2011;84(2):169–72.
101. Goodman LS, Wintrobe MM, Dameshek W, Goodman MJ, Gilman A, McLennan MT. Landmark article Sept. 21, 1946: Nitrogen mustard therapy. Use of methyl-bis(beta-chloroethyl) amine hydrochloride and tris(beta-chloroethyl)amine hydrochloride for Hodgkin's disease, lymphosarcoma, leukemia and certain allied and miscellaneous disorders. By Louis S. Goodman, Maxwell M. Wintrobe, William Dameshek, Morton J. Goodman, Alfred Gilman and Margaret T. McLennan. JAMA. 1984;251(17):2255–61.
102. Criado E, Giron F. Jose Goyanes Capdevila, unsung pioneer of vascular surgery. Ann Vasc Surg. 2006;20(3):422–5.
103. Die-Goyanes A, Die-Trill J. Jose Goyanes. Surgeon and humanist. Cir Esp. 2008;83(1):8–11.
104. Vaca Miguel JM, Granda Juesas J, Garcia Camarero EJ, Alaejos Estebanez A, Llorente de la Fuente A, Tamayo Gomez E. Intra-arterial regional anesthesia. Rev Esp Anestesiol Reanim. 1990;37(6):356–9.
105. Gilsanz F. Intraarterial regional anaesthesia. Br J Anaesth. 1991;67:804.
106. Fiolle J, Fiolle P. Essais d'hematose artificielle et d angeiotherapie arterielle. Mars Med. 1914;51:597–603.
107. Heddaus A. Beitriige zur Heilserumbehandlung des Tetanus (Contributions to the medicinal serum treatment of tetanus). Miinchen Med Wchnschr. 1914;61:2186–9.
108. Glasser TS, Herrlin J, Pollocks B. Intra-arterial injection of penicillin for infections of the extremities. JAMA. 1945;128(11):796–802.
109. Donovan TJ. The uses of plastic tubes in the reparative surgery of battle injuries to arteries with and without intra-arterial heparin administration. Ann Surg. 1949;130:1024.
110. Kappert A. Untersuchungen über intraarterielle Therapie [Studies on intra-arterial therapy]. Helv Med Acta. 1947;14:533–9.
111. Nakstad P, Sortland O, Aaserud O, Lundervold A. Cerebral angiography with the non-ionic water-soluble contrast medium iohexol and meglumine-Ca-metrizoate. A randomized double blind parallel study in man. Neuroradiology. 1982;23(4):199–202.
112. Nakstad PH. The reaction of cerebral arteries to non-ionic contrast media during cerebral angiography. Neuroradiology. 1989;31(3):247–9.
113. Skalpe IO, Anke IM. Complications in cerebral angiography. A comparison between the non-ionic contrast medium iohexol and meglumine metrizoate (Isopaque Cerebral). Neuroradiology. 1983;25(3):157–60.
114. Skalpe IO, Lundervold A, Tjorstad K. Cerebral angiography with non-ionic (metrizamide) and ionic (meglumine metrizoate) water-soluble contrast media. A comparative study with double blind technic. Neuroradiology. 1977;14(1):15–9.
115. Fuhrman FA. Muscle electrolytes and water following intra-arterial injection of thiopental sodium. Am J Phys. 1951;167(2):298–304.
116. Johnson BD. A case of intra-arterial injection of pentothal sodium. Guys Hosp Gaz. 1946;60(1523):336–40.
117. Bennetts FE. Thiopentone anaesthesia at Pearl Harbor. Br J Anaesth. 1995;75(3):366–8.
118. Stone HH, Donnelly CC. The accidental intraarterial injection of thiopental. Anesthesiology. 1961;22:995–1006.
119. Lokoff A, Maynes JT. The incidence, significance, and management of accidental intra-arterial injection: a narrative review. Can J Anaesth. 2019;66(5):576–92.
120. Sen S, Chini EN, Brown MJ. Complications after unintentional intra-arterial injection of drugs: risks, outcomes, and management strategies. Mayo Clin Proc. 2005;80(6):783–95.
121. Wada JA. A fateful encounter: sixty years later—reflections on the Wada test. Epilepsia. 2008;49(4):726–7.

122. Loddenkemper T, Morris HH, Moddel G. Complications during the Wada test. Epilepsy Behav. 2008;13(3):551–3.
123. Loring DW, Meador KJ. History of the Wada test. In: Barr WB, Bieliauskas LA, editors. The Oxford handbook of history of clinical neuropsychology; 2019. p. 1–19.
124. Klopp CT, Alford TC, Bateman J, Berry GN, Winship T. Fractionated intra-arterial cancer; chemotherapy with methyl bis amine hydrochloride; a preliminary report. Ann Surg. 1950;132(4):811–32.
125. Barberio JR, Klopp CT, Ayres WW, Gross HA. Effects of intra-arterial administration of nitrogen mustard. Cancer. 1951;4(6):1341–63.
126. Klopp CT. Regional intra-arterial nitrogen mustard as an adjunct to radiation therapy. Am J Roentgenol Radium Therapy, Nucl Med. 1953;70(6):1005–14.
127. Bierman HR, Byron RL Jr, Miller ER, Shimkin MB. Effects of intra-arterial administration of nitrogen mustard. Am J Med. 1950;8(4):535.
128. French JD, West PM, Von Amerongen FK, Magoun HW. Effects of intracarotid administration of nitrogen mustard on normal brain and brain tumors. J Neurosurg. 1952;9(4):378–89.
129. Reese AB, Hyman GA, Merriam GR Jr, Forrest AW, Kligerman MM. Treatment of retinoblastoma by radiation and triethylenemelamine. AMA Arch Ophthalmol. 1954;53(4):505–13.
130. Cromer JK, Bateman JC, Berry GN, Kennelly JM, Klopp CT, Platt LI. Use of intra-arterial nitrogen mustard therapy in the treatment of cervical and vaginal cancer. Am J Obstet Gynecol. 1952;63(3):538–48.
131. Sullivan RD, Miller E, Sikes MP. Antimetabolite-metabolite combination cancer chemotherapy. Effects of intraarterial methotrexate-intramuscular Citrovorum factor therapy in human cancer. Cancer. 1959;12:1248–62.
132. Byron RL Jr, Yonemoto RH, Hallauer WC, Bierman HR. Radical mastectomy with arterial regional chemotherapy. Surgery. 1961;49:681–6.
133. Byron RL Jr, Perez FM, Yonemoto RH, Bierman HR, Gildenhorn HL, Kelly KH. Left brachial arterial catheterization for chemotherapy in advanced intra-abdominal malignant neoplasms. Surg Gynecol Obstet. 1961;112:689–96.
134. Tarquini A, Di Martino L, Caporelli S. Treatment of penile neoplasms by means of loco-regional intra-arterial therapy. Minerva Chir. 1975;30(13–14):817–24.
135. Aigner KR, Gailhofer S, Kopp S. Regional versus systemic chemotherapy for advanced pancreatic cancer: a randomized study. Hepato-Gastroenterology. 1998;45(22):1125–9.
136. Lefebvre P, De Martelaere R. Repeated intra-arterial injections of heparin in thrombolic disease. Acta Clin Belg. 1954;9(2):164–8.
137. Olesen J, Paulson OB. The effect of intra-arterial papaverine on the regional cerebral blood flow in patients with stroke or intracranial tumor. Stroke. 1971;2(2):148–59.
138. Rentrop KP, Blanke H, Karsch KR, Wiegand V, Kostering H, Oster H, et al. Acute myocardial infarction: intracoronary application of nitroglycerin and streptokinase. Clin Cardiol. 1979;2(5):354–63.
139. Neuwelt EA. Reversible osmotic blood-brain barrier disruption in humans: implications for the chemotherapy of malignant brain tumors. Neurosurgery. 1980;7(2):204.
140. Neuwelt EA, Frenkel EP, Rapoport S, Barnett P. Effect of osmotic blood-brain barrier disruption on methotrexate pharmacokinetics in the dog. Neurosurgery. 1980;7(1):36–43.
141. Kaku Y, Yonekawa Y, Tsukahara T, Kazekawa K. Superselective intra-arterial infusion of papaverine for the treatment of cerebral vasospasm after subarachnoid hemorrhage. J Neurosurg. 1992;77(6):842–7.
142. Isner JM, Walsh K, Symes J, Pieczek A, Takeshita S, Lowry J, et al. Arterial gene transfer for therapeutic angiogenesis in patients with peripheral artery disease. Hum Gene Ther. 1996;7(8):959–88.
143. Correa PL, Mesquita CT, Felix RM, Azevedo JC, Barbirato GB, Falcao CH, et al. Assessment of intra-arterial injected autologous bone marrow mononuclear cell distribution by radioactive labeling in acute ischemic stroke. Clin Nucl Med. 2007;32(11):839–4.
144. Eckman WW, Patlak CS, Fenstermacher JD. A critical evaluation of the principles governing the advantages of intra-arterial infusions. J Pharmacokinet Biopharm. 1974;2(3):257–85.
145. Dedrick RL. Interspecies scaling of regional drug delivery. J Pharm Sci. 1986;75(11):1047–52.
146. Dedrick RL. Arterial drug infusion: pharmacokinetic problems and pitfalls. J Natl Cancer Inst. 1988;80(2):84–9.
147. Cooke JN, Ellis JA, Hossain S, Nguyen J, Bruce JN, Joshi S. Computational pharmacokinetic rationale for intra-arterial delivery to the brain. Drug Deliv Transl Res. 2016;6(5):622–9.
148. Saris SC, Blasberg RG, Carson RE, deVroom HL, Lutz R, Dedrick RL, et al. Intravascular streaming during carotid artery infusions. Demonstration in humans and reduction using diastole-phased pulsatile administration. J Neurosurg. 1991;74(5):763–72.
149. Lutz RJ, Epstein AH, Cook JA, Dedrick RL. An in vitro flow model to study streaming during pelvic intra-arterial drug infusions. Gynecol Oncol. 1995;59(2):288–96.
150. Lutz RJ, Warren K, Balis F, Patronas N, Dedrick RL. Mixing during intravertebral arterial infusions in an in vitro model. J Neurooncol. 2002;58(2):95–106.
151. Hossain SS, Zhang Y, Liang X, Hussain F, Ferrari M, Hughes TJ, et al. In silico vascular modeling for personalized nanoparticle delivery. Nanomedicine (Lond). 2013;8(3):343–57.
152. Koyama H, Wada T, Takahashi Y, Iwanaga T, Aoki Y. Intra-arterial infusion chemotherapy as preoperative treatment of locally advanced breast cancer. Cancer. 1975;36(5):1603–12.
153. Cloughesy TF, Gobin YP, Black KL, Vinuela F, Taft F, Kadkhoda B, et al. Intra-arterial carboplatin chemotherapy for brain tumors: a dose escalation study based on cerebral blood flow. J Neurooncol. 1997;35(2):121–31.
154. Neuwelt EA, Brummett RE, Doolittle ND, Muldoon LL, Kroll RA, Pagel MA, et al. First evidence of otoprotection against carboplatin-induced hearing loss with a two-compartment system in patients with central nervous system malignancy using sodium thiosulfate. J Pharmacol Exp Ther. 1998;286(1):77–84.
155. Oldfield EH, Dedrick RL, Yeager RL, Clark WC, DeVroom HL, Chatterji DC, et al. Reduced systemic drug exposure by combining intra-arterial chemotherapy with hemoperfusion of regional venous drainage. J Neurosurg. 1985;63(5):726–32.
156. Oldfield EH, Clark WC, Dedrick RL, Egorin MJ, Austin HA, DeVroom HD, et al. Reduced systemic drug exposure by combining intraarterial cis-diamminedichloroplatinum(II) with hemodialysis of regional venous drainage. Cancer Res. 1987;47(7):1962–7.
157. Aigner KR. Intra-arterial infusion: overview and novel approaches. Semin Surg Oncol. 1998;14(3):248–53.
158. Pile-Spellman J, Young WL, Joshi S, Duong H, Vang MC, Hartmann A, et al. Adenosine-induced cardiac pause for endovascular embolization of cerebral arteriovenous malformations: technical case report. Neurosurgery. 1999;44(4):881–6; discussion 6–7.
159. Joshi S, Wang M, Etu JJ, Suckow RF, Cooper TB, Feinmark SJ, et al. Transient cerebral hypoperfusion enhances intraarterial carmustine deposition into brain tissue. J Neurooncol. 2008;86(2):123–32.
160. Riina HA, Knopman J, Greenfield JP, Fralin S, Gobin YP, Tsiouris AJ, et al. Balloon-assisted superselective intra-arterial cerebral infusion of bevacizumab for malignant brainstem glioma. A technical note. Interv Neuroradiol. 2010;16(1):71–6.
161. Parker RB, McCollam PL. Adenosine in the episodic treatment of paroxysmal supraventricular tachycardia. Clin Pharm. 1990;9(4):261–71.

162. Joshi S, Duong H, Mangla S, Wang M, Libow AD, Popilskis SJ, et al. In nonhuman primates intracarotid adenosine, but not sodium nitroprusside, increases cerebral blood flow. Anesth Analg. 2002;94(2):393–9, table of contents.
163. Laface C, Laforgia M, Molinari P, Ugenti I, Gadaleta CD, Porta C, et al. Hepatic arterial infusion of chemotherapy for advanced hepatobiliary cancers: state of the art. Cancers (Basel). 2021;13(12):3091.
164. Rapoport SI. Effect of concentrated solutions on blood-brain barrier. Am J Phys. 1970;219(1):270–4.
165. Rapoport SI, Hori M, Klatzo I. Reversible osmotic opening of the blood-brain barrier. Science. 1971;173(4001):1026–8.
166. Rapoport SI, Hori M, Klatzo I. Testing of a hypothesis for osmotic opening of the blood-brain barrier. Am J Phys. 1972;223(2):323–31.
167. Rosenblum MK, Delattre JY, Walker RW, Shapiro WR. Fatal necrotizing encephalopathy complicating treatment of malignant gliomas with intra-arterial BCNU and irradiation: a pathological study. J Neurooncol. 1989;7(3):269–81.
168. Neuwelt EA, Barnett PA, McCormick CI, Frenkel EP, Minna JD. Osmotic blood-brain barrier modification: monoclonal antibody, albumin, and methotrexate delivery to cerebrospinal fluid and brain. Neurosurgery. 1985;17(3):419–23.
169. Zylber-Katz E, Gomori J, Schwartz A, Lossos A, Bokstein F, Siegal T. Pharmacokinetics of methotrexate in cerebrospinal fluid and serum after osmotic blood-brain barrier disruption in patients with brain lymphoma. Clin Pharmacol Ther. 2000;67:631–41.
170. Uluc K, Neuwelt EA, Ambady P. Advances in intraarterial chemotherapy delivery strategies and blood-brain barrier disruption. Neurosurg Clin N Am. 2022;33(2):219–23.
171. Doolittle ND, Muldoon LL, Culp AY, Neuwelt EA. Delivery of chemotherapeutics across the blood-brain barrier: challenges and advances. Adv Pharmacol. 2014;71:203–43.
172. McCrea HJ, Ivanidze J, O'Connor A, Hersh EH, Boockvar JA, Gobin YP, et al. Intraarterial delivery of bevacizumab and cetuximab utilizing blood-brain barrier disruption in children with high-grade glioma and diffuse intrinsic pontine glioma: results of a phase I trial. J Neurosurg Pediatr. 2021;28(4):371–9.
173. Patel NV, Wong T, Fralin SR, Li M, McKeown A, Gruber D, et al. Repeated superselective intraarterial bevacizumab after blood brain barrier disruption for newly diagnosed glioblastoma: a phase I/II clinical trial. J Neurooncol. 2021;155(2):117–24.
174. Greig NH, Daly EM, Sweeney DJ, Rapoport SI. Pharmacokinetics of chlorambucil-tertiary butyl ester, a lipophilic chlorambucil derivative that achieves and maintains high concentrations in brain. Cancer Chemother Pharmacol. 1990;25(5):320–5.
175. Pardridge WM. Blood-brain barrier and delivery of protein and gene therapeutics to brain. Front Aging Neurosci. 2019;11:373.
176. Tyler JL, Yamamoto YL, Diksic M, Theron J, Villemure JG, Worthington C, et al. Pharmacokinetics of superselective intra-arterial and intravenous [11C]BCNU evaluated by PET. J Nucl Med. 1986;27(6):775–80.
177. Wang M, Joshi S, Emerson RG. Comparison of intracarotid and intravenous propofol for electrocerebral silence in rabbits. Anesthesiology. 2003;99(4):904–10.
178. Joshi S, Wang M, Etu JJ, Nishanian EV, Pile-Spellman J. Cerebral blood flow affects dose requirements of intracarotid propofol for electrocerebral silence. Anesthesiology. 2006;104(2):290–8, discussion 5A.
179. Joshi S, Wang M, Etu JJ, Pile-Spellman J. Bolus configuration affects dose requirements of intracarotid propofol for electroencephalographic silence. Anesth Analg. 2006;102(6):1816–22.
180. Mourant JR, Bigio IJ, Boyer JD, Johnson TM, Lacey J, Bohorfoush Iii AG, et al. Elastic scattering spectroscopy as a diagnostic tool for differentiating pathologies in the gastrointestinal tract: preliminary testing. J Biomed Opt. 1996;1(2):192–9.
181. Bigio IJ, Mourant JR, Los G. Noninvasive, in-situ measurement of drug concentrations in tissue using optical spectroscopy. J Gravit Physiol. 1999;6(1):P173–5.
182. Mourant JR, Johnson TM, Los G, Bigio IJ. Non-invasive measurement of chemotherapy drug concentrations in tissue: preliminary demonstrations of in vivo measurements. Phys Med Biol. 1999;44(5):1397–417.
183. Nguyen J, Hossain SS, Cooke JRN, Ellis JA, Deci MB, Emala CW, et al. Flow arrest intra-arterial delivery of small TAT-decorated and neutral micelles to gliomas. J Neurooncol. 2017;133(1):77–85.
184. Nguyen J, Cooke JRN, Ellis JA, Deci M, Emala CW, Bruce JN, et al. Cationizable lipid micelles as vehicles for intraarterial glioma treatment. J Neurooncol. 2016;128(1):21–8.
185. Joshi S, Singh-Moon RP, Wang M, Chaudhuri DB, Holcomb M, Straubinger NL, et al. Transient cerebral hypoperfusion assisted intraarterial cationic liposome delivery to brain tissue. J Neurooncol. 2014;118(1):73–82.
186. Joshi S, Singh-Moon RP, Ellis JA, Chaudhuri DB, Wang M, Reif R, et al. Cerebral hypoperfusion-assisted intra-arterial deposition of liposomes in normal and glioma-bearing rats. Neurosurgery. 2015;76(1):92–100.
187. Joshi S, Singh-Moon R, Wang M, Chaudhuri DB, Ellis JA, Bruce JN, et al. Cationic surface charge enhances early regional deposition of liposomes after intracarotid injection. J Neurooncol. 2014;120(3):489–97.
188. Joshi S, Cooke JR, Chan DK, Ellis JA, Hossain SS, Singh-Moon RP, et al. Liposome size and charge optimization for intraarterial delivery to gliomas. Drug Deliv Transl Res. 2016;6(3):225–33.
189. Joshi S, Cooke JRN, Ellis JA, Emala CW, Bruce JN. Targeting brain tumors by intra-arterial delivery of cell-penetrating peptides: a novel approach for primary and metastatic brain malignancy. J Neurooncol. 2017;135(3):497–506.

Conceptual Justification of Intra-arterial Drug Delivery

2

Jason A. Ellis, Souvik Singha, and Shailendra Joshi

All truths are easy to understand once they are discovered; the point is to discover them.

Galileo Galilei (1564–1642), Astronomer, Physicist, and Engineer

Introduction

The idea of injecting drugs into arteries to improve local drug delivery is intuitively appealing but is enormously misinformed. No doubt, injecting drugs into arteries can transiently achieve high regional concentrations at the target sites but the peak concentrations decline rapidly. For example, ^{11}C-labeled BCNU (1,3-bis(2-chloroethyl)-l-nitrosourea) achieves 50 times greater peak concentration in the brain after arterial injection than intravenous injection [1]. However, those concentrations rapidly decline, and there is only a two times improvement in drug delivery. Furthermore, due to "streaming," tissue drug concentrations can be very unpredictable, risking tissue injury due to excessive concentrations or therapeutic failure due to inadequate concentrations [2–6]. For treatments to be effective, drug delivery must be predictable and in the desired concentration range. In 1908, José Goyanes Capdevila, a Spanish vascular surgeon, first experimented with intra-arterial drug delivery. He successfully delivered local anesthetic drugs to enable regional surgery in about 70 patients, with 2 failures. Little is known about his experiments with intra-arterial cancer treatments, which are mentioned in his biography [7, 8]. By the 1940s, José Goyanes Capdevila and his experiments were largely forgotten. Capdevila's forgotten efforts warn that without a proper understanding of the underlying arterial pharmacokinetic concepts, the applications of arterial drug delivery will remain a curiosity, and their vast potential will remain untapped.

J. A. Ellis (✉) · S. Singha
Department of Neurosurgery, Zuker School of Medicine, Lenox Hill Hospital, New York, NY, USA
e-mail: jellis2@northwell.edu; ssingha3@northwell.edu

S. Joshi
Department of Anesthesiology, Columbia University Irving Medical Center, New York, NY, USA
e-mail: sj121@cumc.columbia.edu

Computational Models of Arterial Drug Delivery

The conceptual foundations of arterial drug delivery were laid at the National Institute of Health in the 1980s. A concerted effort was made to optimize arterial drug delivery. Central to that effort was a core group of researchers who explored the pharmacokinetic aspects of arterial drug delivery. The group primarily focused on the treatment of brain tumors. However, such treatment had little impact on clinical outcomes, and by the mid-1990s, they had largely abandoned the effort. Simulations by Eckman [9], Fenstermacher [10, 11], Collins [12, 13], Dedrick [14–16], and Chen [17] are highly relevant to understanding arterial drug delivery, its scope and application, drug selection, optimum carriers, drug infusion protocol development, and assessing the need for blood-brain barrier (BBB) disruption.

Eckman Model 1974

Represented one of the first attempts to investigate the theoretical advantages of arterial drug injections [9]. It assumed:

- The drug is delivered to the target site only by the artery.
- Individual linear compartments can describe drug distribution.

S. Joshi (ed.), *Arterial Treatment of Neurological Diseases*, https://doi.org/10.1007/978-3-031-80173-0_2

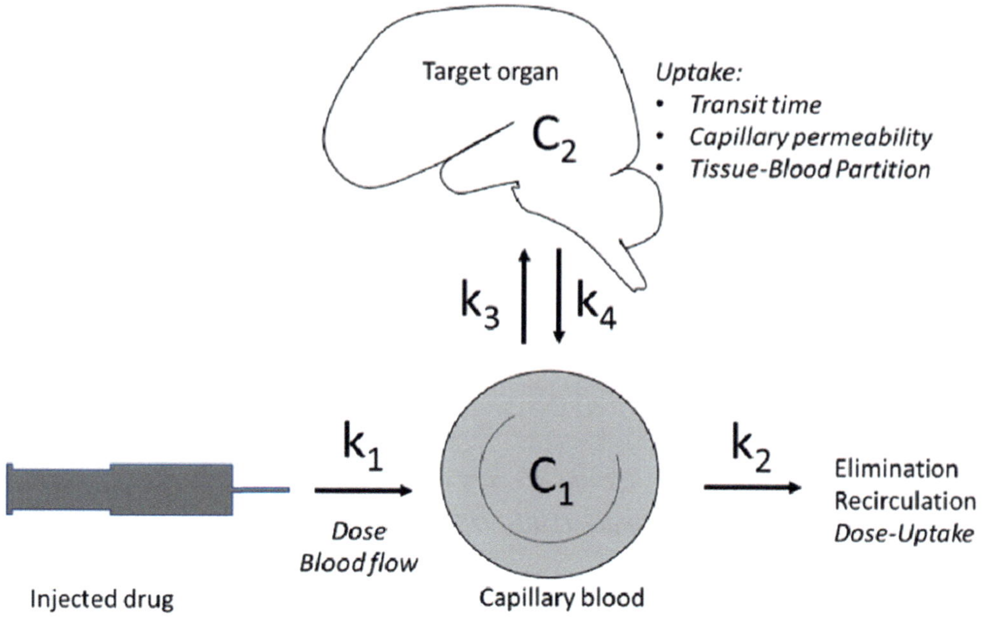

$$R_d = \left[\int_0^{\infty} C_2(t)\,dt\right]_{ART} \Big/ \left[\int_0^{\infty} C_2(t)\,dt\right]_{VEN}$$

Fig. 2.1 Elements of Eckman model: R_d is defined as the concentration ratio in the arterial compartment relative to that in the venous blood [9]

- The rate coefficients, such as blood flow, blood-tissue partition, and elimination, are constant.
- Concentrations directly determine the effects of drugs.
- The initial drug concentration and the concentration at the infinite time are 0.

The model characteristics are summarized in Fig. 2.1. Eckman assessed the benefits of arterial delivery by calculating the ratios of the concentrations achieved in blood or a target compartment after arterial and intravenous injections. The model revealed that arterial drug injections achieved greater (10×) first-pass concentrations than intravenous injections. However, there was little sustained benefit compared to intravenous injections when total body clearance was low (Fig. 2.2). Furthermore, the model showed that increased systemic clearance benefited arterial drug injections. The benefits of arterial injections were also evident when the regional blood flow was low and a smaller proportion of the cardiac output was perfusing the target site. However, the model found that the net blood flow to the target site did not affect drug delivery since the model estimated the probability of individual drug particles taken up by the target; hence, it was independent of the dilution by blood flow. The model was biased by the uptake of the drug during recirculation; therefore, it was significantly influenced by the elimination kinetics of the drug.

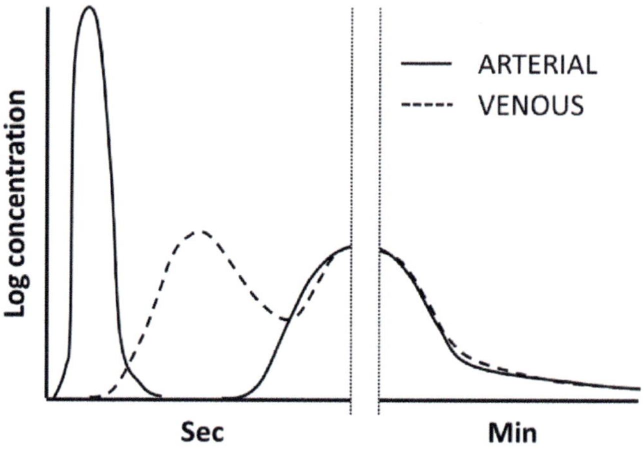

Fig. 2.2 Eckman simulations showed that arterial bolus injections achieved higher first-pass concentrations than venous bolus injections. The benefits of an arterial injection would be minimal if the drug were eliminated from systemic circulation. The benefits of arterial delivery in this model were due to the recirculating drug [9]

Dedrick Model 1986

The 1986 Dedrick model attempted to explain regional drug delivery across experimental animal models [14]. The effort was to scale experimental data across animal species and apply them to human subjects. The model described arterial,

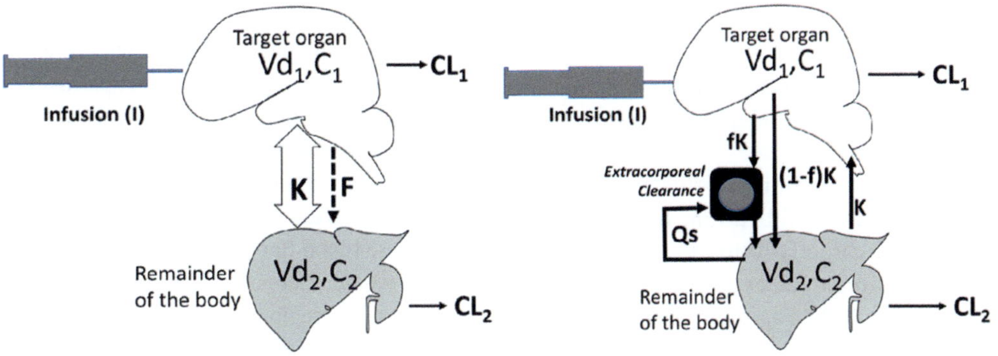

Fig. 2.3 Dedrick's 1986 model with and without extracorporeal clearance: Vd_1, C_1, CL_1, and Vd_2, C_2, CL_2 are the volume of distribution, the concentrations, and the clearances of compartments 1 and 2, respectively; K is the intercompartmental transport parameter; F is the transport term to account for convection if any. The model was developed for intra-arterial, intraperitoneal, and intrathecal drug delivery [14]

intraperitoneal, and intrathecal drug administration. The model also simulated the impact of the extracorporeal removal of drugs. The key parameters of this model are listed in Fig. 2.3. The model had two configurations, one with and the other without extracorporeal removal as an additional drug elimination pathway. The assumptions were:

- The body could be described as a two-compartmental model (the target site and the remainder of the body).
- The characteristics of tissues constituting the remainder of the body are similar, such that they could be lumped together.
- The drug is steadily infused and mixes homogeneously in both compartments.
- The injection rate (I), the intercompartment transfer parameter (K), and the convective transport factor (F) are constant.
- Compartmental clearances (CL) are constant.
- There is no regional clearance during the first pass of the drug.

This is a general model of regional drug delivery that derives the advantages of such delivery based on the concentrations generated by arterial vs. intravenous injection. It compares the pharmacokinetic advantage of regional drug delivery (R_d) as a ratio of C_1/C_2 by a given drug delivery method, where C is the concentration in compartment 1 (C_1) and compartment 2 (C_2), I is the infusion rate, CL is the clearance, Vd is the volume of distribution, K is an intercompartment transport factor, F is an optional transport function related to convection, and I, K, and F are assumed constant, while CL is a function of concentration.

For assessing the benefits of arterial injections, the model compares the C_1/C_2 ratio by the two methods: arterial vs. venous $R_d = R_{art}/R_{iv}$. For intra-arterial drug delivery:

$$\frac{d}{dt}(Vd_1C_1) = I + K(C_2 - C_1) - FC_1 - CL_1C_1$$

$$\frac{d}{dt}(Vd_2C_2) = K(C_1 - C_2) - FC_1 - CL_2C_2$$

To calculate R_d, the model determines the amount of drug in compartments C_1 and C_2 by:

In steady state, $R_{art} = (C_1/C_2)_{art} = (K + CL_2)/(K + F)$

While for intravenous infusion $R_{iv} = (C_1/C_2)_{iv} = K/(K + F + CL_1)$.

The advantage of regional delivery $R_d = R_{art}/R_{iv} = (K + CL_2)(K + F + CL_1)/(K + F)K$

Deriving from which $R_d = 1 + CL_{TB}/K(1 - E)$.

E is the first pass regional elimination (metabolism or removal), and CL_{TB} is total body clearance after IV administration.

Furthermore, for arterial delivery, $F = Q$ or the regional blood flow. If the infused compartment does not metabolize the drug, then $E = 0$. Hence, the formula is reduced to:

$$R_d = 1 + CL_{TB}/K$$

In the second version of the model, extracorporeal removal is added. Increased total body clearance also occurs with intraperitoneal injections when the liver metabolizes more drugs. In these situations, R_d equals:

$$R_d = \frac{1 + \frac{EQ_s + CL_2}{K}}{1 - fE}$$

where E is the irreversible elimination of the drug through metabolism or removal, Q_s is the flow through the extracorporeal device, f is the fraction of the drug returning from the perfused region to the device, and K is the intercompartment transport parameter, the regional blood flow (Q). Removing the drug by an extracorporeal device can significantly increase the $E{\cdot}Q_s$ product and the benefits of arterial drug delivery.

This model showed the significance of drug systemic clearance in improving regional arterial delivery. However, it also described the hazards of scaling animal models across species due to differences in metabolism, brain size, and predisposition to neurotoxicity.

Dedrick Model 1988

While the earlier model [14] focused on drug elimination, the follow-up model focused on blood flow and introduced a tumor compartment (Fig. 2.4) [14].

The parameters and assumptions in this model were similar to those in the earlier publication. In this model, the drugs were injected directly into the artery or its branches. Here, E is the regional extraction of the drug during its first pass through the regional circulation. The flow to and from the infused site was Q. The pharmacokinetic advantage was also described as R_d. R_d was the ratio of the concentrations achieved in compartments C_1 and C_2 by arterial injection relative to the venous injection:

$$R_d = (C_1 / C_2)\text{arterial} / (C_1 / C_2)\text{intravenous}$$
$$R_d = 1 + \mathrm{CL_{TB}} / Q(1 - E)$$

This equation reveals three situations in which arterial injections are specifically advantageous:

- When the body rapidly clears the drug, $\mathrm{CL_{TB}}$ has a high value.
- When the regional blood flow is low. Although the model showed the benefit of regional drug delivery by decreasing the blood flow, there are many additional advantages to regional hypoperfusion, such as:
  - It increases the initial arterial drug concentration.
  - It decreases the washout of the drug after uptake.
  - It also increases the transit time.
  - It decreases the variation in tissue concentrations due to streaming.
  - It decreases the sheer stress of larger molecules and nanoparticles to increase the probability of adhesion to the endothelium.
- When regional extraction (E) is high and there is no regional elimination through either metabolism or secretion.

The authors themselves pointed to the limitations of the model, which included:

- Perfusion variations within the infused region such as due to tumor or tissue compartments (Fig. 2.4, right). Subcompartments may have distinct perfusion and tissue characteristics in an organ like the brain. Thus, if a sub-compartment blood flow responds differently to a challenge, it could affect regional drug delivery. For example, angiotensin II infusion could decrease normal brain blood flow and relatively increase blood flow to the tumor. An increase in tumor blood flow would decrease R_d. Similarly, differences in extraction might affect regional drug delivery.
- They found that the benefits of intra-arterial infusion varied with time. The maximum (R_d) benefits were seen with shorted infusion compared to the longer ones. Keeping the simulation and drug properties the same, the maximum R_d with a 2-h infusion was 5.5, and a 10-h infusion was 3.1. In this context, they reported the problem with obtaining blood samples to test the model, a lack of information about drug-binding properties, and applying the model to nonsteady-state conditions.
- They also raised concerns that while the model reflected data in some studies, it was inconsistent with other studies. They attributed the difference to the type of drug that was being evaluated.
- There was concern about calculating concentration from whole blood. Drug uptake by blood cells can vary depending on lipid or aqueous solubility or by specific mechanisms [18]. The authors assumed that the drug was mixed evenly with blood cells and plasma, which accounts for the net blood flow (Q). The authors were concerned that concentrations based on Q could lead to errors in the model.
- The model did not account for the effect of streaming: Streaming is the variations in arterial blood drug concentrations within a given vascular irrigation [19]. When drugs are infused into an artery, they do not homogeneously mix with blood and are distributed unevenly within arterial irrigation. Streaming can result in excessive concentrations in some regions and inadequate concentrations in others. Streaming has been observed in in vivo primate experiments [4] and human PET studies [3]. *Streaming can be decreased by*:

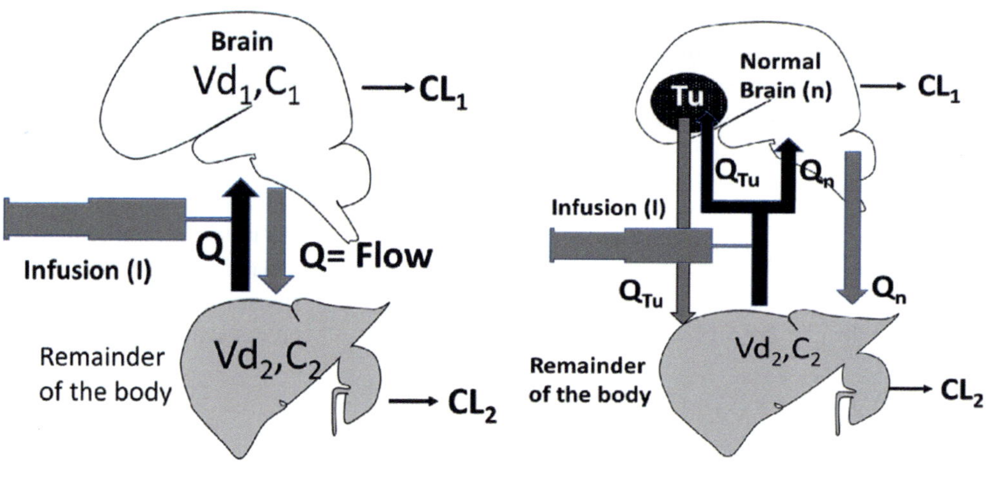

Fig. 2.4 Dedrick's 1988 model was specific to arterial delivery (left). The right image shows the distribution of the blood flow to the tumor (Tu) and the normal brain (n) [15]

– Proximal infusion into larger arteries.
– High drug infusion volume.
– Decreased arterial blood flow.
– Side port catheter injections.
– Injections during the diastole.

The model offered no solution to the problem of streaming.

Updated Dedrick Model 2016

Need to Update the Dedrick Model

Although the Dedrick model provided a robust framework to address arterial drug delivery, arterial drug delivery technology had considerably advanced in the ensuing 30 years. Optical methods had emerged that could track drug and nanoparticle concentrations after arterial injections [20, 21]. Optical pharmacokinetic methods rapidly helped track drug delivery to the target site [22–24]. Thus, the Dedrick model was updated in 2016 and replicated using the MATLAB software [25]. The new model aimed to address some of the technical developments since. These included the role of blood-brain barrier disruption [26], the benefits of reducing blood flow [27–32], and the effect of pulsed injections [33, 34]. The pulsed injections offered the following advantages:

- Pulse injections momentarily disrupt the flow stream to achieve even concentration.
- Pulse injections can exceed the blood flow to deliver the pure drug to the target site.
- When drug pulses are injected during diastole, they reduce the effect of streaming.

The first of the two approaches, using pulsed injection, steady-state, and flow arrest injections, maximizes arterial drug delivery by dosing based on regional blood flow [34]. This approach injects greater doses in an artery with greater flow. Such dose optimization helps deliver the systemic dose safely in relatively small arterial irrigation. The second approach to improving arterial drug delivery is injecting drugs when the blood flow has momentarily stopped for 30–60 s. In the case of the human brain, transient arrest of blood flow can be tolerated for up to 3 min. Flow arrest in human subjects can be achieved by bolus injection of adenosine or balloon-occluding catheters. Repeated balloon occlusion-reperfusion cycles have been used to treat brain tumors safely. The advantages of stopping blood flow are similar to those of decreasing blood flow. However, there are some additional benefits:

- Control the distribution of the drugs and localize them to the target site.
- Deliver pure drug to the target site that avoids binding to blood proteins and cells.
- Permit better shielding of a drug if an antidote is concurrently given to minimize systemic side effects.
- Increase the intravascular drug reserve due to autoregulatory vasodilation.

Thus, compared to arterial infusions, flow arrest drug delivery increases the drug concentration in the tissue by several folds [30].

Model Development

The updated Dedrick model (Figs. 2.5 and 2.6) aimed to test the effects of flow arrest on arterial drug delivery and better understand the effect of drug characteristics and how these parameters interacted with each other (Table 2.1) [25]. The basic model shared the same parameters as those used by Dedrick earlier: V_1 = 1 L; Q = 100 mL/min; CL_1 = 0; V_2 = 40 L; CL_2 = 200 mL/min. Two more sub-compartments were added to V_1, V_3, and V_4. The three sub-compartments now represent V_1, a fast perivascular compartment representing the vascular/endothelial compartment of drug delivery and luminal binding. A fast tissue (V_3) and a slow tissue compartment (V_4) were added to the model to simulate BBB drug transfer and diffusion in the tissues. The rate constants K_1, K_2, K_3, and K_4 reflected the characteristics of the drug. A high K value indicated diffusivity of the drug, while the ratios of K_1/K_2 reflected diffusion and transport across the BBB, while K_3/K_4 represented net reversible and irreversible drug binding. As in the Dedrick model, the drug was not metabolized; hence, CL_1 was 0. The blood flow was decreased to 100 mL/min, or 10% of the baseline value, for 1 min to test for flow arrest delivery. For simulating hyperemia, the blood flow was increased by 150% for 3 min. Three modes of drug delivery were tested: intra-arterial (IA) injection, IA injec-

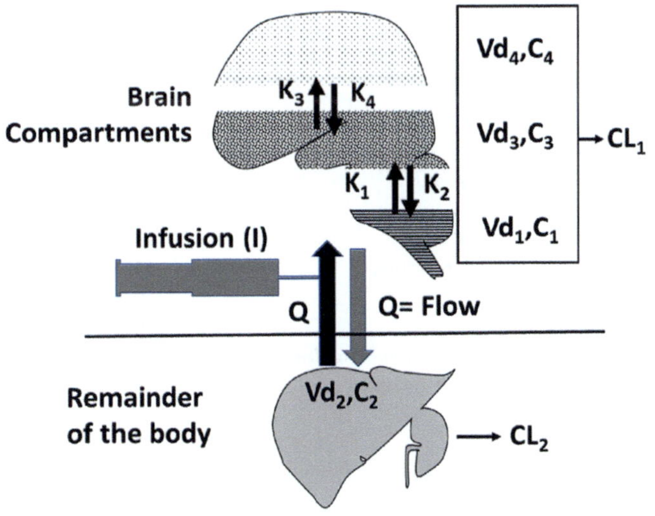

Fig. 2.5 The updated Dedrick model 2016 divided the brain into three compartments, V_1, V_3, and V_4, to explore the effect of a fast compartment in vascular proximity, a compartment like gray matter, and a slower compartment like white matter [25]

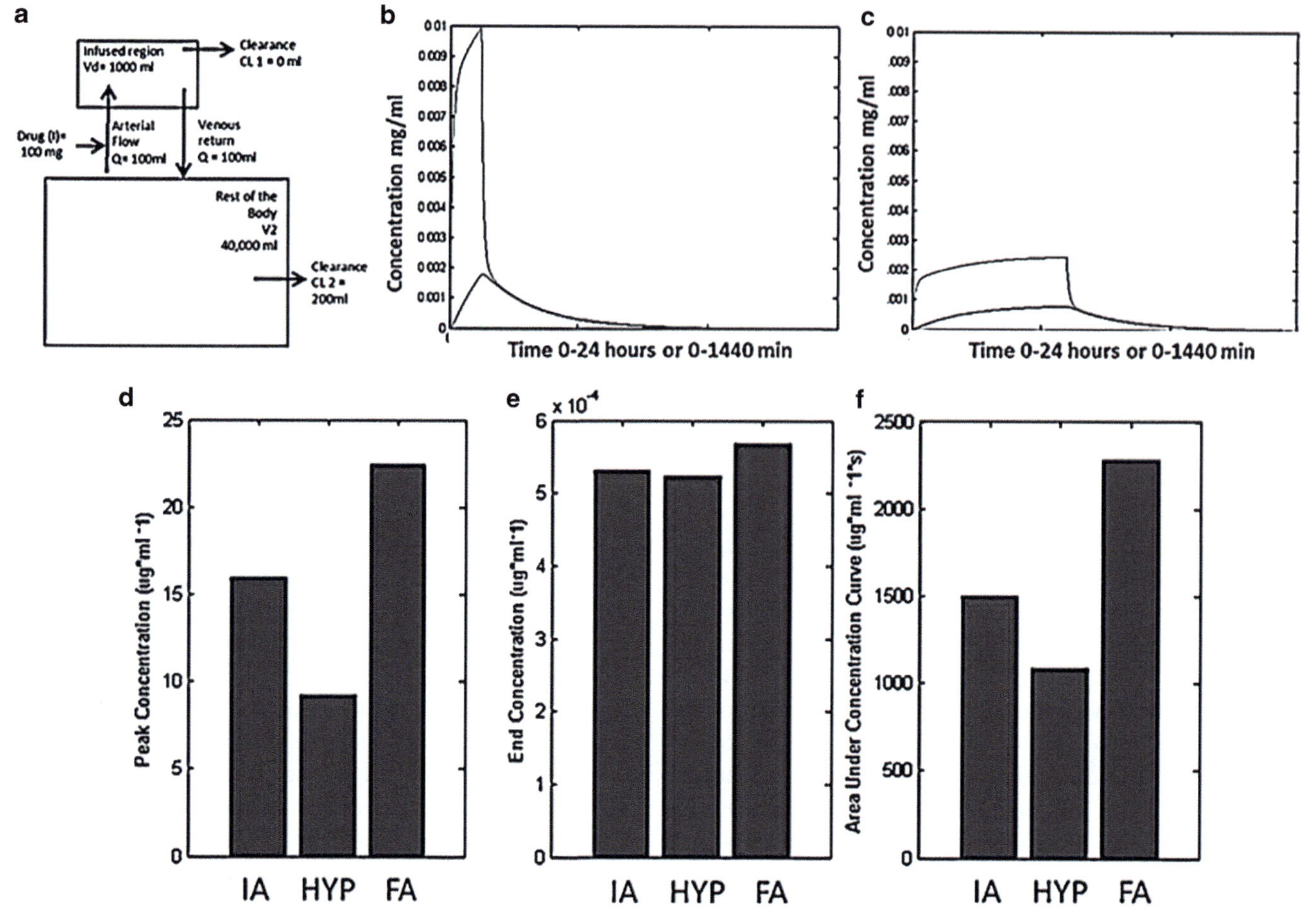

Fig. 2.6 Updated Dedrick model 2016: using the original parameters (**a**), the published results for 2 (**b**) and 10 (**c**) hours of arterial infusion could be recreated. When flow conditions were changed, flow arrest (FA) increased peak concentrations (**d**) and the area under the concentration-time curve (**f**) but did not affect the end concentrations (**e**) [25]

Table 2.1 Parameters used in simulations using the updated Dedrick model [25]

Condition	Compartmental kinetics parameters						Rationale
	K_1	K_2	K_3	K_4	CL_2 (mL/min)	Q (L/min)	
Effect of flow conditions							
Baseline	50	50	50	50	200	1.0	Validation of the model
Flow arrest	50	50	50	50	200	0.1	Adenosine, balloon occlusion
Hyperemia	50	50	50	50	200	1.5	Hypercapnia
Effect of drug properties							
Increased diffusivity	150	150	150	150	200	1.0	Simulate small molecules
BBB disruption (BBBD)	150	150	50	50	200	1.0	Mannitol effect
Preferential BBB penetration	150	50	50	50	200	1.0	Monoclonal antibodies
Increased retention	50	50	50	10	200	1.0	pH trapping methods
Increased CL_2	50	50	50	50	2000	1.0	Dialysis
Combined effects of manipulating drugs and flow conditions							
Increased diffusivity + retention	150	150	150	30	200	1.0	High-tissue affinity rapidly diffusing compounds
BBBD + retention	150	150	50	10	200	1.0	Effect of BBB disruption
Preferential BBB penetration + retention	150	30	50	10	200	1.0	Carriers with tissue avidity
Preferential BBB penetration + retention + increased CL_2	150	30	50	10	2000	1.0	Carriers with tissue avidity and high systemic clearance

BBB blood-brain barrier, *BBBD* BBB disruption, *Lpm* liter per min
Systemic clearance or CL2 units, mL/min; *Q* is regional blood flow

tion during flow arrest (IA-FA), and intravenous (IV) injections. The drug was injected at a constant rate of 100 mg/min in the regional artery or the returning vein for 1 min. The total duration of the simulation was 30 min [25].

Using the parameters in the original publication in a MATLAB simulation, it was possible to recreate the reported results for 2 and 10 h of intra-arterial infusion [15]. Simulations of how blood flow changes affected regional drug delivery revealed that the peak drug concentrations and the area under the concentration-time curve increased by decreasing blood flow and decreased by increasing the blood flow. The end concentrations were not affected by flow manipulation. These results suggest that flow can affect regional drug delivery. Unless the tissues retain the drug, the pharmacokinetic benefits of flow manipulation during arterial injections are transient.

The updated model permits exploring the factors that affect intra-arterial drug delivery (Fig. 2.7). Simulations

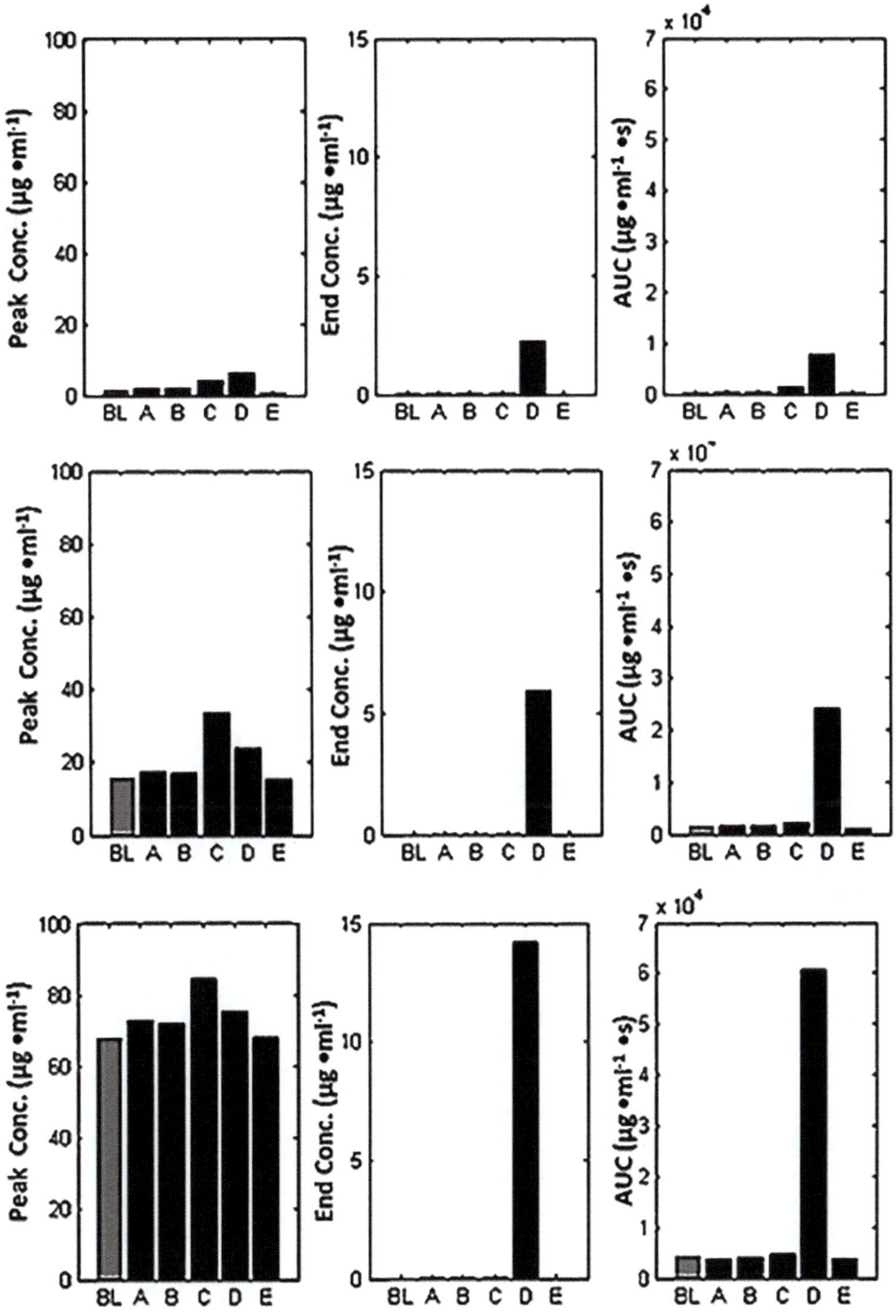

Fig. 2.7 The effects of individual drug properties on peak concentrations, end concentrations, and the area under the concentration-time curve (AUC). The three methods of delivery were intravenous (top panel), intra-arterial (middle panel), and flow arrest intra-arterial delivery (bottom panel). The most essential drug property was the retention by the target site (D). Other properties such as drug diffusivity (A), blood-brain barrier (BBB) penetration (B), preferential BBB penetration (C), and high total body clearance (E) had transient effects compared to baseline (BL). Although flow arrest delivery was superior to arterial delivery, both were superior to intravenous delivery. Tissue retention of the drug is more important than optimizing arterial delivery with flow arrest [25]

compared the five individual factors that influence regional drug deposition, which were:

- *Drug diffusivity* or the free movement of the drug in the target compartment to ensure uniform uptake. Drug diffusivity is an essential characteristic of small molecular weight compounds such as temozolomide. These compounds can easily cross the BBB and move across the brain compartments. Thus, they have a uniformly high K_{1-4} value. Easy drug diffusion can benefit drug uptake when the arterial concentrations are high, but tissue concentrations could also rapidly decrease when arterial concentrations decline.
- BBB disruption: The BBB sev restricts the entry of molecules to impede drug delivery. It is significant for large molecules such as therapeutic monoclonal antibodies. It also limits the movement of polar compounds and molecules with weights exceeding 400 Da. To simulate BBB disruption, K_1 and K_2 values were altered to reflect it. BBB disruption increased drug uptake and area under the concentration-time curve.
- Preferential BBB penetration: It describes a biased transport across the BBB such that the K_1 exceeds K_2, resulting in net tissue uptake of the drug. Preferential BBB penetration can be due to unidirectional transport and drug trapping due to differences in tissue pH or by cationic entities, peptides, albumin, and nanoparticles.
- Increased tissue retention: The ratio of K_3 to K_4 determines the avidity of the drug retained in the target tissue. Increased tissue retention was the most critical factor in drug delivery. Unless the drug is bound to the target site, the benefits of intra-arterial drug delivery are transient.
- Increased total body clearance: Rapid drug clearance from the body helps augment the benefits of arterial delivery. However, with all modes of drug delivery, the ten times increase in drug clearance had a deleterious effect on drug delivery compared to the baseline.

Effects of Combining Factors to Maximize Arterial Drug Delivery

Simulation of how other factors affect drug delivery with high retention, i.e., with a K_3/K_4 ratio, revealed (Fig. 2.8):

- Across the three modes of drug delivery, peak concentrations, end concentrations, and area under the concentration-time curves, there was a consistent pattern: intravenous < intra-arterial < flow arrest-intra-arterial.
- At baseline, without BBBD, the transient rise in concentration did not result in significant tissue concentrations.
- BBB disruption combined with retention significantly increased tissue uptake.
- With preferential BBB penetration and drug retention, there was a dramatic increase in tissue concentrations with intravenous drugs, while the other two modes of drug delivery also increased tissue deposition. Preferential tissue penetration resulted in higher concentrations than BBB disruption due to the greater K_1/K_2 ratios that favored drug uptake by the target site.
- Finally, total body clearance was not helpful in this case, even when combined with preferential BBB penetration and drug retention. The result was similar to the trend seen when these parameters were tested in isolation with all three delivery modes. The mathematical model predicted that a higher total body clearance would directly increase the benefits of arterial injection ($R_d = 1 + CL_{TB}/Q$). This simulation suggests excessive clearance could be deleterious to regional drug delivery when the uptake was maximized.

Limitations of the Updated Model

The updated model's principal limitations are the same as those of previous models. The parameters are the same as Dedrick's 1988 model with sub-compartmentalization of the regional compartment [15]. Thus, if the parameters are altered, the simulations could yield different results. However, the updated model's goal was to expand on a widely cited model. While many other publications describe regional drug delivery, only a few models address arterial injections. None of them address arterial drug delivery in the context of systemic circulation. Furthermore, this model provides an excellent conceptual framework to understand how significant parameters affect arterial drug delivery.

Key Results:

The conclusion from the updated Dedrick models are:

- Flow arrest drug delivery produces significantly higher peak tissue concentrations than arterial infusion. Both of these arterial infusions produce higher concentrations than intravenous delivery.
- Drug retention by the target site is the most significant factor in improving regional drug delivery by arterial or intravenous delivery.
- In the case of drug delivery to the brain, disruption or preferential penetration of the BBB significantly improves drug delivery.
- Increasing the drug's diffusivity to overcome the BBB and rapidly diffuse in brain tissue is effective when combined with tissue retention.
- Arterial drug delivery is most effective when the target site retains a drug after preferential BBB penetration.
- With avid drug retention at the target site, increasing total body clearance does not augment regional drug delivery.

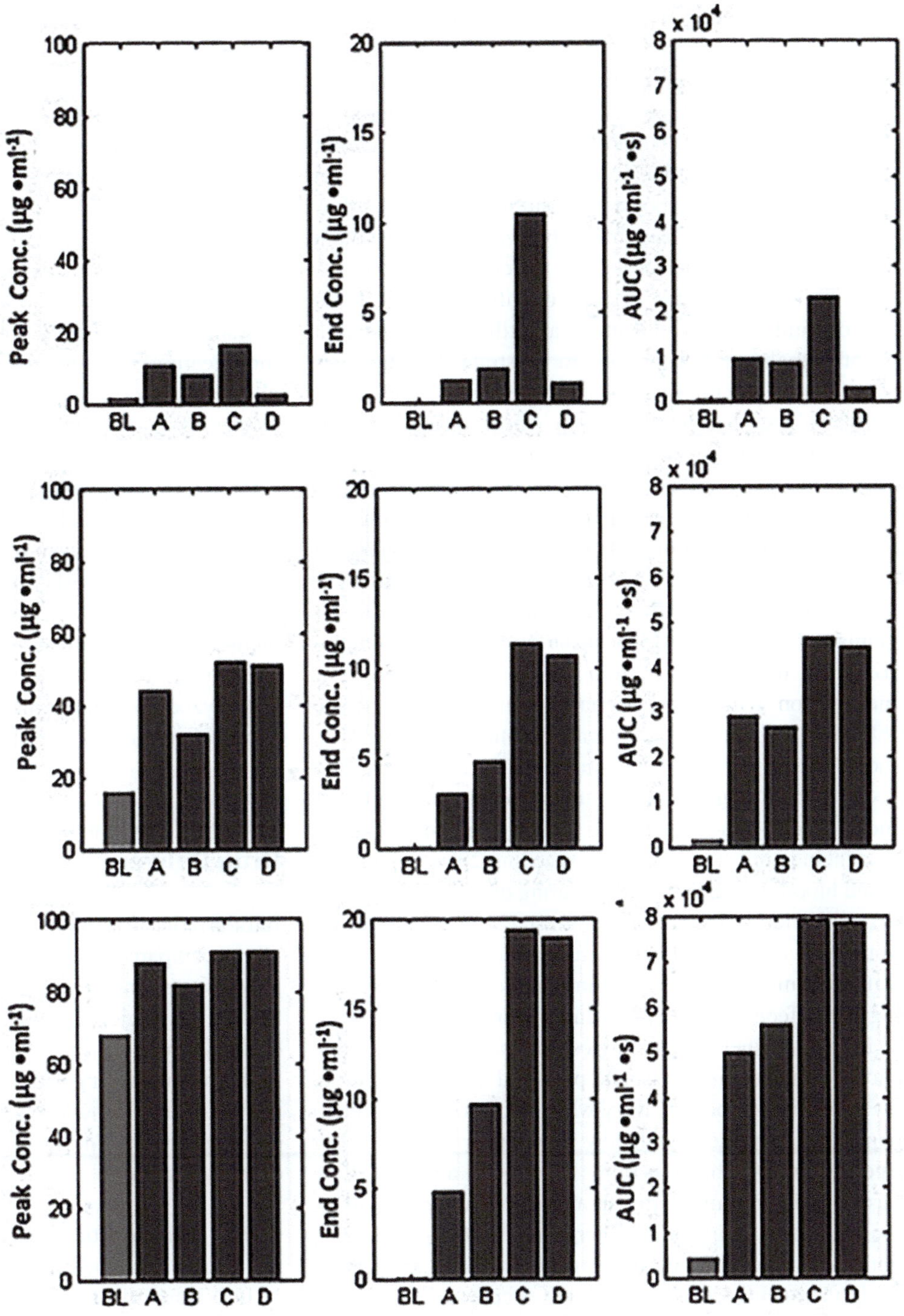

Fig. 2.8 The effects of combining drug properties on peak concentrations, end concentrations, and the area under the concentration-time curve (AUC). The three methods of delivery were intravenous (top panel), intra-arterial (middle panel), and flow arrest intra-arterial delivery (bottom panel). In all these simulations, high retention by the target site was assumed. Conditions: [BL]: Baseline, (A) increased diffusivity with retention, (B) BBB disruption with retention, (C) preferential BBB penetration with retention, (D) preferential BBB penetration with retention and increased systemic clearance [25]

Clinical Significance

The primary concern these simulations raise is a clinical one. Although arterial drug injections are clinically used for treating various neurological diseases, they are essentially an off-label use of their intravenous formulations. The use of intravenous drugs might be appropriate for applications such as thrombolysis or treatment of vasospasm where the site of action of drugs is within the lumen or on the vessel wall or when the drugs are freely diffusible. However, for other applications, such as cancer treatment, where the tissue must take up the drug, drug selection should be based on the uptake and retention of the drugs. The retention in the tissue has to be for a sufficient time to have the desired effect. Perhaps the uptake of 5-fluorouracil (5FU) by liver cells may explain the effectiveness of intra-arterial treatment of liver cancer [35]. The result of this concern is that when drugs are not taken up and retained by the target site, they should be conjugated to carriers that can do so.

Streaming During Intra-arterial Injection

Streaming of drugs refers to the uneven distribution of drugs in the arterial bloodstream, leading to varying concentrations within the arterial distribution [2, 14]. The role of cerebral blood flow in intra-arterial (IA) drug delivery is crucial. Yet, clinical studies often do not monitor or modify flow. Streaming phenomena have been observed both in vivo and in vitro, explaining the focal drug toxicity of chemotherapeutic agents within the arterial distribution [19]. In an in vitro simulation model, Lutz et al. utilized a polystyrene cast of human cerebral arteries to illustrate the impact of streaming and potential mitigation strategies [2]. By placing a P-100 catheter in a supra-ophthalmic position and injecting dyes at 2 mL/min, they observed a distinct flow of dyes to the anterior choroidal artery but not to the anterior cerebral artery. Conversely, injecting the same dye at 17 mL/min in an infra-ophthalmic location resulted in more homogeneous dispersion. This in vitro model indicates that streaming can lead to nearly fivefold differences in drug concentrations. In a human study using O15 positron emission tomography, Saris et al. revealed an 11-fold variation in regional drug concentration within the arterial irrigation of the supra-ophthalmic segment of the internal carotid artery [3]. They concluded that proximal injections at a high rate decrease the effects of streaming, thereby reducing the variability of drug concentration. Other strategies to mitigate the streaming effect include injecting volumes exceeding 20% of the background blood flow rate, injecting during diastole, using catheters with side ports, and flow arrest [2, 30]. Flow arrest through downstream balloon occlusion has been proposed to localize chemotherapies to the tumor region, potentially limiting the effects of streaming and enhancing IA delivery. Advances in catheter technologies, such as single or double balloon catheters, aim to isolate proximal and distal arterial flow to maximize local delivery while minimizing complications [32]. As tumors with low blood flow exhibit better responses to IA chemotherapy, techniques allowing flow arrest or reduction may offer an alternative to increasing IA doses, thereby augmenting therapeutic effects [36, 37]. Subtle variations in injection protocols can significantly impact therapeutic responses and the occurrence of adverse events. Standardizing delivery protocols and defining concurrent blood flow conditions could significantly influence the outcomes of clinical studies [37].

Enhancing Regional Retention of Drugs

The conventional approach to drug design focuses on pharmacokinetic properties for optimal uptake by the target site. However, when drugs are directly delivered to the target site through intra-arterial (IA) injections, traditional considerations become less relevant. Preclinical screening for drug isomers may not effectively identify candidates for IA use, as formulations for IA delivery differ from those administered systemically. In IA drug design, the priority is to ensure maximum tumor uptake and sufficient drug retention to achieve therapeutic effects while minimizing regional toxicity. Rapid uptake is crucial, especially considering the restricted permeability of the BBB [25, 38].

Various methods can be employed to enhance IA drug delivery. Small molecule chemotherapy (<400 Da) aids in crossing the BBB [39]. Increasing lipid solubility through modifications like adding methyl groups or halogenated alkane chains can enhance diffusivity [40, 41]. Liposomal carrier systems with optimized size and surface charge, designed for rapid drug release, have been developed. Immunoliposomes targeting vascular endothelium (ACE, CD 31, or factor VIII/vWF-Ag), transport systems (OX-26 antibody to transferrin receptor), or pathology-specific antigens (ICAMs) offer a novel alternative [42–44]. Immuno-conjugated drugs (OX26-daunorubicin and OX26-methotrexate), chimeric drugs utilizing high-capacity transporter systems, or drugs with brief durations of action hydrolyzed by ubiquitous enzymes during circulation are intriguing options for IA delivery [45].

Future Consideration for Arterial Drug Delivery

Intra-arterial drug delivery models are relatively primitive stages compared to other biological models. However, circulatory system models are rapidly evolving, including those that model regional blood flows. Models of arterial drug delivery could be derived from such models, but they will be far more challenging. The key to developing reliable arterial pharmacokinetic models is first to understand the complexity of the problem. The factors that could affect arterial drug delivery include:

- The characteristics of drug injection:
  - Site of infusion, proximal or distal [2, 46]
  - Nature of catheter, end-on port, or side ports [2]
  - Timing of injection, such as during diastole [3, 4]
  - The volume of injection, concentration, and frequency [33]
- Physiological factors:
  - Of the tissue, such as vessel sizes, pressure gradients, and branching pattern [47]
  - The background flow conditions: Volume flow rate, normal flow or flow arrest [29, 30, 33]
  - Physiological reactivity of the tissue, such as the duration and severity of hyperemia if the flow is arrested or BBB disruption by mannitol [48]
  - Possibility of no-reflow after arrest

  - Permeability of the BBB [49]
- Pharmacological and physiological manipulation of blood flow to target pathologies:
  - The direct and indirect effects of the drug on the regional blood flow [15]
  - Measures to enhance blood flow to pathology using hyperventilation and deep anesthesia [50]
  - Type and depth of anesthesia volatile agents vs. intravenous drugs [51]
  - Deep hypothermia to decrease blood flow and safely increase the duration of flow arrest [52]
- Compartmental characteristics: Differential uptake by gray matter, white matter, pathological lesion, or subcompartments within the brain [53]
- Nature of drug or drug carrier, the extent of BBB penetration, and tissue retention [54]
- Microscopic characteristics of the pathological tissue affect drug and carrier uptake and retention [55]:
  - Vascularity and angiogenesis and its modulation of blood flow by drugs [56, 57]
  - Permeability: The state of the BBB and the extent of iatrogenic disruption [58]
  - Heterogeneity: Tumors with the same histological diagnosis may have different characteristics regarding angioarchitecture, permeability, and cellularity [59]
  - Extracellular fluid volume and pH: Tumors such as CNS lymphomas and medulloblastomas are exceedingly cell-dense with minimal extracellular fluid (ECF) volume. At the same time, gliomas are less cell-dense with significant ECF volume [60]
  - Hydrostatic pressure gradients: Usually greater in the core of large tumors than in the periphery [61–63]. Thus, drugs tend to be pushed from the center to the periphery of the tumors
  - Target specificity of the drug/carrier relative to normal brain tissue [64]

The arterial blood flow and injection parameters determine the effective concentration of the drug at the endothelium. The pharmacokinetic modeling will be derived from endothelial drug concentrations. Unless the biomechanics of events in the vascular compartment can be reliably predicted, downstream pharmacokinetic modeling will be challenging. A lack of experimental data further compounds that difficulty. Current pharmacokinetics modeling is based on tissue sampling and chemical analysis. The capillary transit time in the circulation is between 1 and 5 s in rats and humans, respectively [65, 66]. Tracking pharmacokinetic events in a sub-second time frame is challenging with conventional pharmacokinetic tools using tissue sampling [67].

However, emerging technologies can help us generate pharmacokinetic data needed for future models. In preclinical whole animal studies, one can track changes in tissue concentrations in a sub-second time frame by optical means with suitable drugs, optical tracers, and optically tagged particles. The visual methods are discussed in detail in a later chapter. Optical techniques are safe, tissue-noninvasive, site-specific, and highly cost-effective. The additional advantage of optical methods is that they permit real-time assessment of tissue blood flow. One can also see that for the clinical translation of these models with MR guidance. MR imaging describes patient-specific nanoparticle delivery and guides stem cell delivery in human subjects. How we arrive at better models of intra-arterial drug delivery can be debated, but they are sorely needed to advance and guide future treatments.

Tools that can help make arterial delivery more effective based on current models include:

- Super-selective delivery with angiographic or MR guidance [68–71]
- Injection when perfusion is stopped or transiently reduced by balloon occlusion or pharmacologically [27, 28, 72, 73]
- Injection of drugs as boluses to avoid streaming [3, 4, 34, 70]
- Rapid uptake of the drugs by the target tissue:
  - Adequate and safe permeabilization of the BBB [74–78]
  - Conjugation with carriers capable of rapidly penetrating the barrier [64]
- Development of drug and carriers that are retained by the target tissue for sufficient time after delivery [21, 79]
- Minimizing systemic effects of arterial drugs by:
  - Concurrent administration of systemic antidote [80]
  - Enhanced systemic elimination [81–83]

Conclusion

Arterial drug delivery models require many questionable assumptions due to the lack of critical experimental data. An updated version of a conceptual model was used in the simulations. The simulation reveals that optimum intra-arterial drug delivery is greatly improved when the injections are made during reduced blood flow or flow arrest. Delivery is improved when the drugs can cross the BBB, and the target site retains *them.* Unless the tissue retains drugs, the tissue concentration will decline rapidly, and arterial drug delivery will offer little advantages. Therefore, it is necessary to develop drugs and carriers that have rapid uptake and are retained by the target tissue to improve arterial drug delivery. Much of the next-generation research must focus on identifying effective drug cargoes for arterial delivery. The current models only provide a conceptual overview of arterial delivery. Bench research has to provide data to develop better models. Most tools for effective arterial drug delivery have already been developed. The next generation of arterial drug development research will require identifying and developing drugs or drug-carrier conjugates that are taken up and retained for sufficient time to have the desired effect. Models show that effective regional extraction by rapid uptake and sustained retention of the compounds is the critical step in improving arterial delivery.

References

1. Tyler JL, Yamamoto YL, Diksic M, Theron J, Villemure JG, Worthington C, et al. Pharmacokinetics of superselective intra-arterial and intravenous [11C]BCNU evaluated by PET. J Nucl Med. 1986;27(6):775–80.
2. Lutz RJ, Dedrick RL, Boretos JW, Oldfield EH, Blacklock JB, Doppman JL. Mixing studies during intracarotid artery infusions in an in vitro model. J Neurosurg. 1986;64(2):277–83.
3. Saris SC, Blasberg RG, Carson RE, deVroom HL, Lutz R, Dedrick RL, et al. Intravascular streaming during carotid artery infusions. Demonstration in humans and reduction using diastole-phased pulsatile administration. J Neurosurg. 1991;74(5):763–72.
4. Saris SC, Shook DR, Blasberg RG, Dedrick RL, Doppman JL, Bankiewicz KS, et al. Carotid artery mixing with diastole-phased pulsed drug infusion. J Neurosurg. 1987;67(5):721–5.
5. Blacklock JB, Wright DC, Dedrick RL, Blasberg RG, Lutz RJ, Doppman JL, et al. Drug streaming during intra-arterial chemotherapy. J Neurosurg. 1986;64(2):284–91.
6. Saris SC, Wright DC, Oldfield EH, Blasberg RG. Intravascular streaming and variable delivery to brain following carotid artery infusions in the Sprague-Dawley rat. J Cereb Blood Flow Metab. 1988;8(1):116–20.
7. Criado E, Giron F. Jose Goyanes Capdevila, unsung pioneer of vascular surgery. Ann Vasc Surg. 2006;20(3):422–5.
8. Die-Goyanes A, Die-Trill J. Jose Goyanes. Surgeon and humanist. Cir Esp. 2008;83(1):8–11.
9. Eckman WW, Patlak CS, Fenstermacher JD. A critical evaluation of the principles governing the advantages of intra-arterial infusions. J Pharmacokinet Biopharm. 1974;2(3):257–85.
10. Fenstermacher J, Gazendam J. Intra-arterial infusions of drugs and hyperosmotic solutions as ways of enhancing CNS chemotherapy. Cancer Treat Rep. 1981;65(Suppl 2):27–37.
11. Fenstermacher JD, Cowles AL. Theoretic limitations of intracarotid infusions in brain tumor chemotherapy. Cancer Treat Rep. 1977;61(4):519–26.
12. Collins JM. Pharmacologic rationale for regional drug delivery. J Clin Oncol. 1984;2(5):498–504.
13. Collins JM, Dedrick RL, Flessner MF, Guarino AM. Concentration-dependent disappearance of fluorouracil from peritoneal fluid in the rat: experimental observations and distributed modeling. J Pharm Sci. 1982;71(7):735–8.
14. Dedrick RL. Interspecies scaling of regional drug delivery. J Pharm Sci. 1986;75(11):1047–52.
15. Dedrick RL. Arterial drug infusion: pharmacokinetic problems and pitfalls. J Natl Cancer Inst. 1988;80(2):84–9.
16. Dedrick RL, Oldfield EH, Collins JM. Arterial drug infusion with extracorporeal removal. I. Theoretic basis with particular reference to the brain. Cancer Treat Rep. 1984;68(2):373–80.
17. Chen HS, Gross JF. Intra-arterial infusion of anticancer drugs: theoretic aspects of drug delivery and review of responses. Cancer Treat Rep. 1980;64(1):31–40.
18. Biagiotti S, Pirla E, Magnani M. Drug transport by red blood cells. Front Physiol. 2023;14:1308632.
19. Joshi S, Meyers PM, Ornstein E. Intracarotid delivery of drugs: the potential and the pitfalls. Anesthesiology. 2008;109(3):543–64.
20. Joshi S, Reif R, Wang M, Zhang J, Ergin A, Bruce JN, et al. Intra-arterial mitoxantrone delivery in rabbits: an optical pharmacokinetic study. Neurosurgery. 2011;69(3):706–12; discussion 12.
21. Joshi S, Singh-Moon R, Wang M, Chaudhuri DB, Ellis JA, Bruce JN, et al. Cationic surface charge enhances early regional deposition of liposomes after intracarotid injection. J Neurooncol. 2014;120(3):489–97.
22. Reif R, Wang M, Joshi S, A'Amar O, Bigio IJ. Optical method for real-time monitoring of drug concentrations facilitates the development of novel methods for drug delivery to brain tissue. J Biomed Opt. 2007;12(3):034036.
23. Mourant JR, Johnson TM, Los G, Bigio IJ. Non-invasive measurement of chemotherapy drug concentrations in tissue: preliminary demonstrations of in vivo measurements. Phys Med Biol. 1999;44(5):1397–417.
24. Bigio IJ, Mourant JR, Los G. Noninvasive, in-situ measurement of drug concentrations in tissue using optical spectroscopy. J Gravit Physiol. 1999;6(1):P173–5.
25. Cooke JN, Ellis JA, Hossain S, Nguyen J, Bruce JN, Joshi S. Computational pharmacokinetic rationale for intra-arterial delivery to the brain. Drug Deliv Transl Res. 2016;6(5):622–9.
26. Neuwelt E. Implications of the blood-brain-barrier and its manipulation. New York: Plenum; 1988. p. 223–60.
27. Hashimoto T, Young WL, Aagaard BD, Joshi S, Ostapkovich ND, Pile-Spellman J. Adenosine-induced ventricular asystole to induce transient profound systemic hypotension in patients undergoing endovascular therapy. Dose-response characteristics. Anesthesiology. 2000;93(4):998–1001.
28. Pile-Spellman J, Young WL, Joshi S, Duong H, Vang MC, Hartmann A, et al. Adenosine-induced cardiac pause for endovascular embolization of cerebral arteriovenous malformations: technical case report. Neurosurgery. 1999;44(4):881–6; discussion 6–7.
29. Joshi S, Wang M, Etu JJ, Nishanian EV, Pile-Spellman J. Cerebral blood flow affects dose requirements of intracarotid propofol for electrocerebral silence. Anesthesiology. 2006;104(2):290–8, discussion 5A.
30. Joshi S, Wang M, Etu JJ, Suckow RF, Cooper TB, Feinmark SJ, et al. Transient cerebral hypoperfusion enhances intraarterial carmustine deposition into brain tissue. J Neurooncol. 2008;86(2):123–32.
31. Stephens FO. Induction (neo-adjuvant) chemotherapy: systemic and arterial delivery techniques and their clinical applications. Aust N Z J Surg. 1995;65(10):699–707.
32. Riina HA, Knopman J, Greenfield JP, Fralin S, Gobin YP, Tsiouris AJ, et al. Balloon-assisted superselective intra-arterial cerebral infusion of bevacizumab for malignant brainstem glioma. A technical note. Interv Neuroradiol. 2010;16(1):71–6.
33. Joshi S, Wang M, Etu JJ, Pile-Spellman J. Bolus configuration affects dose requirements of intracarotid propofol for electroencephalographic silence. Anesth Analg. 2006;102(6):1816–22.
34. Gobin YP, Cloughesy TF, Chow KL, Duckwiler GR, Sayre JW, Milanese K, et al. Intraarterial chemotherapy for brain tumors by using a spatial dose fractionation algorithm and pulsatile delivery. Radiology. 2001;218(3):724–32.
35. Speyer JL, Sugarbaker PH, Collins JM, Dedrick RL, Klecker RW Jr, Myers CE. Portal levels and hepatic clearance of 5-fluorouracil after intraperitoneal administration in humans. Cancer Res. 1981;41(5):1916–22.
36. D'Amico RS, Khatri D, Reichman N, Patel NV, Wong T, Fralin SR, et al. Correction to: Super selective intra-arterial cerebral infusion of modern chemotherapeutics after blood-brain barrier disruption: where are we now, and where we are going. J Neurooncol. 2020;147(2):279.
37. D'Amico RS, Khatri D, Reichman N, Patel NV, Wong T, Fralin SR, et al. Super selective intra-arterial cerebral infusion of modern chemotherapeutics after blood-brain barrier disruption: where are we now, and where we are going. J Neurooncol. 2020;147(2):261–78.

38. Ellis JA, Banu M, Hossain SS, Singh-Moon R, Lavine SD, Bruce JN, et al. Reassessing the role of intra-arterial drug delivery for glioblastoma multiforme treatment. J Drug Deliv. 2015;2015:405735.
39. Hoelder S, Clarke PA, Workman P. Discovery of small molecule cancer drugs: successes, challenges and opportunities. Mol Oncol. 2012;6(2):155–76.
40. Greig NH, Daly EM, Sweeney DJ, Rapoport SI. Pharmacokinetics of chlorambucil-tertiary butyl ester, a lipophilic chlorambucil derivative that achieves and maintains high concentrations in brain. Cancer Chemother Pharmacol. 1990;25(5):320–5.
41. Greig NH, Genka S, Daly EM, Sweeney DJ, Rapoport SI. Physicochemical and pharmacokinetic parameters of seven lipophilic chlorambucil esters designed for brain penetration. Cancer Chemother Pharmacol. 1990;25(5):311–9.
42. Chan AS, Leung SY, Wong MP, Yuen ST, Cheung N, Fan YW, et al. Expression of vascular endothelial growth factor and its receptors in the anaplastic progression of astrocytoma, oligodendroglioma, and ependymoma. Am J Surg Pathol. 1998;22(7):816–26.
43. Chen YS, Chen ZP. Vasculogenic mimicry: a novel target for glioma therapy. Chin J Cancer. 2014;33(2):74–9.
44. Friden PM, Walus LR, Musso GF, Taylor MA, Malfroy B, Starzyk RM. Anti-transferrin receptor antibody and antibody-drug conjugates cross the blood-brain barrier. Proc Natl Acad Sci USA. 1991;88(11):4771–5.
45. Friden PM, Olson TS, Obar R, Walus LR, Putney SD. Characterization, receptor mapping and blood-brain barrier transcytosis of antibodies to the human transferrin receptor. J Pharmacol Exp Ther. 1996;278(3):1491–8.
46. Lutz RJ, Warren K, Balis F, Patronas N, Dedrick RL. Mixing during intravertebral arterial infusions in an in vitro model. J Neurooncol. 2002;58(2):95–106.
47. Hossain SS, Zhang Y, Fu X, Brunner G, Singh J, Hughes TJ, et al. Magnetic resonance imaging-based computational modelling of blood flow and nanomedicine deposition in patients with peripheral arterial disease. J R Soc Interface. 2015;12(106):20150001.
48. Joshi S, Singh-Moon R, Wang M, Bruce JN, Bigio IJ, Mayevsky A. Real-time hemodynamic response and mitochondrial function changes with intracarotid mannitol injection. Brain Res. 2014;1549:42–51.
49. Guillaume DJ, Doolittle ND, Gahramanov S, Hedrick NA, Delashaw JB, Neuwelt EA. Intra-arterial chemotherapy with osmotic blood-brain barrier disruption for aggressive oligodendroglial tumors: results of a phase I study. Neurosurgery. 2010;66(1):48–58; discussion.
50. Joshi S, Ornstein E, Young W. Cerebral and spinal cord blood flow. In: Cottrell J, Young WL, editors. Cottrell and Young's neuroaesthesia. 5th ed. Philadelphia: Mosby Elsevier; 2010. p. 17–59.
51. Slupe AM, Kirsch JR. Effects of anesthesia on cerebral blood flow, metabolism, and neuroprotection. J Cereb Blood Flow Metab. 2018;38(12):2192–208.
52. Greeley WJ, Kern FH, Meliones JN, Ungerleider RM. Effect of deep hypothermia and circulatory arrest on cerebral blood flow and metabolism. Ann Thorac Surg. 1993;56(6):1464–6.
53. Zakaria Z, Badhan R. Development of a region-specific physiologically based pharmacokinetic brain model to assess hippocampus and frontal cortex pharmacokinetics. Pharmaceutics. 2018;10(1):14.
54. Pardridge WM. A historical review of brain drug delivery. Pharmaceutics. 2022;14(6):1283.
55. Nikmaneshi MR, Jain RK, Munn LL. Computational simulations of tumor growth and treatment response: benefits of high-frequency, low-dose drug regimens and concurrent vascular normalization. PLoS Comput Biol. 2023;19(6):e1011131.
56. Li W, Li S, Chen IX, Liu Y, Ramjiawan RR, Leung CH, et al. Combining losartan with radiotherapy increases tumor control and inhibits lung metastases from a HER2/neu-positive orthotopic breast cancer model. Radiat Oncol. 2021;16(1):48.
57. Voutouri C, Kirkpatrick ND, Chung E, Mpekris F, Baish JW, Munn LL, et al. Experimental and computational analyses reveal dynamics of tumor vessel cooption and optimal treatment strategies. Proc Natl Acad Sci USA. 2019;116(7):2662–71.
58. Arvanitis CD, Askoxylakis V, Guo Y, Datta M, Kloepper J, Ferraro GB, et al. Mechanisms of enhanced drug delivery in brain metastases with focused ultrasound-induced blood-tumor barrier disruption. Proc Natl Acad Sci USA. 2018;115(37):E8717–E26.
59. Haumann R, Videira JC, Kaspers GJL, van Vuurden DG, Hulleman E. Overview of current drug delivery methods across the blood-brain barrier for the treatment of primary brain tumors. CNS Drugs. 2020;34(11):1121–31.
60. Saleh MAA, de Lange ECM. Impact of CNS diseases on drug delivery to brain extracellular and intracellular target sites in human: a "WHAT-IF" simulation study. Pharmaceutics. 2021;13(1):95.
61. Zoi I, Gargalionis AN, Papavassiliou KA, Nasiri-Ansari N, Piperi C, Basdra EK, et al. Polycystin-1 and hydrostatic pressure are implicated in glioblastoma pathogenesis in vitro. J Cell Mol Med. 2022;26(5):1699–709.
62. Wijeratne NS, Hoo KA. Understanding the role of the tumour vasculature in the transport of drugs to solid cancer tumours. Cell Prolif. 2007;40(3):283–301.
63. Pu W, Qiu J, Nassar ZD, Shaw PN, McMahon KA, Ferguson C, et al. A role for caveola-forming proteins caveolin-1 and CAVIN1 in the pro-invasive response of glioblastoma to osmotic and hydrostatic pressure. J Cell Mol Med. 2020;24(6):3724–38.
64. Joshi S, Cooke JRN, Ellis JA, Emala CW, Bruce JN. Targeting brain tumors by intra-arterial delivery of cell-penetrating peptides: a novel approach for primary and metastatic brain malignancy. J Neurooncol. 2017;135(3):497–506.
65. Hirata M, Yoshimine T, Kato A, Ito M, Hirabuki N, Taniguchi M, et al. Computational imaging of cerebral perfusion by real-time processing of DSA images. Clinical applications. Neurol Res. 1998;20(4):327–32.
66. Shockley RP, LaManna JC. Determination of rat cerebral cortical blood volume changes by capillary mean transit time analysis during hypoxia, hypercapnia and hyperventilation. Brain Res. 1988;454(1–2):170–8.
67. Hardebo JE, Nilsson B. Estimation of cerebral extraction of circulating compounds by the brain uptake index method: influence of circulation time, volume injection, and cerebral blood flow. Acta Physiol Scand. 1979;107(2):153–9.
68. Walczak P, Wojtkiewicz J, Nowakowski A, Habich A, Holak P, Xu J, et al. Real-time MRI for precise and predictable intra-arterial stem cell delivery to the central nervous system. J Cereb Blood Flow Metab. 2017;37(7):2346–58.
69. Shin BJ, Burkhardt JK, Riina HA, Boockvar JA. Superselective intra-arterial cerebral infusion of novel agents after blood-brain disruption for the treatment of recurrent glioblastoma multiforme: a technical case series. Neurosurg Clin N Am. 2012;23(2):323–9, ix-x.
70. Cloughesy TF, Gobin YP, Black KL, Vinuela F, Taft F, Kadkhoda B, et al. Intra-arterial carboplatin chemotherapy for brain tumors: a dose escalation study based on cerebral blood flow. J Neurooncol. 1997;35(2):121–31.
71. Chen SR, Chen MM, Ene C, Lang FF, Kan P. Perfusion-guided endovascular super-selective intra-arterial infusion for treatment of malignant brain tumors. J Neurointerv Surg. 2022;14(6):533–8.
72. Riina HA, Burkhardt JK, Santillan A, Bassani L, Patsalides A, Boockvar JA. Short-term clinico-radiographic response to super-selective intra-arterial cerebral infusion of Bevacizumab for the treatment of vestibular schwannomas in Neurofibromatosis type 2. Interv Neuroradiol. 2012;18(2):127–32.
73. Riina HA, Fraser JF, Fralin S, Knopman J, Scheff RJ, Boockvar JA. Superselective intraarterial cerebral infusion of bevacizumab:

a revival of interventional neuro-oncology for malignant glioma. J Exp Ther Oncol. 2009;8(2):145–50.
74. Uluc K, Ambady P, McIntyre MK, Tabb JP, Kersch CN, Nerison CS, et al. Safety of intra-arterial chemotherapy with or without osmotic blood-brain barrier disruption for the treatment of patients with brain tumors. Neurooncol Adv. 2022;4(1):vdac104.
75. Meng Y, Hynynen K, Lipsman N. Applications of focused ultrasound in the brain: from thermoablation to drug delivery. Nat Rev Neurol. 2021;17(1):7–22.
76. Meng Y, Reilly RM, Pezo RC, Trudeau M, Sahgal A, Singnurkar A, et al. MR-guided focused ultrasound enhances delivery of trastuzumab to Her2-positive brain metastases. Sci Transl Med. 2021;13(615):eabj4011.
77. Karmur BS, Philteos J, Abbasian A, Zacharia BE, Lipsman N, Levin V, et al. Blood-brain barrier disruption in neuro-oncology: strategies, failures, and challenges to overcome. Front Oncol. 2020;10:563840.
78. Thanou M, Gedroyc W. MRI-guided focused ultrasound as a new method of drug delivery. J Drug Deliv. 2013;2013:616197.
79. Joshi S, Singh-Moon RP, Ellis JA, Chaudhuri DB, Wang M, Reif R, et al. Cerebral hypoperfusion-assisted intra-arterial deposition of liposomes in normal and glioma-bearing rats. Neurosurgery. 2015;76(1):92–100.
80. Neuwelt EA, Gilmer-Knight K, Lacy C, Nicholson HS, Kraemer DF, Doolittle ND, et al. Toxicity profile of delayed high dose sodium thiosulfate in children treated with carboplatin in conjunction with blood-brain-barrier disruption. Pediatr Blood Cancer. 2006;47(2):174–82.
81. Oldfield EH, Clark WC, Dedrick RL, Egorin MJ, Austin HA, DeVroom HD, et al. Reduced systemic drug exposure by combining intraarterial cis-diamminedichloroplatinum(II) with hemodialysis of regional venous drainage. Cancer Res. 1987;47(7):1962–7.
82. Oldfield EH, Dedrick RL, Chatterji DC, Yeager RL, Girton ME, Kornblith PL, et al. Arterial drug infusion with extracorporeal removal. II. Internal carotid carmustine in the rhesus monkey. Cancer Treat Rep. 1985;69(3):293–303.
83. Oldfield EH, Dedrick RL, Yeager RL, Clark WC, DeVroom HL, Chatterji DC, et al. Reduced systemic drug exposure by combining intra-arterial chemotherapy with hemoperfusion of regional venous drainage. J Neurosurg. 1985;63(5):726–32.

3 Developing Patient-Specific Arterial Drug Delivery Models

Shaolie S. Hossain

The laws of nature are but the mathematical thoughts of God.

Euclid (circa 300 BCE), Greek Mathematician.

Introduction

Intra-arterial (IA) drug delivery, the administration of therapeutic agents directly into an artery, enables the precise delivery of drugs to a specific organ or tissue. It is generally employed in medical interventions where localized and concentrated drug delivery is crucial for maximizing therapeutic effects while minimizing systemic side effects. IA drug delivery remains an active area of research [1], expanding its applications across different medical specialties. These include (1) cancer, chemotherapy through hepatic arterial infusion to treat liver cancer [2]; (2) neurological disorders, IA delivery of thrombolytic drug to dissolve blood clots in acute ischemic stroke [3]; (3) peripheral arterial disease (PAD), IA drug delivery to improve endothelial function and blood flow in the affected artery [4]; and (4) cardiovascular disease, IA delivery of antiproliferative drug to prevent restenosis [5].

In a typical IA drug delivery process, a catheter is inserted through the femoral artery in the groin. Using real-time angiographic images, the physician directs the catheter through the artery into the heart (as an example), precisely reaching the targeted area of the affected coronary artery. The administration of drugs to the region in the target artery is then achieved by releasing a formulation comprising a fluid carrier medium, encapsulated drug, and a drug ("free drug") either freely dissolved or suspended in the carrier medium. Various options exist for encapsulating the drug, including liposomal, micellar, and polymeric nanoparticles and microbubble. In a nanoparticulate drug delivery system, the nanoparticle's surface is typically conjugated with ligand molecules through nanoengineering to enhance specific interaction with vascular targets and enable firm adhesion (Fig. 3.1) [6].

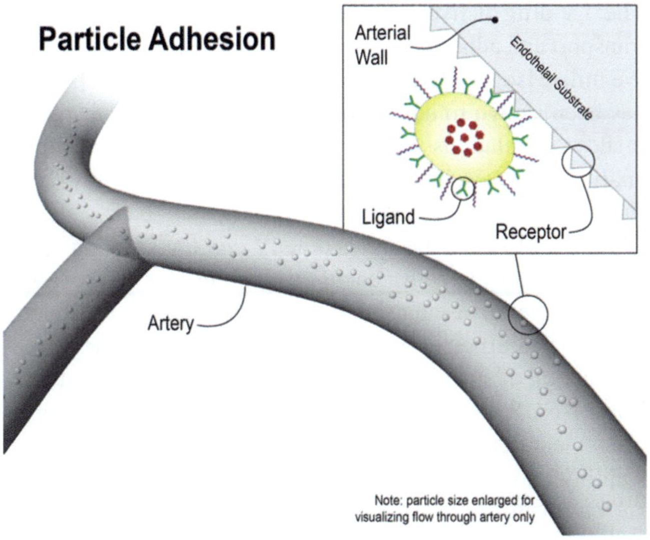

Fig. 3.1 A schematic illustrating the concept of intra-arterial nanoparticulate drug delivery. The nanoparticle surface is typically conjugated with ligand molecules with avidity toward the biological target (receptors). Carried by the blood flow, some of these intravascularly injected nanoparticles drift toward the artery wall. This facilitates specific interactions between the ligands and the receptors overexpressed at the arterial wall, leading to the firm adhesion of nanoparticles through the formation of ligand-receptor bonds, withstanding hydrodynamic forces that tend to dislodge them

S. S. Hossain (✉)
Molecular Cardiology Research Laboratories,
The Texas Heart Institute, Houston, TX, USA

Oden Institute for Computational Engineering and Sciences,
The University of Texas at Austin, Austin, TX, USA
e-mail: shossain@texasheart.org

S. Joshi (ed.), *Arterial Treatment of Neurological Diseases*, https://doi.org/10.1007/978-3-031-80173-0_3

For a given patient, the anatomical features of the vessels, blood flow parameters, and pathological lesions are bound to influence the vascular deposition of nanoparticles and, consequently, treatment efficacy. Important anatomical, physiological, and pathological parameters must be quantified case by case before treatment to ensure optimal delivery [7]. This entails accurately assessing the impact of physiological forces on nanoparticle adhesion and quantifying their deposition in individual patients. Experimental techniques, often relying on trial-and-error approaches, cannot address these crucial design considerations because they are deemed unsafe and impractical to conduct on human subjects. Computational models are particularly advantageous as they allow us to safely test different drug delivery concepts in a virtual environment and predict treatment outcomes with high reliability [8]. They can capture the complexity of biological systems over multiple temporal and spatial scales and incorporate patient information to individualize the analysis results [9]. There is a pressing need for building technologies that use mathematical models to account for IA drug delivery design parameters, in conjunction with patient-specific attributes, to ensure maximum targeting efficiency in an individual patient.

Patient-Specific Modeling of IA Nanoparticle Delivery

The IA drug delivery model uses a flow-coupled particle transport and adhesion model with active targeting (Fig. 3.1). We utilize isogeometric finite element analysis [7, 10], which has been shown to have superior accuracy and convergence in flow simulations compared to traditional finite element analysis. It uses higher-order and higher-continuity basis functions, such as nonuniform rational basis splines (NURBS), to describe the geometry *and* the solution space [10]. It is considered especially well-suited for cardiovascular and cerebrovascular applications because of its smooth, precise, and efficient geometric modeling and accurate representation of stresses [8]. In addition, the parametric definition of NURBS meshes enables automatic boundary layer refinement near the arterial wall, essential for the numerical stability and accurate quantification of near-wall quantities such as the wall shear stress, permeability, and particle adhesion [11]. Below, we describe the main aspects of our modeling approach (see Hossain et al. [12] for further details).

Mathematical Modeling of Flow-Coupled Transport And Adhesion of Particles

Blood is modeled as an incompressible Newtonian fluid with a density (ρ) of 1060 kg/m^3 and a dynamic viscosity (μ) of 0.003 N-s/m^2. The strong form of the continuity and momentum balance equations in the fluid domain Ω with its boundary Γ divided into three nonoverlapping parts, the inflow (Γ_{in}) and outflow (Γ_{out}) boundaries and the vascular wall (Γ_s), can be written as:

$$\rho\frac{\partial \mathbf{u}}{\partial t}+\rho\mathbf{u}\cdot\nabla\mathbf{u}+\nabla p-\nabla\cdot\mu\left(2\nabla^s\mathbf{u}\right)=\mathbf{f}\quad \text{in}\,\Omega\times(0,\,T) \tag{3.1}$$

$$\nabla\cdot\mathbf{u}=0\quad \text{in}\,\Omega\times(0,\,T) \tag{3.2}$$

$$u=g\quad \text{on}\,\Gamma_{in}\times(0,\,T) \tag{3.3}$$

$$u=0\quad \text{on}\,\Gamma_{s}\times(0,\,T) \tag{3.4}$$

$$-pn+\mu\left(2\nabla^s u\right)\cdot n=0\quad \text{on}\,\Gamma_{out}\times(0,\,T) \tag{3.5}$$

$$\mathbf{u}(\mathbf{x},0)=\mathbf{u}_0(\mathbf{x})\quad \text{in}\,\Omega \tag{3.6}$$

where $\mathbf{x}$ is a point in the spatial domain and t is a point in the time domain [0, T]. In these equations, $\mathbf{u}(\mathbf{x};t)$ represents the fluid velocity vector; $p(\mathbf{x};t)$ the pressure; $\mathbf{f}$ the external body force set to zero; $\mathbf{n}$ the unit outward normal to the surface, denoted $\boldsymbol{\Gamma}$; and $\mathbf{u}_0(\mathbf{x};0)$ the initial velocity vector. An inflow velocity vector $\mathbf{g}(\mathbf{x};t)$ is specified at the inlet (Γ_{in}), a no-slip boundary condition is prescribed at the rigid wall (Γ_s), and a traction-free outflow boundary condition is implemented at the branch outlets (Γ_{out}).

The mass transport of nanoparticles released into the bloodstream is modeled to be governed by the unsteady linear scalar-advection-diffusion equation. In the strong form, the transport problem can be stated as:

$$\frac{\partial C}{\partial t}+\mathbf{u}\cdot\nabla C-\nabla\cdot\left(\mathbf{K}\cdot\nabla C\right)+\sigma C=0\quad \text{in}\,\Omega\times(0,\,T) \tag{3.7}$$

$$C=C^0\quad \text{on}\,\Gamma_{in}\times(0,\,T) \tag{3.8}$$

$$\left(K\cdot\nabla C\right)\cdot n=0\quad \text{on}\,\Gamma_{out}\times(0,\,T) \tag{3.9}$$

$$\left(K\cdot\nabla C\right)\cdot n+\Pi C=0\quad \text{on}\,\Gamma_{s}\times(0,\,T) \tag{3.10}$$

$$C(\mathbf{x},0)=0\quad \text{in}\,\Omega \tag{3.11}$$

where $C(\mathbf{x};t)$ is the particle concentration, $\mathbf{K}$ is the diffusivity tensor, and σ is the reaction coefficient. Particle diffusivity is determined by the Einstein-Stokes relation,

$$D=\frac{k_B T}{3\mu d_p}, \tag{3.12}$$

as a function of the particle size, where d_p is the diameter of the particles. Here, k_BT represents the Boltzmann thermal energy. Then,

$$\mathbf{K}=DI \tag{3.13}$$

where $\boldsymbol{I}$ is the 3 × 3 identity matrix. At the inlet Γ_{in}, a Dirichlet boundary condition is prescribed (Eq. 3.8) where C^0 is the particle concentration given as:

$$C^0(x,t) = 1 \text{ for } 0 \le t \le t_i, x \in \Gamma_{\text{in}}$$
$$C^0(x,t) = 0 \text{ for } t > t_i, x \in \Gamma_{\text{in}}. \tag{3.14}$$

Here, t_i denotes the duration of particle injection. A homogenous Neumann boundary condition is specified at the outflow Γ_{out}, and a Robin-type boundary condition is prescribed at the rigid wall interface (Γ_s), where Π is defined as $\Pi = P_a S d_p/2$, accounting for the adhesion of particles to the vessel wall as a function of particle size d_p, local wall shear rate S, and probability of adhesion P_a. The probability of adhesion can be thought of as the propensity to adhere to the vessel wall firmly and a measure of the strength of adhesion. The larger the probability of adhesion, the greater the avidity with which the particle adheres stably to the wall. This probability of adhesion is modeled as follows:

$$P_a \simeq \alpha_1 \alpha_2 \pi a^2 \exp\left[-\beta \frac{\mu S}{\alpha_2}\right] \tag{3.15}$$

where $\alpha_1 = m_l K_A^0$ (= 0.023) and $\alpha_2 = m_r\left[1-\left(1-\frac{\Delta}{a}\right)^2\right]$ ($\approx 1.369 \times 10^{10}$ #/m^2 for $d_p = 0.5$ µm) are two governing parameters and $\beta = \frac{\lambda 6 F^S}{k_B T}$ (= 2.39×10^{11} N^{-1}) is a constant.

In Eq. (3.15), α_1, α_2, the wall shear rate S, and the particle diameter d_p are the independent governing parameters. Here, the uniform surface density of ligand molecules, m_l, decorating the NP surface can specifically interact with counter molecules (i.e., anionic lipids or receptors) expressed on the vessel wall with a surface density m_r. The affinity constant characterizing the molecular interaction between ligands and receptors at zero mechanical load is denoted by K_A^0; the characteristic length of the ligand-receptor bond is λ, generally of the order of 0.1–1 nm; $K_B T$ is the Boltzmann thermal energy (= 4.142×10^{-21} J); F^S(=1.668) is the coefficient of hydrodynamic drag force on a spherical particle; μS is the wall shear stress.

The mass flux of particles ($\partial C\ \partial n$) in the direction $\mathbf{n}$ normal to the vessel wall can be related to the local increase in mass of particles adhering per unit surface $\psi(\mathbf{x};t)$ as:

$$-(\mathbf{K}\cdot\nabla C)\cdot\mathbf{n}\big|_s = -D\frac{\partial C}{\partial n}\bigg|_s = \frac{\partial \psi}{\partial t} \tag{3.16}$$

which is in turn related to the volume concentration of particles at the wall through the equation:

$$-D\frac{\partial C}{\partial n}\bigg|_s = \frac{\partial \psi}{\partial t} = \Pi C\big|_s = P_a S \frac{d_p}{2} C\bigg|_s. \tag{3.17}$$

The term $\Pi = P_a S d_p/2$ is called the vascular deposition parameter, in that the larger the Π, the more significant the number of particles stably adhering to the vessel walls under flow.

Generation of a Patient-Specific Arterial Model from Imaging Data

First, the images are segmented, generating a triangulated surface mesh of the segmented arteries. The 2D triangulated surface mesh is processed through an in-house template-based vascular modeling pipeline that leverages an advanced computer-aided design (CAD) framework to generate a 3D NURBS mesh [13]. The procedure is detailed in previous reports [14, 15]. The process starts with extracting centerlines from the triangulated surface mesh through a skeletonization algorithm. Then, leveraging a CAD geometry library, an algorithm samples the surface mesh around the centerlines. This involves evenly spacing sampling frames along the centerline of each branch and determining their intersections with the triangulated surface mesh. Special consideration is given to placing sampling frames near points where arteries bifurcate or trifurcate, ensuring conformality at these junctions. The polyline intersection of the sampling frames with the triangulated surface mesh is then interpolated by a NURBS curve on each frame. Following this, the NURBS curves are lofted along the appropriate centerline, resulting in a NURBS representation of the 2D triangulated surface mesh geometry parameterized in the circumferential and axial directions. Finally, adding the radial direction to the parameterization completes the process, resulting in a hexahedral NURBS solid mesh. Boundary layer mesh refinement is implemented to accurately compute near-wall hemodynamic quantities, such as wall shear stress. Figure 3.2 shows the main steps of reconstructing a patient-specific coronary artery tree model from a healthy volunteer's 3D computerized tomography (CT) scan to instantiate the process.

Numerical Implementation and Solution Strategy

Within the isogeometric finite element analysis framework, a 3D Navier-Stokes solver simulates blood flow within the patient-specific coronary artery tree model by applying the general solution strategies and numerical procedures described in previous reports [7, 12, 16]. In summary, the system of equations is solved by employing a residual-based variational multiscale (VMS) method using a Newton-Raphson procedure with a multistage predictor-corrector algorithm applied at each time step. The generalized-α method, an implicit second-order, time-accurate, unconditionally stable method, is used for time advancement.

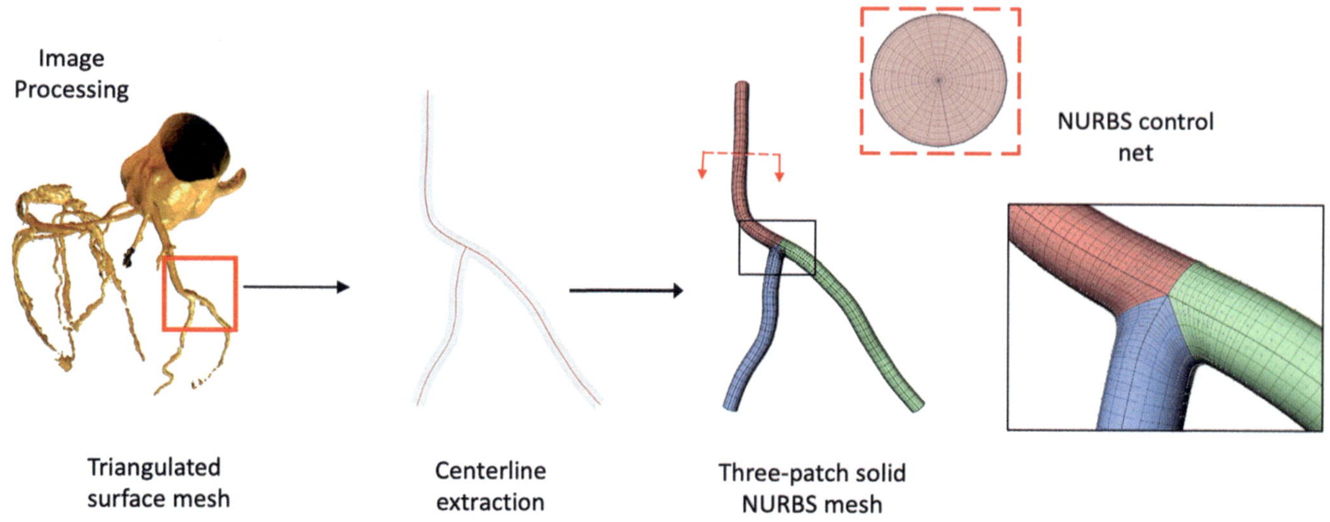

Fig 3.2 Generation of a patient-specific arterial geometry from imaging data. Image segmentation generates a triangulated surface mesh of the left coronary artery tree from patient CT data, from which, centerlines are extracted using a skeletonization algorithm. The centerline and the triangulated surface mesh are then input into an in-house CAD-integrated vascular modeling pipeline to reconstruct a hexahedral solid NURBS mesh using a template-based approach (see previous work by Urick et al. [13]). Quadratic NURBS are used for spatial discretization. A cross-section of the computational mesh is shown to highlight the boundary layer refinement that has been implemented. The inset depicts an enlarged view of the bifurcation region, where three NURBS patches meet

Experimental Validation of Model Predictions:

As detailed in previous work, the coupled particle transport and adhesion model has been validated against in vitro experiments utilizing a parallel plate flow chamber for a range of physiological WSR and particle sizes [12]. Briefly, spherical fluorescent particles (Fluoresbrite® YG Microspheres) were injected into a channel (20 mm in length and 0.274 mm in height) with a rectangular cross-section. The top and bottom plates of the channel were coated with collagen. By controlling the volumetric flow rate within the channel, wall shear rates of 10, 75, and 200 s^{-1} were induced on the plate. The number of particles adhering over the substrate was quantified, and the results were presented in terms of the number of adhering particles (n_{adh}) per unit area (A) normalized by the total number of injected particles (n_{inj}). These experiments were carried out for different-sized spherical particles with a nominal diameter d_p, of 0.75, 3.0, and 6.0 μm. Model predictions were compared with experimental results (Fig. 3.3). Table 3.1 lists the parameter values used in the flow simulations. A biphasic relationship between particle size and the number of adhered particles was observed as a function of the local wall shear rate. The results suggest an optimal particle size for maximum adhesion, and the greater the wall shear rate, the smaller this optimum particle size. These findings indicate that particle adhesion is strongly modulated by the vascular deposition parameter, $\Pi = P_a S d\_p/2$ [12].

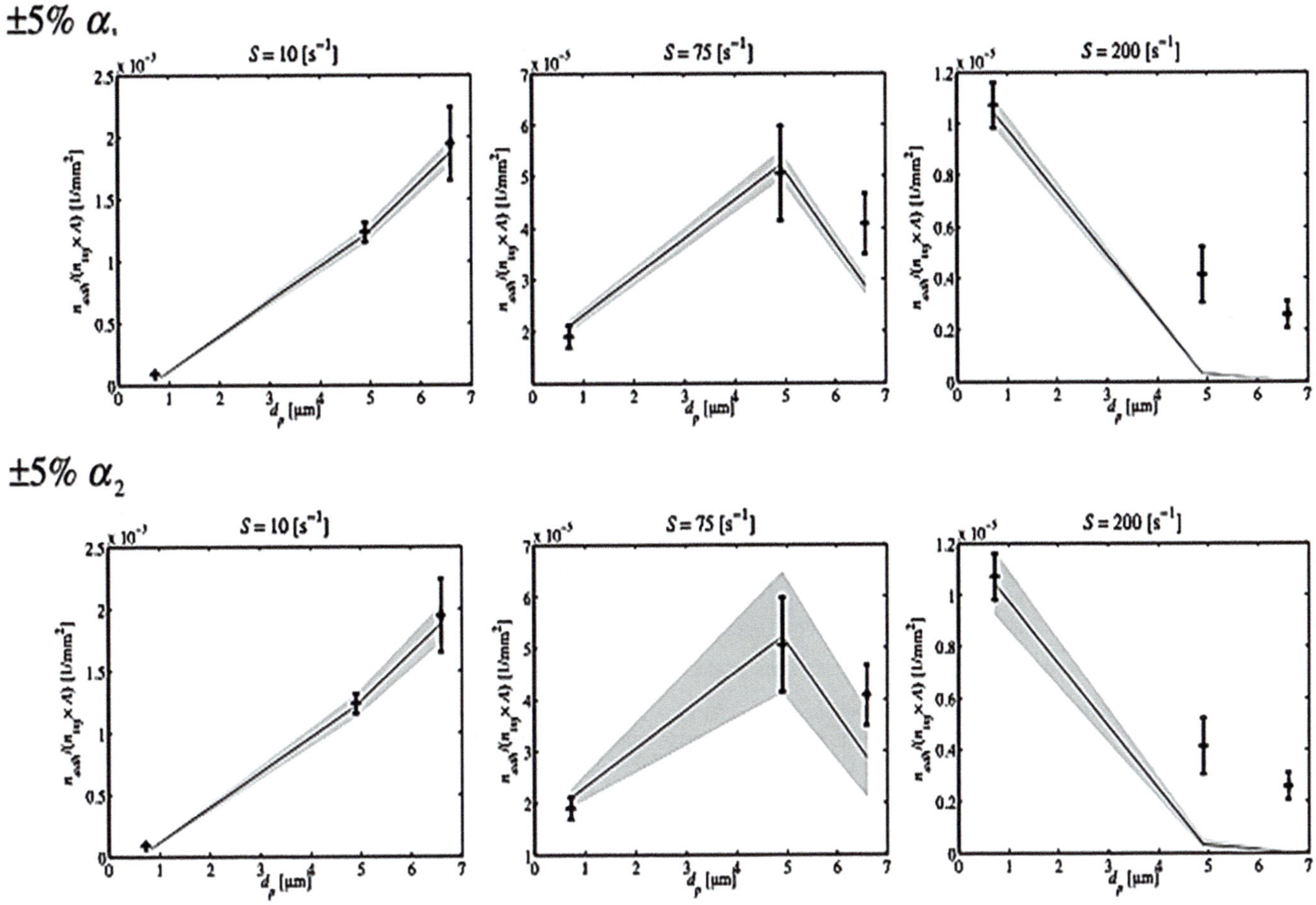

Fig. 3.3 Comparison of model predictions with experimental data. The number of adhering particles n_{adh} per unit surface area A normalized by the total number of injected particles n_{inj} is plotted as a function of particle diameter d_p for three different prevailing wall shear rates: $S = 10\ s^{-1}$, $S = 75\ s^{-1}$, and $S = 200\ s^{-1}$. Black crosses with the standard deviation bars represent the experimental results obtained in a parallel plate flow chamber apparatus. The gray areas represent the in-silico results obtained for values of the parameters α_1 (top) and α_2 (bottom) varying within 5% of their average values

Table 3.1 Model parameters

Parameters	Value
Surface density of ligand molecules	$m_l = 10^{15}$ #/m^2
Surface density of receptor molecules	$m_r = 10^{13}$ #/m^2
Ligand-receptor affinity constant at zero load	$K_A{}^0 = 2.3 \times 10^{-7}$ m^2
Characteristic length of ligand-receptor bond	$\lambda = 1 \times 10^{-10}$ m
Dynamic viscosity of water	$\mu = 0.001$ N-s/m^2
Drag coefficient on the spherical particle	$F^S = 1.668$

Patient-Specific Analysis of IA Nanoparticle Delivery: A Cardiovascular Application

The simulation setup for a patient-specific coronary artery tree model is shown in Fig. 3.4. A time-dependent patient-specific pulsatile inflow condition is imposed with a parabolic profile at the left coronary artery (LCA) inlet [12]. Under a rigid wall approximation, a no-slip boundary condition was prescribed for the vascular wall, and a traction-free outflow boundary condition was implemented at the two branch outlets: the left anterior descending (LAD) artery and the left circumflex (LCX) branch. A catheter was positioned at the inlet of the LCA segment, through which nanoparticles were injected radially and axially at a speed of 4 cm/s over five cardiac cycles. The simulations were run on a computational mesh of quadratic NURBS elements for 14 cardiac cycles (14 s total).

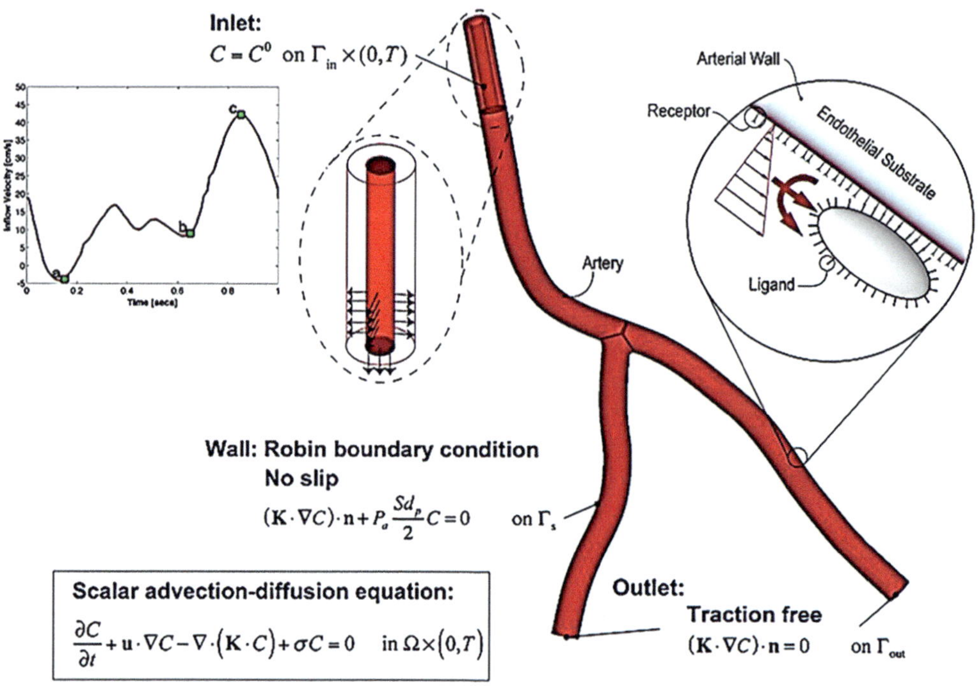

Fig. 3.4 The simulation setup. A patient-specific geometric model of the left coronary artery (LCA) tree is considered. The artery bifurcates into two downstream branches: the left anterior descending (LAD) and the left circumflex (LCX). A Navier-Stokes solver coupled to a scalar advection-diffusion equation, subject to boundary conditions, is used to simulate flow-coupled transport and deposition of nanoparticles in the arterial tree. A pulsatile inflow condition is prescribed at the inlet, a no-slip boundary condition is imposed on the vessel wall, and a traction-free boundary condition is set at the two outlets. A catheter is placed at the inlet through which nanoparticles are injected radially and axially. A Robin-type boundary condition accounts for particle adhesion to the arterial wall, with a zero-flux condition set at the branch outlets

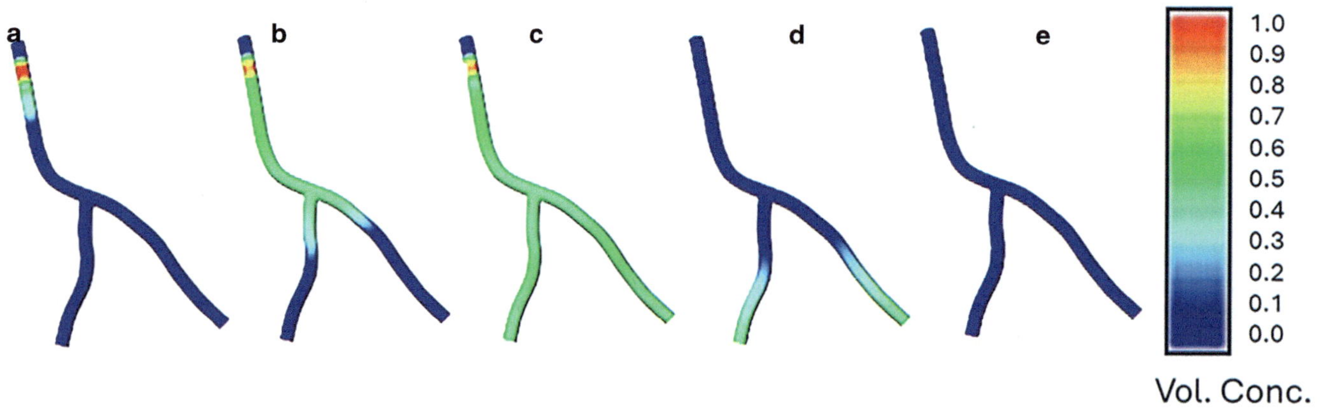

Fig. 3.5 Nanoparticle transport in a patient-specific vascular tree. Volumetric concentration C of nanoparticles, normalized by the concentration at the catheter outlet C^0, at various times t postinjection: (**a**) $t = 0.2$ s, (**b**) $t = 1$ s, (**c**) $t = 5$ s, (**d**) $t = 10$ s, and (**e**) $t = 14$ s

Effect of Particle Size, Arterial Geometry, and Receptor Density on Distribution

Spherical nanoparticles of two sizes were considered: 0.5 and 2.0 μm. As an initial approximation, a uniform distribution of receptor density (m_r) was assumed throughout the arterial tree, representing a nonspecific targeting scenario (see Table 3.1 for a list of parameter values used in the simulation). The time evolution of the particle ($d_p = 0.5$ μm) volumetric concentration within the coronary arteries is presented in Fig. 3.5. With time, the particle distribution front moves from the LCA inlet, where the catheter is located, toward the downstream branch and eventually into the LAD and LCX artery. By 5 s, the particles are uniformly distributed throughout the vascular tree. When the catheter injection stops after 5 s, it takes a while for the particles to leave the domain, and by 14 s, no particles remain within the arterial tree.

The results presented in Fig. 3.6 regarding the surface density of adhered particles suggest that particle adhesion is influenced by local wall shear rate and the particle size and

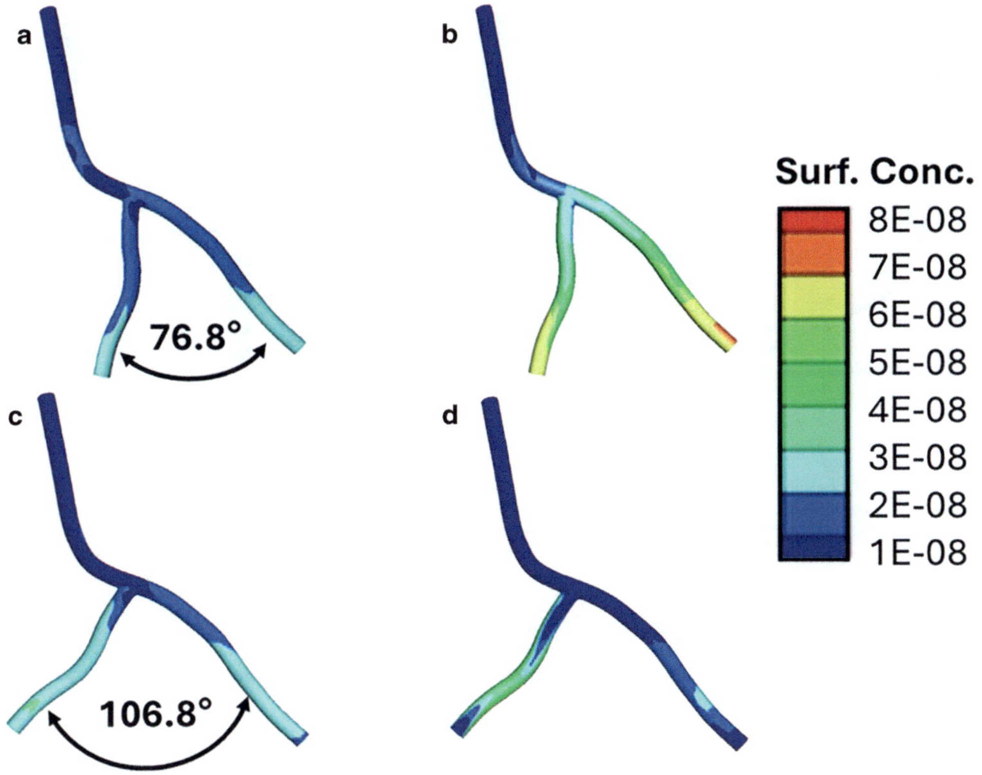

Fig. 3.6 Effect of particle size and vascular architecture on particle distribution pattern of nanoparticles. The normalized surface density of adhering nanoparticles is plotted along the arterial tree at $t = 14$ s, postinjection for (**a**, **c**) the 0.5 µm and (**b**, **d**) 2.0 µm particles. The top and bottom rows present in silico data for the smaller (76.8°) and larger (106.8°) branching angles, respectively. Data are presented as the number of particles adhered per unit area normalized by the injected dose [cm^{-2}]

vascular geometry distribution pattern of the particles vary. Larger particles (2.0 µm in diameter) adhered more in the lower branches of the arterial tree, where the wall shear rates were moderate (<200 s^{-1}). In contrast, smaller particles (0.5 µm in diameter) adhered more in the upper branches, with higher wall shear rates. As the branching angle in the arterial tree increases, the adhesion patterns become more asymmetric between the two downstream branches. Patients with larger branching angles (≈106.8°) received more nanoparticles in the LAD than in the LCX. On the other hand, nanoparticles were distributed equally in the two arterial branches for patients with smaller branching angles (≈76.8°). These findings underscore the importance of incorporating patient-specific information in designing IA drug delivery systems.

A tenfold higher expression of the target receptor was assumed in the LAD branch to study receptor density's effect on nanoparticles' vascular distribution. This resulted in greater nanoparticle adhesion in that region compared to the rest of the domain (results not shown here), indicating that target receptor density strongly modulates particle adhesion [12].

Targeting Inflammation with IA Delivery of Nanoparticles

Inflammation is a precursor to numerous diseases, such as cancer and atherosclerosis, and it induces distinct surface expression patterns of specific vascular molecules. Carried by the blood flow, surface-functionalized nanoparticles, loaded with therapeutic and/or imaging agents, can recognize and utilize these molecules overexpressed at the endothelial surface as docking sites within the vasculature (Fig. 3.1). This facilitates the targeted delivery of a drug and/or imaging agent. In atherosclerosis, low/oscillating wall shear stress is known to prompt an inflammatory reaction leading to an increased expression of specific cell adhesion molecules (CAMs), notably vascular cell adhesion molecule-1 (VCAM-1) and E-selectin [16]. These molecules are indicative of atheroprone conditions. Conversely, a higher shear rate setting, resulting in elevated intercellular adhesion molecule-1 (ICAM-1) expression but a reduction in VCAM-1, is regarded as atheroprotective [17]. We conducted a computational study to predict the vascular distribution patterns of intravascularly injected inflammation-targeted nanoparticles that could provide site-specific delivery of drug imaging and/or therapeutic agents to detect and/or diffuse metabolically active atherosclerotic plaques. These so-called vulnerable plaques are at high risk of rupture, leading to acute coronary syndrome (ACS).

Nanoparticles, ranging in diameter from 500 to 2000 nm, were conjugated with antibodies targeting three CAMs of interest: ICAM-1, VCAM-1, and E-selectin. Local hemodynamics, such as wall shear stress, are known to modulate the upregulation of these molecules. Utilizing the data generated through in vitro experiments conducted by Tsou et al. [12], a functional relationship between local

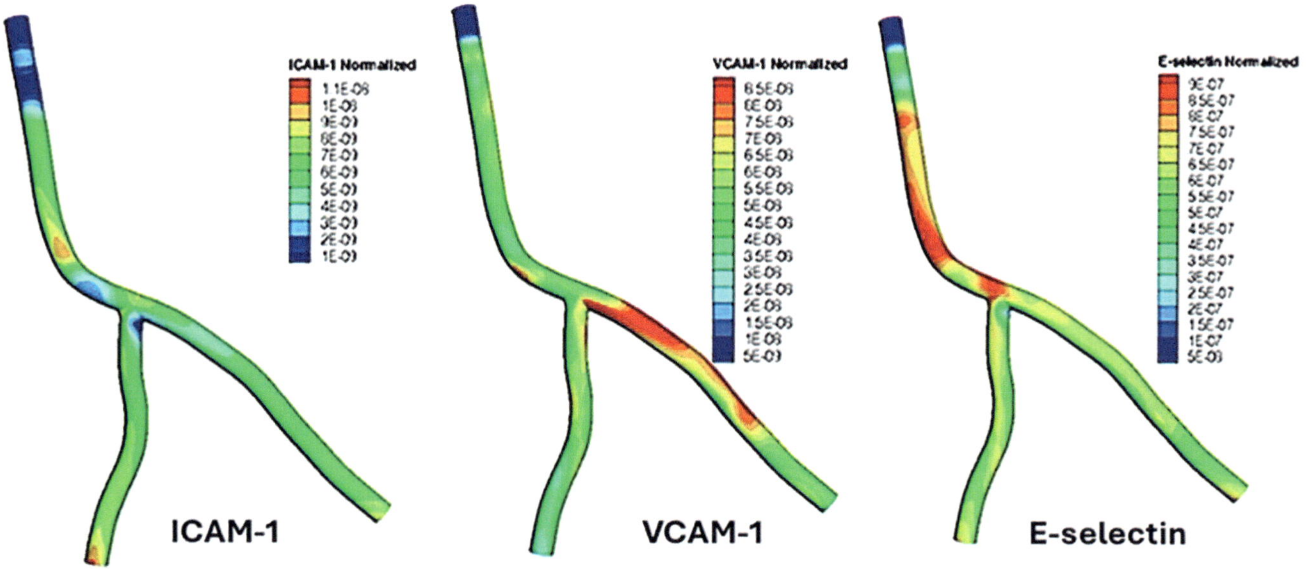

Fig. 3.7 Vascular deposition pattern for inflammation-targeted nanoparticles. Surface density (cm^{-2}) of 0.5 μm particles n_{adh} per unit surface area A normalized by the total number of injected particles n_{inj}, that is, in terms of $n_{adh}/(n_{inj} \times A)$, for the three targeted receptors: (**a**) ICAM-1, (**b**) VCAM-1, and (**c**) E-selectin. Note: color map scales are different

wall shear stress and upregulation of CAMs was devised, and the surface density of ICAM-1, VCAM-1, and E-selectin (target receptors) throughout the coronary artery tree was estimated [18]. Throughout the patient-specific coronary artery tree, flow-coupled transport and adhesion of nanoparticles injected via a catheter (Fig. 3.4) were simulated.

Results show that VCAM-1-targeted nanoparticles exhibited greater adhesion, while ICAM-1-directed nanoparticles showed less efficient adherence, resulting in an approximately one-order-of-magnitude lower-average particle surface density (Fig. 3.7). ICAM-1 and E-selectin-directed 0.5-μm nanoparticles were distributed more uniformly among the bifurcating vascular branches than their VCAM-1 counterparts. When the nanoparticles were coated with antibodies for VCAM-1 and E-selectin in equal proportions, a more uniform vascular distribution was achieved compared with VCAM-1 only targeted particles, thus demonstrating the advantage of nanoparticle multivalency in vascular targeting. Furthermore, larger nanoparticles (2 μm) exhibited increased adhesion (approximately 200%) in the downstream branches.

Therefore, patient-specific modeling of IA delivery offers predictive insights into how particle size, type of ligand, density, and multivalency can be manipulated to improve the vascular adhesion of nanoparticles in an individual patient.

Toward Patient-Specific Modeling of IA Drug Delivery to the Brain

While nanoparticles have been used as drug carriers in IA drug delivery for treating many brain diseases, IA pharmacokinetic models have struggled to predict drug tissue uptake accurately [19]. The failure is attributed to the hydrodynamic complexities that overlay regional pharmacokinetics. Few computational models have explored the relationship between particle adhesion dynamics and local hemodynamics that tend to dislodge the particles after IA injections [20, 21]. No studies have also accounted for patient-specific characteristics known to affect the vascular deposition of nanomedicine. To address these challenges, the patient-specific modeling approach presented in this report can be extended to IA drug delivery of the brain.

In previous work, we developed an image-based patient-specific modeling framework to simulate physiologically realistic blood flow features within the circle of Willis of mice [14] and human subjects [14, 22, 23]. An in silico study involving wild-type (WT) and $ACTA2^{-/-}$ knockout (KO) mice representative of normal and pathological conditions, respectively, was conducted to investigate how cerebrovascular alterations, such as arterial straightening and occlusion, influence local hemodynamics (Fig. 3.8). An occlusion in one of the large vessels changed the flow direction in a

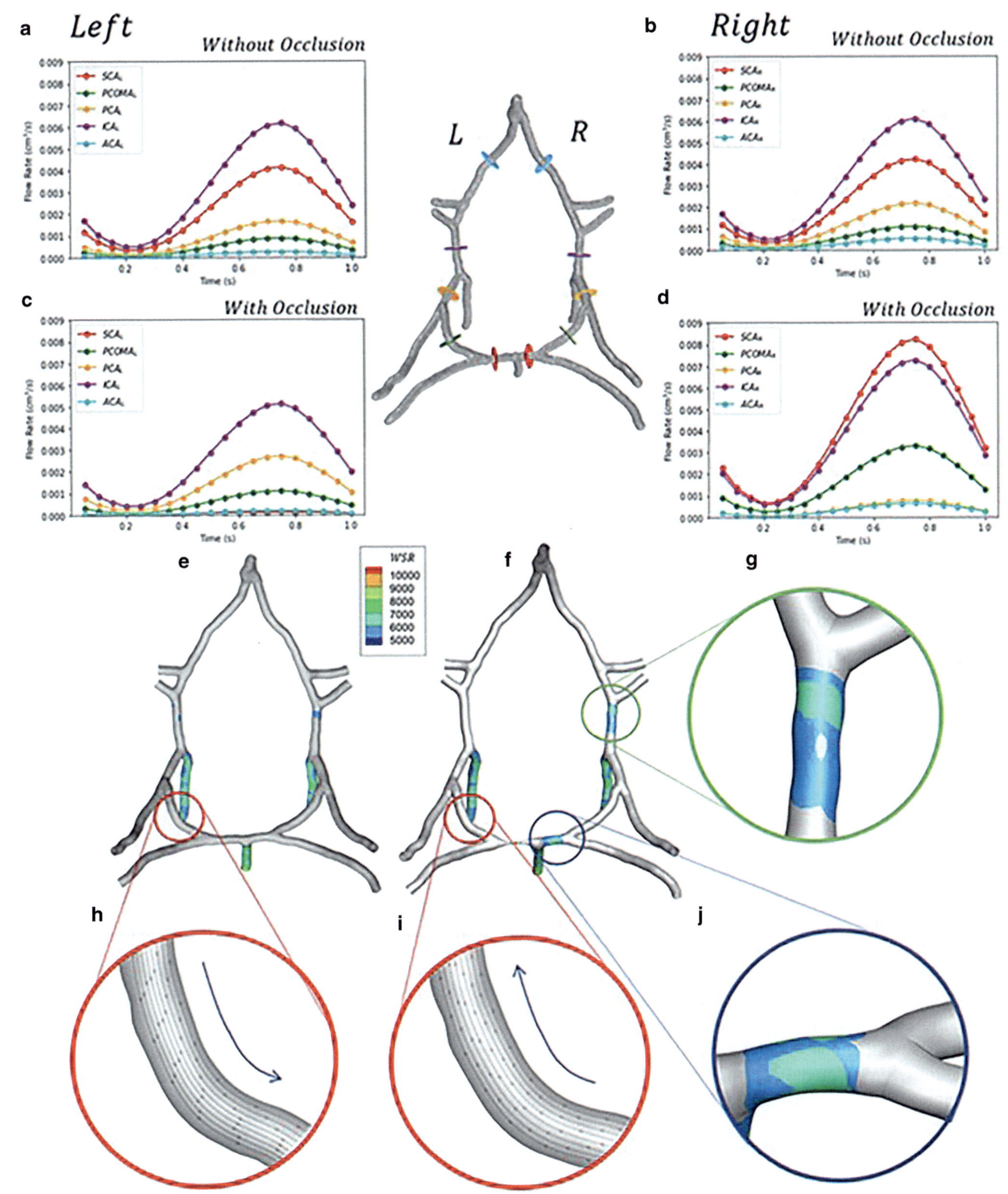

Fig. 3.8 Blood flow rate in cm³/s at various locations within the circle of Willis (CoW) of a ACTA2$^{-/-}$ knockout (KO) mouse model with (**a**, **b**) and without (**c**, **d**) an occlusion indicates that the presence of an occlusion in left superior cerebellar artery (LSCA) results in a flow bias toward the contralateral side. Comparison of critical WSR (>5000 s^{-1}) above the coagulation limit at peak systole in the CoW of a KO mouse model without (**e**) and with (**f**) an occlusion identifies vascular regions (**g** and **j**) contralateral to the occlusion with critically high wall shear rate that are at a higher probability of thrombus formation. Streamline plots within the CoW of the mouse model without (**i**) and with (**h**) occlusion show retrograde flow in the left posterior communicating cerebral artery (LPCOMA) as a consequence of restricted flow in the occluded LSCA

neighboring branch. It increased the hemodynamic burden, raising wall shear rate values in vessels contralateral to the occlusion [14]. These results emphasize that realistic patient-specific 3D modeling of the cerebrovascular is essential for creating physiological flow and transport features necessary for developing IA drug delivery systems for the brain.

Additionally, utilizing the particle adhesion model described previously, a preliminary in silico study was conducted to investigate how two characteristics of liposomes (size and surface charge) affected their near-wall interactions and local adsorption when delivered by the flow arrest (FA)-IA injection technique [24]. The simulations explored various liposome sizes, ranging from 2 to 500 nm, under diverse hemodynamic conditions characterized by local wall shear rates. Notably, particles with a size of 80 nm or larger exhibited enhanced deposition under low wall shear stress, as induced by the flow arrest-IA delivery method. Nevertheless, as wall shear stress escalated, the deposition of larger particles experienced a substantial decrease. Introducing a cationic charge improved the deposition rate. It enhanced the probability of adhesion during FA delivery. Interestingly, the charge had a greater influence in the deposition of larger nanoparticles, and it decreased to negligible levels for <20 nm liposomes. Our modeling indicated that with the FA-IA method for the given endothelial charge density and particle characteristics, the benefits of shear rate reduction are less applicable to particles 20 nm or less. The next step would be to extend these modeling principles to a subject-specific model of the circle of Willis to simulate IA drug delivery to the brain.

Conclusions

In summary, our patient-specific computational modeling approach, capable of accounting for anatomical characteristics, regional blood flow, and drug injection profile, offers a conceptual framework for understanding and enhancing IA delivery. Although the model was developed using coronary angiographic data, it could be applied to the cerebral circulation in the future. Preliminary data on cerebral drug delivery using a mouse model supports developing such applications. Such a modeling approach facilitates the rational design of functionalized nanoparticles, with precise control over sizes, shapes, surface characteristics, and material compositions [25] in conjunction with patient-specific attributes. Through this process, the desired selectivity and adhesion efficiency of nanoparticles tailored to each patient's unique characteristics can be achieved, marking a significant stride toward the realization of precision medicine in IA drug delivery.

References

1. Patra JK, Das G, Fraceto LF, Campos EVR, Rodriguez-Torres MDP, Acosta-Torres LS, et al. Nano based drug delivery systems: recent developments and future prospects. J Nanobiotechnol. 2018;16(1):71.
2. Chapelle N, Matysiak-Budnik T, Douane F, Metairie S, Rougier P, Touchefeu Y. Hepatic arterial infusion in the management of colorectal cancer liver metastasis: current and future perspectives. Dig Liver Dis. 2018;50(3):220–5.
3. Berkhemer OA, Fransen PS, Beumer D, van den Berg LA, Lingsma HF, Yoo AJ, et al. A randomized trial of intraarterial treatment for acute ischemic stroke. N Engl J Med. 2015;372(1):11–20.
4. Kashyap VS, Lakin RO, Campos P, Allemang M, Kim A, Sarac TP, et al. The LargPAD Trial: phase IIA evaluation of l-arginine infusion in patients with peripheral arterial disease. J Vasc Surg. 2017;66(1):187–94.
5. Prabhu S, Hossainy S. Modeling of degradation and drug release from a biodegradable stent coating. J Biomed Mater Res A. 2007;80(3):732–41.
6. Mitchell MJ, Billingsley MM, Haley RM, Wechsler ME, Peppas NA, Langer R. Engineering precision nanoparticles for drug delivery. Nat Rev Drug Discov. 2021;20(2):101–24.
7. Hossain SS, Hossainy SFA, Bazilevs Y, Calo VM, Hughes TJR. Mathematical modeling of coupled drug and drug-encapsulated nanoparticle transport in patient-specific coronary artery walls. Comput Mech. 2012;49(2):213–42.
8. Bao G, Bazilevs Y, Chung JH, Decuzzi P, Espinosa HD, Ferrari M, et al. USNCTAM perspectives on mechanics in medicine. J R Soc Interface. 2014;11(97):20140301.
9. Hossain SS, Kopacz AM, Zhang Y, Lee S-Y, Lee T-R, Ferrari M, et al. Multiscale modeling for the vascular transport of nanoparticles. In: Nano and cell mechanics; 2013. p. 437–59.
10. Hughes TJR, Cottrell JA, Bazilevs Y. Isogeometric analysis: CAD, finite elements, NURBS, exact geometry and mesh refinement. Comput Methods Appl Mech Eng. 2005;194(39):4135–95.
11. Hossain SS, Zhang Y, Fu X, Brunner G, Singh J, Hughes TJ, et al. Magnetic resonance imaging-based computational modelling of blood flow and nanomedicine deposition in patients with peripheral arterial disease. J R Soc Interface. 2015;12(106):20150001.
12. Hossain SS, Zhang Y, Liang X, Hussain F, Ferrari M, Hughes TJ, et al. In silico vascular modeling for personalized nanoparticle delivery. Nanomedicine (Lond). 2013;8(3):343–57.
13. Urick B, Sanders TM, Hossain SS, Zhang YJ, Hughes TJR. Review of patient-specific vascular modeling: template-based isogeometric framework and the case for CAD. Arch Comput Methods Eng. 2019;26(2):381–404.
14. Hossain SS, Starosolski Z, Sanders T, Johnson MJ, Wu MCH, Hsu MC, et al. Image-based patient-specific flow simulations are consistent with stroke in pediatric cerebrovascular disease. Biomech Model Mechanobiol. 2021;20(6):2071–84.
15. Hossain SS, Johnson MJ, Hughes TJR "A parametric study of the effect of 3D plaque shape on local hemodynamics and implications for plaque instability," Biomechanics and Modeling in Mechanobiology Biomechanics, 23(2024);1209–27, https://doi.org/10.1007/s10237-024-01834-6. PMID: 38532042, PMCID: PMC11341608.
16. Cunningham KS, Gotlieb AI. The role of shear stress in the pathogenesis of atherosclerosis. Lab Investig. 2005;85(1):9–23.
17. Chiu JJ, Lee PL, Chen CN, Lee CI, Chang SF, Chen LJ, et al. Shear stress increases ICAM-1 and decreases VCAM-1 and E-selectin expressions induced by tumor necrosis factor-[alpha] in endothelial cells. Arterioscler Thromb Vasc Biol. 2004;24(1):73–9.

18. Hossain SS, Hughes TJ, Decuzzi P. Vascular deposition patterns for nanoparticles in an inflamed patient-specific arterial tree. Biomech Model Mechanobiol. 2014;13(3):585–97.
19. Ellis JA, Banu M, Hossain SS, Singh-Moon R, Lavine SD, Bruce JN, et al. Reassessing the role of intra-arterial drug delivery for glioblastoma multiforme treatment. J Drug Deliv. 2015;2015:405735.
20. Joshi S, Cooke JR, Chan DK, Ellis JA, Hossain SS, Singh-Moon RP, et al. Liposome size and charge optimization for intraarterial delivery to gliomas. Drug Deliv Transl Res. 2016;6(3):225–33.
21. Cooke JN, Ellis JA, Hossain S, Nguyen J, Bruce JN, Joshi S. Computational pharmacokinetic rationale for intra-arterial delivery to the brain. Drug Deliv Transl Res. 2016;6(5):622–9.
22. Horn JD, Johnson MJ, Starosolski Z, Meoded A, Milewicz DM, Annapragada A, et al. Patient-specific modeling could predict occurrence of pediatric stroke. Front Physiol. 2022;13:846404.
23. Horn JD, Starosolski Z, Johnson MJ, Meoded A, Hossain SS. A novel method for improving the accuracy of MR-derived patient-specific vascular models using X-ray angiography. Eng Comput. 2022;38(5):3879–91.
24. Nguyen J, Hossain SS, Cooke JRN, Ellis JA, Deci MB, Emala CW, et al. Flow arrest intra-arterial delivery of small TAT-decorated and neutral micelles to gliomas. J Neurooncol. 2017;133(1):77–85.
25. Choo P, Liu T, Odom TW. Nanoparticle shape determines dynamics of targeting nanoconstructs on cell membranes. J Am Chem Soc. 2021;143(12):4550–5.

Nanocarriers for Transportation Across the Blood-Brain Barrier

4

Howyn Tang, Chao Lu, Hossein Pouri, and Jin Zhang

Trust not the horse, O Trojans. Be it what it may, I fear the Greeks when they offer gifts.

Publius Vergilius Maro (70 to 19 BCE), Roman Poet
The Trojan horse - a sly tool to penetrate a defensive barrier.

Introduction

Brain diseases, including cancers, pose significant challenges to treatment and have notably lower success rates in drug development compared to other diseases [1, 2]. The blood-brain barrier (BBB) is an extensive and exclusive physical barrier that restricts drug entry. The barrier prevents large molecules from crossing into the brain parenchyma while permitting only small lipid-soluble molecules to pass [3, 4]. Despite efforts to synthesize novel drugs such as peptides, proteins, genes, and antisense drugs to combat central nervous system (CNS) diseases, the clinical efficacy of many pharmaceuticals is attenuated in vivo due to inadequate BBB penetration. Central nervous system (CNS) drug delivery also poses additional challenges, such as poor stability in biological fluids, rapid enzymatic degradation, inadequate release profiles, and unfavorable pharmacokinetic properties [5]. The lack of efficient drug delivery technologies across the BBB remains a significant neurotherapeutic obstacle [1]. Current research in CNS drug development primarily centers on optimizing systemic drug delivery to the brain and bypassing the BBB [6]. Thus, various strategies have been devised to effectively release drugs into the brain, such as chemical modification of drugs and prodrugs, temporary disruption of tight junctions, and local delivery through neurosurgery. While these approaches have undergone extensive laboratory and clinical studies, none are universally applicable [3, 7, 8].

A growing focus has recently been on developing effective approaches to deliver therapeutics and macromolecules to the brain [9]. Several promising strategies for targeting and delivering drugs across the BBB have been described, including carrier agents like nanoparticles and immune cells [10]. Nanosized carriers, or nanocarriers, have gained significant attention as they can provide protection and facilitate targeted delivery of drugs that may be ineffective on their own. These carriers enable drugs to associate with nanoparticles through various mechanisms such as adsorption, dissolution, encapsulation, or covalent binding [11]. Utilizing nanoparticles for drug delivery offers numerous advantages, including cost-effectiveness, favorable biodegradability, long-term stability, ease of synthesis, high targeting efficiency, and precise control over drug loading and release across the BBB [7, 12].

In this book chapter, we delve into the mechanisms of BBB permeation and strategies to enhance drug delivery to the brain. We also investigate the potential of various nanocarriers, including inorganic, polymeric, and lipid nanoparticles. Furthermore, we briefly discuss different delivery routes for these carriers. This comprehensive exploration aims to provide valuable insights into the design and optimization of nanocarriers for efficient drug delivery across the BBB, thereby advancing the field of neurotherapeutics relevant to developing arterial drugs for treating neurological diseases.

H. Tang
School of Biomedical Engineering, University of Western Ontario, London, ON, Canada,

C. Lu · H. Pouri
Department of Chemical and Biochemical Engineering, University of Western Ontario, London, ON, Canada

J. Zhang (✉)
Department of Chemical and Biochemical Engineering, University of Western Ontario, London, ON, Canada

School of Biomedical Engineering, University of Western Ontario, London, ON; Canada
e-mail: jzhang@eng.uwo.ca;
http://eng.uwo.ca/chemical/faculty/zhang_j/

S. Joshi (ed.), *Arterial Treatment of Neurological Diseases*, https://doi.org/10.1007/978-3-031-80173-0_4

BBB Permeation Mechanisms

The BBB is a unique and dynamic structure formed by tight junctions among capillary endothelial cells. It creates a monolayer of brain endothelial cells 30–40 mm thick [13, 14]. As a lipophilic barrier, the BBB allows the passive diffusion of lipophilic molecules, small molecules smaller than 400 Da, and gases like carbon dioxide and oxygen [15, 16]. The BBB's tight junctions play a crucial role in regulating the movement of substances between the blood and the brain, effectively controlling paracellular solute movement [15]. Various transmembrane proteins, such as claudins, junctional adhesion molecules, and occludin, form the bicellular and tricellular tight junctions in the BBB [17].

Physiological strategies can improve drug delivery across the BBB, taking advantage of the diverse transporters and receptors expressed on the BBB [18]. Solute carrier systems are responsible for transporting small molecules and peptides, while receptors facilitate the transport of larger molecules. Delivering drugs through solute carriers requires careful consideration of stereochemistry to mimic the natural substrate, presenting a challenge when using peptides as delivery vectors. However, understanding and leveraging these transport mechanisms offer promising opportunities for enhancing drug delivery across the BBB [18, 19]. In general, biomolecule and drug transport involve physiological mechanisms. These mechanisms encompass passive diffusion, carrier-mediated transport, receptor-mediated transcytosis, and adsorptive-mediated transcytosis (Fig. 4.1) [21, 22].

Passive Diffusion

The primary method for drugs to cross the BBB is passive diffusion. Passive diffusion refers to the spontaneous movement of a drug across a cellular lipid bilayer, driven by its concentration gradient [21]. However, tight junctions and efflux transporters can restrict this process, although it can occur through transcellular or paracellular pathways for small, hydrophobic molecules. Factors like molecular weight and lipophilicity influence the passive diffusion of drugs across the BBB, with lipophilic drugs showing better diffusion due to favorable interactions with the lipid bilayer [21, 23]. As a result, solutes and drugs have limited penetration into the CNS. However, efflux transporters, such as P-glycoprotein (ABCB1), multidrug resistance-associated proteins (MRPs), and breast cancer resistance proteins, actively remove substances from the brain endothelium, limiting drug delivery. Although these transporters adversely affect drug delivery, they are critical for preventing the accumulation of harmful substances in the brain [15, 24].

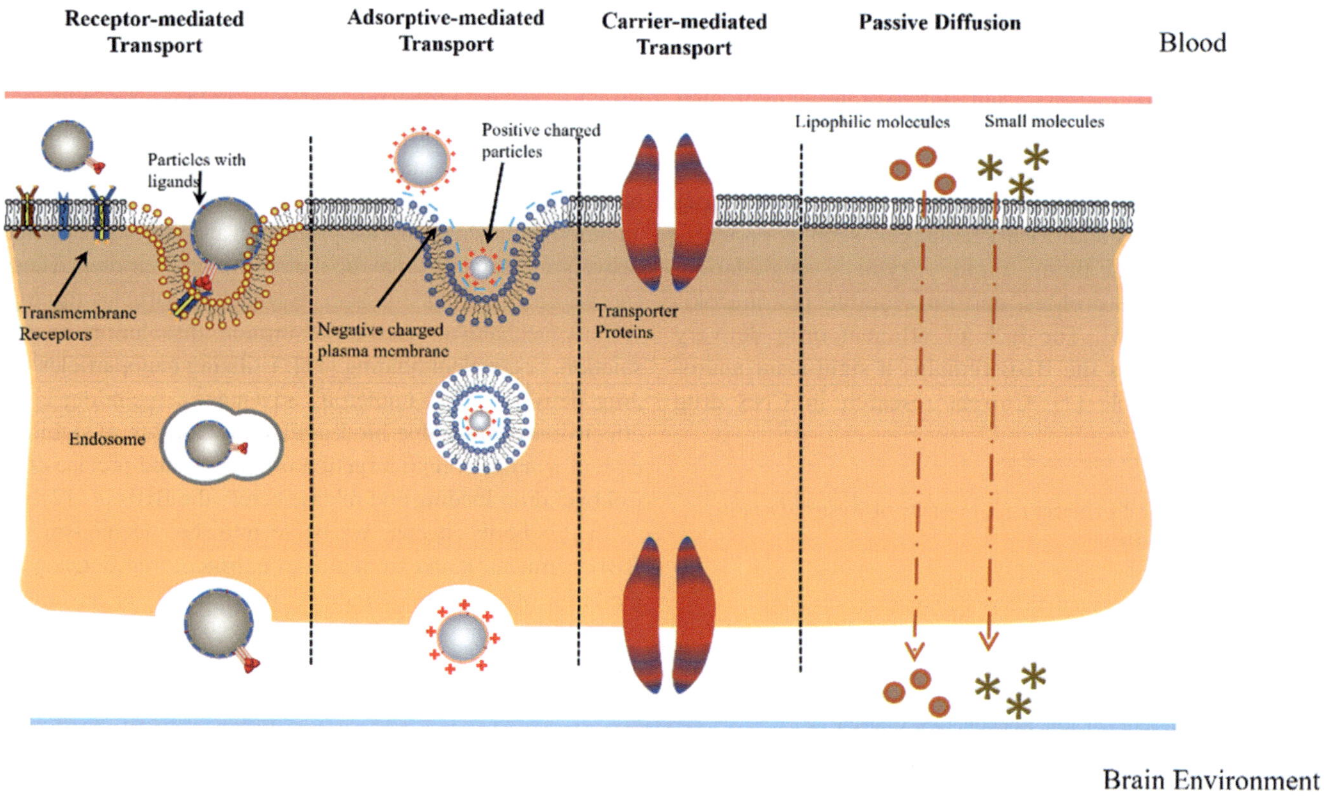

Fig. 4.1 Physiological mechanisms behind transportation across the blood-brain barrier [20]

Drugs may have adequate lipophilicity for passage across the BBB; however, the efflux transporters can reduce tissue retention and efficacy. Understanding these mechanisms offers opportunities to enhance drug delivery and improve therapies for brain disorders [21].

Carrier-Mediated Transport (CMT)

Specialized carrier-mediated transport (CMT) systems expressed in the BBB facilitate the transportation of molecules like amino acids, glucose, neuropeptides, and vitamins into the brain through various transporters [25]. CMT involves molecules binding to specific sites on integral membrane proteins and crossing the cell membrane, either following or counteracting the concentration gradient. The CNS endothelial cells have integral membrane proteins that are responsible for CMT [21, 26]. Glucose transporters, particularly the GLUT protein family, are crucial in transporting glucose, galactose, and fructose across the BBB. Additionally, monocarboxylate transporters facilitate the transportation of short-chain monocarboxylates such as lactate and acetate [21, 27]. Although CMT offers a promising strategy for drug delivery to the brain, many drugs do not target integral membrane proteins, limiting their effectiveness. However, modifying drugs to leverage CMT presents an opportunity to improve their entry into the brain. Currently, CMT-assisted drug delivery includes levodopa and gabapentin, which are delivered to the brain through specific transporter systems like LAT-1 [21, 28].

Receptor-Mediated Transcytosis (RMT)

Drug delivery across the BBB can also be augmented using receptor-mediated transcytosis (RMT) using specific molecules [25, 29]. RMT involves targeting specific receptors present in the BBB endothelial cells. These receptors should have a high expression on the luminal side of endothelial cells, undergo efficient endocytosis or transcytosis with a high turnover rate, and maintain their physiological activity for effective drug delivery [18, 30]. Several highly expressed BBB receptors have been explored as targets for drug delivery, including transferrin receptors (TfR), insulin receptors (IR), and low-density lipoprotein receptors [18, 31]. One of the most commonly targeted BBB receptors is the TfR [32]. TfR is a transmembrane glycoprotein that is only expressed on BBB endothelial cells and not on the endothelial cells that line the rest of the body's vasculature [33]. Hence, TfR-mediated transcytosis has become a popular avenue for delivering agents across the BBB. While the potential of targeting IR is more debated due to its widespread expression in various organs, studies have used antibodies against IR to enhance drug delivery to the brain [18]. Moreover, natural apolipoprotein ligands such as ApoB and ApoE, as well as newer RMT targets such as single-domain llama antibodies (FC5 and FC44) and rabies virus glycoprotein, have been explored for efficiently transporting therapeutic nanoparticles to the brain [25, 34].

During RMT, a drug binds to a specific receptor on the cell surface, triggering an endocytic pathway. This leads to the formation of vesicles within endothelial cells, allowing the drug-receptor complex to traverse the cell and undergo exocytosis on the opposite side. However, most drugs cannot achieve precise binding to transcytosis receptors in their unmodified state. Therefore, specific designs have been developed to enhance drug transport through RMT, similar to strategies for improving drug permeability via CMT [15, 35].

Adsorptive-Mediated Transcytosis

Adsorptive-mediated transcytosis (AMT) facilitates the transport of cationic molecules across the BBB through non-specific electrostatic interactions [25]. The BBB's negative charge, mainly due to negatively charged phosphates in the lipid bilayer, provides sites for attracting cationic substances. Cationic proteins such as albumin and immunoglobulin G (IgG) can undergo increased uptake by brain capillary endothelial cells and are transported to the brain through AMT [25, 36]. In AMT, clathrin, a triangular-shaped protein, plays a crucial role in forming small invaginations that lead to vesicle formation and subsequent transcytosis. Unlike RMT, AMT does not require specific binding to receptors, allowing it to transfer cationic substances across the BBB faster and in higher concentrations. However, a challenge with AMT is its lack of tissue specificity, as it is not a mechanism exclusive to the BBB, leading to potential drug accumulation in other tissues and undesirable side effects [21, 37, 38].

BBB Models

In vitro BBB models have been developed over the last few decades to study nanocarriers' transportation, cytotoxicity, uptake, and distribution. Brain endothelial cells from rodents (bEnd.3, bEnd.5) and humans (HCMEC/D3, HBMEC) are used to build these models. In addition, a simulated BBB cell model can be made with human umbilical vein endothelial cells (HUVECs). The build of this model does not require co-culture with astrocyte cells, unlike others [39, 40], to induce the upregulation of tight junction proteins, taking less time to obtain a fully confluent cellular barrier with high transepithelial electrical resistance (TEER). This model can be used to study the transportation of nanocarriers via AMT and the intercellular route but not via CMT, RMT, or passive diffusion due to the model's lack of the necessary transporters and efflux pumps. These cell models can be cultured on transwell inserts as 2D models to study the change of permeability and response to nanocarriers. The 2D models can be either a monolayer on the upside or a co-culture model (with two layers growing on both sides or one on the transwell and the other on the well plate). 3D models allow cells to grow as microvessels, which can then be used to study angiogenesis and cross-signaling.

Most nanocarriers for neurotherapeutics were studied on animal models, such as rodents and zebrafish, and administrated intravenously, which have shown good BBB permeability and therapeutic effects on brain diseases. However, because of the complexity of the human body, the percentage of administered drugs reaching the brain this way is below 1–4% due to low BBB permeability and selectivity. The electrostatic interaction between cationic carriers and negatively charged cell surfaces by AMT is nonspecific, which may result in a random distribution of carriers in cells or capture by reticuloendothelial cells. AMT affinity is relatively lower compared to RMT. In addition, RMT is the most specific and highest affinity among these three transcytosis mechanisms. However, a receptor-loaded drug carrier can still bind to undesired receptors on different organs. For example, albumin NPs conjugated with low molecular weight protamine are designed to bind to albumin-binding proteins (e.g., SPARC and gp60) on glioma and tumor vessel endothelium. However, results from Lin et al. have shown that other reticuloendothelial systems, such as the lungs and the liver, can capture such albumin-labeled conjugations [41].

Nanocarriers for Drug Delivery Across the BBB

Inorganic Nanomaterials

The treatment of brain diseases is not limited to the transportation of chemotherapy agents, which have nonspecific toxicity and accumulate readily in various organs [42]. Phototherapy (photodynamic and photothermal) agents may have beneficial therapeutic effects and be useful for diagnostic bioimaging. Various materials have been investigated as photothermal agents for brain diseases such as gold nanoparticles [43, 44], graphene, and its derivatives [45, 46], because of their strong visibility to near-infrared (NIR) absorbance and biocompatibility. Photothermally triggered drug delivery has two vital components: a material that can convert light energy to generate heat and a thermally sensitive material that can respond to temperature change [47]. Gold nanomaterials are the most widely studied material because of their size-dependent tailorable optical and photothermal properties, inert properties, and biocompatibility [48]. Similarly, graphene and black phosphorus have attracted more attention as photothermal drug carriers because of their excellent biocompatibility, biodegradability, and high photothermal conversion efficiency [49, 50]. Liposomes can also be integrated with gold nanorods, graphene nanosheets, and black phosphorus nanosheets to form a thermosensitive nanocarrier [49–51]. Under light irradiation, the injected thermosensitive nanocarriers can convert light to heat energy, which may increase the release kinetics of drugs or payloads because of the increased temperature. Such strategies have proven to be effective in controlling drug release. Furthermore, the rate of drug release can also be controlled by adjusting the power of the light source. More recently, semiconducting polymer nanoparticles have attracted more attention to such applications since the delocalized π-electrons of their molecule structures lend them high photostability, significant absorption coefficients, and high photothermal conversion efficiencies [52].

Quantum dots (QDs) have been extensively studied for applications in photodynamic therapy, which is a promising method for brain disease treatment for its noninvasiveness and high spatiotemporal resolution. The interaction between light and photosensitizers (such as Chlorin e6, Ro10, engalgal, and porphyrin) can generate reactive oxygen species (ROS) (including $^1O_2$, $^{\bullet}OH$) to oxidize amino acid residues and inhibit tumor cells. UV and visible light are mainly investigated and are suitable for in vitro study because of their sufficient light energy. However, the challenges of in vivo utilization of radiation below 650 nm are low tissue penetration (less than 1 cm) and the need for expensive high-energy lasers that can cause tissue damage. With its minimal absorption by tissue and deep tissue penetration (up to 10 cm [53]), NIR has been utilized as the excitation light source in bioimaging light-stimulus drug carriers for in vivo applications. Various strategies, such as upconversion nanoparticles (UCNPs) and NIR photosensitizers, have replaced UV light with NIR light [53]. An Er^{3+}-doped NaLnF4 could convert 980 nm light to green and red light for porphyrin to generate ROS, which showed 95% enhanced tumor inhibition [54]. The photochemically triggered drug delivery system is another widely studied system. The covalent bond cleavage facilitates the release of the encapsulated drug under light irradiation. Molecules with ortho-nitrobenzyl moiety and coumarin and pyrene derivatives are readily cleaved upon UV irradiation and suitable for such delivery strategy [55–57]. Model drug capped by various photo-triggerable capping agents, such as coumarin ester derivative and ortho-nitrobenzyl ester derivative [58, 59], can be loaded into the pores of mesoporous silica nanoparticles. The drug was efficiently released by degrading the capping agents via photoirradiation. Lanthanide ion-doped inorganic UCNPs can be used for this photo-responsive drug release and therapy [60–62].

Magnetic nanoparticles (MNPs) are an appealing material as drug carriers. Their magnetization properties can guide the accumulation of MNPs in specific regions. Under the influence of an external magnetic field, MNPs increase the permeability of the BBB, impairing its integrity and accumulating in the brain [63, 64]. MNPs are also an effective contrast enhancement agent for magnetic resonance imaging with tissue-level resolution. Paclitaxel-loaded MNPs exhibited prolonged blood circulation and successful penetration of the BBB into brain tissue [65]. The superparamagnetic properties of MNPs can enable the use of nanocarriers for targeted hyperthermia. When subjected to alternating magnetic fields, such nanoparticles generate heat.

Polymeric Nanomaterials

Polymeric nanomaterials are assembled from biodegradable, biocompatible, low-water-solubility polymers. They can carry encapsulated drugs or be bound to the polymer matrix [66]. Polymeric nanomaterial can improve therapeutic efficacy by preventing degradation, controlling the drug release rate, enhancing drug absorption into specific tissues, and improving circulation time [66, 67]. Furthermore, polymeric nanomaterials can be modified to possess targeting and stimuli-responsive characteristics through surface functional groups [67]. The size, solubility, entrapment efficiency, loading efficiency, and surface charge determine the effectiveness of polymer-based nanoparticles as drug carriers. Polymer-based nanoparticles form through the polymerization reactions of monomer units and are usually about 10–100 nm in size [67]. They can be created with both natural and synthetic polymers [68]. Nanocarriers made of natural polymers have the advantages of biocompatibility, low toxicity, and biodegradability, where they will slowly be metabolized and removed from the body [67]. However, they sometimes suffer from uncontrolled and inconsistent degradation [69]. In contrast, synthetic polymers have tunable physical, chemical, and mechanical features and a controlled degradation rate. Many polymers, such as poly(lactic-co-glycolic acid), chitosan, and gelatin, are used to make polymeric nanomaterials [66, 68].

Among synthetic polymers, polyesters have been well-studied in biomedical applications [69]. The two most commonly used for drug delivery applications are poly(lactic-co-glycolic acid) (PLGA) and poly(lactic acid) (PLA). PLGA is a biodegradable polymer approved by both the European Medicines Agency (EMA) and the US Food and Drug Administration (FDA) [70, 71]. Hydrolysis of PLGA creates lactic acid and glycolic acid, which are quickly metabolized by the body, leading to minimal toxicity [69, 70]. Furthermore, PLGA nanoparticles are highly stable with tunable properties via numerous surface modification options [71]. However, they suffer from disadvantages such as short half-life, immunogenicity, high burst release, and poor drug loading, which can be improved by combining other materials with PLGA to form hybrid PLGA nanoparticles (e.g., PLGA-lipid hybrid nanoparticles). In addition, PLGA lends a negative charge to nanoparticles, resulting in cells' lower internalization rates than nanoparticles with positive charges [70]. This can be remedied through surface modification, such as PEGylation, to shift the overall charge of the PLGA nanoparticles to neutral or positive charges. PLGA nanoparticles can be prepared through many methods, including emulsification-solvent evaporation, nanoprecipitation or interfacial deposition, and spray drying [70]. Loading drugs into PLGA nanoparticles is done either by incorporating the drug during the production of PLGA nanoparticles or by adsorbing the drug onto the surface of prepared nanoparticles [70]. PLGA nanoparticles have been modified with cell-penetrating peptides (CPPs) and ligands for RMT and AMT to cross the BBB [72]. CPPs are short peptides containing 30 or fewer amino acids that have been found to facilitate the translocation of various complexes and have been well-studied for the last three decades [73]. While the mechanisms behind the cellular uptake of CPPs are still under discussion, they aid in cellular uptake through electrostatic interactions or hydrogen bonding with cell membranes and by triggering endocytosis. PLGA nanoparticles can penetrate the BBB when modified with CPPs such as the trans-activating transcriptor (TAT) peptide [72, 74]. Furthermore, polysorbate 80 (tween 80), poloxamer 188, transferrin, lactoferrin, leptin, and peptides such as G7 enabled PLGA nanocarriers to cross the BBB through RMT [72]. Furthermore, PLGA nanocarriers can cross the BBB by AMT when their surfaces are coated with chitosan, polyethylene imine, poly-L-lysine, and other cationic materials.

PLA is an aliphatic polyester used widely in the biomedical field, with desirable properties such as biodegradability, low toxicity, and biocompatibility [75]. Hydrolysis of PLA creates lactic acid, which can be eliminated from the body through Krebs cycle [69]. Furthermore, PLA can be produced with standard, established technologies through step-growth or ring-opening polymerization [75]. Emulsion-based, precipitation-based, and compositing techniques produce PLA nanoparticles [75]. PLA nanoparticles labeled with CPPs, such as penetratin, can cross the BBB [76] and ligands, such as lactoferrin [77] and transferrin [78], for RMT. Other synthetic polymers that have been explored as BBB nanocarriers include poly(alkyl cyanoacrylate) (PACA), poly-ε-caprolactone (PCL), and polyamidoamine dendrimers [79].

Several natural polymers have also been used to create BBB nanocarriers. Chitosan is a linear polysaccharide with a random sequence of *N*-acetyl-D-glucosamine and β-1,4-D-glucosamine units [79, 80]. It is commonly sourced from oysters or as a crustacean by-product from shrimp, crabs, lobster, and crayfish. Chitosan can then be prepared via chemical, enzymatic, and fermentation methods, which all involve the steps of demineralization, deproteinization, and deacetylation [80]. Chitosan has many desirable properties, such as anti-cancer, antioxidant, and antimicrobial characteristics, good biodegradability, and a wide range of molecular weights [79]. Furthermore, chitosan's amine and hydroxyl functional groups have been exploited to modify its properties, such as biodegradability. Chitosan nanoparticles can be formed through ionic gelation and microfluidic synthesis, among other methods [79]. Chitosan nanoparticles cross the BBB through RMT, for example, when modified with an anti-TfR antibody [81, 82] and anti-bradykinin B2 receptor antibody [81]. Furthermore, chitosan's natural positive charge also aids in uptake by BBB endothelial cells [79]. However, chitosan nanocarriers' limitations include low drug loading efficiency, which can be improved through chemical modifications.

Alginate, a linear polysaccharide found in brown seaweed, has been used in food, wound dressings, and tissue regeneration [79, 83]. Alginate is made of repeating and alternating 1,4 α-L-guluronic acid (G) residues and 1,4-linked β-D-mannuronic acid (M), differing in both the composition and the sequence of G and M residues depending on the source of the alginate [83]. Although alginate is usually considered nontoxic, non-immunogenic, biocompatible, and approved by the FDA, higher M content may result in more immunogenicity [79, 83]. Other polymeric materials, both synthetic and natural, and materials such as inorganic nanoparticles may be added to alginate to form alginate composites with better physical properties [83]. Furthermore, alginate possesses carboxylic acid and hydroxyl functional groups that can be used to tune its properties [79]. Alginate nanoparticles can be prepared through complexation with cationic compounds, through water/oil emulsion methods, and by missing with other polymers. Alginate nanoparticles have found success in crossing the BBB when functionalized with polysorbate 80 (tween 80) [84] and mixed with chitosan to form alginate/chitosan nanoparticles [85].

Another natural polymer is gelatin. Gelatin is a denatured protein usually obtained from collagen, and its quality varies depending on its source [86]. Gelatin has been used in food, cosmetics, and pharmaceuticals and has been approved by the FDA [87]. Furthermore, it is cheap and readily available with good biocompatibility and biodegradability [86, 87]. Gelatin-based nanoparticles can be surface functionalized, providing good biological fluid stability [86]. Gelatin nanoparticles are commonly prepared through nanoprecipitation, emulsification-solvent evaporation, double desolvation, and reverse-phase microemulsion, among other methods. There has been some success in using gelatin nanoparticles as BBB carriers. For example, gelatin-siloxane nanoparticles modified with PEG and SynB peptide, a CPP, were found to cross the rat BBB model with higher success when compared to PEG-gelatin-siloxane nanoparticles [88]. However, as of this writing, there has been limited research on the applications of gelatin nanoparticles as BBB carriers. Other natural polymers explored for applications as BBB carriers include zein [89] and albumin [90].

Nanogels

Gels are three-dimensional polymeric networks that undergo physical or chemical cross-linking and swell in certain liquids [91]. Hydrogels can retain a substantial volume of water without dissolving, are excellently biocompatible, and enable drug loading and release [91]. Nanocomposite hydrogels, formed by integrating nanoparticles into the hydrogel matrix, provide a platform for controlled-release drug delivery at the cellular level [92]. Researchers have extensively explored hydrogel applications for drug delivery, especially in the context of nanogels, which are nanoparticles of hydrogels [93].

Nanogels have garnered significant attention over the past decade due to their diverse applications in drug delivery, tissue engineering, biomedical implants, and gene therapy [15, 94]. Their small size and unique properties offer advantages such as improved permeability and efficient crossing of cellular and biological barriers [92]. The hydrophilic nature of nanogels makes them suitable carriers for aqueous-soluble drugs, proteins, and nuclear acids. The type and concentration of polymers used during synthesis can tailor nanogels' properties [91, 94, 95].

The specific transport mechanisms of nanogels offer intriguing opportunities for designing brain-specific drug delivery systems. They can exploit RMT, cell-mediated transcytosis, or AMT to cross the BBB [96, 97]. Various therapeutic strategies have been explored to achieve active targeting, including attaching functionalized ligands, utilizing noninvasive responsiveness to magnetic fields or ultrasound, and employing shutter peptide-mediated BBB crossing [93].

Recent advancements in nanogels have shown promise in enhancing brain drug delivery. Nanogels decorated with polysorbate-80 can penetrate the BBB through the low-density lipoprotein RMT pathway [92, 97]. Insulin-conjugated nanogels efficiently transported insulin across the BBB, showcasing their potential in CNS drug delivery [94, 98]. Nanogels have also enhanced the CNS penetration of oligonucleotide analog transcytosis across the BBB [97, 99].

On the other hand, the limitations of nanogels used as drug carriers have been reported. These include particle size variability, polydispersity, polymer degradation, and premature drug release in response to external stimuli. The impermeability of the BBB remains a significant challenge in CNS drug delivery. Further research and development are necessary to address these limitations and unlock the full potential of nanogels as effective and safe drug carriers for treating CNS diseases [100, 101].

Liposomes

Liposomes comprise one or more phospholipid bilayers encapsulating an aqueous compartment [102, 103]. They range in size from mere nanometers to several micrometers and can encapsulate a variety of different agents within both the lipid membrane and the aqueous compartment. Due to their ability to entrap agents, their similar morphology to cellular membranes, biodegradability, biocompatibility, low toxicity, ease of preparation, and low risk of immunogenicity, liposomes have been heavily researched for use as a delivery system [103–107].

Many liposome production methods can generate liposomes with differing properties, such as size and lamellarity. Unilamellar liposomes are smaller (50–250 nm) and suitable for encapsulating hydrophilic agents, while multilamellar liposomes are larger (1–5 μm) and preferentially trap lipid-soluble agents [108]. Furthermore, increased lamellarity results in slower drug release [103]. The liposome size affects drug release, liposome retention in circulation, and liposome accumulation in target tissues [109]. However, these features are also affected by conjugated surface ligands, polarity, lipid composition, and the use of suitable drugs. For example, surface conjugation with polyethylene glycol (PEG) and polysaccharides prevents liposome opsonization and subsequent clearance, prolonging liposome retention in circulation [32, 106].

Liposomes employ many different strategies to transport drugs across the BBB. The most common strategy for liposome BBB carriers is RMT [106]. Liposomes have been modified with transferrin [110, 111] and anti-TfR [112]. To target the TfR (Fig. 4.2), liposomes can also be adjusted with an aptamer to target receptors. Aptamers are single-stranded oligonucleotides that can selectively and specifically bind to target molecules. They are highly stable and non-immunogenic [113]. For example, aptamer-modified liposomes could deliver obidoxime to the brain to treat paraoxon poisoning in mice by targeting the TfR [113].

Another receptor commonly targeted for crossing the BBB is the lactoferrin receptor. Lactoferrin is a cationic iron-binding glycoprotein closely related to transferrin and is involved in defending against infection and inflammation [114]. The lactoferrin receptor is expressed on the surface of many cells, including platelets, neurons, and the endothelial cells of microvessels in the brain. It is overexpressed on the surface of tumor cells in response to their high nutritional demands, and it is also overexpressed on brain endothelial cells [115]. Hence, the lactoferrin receptor is a popular target for crossing the BBB. For example, lactoferrin-modified liposomes carrying the antitumor drugs honokiol and daunorubicin improved drug transportation across the BBB, inhibiting the invasion of tumor cells and destroying the vasculogenic mimicry channels generated by glioma cells [116]. Some liposomes have also been modified with more than one ligand to target several receptors, overcoming the limitation of receptor saturation.

Another strategy involves cationic liposomes. These liposomes interact with the negatively charged BBB through electrostatic interactions and cross the BBB through AMT [32, 105, 106]. Compared to anionic and neutral liposomes, cationic liposomes have enhanced liposomal delivery into the brain and greater retention in the brain [117]. However, they are subject to nonspecific uptake by peripheral tissues and the binding of serum proteins, which masks their positive charge [32, 106]. Therefore, cationic liposomes require high doses to

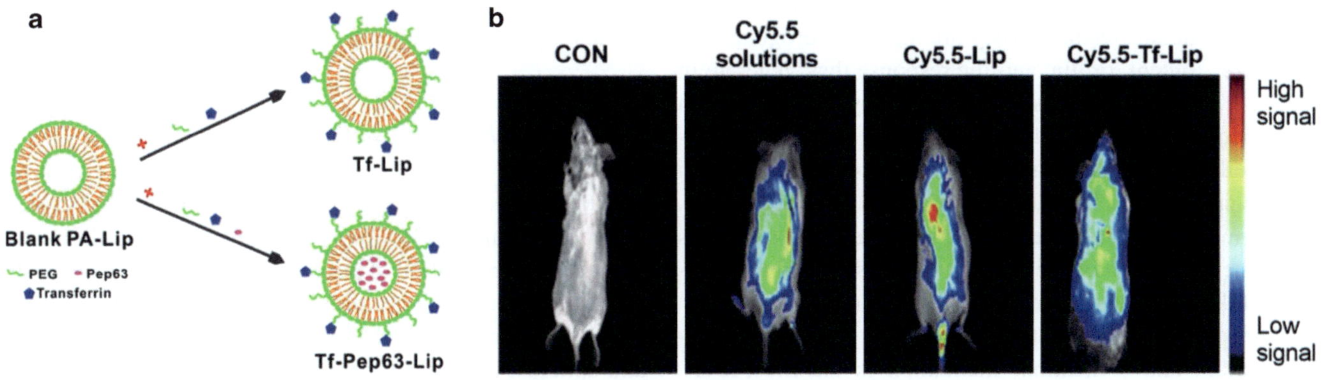

Fig. 4.2 Transferrin-Pep63-liposomes aid clearance of extracellular β-amyloid in early Alzheimer's disease models. (**a**) Schematic of preparing transferrin-liposomes and transferrin-Pep63-liposomes. (**b**) Distribution of unmodified liposomes and transferrin-modified liposomes labeled with Cy5.5 in living mice 2 h after intravenous injection. In comparison, control mice and Cy5.5 solutions in live mice are shown. Transferrin-modified liposomes are shown to be able to enter the brain. (Modified from Yang et al. [111])

reach therapeutic efficacy and are potentially cytotoxic. Cationic liposomes do not require maximum surface charges to be delivered and retained in the brain, thus potentially minimizing some of the adverse, cytotoxic effects of cationic liposomes [117]. To avoid nonspecific uptake by other tissues, cationic liposomes can be modified by targeting ligands on their surface to create dual functionalized liposomes that also take advantage of RMT. For example, cationic liposomes modified with penetratin and transferrin [115] and wheat germ agglutin [116] cross the BBB. Liposomes can also cross the BBB through CMT. For example, Arora et al. developed liposomes modified with mannose and CPPs on their surface to treat Alzheimer's disease [118]. Other transporters targeted for CMT across the BBB include the glutathione transporter [119, 120], the large amino acid transporter 1 [118, 121], and the choline transporter [122].

Exosomes

Exosomes are extracellular vesicles released by all cells and are about 40–160 nm in diameter [123–125]. They are produced from endosomes in eukaryotic cells, formed when intracellular multivesicular bodies invaginate to generate intraluminal vesicles. The multivesicular bodies fuse to the plasma membrane, and the intraluminal vesicles are released into the extracellular environment as exosomes [123]. The interior of the exosome is cytoplasmic in origin and contains various biomolecules, including growth factors, enzymes, and nucleic acids [123, 124]. Exosomes facilitate paracrine cell-to-cell communication by delivering these biomolecules to other recipient cells [124, 125]. Furthermore, exosomes are nontoxic, are well-tolerated by the body, and have low immunogenicity [124]. They can carry many agents, including RNA, and protect their contents from degradation. Hence, they have potential as BBB carriers.

While exosomes are present in most biological fluids, including blood, urine, breast milk, and saliva [123, 126], they are difficult to isolate. They are highly heterogenous in their size, content, origin, and the response they generate in recipient cells [123]. Exosomes are usually separated from the supernatant of cultured cells from cell lines such as dendritic cells and mesenchymal stem cells [124, 126]. They can also be produced from induced pluripotent stem cells [127]. Furthermore, self-exosomes can be produced with host cells to reduce potential adverse immune responses from the presence of the major histocompatibility complex [128].

Drugs can be loaded into exosomes via incubation, electroporation, and sonication. Incubation is the most well-studied method due to its simplicity and cost-effectiveness [129]. It involves incubating exosomes or exosome-producing cells with a drug solution [129]. The first method is more common, as it is usually sufficient in loading drugs into the exosomes, and the exosomes maintain their stability, bioavailability, and low immunogenicity [124, 129]. While the exact method of crossing the BBB is unclear and requires further research, exosomes mainly cross through transcytosis [124, 125, 130, 131]. Since transcytosis decreases when clathrin-dependent and caveolae-dependent endocytosis is inhibited, both are possible routes for the uptake of exosomes by BBB endothelial cells [131]. However, exosomes from different types of cells contain other proteins and lipids on their surfaces, thus possibly interacting with different BBB receptors and altering the mechanism of crossing the BBB. For example, exosomes derived from glioblastoma cells differ in size, morphology, and concentration of surface proteins from those derived from BBB endothelial cells. The specific biomarkers on exosomes derived from BBB endothelial cells may allow for higher transport rates across the BBB, as they could cross via RMT at greater rates than those derived from glioblastoma cells [132]. Furthermore, exosomes tend to express some parent cell-derived markers, some of which may be tissue-specific and influence the performance of exosomes carrying drugs across the BBB.

Exosomes derived from human primary glioma cells were found to upregulate the expression of Lipocalin-2 on BBB endothelial cells [133]. Lipocalin-2 is a protein highly expressed on cancer cell membranes that enables tumor cell-microenvironment interactions. The glioma-derived exosomes activated the JAK-STAT3 pathway in BBB endothelial cells, upregulating the expression of Lipocalin-2. As a result, the fluidity of the BBB increased, allowing significantly more nanocarriers to cross the BBB [133]. Therefore, glioma-derived exosomes can increase the permeability of the BBB, enabling other nanocarriers to cross it more easily.

Targeting the BBB with exosomes has also been investigated. Lamp2b, an abundant protein found on exosome membranes, can have its N-terminus modified to fuse brain-targeting peptides to Lamp2b [128, 134]. For example, fusing rabies virus glycoprotein onto Lamp2b can aid exosomes in crossing the BBB by promoting clathrin and caveolae-mediated energy-depending endocytosis [134, 135].

Polymeric Micelles

Polymeric micelles are micelles formed through the self-assembly of amphiphilic polymers [136]. They are created when the concentration of polymers in a medium reaches the "critical micelle concentration" threshold [136, 137]. Polymeric micelles can take on many forms, such as tubules and spheres, depending on the solvent conditions and their hydrophobic and hydrophilic segments [136]. Their preparation includes solvent evaporation, dialysis, oil-in-water emulsion, lyophilization, and dilution. Polymeric micelles consist of a hydrophobic core with a hydrophilic outer shell.

They usually are 10–200 nm in size [137]. Non-immunogenic, biocompatible, biodegradable polymers such as polyesters, poly(amino acids), and polyethylene oxide generally comprise the micelle core, while PEG blocks typically comprise the outer shell [138].

By exploiting the functional groups of amphiphilic polymers, polymeric micelles can be modified with stimuli-responsive moieties and targeting ligands [138]. When subjected to specific conditions such as temperature and pH or externally applied triggers such as ultrasound and radiation, stimuli-responsive polymeric micelles will undergo alterations to release drugs [138, 139]. Such polymeric micelles can prevent premature drug release in circulation and accumulate in targeted tissues for triggered drug release [139]. For example, ferrocene starts swelling and disassembling the micelles upon applying a current, releasing the encapsulated drug [140].

There are two main techniques to aid polymeric micelles in crossing the BBB. The first involves modifying the polymeric micelles with targeting ligands to cross the BBB through RMT. For example, brain endothelial cells took up transferrin-modified polyphosphoester hybrid micelles almost twice as much as non-modified micelles [141]. The second technique involves using Pluronic® amphiphilic polymers to construct the micelle. These polymers are made of ethylene oxide (EO) and propylene oxide (PO), which form the basic units EO-PO-EO that make up Pluronic® [142]. By changing the number of these basic units present in the polymer, the lipophilicity and hydrophilicity of Pluronic® can change. Pluronic® has been found to inhibit P-glycoprotein [142, 143]. Pluronic® inhibits P-glycoprotein-dependent drug efflux out of the cell by depleting cellular ATP levels and increasing membrane fluidity [142]. Therefore, Pluronic® improves drug transport into the BBB by inhibiting the drug efflux transporter, P-glycoprotein. Furthermore, Pluronic® has been shown to target brain tumors and can also serve as a targeting ligand for glioblastomas [144, 145]. For example, Pluronic®-based micelles modified with chitosan could cross the BBB and improve the cellular uptake of myricetin, thereby improving the drug's antitumor activity [144].

Limitations and Recommendations

The compatibility and biodegradability of polymeric and lipid nanocarriers make them desirable for therapeutic applications. These carriers have shown significant encapsulation efficiency in loading hydrophobic drugs and prolonged circulation time in the blood. The properties of the nanocarrier surface can be designed and engineered to transport BBB by conjugating with ligands, manipulating the surface charge, and controlling lipophilicity. In addition, functional nanocarriers such as gold, graphene, QDs, UCNPs, and MNPs have extra unique properties, including photothermal, magnetic, and light-emitting properties, which makes on-demand delivery and light therapy possible, and combine the therapeutics and imaging for diagnosis. All of these properties of nanocarriers offer alternative methods to overcome BBB.

However, it should be noted that the development of nanocarriers for crossing BBB for diagnosis and therapeutics is in the early stages. The biocompatibility and colloidal stability of nanocarriers should be carefully investigated. Some chemicals, such as oleic acid, trioctylphosphine oxide, and oleylamine, are involved in preparing inorganic nanocarriers, which could cause carriers' hydrophobicity and impose toxic effects on cells. Hence, ligand-exchange biocompatible coatings on these materials have improved their colloidal stability and reduced toxicity [60]. In addition, nanocarriers' suspension ability in aqueous media largely depends on surface modifications, and the ions in the physiological environment may alter the properties of nanocarriers. It is noted that many nanostructures, e.g., gold nanorods, graphene nanosheets, and black phosphorus, have shown good biocompatibility and colloidal stability. However, the effect of tissue accumulation of gold nanorods, graphene, and black phosphorus on the thermal stability of drugs should be carefully investigated to avoid potential toxic effects or local heat generation. Unlike the biodegradable polymeric carriers, inorganic nanomaterials cannot be degraded easily, and their metabolism in vivo is still being investigated.

On the other hand, the light source to trigger these functional nanocarriers can vary from UV to visible light to NIR. UV and visible light under 650 nm have low tissue penetration and may damage tissues. Utilizing these NIR and UCNP systems may cause overheating problems since water has a strong absorption at 980 nm. The alternative is the magnetic field generators usually used for inductive heating. These are expensive and are unsuitable for therapeutical applications due to their geometry. Furthermore, the efficiency in releasing drugs from MNPs is still low.

Administration of nanocarriers for brain diseases via oral, intravenous, direct brain/intrathecal, and intranasal routes has been successful. Intra-arterial (IA) administration is an alternative to systemic administration and can provide higher local drug concentrations and reduced systemic exposure. Furthermore, IA administration is effective in tumor therapy [146]. Studies on IA delivery for brain diseases are still in their early stages. Due to the existence of BBB, the effectiveness of drugs administered via the IA route for brain diseases was restricted. At the time of writing, mannitol and ultrasound disruption of BBB have been investigated with IA administration of drugs to the brain [147]. Few studies combine BBB disruption and IA delivery of nanocarriers. Therefore, it is promising to apply these well-designed nanocarriers with IA injection to obtain adequate BBB transportation and focused drug concentration.

Conclusion and Future Directions

Nanocarriers with good biodegradability have been developed to deliver various payloads, including peptides, proteins, antibodies, nucleic acid, anticancer drugs, and antiretroviral drugs. Studies indicate that nanocarriers can significantly reduce the cost of developing medicine for treating brain diseases and enhance efficiency. Nanocarriers have great potential in treating brain diseases and bypassing the BBB. Over the years, many different nanocarriers have been developed, including inorganic-based nanoparticles, polymeric nanoparticles, nanogels, liposomes, exosomes, and polymeric micelles. These nanocarriers can be surface-modified with positive charges and various ligands such as transferrin and antibodies to cross the BBB. Mechanisms of crossing the BBB include passive diffusion, carrier-mediated transport, receptor-mediated transcytosis, and adsorptive-mediated transcytosis. The administration of nanocarriers through intravenous oral, intranasal, and intrathecal administration has been studied recently, and intra-arterial injections have shown great promise in introducing nanocarriers into the body. Novel techniques of intra-arterial drug delivery, such as injection under flow arrest, can further enhance nanocarrier delivery [148]. The flow arrest drug delivery method involves transient cessation of cerebral circulation for 30–60 s or profound systemic hypotension during drug pulse injection. In clinical settings, this can be achieved by balloon occlusion or intravenous adenosine injection [149–152]. Chapter 2 extensively discusses this method's theoretical basis. One significant advantage of flow arrest delivery is that it delivers virtually pure drugs to the site. This prevents contact with blood cells, circulating proteins, enzymes, or pH changes. Thus, nanoparticles in a pristine state can be delivered to the target site. Recent reports suggest that the flow arrest arterial drug delivery method is highly effective in tumor-selective cationic nanocarrier delivery [153–157]. Nanocarriers have great potential as BBB drug carriers. However, research on the applications of using nanoparticles as drug carriers across the BBB is still in its early stages, and more research needs to be done.

References

1. Dong X. Current strategies for brain drug delivery. Theranostics. 2018;8(6):1481–93.
2. Bahadur S, Pardhi DM, Rautio J, Rosenholm JM, Pathak K. Intranasal nanoemulsions for direct nose-to-brain delivery of actives for CNS disorders. Pharmaceutics. 2020;12(12):1230.
3. Terstappen GC, Meyer AH, Bell RD, Zhang W. Strategies for delivering therapeutics across the blood–brain barrier. Nat Rev Drug Discov. 2021;20(5):362–83.
4. Nair KGS, Ramaiyan V, Sukumaran SK. Enhancement of drug permeability across blood brain barrier using nanoparticles in meningitis. Inflammopharmacology. 2018;26(3):675–84.
5. Furtado D, Björnmalm M, Ayton S, Bush AI, Kempe K, Caruso F. Overcoming the blood–brain barrier: the role of nanomaterials in treating neurological diseases. Adv Mater. 2018;30(46):1801362.
6. Haumann R, Videira JC, Kaspers GJL, van Vuurden DG, Hulleman E. Overview of current drug delivery methods across the blood-brain barrier for the treatment of primary brain tumors. CNS Drugs. 2020;34(11):1121–31.
7. Zhou Y, Peng Z, Seven ES, Leblanc RM. Crossing the blood-brain barrier with nanoparticles. J Control Release. 2018;270:290–303.
8. Dube T, Chibh S, Mishra J, Panda JJ. Receptor targeted polymeric nanostructures capable of navigating across the blood-brain barrier for effective delivery of neural therapeutics. ACS Chem Neurosci. 2017;8(10):2105–17.
9. Ding S, Khan AI, Cai X, Song Y, Lyu Z, Du D, et al. Overcoming blood-brain barrier transport: advances in nanoparticle-based drug delivery strategies. Mater Today (Kidlington). 2020;37:112–25.
10. Hersh DS, Wadajkar AS, Roberts N, Perez JG, Connolly NP, Frenkel V, et al. Evolving drug delivery strategies to overcome the blood brain barrier. Curr Pharm Des. 2016;22(9):1177–93.
11. Furtado D, Bjornmalm M, Ayton S, Bush AI, Kempe K, Caruso F. Overcoming the blood-brain barrier: the role of nanomaterials in treating neurological diseases. Adv Mater. 2018;30(46):e1801362.
12. Raman S, Mahmood S, Hilles AR, Javed MN, Azmana M, Al-Japairai KA. Polymeric nanoparticles for brain drug delivery—a review. Curr Drug Metab. 2020;21(9):649–60.
13. Jagtiani E, Yeolekar M, Naik S, Patravale V. In vitro blood brain barrier models: an overview. J Control Release. 2022;343:13–30.
14. Zhang W, Mehta A, Tong Z, Esser L, Voelcker NH. Development of polymeric nanoparticles for blood-brain barrier transfer-strategies and challenges. Adv Sci (Weinh). 2021;8(10):2003937.
15. Harilal S, Jose J, Parambi DGT, Kumar R, Unnikrishnan MK, Uddin MS, et al. Revisiting the blood-brain barrier: a hard nut to crack in the transportation of drug molecules. Brain Res Bull. 2020;160:121–40.
16. Pandit R, Chen L, Gotz J. The blood-brain barrier: physiology and strategies for drug delivery. Adv Drug Deliv Rev. 2020;165–166:1–14.
17. Wakayama E, Kuzu T, Tachibana K, Hirayama R, Okada Y, Kondoh M. Modifying the blood–brain barrier by targeting claudin-5: safety and risks. Ann N Y Acad Sci. 2022;1514(1):62–9.
18. Kristensen M, Brodin B. Routes for drug translocation across the blood-brain barrier: exploiting peptides as delivery vectors. J Pharm Sci. 2017;106(9):2326–34.
19. Hu C, Tao L, Cao X, Chen L. The solute carrier transporters and the brain: physiological and pharmacological implications. Asian J Pharm Sci. 2020;15(2):131–44.
20. Song J, Lu C, Leszek J, Zhang J. Design and development of nanomaterial-based drug carriers to overcome the blood–brain barrier by using different transport mechanisms. Int J Mol Sci [Internet]. 2021;22(18):10118.
21. Sun Y, Zabihi M, Li Q, Li X, Kim BJ, Ubogu EE, et al. Drug permeability: from the blood–brain barrier to the peripheral nerve barriers. Adv Ther. 2023;6(4):2200150.
22. La Barbera L, Mauri E, D'Amelio M, Gori M. Functionalization strategies of polymeric nanoparticles for drug delivery in Alzheimer's disease: current trends and future perspectives. Front Neurosci. 2022;16:939855.
23. Mansor NI, Nordin N, Mohamed F, Ling KH, Rosli R, Hassan Z. Crossing the blood-brain barrier: a review on drug delivery strategies for treatment of the central nervous system diseases. Curr Drug Deliv. 2019;16(8):698–711.
24. Girardin F. Membrane transporter proteins: a challenge for CNS drug development. Dialogues Clin Neurosci. 2006;8(3):311–21.
25. Choudhari M, Hejmady S, Narayan Saha R, Damle S, Singhvi G, Alexander A, et al. Evolving new-age strategies to transport therapeutics across the blood-brain-barrier. Int J Pharm. 2021;599:120351.

26. Mitusova K, Peltek OO, Karpov TE, Muslimov AR, Zyuzin MV, Timin AS. Overcoming the blood-brain barrier for the therapy of malignant brain tumor: current status and prospects of drug delivery approaches. J Nanobiotechnol. 2022;20(1):412.
27. Nguyen YTK, Ha HTT, Nguyen TH, Nguyen LN. The role of SLC transporters for brain health and disease. Cell Mol Life Sci. 2021;79(1):20.
28. Kim J, Ahn SI, Kim Y. Nanotherapeutics engineered to cross the blood-brain barrier for advanced drug delivery to the central nervous system. J Ind Eng Chem. 2019;73:8–18.
29. Tashima T. Smart strategies for therapeutic agent delivery into brain across the blood–brain barrier using receptor-mediated transcytosis. Chem Pharm Bull. 2020;68(4):316–25.
30. Pulgar VM. Transcytosis to cross the blood brain barrier, new advancements and challenges. Front Neurosci. 2018;12:1019.
31. Fang F, Zou D, Wang W, Yin Y, Yin T, Hao S, et al. Non-invasive approaches for drug delivery to the brain based on the receptor mediated transport. Mater Sci Eng C Mater Biol Appl. 2017;76:1316–27.
32. Agrawal M, Ajazuddin TDK, Saraf S, Saraf S, Antimisiaris SG, et al. Recent advancements in liposomes targeting strategies to cross blood-brain barrier (BBB) for the treatment of Alzheimer's disease. J Control Release. 2017;260:61–77.
33. Johnsen KB, Burkhart A, Thomsen LB, Andresen TL, Moos T. Targeting the transferrin receptor for brain drug delivery. Prog Neurobiol. 2019;181:101665.
34. Mizrahy S, Gutkin A, Decuzzi P, Peer D. Targeting central nervous system pathologies with nanomedicines. J Drug Target. 2019;27(5–6):542–54.
35. Haqqani AS, Stanimirovic DB. Brain delivery of therapeutics via transcytosis: types and mechanisms of vesicle-mediated transport across the BBB. In: de Lange EC, Hammarlund-Udenaes M, Thorne RG, editors. Drug delivery to the brain: physiological concepts, methodologies and approaches, vol. 33. Cham: Springer; 2022. p. 71–91.
36. Poustforoosh A, Nematollahi MH, Hashemipour H, Pardakhty A. Recent advances in bio-conjugated nanocarriers for crossing the blood-brain barrier in (pre-)clinical studies with an emphasis on vesicles. J Control Release. 2022;343:777–97.
37. Matsumoto J, Stewart T, Banks WA, Zhang J. The transport mechanism of extracellular vesicles at the blood-brain barrier. Curr Pharm Des. 2017;23(40):6206–14.
38. Zhou Q, Li J, Xiang J, Shao S, Zhou Z, Tang J, et al. Transcytosis-enabled active extravasation of tumor nanomedicine. Adv Drug Deliv Rev. 2022;189:114480.
39. Kim W, Kim J, Lee S-Y, Kim H-M, Joo KM, Nam D-H. Simplified in vitro 3D co-culture-based blood-brain barrier model using transwell. Biochem Biophys Res Commun. 2022;620:63–8.
40. Xie R, Wu Z, Zeng F, Cai H, Wang D, Gu L, et al. Retro-enantio isomer of angiopep-2 assists nanoprobes across the blood-brain barrier for targeted magnetic resonance/fluorescence imaging of glioblastoma. Signal Transduct Target Ther. 2021;6(1):309.
41. Lin T, Zhao P, Jiang Y, Tang Y, Jin H, Pan Z, et al. Blood–brain-barrier-penetrating albumin nanoparticles for biomimetic drug delivery via albumin-binding protein pathways for antiglioma therapy. ACS Nano. 2016;10(11):9999–10012.
42. Muddineti OS, Kumari P, Ghosh B, Torchilin VP, Biswas S. d-α-Tocopheryl succinate/phosphatidyl ethanolamine conjugated amphiphilic polymer-based nanomicellar system for the efficient delivery of curcumin and to overcome multiple drug resistance in cancer. ACS Appl Mater Interfaces. 2017;9(20):16778–92.
43. Yin T, Xie W, Sun J, Yang L, Liu J. Penetratin peptide-functionalized gold nanostars: enhanced BBB permeability and NIR photothermal treatment of Alzheimer's disease using ultralow irradiance. ACS Appl Mater Interfaces. 2016;8(30):19291–302.
44. Gao Y, Li Y, Chen J, Zhu S, Liu X, Zhou L, et al. Multifunctional gold nanostar-based nanocomposite: synthesis and application for noninvasive MR-SERS imaging-guided photothermal ablation. Biomaterials. 2015;60:31–41.
45. Zhao H, Ding R, Zhao X, Li Y, Qu L, Pei H, et al. Graphene-based nanomaterials for drug and/or gene delivery, bioimaging, and tissue engineering. Drug Discov Today. 2017;22(9):1302–17.
46. Li M, Yang X, Ren J, Qu K, Qu X. Using graphene oxide high near-infrared absorbance for photothermal treatment of Alzheimer's disease. Adv Mater. 2012;24(13):1722–8.
47. Linsley CS, Wu BM. Recent advances in light-responsive on-demand drug-delivery systems. Ther Deliv. 2017;8(2):89–107.
48. Yang Y, Lin Y, Di D, Zhang X, Wang D, Zhao Q, et al. Gold nanoparticle-gated mesoporous silica as redox-triggered drug delivery for chemo-photothermal synergistic therapy. J Colloid Interface Sci. 2017;508:323–31.
49. Chen J, Liu H, Zhao C, Qin G, Xi G, Li T, et al. One-step reduction and PEGylation of graphene oxide for photothermally controlled drug delivery. Biomaterials. 2014;35(18):4986–95.
50. Hai L, Zhang A, Wu X, Cheng H, He D, Wang T, et al. Liposome-stabilized black phosphorus for photothermal drug delivery and oxygen self-enriched photodynamic therapy. ACS Appl Nano Mater. 2020;3(1):563–75.
51. Zhan C, Wang W, McAlvin JB, Guo S, Timko BP, Santamaria C, et al. Phototriggered local anesthesia. Nano Lett. 2016;16(1):177–81.
52. Jiang Y, Pu K. Multimodal biophotonics of semiconducting polymer nanoparticles. Acc Chem Res. 2018;51(8):1840–9.
53. Barhoumi A, Liu Q, Kohane DS. Ultraviolet light-mediated drug delivery: principles, applications, and challenges. J Control Release. 2015;219:31–42.
54. Wang Q-X, Yang Y-F, Yang X-F, Pan Y, Sun L-D, Zhang W-Y, et al. Upconverted/downshifted $NaLnF_4$ and metal-organic framework heterostructures boosting NIR-II imaging-guided photodynamic immunotherapy toward tumors. Nano Today. 2022;43:101439.
55. Zhao H, Sterner ES, Coughlin EB, Theato P. o-Nitrobenzyl alcohol derivatives: opportunities in polymer and materials science. Macromolecules. 2012;45(4):1723–36.
56. Wang H, Zhang W, Gao C. Shape transformation of light-responsive pyrene-containing micelles and their influence on cytoviability. Biomacromolecules. 2015;16(8):2276–81.
57. Pelliccioli AP, Wirz J. Photoremovable protecting groups: reaction mechanisms and applications. Photochem Photobiol Sci. 2002;1(7):441–58.
58. Wu C, Chen C, Lai J, Chen J, Mu X, Zheng J, Zhao Y. Molecule-scale controlled-release system based on light-responsive silica nanoparticles. Chem Commun. 2008;23:2662–4. (1359–7345 (Print)).
59. Wu M, Lin X, Tan X, Li J, Wei Z, Zhang D, et al. Photoresponsive nanovehicle for two independent wavelength light-triggered sequential release of P-gp shRNA and doxorubicin to optimize and enhance synergistic therapy of multidrug-resistant cancer. ACS Appl Mater Interfaces. 2018;10(23):19416–27.
60. Lu C, Joulin E, Tang H, Pouri H, Zhang J. Upconversion nanostructures applied in theranostic systems. Int J Mol Sci. 2022;23(16):9003.
61. Sun F, Shen H, Yang Q, Yuan Z, Chen Y, Guo W, et al. Dual behavior regulation: tether-free deep-brain stimulation by photothermal and upconversion hybrid nanoparticles. Adv Mater. 2023;2023:2210018.
62. Zhou S, Ding C, Wang Y, Jiang W, Fu J. Supramolecular valves functionalized rattle-structured UCNPs@ hm-SiO_2 nanoparticles with controlled drug release triggered by quintuple stimuli and dual-modality imaging functions: a potential theranostic nanomedicine. ACS Biomater Sci Eng. 2019;5(11):6022–35.
63. Chertok B, David AE, Yang VC. Brain tumor targeting of magnetic nanoparticles for potential drug delivery: effect of administration route and magnetic field topography. J Control Release. 2011;155(3):393–9.

64. Hua M-Y, Liu H-L, Yang H-W, Chen P-Y, Tsai R-Y, Huang C-Y, et al. The effectiveness of a magnetic nanoparticle-based delivery system for BCNU in the treatment of gliomas. Biomaterials. 2011;32(2):516–27.
65. Dilnawaz F, Singh A, Mewar S, Sharma U, Jagannathan N, Sahoo SK. The transport of non-surfactant based paclitaxel loaded magnetic nanoparticles across the blood brain barrier in a rat model. Biomaterials. 2012;33(10):2936–51.
66. Pinto M, Silva V, Barreiro S, Silva R, Remião F, Borges F, et al. Brain drug delivery and neurodegenerative diseases: polymeric PLGA-based nanoparticles as a forefront platform. Ageing Res Rev. 2022;79:101658.
67. Herdiana Y, Wathoni N, Shamsuddin S, Muchtaridi M. Scale-up polymeric-based nanoparticles drug delivery systems: development and challenges. OpenNano. 2022;7:100048.
68. Gagliardi A, Giuliano E, Venkateswararao E, Fresta M, Bulotta S, Awasthi V, et al. Biodegradable polymeric nanoparticles for drug delivery to solid tumors. Front Pharmacol. 2021;12:601626.
69. Elmowafy EM, Tiboni M, Soliman ME. Biocompatibility, biodegradation and biomedical applications of poly(lactic acid)/poly(lactic-co-glycolic acid) micro and nanoparticles. J Pharm Investig. 2019;49(4):347–80.
70. Danhier F, Ansorena E, Silva JM, Coco R, Le Breton A, Préat V. PLGA-based nanoparticles: an overview of biomedical applications. J Control Release. 2012;161(2):505–22.
71. Ghitman J, Biru EI, Stan R, Iovu H. Review of hybrid PLGA nanoparticles: future of smart drug delivery and theranostics medicine. Mater Des. 2020;193:108805.
72. Cai Q, Wang L, Deng G, Liu J, Chen Q, Chen Z. Systemic delivery to central nervous system by engineered PLGA nanoparticles. Am J Transl Res. 2016;8(2):749.
73. Xie J, Bi Y, Zhang H, Dong S, Teng L, Lee RJ, et al. Cell-penetrating peptides in diagnosis and treatment of human diseases: from preclinical research to clinical application. Front Pharmacol. 2020;11:697.
74. Vijayan AN, Indrakumar J, Gomathinayagam S, Gothandam KM, Korrapati PS. Bi-functional aspects of peptide decorated PLGA nanocarriers for enhanced translocation across the blood-brain barrier through macropinocytosis. Macromol Res. 2022;30(8):557–70.
75. Casalini T, Rossi F, Castrovinci A, Perale G. A perspective on polylactic acid-based polymers use for nanoparticles synthesis and applications. Front Bioeng Biotechnol. 2019;7:259.
76. Xia H, Gao X, Gu G, Liu Z, Hu Q, Tu Y, et al. Penetratin-functionalized PEG–PLA nanoparticles for brain drug delivery. Int J Pharm. 2012;436(1):840–50.
77. Hu K, Li J, Shen Y, Lu W, Gao X, Zhang Q, et al. Lactoferrin-conjugated PEG–PLA nanoparticles with improved brain delivery: in vitro and in vivo evaluations. J Control Release. 2009;134(1):55–61.
78. Ren W-h, Chang J, Yan C-h, Qian X-m, Long L-x, He B, et al. Development of transferrin functionalized poly(ethylene glycol)/poly(lactic acid) amphiphilic block copolymeric micelles as a potential delivery system targeting brain glioma. J Mater Sci Mater Med. 2010;21(9):2673–81.
79. Zhang W, Mehta A, Tong Z, Esser L, Voelcker NH. Development of polymeric nanoparticles for blood–brain barrier transfer—strategies and challenges. Adv Sci. 2021;8(10):2003937.
80. Kou S, Peters LM, Mucalo MR. Chitosan: a review of sources and preparation methods. Int J Biol Macromol. 2021;169:85–94.
81. Gu J, Al-Bayati K, Ho EA. Development of antibody-modified chitosan nanoparticles for the targeted delivery of siRNA across the blood-brain barrier as a strategy for inhibiting HIV replication in astrocytes. Drug Deliv Transl Res. 2017;7(4):497–506.
82. Sahin A, Yoyen-Ermis D, Caban-Toktas S, Horzum U, Aktas Y, Couvreur P, et al. Evaluation of brain-targeted chitosan nanoparticles through blood–brain barrier cerebral microvessel endothelial cells. J Microencapsul. 2017;34(7):659–66.
83. Ahmad Raus R, Wan Nawawi WMF, Nasaruddin RR. Alginate and alginate composites for biomedical applications. Asian J Pharm Sci. 2021;16(3):280–306.
84. Spadari CC, Lanser DM, Araújo MV, De Jesus DFF, Lopes LB, Gelli A, et al. Oral delivery of brain-targeted miltefosine-loaded alginate nanoparticles functionalized with polysorbate 80 for the treatment of cryptococcal meningitis. J Antimicrob Chemother. 2023;78(4):1092–101.
85. Hagras NA-e, Mogahed NMFH, Sheta E, Darwish AA-e, El-Hawary MA, Hamed MT, et al. The powerful synergistic effect of spiramycin/propolis loaded chitosan/alginate nanoparticles on acute murine toxoplasmosis. PLoS Negl Trop Dis. 2022;16(3):e0010268.
86. Hathout RM, Metwally AA. Gelatin nanoparticles. Methods Mol Biol. 2019;2000:71–8.
87. Su K, Wang C. Recent advances in the use of gelatin in biomedical research. Biotechnol Lett. 2015;37(11):2139–45.
88. Tian X-h, Wei F, Wang T-x, Wang P, Lin X-n, Wang J, et al. In vitro and in vivo studies on gelatin-siloxane nanoparticles conjugated with SynB peptide to increase drug delivery to the brain. Int J Nanomedicine. 2012;7:1031–41.
89. Zhang H, van Os WL, Tian X, Zu G, Ribovski L, Bron R, et al. Development of curcumin-loaded zein nanoparticles for transport across the blood–brain barrier and inhibition of glioblastoma cell growth. Biomater Sci. 2021;9(21):7092–103.
90. Ulbrich K, Hekmatara T, Herbert E, Kreuter J. Transferrin- and transferrin-receptor-antibody-modified nanoparticles enable drug delivery across the blood–brain barrier (BBB). Eur J Pharm Biopharm. 2009;71(2):251–6.
91. Li X, Tsibouklis J, Weng T, Zhang B, Yin G, Feng G, et al. Nano carriers for drug transport across the blood–brain barrier. J Drug Target. 2017;25(1):17–28.
92. Hersh AM, Alomari S, Tyler BM. Crossing the blood-brain barrier: advances in nanoparticle technology for drug delivery in neuro-oncology. Int J Mol Sci. 2022;23(8):4153.
93. Zhang Y, Zou Z, Liu S, Miao S, Liu H. Nanogels as novel nanocarrier systems for efficient delivery of CNS therapeutics. Front Bioeng Biotechnol. 2022;10:954470.
94. Ashfaq A, An JC, Ulanski P, Al-Sheikhly M. On the mechanism and kinetics of synthesizing polymer nanogels by ionizing radiation-induced intramolecular crosslinking of macromolecules. Pharmaceutics. 2021;13(11):1765.
95. Antunes JL, Amado J, Veiga F, Paiva-Santos AC, Pires PC. Nanosystems, drug molecule functionalization and intranasal delivery: an update on the most promising strategies for increasing the therapeutic efficacy of antidepressant and anxiolytic drugs. Pharmaceutics. 2023;15(3):998.
96. Vinogradov SV. Polymeric nanogel formulations of nucleoside analogs. Expert Opin Drug Deliv. 2007;4(1):5–17.
97. Cuggino JC, Blanco ERO, Gugliotta LM, Alvarez Igarzabal CI, Calderon M. Crossing biological barriers with nanogels to improve drug delivery performance. J Control Release. 2019;307:221–46.
98. Paolino D, Cosco D, Molinaro R, Celia C, Fresta M. Supramolecular devices to improve the treatment of brain diseases. Drug Discov Today. 2011;16(7–8):311–24.
99. Gilmore JL, Yi X, Quan L, Kabanov AV. Novel nanomaterials for clinical neuroscience. J Neuroimmune Pharmacol. 2008;3(2):83–94.
100. Stawicki B, Schacher T, Cho H. Nanogels as a versatile drug delivery system for brain cancer. Gels. 2021;7(2):63.
101. De R, Mahata MK, Kim KT. Structure-based varieties of polymeric nanocarriers and influences of their physicochemical properties on drug delivery profiles. Adv Sci (Weinh). 2022;9(10):e2105373.

102. Edwards KA, Baeumner AJ. Analysis of liposomes. Talanta. 2006;68(5):1432–41.
103. Bozzuto G, Molinari A. Liposomes as nanomedical devices. Int J Nanomedicine. 2015;10:975–99.
104. Jain A, Jain SK. In vitro release kinetics model fitting of liposomes: an insight. Chem Phys Lipids. 2016;201:28–40.
105. Simonis B, Vignone D, Gonzalez Paz O, Donati E, Falchetti ML, Bombelli C, et al. Transport of cationic liposomes in a human blood brain barrier model: role of the stereochemistry of the gemini amphiphile on liposome biological features. J Colloid Interface Sci. 2022;627:283–98.
106. Vieira DB, Gamarra LF. Getting into the brain: liposome-based strategies for effective drug delivery across the blood–brain barrier. Int J Nanomedicine. 2016;11:5381–414.
107. Li M, Du C, Guo N, Teng Y, Meng X, Sun H, et al. Composition design and medical application of liposomes. Eur J Med Chem. 2019;164:640–53.
108. Immordino ML, Dosio F, Cattel L. Stealth liposomes: review of the basic science, rationale, and clinical applications, existing and potential. Int J Nanomedicine. 2006;1(3):297–315.
109. Nagayasu A, Uchiyama K, Kiwada H. The size of liposomes: a factor which affects their targeting efficiency to tumors and therapeutic activity of liposomal antitumor drugs. Adv Drug Deliv Rev. 1999;40(1):75–87.
110. Chen Z-L, Huang M, Wang X-R, Fu J, Han M, Shen Y-Q, et al. Transferrin-modified liposome promotes α-mangostin to penetrate the blood–brain barrier. Nanomedicine. 2016;12(2):421–30.
111. Yang X, Li X, Liu L, Chen Y-H, You Y, Gao Y, et al. Transferrin-Pep63-liposomes accelerate the clearance of Aβ and rescue impaired synaptic plasticity in early Alzheimer's disease models. Cell Death Discov. 2021;7(1):256.
112. Mourtas S, Lazar AN, Markoutsa E, Duyckaerts C, Antimisiaris SG. Multifunctional nanoliposomes with curcumin–lipid derivative and brain targeting functionality with potential applications for Alzheimer disease. Eur J Med Chem. 2014;80:175–83.
113. Zhang Y, He J, Shen L, Wang T, Yang J, Li Y, et al. Brain-targeted delivery of obidoxime, using aptamer-modified liposomes, for detoxification of organophosphorus compounds. J Control Release. 2021;329:1117–28.
114. Ji B, Maeda J, Higuchi M, Inoue K, Akita H, Harashima H, et al. Pharmacokinetics and brain uptake of lactoferrin in rats. Life Sci. 2006;78(8):851–5.
115. Sabra S, Agwa MM. Lactoferrin, a unique molecule with diverse therapeutical and nanotechnological applications. Int J Biol Macromol. 2020;164:1046–60.
116. Liu S, Zhang S-m, Ju R-j, Xiao Y, Wang X, Song X-l, et al. Antitumor efficacy of Lf modified daunorubicin plus honokiol liposomes in treatment of brain glioma. Eur J Pharm Sci. 2017;106:185–97.
117. Joshi S, Singh-Moon RP, Ellis JA, Chaudhuri DB, Wang M, Reif R, et al. Cerebral hypoperfusion-assisted intraarterial deposition of liposomes in normal and glioma-bearing rats. Neurosurgery. 2015;76(1):92–100.
118. Li L, Di X, Zhang S, Kan Q, Liu H, Lu T, et al. Large amino acid transporter 1 mediated glutamate modified docetaxel-loaded liposomes for glioma targeting. Colloids Surf B Biointerfaces. 2016;141:260–7.
119. Najmi A, Wang S, Huang Y, Seefeldt T, Alqahtani Y, Guan X. 2-(2-Cholesteroxyethoxyl)ethyl-3′-S-glutathionylpropionate (COXP) for brain-targeting liposomes. J Drug Deliv Sci Technol. 2022;75:103674.
120. Kuo Y-C, Tsai H-C, Rajesh R. Glutathione liposomes carrying ceftriaxone, FK506, and nilotinib to control overexpressed dopamine markers and apoptotic factors in neurons. ACS Biomater Sci Eng. 2021;7(7):3242–55.
121. Bhunia S, Vangala V, Bhattacharya D, Ravuri HG, Kuncha M, Chakravarty S, et al. Large amino acid transporter 1 selective liposomes of l-DOPA functionalized amphiphile for combating glioblastoma. Mol Pharm. 2017;14(11):3834–47.
122. Li J, Guo Y, Kuang Y, An S, Ma H, Jiang C. Choline transporter-targeting and co-delivery system for glioma therapy. Biomaterials. 2013;34(36):9142–8.
123. Kalluri R, LeBleu VS. The biology, function, and biomedical applications of exosomes. Science. 2020;367(6478):eaau6977.
124. Druzhkova TA, Yakovlev AA. Exosome drug delivery through the blood–brain barrier: experimental approaches and potential applications. Neurochem J. 2018;12(3):195–204.
125. Heidarzadeh M, Gürsoy-Özdemir Y, Kaya M, Eslami Abriz A, Zarebkohan A, Rahbarghazi R, et al. Exosomal delivery of therapeutic modulators through the blood–brain barrier; promise and pitfalls. Cell Biosci. 2021;11(1):142.
126. Raposo G, Stoorvogel W. Extracellular vesicles: exosomes, microvesicles, and friends. J Cell Biol. 2013;200(4):373–83.
127. Wang S, Hou Y, Li X, Song Z, Sun B, Li X, et al. Comparison of exosomes derived from induced pluripotent stem cells and mesenchymal stem cells as therapeutic nanoparticles for treatment of corneal epithelial defects. Aging. 2020;12(19):19546–62.
128. Alvarez-Erviti L, Seow Y, Yin H, Betts C, Lakhal S, Wood MJA. Delivery of siRNA to the mouse brain by systemic injection of targeted exosomes. Nat Biotechnol. 2011;29(4):341–5.
129. Mehryab F, Rabbani S, Shahhosseini S, Shekari F, Fatahi Y, Baharvand H, et al. Exosomes as a next-generation drug delivery system: an update on drug loading approaches, characterization, and clinical application challenges. Acta Biomater. 2020;113:42–62.
130. Abdelsalam M, Ahmed M, Osaid Z, Hamoudi R, Harati R. Insights into exosome transport through the blood–brain barrier and the potential therapeutical applications in brain diseases. Pharmaceuticals. 2023;16(4):571.
131. Saeedi S, Israel S, Nagy C, Turecki G. The emerging role of exosomes in mental disorders. Transl Psychiatry. 2019;9(1):122.
132. Yang T, Martin P, Fogarty B, Brown A, Schurman K, Phipps R, et al. Exosome delivered anticancer drugs across the blood-brain barrier for brain cancer therapy in Danio rerio. Pharm Res. 2015;32(6):2003–14.
133. Yang C, Wu Y, Wang L, Li S, Zhou J, Tan Y, et al. Glioma-derived exosomes hijack the blood–brain barrier to facilitate nanocapsule delivery via LCN2. J Control Release. 2022;345:537–48.
134. Yang J, Zhang X, Chen X, Wang L, Yang G. Exosome mediated delivery of miR-124 promotes neurogenesis after ischemia. Mol Ther Nucleic Acids. 2017;7:278–87.
135. Liu Y, Huang R, Han L, Ke W, Shao K, Ye L, et al. Brain-targeting gene delivery and cellular internalization mechanisms for modified rabies virus glycoprotein RVG29 nanoparticles. Biomaterials. 2009;30(25):4195–202.
136. Perumal S, Atchudan R, Lee W. A review of polymeric micelles and their applications. Polymers. 2022;14(12):2510.
137. Almeida M, Magalhães M, Veiga F, Figueiras A. Poloxamers, poloxamines and polymeric micelles: definition, structure and therapeutic applications in cancer. J Polym Res. 2017;25(1):31.
138. Kaur J, Gulati M, Kapoor B, Jha NK, Gupta PK, Gupta G, et al. Advances in designing of polymeric micelles for biomedical application in brain related diseases. Chem Biol Interact. 2022;361:109960.
139. Hari SK, Gauba A, Shrivastava N, Tripathi RM, Jain SK, Pandey AK. Polymeric micelles and cancer therapy: an ingenious multimodal tumor-targeted drug delivery system. Drug Deliv Transl Res. 2023;13(1):135–63.
140. Meng X-y, Li J-j, Ni T-j, Xiao-tong L, He T, Men Z-n, et al. Electro-responsive brain-targeting mixed micelles based on Pluronic F127

and d-α-tocopherol polyethylene glycol succinate–ferrocene. Colloids Surf A Physicochem Eng Asp. 2020;601:124986.
141. Zhang P, Hu L, Yin Q, Zhang Z, Feng L, Li Y. Transferrin-conjugated polyphosphoester hybrid micelle loading paclitaxel for brain-targeting delivery: synthesis, preparation and in vivo evaluation. J Control Release. 2012;159(3):429–34.
142. Kabanov AV, Batrakova EV, Miller DW. Pluronic® block copolymers as modulators of drug efflux transporter activity in the blood–brain barrier. Adv Drug Deliv Rev. 2003;55(1):151–64.
143. Seelig A. P-glycoprotein: one mechanism, many tasks and the consequences for pharmacotherapy of cancers. Front Oncol. 2020;10:576559.
144. Wang G, Wang J-J, Tang X-J, Du L, Li F. In vitro and in vivo evaluation of functionalized chitosan–Pluronic micelles loaded with myricetin on glioblastoma cancer. Nanomedicine. 2016;12(5):1263–78.
145. Niu J, Wang A, Ke Z, Zheng Z. Glucose transporter and folic acid receptor-mediated Pluronic P105 polymeric micelles loaded with doxorubicin for brain tumor treating. J Drug Target. 2014;22(8):712–23.
146. Joshi S, Ellis JA, Ornstein E, Bruce JN. Intraarterial drug delivery for glioblastoma mutiforme: will the phoenix rise again? J Neuro-Oncol. 2015;124:333–43.
147. Angelov L, Doolittle ND, Siegal T, Kraemer DF, Peereboom D, Jahnke K, et al. Blood brain barrier disruption (BBBD) and intra-arterial methotrexate based therapy for newly diagnosed primary CNS lymphoma: the BBBD Consortium experience. J Clin Oncol. 2007;25(18_Suppl):2014.
148. Joshi S, Wang M, Etu JJ, Suckow RF, Cooper TB, Feinmark SJ, et al. Transient cerebral hypoperfusion enhances intraarterial carmustine deposition into brain tissue. J Neuro-Oncol. 2008;86(2):123–32.
149. Riina HA, Fraser JF, Fralin S, Knopman J, Scheff RJ, Boockvar JA. Superselective intraarterial cerebral infusion of bevacizumab: a revival of interventional neuro-oncology for malignant glioma. J Exp Ther Oncol. 2009;8(2):145–50.
150. Riina HA, Knopman J, Greenfield JP, Fralin S, Gobin YP, Tsiouris AJ, et al. Balloon-assisted superselective intra-arterial cerebral infusion of bevacizumab for malignant brainstem glioma. A technical note. Interv Neuroradiol. 2010;16(1):71–6.
151. Hashimoto T, Young WL, Aagaard BD, Joshi S, Ostapkovich ND, Pile-Spellman J. Adenosine-induced ventricular asystole to induce transient profound systemic hypotension in patients undergoing endovascular therapy: dose-response characteristics [in process citation]. Anesthesiology. 2000;93(4):998–1001.
152. Pile-Spellman J, Young WL, Joshi S, Duong DH, Vang MC, Hartmann A, et al. Adenosine-induced cardiac pause for endovascular embolization of cerebral arteriovenous malformations: technical case report. Neurosurgery. 1999;44(4):881–6; discussion 6–7.
153. Joshi S, Cooke JRN, Ellis JA, Emala CW, Bruce JN. Targeting brain tumors by intra-arterial delivery of cell-penetrating peptides: a novel approach for primary and metastatic brain malignancy. J Neurooncol. 2017;135(3):497–506.
154. Joshi S, Singh-Moon R, Wang M, Chaudhuri DB, Ellis JA, Bruce JN, et al. Cationic surface charge enhances early regional deposition of liposomes after intracarotid injection. J Neurooncol. 2014;120(3):489–97.
155. Joshi S, Singh-Moon RP, Wang M, Chaudhuri DB, Holcomb M, Straubinger NL, et al. Transient cerebral hypoperfusion assisted intraarterial cationic liposome delivery to brain tissue. J Neurooncol. 2014;118(1):73–82.
156. Nguyen J, Cooke JRN, Ellis JA, Deci M, Emala CW, Bruce JN, et al. Cationizable lipid micelles as vehicles for intraarterial glioma treatment. J Neurooncol. 2016;128(1):21–8.
157. Nguyen J, Hossain SS, Cooke JRN, Ellis JA, Deci MB, Emala CW, et al. Flow arrest intra-arterial delivery of small TAT-decorated and neutral micelles to gliomas. J Neuro-Oncol. 2017;133(1):77–85.

The Blood-Brain Barrier Disruption Methods for Drug Delivery

5

Misha Amini and Matei A. Banu

Extreme remedies are very appropriate for extreme diseases.

Hippocrates (c. 450-380 BCE), Greek Physician and Philosopher

Introduction

The blood-brain barrier (BBB) is a unique property of the differentiated central nervous system vasculature that tightly regulates the movement of ions, molecules, and cells between the blood and the tissue. The brain is separated from the bloodstream at three sites: the epithelium of the choroid plexus, the epithelium of the arachnoid mater, and the endothelium of capillaries within the brain parenchyma [1–3]. The latter represents the BBB and constitutes the most significant component. The brain capillary endothelium accounts for the largest surface area of blood-brain separation and is thus the primary site for exchange between the bloodstream and the brain parenchyma [4].

The blood-brain barrier (BBB) was first described at the turn of the twentieth century following a series of experiments that showed a distinct isolation of the central nervous system (CNS) from its supplying vasculature following parenteral and intrathecal injection of various toxins and dyes. Since then, studies have shown that the BBB is integral to brain physiology. The barrier severely restricts the movement of ions, molecules, and cells between the tissue and the blood. Its integrity is critical to the physiological functioning of the nervous system, and its disruption leads to a wide variety of pathologies that severely affect neurological functioning. Notably, the BBB remains a hurdle for effective delivery of therapeutics to the brain, and endeavors to purposely manipulate its integrity are in high clinical demand. This chapter describes the current state of knowledge regarding the BBB while focusing on the methods used to disrupt it.

M. Amini
Department of Neurosurgery, Columbia University Irving Medical Center, New York, NY, USA
e-mail: ma4557@cumc.columbia.edu

M. A. Banu (✉)
Department of Neurosurgery, Columbia University Irving Medical Center, New York, NY, USA

Department of Neurosurgery, Stanford University School of Medicine, Stanford, California, USA
e-mail: mbanu@stanford.edu

Components of the BBB

The "neurovascular unit" represents the intersection between the brain and its vasculature. Essentially, the unit merges the brain's and vasculature's physiological functioning into a single entity. It consists of cells, linking proteins and signaling molecules. The principal cells of the neurovascular unit are endothelial cells, astrocytes, pericytes, and neurons [5]. Tight junctions, gap junctions, adherens junctions, membrane transport proteins, and the basal lamina are essential structures that maintain the BBB's integrity and functions [5]. Each is made up of smaller components with specialized functions. This section dissects the main elements of the neurovascular unit and their specific roles in the BBB's integrity and functioning.

Endothelial Cells

The walls of brain capillaries are composed of a single layer of endothelial cells (ECs). This layer forms the immediate barrier to the blood [6]. The endothelial cells are nonfenestrated and adhere via junctional complexes, which limits paracellular diffusion [7]. These junctional complexes include tight junctions, gap junctions, and adherens junc-

S. Joshi (ed.), *Arterial Treatment of Neurological Diseases*, https://doi.org/10.1007/978-3-031-80173-0_5

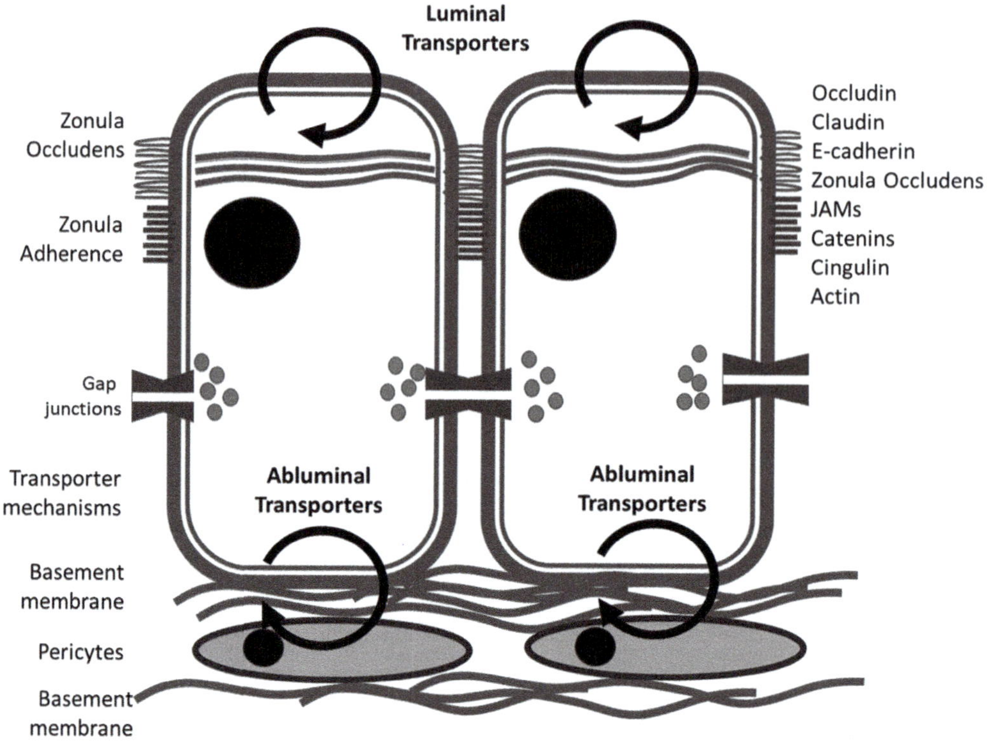

Fig. 5.1 Structural barriers and mechanisms that provide potential BBB disruption targets

tions. Given the limited transport between cells, regulated transcellular transport becomes the major transport route across the endothelium. Figure 5.1 illustrates the major EC-associated structures that have been studied extensively and are described below.

Tight Junctions

As the ECs constitute the foundational component of the BBB, their integrity and paracellular impermeability are essential. Tight junctions are vital to maintaining an intact capillary wall. Tight junctions are specific adherence structures between neighboring cells that result from interactions between transmembrane proteins and cytoskeletal components. The major transmembrane proteins include claudins (mainly claudin-5), occludins, and junctional adhesion molecules (JAM-A, JAM-B, and JAM-C) (Fig. 5.2) [8]. Each membrane protein has a specific function in ensuring paracellular impermeability. Claudins are the primary "tighteners" of the tight junctions. Knockout of claudin-5 has been shown to increase BBB permeability and lead to incompatibility with life in mice [9]. Occludins regulate the development of the tight junction seal [10]. The junctional adhesion molecules, related to immunoglobulin proteins, modulate leukocyte extravasation into the brain [11].

The transmembrane proteins attach to cytoskeletal proteins inside neighboring cells through adaptor proteins, which both have structural and functional implications for the tight junctions [12]. The connections between transmembrane protein and cytoskeletal component are possible, partly due to binding at PDZ domains on the transmembrane proteins [13]. PDZ is an acronym derived from the first letters of three proteins in which the protein was observed: the postsynaptic density protein, the *Drosophila* disc large tumor suppressor, and the zona occludens. The PDZ protein domains provide structural connections between transmembrane proteins and cytoskeletal proteins.

PDZ domains on the zona occludens (ZO) enable the structural bindings between tight junctions and the cytoskeleton. ZOs generally have three different PDZ domains that may interact with the components of tight junctions and surrounding cellular structures [14]. ZOs play an integral role in the function and assembly of claudins, occludins, and JAM-As within the tight junctions [15]. Depletion of ZO-1 leads to disruption of tight junctions [16]. ZO-1 establishes direct connections between occludins and cytoskeletal actin (Fig. 5.2) [17]. Furthermore, ZO-1 and ZO-2 play a role in the polymerization of claudins [18]. ZO-1 has also been shown to play a role in connections between JAMs and claudins, enabling interactions between JAMs and proteinase-activated receptor 3 (PAR-3), another adaptor protein [19]. Given the importance of ZO-1 in maintaining endothelial composition, it plays an essential role in maintaining the integrity of the BBB. Tornavaca et al. showed that ZO-1 indirectly regulates angiogenesis by regulating cell migration. In their study, depletion of ZO-1 led to reduced endothelial sprouting. In vivo mouse experiments and studies on human dermal microvascular endothelial cells with siRNAs knockdown of ZO-1 showed a

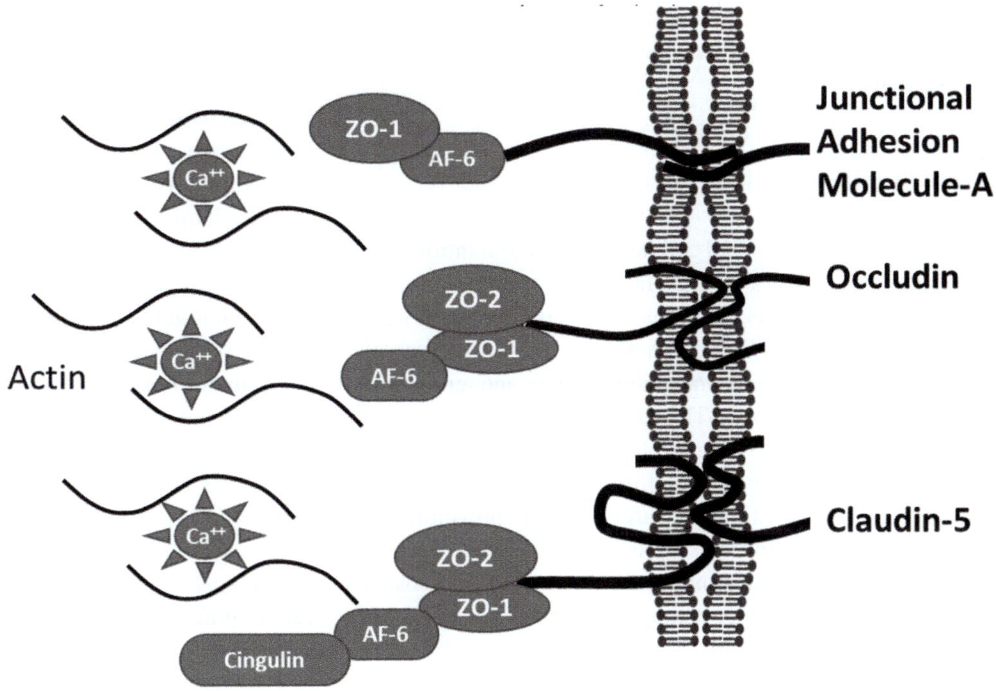

Fig. 5.2 Tight junction components underlying the BBB. See text for abbreviations

significantly decreased number of vessels [16]. ZO-1 is thus a target for BBB disruption.

Other tight junction adaptor proteins with PDZ domains include membrane-associated guanylate kinase (MAGIs), multi-PDZ domain protein 1 (MUPP1), and afadin [20]. MAGI-1 is required for vascular endothelial cadherin-mediated cell adhesion [21]. Although its exact role is unclear, MUPP1 has been shown to interact with claudin-1 and JAMs at tight junctions [22]. Afadin-6 (AF-6) is essential for many cellular functions, including cell-cell adhesions, migration, differentiation, and polarity [23].

Several proteins related to the tight junctions also make connections without the PDZ domains. One such protein is cingulin (Fig. 5.2). Cingulin is expressed at the ECs in the brain, where it interacts with ZO-1. Its knockdown in mice has been shown to increase the uptake of tracers in the brain [24].

The cytoskeleton is the final component of the tight junction complex. Microtubules and actin-binding proteins are the most important constituents. The strength of adhesion is dependent on the organization of the cytoskeletal actin. The organization of actin is, in turn, highly regulated by actin-binding proteins, which modulate the interaction of actin cytoskeleton with the adaptor proteins, predominantly through polymerization [25]. Major polymerizing proteins include actin-related protein 2/3 complex, cortactin, and vasodilator-stimulated phosphoprotein [26]. Microtubules, in turn, interact with the actin filament and influence focal adhesion, cellular contraction, and leukocyte migration across the endothelium [27].

Gap Junctions

Intercellular communication in the BBB is mediated through gap junctions. Two connexons, also known as hemichannels, make up a gap junction. Connexons are protein hexamers located at the plasma membrane. Each connexon is made from the assembly of six connexins (Cx). Major connexins of the endothelial cells include Cx37, Cx40, and Cx43 [12]. The gap junctions mediate cellular communication by allowing the passage of ions between neighboring cells. Beyond cell-cell communication, connexins are also suggested to be involved in cell proliferation and migration [28].

Adherence Junctions

Adherens junctions are another critical component of the BBB. Their function is to supply cohesion to the BBB. The major constituents of adherens junctions are cadherins and catenins [29]. Specifically, vascular endothelial cadherin (VE-cadherin) is a significant type of cadherin in the brain and integral to forming adherens junctions. VE-cadherin binds to the actin cytoskeleton via β-catenins, γ-catenins, and p120-catenin intracellularly and to other VE-cadherins extracellularly. Together, they form adherens junctions [30]. The VE-cadherins are suggested to be involved in cellular processes such as forming vascular connections [31], intracellular signaling [32], and cytoskeletal organization [33]. Furthermore, VE-cadherin initiates the expression of tight junction protein claudin-5 through modulation of Wnt/β--catenin signaling [34]. Morini et al. compared a VE-cadherin null cell line with a VE-cadherin wild type. They found that VE-cadherin expression leads to upregulation of claudin-5 via inhibition of polycomb protein activity on claudin-5 promoter regions [35]. These findings suggest that VE-cadherin has direct epigenetic influences on other tight junction components.

Basal Lamina

Adjacent to the endothelial cell layer is the basal lamina. The basal lamina separates the ECs from the underlying neurons and glial cells. It forms two sides: one facing the brain's glial cells and another facing the endothelial cells of the vessels; these are referred to as the parenchymal and endothelial basal lamina, respectively. The basal lamina comprises extracellular matrix (ECM) glycoproteins synthesized mainly by ECs, astrocytes, and pericytes [36]. It adds to the physical barrier between the brain and circulation by preventing the infiltration of undesired substances and leukocytes. Thus, the basal lamina is a significant regulator of brain homeostasis [37]. The major ECM proteins that form the basal lamina include collagen IV, laminins, and glycoproteins [38].

Collagen IV

Collagen IV and laminin comprise the bulk of the ECM. The collagen IV isoform most abundant in the brain is made from assembling two α1 and one α2 chain polypeptides. Together, they form the collagen IV $[\alpha1(IV)]_2\alpha2(IV)$ isoform [39]. ECs, astrocytes, and pericytes secrete collagen IV, essential for maintaining and functioning the BBB [40]. Jeanne et al. showed that disruption of collagen IV from ECs and pericytes leads to more significant intracerebral hemorrhage in mice than from astrocytes [41]. Interactions between integrins of the ECs with collagen IV of the basal lamina directly affect the expression of tight junction proteins, indicating that collagen IV has a broader influence over the BBB [42]. Furthermore, the knockout of collagen IV in mice has been shown to affect the stability of the basal lamina and is incompatible with life [43].

Laminin

ECs, pericytes, and astrocytes also produce laminin. The specific laminin isoforms in the basal lamina differ depending on which cell produces it. Astrocytes produce laminin-211, which is mainly found on the parenchymal side of the basal lamina, whereas laminin-411 and laminin-511 are produced by ECs and found on the endothelial side of the basal lamina [44]. Pericytes seem to generate laminin subunits found in several different laminin isoforms [45, 46]. Disruption of different laminin subunits leads to varied effects on the BBB. For example, disrupting the laminin-α2 subunit of laminin-211 in mice, which is produced by astrocytes and pericytes, has been shown to cause BBB disruption with increased infiltration of immune cells into the brain parenchyma, changes in tight junction organization, and decreases in pericyte populations [47]. Knockdown of laminin-α4 and laminin-α5 in ECs demonstrates moderate BBB breakdown [37].

Glycoproteins

Nidogens are another essential component of the basal lamina. Nidogens are glycoproteins that stabilize and cross-link the laminin and collagen IV of the basal lamina [48]. Similar to laminin and collagen IV, nidogens are produced by ECs, astrocytes, and pericytes. There are two main isotypes, nidogen-1 and nidogen-2 [49]. Knockout experiments targeting the two nidogen isoforms have been performed in mice. Individual knockout of each isoform is compatible with life and has no significant adverse effects. In the case of nidogen-1 knockout, an upregulation of nidogen-2 was seen [50]. This type of compensation was not observed in nidogen-2 knockout [51]. Simultaneous knockout of both isoforms is incompatible with life, resulting in severe basal lamina defects [52]. These experiments indicate that nidogens are crucial for the basal lamina and BBB function.

Large heparan sulfate proteoglycans such as agrin and perlecan are also featured in the basal lamina. Agrin interacts with laminin and is believed to play a role in early BBB development [53, 54]. Perlecans are found within the collagen IV and laminin network and help maintain basal lamina integrity [55], binding of growth factors [56], and recruitment of pericytes in injury [57]. Some data suggest that perlecan is dispensable in the healthy BBB and that perlecan knockout only has significant consequences in the context of injury [58].

Pericytes

Pericytes are located on the outer margins of the brain capillaries, either adjacent to ECs or enveloped within the basal lamina [59]. Their exact identity is debated. In some studies, the term is used broadly to include any peri-endothelial mesenchymal cell, including vascular smooth muscle cells. Anatomically, pericytes have circular soma and primary cytoplasmic processes extending along the adjacent endothelium's abluminal surface. The primary processes may further extend secondary processes that attach to the endothelium. Such connections between pericytes and endothelial cells make communication between them possible. Several pericyte-endothelial cell connections, including the "peg-socket" type, direct membrane contact, gap junctions, and adhesion plaques (resembling adherence junctions), have been identified. Pericytes are found on arterioles, capillaries, and venules. The number of ECs is estimated to be greater than the number of pericytes, with an approximate 10:1 ratio [60].

Pericytes play a structural role in the BBB. They provide structural support and stability to the capillaries. Furthermore, pericytes are involved in regulating cerebral blood flow. For example, they help redirect blood flow toward areas of increased neuronal activity [61]. This function is mainly possessed by the pericytes of the arterioles, which contain higher levels of alpha-smooth muscle actin, a protein involved in contraction [62]. The communication between pericytes and ECs can be achieved through direct cell-cell contact via cell processes, as described, or through autocrine and paracrine signaling. Paracrine and autocrine signaling have been seen in angiogenesis, vascular remodeling, and development. The angiopoietin (Ang)/Tie-2 system is an example of such communication. Ang-1, secreted by pericytes, phosphorylates the receptor tyrosine kinase Tie-2 on ECs and promotes vessel maturation and stabilization. ECs, on the other hand, promote angiogenesis in an autocrine manner by secreting Ang-2, which antagonizes the process [63]. Similar signaling mechanisms have been seen in the vascular endothelial growth factor A (VEGFA)-VEGFR2 pathway, which is believed to promote EC survival in tumors [64]. Furthermore, a decrease in pericytes is correlated with increased BBB permeability through loss of tight junctions in ECs [65], indicating the importance of pericyte-EC cross talk for BBB function. Lastly, there is increasing evidence that pericytes serve an immune function by harboring responsivity and an intrinsic ability to secrete inflammatory molecules such as cytokines. The pericytes also possess the potential for phagocytosis and are involved in the recruitment of leukocytes into the brain [66, 67].

Astrocytes

Astrocytes are the most abundant cells in the brain and a critical component of the BBB. Astrocytic processes extend to the capillaries and ensheath vessels with their end feet [68]. Similarly, astrocytic processes also ensheath neuronal processes. Thus, astrocytes act as a bridge, linking neurons to blood vessels and allowing neural control over the blood supply [69]. Astrocytes are integral to the development and function of the BBB. Several studies have demonstrated this by comparing ECs in the presence and absence of astrocytes, and they have found a lack of barrier capacity in the absence of astrocytes [70, 71].

A range of mechanisms for astrocytic influence upon the BBB have been identified. Astrocytes anchor transmembrane proteins such as aquaporin 4 (AQP4) and inward rectifying potassium channel 4.1 (KIR4.1) to the vasculature through adaptor molecules like syntrophin, dystrophin, and dystrobrevin [72–74]. AQP4 regulates water influx at the BBB. Knockout studies suggest that AQP4 deficiency reduces brain water uptake across the BBB [75]. Similarly, astrocytic KIR4.1, co-localized with AQP4, maintains potassium and water balance [76]. Astrocytes communicate through gap junctions. The disruption in the astrocytic gap junction proteins results in BBB dysfunction [77]. Additionally, astrocytes supply energy to neurons through the astrocyte-neuron lactate shuttle, where glucose from endothelial cells fuels lactate production for neuronal energy [78].

Astrocytes are also involved in the development of the BBB. The sonic hedgehog (Shh) and Wnt signaling pathways are critical pathways for astrocytic influence on the BBB. Shh secreted from astrocytes acts on hedgehog receptors on ECs and promotes barrier functions and expression of inflammatory mediators at ECs [79, 80]. The Wnt/β-catenin signaling pathway is essential for angiogenesis and BBB development [81–83]. Recent studies have shown that Wnt signaling in astrocytes is crucial for maintaining the integrity and function of the BBB and that its suppression results in astrocytic end-feet alterations and AQP4 disruption [84]. Furthermore, astrocytes promote angiogenesis by releasing VEGF and transforming growth factor β (TGF-β) [85, 86]. TGF-β also maintains the expression of P-glycoprotein (P-gp), a critical efflux protein in the BBB [87]. Src-suppressed C kinase substrate and angiotensin II are astrocytic substrates that have been shown to promote the generation of tight junction components [88, 89]. Astrocytes play a multifactorial role by regulating, supporting, and contributing to the BBB.

BBB Transport Mechanisms

Passive Diffusion

Some molecules and compounds can diffuse passively along their concentration gradients across the BBB without the aid of transporters. O_2 and CO_2 are two classic examples of such molecules. Passive diffusion of such molecules mainly occurs at the cell membrane. Molecular size and lipid solubility are the critical determinants of whether a compound can passively diffuse across the cell membrane [90]. Generally, molecules with a molecular weight below 500 Daltons (Da) and lipophilic/hydrophobic properties can cross the BBB through passive diffusion [91].

Carrier-Mediated Transport

Membrane transport proteins can also facilitate the transport of small compounds [92]. Four types of membrane transport proteins exist in the BBB. These include ion channels, solute-carrier (SLC) transporters, aquaporins, and ATP-powered pumps [93]. These transporters constitute the main route for the influx of nutrients, ions, and smaller drug molecules and the efflux of waste products to and from the brain [94]. The membrane transporters at the ECs can be involved in three modes of transport: influx, efflux, or bidirectional transport [95]. Transport can be divided into passive, where the substrate follows its electrochemical gradient, and active, where energy from ATP is used and the substrate is transported against its electrochemical gradient.

The SLC superfamily of transporters is a prominent class of transporters in the brain that facilitates the movement of substrates and plays a vital role in transporting nutrients such as glucose, amino acids, metabolites, and certain drug compounds. These may either facilitate the transport of a single substrate passively along its electrochemical gradient or cotransport multiple substrates. Cotransportation can either be in the same direction (symporters) or the opposite direction (anti-porters) [93]. As of 2020, 287 SLC genes had been identified in the brain [96]. Their malfunction is believed to play a role in brain disorders such as epilepsy, neurodegenerative diseases, and autism, and recently, they have become an attractive target for drug delivery [96].

Aquaporins are another class of transporters specialized in transporting water molecules along their osmotic gradient. Eight different types of aquaporins are expressed in the CNS. Aquaporin 4 is expressed at the highest concentrations in the brain, often found at the astrocytic end feet in the BBB [97].

Lastly, the ATP-binding cassette (ABC) pumps are a significant transport protein group that uses energy from ATP to transport substrates against an electrochemical gradient [93]. They make up a wide range of efflux pumps in the brain, which protect it against xenobiotics and toxic metabolites by pumping them back into circulation. The efflux pumps limit drug uptake in the brain and some cancer cells. Significant efflux transporters include P-gp, breast cancer resistance protein (BCRP), and multidrug resistance-associated proteins (MRP) [98].

Transcytosis

Vesicular transportation, or transcytosis, is another form of transcellular transport. This method involves engulfing a compound in a vesicle created at the cell membrane, intracellular transport to the abluminal membrane, and releasing the contents via exocytosis. It often involves larger molecules of particles. There are two primary transcytosis mechanisms: receptor-mediated and adsorption-mediated transcytosis.

Receptor-mediated transcytosis is specific and pertains to select interactions between established ligands and their receptors. The compound is internalized following ligand-receptor interaction. Receptors that are involved in this type of transcytosis include the transferrin receptor [99], insulin and insulin-like growth factor receptors [100], and lipoprotein receptors [101].

Unlike receptor-mediated transcytosis, adsorption-mediated transcytosis is an unspecific mechanism for vesicle transport. It occurs when molecules interact directly with clathrin-coated or caveolar vesicle membranes [102]. Cationic proteins, including histones [103], along with protamine [104], and avidin [105], can trigger such uptake. Biochemical properties of the BBB that enhance adsorption-mediated transcytosis of cationic proteins include negative charges at the surface from heparan sulfate proteoglycans such as syndecans and glypicans [106].

Transcytosis, through the methods mentioned above, is an energy-consuming process. Consequently, brain ECs contain more mitochondria than peripheral ECs, where passive transport is more common [107].

Blood-Tumor Barrier

When addressing BBB penetration in disease, particularly in neuro-oncology, the effects of the underlying pathology on the BBB are essential to consider. Increasing evidence shows that brain tumors have a disrupting effect on the BBB. The barrier between circulation and tumor at these vessels is often called the "blood-tumor barrier" (BTB). The BTB is highly variable between different tumors and within a single tumor. A critical step in enhancing drug delivery is understanding how a brain tumor affects the exchange between the blood and the brain/tumor tissue.

Gliomas

Disruption of the BBB by gliomas has primarily been evidenced by the increased uptake of gadolinium contrast as seen on magnetic resonance imaging (MRI) [108]. High-grade gliomas (HGG) are highly vascularized tumors, and the degree of vascularization in GBM correlates with the severity of the disease [109]. Hypoxia in highly proliferative and oxygen-demanding glioma cells activates the transcription factor hypoxia-inducible factor-1 (HIF-1), which induces the generation of angiogenesis-promoting factors and components needed to build new vessels [110–112]. Tumor-promoted angiogenesis in HGG is mainly driven by VEGF, basic fibroblast growth factor (bFGF), hepatocyte growth factor (HGF), platelet-derived growth factor (PDGF), TGF-β, matrix metalloproteases (MMPs), and angiopoietins (Angs) [113]. Extensive angiogenesis in gliomas results in dysmorphic vessels. Glioma-related angiogenesis creates aberrant blood vessels that differ from their healthy counterparts. For example, upregulation of VEGF expression induces activation of protein kinase C, which may disrupt occludins in tight junctions through phosphorylation [114]. Similarly, MMPs in tumor angiogenesis degrade claudin-5, which is, as mentioned, an essential component of tight junctions [115]. The process is inexact and less regulated than typical angiogenesis, creating dysfunctional, immature, and leaky vessels [116, 117].

Histologically, the BTB's endothelium is heterogeneously distributed, with greater variety in vessel diameter and a defective basal lamina [118, 119]. Furthermore, the endothelial cells of the BTB have altered expression of tight junction proteins such as claudin-5 [120]. Advanced gliomas show increased fenestrations between the endothelial cells and widened intercellular junctions [121]. The defective barrier leads to fluid leakage and may also enhance the hematogenous spread of tumor cells [122]. In addition to the endothelial cells, pericytes of the BTB in gliomas have been shown to have a changed distribution with a nonuniform coverage. Pericytes are innate in the normal BBB yet are also commonly displayed, harboring a pro-tumorigenic role in gliomas [123]. Evidence shows that BTB pericytes are derived from glioma stem cells and support the vessels supplying the tumor [124]. In support of this role, studies have found that targeting these pericytes leads to disruption of the BTB and increased drug delivery [125].

Beyond abnormal angiogenesis, the glioma cells also cause damage to existing healthy vessels. The invading glioma cells travel along healthy vessels before invading and growing into new spaces. They may be guided by signaling peptides from ECs; one such signaling peptide is bradykinin [126]. During this process, the glioma cells disrupt the astrocytic end feet, which mediate communication between the astrocytes, neurons, and the ECs. Loss of the integrity of the astrocytic end feet entails disruption of the neurovascular unit and impairs neurovascular coupling [127]. Besides disrupting these interactions, glioma cells have been shown to hijack the regulation of the vessel tone [128]. Montgomery et al. have studied the effects of gliomas on vascular dynamics using longitudinal in vivo, wide-field optical mapping. They saw a decreased perfusion in glioma regions associated with seizures compared to healthy brain regions, perhaps attributed to abnormal neurovascular coupling. An abnormal vasoconstricting neurovascular response to seizures in gliomas may thus accentuate abnormal angiogenesis [129]. Recent studies have shown that gliomas also may perturb neuronal components [130]. Such neuronal interactions can influence tumor progression and disrupt neural circuits in the brain, affecting cognition [130]. Furthermore, the interplay between astrocytic end feet and ECs is essential for maintaining the basal lamina. As both astrocytic end feet and the ECs are dysregulated by glioma, the underlying basal lamina is often degraded or compromised [127, 131]. Consequentially, a vicious cycle is created where disruption of normal blood supply by healthy blood vessels leads to hypoxia, which, as previously mentioned, increases faulty angiogenesis [132].

Despite compromise to the BBB and a faulty BTB following tumor invasion, the disorganized and heterogeneous BTB is not optimized for drug delivery. HGGs develop additional strategies to decrease susceptibility to pharmacological agents. For example, glioblastomas may synthesize specific efflux proteins that counteract and complicate cancer drugs' penetration of the BBB, including P-gp, breast cancer resistance protein (BCRP), and multidrug resistance protein 1 (MRP1) [133, 134]. As such, there is a need for approaches to manipulate these barriers to drug delivery.

Metastasis

The mechanisms of BBB disruption are different in brain metastases compared to gliomas. Brain metastases are a heterogeneous group originating from a variety of primary tumors. Common metastases to the brain include adenocarcinomas of the lung, breast, and colon, as well as melanomas [135]. Each has a slightly different impact on the brain and the BBB.

Importantly, all metastases, which metastasize through the circulatory system to the brain, need to breach the blood-brain barrier to infiltrate the brain. Still a relatively unexplored field, the exact mechanisms of brain infiltration vary depending on the cancer type. Bos et al. performed genetic analysis on breast cancers and identified 17 genes associated with brain metastasis, with ST6GALNAC5 identified as a critical gene facilitating infiltration through the BBB. Moreover, COX2 and EGFR ligands were found to enhance cancer cell motility, aiding in brain metastasis [136]. Another study on triple-negative breast cancer metastases found that elevated Ang-2 expression in ECs correlated with BBB disruption and that treatment with the Ang-2 inhibitor trebananib prevented these changes—suggesting Ang-2 as a potential therapeutic target for brain metastasis [137]. It has also been shown that breast metastases transmigrate across the BBB using proteases such as cathepsin-S to degrade JAM-B proteolytically [138]. Real-time imaging of lung and melanoma metastasis formation in the brain using mouse models showed that metastatic tumor infiltration depends on motility arrest to extravasate to the brain [139]. Furthermore, the metastatic tumors in the real-time imaging study depended on angiogenesis and nutrient supply from the same vessel [139]. Perhaps this is an explanation for their perivascular location in the brain. Other benefits of being located perivascularly include access to survival factors from endothelial cells and the basal lamina [140–142]. Studying the mechanisms of BBB invasion by the metastases may provide clues to potential targets for BBB disruption.

Brain metastases also utilize vascular cooption, meaning interaction with preexisting vasculature [143, 144]. The CNS has specific safety guards in place to deter cooption. For example, plasmin from the brain stroma can avert vascular cooption. However, metastatic lung and breast cancers have been shown to bypass this mechanism by expressing serpins that prevent plasmin production [142].

Several mechanisms within the brain metastases have been identified that are associated with an increased BTB permeability. For example, astrocytic alterations have been shown to enhance BTB permeability in breast metastases. Specifically, the upregulation of sphingosine-1 phosphate receptor 3 (S1P3) mediates permeability through astrocytic secretion of the inflammatory mediators [145]. Pericytes have also been shown to play a role in BTB permeability in brain metastases. Desmin-positivity in pericytes correlated with increased drug permeability breast cancer metastases in the brain [146].

As described, BBB disruption in brain metastases is part of the pathogenesis. However, drug delivery to the metastases remains a challenge. Further studies are needed into the BBB and BTB vulnerabilities in brain metastases.

Primary Central Nervous System Lymphomas

As with gliomas and brain metastases, primary central nervous system lymphomas (PCNSL) also change the BBB properties. In a 1999 study, Molnár et al. set out to understand the "ghost phenomenon," the increased contrast extravasation that does not correlate to surgical findings in lymphoma. Using electron microscopy imaging, they described the thinning of endothelial cells, with fenestrations and sometimes even endothelial discontinuation, indicating a disrupted BBB/BTB in PCNSL. They attributed this to selective apoptosis in the ECs [147].

Despite this weakened barrier, therapies that successfully target extra-CNS lymphomas have difficulty penetrating PCNSL. Effective methods of opening the BBB in PCNSL may allow for new and emerging treatments such as immunotherapy, which entails high weight molecules such as monoclonal antibodies, currently with significant limitations in reaching the CNS pathology at a cellular level [148].

Additional Barriers to Drug Delivery

The vascular hydrodynamics and physiology in the brain, specifically within the brain tumor, add another layer of complexity to the delivery of therapeutics to tumors. It has been shown that the angiogenesis within tumors such as HGGs is highly heterogeneous, with a great variety of hypoperfused and hyperperfused regions within a single tumor [149]. As such, therapeutics may be unable to reach certain tumor areas. Tumor-related consequences such as necrosis, hemorrhage, mass effect, and thrombosis around tumors are other factors that impact drug delivery on a microcirculatory level [150]. The brain is a highly perfused organ, receiving around 15–20% of the body's cardiac output, which may be a limiting factor for localized drug delivery. This especially comes into play in the context of intra-arterial delivery, where "streaming" may result in the maldistribution of the infused drugs due to a superior background flow rate [151–153]. However, the true impact of streaming remains disputed [152]. Procedure-related factors, such as using anesthetic agents or other concomitantly used pharmaceuticals, may also change the regional pharmacokinetics and drug delivery [154, 155].

The Dedrick pharmacokinetics model of intra-arterial (IA) drug delivery shows that IA drug delivery is most efficient when the regional flow is low, regional extraction is high, and systemic clearance is high [156]. However, it fails to address blood flow hydrodynamics and efflux transporters, which both have implications for drug delivery [151]. Novel experimental models that allow for high-quality real-time in vivo assessment are needed to understand the capillary dynamics of drug delivery better. Advanced optical imaging methods like intravital microscopy could observe capillary-level dynamics [150].

Recent advances in microcatheterization techniques have allowed manipulations that counteract the unfavorable flow dynamics in a clinical setting. For example, flow arrest during local drug delivery can decrease the washout of therapeutics by blood flow. The two main methods for flow arrest that have been employed in IA drug delivery are local balloon occlusions and systemic arrest of blood flow [157, 158].

Although often an overlooked aspect of drug delivery to the brain, capillary hydrodynamics certainly has implications for the chances of delivering drugs, both IA and intravenously (IV). As such, there is much more to learn about this aspect of drug delivery.

Methods for BBB Disruption

A variety of methods have been developed to disrupt the BBB. While some of these approaches have progressed to clinical trials, others remain in the preclinical stage or have very few supporting clinical studies. The basis for disruption builds on subverting and disturbing key points upholding the sanctity of the neurovascular unit. The most common compounds used in drug-based methodology and the most studied device-based techniques will be covered in this section. Figure 5.3 presents an overview of the methods discussed in this section, together with some of the more emerging methods described in the final section of this chapter.

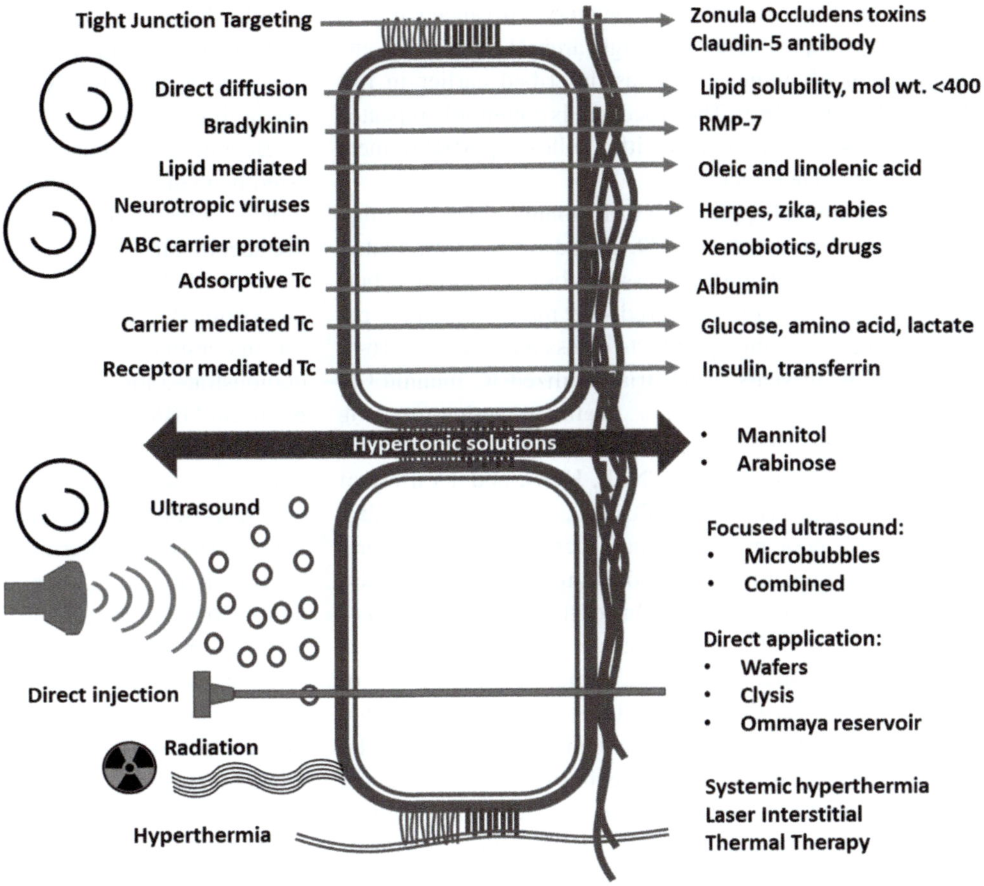

Fig. 5.3 Strategies for delivering drugs across the BBB

Intracarotid Osmotic Disruption

The concept of disruption of the BBB using intra-arterial (IA) or intracarotid (IC) hypertonic agents is based on the osmotic effects on intracellular fluid. Osmosis, a phenomenon for maintaining tonicity equilibrium, describes the diffusion of water molecules from areas of low to high solute concentration. Hypertonic agents contain higher levels of solutes than the body's regular fluid spaces. As such, they may cause shrinkage of the endothelial cells as they draw liquid out of the cells and into the interstitial space. This disrupts the tight junctions, allowing for increased paracellular transport of solutes. This method for BBB disruption was first described in 1972 by Rapoport et al. Their study showed that electrolytes and nonelectrolyte, lipid-insoluble solutions could increase the permeability of Evans blue-albumin into the BBB in rabbits in a reversible manner [159]. Following this landmark study, others showed that tight junction openings can be directly visualized using methods similar to electron microscopy [160]. Apart from the tight junction manipulation that occurs secondary to decreased endothelial cell size, osmotic agents also increase the intravascular volume. This increase in volume decreases viscosity, which results in vasodilation, further contributing to the opening of the tight junctions. A range of osmotic agents have been tested for hypertonic disruption of the BBB; mannitol is the agent that has gained the most traction [159, 161, 162].

In parallel with customary treatment, the use of hyperosmolar mannitol has shown clinical therapeutic significance. Neuwelt and colleagues' animal studies on disruption of the BBB with mannitol laid the foundation for the many human trials that followed [163, 164]. Most trials in humans follow a similar setup developed by the abovementioned group. MR or CT imaging with contrast is performed before the procedure to establish a baseline. The procedure is most often performed under general anesthesia for better control in case of adverse events. Cerebral angiography is utilized for visualization during the procedure. Percutaneous catheterization of the femoral artery is followed by access to an intracranial artery using microcatheters. The procedure involves infusing 20–25% mannitol into the carotid or vertebral arteries, depending on the location of the lesion, for 30–60 s. The flow rate is carefully adjusted to exceed the cerebral blood flow, as determined by fluoroscopy. The infusion rate is typically 3–12 mL/s [165]. The desired chemotherapeutic agent is also infused intra-arterially over several minutes, starting immediately after IC mannitol delivery. Advanced microcatheter techniques allow for high arterial selectivity and optimization of tissue uptake, as described earlier in this chapter [152, 157, 166]. The procedure is commonly repeated every 4 weeks for 12 months with a follow-up MRI to measure the treatment effect [165].

The first clinical application of IC mannitol for BBB disruption was conducted in 1979. Based on the flow that is necessary to blanch surface vessels observed through burr holes, the investigators delivered 4–8 mL of mannitol per 30 s, and they used angiography to assess the flow rate [164]. In the following years, many trials utilized IC mannitol to open the BBB in brain tumor treatment with promising results. IC mannitol has been used to deliver therapy for several tumor types, including PCNSL, HGG, and a variety of brain metastases [167, 168]. PCNSL, a rare brain malignancy with a poor prognosis, has been studied by several groups and is one of the most promising areas of drug delivery using this technique [169]. One of the mainstay therapies for PCNSL is high-dose methotrexate. However, methotrexate has limited BBB penetrance, displaying around 5% of plasma levels [152, 170]. In a multicenter analysis, Angelov et al. published the results of IC mannitol disruption and IA methotrexate therapy in 149 patients over 23 years. Focal seizures without long-term sequelae were the most common side effect, occurring in 9.2%. Nevertheless, the study demonstrated the safety and efficiency of this treatment with an overall response rate of 81.9% [171]. Another two-arm phase II trial examines IC mannitol for IA delivery of high-dose methotrexate and carboplatin in patients with refractory PCNSL. The BBB disruption treatment combines induction courses of IV and intrathecal cytoreductive regimens and autologous stem cell transplantations. The study's early results were published recently and reported a treatment response in 88% of patients and a 2-year overall survival rate of 81.0%. Acute grade III–IV hematological toxicity was the major adverse event related to the BBB disruption [172]. Furthermore, studies have used IC mannitol to enhance the delivery of other chemotherapeutic agents in HGG [173]. In HGG, disruption of the BBB, using IC mannitol, may provide an opportunity to expose and target the tumor stem cell within the perivascular niche [174]. A study on the mainstay chemotherapeutic agent temozolomide, administered intra-arterially (IA) in a rat model, concluded that temozolomide is unsafe for IA infusion due to toxicity [175]. Nevertheless, several clinical studies using other chemotherapeutic agents, such as platinum analogs (carboplatin) [176, 177], nitrosourea derivatives (nimustine) [178], and vinca alkaloids (vincristine) [179], have been published. In summary, the efficacy of these therapies has been questionable, and toxicity is a concern [152, 165]. The complexity and profound treatment resistance of high-grade gliomas (HGG) and the potential damage that cytotoxic chemotherapy poses to the healthy brain may contribute to these findings. Therefore, further studies are warranted to explore the efficacy and safety of intracarotid (IC) mannitol and chemotherapy delivery in this context.

Beyond chemotherapeutic agents, other trials have utilized IC mannitol to enhance IA delivery of emerging monoclonal antibody therapies in HGG. Monoclonal antibodies are specifically challenging to deliver IV due to their larger size, which limits BBB penetration [180]. Boockvar et al. have studied the IA delivery of bevacizumab, a VEGF inhibitor, in conjunction with IC mannitol. In a phase I trial, they demonstrated the safety and tolerability of this procedure in recurrent GBM [181]. This has been followed by several trials indicating promising effects of IC mannitol combined with IA bevacizumab therapy [182, 183]. Jeon et al. reported a progression-free survival of 10 months with IA bevacizumab [182]. The interim results from a phase I/II trial on IA bevacizumab and IC mannitol, in conjunction with standard temozolomide therapy and radiation for GBM, showed progression-free survival of 29.5 months and overall survival rates of 38.2 months [184]. A phase I study used another monoclonal antibody, cetuximab, in conjunction with IC mannitol; this combination was also deemed safe and well-tolerated [185].

BBB disruption using IC mannitol is a complex and multidimensional procedure, and several factors can affect its efficiency. Animal studies with hyperosmotic therapy in brain tumor models concluded that the effect of IC mannitol is highly variable depending on tumor type, brain region, and the tumor's innate permeability before disruption [164]. Each variable affects the degree to which mannitol can induce BBB disruption. In addition to the physiological circumstances of the tumor and the patient, several procedural aspects may influence the outcome. If anesthesia is used, the type of anesthetic agent and the partial carbon dioxide pressure have been shown to impact the efficiency of BBB disruption with IC mannitol in animal studies [164]. Moreover, the concentration and duration of the mannitol infusion, the time between mannitol and the therapeutic agent delivery, and the type of therapeutic agent can all impact the results [164]. It is crucial to consider the modality used to assess the opening of the BBB. As will be described later in this chapter, various methods are used to monitor BBB disruption, and each can impact the interpretation of the procedure [186]. More studies are needed to assess the hydrodynamic aspects of IA delivery, including maximizing drug concentration in the feeding artery and increasing tumor selective uptake while limiting spread to the remaining brain or washout from the brain to the body [151]. Another important aspect is the timing of the BBB opening and drug delivery. Al-Sarraf et al. studied this using a radiolabeled sucrose marker to measure BBB permeability in rats. They reported that it took 2 min for the radiolabeled sucrose to reach significant levels following hyperosmolar mannitol infusion and that the length of these effects was different between CSF-normotensive rats (30 min) and CSF-hypertensive rats (20 min) [187]. Although the implications of some patient-dependent factors are understood, other factors need more exploration. For example, the effects of radiation and surgery and their timing on IA drug delivery must be assessed. Radiation as an independent BBB disruptor will be discussed later. Joshi et al. have shown the variability and inconsistency of BBB opening with IC mannitol in rabbits. Thus, they emphasized the importance of real-time assessment and monitoring of the BBB opening [188, 189]. The damaging effects of BBB opening with IC mannitol also need further exploration. Preclinical studies have found that IC mannitol can damage the brain's white matter [190]. The immunogenic effects of hyperosmolar disruption may also have implications for tumor treatment. Burks et al. found that BBB disruption with IC mannitol induces sterile inflammatory and innate immune responses in rats [191]. This may be utilized to achieve an immunogenic therapeutic effect. Overall, osmotic BBB disruption provides various opportunities and challenges that necessitate further study and development.

Alkylglycerol

Hydrophobic, nonpolar, and small (<500 Da) molecules can diffuse passively across the BBB. This passive diffusion of hydrophobic/lipophilic substances can be leveraged therapeutically. Alkylglycerols are found naturally in a variety of biological tissues [192]. Alkylglycerols are a class of lipids characterized by one or more alkyl chains linked to a glycerol backbone. In high concentrations, alkylglycerol molecules form vesicles, and these lipophilic vesicles are believed to disrupt the BBB [193].

It has long been known that alkylglycerols can disrupt biological membranes [194]. In 1985, Unger et al. showed that the BBB penetration of chemotherapeutics was significantly increased in rats if short-chain alkylglycerols were added to the solution mix and given IC [195]. In later years, Erdlenbruch et al. extensively studied the effects of alkylglycerol on the BBB at the same institution. In a study published in 2000, they showed increased delivery of cisplatin and methotrexate, as well as vancomycin and gentamycin, when given IC in conjunction with short-chain alkylglycerols in a rat glioma model. They saw that 0.01–0.3 M alkylglycerol resulted in a transient disruption of the BBB, which was restored within 3–15 min of the injection. The drug permeability depended on the alkylglycerol's chemical structure, and they saw an increased permeability with increased chain length of the alkyl group and decreased glycerol content. Interestingly, they observed a homogenous distribution of the enhanced BBB penetration, both in glioma models and normal rats. Furthermore, the study showed that the permeability of vancomycin and gentamicin, which have higher molecular weights, were lower than those of methotrexate and cisplatin [196].

This study prompted several preclinical studies further dissecting the effects of alkylglycerols on BBB disruption. A 2005 study aimed to explore the biodistribution and elimination of 1-*O*-pentylglycerol, a short-chain alkylglycerol, when given IA and IV with radioactive markers. IC injections of 1-*O*-pentylglycerol lead to significant radioactive detection within the brains of rats within 5 min of injection, with a dramatic decrease after 30 min. However, IV injections failed to accumulate in the brain [197]. Similar limitations in IV delivery have been seen in other studies [193]. This could be due to inadequate concentrations in the brain capillaries. Hülper et al. further dissected the mechanisms of alkylglycerols in vitro. They found that alkylglycerols resulted in a decrease in transendothelial electrical resistance (TEER) values, a measure considered to be associated with increased paracellular permeability. In addition, using a fluorescein dye, they confirmed increased paracellular passage across tight junctions. Interestingly, albumin passage, commonly transported through the transcellular route at low levels in the BBB, was not increased. These findings strengthen the theory that alkylglycerols target tight junctions and their related structures [198].

Although alkylglycerol has yet to reach clinical studies, the evidence suggests that such nonionic, amphipathic molecules may be utilized to disrupt the BBB.

Lipids and Triglycerides

Oleic Acid

Oleic acid is a monounsaturated omega-9 fatty acid. It is one of the most common unsaturated fatty acids found in nature and is abundant in various dietary sources, particularly vegetable oils [199]. At high concentrations, fatty acids like oleic acid can aggregate into micelles, which could penetrate membrane lipids and disrupt their structure [200]. In 1991, Sztriha and Betz saw that IC oleic acid infusion in rats transiently increased BBB permeability in a dose-dependent and reversible manner, measured by Evans blue staining [201]. Sztriha and Betz theorized that in addition to structural disruption, biochemical changes such as protein kinase C activation, modulation of Na^+ K^+-ATPase activity, inhibition of mitochondrial phosphorylation, and increased reactive oxygen species might also contribute to the BBB disruption from oleic acid [201]. Han et al. suggested that the effects of IA oleic acid in rats are mediated by nitric oxide, which induces MMP-2 and MMP-13 [202]. This was supported by a loss of laminin in the affected area. The sequence that oleic acid induces is believed to start with the upregulation of intracellular adhesion molecule-1 (ICAM-1), which recruits neutrophils that express nitric oxide synthase, thus producing nitric oxide. Experiments supported this by demonstrating that inhibition of nitric oxide synthase suppressed the loss of laminin [202].

Triolein

Triolein is a triglyceride composed of three molecules of oleic acid, esterified to a glycerol backbone. It is believed to be involved in cerebral fat embolism, in which fat particles from bone marrow or adipose tissue enter the cerebral vasculature and cause neurological deficits. These deficits can be permanent and fatal due to mechanical blood flow obstruction causing strokes. However, mild cases are often reversible [203–205]. As such, triolein has been studied in preclinical models of cerebral fat embolism [206, 207]. Interestingly, these studies have shown that IA triolein causes a transient BBB disruption in cats, measured by contrast enhancement on MRI, which may last several hours to 3 days [206, 207]. A 2016 study investigated the permeability of IA doxorubicin in rabbits and IA cisplatin in rats in conjunction with triolein-mediated BBB disruption. The drugs were injected IA via microcatheters immediately after IC triolein was given. Fluorometric assessment of the brain tissues showed that both drugs were increased ipsilaterally compared to the contralateral hemisphere. As both drugs have a limited penetrance to the BBB in normal conditions, this study demonstrates the potential triolein [208]. In another study, Seung et al. examined the effects of IA/IC triolein emulsion followed by IV delivery of the standard HGG therapy, temozolomide. They concluded that the temozolomide concentration in the rat brain was approximately two times higher with the triolein emulsion than without it [209]. The exact mechanism behind triolein-mediated BBB disruption has not been fully comprehended.

Other Fatty Acids

Kim et al. compared the delivery-enhancing effects of IC oleic, linoleic, and linolenic acid emulsions. Each emulsion was given IC, followed by IV therapeutics. Measuring the drugs with desorption electrospray ionization-mass spectrometry imaging showed increased drug delivery with all three emulsions. Furthermore, staining with trypan blue showed that the staining weakened in the linoleic and linolenic acid groups over time. In terms of mechanism of action, electron microscopy revealed that the tight junctions were filled with contrast medium, suggesting enhancement of paracellular transport. Interestingly, the linolenic group resulted in the widening of perivascular space [210].

Recently, Jatyan et al. studied separate conjugates of oleic acid, the polyunsaturated fatty acid linoleic acid and the saturated fatty acid palmitic acid, with temozolomide. The conjugates were given intravenously to a rat orthotropic glioma model. They saw many benefits over free temozolomide, including increased efficiency, overcoming methyl guanine methyl transferase resistance, and a synergistic therapeutic effect [211]. In vivo studies in rats resulted in better survival rates and decreased tumor burden [211]. This study demonstrates the promise of fatty acids in BBB disruption and enhancing drug effects.

No clinical trials have been performed using these intracarotid fatty acids or triglycerides. The risks, with an emphasis on neurological strokes, need to be further explored, and the preparation and dosages of the emulsions need to be optimized. Additionally, there is a lack of studies on brain tumor models that provide a better understanding of how these emulsions interact with tumor tissue, an aspect of importance for the move to a clinical setting. Nevertheless, the preclinical data gives cause for optimism.

Bradykinin B2

Bradykinin, a peptide hormone involved in various body processes, mainly related to the cardiovascular system, inflammation, and pain signaling, has been shown to disrupt the BBB [212]. It has long been known that bradykinin can increase the permeability of systemic capillaries [213]. Inamura et al. were among the first to extensively study the effects of IC bradykinin and the synthetic bradykinin analog RMP-7 on the BBB in preclinical glioma rat models [214, 215]. Their studies used a bradykinin dose that did not affect systemic blood pressure or alter blood volumes. They saw an increased BBB permeability of IV radiolabeled tracers, including radiolabeled α-aminoisobutyric acid, sucrose, dextran, inulin, horseradish peroxidase, and Evans blue in a reversible manner. The effects lasted for no longer than 20 min. Despite continued infusion, a return to baseline permeability was seen within this time frame [216]. Interestingly, the disruption had a higher selectivity for the tumor tissue than the normal brain tissue [214, 215]. The same group also saw a similar effect from IC delivery of the bradykinin analog RMP-7 with the therapeutic agent carboplatin. They saw an increased uptake in the brain tumor tissue specifically and longer survival compared to when the drugs were given without IC RMP-7. Notably, the enhanced delivery was not seen with IV delivery of RMP-7 [217].

The preclinical results led to a clinical trial on RMP-7-enhanced delivery of gallium-68 ethylenediamine tetraacetic acid (Ga-EDTA) and carboplatin in nine adult patients with malignant gliomas. Under angiographic guidance, catheterization of the carotid artery was done. Subsequently, the patients were moved into a positron emission tomography scatter, and RMP-7 was injected for 15 min, alternating with a 5-min IC infusion of carboplatin. Four doses of RMP-7

(10, 30, 100, or 300 ng/kg) were tested with 100-mg carboplatin. For the PET scan and measurement of BBB disruption, Ga-EDTA was injected intravenously 5 min after RMP-7 infusion. The authors suggest that Ga-EDTA's permeability reflects carboplatin's permeability due to similarities in their molecular attributes. The PET scans showed that IC infusion of RMP-7 increased the permeability of Ga-EDTA to the tumor regions 2.7-fold. A significant increase in permeability was not observed in the normal brain tissue [218].

The exact mechanism through which bradykinin B2 agonists increase BBB permeability is still debatable. As mentioned, the permeability of the tumor-associated BBB only lasted for 20 min despite continuous infusion of RMP-7. This suggests that the effects might have been mediated by a secondary messenger, which was exhausted [216, 218]. Early on, it was suggested that nitric oxide mediates the effects of bradykinin. This was based on rat experiments in which the effects of nitric oxide synthase inhibitors in conjunction with bradykinin were assessed [219]. The same study demonstrated that tumors possess higher levels of nitric oxide synthase than normal brain tissue, which could explain the tumor-BBB/BTB specificity [219]. Another explanation for BTB specificity in bradykinin-enhanced drug delivery lies in the expression of bradykinin B2 receptors. Liu et al. showed that the level of B2-receptor expression in different glioma models correlated with the increase in permeability caused by bradykinin treatment [220]. Others have suggested that the expression of bradykinin B1 receptors also may play a role [221, 222]. In a rat glioma model, Liu et al. demonstrated that bradykinin causes downregulation of critical tight junction proteins, including zonula occludens-1, occludin, and claudin-5. Furthermore, they saw a rearrangement of cytoskeletal F-actin. Radioimmunity and Western blot assays showed a decrease of cAMP and the catalytic subunit of protein kinase A (PKAcs) in the tumor tissue, suggesting that the cAMP/PKA signaling system may mediate these effects [223]. Another study suggested that increases in nitric oxide synthases nNOS and eNOS decreased the expression of claudin-5 and occludin [224].

In summary, bradykinin disrupts the blood-brain barrier (BBB), enhancing its permeability selectively in tumor tissue. However, the mechanisms for this are yet to be entirely understood.

Zonula Occludens Toxin

As mentioned in the first section of this chapter, zonula occludens (ZO) is a crucial adaptor protein in tight junctions. It helps stabilize and bridge transmembrane proteins and intracellular cytoskeletal components. Specifically, ZO is involved in the function and assembly of claudins, occludins, and JAM-As [225]. Due to their inherent importance in the integrity of tight junctions, ZO presents a target for BBB disruption. ZOT is a protein produced by certain strains of *Vibrio cholerae*. In addition to cholera toxin, ZOT is also believed to contribute to the pathogenicity of cholera by disrupting the tight junctions between epithelial cells in the intestinal lining [226]. It has been suggested that ZOT exerts its effects on ZO permeability in the intestine through protein kinase C-dependent polymerization and rearrangement of F-actin [227]. Specifically, actin monomers that are involved in the regulation of the paracellular pathway are targeted [228]. In addition, it has also been suggested that ZOT exerts its effects by mimicking the mannose-binding lectin-associated serine protease zonulin, a structure believed to be involved in tight junction regulation [229, 230]. Contradictory to this, Stuart et al. argued that zonulin does not have a role in human BBB regulation. They measured serum zonulin levels in healthy individuals and patients with neurological diseases. To measure BBB permeability, they obtained dynamic contrast-enhanced MR imaging and measured the quotient of cerebrospinal fluid to serum albumin in the subjects. They saw no significant association between serum zonulin and BBB permeability in the cohorts [231].

Several studies have examined the effects of ZOT and its active fragment, ΔG, on the BBB. Karyekar et al. studied the effects of ZOT in bovine brain endothelial cells. In vitro, they demonstrated that the permeability of sucrose, inulin, doxorubicin, and paclitaxel all significantly increased when the endothelial cells were treated with 4 μg/mL of ZOT [232]. Menon et al. looked at the effects of ΔG on the BBB permeability of methotrexate and paclitaxel in rats. After estimating the effective dose of ΔG using a paracellular sucrose marker, they co-administered ΔG with methotrexate and paclitaxel through IC cannulas. At specific doses, they observed a sevenfold and 2.5-fold increase in the brain distributions of methotrexate and paclitaxel, respectively [233]. In a 2016 study, Bocsik et al. looked at six different tight junction-modulating peptides, including the AT-1002 peptide, an active fragment of ZOT. In vitro experiments in cultured endothelial rat cell models of the BBB showed that AT-1002 reversibly opened tight junctions [234]. Although the exact mechanism by which ZOT affects the BBB is not certain, preclinical data suggest that the disruption is reversible.

Claudin-5 Targeting

As mentioned previously, claudins are sealants of tight junctions. Knockout of dominant claudin-5 increases BBB permeability in mice [9]. Significantly, claudin-5 knockout in mice has been associated with death within days of birth [9]. As such, targeting claudin-5 provides an opportunity to increase drug delivery. However, studies on its damaging effects are needed. Short-interfering RNA sequences (siRNA), antibodies, and peptidomimetics have all been employed in this approach in preclinical settings. These methods and the evidence so far are discussed below:

Claudin-5 siRNAs

siRNAs are short, double-stranded RNA molecules that silence specific genes by targeting and degrading their complementary messenger RNA (mRNA) molecules [235]. Campbell et al. conducted systemic infusions of siRNA targeting claudin-5 in a murine model. They achieved a high specificity for brain endothelial claudin-5 with a maximum suppression of claudin-5 mRNA after 48 h, and levels returned to baseline between 72 h and 1 week. Assessing the BBB permeability with EZ-Link TM Sulfo-NHS-Biotin (443 Da), they saw an increased permeability for up to 72 h after siRNA delivery. They also tested the permeability of nuclear stain Hoechst H33342 (562 Da) and the FITC-labelled dextran FD-4 (4400 Da), observing an increased permeability of Hoechst for up to 48 h postdelivery but not for FD-4. Furthermore, MR imaging with contrast agent gadolinium diethylenetriamine *N,N,N′,N′,N′*-pentaacetic acid (Gd-DTPA), with a molecular weight of 724 Da, showed increased permeability up to 48 h post-siRNA delivery [236].

Claudin-5 Peptidomimetics

Two essential components of the claudin structures are their two extracellular loops (ECLs), ECL1 and ECL2. These ECLs connect to the claudins and, specifically, the ECLs of adjacent cells to seal tight junctions [237]. Dithmer et al. targeted claudin-5 ECLs using peptidomimetics, synthetic compounds designed to mimic their structure and function [238]. They developed an ECL1-derived peptide, C5C2, and studied the effects on BBB permeability in vitro and in vivo. The group demonstrated that C5C2 significantly increases the BBB permeability in a dose-dependent manner for molecules from 457 Da up to 10 kDa, including for doxorubicin, in vitro. In vivo, they demonstrated that IV administration of C5C2 results in increased BBB permeability of contrast agents on MRI and increased brain accumulation of fluorescein in brain specimens. The effects were reversible, and a return to baseline was seen after 12–48 h [239]. Furthermore, they observed that the effects of C5C2 were mediated by downregulation and redistribution of claudin-5, occludin, and ZO-1 [239]. Specifically, claudin-5 and its peptides were internalized by the ECs, as observed through laser scanning microscopy of living brain endothelial cells following C5C2 treatment [239].

Claudin-5 Antibodies

Others have studied anti-claudin-5 antibodies for targeting the BBB. Hashimoto et al. generated anti-claudin-5 monoclonal antibodies by immunizing mice and rats. When testing the antibodies on an in vitro BBB model composed of monkey brain microvasculature endothelial cells, rat pericytes, and rat astrocytes, they saw a time-dependent reduction in TEER and an increased permeability of fluorescein dye without cytotoxicity [240]. Using the same technology to generate antibodies, the group conducted in vivo studies in male cynomolgus monkeys. Claudin-5 antibodies were delivered IV, and the permeability of fluorescein was examined by measuring concentrations in the cerebrospinal fluid (CSF). Measurements were performed 24 h after antibody delivery and 30 min after IV fluorescein administration. At 3.0 mg/kg of anti-claudin-5-antibodies, they saw an increased dye concentration in the CSF. Interestingly, an antibody dose of 6 mg/kg resulted in severe side effects, including convulsions, lung hemorrhage, and brain edema. As such, they concluded that anti-claudin-5-antibodies do increase BBB permeability, although it has a narrow therapeutic window with the risk for severe side effects [241].

Nitrone OKN-007

Nitrone OKN-007 (Oklahoma Nitrone-007; 2,4-disulfophenyl-PBNA) is known to have anticancer effects in gliomas. Preclinical studies have shown that OKN-007 significantly reduces tumor volumes and increases survival in animal and orthotopic glioma models [242–247]. Mechanisms of the therapeutic effect have not been fully unraveled. Suggested mechanisms include suppression of nitric oxide synthase [248], modulation of ECM-related genes through the TGF-B1 and mTOR pathways [249], modulation of the PDGFRα pathway [247], decreased free radicals [245], and decreased VEGFR-2 [244]. A similar nitrone compound, NXY-059, has been studied in clinical trials with acute ischemic stroke patients for its neuroprotective effects, focusing on decreasing oxidative stress [250, 251]. Although the therapeutic effects in the stroke context have been disproved, it is safe for human use [251]. As such, Nitrone OKN-007 is used in an ongoing clinical trial to assess its therapeutic effects in gliomas (NCT04388475).

Interestingly, OKN-007 has also been shown to affect BBB permeability in preclinical models. Recently, Towner et al. showed that intravenous OKN-007 can reversibly open the BBB in mice. The group saw increased permeabilities of two gadolinium-based contrast agents, β-galactosidase-Gd-DOTA and Gd-DTPA. They also looked at Gd-DOTA attached to an antibody against the neuron-specific marker EphB (anti-EphB2-Gd-DOTA) and albumin and biotin (albumin-Gd-DTPA-biotin). The BBB permeability was examined both in vivo and ex vivo. They found that OKN-007 was cleared from the blood in less than 4 h. Based on MRI, they saw that it increases the permeability of Gd-DTPA for 1–3 h following IV administration. Furthermore, they saw that the larger Gd-DOTA-labeled β-galactosidase, which has a molecular weight of 465 kDa, can cross the BBB up to 1 h after OKN-007 delivery. They also saw that both the anti-EphB2-Gd-DOTA and albumin-Gd-DTPA-biotin had significantly increased BBB permeabilities [252].

Given its safety in humans, therapeutic effects, and preclinical data demonstrating its capacity for BBB disruption, OKN-007 has the potential for human trials in BBB disruption and drug delivery. However, more studies are needed to dissect the exact mechanism of BBB opening with OKN-007.

Focused Ultrasound with Microbubbles

Since the 1970s, ultrasound has been one of the most well-known and widely used imaging modalities [253]. Studies on the effects of exposing rabbit brains to increased intensities of ultrasound pulses were conducted in the mid-1990s. Vykhodtseva et al. showed in 1994 that increased ultrasound intensities may be used to ablate brain tissue [254]. After that, they studied the effects of decreasing focused ultrasound intensities by reducing exposure time, pulse frequency (Hz), and power (W) to find a level of "subharmonic" exposure. They found that at specific intensities, the BBB could be safely disrupted [255]. Hynynen et al. employed MR-guided focused ultrasound (FUS) in a rabbit study. Before sonification with FUS, an ultrasonographic contrast agent (Optison) that contained microbubbles with a diameter of 2.0–4.5 μm at a concentration of 5–8 × 10^8 bubbles per milliliter was given IV. Sonification was performed for 20 s, and the gadolinium-based MRI contrast agent gadopentetate dimeglumine (Magnevist) was given IV. The BBB opening was visualized on MR imaging in the targeted areas, evidenced by increased contrast uptake. Gadopentetate dimeglumine has a molecular weight of 928 Da. As such, it was theorized that the permeability of chemotherapeutic agents, which generally have molecular weights between 200 and 1200 Da, also would be enhanced by this procedure. The study opened an avenue into investigating FUS with microbubbles to improve drug delivery into brain tumors [256].

FUS with microbubbles as a mode of BBB disruption relies on pulsatile stress to the endothelium. Low-intensity pulses with ultrasound cause oscillations in gas-filled particles, and these oscillations lead to a reversible disruption of BBB by causing shear stress on the vessel walls [257]. This energy transfer from ultrasound to microbubbles to endothelium has shown that it results in transient disruption of junctional complexes and cellular membranes. Additionally, FUS has been shown to reduce gap junctions and P-gp, and increase transcytosis [258–260]. Notably, FUS with microbubbles directly impacts the targeted area's immune response. Kovacs et al. showed a sterile inflammatory response in the affected brain parenchyma. Specifically, they observed an upregulation of proinflammatory cytokines and intercellular adhesion molecules, transcriptomic changes related to the NFkB pathway, and an increased presence of microglia on histology [261]. Sheybani et al. showed increased penetration of dendritic cells and increased activation of CD8+ T cells following FUS treatment [262]. As such, FUS appears to have potential therapeutic effects which may be synergistic with novel immunotherapies.

Englander et al. showed enhancement of Evans blue dye using FUS with microbubbles in a primary pontine glioma mouse model. They showed that the method is safe in mice and does not change survival compared to sham control [263]. Furthermore, the same group showed that FUS with microbubbles could be utilized to increase the concentration of etoposide, a chemotherapeutic drug, in a glioblastoma model and, in turn, improve survival [264]. Studies in murine models have shown increased temozolomide, cisplatin, and carboplatin delivery with this technique [265–267]. FUS with microbubble treatment has also increased the BBB permeability of non-chemotherapeutic agents such as immunotherapy and siRNA [268]. Samiotaki et al. studied the duration of the BBB opening in FUS. MRI in mice showed that the duration from opening to closure following the procedure was proportional to the volume of opening, which in turn was dependent on FUS pressure (peak rarefactional pressure) and microbubble diameter. Thus, in their study, the time lapsed for the BBB to close varied from 24 h for smaller microbubbles to 5 days for the high peak rarefactional pressures [269]. Several studies have reported that the effects of FUS are transient and that the BBB functions are restored after the treatment [270].

Recently, a range of clinical trials have started testing the feasibility of FUS with microbubbles for enhancing drug delivery in humans. Three different technologies have been prominent for in-human use: Exablate Neuro, Sonocloud-1/Sonocloud-9, and NaviFUS. Of the three, Sonocloud is the only invasive method requiring the implantation of the transducer [271]. Exblate is a hemispheric transducer placed on top of the skull [272]. NaviFUS is a portable transducer similar to conventional imaging-ultrasound probes [273]. Idbaih et al. published the first-in-human trial in 2019. They studied the use of implantable Sonocloud-1 device to increase the delivery of intravenous carboplatin. They reported no severe treatment-related adverse events other than transient edema. Their results indicated that patients with more BBB permeability visible on MR imaging had a longer progression-free and overall survival [274]. Sonabend et al. recently published a phase 1 trial using the Sonocloud-9 device to increase the delivery of albumin-bound paclitaxel and carboplatin. Interestingly, they used nine times larger sonification fields compared to the 2019 study and reported no other significant adverse effects. A minor adverse effect in most patients was a transient grade 1–2 headache. Neutropenia, leukopenia, and hypertension were adverse effects attributed to the chemotherapeutic substances used rather than FUS. They showed a threefold to sevenfold increase in brain parenchymal concentrations of albumin-bound paclitaxel in the FUS group compared to the control group. They also showed that their technique restored the BBB function as early as 1 h after treatment [275]. This study is being followed up with an ongoing phase 2 study (NCT04528680). Various other FUS-related clinical trials in treating gliomas, including pediatric DIPG (NCT04805709), are in process.

Several aspects of FUS make it a promising method for disrupting the BBB. However, the long-term physiological effects on the BBB must be further explored. For example, a 2019 study found that FUS causes changes in functional brain connectivity in patients with Alzheimer's disease [276]. Furthermore, the immunological effects of FUS are of specific interest as these changes may affect the tumor microenvironment and treatment response. In addition, more precise and less invasive technologies should be developed. Current clinical trials have looked at implantable devices [274]. More studies need to be performed on noninvasive and user-friendly devices. Precision within FUS also has room for improvement. For example, combining FUS with local IA drug delivery instead of systemic delivery would permit increased precision. As with all emerging procedures, FUS must be optimized and tailored for the specific tumor types.

Radiation

The notion that radiation may affect the integrity of the brain microcirculation was raised as early as 1968 by Rubin and Casarett [277]. In a 1994 study, Rubin et al. showed an increased BBB permeability measured by Gd-DTPA leakage on MRI and horseradish peroxidase perfusion in rats that received 60 Gy of irradiation. At 6–12 weeks, there were signs of reversal of the BBB insult. However, late injury manifested as diffuse vascular leakage, cortical atrophy, and white matter necrosis, also observed at 24 weeks. This suggests that BBB radiation damage occurs in acute and chronic phases [278]. Subsequent studies suggested that the acute phase is caused by direct damage causing apoptosis of ECs [279]. The late phase of the BBB breakdown is caused by secondary injury from microenvironmental changes and inflammation [280]. Specifically, hypoxia is believed to alter VEGF expression via HIF-alfa upregulation, leading to more leaky vessels [280, 281]. Furthermore, the leukocyte adhesion molecule ICAM-1, regulated by VEGF, has been shown to increase following irradiation of the mouse brain, attracting leukocytes [282]. Blethen et al. performed 15.5 Gy whole-brain radiations in immunocompetent and athymic mouse models. They showed that the BBB permeability was altered in the immunocompetent model as early as 12 h after whole-brain radiation but not in the immunocompromised, suggesting that functional T-cells may have a role in irradiation-induced BBB disruption [283]. They hypothesize that TNF-α, Th17 cells, and IL-17 mediate the effect on the BBB. Their theory was supported by measurements of increased TNF-α acutely following radiation in the immunocompetent group [283]. Interestingly, another study has shown that anti-TNF treatment decreases the BBB disruption caused by radiation in mice, strengthening the role of TNF in radiation-induced BBB disruption [284]. Blethen et al. also observed a significant decrease in efflux protein activity in the immunocompetent mice; however, this returned to normal 24 h postradiation. They speculate that there is an immune response-dependent time window when efflux transporter activity is decreased following whole-brain radiation therapy [283]. Based on these findings, the group conducted experiments demonstrating that administering α-CTLA-4 immunotherapy in a mouse model of lung cancer brain metastases 12 h postradiation gave a significantly decreased tumor burden compared to administration 24 h before radiation [285]. These findings may have implications for understanding the optimal timing for immunomodulating therapies combined with radiation and delivery of other therapeutic agents.

Radiotherapy is used for many malignant brain lesions [286]. The effects of radiation on the BBB have, though, been explored scarcely in a clinical setting, and the optimal timing for drug delivery in light of radiation-induced BBB disruption is currently unclear. Lim et al. showed that gadolinium accumulation in supratentorial glioblastomas was significantly higher on MR imaging postradiation therapy as compared to before radiation [287]. Teng et al. showed that patients who received whole-brain radiotherapy or stereotactic radiosurgery for metastatic brain cancer had lesions showing greater permeability on dynamic contrast-enhanced (DCE) MR imaging compared to controls. They suggest that DCE MRI may be used to select and personalize the optimal time of drug administration in patients following radiotherapy. They observed that the change in BBB permeability was highly heterogeneous and dependent on the baseline permeability of the tumor, the type and dosage of radiation, and the type of tumor. Nevertheless, they concluded that the increased BBB permeability postradiation lasts for at least 1 month for low-permeability metastatic lesions and may peak at 2–4 weeks [288]. More studies are needed to understand how the timing of drug delivery can be optimized after radiation in brain tumors.

Hyperthermia

Using heat to treat cancers has been theorized since the nineteenth century [289]. Initially, systemic hyperthermia was believed to invoke tumor regression [290]. In modern medicine, this has evolved into localized heat-based ablation of tumors [291]. Several mechanisms for cell and tumor vulnerability to locally delivered heat have been suggested. For example, it has been speculated that tumor tissue is more vulnerable to heat than healthy tissue due to a decreased heat-dissipating ability and an increased baseline acidic environment [292]. Excessive heat can induce necrosis and/or apoptosis on a cellular level. This occurs through damaging effects on cellular components such as the cell membrane, the mitochondria, the cytoskeleton, and a range of proteins involved in cell cycle regulation [292].

In the field of brain tumors, laser interstitial thermal therapy (LITT) is a heat-based method that has been utilized to ablate brain tumors [293]. In LITT, a laser probe is delivered through a burr hole in the skull, localizing to the tumor intracranially using stereotactic navigation and intraoperative MRI [292]. The mechanism entails delivering laser photons to the tumor tissue; photons are converted into thermal energy, which subsequently damages the surrounding cells [289]. More recent studies using LITT and advanced MRI-based imaging methods have confirmed that LITT increases human BBB permeability. Bartlett et al. used DCE-MRI and serum neuron-specific enolase (NSE) levels to assess BBB permeability following LITT delivery in recurrent glioblastomas. They saw that serum NSE significantly increased, peaking at 2 weeks following ablation and returning to baseline at 8 weeks post-LITT. The same pattern was seen in DCE-MRI [294]. Similarly, Leuthardt et al. found an increased BBB permeability in recurrent glioblastomas following LITT as measured by DCE-MRI, with the permeability peaking in 1–3 weeks post-LITT and reaching baseline by 6 weeks [295]. Butt et al. studied the effects of survival when doxorubicin was delivered following LITT in recurrent glioblastomas, comparing it to historical data from standard salvage therapy with bevacizumab with or without LITT. The overall survival was significantly improved in the group receiving LITT, followed by doxorubicin [296].

In preclinical settings, it has long been known that the delivery of heat to the brain induces increased BBB permeability and, thus, potentially enhances the effects of chemotherapeutic agents [297–299]. Salehi et al. sought to dissect the mechanisms of increased BBB permeability following LITT in a preclinical in vivo setting. They saw an increased endothelial transcytosis across the BBB following LITT treatment. Furthermore, they saw a decrease in claudin-5 levels in the plasma levels following heat therapy, suggesting an effect on the tight junction function [300].

Heating tumors also affect the immunoenvironment, inducing adaptive and innate immune responses. These effects are partly mediated by heat shock proteins (HSPs), chaperone proteins expressed during increased environmental stress. In addition to acting as chaperon proteins, HSPs act as signaling molecules engaging dendritic cells and macrophages [301]. Preclinical in vivo studies have shown that HSP proteins produced by tumors following heat delivery may increase the chemoattraction of dendritic cells and T cells, inducing antitumoral immunity [302]. Perhaps these immunogenic changes could be utilized to enhance immunotherapy in brain tumors [303].

In summary, thermal therapies can be directly tumor cytoablative and enhance the effectiveness of other treatments. More studies are needed to understand the dynamics of BBB opening following LITT and the best-suited combinatory therapies.

Monitoring BBB Disruption

Monitoring blood-brain barrier disruption is crucial in both clinical and preclinical contexts. High-quality monitoring is necessary to assess the procedure's effectiveness and potential harms and to understand disruption dynamics. Excessive disruption can lead to vasogenic edema and ensuing neurological damage, such as secondary infarction. Suboptimal disruption can make the treatment an unnecessary cost without benefit. Several methods may be used to monitor BBB disruption. These methods are summarized below:

Contrast Extravasation

One of the most common methods used to study BBB disruption, both in a clinical and a preclinical setting, is the imaging of contrast that extravasates from the blood vessels and into the brain parenchyma or the tumor. Although CT and MRI have been used for this technique, most studies use MRI with gadolinium-based contrast agents as a standard method. This technique is used in the laboratory with animal models and in the clinic with patients [206, 304].

The movement of gadolinium-based contrast agents across the BBB and into brain and tumor tissue is foundational for contrast enhancement and, thus, a metric for BBB permeability. Several studies mentioned in the previous section used gadolinium-based contrast, including Gd-DTPA and Gd-DOTA, to measure BBB permeability [206, 236, 252]. These types of contrast agents generally have molecular weights of 500–1000 Da. The BBB is generally permeable to small lipophilic molecules with molecular weights <500 Da. Therefore, disruptions in the BBB caused either by the tumor itself or through the variety of methods described will increase their permeability and show contrast enhancement on the MR image.

All techniques mentioned in this chapter cause a transient opening of the BBB. As such, it is crucial that the timing of the drug delivery is within the window of BBB opening. The temporal aspects of BBB opening seem highly variable and dependent on many factors such as patient, tumor type, technique used, and periprocedural circumstances. Therefore, individualized monitoring is needed. Detection of contrast extravasation through MRI provides an opportunity to study the BBB opening and optimize therapy delivery in each patient. It also allows for recovery assessment and return to baseline BBB function following a procedure. As such, contrast extravasation and its capture through MRI will be vital in implementing BBB disruption techniques.

Certain limitations exist regarding contrast extravasation. Contrast extravasation is limited to a level of BBB disruption that allows for the passage of gadolinium-based agents, generally >500 Da. Thus, the sensitivity to minor permeability changes is not high. Furthermore, contrast-based imaging is invasive (requiring an injection of the contrast agent), and repeated permeability measurements are restricted to the systemic clearance of the contrast agent and cannot be performed continuously [305]. The contrast agents used in MRI are believed to cross the BBB only through the paracellular route. Therefore, this method does not adequately quantify other routes of BBB passage, such as through transporters and the transcellular route [306]. In addition, MRI with contrast can be complicated by artifacts that lead to the misinterpretation of BBB leakage due to background noise [306].

Fluid Shift

Fluid shift, a measure of BBB permeability, utilizes MRI to measure water exchange from the intravascular space to the extravascular space across the BBB. There are several benefits to using water as a proxy for BBB permeability instead of gadolinium-based contrast agents. The water molecule is smaller and more permeable, resulting in faster transport across the BBB [307]. Beyond paracellular transport in BBB disruption, water is transported transcellularly across the BBB via passive diffusion, aquaporins, and carrier-mediated transport through transporter proteins of other substrates where it is cotransported (e.g., glucose transporters) [308]. This means more subtle changes in the barrier environment that affect the natural water transport mechanisms can be detected. For example, it has been suggested that altered expression of aquaporin 4 is a common phenomenon in gliomas [309]. Imaging water exchange with MRI permits early observation of such changes.

MRI can measure water exchange with or without contrast agents. Contrast agent-based techniques increase the difference in intravascular and extravascular signals, making it easier to differentiate between the water inside the vessels and the water that has shifted into the tissue [306]. One benefit of using contrast agents is that they allow for estimations of the total cerebral volume, which can be used to calculate the amount of water exchanged per unit of time. In contrast, the non-contrast techniques only convey information about the exchange frequency of each water molecule [310]. Non-contrast MRI techniques include arterial spin-labeling and double-diffusion encoding MRI [306]. The arterial spin-labeling technique is noninvasive and examines the movement of labeled water from inside the arteries through the vasculature and into the tissue [306]. The double-diffusion encoding MRI uses filter-exchange imaging to measure water exchange by harnessing natural differences in water diffusion between extravascular and intravascular compartments [310].

The challenges of water exchange imaging include accurately distinguishing signals from each compartment, accurately modeling compartmental water dynamics, and interpreting data in the context of overall BBB permeability [310].

Nuclear Imaging

Radiotracers are compounds with a radioactive isotope linked to a carrier molecule [311].The two techniques frequently used for measuring radiotracers in the brain are single-photon emission computed tomography (SPECT) and positron emission tomography (PET):

- SPECT is the oldest of these, and it has classically been used with Technetium-99m (Tc-99m)-based radiotracers to measure cerebral blood flow [312]. A gamma camera captures the emission of single gamma rays by the Tc-99m and reconstructs them into 3D images [313]. It has been shown that Tc-99m tracers can passively diffuse across the BBB [314]. As such, Tc-99m compounds have been used to measure BBB permeability. For example, Lin et al. showed that TC-99m-DTPA can be used with SPECT to measure FUS-induced BBB opening in rats [315].
- PET imaging: Unlike SPECT, the radiotracers used in PET emit positrons. These positrons engage with nearby structures, and each interaction results in the emission of two photons in opposite directions, which are detected by a PET scanner. Generally, PET scanning has higher spatial resolution, better quantification, and uses radiotracers with shorter half-lives. As such, it is considered more suitable for BBB permeability measurement [316].

Okada et al. compared the detection of BBB permeability through PET imaging using the radiotracer 2-amino-isobutyric acid [3-11C]-AIB, with Evans blue ex vivo and with Gd-DTPA enhanced MRI in vivo in rats. They used FUS and lipopolysaccharides to disrupt the BBB. The ex vivo studies showed a linear correlation between the [3-11C]-AIB and Evans blue, demonstrating its feasibility. Furthermore, in vivo, they saw that Gd-DTPA intensity in MR imaging reached its maximum after 10 min, whereas [3-11C]-AIB showed an increase during the session, which lasted for 60 min. They attributed this to the transport mechanisms of the two compounds, Gd-DTPA being transported bidirectionally, whereas ([3-11C]-AIB) is transported unidirectionally and irreversibly. In addition, they considered the higher spatial resolution of PET to serve as explanation for this result. The authors argue that [3-11C]-AIB PET can monitor temporal changes in BBB permeability in a way not achievable by Gd-DTPA MR imaging [316]. Furthermore, PET imaging can be used to measure the function of efflux transporters, which, as mentioned previously in this chapter, are vital components of the BBB. For example, PET with [11C]-verapamil, [11C]-*N*-desmethyl-loperamide, and [11C]-metoclopramide have been used to measure the function of the efflux transporter P-gp [317]. Also, PET imaging has the potential to measure glucose transport across the BBB. Using fludeoxyglucose (FDG) PET is significant as it can provide insights into the brain's metabolic activity. In the case of tumors, this can be used to measure the metabolism of the tumor cells [318]. PET imaging with radiolabeled albumin may be used to measure more extensive disruptions in the BBB [319].

The varied routes that radiotracers can take across the BBB and their interactions with BBB components make an opportunity to measure aspects of BBB permeability that contrast extravasation does not. However, more studies are needed to understand when nuclear imaging can be beneficial compared to the more common and widely available contrast extravasation MRI [310].

Electroencephalography

Kiviniemi et al. used direct current electroencephalography (DC-EEG) to monitor the effects of BBB disruption with IC mannitol before chemotherapy administration in primary CNS lymphomas. Forty-seven patients receiving routine IC mannitol before their chemotherapy saw a real-time robust and multiphasic response in the EEG channels that monitored the treated arterial territory [320]. The changes in DC-EEG are believed to represent the voltage changes across the BBB [321]. Thus, DC-EEG may have the potential for a real-time, noninvasive monitoring technique for BBB disruption.

Somatosensory Evoked Potentials

Several studies have utilized somatosensory evoked potentials (SSEP) to measure BBB permeability. SSEP depicts neuromodulation in the brain. It measures the brain's electrical activity in response to sensory stimuli applied to the body, particularly to peripheral nerves. Chu et al. investigated changes in SSEP in rats following manipulation of the BBB with MB-FUS. They found that SSEP suppression occurred with higher intensities of FUS and that the effects lasted 7 days, suggesting that FUS-induced opening of the BBB causes reversible changes in neuron responses [322]. A 1989 study on dogs showed that suppression of SSEPs is also seen with intracarotid hypertonic infusion of saline and mannitol [323]. SSEP is already an established neuromodulation measurement technique, therefore it has excellent potential for use in clinical BBB disruption monitoring and it should be further explored.

Intravital Microscopy

Intravital microscopy is a technique for observing biological processes in vivo at high resolution and in real time. It involves using specialized microscopes with imaging systems to penetrate tissues and visualize cellular dynamics within living organisms [324]. This technique is valuable for studying various physiological and pathological processes in vivo in a laboratory setting.

Intravital microscopy utilizes multiphoton imaging and near-infrared lasers to excite and detect fluorophores. With BBB permeability, this can be done using either dyes such as fluorescent dextran or cell-specific fluorescent markers [310]. Intravital microscopy has helped us understand several BBB-related processes, including the physiology of functional hyperemia, increased permeability of liposomes in stroke, visualizing leukocyte diapedesis, and glial scarring following brain injury [310].

Poon et al. developed a protocol for creating a cranial window in mouse models, through which increased BBB permeability during FUS can be visualized using fluorescent dextran and intravital multiphoton microscopy. This protocol allows for real-time visualization of the effects of FUS on the BBB [325]. Waithe et al. developed a similar protocol for visualization of the BBB in traumatic brain injury models [326]. However, the authors do report certain limitations and challenges. Intravital microscopy requires exposure of the brain parenchyma, and invasive surgery can disrupt the tissue microenvironment through inflammation [327]. Furthermore, the microscopes increase the brain temperature, which may cause cellular damage [328]. Microscopes also have limitations regarding the depth of the brain, requiring further invasive procedures to visualize deeper cortical structures [325].

In summary, intravital microscopy is a promising technique for obtaining real-time high-resolution visualization of cellular processes at the BBB. However, its dependency on invasive procedures to expose the brain makes it mainly applicable in a preclinical setting.

Other Markers

Evans Blue

Evans blue was first used to measure BBB permeability in the 1960s and has been widely employed in the laboratory. Evans blue binds to serum albumin, which does not cross the BBB in normal healthy conditions. Thus, the entry of Evans blue-bound albumin into the CNS indicates increased BBB permeability. However, Evans blue has several limitations, including a lack of specificity in binding, inappropriate quantitative methods, and a lack of appropriate carrier solutions that do not affect the structure of the dye [319].

Radiolabeled Sucrose

Sucrose is a molecule with low molecular weight (342 Da), neutral charge, and hydrophilicity. Additionally, sucrose does not bind to proteins. Given its characteristics, the penetration of sucrose across the BBB is limited in healthy conditions but increases with greater disruption. 14C sucrose, a radiolabeled type of sucrose, has been recognized as one of the most accurate and widely established dyes for measuring BBB permeability in a laboratory setting. It is given intravenously, and the BBB permeability is measured by assessing the brain's radioactivity level. More recent studies have refined the use of sucrose and generated new versions of radiolabeled sucrose [329].

Radiolabeled Inulin

Inulin, a polymer of a variable number of fructose molecules, displays great size and molecular weight heterogeneity. Intrinsic BBB permeability hence varies between inulin batches. Although radiolabeled inulin can be used to quantify BBB permeability, its size and size variability limit its ability to assess permeability and integrity for smaller molecules [330].

Sodium Fluorescein

Sodium fluorescein is slightly larger than sucrose (376 Da) and displays only weak protein binding. Compared to the radiolabeled tracers, sodium fluorescein is more sensitive to more discrete changes in BBB permeability [331]. Furthermore, unlike Evans blue, sodium fluorescein has not displayed toxic effects in vivo [332]. As such, it has become one of the more popular markers for measuring BBB integrity [332].

Dextrans

Dextrans are polysaccharides with glucose molecule branches. They can be labeled with different entities, most commonly fluorophores or biotin. The biotin-labeled dextrans are visible on both light and electron microscopy [333]. There have been varied results regarding toxicity using dextrans, specifically anaphylaxis, which appears to be dose-dependent [334–336].

Complications of BBB Disruption

It is essential to assess the safety and impact of BBB disruption. The complications and risks are diverse and depend on the method used. Complications can be procedure-related or secondary to the actual disruption mechanism:

Procedure-Related Complications

Procedure-related complications include issues related to catheterization from the femoral artery to the targeted cranial artery. These issues involve tears in the subintimal tissue during catheterization, thrombosis in the associated parent vessel, and groin hematoma at the arterial access site. Thrombosis can lead to ischemic injury in the affected vascular distribution and related neurological deficits. Judicious anticoagulation and antiplatelet treatment can minimize this risk [337].

Seizures

Disruption of the BBB is a contributing factor in the pathogenesis of several neurological conditions. It has been suggested that BBB disruption contributes to seizure activity in the brain. Greene et al. showed a correlation between epilepsy and BBB dysfunction, specifically claudin-5 dysfunction [338]. In temporal lobe tissue resected from patients with temporal lobe epilepsy, claudin-5 expression was decreased. In these same epileptic patients, BBB disruption was also evidenced by increased pre-surgical gadolinium extravasation on DCE-MRI as compared to control. Furthermore, mice with heterogeneous expression of claudin-5 had a higher susceptibility to seizures from kainic acid than wild-type mice. The mice also showed more CNS inflammation, possibly through increased expression of cell adhesion molecules such as ICAM-1. These findings suggest that modulation of the BBB permeability, specifically via claudin-5, consequentially leads to increased susceptibility to seizure activity [338]. Another study on rats showed that increased BBB permeability visualized on MRI is a significant predictor for the occurrence of seizure activity 4–8 weeks later [339]. The link between epileptogenic mechanism and BBB disruption has not been fully uncovered. A potential mechanistic link between BBB disruption and increased seizure activity is the downstream result of serum albumin extravasation into the brain tissue following its binding to TGF-β receptors in astrocytes, which leads to a range of microenvironmental changes known to increase the likelihood of seizure [340, 341].

In a clinical trial with IC mannitol for increased delivery of chemotherapy in a range of different types of brain tumors, 16.1% of patients had a seizure within 3 days after the procedure. There was a significantly higher seizure rate in patients receiving IA chemotherapeutic delivery with osmotic disruption as compared to patients with IA chemotherapeutic delivery without osmotic disruption [342]. These findings have been consistent with those of other trials [181, 185]. In the context of induced BBB disruption for therapeutic purposes, it is essential to study the relationship between seizure and increased BBB permeability, as this can be a source of misinterpretation.

Focal Neurological Deficits

Focal neurological deficits in the context of BBB disruption can theoretically arise due to damage and irritation in localized areas or as the result of global edema accentuating stress on eloquent brain regions and/or tissue compromised by tumors. One early study by Doolittle et al. studying the effect of IA mannitol and chemotherapy for several malignant brain tumors reported transient neurological deficits, such as hemiparesis and aphasia, in a minority of patients [167]. Doolittle et al. correlated this to the known BBB disruption-induced increase in total brain water, estimated at least 1.5% [343, 344]. Patients were treated with steroids, and symptoms resolved within 48 h. In a study with long-term follow-up for patients with PCNSL treated with IA mannitol and chemotherapy, similar deficits were noted in the minority. 1.1% of patients had symptoms that lasted longer than 48 h, and all eventually returned to their baseline [345]. Multiple studies on the safety and efficacy of FUS, a localized modality for disruption, have all reported no incidence of BBB disruption-related focal neurological deficits, even when applied near eloquent regions [346–348]. Continued monitoring for focal deficits is essential to ensure the safety of BBB disruption methods.

Cerebral Edema

There is a link between BBB disruption and cerebral edema. Studies on osmotic BBB disruption in rats have shown that total brain water increases by approximately 1.5% [343, 344]. This has been described in the context of ischemic stroke, which also accentuates the link between BBB disruption and cerebral edema. Following ischemic insult in the brain, there is evidence of increased transcellular and paracellular transport of fluids across the BBB. The opening of the BBB in ischemic stroke leads to both cytogenic and vasogenic edema [349]. Giraud et al. have reported evidence of BBB disruption in ischemic stroke on MRI, using post-contrast T1-weighted images to discern enhancement of leptomeninges and parenchyma within areas where diffusion-weighted imaging was consistent with stroke [350]. Ionic homeostasis disruption following BBB disruption in ischemia contributes to disturbed paracellular transport. This disruption is mediated by increased activity of BBB transporters, which enhance the transcellular transport of Na^+ and Cl—from the blood into the brain [351]. After ischemic insult, a structural disruption of tight junction proteins from oxidative stress is also present. Molecular changes to tight junction proteins, such as phosphorylation and MMP activity, contribute to the tight junction alteration by degrading vital TJ proteins. The weakening of tight junction proteins leads to increased paracellular transport and contributes to edema [352, 353].

Similarly, brain tumor-related edema is believed to result from the disruption of healthy BBB functions. Unlike the artificially induced BBB disruption methods suggested in this text, ischemic stroke and brain tumors cause disruption from a pathologic insult to the brain. However, there are similarities in some of the affected structures, such as tight junction disruption. Thus, studies on the effects of ischemic stroke and tumors and the resultant BBB disruption may help to understand how cerebral edema can occur as a consequence of therapeutic BBB disruption.

Increased ICP

Increased intracranial pressure (ICP) due to BBB disruption is a well-documented adverse effect that has been documented in many different contexts. It is intrinsically connected to mechanisms of cerebral edema. Specifically, it has been extensively studied in traumatic brain injury. Increased leakiness of the BBB results in vasogenic edema in the brain, elevating the ICP. Furthermore, dysfunction of BBB structures that maintain the homeostasis of the brain, such as ion pumps, results in cytotoxic edema [354]. If severe, this may result in fatal consequences such as herniation of the brain. Doolittle et al. studied the safety of the osmotic opening of the BBB in conjunction with chemotherapy for brain tumors. In the paper, they report brain herniation as a significant adverse event, occurring in 4 of 221 patients, 3 of whom died [346]. Of the three fatalities, only one had received BBB disruption. The other two received intra-arterial chemotherapy without disruption of the BBB. An image review of these cases demonstrated high-volume, infiltrating gliomas with rapid growth patterns. As such, the danger of mass effect should be considered for intra-arterial BBB disruption and intra-arterial chemotherapy. The authors concluded that both treatments, alone or together, are safest when given before the tumor burden leaves little margin for brain swelling.

Maculopathy

Maculopathy was first reported in patients who underwent IC mannitol treatment in 1986 by Millay et al. [355]. This correlation has often been reported in the context of PCNSL treatment, where hypertonic mannitol has been utilized to increase drug delivery. The intracarotid administration of hypertonic solutes not only affects the BBB but also impacts the blood-retinal barrier, leading to an increased susceptibility of the retina to therapeutic agents, which may cause direct damage. However, whether the mechanism of the maculopathy is a consequence of the chemotherapy agents or the BBB disruption is not entirely known. Simonett et al. recently reported a correlation between the number of osmotic BBB disruption sessions and maculopathy. In a case series of 68 patients who were treated with IA mannitol and systemic chemotherapy for different brain tumors and who underwent ophthalmic examination after their procedure, 49.2% of the patients were found to have pigmentary maculopathy. The number of treatment sessions was shown to be correlated with maculopathy development [356].

Enhanced Contrast Toxicity

As described earlier in this chapter, one of the most established methods of measuring the degree of BBB disruption is increased extravasation of contrast agents on imaging. Radiocontrast or gadolinium are two commonly utilized agents [357]. Although contrast agents are commonly associated with adverse effects on other organ systems than the brain, most prominently nephrotoxicity, understanding their effects on the brain is essential in BBB disruption monitoring [358, 359].

The effect of gadolinium on the brain is a topic of debate [360]. In 2014, Kanda et al. first reported a correlation between high signal intensity in the dentate nucleus and the globus pallidus on unenhanced T1-weighted MR imaging and the number of previous gadolinium-based contrast administrations, suggesting retention of gadolinium in these areas [361]. Other case reports have supported this finding [362]. Although a source of concern, there is no clear evidence that this finding has clinical implications. BBB disruption may enhance this phenomenon. Thus, further investigation is needed.

Contrast-induced neurotoxicity, also known as contrast-induced encephalopathy or acute transient contrast-induced neurological deficit, is a typically transient condition associated with the intra-arterial administration of iodinated contrast agents. Although rare, it has been described in the literature since 1970 [363]. It is most often characterized by visual deficits; however, other focal neurological deficits, such as motor or sensory loss, aphasia, and even affected consciousness, have also been reported [364, 365]. One hypothesis regarding the pathophysiology of this condition attributes it to a weakening of the BBB, which leads to extravasation of the contrast agent into the brain parenchyma [366, 367]. Thus, it is increasingly seen in the neuro-interventional field, where iodinated contrast is directly injected into the diseased brain under angiographic guidance [367]. In BBB disruption, this becomes relevant in the intra-arterial drug delivery methods, where iodinated contrast agents are used.

Other agents, such as tracers used in positron emission tomography (PET), are also subject to changes in permeability post-BBB disruption. The most common PET tracers include Tc-99m-based agents, fluorodeoxyglucose, and radiolabeled albumin. Of these, albumin has documented neurotoxicity and risks intraparenchymal accumulation and toxicity with increased BBB permeability [368].

Enhanced Chemotherapeutic Toxicity

BBB disruption increases chemotherapeutic penetration to tumor cells and healthy brain tissue, increasing the risk for neurotoxicity. Notably, several chemotherapeutic agents, including carboplatin, cisplatin, doxorubicin, etoposide phosphate, and 5-fluorouracil, have displayed substantial neurotoxicity in the context of BBB disruption in preclinical experiments. This showcases the need for targeted as opposed to general BBB disruption and the importance of recalibrating therapeutic regimens for BBB-disrupted milieus [369–371]. Nonetheless, in diffusely infiltrating gliomas, such recalibrations may also decrease therapeutic efficacy by preventing the targeting of tumor cells in areas with intact BBB.

Accelerating Pathogenesis

As discussed previously, aggressive tumors display their own BBB disruption. This disruption partly allows for increased uptake of systemic metabolites, aiding tumor progression [372]. Currently, there are no studies on the direct effects of induced, artificial BBB disruption on the proliferation of gliomas. Conceivably, BBB disruption paired with antiproliferative treatment can overcome any metabolic advantage the tumor receives secondary to increased BBB permeability. Short-lived BBB disruption also diminishes these risks.

Emerging Methods for Drug Delivery across the BBB

Recent advancements in BBB drug delivery have stimulated interest in nanomedical developments, leveraging natural transport mechanisms across the BBB. Additionally, minimally invasive techniques to bypass the BBB are under development. This section delves into some of these emerging methods:

Coopting Natural Transport Mechanisms

The BBB has developed various mechanisms to transport substances such as nutrients, metabolites, ions, and waste products from the blood to the brain and vice versa. These are generally either carrier-mediated transport or transcytosis, as described earlier [95]. Both mechanisms have been manipulated to deliver drugs to the brain and brain tumors.

Carrier-Mediated Transport

Efforts are being made to utilize membrane transport proteins to deliver drugs into the brain. Principally, this can be done through three different methods: (1) modifying the drug so that it engages directly with the transporter in the shape of a prodrug, (2) conjugating the drug with a molecule that naturally engages with the transporter, or (3) coating the drug with a nanoparticle that is similar to the substrate of the transporter [95].

Several of the SLC family of transport proteins have been targeted in glioma models. For example, Li et al. targeted the large amino acid transporter 1 (LAT1) in glioma cells using docetaxel-loaded liposomes with modified glutamate. In vivo, fluorescent imaging demonstrated that the glutamate-modified liposomes had higher BBB penetration than the unmodified liposomes [373]. Bhunia et al. showed that targeting LAT1 with liposomes conjugated with L-dopa can increase delivery of the JAK2/STAT3 inhibitor WP1066, and increase survival in mice with orthotopic glioblastoma [374]. Some other transporters targeted to deliver anticancer drugs to brain glioma models include glucose transporters [375, 376], sodium ascorbic acid cotransporters [376, 377], and carnitine transporters [378].

Targeting SLC transporter proteins mainly applies to smaller hydrophilic molecules with specific molecular selectivity and size [379]. However, even for such molecules, mechanistic and pharmacokinetic studies are needed to move from preclinical studies to successful clinical trials [95].

Receptor-Mediated Transcytosis

Transcytosis, a transport mechanism across the BBB for larger solutes, can be initiated by receptor ligand interactions (receptor-mediated transcytosis) or cationic proteins encountering the anionic cell membrane (adsorption-mediated transcytosis). Studies have looked at modifying drugs to breach the BBB using these mechanisms.

Drugs can be modified to target receptor-mediated transcytosis using a receptor-targeting compound. The receptor ligand can be conjugated directly with the drug, through a linker, or on the surface of a nanoparticle [92]. Ligands for receptor-mediated transcytosis include monoclonal antibodies, endogenous receptor ligands, and peptides that mimic ligands [91]. For receptor-mediated transcytosis to work, receptors with endocytic capability must be targeted. Some of the most studied targets in the brain include the low-density lipoprotein receptor, the transferrin receptor, and the insulin receptor [380].

Adsorption-Mediated Transcytosis

Targeting adsorption-mediated transcytosis is based on coating/linking the drug with cationic components, which may induce transcytosis when in contact with the cell membrane. Cationic components can be obtained through protein cationization or by using cell-penetrating peptides [106]. Protein cationization is achieved by chemically modifying the carboxylic acid group of a protein with diamines and polyamines [106]. This method has been used to modify and increase the delivery of antibodies across the BBB [381].

One limitation of the adsorption-mediated transcytosis techniques is that they are relatively unspecific and can target any cell membrane once administered. More targeted versions are under development [106].

Cell-Penetrating Peptides

Cell-penetrating peptides (CPPs), also known as protein transduction domains, were discovered when studying the

HIV Tat protein's ability to penetrate cell membranes and deliver cargo into cells [382, 383]. The CPPs are short peptides with a length of 10–30 amino acids, either derived from natural proteins, synthetically engineered, or a mix of both (chimeric) [384]. The cationic CPPs contain positive charges from residues such as arginine and lysine that can interact with negative charges on the cell membrane. They can also contain an amphipathic sequence that engages with the lipid membrane [106]. CPPs can directly either penetrate the cells themselves or translocate a "cargo" across cell membranes in lipid rafts [384]. Interestingly, the exact transport mechanism via cell-penetrating peptides is a topic of debate [385]. It is believed that they can permeate the cell membrane in either an energy-independent way, also referred to as direct translocation, or in an energy-dependent way, with mechanisms similar to adsorption-based endocytosis [386]. As of now, 1855 different types of CPPs have been discovered [387]. They deliver fluorophores, nucleic acids, proteins, nanoparticles, peptides, and drug compounds [387].

Bypassing the BBB

Several techniques under investigation are aimed at bypassing the BBB without the need to disrupt it. These techniques aim to deliver the drugs through routes other than the blood. Some of these are discussed below:

Intrathecal Delivery

Intrathecal delivery is a method that allows for direct drug injections into the CSF space. This can be performed at several locations, including in the spinal cord, cerebral ventricles, or large brain cisterns such as cisterna magna [388]. The latter is more commonly used in animal models. This is an invasive procedure that requires surgical access to intrathecal space. It often involves placing a pump or catheter system, allowing continuous therapeutic administration [388]. Intrathecal therapy can achieve higher drug concentrations in the CNS with lower systemic exposure, potentially reducing systemic side effects and improving therapeutic efficacy. In clinical practice, intrathecal lumbar delivery has been used to administer narcotics and baclofen to patients with chronic pain or movement problems [389, 390]. Furthermore, the delivery of antitumor agents in the brain ventricles is also being explored [391].

Biodegradable Materials

Hydrogels and polymeric implants have long been studied for the local delivery of chemotherapeutic agents in brain tumors. One prominently studied biodegradable wafer is the carmustine-releasing Gliadel wafer, which was introduced in the early 1990s [392]. In a range of clinical trials, the Gliadel wafer showed increased survival compared to placebo wafers, and as such, the FDA approved it for both recurrent and primary gliomas [393]. Following the introduction of the Stupp protocol in 2005 [394], the Gliadel wafers ended up in the shadow of temozolomide and radiotherapy.

Recently, there has been a renewed interest in biodegradable materials. Several groups explored the local placement of new biodegradable materials loaded with therapeutic compounds [395]. These include biodegradable microneedles, which have allowed for increased precision for local delivery. Microneedles have a minimal shaft length of <1000 μm and can be either solid, hollow, coated, dissolving, or hydrogel-forming [396]. They are placed into the tissue of interest, and therapeutics are slowly delivered through them [397]. Most microneedles studies have focused on transdermal drug delivery systems. However, they are also being employed to bypass the BBB. For example, Lee et al. demonstrated the localized delivery of nanoparticles in in vivo mouse tumor models using bioresorbable microneedles, followed by the delivery of high-energy photons using light-guiding/spreading microneedles [398].

Intranasal Administration

Drugs administered intranasally are believed to reach the brain through three different paths. These include (1) the olfactory nerve, (2) the trigeminal nerve, and (3) the blood (via the lungs or the gastrointestinal system) [399, 400]. The neuronal pathways are believed to be the major contributors [400, 401]. Transport toward the brain occurs both extracellularly and intracellularly [399]. In the olfactory nerve path, once the drug has passed the cribriform plate, it spreads out within the CNS through the perivascular spaces [399]. One of the main benefits of intranasal delivery is that it is the only noninvasive method for direct delivery into the brain. Furthermore, the proximity to the brain allows for a relatively fast delivery [400]. Limitations to intranasal delivery include poor permeability to the nasal mucosa, mucociliary clearance, degradation, and nasomucosal toxicity [399]. Furthermore, the notion that the route from the nose to the brain is direct has been questioned. For example, van den Berg et al. demonstrated no difference in the CSF-to-plasma ratio of hydroxocobalamin in rats when they compared intranasal delivery with IV delivery [402]. However, another group showed an enhanced delivery of 17 beta-estradiol intranasally compared to IV administration [403]. Other compounds that have been delivered to the brain through intranasal administration in preclinical models include siRNAs [404], mesenchymal stem cells [405], and polymer nanoparticles [406].

What Is the Future of BBB Disruption?

This chapter has touched upon some key aspects of BBB disruption, particularly its implications in brain tumor therapy. As emphasized, leveraging BBB disruption to augment drug permeability within brain and tumor tissues represents a promising avenue of research that has been translated into various clinical trials. Here, some pivotal considerations necessary for further advancing this field are lifted.

Further efforts are needed to understand and mitigate the potential damages inflicted by BBB disruption on the healthy brain. Some of these complications have been raised in this chapter. Given the role of BBB breakdown in numerous neurological diseases [407], understanding the long-term consequences of BBB disruption is clinically highly relevant. As such, robust preclinical models to study pathobiological mechanisms are necessary. While most preclinical studies are conducted on rodents, differences in brain vasculature dynamics and BBB physiology between rodents and humans underscore the importance of caution when translating such research into clinical practice [408]. Developing technologies with higher precision is essential to mitigate the damaging effects of BBB disruption. By achieving a localized BBB disruption, collateral damage to healthy brain tissue will be minimized. Moreover, aside from the potential inherent damage that BBB disruption does to the healthy brain, it may also enhance drug toxicity due to the higher and more penetrable concentrations. Consequently, a reassessment of pharmacodynamics in the light of a manipulated BBB is required. Furthermore, the influence of BBB disruption on the hematogenous spread of tumor cells and tumor multifocality needs to be explored.

Several methods for monitoring BBB permeability are discussed in this chapter, with MRI (contrast extravasation/fluid shift measurement) and PET emerging as potentially clinically scalable methods. Neuromonitoring with EEG and SSEPs may also play a role in a clinical setting. Intravital microscopy has opened an avenue to a deeper understanding of the mechanisms of BBB disruption in preclinical models. These methods will play a role in understanding the duration and character of the BBB disruption, i.e., the therapeutic window. The BBB/BTB physiology is highly complex and heterogeneous with interindividual variation. Various factors, including tumor type, tumor location, vascular hydrodynamics, concomitant vascular or neurological diseases, and the specific therapy delivered, can influence the effects of disruption. As such, real-time monitoring of the BBB permeability will allow for a personalized procedure, guiding the optimal timing of drug delivery. In addition, monitoring the BBB will allow for the detection of barrier recovery following a procedure, thereby increasing the procedure's safety.

Lastly, developing intra-arterial drug delivery will play a key role in therapeutic delivery following BBB disruption. As highlighted in this chapter, many BBB disruption studies utilize concomitant drug delivery through the IA route. IA drug delivery may result in up to 50-fold increases in tumor tissue drug concentrations compared to IV delivery [151]. Advances in microcatheterization techniques allow for an even higher selectivity and precision of drug delivery with BBB disruption. IA delivery, in combination with BBB disruption, provides an excellent opportunity for enhanced drug delivery into the brain.

In summary, BBB disruption may play a pivotal role in the delivery of drugs to the brain. Not least in the field of neuro-oncology, where restricted drug access has remained a significant hurdle for effective treatments, resulting in dire outcomes for patients. Increased efforts are needed to understand the physiological effects of BBB disruption and its consequences. Furthermore, improved monitoring techniques used during BBB disruption procedures will help increase safety and efficiency. Lastly, transient localized BBB disruption technologies could play an essential role in improving the outcome.

Conclusion

In conclusion, this chapter reviewed the current state of BBB disruption to enhance drug delivery. The BBB remains a significant limiting factor for effectively delivering several chemotherapeutic drugs and novel antibodies used in cancer treatments. Ineffective drug delivery has impeded treatment advances for cancer and other neurological diseases. A deeper understanding of the anatomy and physiology of the BBB is necessary for effective manipulation of it. The roles of various components, how they limit drug delivery, and how they can be manipulated must be better understood. Several methods for disrupting the BBB, including both drug- and device-based methods, are emerging. In addition, techniques to monitor BBB disruption are evolving for bench and clinical research. Monitoring will be essential to ensure timely, safe, and effective BBB disruption while avoiding potential complications. A wide range of BBB penetrating methods are now in development. These innovative strategies could safely overcome the most stubborn barrier to drug delivery to the central nervous system.

References

1. Becker NH, Novikoff AB, Zimmerman HM. Fine structure observations of the uptake of intravenously injected peroxidase by the rat choroid plexus. J Histochem Cytochem. 1967;15(3):160–5.
2. Nabeshima S, Reese TS, Landis DM, Brightman MW. Junctions in the meninges and marginal glia. J Comp Neurol. 1975;164(2):127–69.
3. Kadry H, Noorani B, Cucullo L. A blood–brain barrier overview on structure, function, impairment, and biomarkers of integrity. Fluids Barriers CNS. 2020;17(1):69.
4. Cecchelli R, Berezowski V, Lundquist S, Culot M, Renftel M, Dehouck M-P, et al. Modelling of the blood–brain bar-

rier in drug discovery and development. Nat Rev Drug Discov. 2007;6(8):650–61.
5. Abbott NJ, Friedman A. Overview and introduction: the blood-brain barrier in health and disease. Epilepsia. 2012;53(Suppl 6):1–6.
6. Aird WC. Phenotypic heterogeneity of the endothelium. Circ Res. 2007;100(2):158–73.
7. Coomber BL, Stewart PA. Morphometric analysis of CNS microvascular endothelium. Microvasc Res. 1985;30(1):99–115.
8. Kakogiannos N, Ferrari L, Giampietro C, Scalise AA, Maderna C, Ravà M, et al. JAM-A acts via C/EBP-α to promote claudin-5 expression and enhance endothelial barrier function. Circ Res. 2020;127(8):1056–73.
9. Nitta T, Hata M, Gotoh S, Seo Y, Sasaki H, Hashimoto N, et al. Size-selective loosening of the blood-brain barrier in claudin-5–deficient mice. J Cell Biol. 2003;161(3):653–60.
10. Wong V, Gumbiner BM. A synthetic peptide corresponding to the extracellular domain of occludin perturbs the tight junction permeability barrier. J Cell Biol. 1997;136(2):399–409.
11. Sladojevic N, Stamatovic SM, Keep RF, Grailer JJ, Sarma JV, Ward PA, et al. Inhibition of junctional adhesion molecule-A/LFA interaction attenuates leukocyte trafficking and inflammation in brain ischemia/reperfusion injury. Neurobiol Dis. 2014;67:57–70.
12. Stamatovic SM, Johnson AM, Keep RF, Andjelkovic AV. Junctional proteins of the blood-brain barrier: new insights into function and dysfunction. Tissue Barriers. 2016;4(1):e1154641.
13. Aijaz S, Balda MS, Matter K. Tight junctions: molecular architecture and function. Int Rev Cytol. 2006;248:261–98.
14. Itoh M, Furuse M, Morita K, Kubota K, Saitou M, Tsukita S. Direct binding of three tight junction-associated MAGUKs, ZO-1, ZO-2, and ZO-3, with the COOH termini of Claudins. J Cell Biol. 1999;147(6):1351–63.
15. Fanning AS, Little BP, Rahner C, Utepbergenov D, Walther Z, Anderson JM. The Unique-5 and -6 motifs of ZO-1 regulate tight junction strand localization and scaffolding properties. Mol Biol Cell. 2007;18(3):721–31.
16. Tornavaca O, Chia M, Dufton N, Almagro LO, Conway DE, Randi AM, et al. ZO-1 controls endothelial adherens junctions, cell–cell tension, angiogenesis, and barrier formation. J Cell Biol. 2015;208(6):821–38.
17. Fanning AS, Jameson BJ, Jesaitis LA, Anderson JM. The tight junction protein ZO-1 establishes a link between the transmembrane protein occludin and the actin cytoskeleton. J Biol Chem. 1998;273(45):29745–53.
18. Umeda K, Ikenouchi J, Katahira-Tayama S, Furuse K, Sasaki H, Nakayama M, et al. ZO-1 and ZO-2 independently determine where claudins are polymerized in tight-junction strand formation. Cell. 2006;126(4):741–54.
19. Itoh M, Sasaki H, Furuse M, Ozaki H, Kita T, Tsukita S. Junctional adhesion molecule (JAM) binds to PAR-3. J Cell Biol. 2001;154(3):491–8.
20. Günzel D, Yu AS. Claudins and the modulation of tight junction permeability. Physiol Rev. 2013;93(2):525–69.
21. Sakurai A, Fukuhara S, Yamagishi A, Sako K, Kamioka Y, Masuda M, et al. MAGI-1 is required for Rap1 activation upon cell-cell contact and for enhancement of vascular endothelial cadherin-mediated cell adhesion. Mol Biol Cell. 2006;17(2):966–76.
22. Hamazaki Y, Itoh M, Sasaki H, Furuse M, Tsukita S. Multi-PDZ domain protein 1 (MUPP1) is concentrated at tight junctions through its possible interaction with claudin-1 and junctional adhesion molecule. J Biol Chem. 2002;277(1):455–61.
23. Luo Y, Fukuhara M, Weitzman M, Rizzolo LJ. Expression of JAM-A, AF-6, PAR-3 and PAR-6 during the assembly and remodeling of RPE tight junctions. Brain Res. 2006;1110(1):55–63.
24. Schossleitner K, Rauscher S, Gröger M, Friedl HP, Finsterwalder R, Habertheuer A, et al. Evidence that cingulin regulates endothelial barrier function in vitro and in vivo. Arterioscler Thromb Vasc Biol. 2016;36(4):647–54.
25. Zhou F, Li F, Hou Y, Yang B. HSPB8-mediated actin filament reorganization by promoting autophagic flux confers resilience to blood-brain barrier (BBB) injury in an in vitro model of ischemic stroke. ACS Chem Neurosci. 2023;14(16):2868–75.
26. Pollard TD. Actin and actin-binding proteins. Cold Spring Harb Perspect Biol. 2016;8(8):a018226.
27. Honore S, Pasquier E, Braguer D. Understanding microtubule dynamics for improved cancer therapy. Cell Mol Life Sci. 2005;62(24):3039–56.
28. Lagos-Cabré R, Burgos-Bravo F, Avalos AM, Leyton L. Connexins in astrocyte migration. Front Pharmacol. 2020;10:1546.
29. Hartsock A, Nelson WJ. Adherens and tight junctions: structure, function and connections to the actin cytoskeleton. Biochim Biophys Acta Biomembranes. 2008;1778(3):660–9.
30. Li W, Chen Z, Chin I, Chen Z, Dai H. The role of VE-cadherin in blood-brain barrier integrity under central nervous system pathological conditions. Curr Neuropharmacol. 2018;16(9):1375–84.
31. Montero-Balaguer M, Swirsding K, Orsenigo F, Cotelli F, Mione M, Dejana E. Stable vascular connections and remodeling require full expression of VE-cadherin in zebrafish embryos. PLoS One. 2009;4(6):e5772.
32. Mccrea PD, Gu D, Balda MS. Junctional music that the nucleus hears: cell-cell contact signaling and the modulation of gene activity. Cold Spring Harb Perspect Biol. 2009;1(4):a002923.
33. Vestweber D. VE-cadherin: the major endothelial adhesion molecule controlling cellular junctions and blood vessel formation. Arterioscler Thromb Vasc Biol. 2008;28(2):223–32.
34. Taddei A, Giampietro C, Conti A, Orsenigo F, Breviario F, Pirazzoli V, et al. Endothelial adherens junctions control tight junctions by VE-cadherin-mediated upregulation of claudin-5. Nat Cell Biol. 2008;10(8):923–34.
35. Morini MF, Giampietro C, Corada M, Pisati F, Lavarone E, Cunha SI, et al. VE-cadherin–mediated epigenetic regulation of endothelial gene expression. Circ Res. 2018;122(2):231–45.
36. Baeten KM, Akassoglou K. Extracellular matrix and matrix receptors in blood–brain barrier formation and stroke. Dev Neurobiol. 2011;71(11):1018–39.
37. Nguyen B, Bix G, Yao Y. Basal lamina changes in neurodegenerative disorders. Mol Neurodegener. 2021;16(1):81.
38. Xu L, Nirwane A, Yao Y. Basement membrane and blood-brain barrier. Stroke Vasc Neurol. 2019;4(2):78–82.
39. Thomsen MS, Routhe LJ, Moos T. The vascular basement membrane in the healthy and pathological brain. J Cereb Blood Flow Metab. 2017;37(10):3300–17.
40. PöSchl E, Schlötzer-Schrehardt U, Brachvogel B, Saito K, Ninomiya Y, Mayer U. Collagen IV is essential for basement membrane stability but dispensable for initiation of its assembly during early development. Development. 2004;131(7):1619–28.
41. Jeanne M, Labelle-Dumais C, Jorgensen J, Kauffman WB, Mancini M, Grazia FJ, et al. COL4A2 mutations impair COL4A1 and COL4A2 secretion and cause hemorrhagic stroke. Am J Hum Genet. 2012;90(1):91–101.
42. Osada T, Gu Y-H, Kanazawa M, Tsubota Y, Hawkins BT, Spatz M, et al. Interendothelial claudin-5 expression depends on cerebral endothelial cell–matrix adhesion by β_1-Integrins. J Cereb Blood Flow Metab. 2011;31(10):1972–85.
43. Gould DB, Phalan FC, Breedveld GJ, van Mil SE, Smith RS, Schimenti JC, et al. Mutations in Col4a1 cause perinatal cerebral hemorrhage and porencephaly. Science. 2005;308(5725):1167–71.

44. Hallmann R, Horn N, Selg M, Wendler O, Pausch F, Sorokin LM. Expression and function of laminins in the embryonic and mature vasculature. Physiol Rev. 2005;85(3):979–1000.
45. Gautam J, Zhang X, Yao Y. The role of pericytic laminin in blood brain barrier integrity maintenance. Sci Rep. 2016;6(1):36450.
46. Vanlandewijck M, He L, Mäe MA, Andrae J, Ando K, Del Gaudio F, et al. A molecular atlas of cell types and zonation in the brain vasculature. Nature. 2018;554(7693):475–80.
47. Menezes MJ, Mcclenahan FK, Leiton CV, Aranmolate A, Shan X, Colognato H. The extracellular matrix protein laminin α2 regulates the maturation and function of the blood–brain barrier. J Neurosci. 2014;34(46):15260–80.
48. Yurchenco PD, Schittny JC. Molecular architecture of basement membranes. FASEB J. 1990;4(6):1577–90.
49. Kang SH, Kramer JM. Nidogen is nonessential and not required for normal type IV collagen localization in *Caenorhabditis elegans*. Mol Biol Cell. 2000;11(11):3911–23.
50. Miosge N, Sasaki T, Timpl R. Evidence of nidogen-2 compensation for nidogen-1 deficiency in transgenic mice. Matrix Biol. 2002;21(7):611–21.
51. Schymeinsky J, Nedbal S, Miosge N, Pöschl E, Rao C, Beier DR, et al. Gene structure and functional analysis of the mouse Nidogen-2 gene: Nidogen-2 is not essential for basement membrane formation in mice. Mol Cell Biol. 2002;22(19):6820–30.
52. Bader BL, Smyth N, Nedbal S, Miosge N, Baranowsky A, Mokkapati S, et al. Compound genetic ablation of Nidogen 1 and 2 causes basement membrane defects and perinatal lethality in mice. Mol Cell Biol. 2005;25(15):6846–56.
53. Denzer AJ, Brandenberger R, Gesemann M, Chiquet M, Ruegg MA. Agrin binds to the nerve–muscle basal lamina via laminin. J Cell Biol. 1997;137(3):671–83.
54. Gautam M, Noakes PG, Moscoso L, Rupp F, Scheller RH, Merlie JP, et al. Defective neuromuscular synaptogenesis in agrin-deficient mutant mice. Cell. 1996;85(4):525–35.
55. Farach-Carson MC, Warren CR, Harrington DA, Carson DD. Border patrol: insights into the unique role of perlecan/heparan sulfate proteoglycan 2 at cell and tissue borders. Matrix Biol. 2014;34:64–79.
56. Göhring W, Sasaki T, Heldin CH, Timpl R. Mapping of the binding of platelet-derived growth factor to distinct domains of the basement membrane proteins BM-40 and perlecan and distinction from the BM-40 collagen-binding epitope. Eur J Biochem. 1998;255(1):60–6.
57. Nakamura K, Ikeuchi T, Nara K, Rhodes CS, Zhang P, Chiba Y, et al. Perlecan regulates pericyte dynamics in the maintenance and repair of the blood–brain barrier. J Cell Biol. 2019;218(10):3506–25.
58. Costell M, Gustafsson E, Aszódi A, Mörgelin M, Bloch W, Hunziker E, et al. Perlecan maintains the integrity of cartilage and some basement membranes. J Cell Biol. 1999;147(5):1109–22.
59. Díaz-Flores L, Gutiérrez R, Madrid JF, Varela H, Valladares F, Acosta E, et al. Pericytes. Morphofunction, interactions and pathology in a quiescent and activated mesenchymal cell niche. Histol Histopathol. 2009;24(7):909–69.
60. Armulik A, Genové G, Betsholtz C. Pericytes: developmental, physiological, and pathological perspectives, problems, and promises. Dev Cell. 2011;21(2):193–215.
61. Cai C, Fordsmann JC, Jensen SH, Gesslein B, Lønstrup M, Hald BO, et al. Stimulation-induced increases in cerebral blood flow and local capillary vasoconstriction depend on conducted vascular responses. Proc Natl Acad Sci USA. 2018;115(25):E5796–E804.
62. Alarcon-Martinez L, Yilmaz-Ozcan S, Yemisci M, Schallek J, Kılıç K, Can A, et al. Capillary pericytes express α-smooth muscle actin, which requires prevention of filamentous-actin depolymerization for detection. Elife. 2018;7:e34861.
63. Wakui S, Yokoo K, Muto T, Suzuki Y, Takahashi H, Furusato M, et al. Localization of Ang-1, -2, Tie-2, and VEGF expression at endothelial-pericyte interdigitation in rat angiogenesis. Lab Investig. 2006;86(11):1172–84.
64. Franco M, Roswall P, Cortez E, Hanahan D, Pietras K. Pericytes promote endothelial cell survival through induction of autocrine VEGF-A signaling and Bcl-w expression. Blood. 2011;118(10):2906–17.
65. Sengillo JD, Winkler EA, Walker CT, Sullivan JS, Johnson M, Zlokovic BV. Deficiency in mural vascular cells coincides with blood–brain barrier disruption in Alzheimer's Disease. Brain Pathol. 2013;23(3):303–10.
66. Rustenhoven J, Jansson D, Smyth LC, Dragunow M. Brain pericytes as mediators of neuroinflammation. Trends Pharmacol Sci. 2017;38(3):291–304.
67. Wang S, Voisin M-B, Larbi KY, Dangerfield J, Scheiermann C, Tran M, et al. Venular basement membranes contain specific matrix protein low expression regions that act as exit points for emigrating neutrophils. J Exp Med. 2006;203(6):1519–32.
68. Abbott NJ, Rönnbäck L, Hansson E. Astrocyte-endothelial interactions at the blood-brain barrier. Nat Rev Neurosci. 2006;7(1):41–53.
69. Attwell D, Buchan AM, Charpak S, Lauritzen M, Macvicar BA, Newman EA. Glial and neuronal control of brain blood flow. Nature. 2010;468(7321):232–43.
70. Rubin LL, Hall DE, Porter S, Barbu K, Cannon C, Horner HC, et al. A cell culture model of the blood-brain barrier. J Cell Biol. 1991;115(6):1725–35.
71. Neuhaus J, Risau W, Wolburg H. Induction of blood-brain barrier characteristics in bovine brain endothelial cells by rat astroglial cells in transfilter coculture. Ann N Y Acad Sci. 1991;633:578–80.
72. Higashi K, Fujita A, Inanobe A, Tanemoto M, Doi K, Kubo T, et al. An inwardly rectifying K(+) channel, Kir4.1, expressed in astrocytes surrounds synapses and blood vessels in brain. Am J Physiol Cell Physiol. 2001;281(3):C922–31.
73. Lien CF, Hazai D, Yeung D, Tan J, Füchtbauer EM, Jancsik V, et al. Expression of alpha-dystrobrevin in blood-tissue barriers: sub-cellular localisation and molecular characterisation in normal and dystrophic mice. Cell Tissue Res. 2007;327(1):67–82.
74. Nielsen S, Nagelhus EA, Amiry-Moghaddam M, Bourque C, Agre P, Ottersen OP. Specialized membrane domains for water transport in glial cells: high-resolution immunogold cytochemistry of aquaporin-4 in rat brain. J Neurosci. 1997;17(1):171–80.
75. Haj-Yasein NN, Vindedal GF, Eilert-Olsen M, Gundersen GA, Skare Ø, Laake P, et al. Glial-conditional deletion of aquaporin-4 (Aqp4) reduces blood-brain water uptake and confers barrier function on perivascular astrocyte endfeet. Proc Natl Acad Sci USA. 2011;108(43):17815–20.
76. Nwaobi SE, Cuddapah VA, Patterson KC, Randolph AC, Olsen ML. The role of glial-specific Kir4.1 in normal and pathological states of the CNS. Acta Neuropathol. 2016;132(1):1–21.
77. Ezan P, André P, Cisternino S, Saubaméa B, Boulay AC, Doutremer S, et al. Deletion of astroglial connexins weakens the blood-brain barrier. J Cereb Blood Flow Metab. 2012;32(8):1457–67.
78. Giaume C, Koulakoff A, Roux L, Holcman D, Rouach N. Astroglial networks: a step further in neuroglial and gliovascular interactions. Nat Rev Neurosci. 2010;11(2):87–99.
79. Alvarez JI, Dodelet-Devillers A, Kebir H, Ifergan I, Fabre PJ, Terouz S, et al. The Hedgehog pathway promotes blood-brain barrier integrity and CNS immune quiescence. Science. 2011;334(6063):1727–31.
80. Wang H, Xu Z, Xia Z, Rallo M, Duffy A, Matise MP. Inactivation of Hedgehog signal transduction in adult astrocytes results in region-specific blood-brain barrier defects. Proc Natl Acad Sci USA. 2021;118(34):e2017779118.

81. Daneman R, Agalliu D, Zhou L, Kuhnert F, Kuo CJ, Barres BA. Wnt/beta-catenin signaling is required for CNS, but not non-CNS, angiogenesis. Proc Natl Acad Sci USA. 2009;106(2):641–6.
82. Liebner S, Corada M, Bangsow T, Babbage J, Taddei A, Czupalla CJ, et al. Wnt/beta-catenin signaling controls development of the blood-brain barrier. J Cell Biol. 2008;183(3):409–17.
83. Zhou Y, Wang Y, Tischfield M, Williams J, Smallwood PM, Rattner A, et al. Canonical WNT signaling components in vascular development and barrier formation. J Clin Invest. 2014;124(9):3825–46.
84. Guérit S, Fidan E, Macas J, Czupalla CJ, Figueiredo R, Vijikumar A, et al. Astrocyte-derived Wnt growth factors are required for endothelial blood-brain barrier maintenance. Prog Neurobiol. 2021;199:101937.
85. Lee S, Chen TT, Barber CL, Jordan MC, Murdock J, Desai S, et al. Autocrine VEGF signaling is required for vascular homeostasis. Cell. 2007;130(4):691–703.
86. Puebla M, Tapia PJ, Espinoza H. Key role of astrocytes in postnatal brain and retinal angiogenesis. Int J Mol Sci. 2022;23(5):2646.
87. Baello S, Iqbal M, Bloise E, Javam M, Gibb W, Matthews SG. TGF-β1 regulation of multidrug resistance P-glycoprotein in the developing male blood-brain barrier. Endocrinology. 2014;155(2):475–84.
88. Lee SW, Kim WJ, Choi YK, Song HS, Son MJ, Gelman IH, et al. SSeCKS regulates angiogenesis and tight junction formation in blood-brain barrier. Nat Med. 2003;9(7):900–6.
89. Wosik K, Cayrol R, Dodelet-Devillers A, Berthelet F, Bernard M, Moumdjian R, et al. Angiotensin II controls occludin function and is required for blood brain barrier maintenance: relevance to multiple sclerosis. J Neurosci. 2007;27(34):9032–42.
90. Habgood MD, Begley DJ, Abbott NJ. Determinants of passive drug entry into the central nervous system. Cell Mol Neurobiol. 2000;20(2):231–53.
91. Pulgar VM. Transcytosis to cross the blood brain barrier, new advancements and challenges. Front Neurosci. 2018;12:1019.
92. Tashima T. Smart strategies for therapeutic agent delivery into brain across the blood-brain barrier using receptor-mediated transcytosis. Chem Pharm Bull (Tokyo). 2020;68(4):316–25.
93. Vasiliou V, Vasiliou K, Nebert DW. Human ATP-binding cassette (ABC) transporter family. Hum Genomics. 2009;3(3):281–90.
94. Fu BM. Transport across the blood-brain barrier. Adv Exp Med Biol. 2018;1097:235–59.
95. Puris E, Fricker G, Gynther M. Targeting transporters for drug delivery to the brain: can we do better? Pharm Res. 2022;39(7):1415–55.
96. Hu C, Tao L, Cao X, Chen L. The solute carrier transporters and the brain: physiological and pharmacological implications. Asian J Pharm Sci. 2020;15(2):131–44.
97. Filippidis AS, Carozza RB, Rekate HL. Aquaporins in brain edema and neuropathological conditions. Int J Mol Sci. 2016;18(1):55.
98. Begley DJ. ABC transporters and the blood-brain barrier. Curr Pharm Des. 2004;10(12):1295–312.
99. Bien-Ly N, Yu YJ, Bumbaca D, Elstrott J, Boswell CA, Zhang Y, et al. Transferrin receptor (TfR) trafficking determines brain uptake of TfR antibody affinity variants. J Exp Med. 2014;211(2):233–44.
100. Wu J, Park SH, Choi E. The insulin receptor endocytosis. Prog Mol Biol Transl Sci. 2023;194:79–107.
101. Ewers H, Helenius A. Lipid-mediated endocytosis. Cold Spring Harb Perspect Biol. 2011;3(8):a004721.
102. Mousavi SA, Malerød L, Berg T, Kjeken R. Clathrin-dependent endocytosis. Biochem J. 2004;377(1):1–16.
103. Pardridge WM, Triguero D, Buciak J. Transport of histone through the blood-brain barrier. J Pharmacol Exp Ther. 1989;251(3):821–6.
104. Pardridge WM, Buciak JL, Kang YS, Boado RJ. Protamine-mediated transport of albumin into brain and other organs of the rat. Binding and endocytosis of protamine-albumin complex by microvascular endothelium. J Clin Invest. 1993;92(5):2224–9.
105. Pardridge WM, Boado RJ. Enhanced cellular uptake of biotinylated antisense oligonucleotide or peptide mediated by avidin, a cationic protein. FEBS Lett. 1991;288(1–2):30–2.
106. Hervé F, Ghinea N, Scherrmann J-M. CNS delivery via adsorptive transcytosis. AAPS J. 2008;10(3):455–72.
107. Oldendorf WH, Cornford ME, Brown WJ. The large apparent work capability of the blood-brain barrier: a study of the mitochondrial content of capillary endothelial cells in brain and other tissues of the rat. Ann Neurol. 1977;1(5):409–17.
108. Cao Y, Sundgren PC, Tsien CI, Chenevert TT, Junck L. Physiologic and metabolic magnetic resonance imaging in gliomas. J Clin Oncol. 2006;24(8):1228–35.
109. Hanif F, Muzaffar K, Perveen K, Malhi SM, Simjee SU. Glioblastoma multiforme: a review of its epidemiology and pathogenesis through clinical presentation and treatment. Asian Pac J Cancer Prev. 2017;18(1):3–9.
110. Liao D, Johnson RS. Hypoxia: a key regulator of angiogenesis in cancer. Cancer Metastasis Rev. 2007;26(2):281–90.
111. Lin JL, Wang MJ, Lee D, Liang CC, Lin S. Hypoxia-inducible factor-1alpha regulates matrix metalloproteinase-1 activity in human bone marrow-derived mesenchymal stem cells. FEBS Lett. 2008;582(17):2615–9.
112. Fitsialos G, Bourget I, Augier S, Ginouvès A, Rezzonico R, Odorisio T, et al. HIF1 transcription factor regulates laminin-332 expression and keratinocyte migration. J Cell Sci. 2008;121(Pt 18):2992–3001.
113. Ahir BK, Engelhard HH, Lakka SS. Tumor development and angiogenesis in adult brain tumor: glioblastoma. Mol Neurobiol. 2020;57(5):2461–78.
114. Saitou M, Furuse M, Sasaki H, Schulzke JD, Fromm M, Takano H, et al. Complex phenotype of mice lacking occludin, a component of tight junction strands. Mol Biol Cell. 2000;11(12):4131–42.
115. Yang Y, Rosenberg GA. MMP-mediated disruption of claudin-5 in the blood-brain barrier of rat brain after cerebral ischemia. Methods Mol Biol. 2011;762:333–45.
116. Carmeliet P, Jain RK. Molecular mechanisms and clinical applications of angiogenesis. Nature. 2011;473(7347):298–307.
117. Engelhardt S, Patkar S, Ogunshola OO. Cell-specific blood–brain barrier regulation in health and disease: a focus on hypoxia. Br J Pharmacol. 2014;171(5):1210–30.
118. Dvorak HF. How tumors make bad blood vessels and stroma. Am J Pathol. 2003;162(6):1747–57.
119. De Bock K, Cauwenberghs S, Carmeliet P. Vessel abnormalization: another hallmark of cancer? Molecular mechanisms and therapeutic implications. Curr Opin Genet Dev. 2011;21(1):73–9.
120. Liebner S, Fischmann A, Rascher G, Duffner F, Grote EH, Kalbacher H, et al. Claudin-1 and claudin-5 expression and tight junction morphology are altered in blood vessels of human glioblastoma multiforme. Acta Neuropathol. 2000;100(3):323–31.
121. Hirano A, Matsui T. Vascular structures in brain tumors. Hum Pathol. 1975;6(5):611–21.
122. Papetti M, Herman IM. Mechanisms of normal and tumor-derived angiogenesis. Am J Physiol Cell Physiol. 2002;282(5):C947–70.
123. Caspani EM, Crossley PH, Redondo-Garcia C, Martinez S. Glioblastoma: a pathogenic crosstalk between tumor cells and pericytes. PLoS One. 2014;9(7):e101402.

124. Cheng L, Huang Z, Zhou W, Wu Q, Donnola S, Liu JK, et al. Glioblastoma stem cells generate vascular pericytes to support vessel function and tumor growth. Cell. 2013;153(1):139–52.
125. Zhou W, Chen C, Shi Y, Wu Q, Gimple RC, Fang X, et al. Targeting glioma stem cell-derived pericytes disrupts the blood-tumor barrier and improves chemotherapeutic efficacy. Cell Stem Cell. 2017;21(5):591–603.e4.
126. Montana V, Sontheimer H. Bradykinin promotes the chemotactic invasion of primary brain tumors. J Neurosci. 2011;31(13):4858–67.
127. Watkins S, Robel S, Kimbrough IF, Robert SM, Ellis-Davies G, Sontheimer H. Disruption of astrocyte-vascular coupling and the blood-brain barrier by invading glioma cells. Nat Commun. 2014;5:4196.
128. Winkler F, Kienast Y, Fuhrmann M, Von Baumgarten L, Burgold S, Mitteregger G, et al. Imaging glioma cell invasion in vivo reveals mechanisms of dissemination and peritumoral angiogenesis. Glia. 2009;57(12):1306–15.
129. Montgomery MK, Kim SH, Dovas A, Zhao HT, Goldberg AR, Xu W, et al. Glioma-induced alterations in neuronal activity and neurovascular coupling during disease progression. Cell Rep. 2020;31(2):107500.
130. Krishna S, Choudhury A, Keough MB, Seo K, Ni L, Kakaizada S, et al. Glioblastoma remodelling of human neural circuits decreases survival. Nature. 2023;617(7961):599–607.
131. Cuddapah VA, Robel S, Watkins S, Sontheimer H. A neurocentric perspective on glioma invasion. Nat Rev Neurosci. 2014;15(7):455–65.
132. Jain RK, di Tomaso E, Duda DG, Loeffler JS, Sorensen AG, Batchelor TT. Angiogenesis in brain tumours. Nat Rev Neurosci. 2007;8(8):610–22.
133. van Tellingen O, Yetkin-Arik B, de Gooijer MC, Wesseling P, Wurdinger T, de Vries HE. Overcoming the blood-brain tumor barrier for effective glioblastoma treatment. Drug Resist Updat. 2015;19:1–12.
134. Veringa SJE, Biesmans D, Van Vuurden DG, Jansen MHA, Wedekind LE, Horsman I, et al. In vitro drug response and efflux transporters associated with drug resistance in pediatric high grade glioma and diffuse intrinsic pontine glioma. PLoS One. 2013;8(4):e61512.
135. Amsbaugh MJ, Kim CS. Brain metastasis. In: StatPearls. Treasure Island, FL: StatPearls Publishing; 2024.
136. Bos PD, Zhang XH, Nadal C, Shu W, Gomis RR, Nguyen DX, et al. Genes that mediate breast cancer metastasis to the brain. Nature. 2009;459(7249):1005–9.
137. Avraham HK, Jiang S, Fu Y, Nakshatri H, Ovadia H, Avraham S. Angiopoietin-2 mediates blood-brain barrier impairment and colonization of triple-negative breast cancer cells in brain. J Pathol. 2014;232(3):369–81.
138. Sevenich L, Bowman RL, Mason SD, Quail DF, Rapaport F, Elie BT, et al. Analysis of tumour- and stroma-supplied proteolytic networks reveals a brain-metastasis-promoting role for cathepsin S. Nat Cell Biol. 2014;16(9):876–88.
139. Kienast Y, von Baumgarten L, Fuhrmann M, Klinkert WE, Goldbrunner R, Herms J, et al. Real-time imaging reveals the single steps of brain metastasis formation. Nat Med. 2010;16(1):116–22.
140. Rafii S, Butler JM, Ding BS. Angiocrine functions of organ-specific endothelial cells. Nature. 2016;529(7586):316–25.
141. Carbonell WS, Ansorge O, Sibson N, Muschel R. The vascular basement membrane as "soil" in brain metastasis. PLoS One. 2009;4(6):e5857.
142. Valiente M, Obenauf AC, Jin X, Chen Q, Zhang XH, Lee DJ, et al. Serpins promote cancer cell survival and vascular co-option in brain metastasis. Cell. 2014;156(5):1002–16.
143. Berghoff AS, Rajky O, Winkler F, Bartsch R, Furtner J, Hainfellner JA, et al. Invasion patterns in brain metastases of solid cancers. Neuro Oncol. 2013;15(12):1664–72.
144. Nguyen DX, Chiang AC, Zhang XH, Kim JY, Kris MG, Ladanyi M, et al. WNT/TCF signaling through LEF1 and HOXB9 mediates lung adenocarcinoma metastasis. Cell. 2009;138(1):51–62.
145. Gril B, Paranjape AN, Woditschka S, Hua E, Dolan EL, Hanson J, et al. Reactive astrocytic S1P3 signaling modulates the blood-tumor barrier in brain metastases. Nat Commun. 2018;9(1):2705.
146. Lyle LT, Lockman PR, Adkins CE, Mohammad AS, Sechrest E, Hua E, et al. Alterations in pericyte subpopulations are associated with elevated blood-tumor barrier permeability in experimental brain metastasis of breast cancer. Clin Cancer Res. 2016;22(21):5287–99.
147. Molnár PP, O'Neill BP, Scheithauer BW, Groothuis DR. The blood-brain barrier in primary CNS lymphomas: ultrastructural evidence of endothelial cell death. Neuro Oncol. 1999;1(2):89–100.
148. Jahnke K, Doolittle ND, Muldoon LL, Neuwelt EA. Implications of the blood–brain barrier in primary central nervous system lymphoma. Neurosurg Focus. 2006;21(5):1–11.
149. Mosteiro A, Pedrosa L, Ferrés A, Diao D, Sierra À, González JJ. The vascular microenvironment in glioblastoma: a comprehensive review. Biomedicines. 2022;10(6):1285.
150. Ellis JA, Banu M, Hossain SS, Singh-Moon R, Lavine SD, Bruce JN, et al. Reassessing the role of intra-arterial drug delivery for glioblastoma multiforme treatment. J Drug Deliv. 2015;2015:405735.
151. Joshi S, Ellis JA, Ornstein E, Bruce JN. Intraarterial drug delivery for glioblastoma mutiforme: will the phoenix rise again? J Neurooncol. 2015;124(3):333–43.
152. D'Amico RS, Khatri D, Reichman N, Patel NV, Wong T, Fralin SR, et al. Super selective intra-arterial cerebral infusion of modern chemotherapeutics after blood-brain barrier disruption: where are we now, and where we are going. J Neurooncol. 2020;147(2):261–78.
153. Saris SC, Blasberg RG, Carson RE, deVroom HL, Lutz R, Dedrick RL, et al. Intravascular streaming during carotid artery infusions. Demonstration in humans and reduction using diastole-phased pulsatile administration. J Neurosurg. 1991;74(5):763–72.
154. Joshi S, Wang M, Etu JJ, Pile-Spellman J. Reducing cerebral blood flow increases the duration of electroencephalographic silence by intracarotid thiopental. Anesth Analg. 2005;101(3):851–8.
155. Wang M, Joshi S. Electrocerebral silence after intracarotid propofol injection is a function of transit time. Anesth Analg. 2007;104(6):1498–503, table of contents.
156. Dedrick RL. Arterial drug infusion: pharmacokinetic problems and pitfalls. J Natl Cancer Inst. 1988;80(2):84–9.
157. Riina HA, Knopman J, Greenfield JP, Fralin S, Gobin YP, Tsiouris AJ, et al. Balloon-assisted superselective intra-arterial cerebral infusion of bevacizumab for malignant brainstem glioma. A technical note. Interv Neuroradiol. 2010;16(1):71–6.
158. Pile-Spellman J, Young WL, Joshi S, Duong H, Vang MC, Hartmann A, et al. Adenosine-induced cardiac pause for endovascular embolization of cerebral arteriovenous malformations: technical case report. Neurosurgery. 1999;44(4):881–6; discussion 6–7.
159. Rapoport SI, Hori M, Klatzo I. Testing of a hypothesis for osmotic opening of the blood-brain barrier. Am J Phys. 1972;223(2):323–31.
160. Brightman MW, Hori M, Rapoport SI, Reese TS, Westergaard E. Osmotic opening of tight junctions in cerebral endothelium. J Comp Neurol. 1973;152(4):317–25.
161. Neuwelt EA, Frenkel EP, Rapoport S, Barnett P. Effect of osmotic blood-brain barrier disruption on methotrexate pharmacokinetics in the dog. Neurosurgery. 1980;7(1):36–43.

162. Rapoport SI, Thompson HK. Osmotic opening of the blood-brain barrier in the monkey without associated neurological deficits. Science. 1973;180(4089):971.
163. Neuwelt EA. Mechanisms of disease: the blood-brain barrier. Neurosurgery. 2004;54(1):131–40; discussion 41–2.
164. Kroll RA, Neuwelt EA. Outwitting the blood-brain barrier for therapeutic purposes: osmotic opening and other means. Neurosurgery. 1998;42(5):1083–99; discussion 99–100.
165. Doolittle ND, Muldoon LL, Culp AY, Neuwelt EA. Delivery of chemotherapeutics across the blood-brain barrier: challenges and advances. Adv Pharmacol. 2014;71:203–43.
166. Joshi S, Singh-Moon RP, Wang M, Chaudhuri DB, Holcomb M, Straubinger NL, et al. Transient cerebral hypoperfusion assisted intraarterial cationic liposome delivery to brain tissue. J Neurooncol. 2014;118(1):73–82.
167. Doolittle ND, Miner ME, Hall WA, Siegal T, Jerome E, Osztie E, et al. Safety and efficacy of a multicenter study using intraarterial chemotherapy in conjunction with osmotic opening of the blood-brain barrier for the treatment of patients with malignant brain tumors. Cancer. 2000;88(3):637–47.
168. Fortin D, Gendron C, Boudrias M, Garant MP. Enhanced chemotherapy delivery by intraarterial infusion and blood-brain barrier disruption in the treatment of cerebral metastasis. Cancer. 2007;109(4):751–60.
169. Haldorsen IS, Krossnes BK, Aarseth JH, Scheie D, Johannesen TB, Mella O, et al. Increasing incidence and continued dismal outcome of primary central nervous system lymphoma in Norway 1989–2003: time trends in a 15-year national survey. Cancer. 2007;110(8):1803–14.
170. Neuwelt E, Abbott NJ, Abrey L, Banks WA, Blakley B, Davis T, et al. Strategies to advance translational research into brain barriers. Lancet Neurol. 2008;7(1):84–96.
171. Angelov L, Doolittle ND, Kraemer DF, Siegal T, Barnett GH, Peereboom DM, et al. Blood-brain barrier disruption and intraarterial methotrexate-based therapy for newly diagnosed primary CNS lymphoma: a multi-institutional experience. J Clin Oncol. 2009;27(21):3503–9.
172. Kuitunen HK, Rönkä ALK, Sonkajärvi EM, Isokangas JM, Pyörälä M, Palosaari KAA, et al. Blood-brain barrier disruption (BBBD)-based immunochemotherapy for primary central nervous system lymphoma (PCNSL), early results of a phase II study. Cancers (Basel). 2023;15(4):1341.
173. Fortin D, Desjardins A, Benko A, Niyonsega T, Boudrias M. Enhanced chemotherapy delivery by intraarterial infusion and blood-brain barrier disruption in malignant brain tumors: the Sherbrooke experience. Cancer. 2005;103(12):2606–15.
174. Calabrese C, Poppleton H, Kocak M, Hogg TL, Fuller C, Hamner B, et al. A perivascular niche for brain tumor stem cells. Cancer Cell. 2007;11(1):69–82.
175. Muldoon LL, Pagel MA, Netto JP, Neuwelt EA. Intra-arterial administration improves temozolomide delivery and efficacy in a model of intracerebral metastasis, but has unexpected brain toxicity. J Neurooncol. 2016;126(3):447–54.
176. Fortin D, Morin PA, Belzile F, Mathieu D, Paré FM. Intra-arterial carboplatin as a salvage strategy in the treatment of recurrent glioblastoma multiforme. J Neurooncol. 2014;119(2):397–403.
177. Hall WA, Doolittle ND, Daman M, Bruns PK, Muldoon L, Fortin D, et al. Osmotic blood-brain barrier disruption chemotherapy for diffuse pontine gliomas. J Neurooncol. 2006;77(3):279–84.
178. Imbesi F, Marchioni E, Benericetti E, Zappoli F, Galli A, Corato M, et al. A randomized phase III study: comparison between intravenous and intraarterial ACNU administration in newly diagnosed primary glioblastomas. Anticancer Res. 2006;26(1b):553–8.
179. Owens G, Javid R, Belmusto L, Bender M, Blau M. Intra-arterial vincristine therapy of primary gliomas. Cancer. 1965;18:756–60.
180. Kouhi A, Pachipulusu V, Kapenstein T, Hu P, Epstein AL, Khawli LA. Brain disposition of antibody-based therapeutics: dogma, approaches and perspectives. Int J Mol Sci. 2021;22(12):6442.
181. Boockvar JA, Tsiouris AJ, Hofstetter CP, Kovanlikaya I, Fralin S, Kesavabhotla K, et al. Safety and maximum tolerated dose of superselective intraarterial cerebral infusion of bevacizumab after osmotic blood-brain barrier disruption for recurrent malignant glioma. J Neurosurg. 2011;114(3):624–32.
182. Jeon JY, Kovanlikaya I, Boockvar JA, Mao X, Shin B, Burkhardt JK, et al. Metabolic response of glioblastoma to superselective intra-arterial cerebral infusion of bevacizumab: a proton MR spectroscopic imaging study. AJNR Am J Neuroradiol. 2012;33(11):2095–102.
183. Galla N, Chiang G, Chakraborty S, Singh R, John Tsiouris A, Boockvar J, et al. Apparent diffusion coefficient changes predict survival after intra-arterial bevacizumab treatment in recurrent glioblastoma. Neuroradiology. 2017;59(5):499–505.
184. Patel NV, Wong T, Fralin SR, Li M, McKeown A, Gruber D, et al. Repeated superselective intraarterial bevacizumab after blood brain barrier disruption for newly diagnosed glioblastoma: a phase I/II clinical trial. J Neurooncol. 2021;155(2):117–24.
185. Chakraborty S, Filippi CG, Wong T, Ray A, Fralin S, Tsiouris AJ, et al. Superselective intraarterial cerebral infusion of cetuximab after osmotic blood/brain barrier disruption for recurrent malignant glioma: phase I study. J Neurooncol. 2016;128(3):405–15.
186. Moyaert P, Padrela BE, Morgan CA, Petr J, Versijpt J, Barkhof F, et al. Imaging blood-brain barrier dysfunction: a state-of-the-art review from a clinical perspective. Front Aging Neurosci. 2023;15:1132077.
187. Al-Sarraf H, Ghaaedi F, Redzic Z. Time course of hyperosmolar opening of the blood-brain and blood-CSF barriers in spontaneously hypertensive rats. J Vasc Res. 2007;44(2):99–109.
188. Joshi S, Ergin A, Wang M, Reif R, Zhang J, Bruce JN, et al. Inconsistent blood brain barrier disruption by intraarterial mannitol in rabbits: implications for chemotherapy. J Neurooncol. 2011;104(1):11–9.
189. Chu C, Jablonska A, Gao Y, Lan X, Lesniak WG, Liang Y, et al. Hyperosmolar blood-brain barrier opening using intra-arterial injection of hyperosmotic mannitol in mice under real-time MRI guidance. Nat Protoc. 2022;17(1):76–94.
190. Foley CP, Rubin DG, Santillan A, Sondhi D, Dyke JP, Crystal RG, et al. Intra-arterial delivery of AAV vectors to the mouse brain after mannitol mediated blood brain barrier disruption. J Control Release. 2014;196:71–8.
191. Burks SR, Kersch CN, Witko JA, Pagel MA, Sundby M, Muldoon LL, et al. Blood-brain barrier opening by intracarotid artery hyperosmolar mannitol induces sterile inflammatory and innate immune responses. Proc Natl Acad Sci USA. 2021;118(18):e2021915118.
192. Iannitti T, Palmieri B. An update on the therapeutic role of alkylglycerols. Mar Drugs. 2010;8(8):2267–300.
193. Lee HJ, Zhang Y, Pardridge WM. Blood-brain barrier disruption following the internal carotid arterial perfusion of alkyl glycerols. J Drug Target. 2002;10(6):463–7.
194. Schuff-Werner P, Müller U, Unger C, Nagel GA, Eibl H. 1-O-methyl-rac-glycerol: a new agent for the cryopreservation of mononuclear cells. Cryobiology. 1988;25(6):487–94.
195. Unger C, Eibl H, von Heyden HW, Krisch B, Nagel GA. Blood-brain barrier and the penetration of cytostatic drugs. Klin Wochenschr. 1985;63(12):565–71.
196. Erdlenbruch B, Jendrossek V, Eibl H, Lakomek M. Transient and controllable opening of the blood-brain barrier to cytostatic and antibiotic agents by alkylglycerols in rats. Exp Brain Res. 2000;135(3):417–22.

197. Erdlenbruch B, Kugler W, Schinkhof C, Neurath H, Eibl H, Lakomek M. Blood-brain barrier opening with alkylglycerols: biodistribution of 1-O-pentylglycerol after intravenous and intracarotid administration in rats. J Drug Target. 2005;13(3):143–50.
198. Hülper P, Veszelka S, Walter FR, Wolburg H, Fallier-Becker P, Piontek J, et al. Acute effects of short-chain alkylglycerols on blood-brain barrier properties of cultured brain endothelial cells. Br J Pharmacol. 2013;169(7):1561–73.
199. Belury MA, Raatz S, Conrad Z. Modeled substitution of traditional oils with high-oleic acid oils decreases essential fatty acid intake in children. Am J Clin Nutr. 2022;115(4):1180–8.
200. Demirbolat GM, Coskun GP, Erdogan O, Cevik O. Long chain fatty acids can form aggregates and affect the membrane integrity. Colloids Surf B Biointerfaces. 2021;204:111795.
201. Sztriha LS, Betz AL. Oleic acid reversibly opens the blood-brain barrier. Brain Res. 1991;550(2):257–62.
202. Han HS, Jang JH, Park JS, Kim HJ, Kim JK. Transient blood brain barrier disruption induced by oleic acid is mediated by nitric oxide. Curr Neurovasc Res. 2013;10(4):287–96.
203. Bouaggad A, Harti A, Elmouknia M, Bouderka MA, Barrou H, Abassi O, et al. Neurologic manifestations of fat embolism. Cah Anesthesiol. 1995;43(5):441–3.
204. George J, George R, Dixit R, Gupta RC, Gupta N. Fat embolism syndrome. Lung India. 2013;30(1):47–53.
205. Kim HJ, Lee CH, Lee SH, Moon TY. Magnetic resonance imaging and histologic findings of experimental cerebral fat embolism. Investig Radiol. 2003;38(10):625–34.
206. Kim HJ, Lee CH, Kim HG, Lee SD, Son SM, Kim YW, et al. Reversible MR changes in the cat brain after cerebral fat embolism induced by triolein emulsion. AJNR Am J Neuroradiol. 2004;25(6):958–63.
207. Kim HJ, Lee CH, Lee SH, Cho BM, Kim HK, Park BR, et al. Early development of vasogenic edema in experimental cerebral fat embolism in cats: correlation with MRI and electron microscopic findings. Investig Radiol. 2001;36(8):460–9.
208. Kim HJ, Kim YW, Choi SH, Cho BM, Bandu R, Ahn HS, et al. Triolein emulsion infusion into the carotid artery increases brain permeability to anticancer agents. Neurosurgery. 2016;78(5):726–33.
209. Seung WB, Cha SH, Kim HJ, Choi SH, Lee J, Kwak D, et al. Triolein emulsion enhances temozolomide brain delivery: an experimental study in rats. Drug Deliv. 2021;28(1):2373–82.
210. Kim YW, Choi SH, Choi KJ, Kim HJ, Kang JS, Hong DJ. Unsaturated free fatty acid emulsion infusion into carotid artery enhances drug delivery to the rat brain. Brain Behav. 2023;13(6):e2994.
211. Jatyan R, Sahel DK, Singh P, Sakhuja R, Mittal A, Chitkara D. Temozolomide-fatty acid conjugates for glioblastoma multiforme: in vitro and in vivo evaluation. J Control Release. 2023;359:161–74.
212. Rodríguez-Massó SR, Erickson MA, Banks WA, Ulrich H, Martins AH. The bradykinin B2 receptor agonist (NG291) causes rapid onset of transient blood-brain barrier disruption without evidence of early brain injury. Front Neurosci. 2021;15:791709.
213. Alvarez AL, Delorenzi A, Santajuliana D, Finkielman S, Nahmod VE, Pirola CJ. Central bradykininergic system in normotensive and hypertensive rats. Clin Sci (Lond). 1992;82(5):513–9.
214. Inamura T, Black KL. Bradykinin selectively opens blood-tumor barrier in experimental brain tumors. J Cereb Blood Flow Metab. 1994;14(5):862–70.
215. Nomura T, Inamura T, Black KL. Intracarotid infusion of bradykinin selectively increases blood-tumor permeability in 9L and C6 brain tumors. Brain Res. 1994;659(1–2):62–6.
216. Black KL. Biochemical opening of the blood-brain barrier. Adv Drug Deliv Rev. 1995;15(1–3):37–52.
217. Matsukado K, Inamura T, Nakano S, Fukui M, Bartus RT, Black KL. Enhanced tumor uptake of carboplatin and survival in glioma-bearing rats by intracarotid infusion of bradykinin analog, RMP-7. Neurosurgery. 1996;39(1):125–33; discussion 33–4.
218. Black KL, Cloughesy T, Huang SC, Gobin YP, Zhou Y, Grous J, et al. Intracarotid infusion of RMP-7, a bradykinin analog, and transport of gallium-68 ethylenediamine tetraacetic acid into human gliomas. J Neurosurg. 1997;86(4):603–9.
219. Nakano S, Matsukado K, Black KL. Increased brain tumor microvessel permeability after intracarotid bradykinin infusion is mediated by nitric oxide. Cancer Res. 1996;56(17):4027–31.
220. Liu Y, Hashizume K, Chen Z, Samoto K, Ningaraj N, Asotra K, et al. Correlation between bradykinin-induced blood-tumor barrier permeability and B2 receptor expression in experimental brain tumors. Neurol Res. 2001;23(4):379–87.
221. Zhang Q, Tan J, Wan L, Chen C, Wu B, Ke X, et al. Increase in blood-brain barrier permeability is modulated by tissue kallikrein via activation of bradykinin B1 and B2 receptor-mediated signaling. J Inflamm Res. 2021;14:4283–97.
222. Wang H, Sun W, Li F, Jiang P, Wang L, Zhou N, et al. Bradykinin-bradykinin receptor (B1R) signalling is involved in the blood-brain barrier disruption in moyamoya disease. J Cell Mol Med. 2023;27(24):4069–79.
223. Liu LB, Xue YX, Liu YH, Wang YB. Bradykinin increases blood-tumor barrier permeability by down-regulating the expression levels of ZO-1, occludin, and claudin-5 and rearranging actin cytoskeleton. J Neurosci Res. 2008;86(5):1153–68.
224. Liu LB, Liu XB, Ma J, Liu YH, Li ZQ, Ma T, et al. Bradykinin increased the permeability of BTB via NOS/NO/ZONAB-mediating down-regulation of claudin-5 and occludin. Biochem Biophys Res Commun. 2015;464(1):118–25.
225. Haas AJ, Zihni C, Krug SM, Maraspini R, Otani T, Furuse M, et al. ZO-1 guides tight junction assembly and epithelial morphogenesis via cytoskeletal tension-dependent and -independent functions. Cells. 2022;11(23):3775.
226. Fasano A, Baudry B, Pumplin DW, Wasserman SS, Tall BD, Ketley JM, et al. Vibrio cholerae produces a second enterotoxin, which affects intestinal tight junctions. Proc Natl Acad Sci USA. 1991;88(12):5242–6.
227. Fasano A, Fiorentini C, Donelli G, Uzzau S, Kaper JB, Margaretten K, et al. Zonula occludens toxin modulates tight junctions through protein kinase C-dependent actin reorganization, in vitro. J Clin Invest. 1995;96(2):710–20.
228. Fasano A, Uzzau S, Fiore C, Margaretten K. The enterotoxic effect of zonula occludens toxin on rabbit small intestine involves the paracellular pathway. Gastroenterology. 1997;112(3):839–46.
229. Di Pierro M, Lu R, Uzzau S, Wang W, Margaretten K, Pazzani C, et al. Zonula occludens toxin structure-function analysis. Identification of the fragment biologically active on tight junctions and of the zonulin receptor binding domain. J Biol Chem. 2001;276(22):19160–5.
230. Lu R, Wang W, Uzzau S, Vigorito R, Zielke HR, Fasano A. Affinity purification and partial characterization of the zonulin/zonula occludens toxin (Zot) receptor from human brain. J Neurochem. 2000;74(1):320–6.
231. Stuart CM, Varatharaj A, Winberg ME, Galea P, Larsson HBW, Cramer SP, et al. Zonulin and blood-brain barrier permeability are dissociated in humans. Clin Transl Med. 2022;12:e965.
232. Karyekar CS, Fasano A, Raje S, Lu R, Dowling TC, Eddington ND. Zonula occludens toxin increases the permeability of molecular weight markers and chemotherapeutic agents across the bovine brain microvessel endothelial cells. J Pharm Sci. 2003;92(2):414–23.
233. Menon D, Karyekar CS, Fasano A, Lu R, Eddington ND. Enhancement of brain distribution of anticancer agents using DeltaG, the 12 kDa active fragment of ZOT. Int J Pharm. 2005;306(1–2):122–31.

234. Bocsik A, Walter FR, Gyebrovszki A, Fülöp L, Blasig I, Dabrowski S, et al. Reversible opening of intercellular junctions of intestinal epithelial and brain endothelial cells with tight junction modulator peptides. J Pharm Sci. 2016;105(2):754–65.
235. Dana H, Chalbatani GM, Mahmoodzadeh H, Karimloo R, Rezaiean O, Moradzadeh A, et al. Molecular mechanisms and biological functions of siRNA. Int J Biomed Sci. 2017;13(2):48–57.
236. Campbell M, Kiang AS, Kenna PF, Kerskens C, Blau C, O'Dwyer L, et al. RNAi-mediated reversible opening of the blood-brain barrier. J Gene Med. 2008;10(8):930–47.
237. Krause G, Winkler L, Piehl C, Blasig I, Piontek J, Müller SL. Structure and function of extracellular claudin domains. Ann N Y Acad Sci. 2009;1165:34–43.
238. Vagner J, Qu H, Hruby VJ. Peptidomimetics, a synthetic tool of drug discovery. Curr Opin Chem Biol. 2008;12(3):292–6.
239. Dithmer S, Staat C, Müller C, Ku MC, Pohlmann A, Niendorf T, et al. Claudin peptidomimetics modulate tissue barriers for enhanced drug delivery. Ann N Y Acad Sci. 2017;1397(1):169–84.
240. Hashimoto Y, Shirakura K, Okada Y, Takeda H, Endo K, Tamura M, et al. Claudin-5-binders enhance permeation of solutes across the blood-brain barrier in a mammalian model. J Pharmacol Exp Ther. 2017;363(2):275–83.
241. Tachibana K, Hashimoto Y, Shirakura K, Okada Y, Hirayama R, Iwashita Y, et al. Safety and efficacy of an anti-claudin-5 monoclonal antibody to increase blood-brain barrier permeability for drug delivery to the brain in a non-human primate. J Control Release. 2021;336:105–11.
242. Garteiser P, Doblas S, Watanabe Y, Saunders D, Hoyle J, Lerner M, et al. Multiparametric assessment of the anti-glioma properties of OKN007 by magnetic resonance imaging. J Magn Reson Imaging. 2010;31(4):796–806.
243. Towner RA, Gillespie DL, Schwager A, Saunders DG, Smith N, Njoku CE, et al. Regression of glioma tumor growth in F98 and U87 rat glioma models by the Nitrone OKN-007. Neuro Oncol. 2013;15(3):330–40.
244. de Souza PC, Smith N, Pody R, He T, Njoku C, Silasi-Mansat R, et al. OKN-007 decreases VEGFR-2 levels in a preclinical GL261 mouse glioma model. Am J Nucl Med Mol Imaging. 2015;5(4):363–78.
245. Coutinho de Souza P, Smith N, Atolagbe O, Ziegler J, Njoku C, Lerner M, et al. OKN-007 decreases free radical levels in a preclinical F98 rat glioma model. Free Radic Biol Med. 2015;87:157–68.
246. Towner RA, Smith N, Saunders D, Brown CA, Cai X, Ziegler J, et al. OKN-007 increases temozolomide (TMZ) sensitivity and suppresses TMZ-resistant glioblastoma (GBM) tumor growth. Transl Oncol. 2019;12(2):320–35.
247. Coutinho de Souza P, Mallory S, Smith N, Saunders D, Li XN, McNall-Knapp RY, et al. Inhibition of pediatric glioblastoma tumor growth by the anti-cancer agent OKN-007 in orthotopic mouse xenografts. PLoS One. 2015;10(8):e0134276.
248. Floyd RA, Chandru HK, He T, Towner R. Anti-cancer activity of nitrones and observations on mechanism of action. Anti Cancer Agents Med Chem. 2011;11(4):373–9.
249. Towner RA, Hocker J, Smith N, Saunders D, Battiste J, Hanas J. OKN-007 alters protein expression profiles in high-grade gliomas: mass spectral analysis of blood sera. Brain Sci. 2022;12(1):100.
250. Lees KR, Zivin JA, Ashwood T, Davalos A, Davis SM, Diener HC, et al. NXY-059 for acute ischemic stroke. N Engl J Med. 2006;354(6):588–600.
251. Shuaib A, Lees KR, Lyden P, Grotta J, Davalos A, Davis SM, et al. NXY-059 for the treatment of acute ischemic stroke. N Engl J Med. 2007;357(6):562–71.
252. Towner RA, Saunders D, Lerner M, Silasi Mansat R, Yuan T, Barber D, et al. Temporary opening of the blood-brain barrier with the nitrone compound OKN-007. Am J Nucl Med Mol Imaging. 2021;11(5):363–73.
253. Deffieux T, Demené C, Tanter M. Functional ultrasound imaging: a new imaging modality for neuroscience. Neuroscience. 2021;474:110–21.
254. Vykhodtseva NI, Hynynen K, Damianou C. Pulse duration and peak intensity during focused ultrasound surgery: theoretical and experimental effects in rabbit brain in vivo. Ultrasound Med Biol. 1994;20(9):987–1000.
255. Vykhodtseva NI, Hynynen K, Damianou C. Histologic effects of high intensity pulsed ultrasound exposure with subharmonic emission in rabbit brain in vivo. Ultrasound Med Biol. 1995;21(7):969–79.
256. Hynynen K, McDannold N, Vykhodtseva N, Jolesz FA. Noninvasive MR imaging-guided focal opening of the blood-brain barrier in rabbits. Radiology. 2001;220(3):640–6.
257. Stride E, Segers T, Lajoinie G, Cherkaoui S, Bettinger T, Versluis M, et al. Microbubble agents: new directions. Ultrasound Med Biol. 2020;46(6):1326–43.
258. Olsman M, Sereti V, Mühlenpfordt M, Johnsen KB, Andresen TL, Urquhart AJ, et al. Focused ultrasound and microbubble treatment increases delivery of transferrin receptor-targeting liposomes to the brain. Ultrasound Med Biol. 2021;47(5):1343–55.
259. Cho H, Lee H-Y, Han M, Choi J-R, Ahn S, Lee T, et al. Localized down-regulation of P-glycoprotein by focused ultrasound and microbubbles induced blood-brain barrier disruption in rat brain. Sci Rep. 2016;6(1):31201.
260. Alonso A, Reinz E, Jenne JW, Fatar M, Schmidt-Glenewinkel H, Hennerici MG, et al. Reorganization of gap junctions after focused ultrasound blood–brain barrier opening in the rat brain. J Cereb Blood Flow Metab. 2010;30(7):1394–402.
261. Kovacs ZI, Kim S, Jikaria N, Qureshi F, Milo B, Lewis BK, et al. Disrupting the blood-brain barrier by focused ultrasound induces sterile inflammation. Proc Natl Acad Sci USA. 2017;114(1):E75–e84.
262. Sheybani ND, Witter AR, Garrison WJ, Miller GW, Price RJ, Bullock TNJ. Profiling of the immune landscape in murine glioblastoma following blood brain/tumor barrier disruption with MR image-guided focused ultrasound. J Neurooncol. 2022;156(1):109–22.
263. Englander ZK, Wei H-J, Pouliopoulos AN, Bendau E, Upadhyayula P, Jan C-I, et al. Focused ultrasound mediated blood–brain barrier opening is safe and feasible in a murine pontine glioma model. Sci Rep. 2021;11(1):6521.
264. Wei HJ, Upadhyayula PS, Pouliopoulos AN, Englander ZK, Zhang X, Jan CI, et al. Focused ultrasound-mediated blood-brain barrier opening increases delivery and efficacy of etoposide for glioblastoma treatment. Int J Radiat Oncol Biol Phys. 2021;110(2):539–50.
265. Mcdannold N, Zhang Y, Supko JG, Power C, Sun T, Peng C, et al. Acoustic feedback enables safe and reliable carboplatin delivery across the blood-brain barrier with a clinical focused ultrasound system and improves survival in a rat glioma model. Theranostics. 2019;9(21):6284–99.
266. Timbie KF, Afzal U, Date A, Zhang C, Song J, Wilson Miller G, et al. MR image-guided delivery of cisplatin-loaded brain-penetrating nanoparticles to invasive glioma with focused ultrasound. J Control Release. 2017;263:120–31.
267. Wei K-C, Chu P-C, Wang H-YJ, Huang C-Y, Chen P-Y, Tsai H-C, et al. Focused ultrasound-induced blood–brain barrier opening to enhance temozolomide delivery for glioblastoma treatment: a preclinical study. PLoS One. 2013;8(3):e58995.

268. Sabbagh A, Beccaria K, Ling X, Marisetty A, Ott M, Caruso H, et al. Opening of the blood–brain barrier using low-intensity pulsed ultrasound enhances responses to immunotherapy in preclinical glioma models. Clin Cancer Res. 2021;27(15):4325–37.
269. Samiotaki G, Vlachos F, Tung YS, Konofagou EE. A quantitative pressure and microbubble-size dependence study of focused ultrasound-induced blood-brain barrier opening reversibility in vivo using MRI. Magn Reson Med. 2012;67(3):769–77.
270. Burgess A, Shah K, Hough O, Hynynen K. Focused ultrasound-mediated drug delivery through the blood-brain barrier. Expert Rev Neurother. 2015;15(5):477–91.
271. Carpentier A, Canney M, Vignot A, Reina V, Beccaria K, Horodyckid C, et al. Clinical trial of blood-brain barrier disruption by pulsed ultrasound. Sci Transl Med. 2016;8(343):343re2.
272. Kyriakou A, Neufeld E, Werner B, Székely G, Kuster N. Full-wave acoustic and thermal modeling of transcranial ultrasound propagation and investigation of skull-induced aberration correction techniques: a feasibility study. J Ther Ultrasound. 2015;3(1):11.
273. Chen KT, Lin YJ, Chai WY, Lin CJ, Chen PY, Huang CY, et al. Neuronavigation-guided focused ultrasound (NaviFUS) for transcranial blood-brain barrier opening in recurrent glioblastoma patients: clinical trial protocol. Ann Transl Med. 2020;8(11):673.
274. Idbaih A, Canney M, Belin L, Desseaux C, Vignot A, Bouchoux G, et al. Safety and feasibility of repeated and transient blood–brain barrier disruption by pulsed ultrasound in patients with recurrent glioblastoma. Clin Cancer Res. 2019;25(13):3793–801.
275. Sonabend AM, Gould A, Amidei C, Ward R, Schmidt KA, Zhang DY, et al. Repeated blood-brain barrier opening with an implantable ultrasound device for delivery of albumin-bound paclitaxel in patients with recurrent glioblastoma: a phase 1 trial. Lancet Oncol. 2023;24(5):509–22.
276. Meng Y, MacIntosh BJ, Shirzadi Z, Kiss A, Bethune A, Heyn C, et al. Resting state functional connectivity changes after MR-guided focused ultrasound mediated blood-brain barrier opening in patients with Alzheimer's disease. Neuroimage. 2019;200:275–80.
277. Rubin P, Casarett GW. Clinical radiation pathology as applied to curative radiotherapy. Cancer. 1968;22(4):767–78.
278. Rubin P, Gash DM, Hansen JT, Nelson DF, Williams JP. Disruption of the blood-brain barrier as the primary effect of CNS irradiation. Radiother Oncol. 1994;31(1):51–60.
279. Peña LA, Fuks Z, Kolesnick RN. Radiation-induced apoptosis of endothelial cells in the murine central nervous system: protection by fibroblast growth factor and sphingomyelinase deficiency. Cancer Res. 2000;60(2):321–7.
280. Nordal RA, Wong CS. Molecular targets in radiation-induced blood-brain barrier disruption. Int J Radiat Oncol Biol Phys. 2005;62(1):279–87.
281. Tsao MN, Li YQ, Lu G, Xu Y, Wong CS. Upregulation of vascular endothelial growth factor is associated with radiation-induced blood-spinal cord barrier breakdown. J Neuropathol Exp Neurol. 1999;58(10):1051–60.
282. Olschowka JA, Kyrkanides S, Harvey BK, O'Banion MK, Williams JP, Rubin P, et al. ICAM-1 induction in the mouse CNS following irradiation. Brain Behav Immun. 1997;11(4):273–85.
283. Blethen KE, Sprowls SA, Arsiwala TA, Wolford CP, Panchal DM, Fladeland RA, et al. Effects of whole-brain radiation therapy on the blood–brain barrier in immunocompetent and immunocompromised mouse models. Radiat Oncol. 2023;18(1):22.
284. Wilson CM, Gaber MW, Sabek OM, Zawaski JA, Merchant TE. Radiation-induced astrogliosis and blood-brain barrier damage can be abrogated using anti-TNF treatment. Int J Radiat Oncol Biol Phys. 2009;74(3):934–41.
285. Blethen KE, Wolford CP, Pecar GL, Arsiwala TA, Adjeroh E, Dykstra LP, et al. Coordination of anti-CTLA-4 with whole-brain radiation therapy decreases tumor burden during treatment in a novel syngeneic model of lung cancer brain metastasis. Cancer Immunol Immunother. 2024;73(1):20.
286. Grunert M, Kassubek R, Danz B, Klemenz B, Hasslacher S, Stroh S, et al. Radiation and brain tumors: an overview. Crit Rev Oncog. 2018;23(1–2):119–38.
287. Lim WH, Choi SH, Yoo R-E, Kang KM, Yun TJ, Kim J-H, et al. Does radiation therapy increase gadolinium accumulation in the brain?: quantitative analysis of T1 shortening using R1 relaxometry in glioblastoma multiforme patients. PLoS One. 2018;13(2):e0192838.
288. Teng F, Tsien CI, Lawrence TS, Cao Y. Blood-tumor barrier opening changes in brain metastases from pre to one-month post radiation therapy. Radiother Oncol. 2017;125(1):89–93.
289. Patel B, Yang PH, Kim AH. The effect of thermal therapy on the blood-brain barrier and blood-tumor barrier. Int J Hyperth. 2020;37(2):35–43.
290. Coley WB. The treatment of malignant tumors by repeated inoculations of erysipelas. With a report of ten original cases. 1893. Clin Orthop Relat Res. 1991;262:3–11.
291. Stafford RJ, Fuentes D, Elliott AA, Weinberg JS, Ahrar K. Laser-induced thermal therapy for tumor ablation. Crit Rev Biomed Eng. 2010;38(1):79–100.
292. Skandalakis GP, Rivera DR, Rizea CD, Bouras A, Jesu Raj JG, Bozec D, et al. Hyperthermia treatment advances for brain tumors. Int J Hyperth. 2020;37(2):3–19.
293. Rahmathulla G, Recinos PF, Kamian K, Mohammadi AM, Ahluwalia MS, Barnett GH. MRI-guided laser interstitial thermal therapy in neuro-oncology: a review of its current clinical applications. Oncology. 2014;87(2):67–82.
294. Bartlett S, Nagaraja TN, Griffith B, Farmer KG, Van Harn M, Haider S, et al. Persistent peri-ablation blood-brain barrier opening after laser interstitial thermal therapy for brain tumors. Cureus. 2023;15(4):e37397.
295. Leuthardt EC, Duan C, Kim MJ, Campian JL, Kim AH, Miller-Thomas MM, et al. Hyperthermic laser ablation of recurrent glioblastoma leads to temporary disruption of the peritumoral blood brain barrier. PLoS One. 2016;11(2):e0148613.
296. Butt OH, Zhou AY, Huang J, Leidig WA, Silberstein AE, Chheda MG, et al. A phase II study of laser interstitial thermal therapy combined with doxorubicin in patients with recurrent glioblastoma. Neurooncol Adv. 2021;3(1):vdab164.
297. Urakawa M, Yamaguchi K, Tsuchida E, Kashiwagi S, Ito H, Matsuda T. Blood-brain barrier disturbance following localized hyperthermia in rats. Int J Hyperth. 1995;11(5):709–18.
298. Oscar KJ, Hawkins TD. Microwave alteration of the blood-brain barrier system of rats. Brain Res. 1977;126(2):281–93.
299. Allen IV. Cerebral changes in experimental heatstroke. Ir J Med Sci. 1964;465:413–22.
300. Salehi A, Paturu MR, Patel B, Cain MD, Mahlokozera T, Yang AB, et al. Therapeutic enhancement of blood-brain and blood-tumor barriers permeability by laser interstitial thermal therapy. Neurooncol Adv. 2020;2(1):vdaa071.
301. Lee S, Son B, Park G, Kim H, Kang H, Jeon J, et al. Immunogenic effect of hyperthermia on enhancing radiotherapeutic efficacy. Int J Mol Sci. 2018;19(9):2795.
302. Chen T, Guo J, Han C, Yang M, Cao X. Heat shock protein 70, released from heat-stressed tumor cells, initiates antitumor immunity by inducing tumor cell chemokine production and activating dendritic cells via TLR4 pathway. J Immunol. 2009;182(3):1449–59.
303. Chandar JS, Bhatia S, Ingle S, Mendez Valdez MJ, Maric D, Seetharam D, et al. Laser interstitial thermal therapy induces robust local immune response for newly diagnosed glioblastoma with long-term survival and disease control. J Immunother. 2023;46(9):351–4.

304. Varatharaj A, Liljeroth M, Darekar A, Larsson HBW, Galea I, Cramer SP. Blood-brain barrier permeability measured using dynamic contrast-enhanced magnetic resonance imaging: a validation study. J Physiol. 2019;597(3):699–709.
305. Huang S, Farrar CT, Dai G, Kwon SJ, Bogdanov AA Jr, Rosen BR, et al. Dynamic monitoring of blood-brain barrier integrity using water exchange index (WEI) during mannitol and CO_2 challenges in mouse brain. NMR Biomed. 2013;26(4):376–85.
306. Dickie BR, Parker GJM, Parkes LM. Measuring water exchange across the blood-brain barrier using MRI. Prog Nucl Magn Reson Spectrosc. 2020;116:19–39.
307. Shao X, Jann K, Ma SJ, Yan L, Montagne A, Ringman JM, et al. Comparison between blood-brain barrier water exchange rate and permeability to gadolinium-based contrast agent in an elderly cohort. Front Neurosci. 2020;14:571480.
308. Zeuthen T. Water-transporting proteins. J Membr Biol. 2010;234(2):57–73.
309. Lan YL, Wang X, Lou JC, Ma XC, Zhang B. The potential roles of aquaporin 4 in malignant gliomas. Oncotarget. 2017;8(19):32345–55.
310. Harris WJ, Asselin MC, Hinz R, Parkes LM, Allan S, Schiessl I, et al. In vivo methods for imaging blood-brain barrier function and dysfunction. Eur J Nucl Med Mol Imaging. 2023;50(4):1051–83.
311. Johannsen B. The usefulness of radiotracers to make the body biochemically transparent. Amino Acids. 2005;29(4):307–11.
312. Umemura A, Suzuka T, Yamada K. Quantitative measurement of cerebral blood flow by (99m)Tc-HMPAO SPECT in acute ischaemic stroke: usefulness in determining therapeutic options. J Neurol Neurosurg Psychiatry. 2000;69(4):472–8.
313. Kane SM, Padda IS, Davis DD. Technetium-99m. In: StatPearls. Treasure Island, FL: StatPearls Publishing; 2024.
314. Loberg MD, Corder EH, Fields AT, Callery PS. Membrane transport of Tc-99m-labeled radiopharmaceuticals, I. Brain uptake by passive transport. J Nucl Med. 1979;20(11):1181–8.
315. Lin KJ, Liu HL, Hsu PH, Chung YH, Huang WC, Chen JC, et al. Quantitative micro-SPECT/CT for detecting focused ultrasound-induced blood-brain barrier opening in the rat. Nucl Med Biol. 2009;36(7):853–61.
316. Okada M, Kikuchi T, Okamura T, Ikoma Y, Tsuji AB, Wakizaka H, et al. In-vivo imaging of blood-brain barrier permeability using positron emission tomography with 2-amino-[3-11C]isobutyric acid. Nucl Med Commun. 2015;36(12):1239–48.
317. Marie S, Tournier N. PET imaging to study the functional impact of P-glycoprotein in neuropharmacokinetics. Therapie. 2020;75(6):623–32.
318. Verger A, Langen KJ. PET imaging in glioblastoma: use in clinical practice. In: De Vleeschouwer S, editor. Glioblastoma. Brisbane: Codon Publications; 2017.
319. Saunders NR, Dziegielewska KM, Møllgård K, Habgood MD. Markers for blood-brain barrier integrity: how appropriate is Evans blue in the twenty-first century and what are the alternatives? Front Neurosci. 2015;9:385.
320. Kiviniemi V, Korhonen V, Kortelainen J, Rytky S, Keinänen T, Tuovinen T, et al. Real-time monitoring of human blood-brain barrier disruption. PLoS One. 2017;12(3):e0174072.
321. Nita DA, Vanhatalo S, Lafortune FD, Voipio J, Kaila K, Amzica F. Nonneuronal origin of CO_2-related DC EEG shifts: an in vivo study in the cat. J Neurophysiol. 2004;92(2):1011–22.
322. Chu P-C, Liu H-L, Lai H-Y, Lin C-Y, Tsai H-C, Pei Y-C. Neuromodulation accompanying focused ultrasound-induced blood-brain barrier opening. Sci Rep. 2015;5(1):15477.
323. Warnke PC, Phillips A, Bernstein LP, Groothuis DR. The somatosensory evoked potential as a noninvasive method to determine flow rates for hyperosmotic disruption of the blood-brain barrier. Neurosurgery. 1989;25(3):405–11.
324. Momoh J, Kapsokalyvas D, Vogt M, Hak S, Kiessling F, van Zandvoort M, et al. Intravital microscopy for real-time monitoring of drug delivery and nanobiological processes. Adv Drug Deliv Rev. 2022;189:114528.
325. Poon C, Mühlenpfordt M, Olsman M, Kotopoulis S, de Lange Davies C, Hynynen K. Real-time intravital multiphoton microscopy to visualize focused ultrasound and microbubble treatments to increase blood-brain barrier permeability. J Vis Exp. 2022;(180).
326. Waithe OY, Shaji CA, Childs EW, Tharakan B. Determination of blood-brain barrier hyperpermeability using intravital microscopy. Methods Mol Biol. 2024;2711:117–27.
327. Denes A, Pradillo JM, Drake C, Buggey H, Rothwell NJ, Allan SM. Surgical manipulation compromises leukocyte mobilization responses and inflammation after experimental cerebral ischemia in mice. Front Neurosci. 2013;7:271.
328. Podgorski K, Ranganathan G. Brain heating induced by near-infrared lasers during multiphoton microscopy. J Neurophysiol. 2016;116(3):1012–23.
329. Chowdhury EA, Alqahtani F, Bhattacharya R, Mehvar R, Bickel U. Simultaneous UPLC–MS/MS analysis of two stable isotope labeled versions of sucrose in mouse plasma and brain samples as markers of blood-brain barrier permeability and brain vascular space. J Chromatogr B. 2018;1073:19–26.
330. Chowdhury EA, Noorani B, Alqahtani F, Bhalerao A, Raut S, Sivandzade F, et al. Understanding the brain uptake and permeability of small molecules through the BBB: a technical overview. J Cereb Blood Flow Metab. 2021;41(8):1797–820.
331. Kaya M, Ahishali B. Assessment of permeability in barrier type of endothelium in brain using tracers: Evans blue, sodium fluorescein, and horseradish peroxidase. Methods Mol Biol. 2011;763:369–82.
332. Salem H, Loux JJ, Smith S, Nichols CW. Evaluation of the toxicologic and teratogenic potentials of sodium fluorescein in the rat. Toxicology. 1979;12(2):143–50.
333. Ek CJ, Dziegielewska KM, Stolp H, Saunders NR. Functional effectiveness of the blood-brain barrier to small water-soluble molecules in developing and adult opossum (Monodelphis domestica). J Comp Neurol. 2006;496(1):13–26.
334. Rowley DA, Benditt EP. 5-Hydroxytryptamine and histamine as mediators of the vascular injury produced by agents which damage mast cells in rats. J Exp Med. 1956;103(4):399–412.
335. Lundsgaard-Hansen P. Treatment of shock with dextrans and gelatins. Effects and side effects. Vox Sang. 1969;17(3):161–93.
336. Ek CJ, Habgood MD, Dziegielewska KM, Potter A, Saunders NR. Permeability and route of entry for lipid-insoluble molecules across brain barriers in developing Monodelphis domestica. J Physiol. 2001;536(Pt 3):841–53.
337. Bellavance MA, Blanchette M, Fortin D. Recent advances in blood-brain barrier disruption as a CNS delivery strategy. AAPS J. 2008;10(1):166–77.
338. Greene C, Hanley N, Reschke CR, Reddy A, Mäe MA, Connolly R, et al. Microvascular stabilization via blood-brain barrier regulation prevents seizure activity. Nat Commun. 2022;13(1):2003.
339. Bar-Klein G, Lublinsky S, Kamintsky L, Noyman I, Veksler R, Dalipaj H, et al. Imaging blood–brain barrier dysfunction as a biomarker for epileptogenesis. Brain. 2017;140(6):1692–705.
340. Cacheaux LP, Ivens S, David Y, Lakhter AJ, Bar-Klein G, Shapira M, et al. Transcriptome profiling reveals TGF-signaling involvement in epileptogenesis. J Neurosci. 2009;29(28):8927–35.
341. Swissa E, Serlin Y, Vazana U, Prager O, Friedman A. Blood-brain barrier dysfunction in status epileptics: mechanisms and role in epileptogenesis. Epilepsy Behav. 2019;101(Pt B):106285.
342. Uluc K, Ambady P, Mcintyre MK, Tabb JP, Kersch CN, Nerison CS, et al. Safety of intra-arterial chemotherapy with or without osmotic blood–brain barrier disruption for the treatment of patients with brain tumors. Neurooncol Adv. 2022;4(1):vdac104.

343. Scott RE. Undifferentiated and differentiated L6 myoblast plasma membranes. II: Comparison of the morphological and biochemical characteristics of isolated plasma membranes. Cell Differ. 1978;7(6):335–43.
344. Kaya M, Gulturk S, Elmas I, Kalayci R, Arican N, Kocyildiz ZC, et al. The effects of magnesium sulfate on blood-brain barrier disruption caused by intracarotid injection of hyperosmolar mannitol in rats. Life Sci. 2004;76(2):201–12.
345. McAllister LD, Doolittle ND, Guastadisegni PE, Kraemer DF, Lacy CA, Crossen JR, et al. Cognitive outcomes and long-term follow-up results after enhanced chemotherapy delivery for primary central nervous system lymphoma. Neurosurgery. 2000;46(1):51–60; discussion 61.
346. Park SH, Kim MJ, Jung HH, Chang WS, Choi HS, Rachmilevitch I, et al. Safety and feasibility of multiple blood-brain barrier disruptions for the treatment of glioblastoma in patients undergoing standard adjuvant chemotherapy. J Neurosurg. 2021;134(2):475–83.
347. Chen KT, Chai WY, Lin YJ, Lin CJ, Chen PY, Tsai HC, et al. Neuronavigation-guided focused ultrasound for transcranial blood-brain barrier opening and immunostimulation in brain tumors. Sci Adv. 2021;7(6):eabd0772.
348. Park SH, Kim MJ, Jung HH, Chang WS, Choi HS, Rachmilevitch I, et al. One-year outcome of multiple blood-brain barrier disruptions with temozolomide for the treatment of glioblastoma. Front Oncol. 2020;10:1663.
349. Dharmasaroja PA. Fluid intake related to brain edema in acute middle cerebral artery infarction. Transl Stroke Res. 2016;7(1):49–53.
350. Giraud M, Cho TH, Nighoghossian N, Maucort-Boulch D, Deiana G, Østergaard L, et al. Early blood brain barrier changes in acute ischemic stroke: a sequential MRI study. J Neuroimaging. 2015;25(6):959–63.
351. O'Donnell ME. Blood-brain barrier Na transporters in ischemic stroke. Adv Pharmacol. 2014;71:113–46.
352. Asahi M, Wang X, Mori T, Sumii T, Jung J-C, Moskowitz MA, et al. Effects of matrix metalloproteinase-9 gene knock-out on the proteolysis of blood–brain barrier and white matter components after cerebral ischemia. J Neurosci. 2001;21(19):7724–32.
353. Kago T, Takagi N, Date I, Takenaga Y, Takagi K, Takeo S. Cerebral ischemia enhances tyrosine phosphorylation of occludin in brain capillaries. Biochem Biophys Res Commun. 2006;339(4):1197–203.
354. Jha RM, Kochanek PM, Simard JM. Pathophysiology and treatment of cerebral edema in traumatic brain injury. Neuropharmacology. 2019;145(Pt B):230–46.
355. Millay RH, Klein ML, Shults WT, Dahlborg SA, Neuwelt EA. Maculopathy associated with combination chemotherapy and osmotic opening of the blood-brain barrier. Am J Ophthalmol. 1986;102(5):626–32.
356. Simonett JM, Skalet AH, Lujan BJ, Neuwelt EA, Ambady P, Lin P. Risk factors and disease course for blood-brain barrier disruption-associated maculopathy. JAMA Ophthalmol. 2021;139(2):143–9.
357. Heye AK, Culling RD, Valdés Hernández Mdel C, Thrippleton MJ, Wardlaw JM. Assessment of blood-brain barrier disruption using dynamic contrast-enhanced MRI. A systematic review. Neuroimage Clin. 2014;6:262–74.
358. Martino F, Amici G, Rosner M, Ronco C, Novara G. Gadolinium-based contrast media nephrotoxicity in kidney impairment: the physio-pathological conditions for the perfect murder. J Clin Med. 2021;10(2):271.
359. Rundback JH, Nahl D, Yoo V. Contrast-induced nephropathy. J Vasc Surg. 2011;54(2):575–9.
360. Layne KA, Wood DM, Dargan PI. Gadolinium-based contrast agents—what is the evidence for 'gadolinium deposition disease' and the use of chelation therapy? Clin Toxicol (Phila). 2020;58(3):151–60.
361. Kanda T, Ishii K, Kawaguchi H, Kitajima K, Takenaka D. High signal intensity in the dentate nucleus and globus pallidus on unenhanced T1-weighted MR images: relationship with increasing cumulative dose of a gadolinium-based contrast material. Radiology. 2014;270(3):834–41.
362. Miller JH, Hu HH, Pokorney A, Cornejo P, Towbin R. MRI brain signal intensity changes of a child during the course of 35 gadolinium contrast examinations. Pediatrics. 2015;136(6):e1637–40.
363. Fischer-Williams M, Gottschalk PG, Browell JN. Transient cortical blindness. An unusual complication of coronary angiography. Neurology. 1970;20(4):353–5.
364. Li J, Qi G, Zhang H, Chen G, Wang S, Yan M, et al. Contrast-induced encephalopathy mimicking stroke after a second cerebral DSA: an unusual case report. BMC Neurol. 2021;21(1):430.
365. Andone S, Balasa R, Barcutean L, Bajko Z, Ion V, Motataianu A, et al. Contrast medium-induced encephalopathy after coronary angiography—case report. J Crit Care Med (Targu Mures). 2021;7(2):145–9.
366. Torvik A, Walday P. Neurotoxicity of water-soluble contrast media. Acta Radiol Suppl. 1995;399:221–9.
367. Yu J, Dangas G. Commentary: New insights into the risk factors of contrast-induced encephalopathy. J Endovasc Ther. 2011;18(4):545–6.
368. Hassel B, Iversen EG, Fonnum F. Neurotoxicity of albumin in vivo. Neurosci Lett. 1994;167(1–2):29–32.
369. Neuwelt EA, Glasberg M, Frenkel E, Barnett P. Neurotoxicity of chemotherapeutic agents after blood-brain barrier modification: neuropathological studies. Ann Neurol. 1983;14(3):316–24.
370. Neuwelt EA, Barnett PA, Glasberg M, Frenkel EP. Pharmacology and neurotoxicity of cis-diamminedichloroplatinum, bleomycin, 5-fluorouracil, and cyclophosphamide administration following osmotic blood-brain barrier modification. Cancer Res. 1983;43(11):5278–85.
371. Fortin D, McCormick CI, Remsen LG, Nixon R, Neuwelt EA. Unexpected neurotoxicity of etoposide phosphate administered in combination with other chemotherapeutic agents after blood-brain barrier modification to enhance delivery, using propofol for general anesthesia, in a rat model. Neurosurgery. 2000;47(1):199–207.
372. Riviere-Cazaux C, Carlstrom LP, Rajani K, Munoz-Casabella A, Rahman M, Gharibi-Loron A, et al. Blood-brain barrier disruption defines the extracellular metabolome of live human high-grade gliomas. Commun Biol. 2023;6(1):653.
373. Li L, Di X, Zhang S, Kan Q, Liu H, Lu T, et al. Large amino acid transporter 1 mediated glutamate modified docetaxel-loaded liposomes for glioma targeting. Colloids Surf B Biointerfaces. 2016;141:260–7.
374. Bhunia S, Vangala V, Bhattacharya D, Ravuri HG, Kuncha M, Chakravarty S, et al. Large amino acid transporter 1 selective liposomes of l-DOPA functionalized amphiphile for combating glioblastoma. Mol Pharm. 2017;14(11):3834–47.
375. Ying X, Wen H, Lu WL, Du J, Guo J, Tian W, et al. Dual-targeting daunorubicin liposomes improve the therapeutic efficacy of brain glioma in animals. J Control Release. 2010;141(2):183–92.
376. Peng Y, Zhao Y, Chen Y, Yang Z, Zhang L, Xiao W, et al. Dual-targeting for brain-specific liposomes drug delivery system: synthesis and preliminary evaluation. Bioorg Med Chem. 2018;26(16):4677–86.
377. Shao K, Ding N, Huang S, Ren S, Zhang Y, Kuang Y, et al. Smart nanodevice combined tumor-specific vector with cellular microenvironment-triggered property for highly effective antiglioma therapy. ACS Nano. 2014;8(2):1191–203.
378. Kou L, Hou Y, Yao Q, Guo W, Wang G, Wang M, et al. L-Carnitine-conjugated nanoparticles to promote permeation across blood-

brain barrier and to target glioma cells for drug delivery via the novel organic cation/carnitine transporter OCTN2. Artif Cells Nanomed Biotechnol. 2018;46(8):1605–16.
379. Ohtsuki S, Terasaki T. Contribution of carrier-mediated transport systems to the blood-brain barrier as a supporting and protecting interface for the brain; importance for CNS drug discovery and development. Pharm Res. 2007;24(9):1745–58.
380. Lajoie JM, Shusta EV. Targeting receptor-mediated transport for delivery of biologics across the blood-brain barrier. Annu Rev Pharmacol Toxicol. 2015;55:613–31.
381. Bickel U. Antibody delivery through the blood-brain barrier. Adv Drug Deliv Rev. 1995;15(1–3):53–72.
382. Frankel AD, Pabo CO. Cellular uptake of the tat protein from human immunodeficiency virus. Cell. 1988;55(6):1189–93.
383. Green M, Loewenstein PM. Autonomous functional domains of chemically synthesized human immunodeficiency virus tat trans-activator protein. Cell. 1988;55(6):1179–88.
384. Xie J, Bi Y, Zhang H, Dong S, Teng L, Lee RJ, et al. Cell-penetrating peptides in diagnosis and treatment of human diseases: from preclinical research to clinical application. Front Pharmacol. 2020;11:697.
385. Vivès E, Richard JP, Rispal C, Lebleu B. TAT peptide internalization: seeking the mechanism of entry. Curr Protein Pept Sci. 2003;4(2):125–32.
386. Kauffman WB, Fuselier T, He J, Wimley WC. Mechanism matters: a taxonomy of cell penetrating peptides. Trends Biochem Sci. 2015;40(12):749–64.
387. Usmani PASS. CPPsite 2.0: a database of cell penetrating peptides. 2024. https://webs.iiitd.edu.in/raghava/cppsite/stats1.php.
388. Fowler MJ, Cotter JD, Knight BE, Sevick-Muraca EM, Sandberg DI, Sirianni RW. Intrathecal drug delivery in the era of nanomedicine. Adv Drug Deliv Rev. 2020;165–166:77–95.
389. Gehling M, Tryba M. Risks and side-effects of intrathecal morphine combined with spinal anaesthesia: a meta-analysis. Anaesthesia. 2009;64(6):643–51.
390. Lake W, Shah H. Intrathecal baclofen infusion for the treatment of movement disorders. Neurosurg Clin N Am. 2019;30(2):203–9.
391. Sandberg DI, Yu B, Patel R, Hagan J, Miesner E, Sabin J, et al. Infusion of 5-Azacytidine (5-AZA) into the fourth ventricle or resection cavity in children with recurrent posterior fossa ependymoma: a pilot clinical trial. J Neurooncol. 2019;141(2):449–57.
392. Brem H, Mahaley MS Jr, Vick NA, Black KL, Schold SC Jr, Burger PC, et al. Interstitial chemotherapy with drug polymer implants for the treatment of recurrent gliomas. J Neurosurg. 1991;74(3):441–6.
393. Ashby LS, Smith KA, Stea B. Gliadel wafer implantation combined with standard radiotherapy and concurrent followed by adjuvant temozolomide for treatment of newly diagnosed high-grade glioma: a systematic literature review. World J Surg Oncol. 2016;14(1):225.
394. Stupp R, Mason WP, van den Bent MJ, Weller M, Fisher B, Taphoorn MJ, et al. Radiotherapy plus concomitant and adjuvant temozolomide for glioblastoma. N Engl J Med. 2005;352(10):987–96.
395. Puente P, Fettig N, Luderer MJ, Jin A, Shah S, Muz B, et al. Injectable hydrogels for localized chemotherapy and radiotherapy in brain tumors. J Pharm Sci. 2018;107(3):922–33.
396. Dugam S, Tade R, Dhole R, Nangare S. Emerging era of microneedle array for pharmaceutical and biomedical applications: recent advances and toxicological perspectives. Fut J Pharm Sci. 2021;7(1):19.
397. Muresan P, McCrorie P, Smith F, Vasey C, Taresco V, Scurr DJ, et al. Development of nanoparticle loaded microneedles for drug delivery to a brain tumour resection site. Eur J Pharm Biopharm. 2023;182:53–61.
398. Lee Y, Kang T, Cho HR, Lee GJ, Park OK, Kim S, et al. Localized delivery of theranostic nanoparticles and high-energy photons using microneedles-on-bioelectronics. Adv Mater. 2021;33(24):e2100425.
399. Agrawal M, Saraf S, Antimisiaris SG, Chougule MB, Shoyele SA, Alexander A. Nose-to-brain drug delivery: an update on clinical challenges and progress towards approval of anti-Alzheimer drugs. J Control Release. 2018;281:139–77.
400. Wu D, Chen Q, Chen X, Han F, Chen Z, Wang Y. The blood-brain barrier: structure, regulation, and drug delivery. Signal Transduct Target Ther. 2023;8(1):217.
401. Hanson LR, Frey WH II. Intranasal delivery bypasses the blood-brain barrier to target therapeutic agents to the central nervous system and treat neurodegenerative disease. BMC Neurosci. 2008;9(Suppl 3):S5.
402. Van den Berg MP, Merkus P, Romeijn SG, Verhoef JC, Merkus FW. Hydroxocobalamin uptake into the cerebrospinal fluid after nasal and intravenous delivery in rats and humans. J Drug Target. 2003;11(6):325–31.
403. Al-Ghananeem AM, Traboulsi AA, Dittert LW, Hussain AA. Targeted brain delivery of 17 beta-estradiol via nasally administered water soluble prodrugs. AAPS PharmSciTech. 2002;3(1):E5.
404. Kanazawa T, Akiyama F, Kakizaki S, Takashima Y, Seta Y. Delivery of siRNA to the brain using a combination of nose-to-brain delivery and cell-penetrating peptide-modified nano-micelles. Biomaterials. 2013;34(36):9220–6.
405. Danielyan L, Schäfer R, von Ameln-Mayerhofer A, Bernhard F, Verleysdonk S, Buadze M, et al. Therapeutic efficacy of intranasally delivered mesenchymal stem cells in a rat model of Parkinson disease. Rejuvenation Res. 2011;14(1):3–16.
406. Godfrey L, Iannitelli A, Garrett NL, Moger J, Imbert I, King T, et al. Nanoparticulate peptide delivery exclusively to the brain produces tolerance free analgesia. J Control Release. 2018;270:135–44.
407. Rosenberg GA. Neurological diseases in relation to the blood-brain barrier. J Cereb Blood Flow Metab. 2012;32(7):1139–51.
408. Verscheijden LFM, Koenderink JB, de Wildt SN, Russel FGM. Differences in P-glycoprotein activity in human and rodent blood-brain barrier assessed by mechanistic modelling. Arch Toxicol. 2021;95(9):3015–29.

Magnetic Resonance-Guided Focused Ultrasound Blood-Brain Barrier Disruption for Targeted Delivery of Therapeutics to the Central Nervous System

6

Christopher B. Pople, Yuexi Huang, Ying Meng, and Nir Lipsman

"Science cannot progress without reliable and accurate measurements of what you are trying to study. The key is measurement, simple as that."

Robert D. Hare, (born 1934), Canadian Psychologist

Introduction

Disorders of the central nervous system (CNS) are highly prevalent and significantly degrade the quality of life, productivity, and survival. Data from the Global Burden of Disease study suggests that neurological disorders are the largest source of disability-adjusted life-years and the second largest cause of mortality worldwide, with increasing prevalence in aging populations [1, 2]. In the USA alone, it has been estimated that neurological disorders cost nearly $800 billion US dollars (2014) per year [3]. Additionally, progression of many peripheral diseases into the CNS is associated with a higher risk of mortality. For example, a retrospective analysis of patients with stage IV breast cancer identified the brain as the metastatic site with the poorest prognosis [4]. As such, the development and iterative improvement of treatment for CNS disorders present significant opportunities to improve individual health outcomes, quality of life, and societal well-being.

Considerable private and public funds and research efforts have been directed to CNS drug development. For example, categorizing the NIH grant portfolio by research area, neuroscience represented the most significant portion of funding and grew by nearly 50% between 2016 and 2019 [5]. Despite this, CNS drug development is associated with a substantially higher failure rate, particularly in phase 3 clinical trials, relative to translational research in other areas [6, 7]. Drugs intended for CNS indications face numerous barriers to success. In particular, poor mechanistic understanding of pathobiology and/or drug action and pharmacokinetic shortcomings, including lack of target engagement, have been identified as likely explanations for failed trials in CNS disorders [8]. Additionally, neurotoxicity and off-target CNS effects are significant concerns that contribute significantly to adverse drug effects [7, 9]. While improving mechanistic understanding of CNS pathobiology and pharmacodynamics are broad goals, optimizing and improving drug delivery platforms represent an opportunity to increase the efficacy and translational success of novel CNS-targeted therapies [8, 10].

An important limiting factor in discovering new CNS drug candidates is the relative rarity and substantial constraints on their structure relative to drugs with peripheral targets [10, 11]. For example, it's been estimated that 98% of all drug candidates do not enter the brain parenchyma to a significant extent due to limitations on size and sufficient lipid solubility imposed by the blood-brain barrier (BBB) and blood-cerebrospinal fluid (CSF) barrier [10, 11]. Furthermore, virtually all large molecules, particularly biological therapies, including monoclonal antibodies, cannot cross the BBB [10]. In addition, while many small lipophilic drugs may readily cross the BBB, protein binding and the tendency to accumulate in lipid-rich environments in the periphery may still limit CNS exposure and parenchymal penetrance [9, 10]. When injected directly into the brain parenchyma, many drugs travel only a few millimeters from the site of administration [10]. Lastly, many drugs possess an affinity for efflux pumps located at the BBB, such as the

C. B. Pople · Y. Huang · Y. Meng · N. Lipsman (✉)
Sunnybrook Health Sciences Centre, Department of Surgery, University of Toronto, Toronto, ON, Canada
e-mail: nir.lipsman@sunnybrook.ca

S. Joshi (ed.), *Arterial Treatment of Neurological Diseases*, https://doi.org/10.1007/978-3-031-80173-0_6

ATP-binding cassette transporter P-glycoprotein (P-gp), which actively transports substrates out of the brain and thereby limits CNS penetrance [9, 10].

As a result, vectors for successful CNS drug delivery are an area of great interest. Many approaches (and combinations thereof) are being explored to optimize drug delivery to the CNS. These include molecules functionalized to be transported via active processes, various nanoparticles, and mechanisms to physically disrupt the BBB [10, 12]. Intra-arterial hyperosmotic mannitol can open the BBB by exploiting osmotic pressures induced at downstream capillaries. However, its use has been limited by its lack of spatial specificity and incidence of associated seizures [13]. Low-intensity focused ultrasound (FUS) with intravascular microbubbles is an emerging intervention intended to temporarily disrupt the BBB for enhanced drug delivery with excellent spatial and temporal control [14]. The benefits of FUS BBB opening include the ability to (1) use unmodified drugs, (2) deliver a wide variety of therapeutics, including those with poor lipid solubility and large molecules such as nanoparticles and viruses, (3) target sites of pathology while sparing other brain tissue, and (4) flexibly augment other drug delivery strategies [15–17]. Initial safety and feasibility data from FUS BBB opening clinical trials have been encouraging for several indications, and many additional clinical trials are ongoing or planned.

The Blood-Brain Barrier (BBB)

The BBB is a series of features of brain capillaries, choroid plexus, and meninges that limit their permeability to molecules in the blood through various passive structural features and active molecular processes [18, 19]. Along with the blood-cerebrospinal fluid barrier, composed of choroid plexus ependymal cells, the BBB maintains a tightly regulated separation of peripheral and central systems [18, 19]. These barriers maintain the distinct composition of CSF and brain interstitial fluid relative to blood, protect the CNS from peripheral toxins, infection, and the host immune system, and isolate many central and peripheral signaling molecules, allowing divergent functions [18, 19]. It also poses a considerable barrier to the delivery and efficacy of most potential therapeutics [10].

In healthy brain tissue, capillary endothelial cells of the BBB are lined by a dense, negatively charged glycocalyx and joined by tight junction complexes and adherens junctions, which profoundly limit passive paracellular diffusion [12, 19]. These capillary endothelial cells are additionally surrounded by basal lamina, pericytes, and astrocyte end-feet, which contribute to maintaining the BBB's structural and functional integrity [12, 19]. As a result of these structural features, the BBB profoundly limits the permeability of small (<500 Da) water-soluble molecules and prohibits the passage of larger molecules [12, 19]. Specific brain regions (e.g., the ventromedial hypothalamus) lack a proper BBB, with tanycytes providing a more permeable barrier [12, 18].

Various active transport mechanisms are also localized to the BBB, including drug efflux pumps that remove substances from the CNS and transport systems for specific molecules in the peripheral circulation [10, 19, 20]. Drugs with an affinity for efflux transporters, such as P-gp, are transported from the CNS back into the peripheral circulation, limiting their ability to act in the brain [10, 20]. Conversely, some channels, transporters, and receptors associated with vesicular transcytosis pathways localized to the BBB act to transport their substrates selectively from peripheral circulation into the CNS [10, 12]. Examples include glucose transport via the solute carrier transporter GLUT1 and transferrin via the transferrin receptor (TfR) [12].

In healthy individuals, the BBB is predominantly intact through CNS and is a robust barrier to most peripheral substances. However, variations in circadian rhythm, psychosocial stress, and changes in diet do occur [21]. In disease states, BBB function can be disrupted, or in some cases enhanced, to alter permeability in manners that may contribute to pathology or interfere with treatment [19, 22, 23]. For example, BBB integrity decreases with age and is sparsely compromised in many neurodegenerative diseases [19]. In contrast, the BBB is often compromised focally within brain tumors, although considerable function remains even in lesions enhancing with BBB-impermeable contrast agents [24]. In particular, efflux transporters can be upregulated in some solid tumors and confer chemoresistance even when brain tumors disrupt the BBB [23, 24]. Furthermore, such efflux transporters have also been implicated in drug resistance in epilepsy [22].

Thus, although the BBB is not always perfectly intact, it represents a considerable barrier to brain delivery and CNS target engagement by diverse classes of therapeutics. As such, there is great interest in approaches to modulate BBB permeability to improve drug delivery across various indications. Much work has focused on developing novel formulations for drug delivery across the BBB, such as novel pro-drugs, various lipid and polymer nanoparticles, and antibody-drug conjugates targeting transport systems such as the TfR [25–27]. These platforms offer many advantages, including the possibility of creating oral or intranasal formulations and controlling the kinetics of drug delivery and release [26, 27]. Additionally, they may provide better safety and scalability relative to many alternative approaches. Nonetheless, they are hindered by limitations on the physical properties of therapeutics with which they can be combined and the additional regulatory burden of testing novel formulations.

Due to these limitations, modalities for drug delivery to the CNS that do not require modification of the existing therapeutic are of particular interest. Existing surgical interventions such as convection-enhanced delivery allow focal delivery of the maximum possible dose but require intracranial access. Drug-infused wafers yield similar benefits with minimal limitations on the therapeutic involved but similarly carry an intrinsic risk of intracranial hemorrhage, swelling, infection, and other neurological sequelae associated with the related surgical intervention. Intra-arterial mannitol allows relatively less spatial specificity and avoids much of the risk of a craniotomy, but seizures have still been reported [13]. Therefore, considerable value could be derived from safer mechanisms of modulating BBB permeability or improving drug delivery to the CNS that do not necessitate modifying existing therapeutics.

Focused Ultrasound

An emerging modality for BBB disruption is FUS, which combines low-intensity ultrasound emissions with intravascular microbubbles. Intravascular microbubbles are ultrasound contrast agents already approved for human use and are used extensively for diagnostic echocardiograms [28]. FUS achieves BBB opening via a physical mechanism. Ultrasound energy triggers stable cavitation of microbubbles, a phenomenon in which the bubbles exhibit oscillating stretching and contractions. This leads to altered, fluctuating intravascular pressure and reversible separation of tight junctions between endothelial cells of the BBB [15, 29]. Additionally, indirect biological effects of FUS BBB opening also induce downregulation of drug efflux transporters at the BBB [30]. Together, this produces increased permeability of the BBB within the targeted tissue volume where sufficient pressures are reached.

Ultrasound can produce various thermal, mechanical, and downstream biological effects on tissues. In high-intensity FUS, ultrasound alone achieves thermocoagulation lesioning. However, skull heating limits the spatial location of targets, which can be impacted by target depth and skull shape [31, 32]. Specifically, with a hemispherical transducer array design, deeper targets are more readily lesioned as more transducers can focus on the target while remaining perpendicular to the skull, spreading heat deposition across a large area of the skull [29, 33, 34]. Many transducers will have high incident angles for shallower targets, likely resulting in substantial off-target reflection of ultrasound and attenuation by skull heating [29, 32]. In such cases, individual transducers must be turned off, limiting maximum energy deposition and reducing the area of the skull through which all ultrasound energy must pass. A lower-frequency ultrasound reduces skull attenuation and, therefore, skull heating. Still, it is more likely to cause (unwanted) cavitation in vessels and tissues at high intensities, possibly leading to unexpected damage [32]. Skull heating is significant at high intensities despite active water cooling, limiting sonication intensity and duration while requiring breaks between sonications. As a result, this limits the volume of tissue that can be lesioned both at once and over consecutive closely spaced targets. At lower intensities, such as with FUS for BBB opening, skull heating is not a concern; therefore, shallower regions of the cortex and more inferior/posterior regions of the brain can be targeted in addition to the deeper targets.

Although FUS BBB opening was initially observed at the periphery of thermocoagulative lesions from high-intensity FUS [35, 36], the low-intensity FUS BBB opening relies on the cavitation of exogenously supplied microbubbles. BBB opening can be achieved with ultrasound power 2–3 orders of magnitude lower than that used in thermal lesioning [15, 37]. Specifically, ultrasound energy converging at a target achieves BBB opening by stable cavitation of intravascular microbubbles, in which oscillations act on vessel walls. These forces act on capillary endothelial cells, separating tight junctions that provide the fundamental physical barrier to the diffusion of large molecules [15, 31]. When pressure fluctuations are too large due to inertial cavitation, the bubbles burst, resulting in high-intensity shear forces, which can induce unwanted vascular damage. Nonetheless, the magnitude of potential vascular damage is proportional to the intensity of ultrasound. With cavitation feedback monitoring, FUS BBB opening has only been associated with asymptomatic and largely transient microhemorrhage in clinical trials and preclinical investigations [15, 38]. In addition to separating tight junctions, FUS BBB opening can elicit biological effects that may increase drug delivery to the brain, such as reduced expression of multi-drug efflux transporters at the BBB, including P-gp [30]. Notably, such efflux systems have been shown to reduce brain bioavailability of substrate drugs even in cases where the BBB is otherwise disrupted, as is the case with many brain tumors [24].

As the name suggests, focused ultrasound (FUS) exploits converging ultrasound emissions to achieve various biophysical effects at a relatively small target volume. Currently, the only FDA-approved transcranial MR-guided FUS (MRgFUS) system for thermoablation uses 1024 transducers operating at 650 kHz arranged in a hemispherical array around the head (ExAblate Neuro Type 1, Insightec) to spread ultrasound energy across the largest possible area [29]. CT images of the skull bone are aligned to structural MR images, from which ultrasound transducers can be steered to focus on a target, and optimal intensity and phase can be estimated to optimize energy delivery to the target while minimizing effects on the skull and off-target brain regions (Fig. 6.1) [29, 32]. This device is approved for thermal lesioning of the ventral intermediate nucleus of the thalamus to treat medication-refractory essential tremor. In this case, focal heating can be achieved so that the lesion, on the order of 5 mm, can be formed with sub-millimeter accuracy [29].

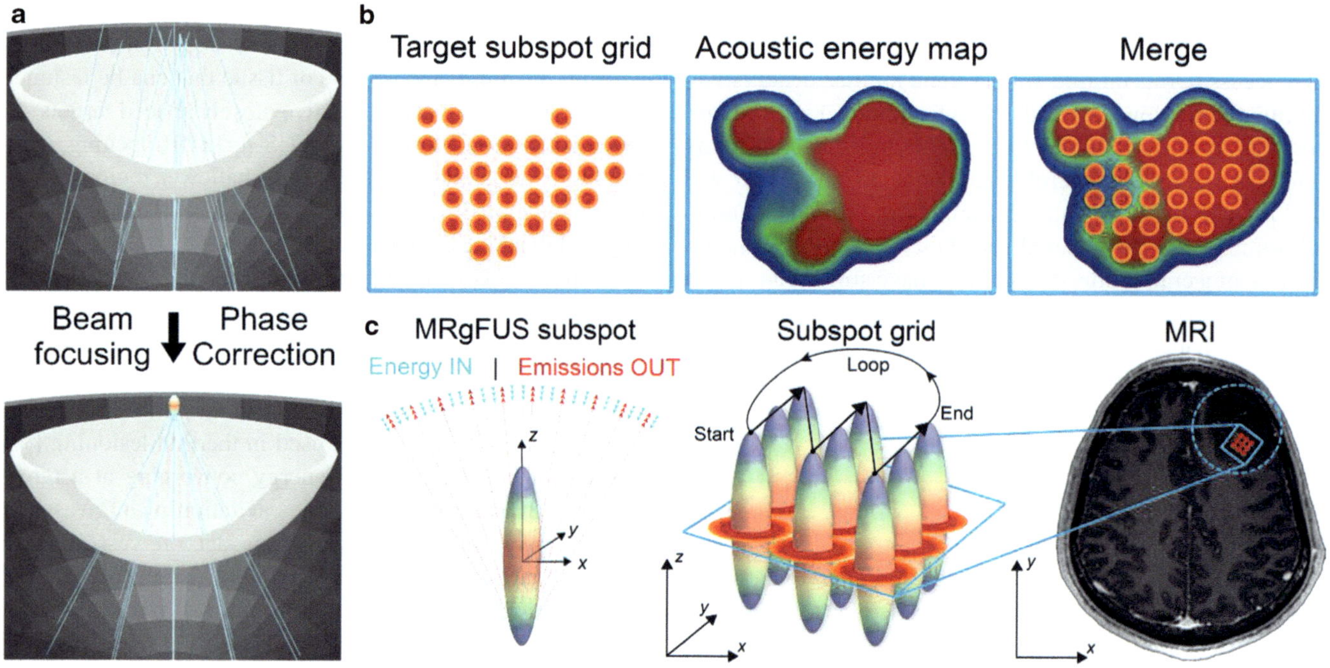

Fig. 6.1 Technical principles of MR-guided focused ultrasound blood-brain barrier disruption. Technical principles of MRgFUS BBB opening. (**a**) Using CT and MR imaging, many ultrasound "beams" (cyan) from transducers in a hemispheric array (dark grey) are focused through the skull, with correction for skull-induced phase aberrations made automatically. (**b**) Targets are selected in a 2D axial plane, arranged in a grid 1–32 subspots. Real-time acoustic feedback allows the estimation of cavitation signals at each individual target within the grid. (**c**) Converging ultrasound energy forms an ovoid target that is longer parallel to the incident beams and most intense towards the center, allowing overlapping axial layers to cover 3D volumes. During sonications, transducers sequentially sonicate each subspot in a grid briefly, looping back through the grid many times over a 60–120 s sonication. (Figures in **b** and **c** were reproduced from Anastasiadis et al. [50])

Such lesioning procedures, termed high-intensity MRgFUS, use 650 kHz ultrasound in transcranial applications to heat tissue at the focus above a target temperature of at least 55 °C to achieve thermal coagulation. Intra-operative MR thermometry is used to measure tissue heating [15, 29, 39].

Low-intensity transcranial FUS, used for BBB opening and neuromodulation, employs ultrasound at much lower intensities to achieve milder mechanical effects with negligible temperature rise [15, 29]. BBB opening can be achieved by combining low-intensity FUS with intravascular microbubble ultrasound contrast agents (e.g., FDA-approved Definity, Sonovue, and Optison) that nucleate mechanical forces within the vessels of the sonicated tissue volume [15, 31]. Intraoperative acoustic feedback via cavitation detection is often used to read out biophysical effects in situ and may improve the safety and reliability of BBB opening [15, 38, 40]. Additional emerging indications for low-frequency FUS include BBB opening for liquid biopsy [41, 42], neuromodulation with or without microbubbles at low sonication intensities [43, 44], and mechanical lesioning of tissue at higher sonication intensities with exogenous microbubbles [45, 46], or by generating them with ultrasound in situ (histotripsy) [47–49].

Without real-time MR guidance, targeted BBB opening has been achieved using neuronavigation systems alongside a single-element FUS transducer (NaviFUS and BrainSonix), providing a scalable and relatively low-cost option for BBB opening. An implantable intracranial transducer facilitates reproducible longitudinal BBB opening (SonoCloud, CarThera). One prototype MRgFUS device for BBB opening (ExAblate Neuro Type 2, Insightec) uses 1024 ultrasound transducers operating at 220 kHz. MRgFUS BBB opening using this device produces a pattern of BBB opening characterized by focal at "subspots" arranged within a grid of up to 32 "subspots." At each subspot, the extent of BBB opening is greatest at the center. It decreases as one moves along the pressure gradient, which typically takes on an oblong, oval shape (approximately 6.5 mm parallel to the transducer elements with a ~1.63 mm radius in the perpendicular plane) due to the angle of incident ultrasound [50]. Grids of subspots can be conformed to a target in 2D space and layered in 3D space to achieve a relatively dense coverage of BBB opening across target of arbitrary shape and size (Fig. 6.2) [50]. When assessed by gadolinium contrast-enhanced T1-weighted MR imaging, this produces a clear BBB opening that lasts approximately 8–24 h [51, 52].

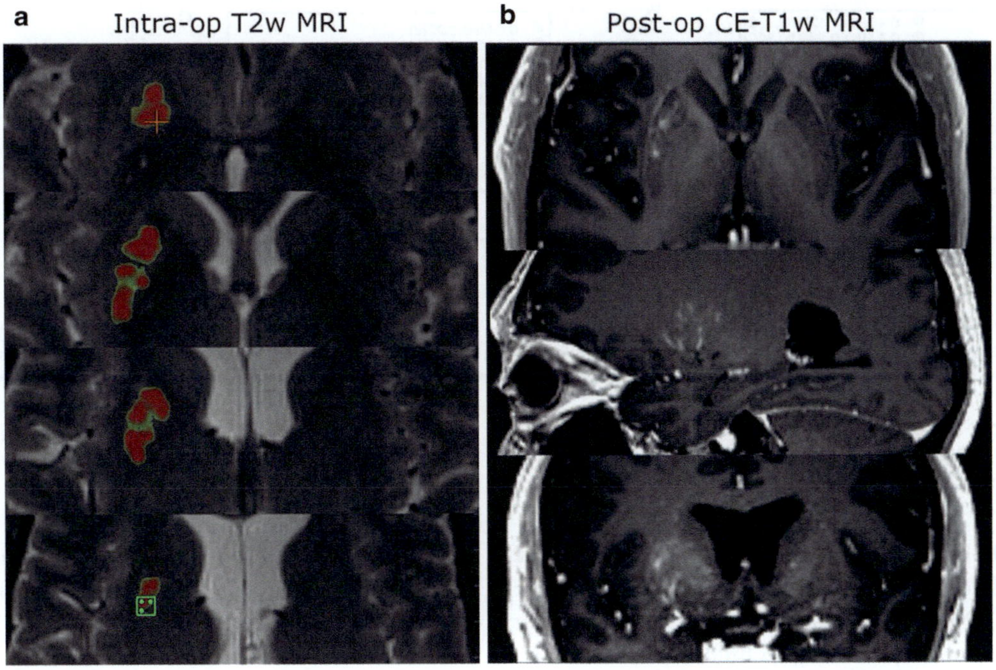

Fig. 6.2 Conformal MRgFUS BBB opening with even cavitation dosing throughout a 3D target. Representative images of three-dimensional conformal BBB opening throughout the putamen in patients with Parkinson's disease undergoing MRgFUS BBB opening of the putamen to facilitate imiglucerase delivery in a clinical trial (NCT04370665). (**a**) Overlayed on axial intra-operative T2-weighted MR images, cavitation maps show retrospective cumulative acoustic feedback acquired in real-time during sonication of many target grids (one shown in the bottom image), demonstrating even distribution of cavitation signal throughout axial layers of the putamen. (**b**) Axial (top), sagittal (middle), and coronal (bottom) slices of the putamen in immediate post-operative gadolinium contrast-enhanced MR imaging showing BBB opening throughout the 3D target volume. (Reproduced from Meng et al. [99])

Focused Ultrasound for Drug Delivery

So far, FUS BBB opening has primarily been investigated as a modality for drug delivery to the brain [15]. In this context, a substantial volume of preclinical research supports the ability of low-intensity FUS in combination with intravascular microbubbles to achieve a biologically significant increase in BBB permeability, substantial increases in drug delivery to the parenchyma or intracranial tumors, and significantly improved therapeutic efficacy [15, 31, 53]. A significant advantage of FUS BBB opening as a drug delivery modality is that it does not require modification of an existing therapeutic for parenchymal delivery, can provide spatially precise delivery, and can be conducted through a transcranial route. Nonetheless, certain ultrasound-sensitive carriers may allow local drug release at the site and time of BBB opening, further improving drug delivery while reducing systemic exposure [16, 54, 55].

FUS BBB opening was initially observed on the peripheries of animal thermocoagulative lesions [35, 56]. Subsequent work combining low-intensity FUS with intravenous delivery of microbubbles as a more reliable, exogenous driver of cavitation was able to achieve BBB opening at substantially lower powers [15, 56]. Over time, parameters have been refined to reliably achieve BBB opening in animal models without histological or other molecular evidence of tissue damage, albeit with occasional extravasation of erythrocytes [15, 57].

Preclinical research has characterized many underlying mechanisms of FUS BBB opening, relationships between sonication or drug parameters, and the extent of drug delivery in animal models. Electron microscopy has been used to visualize disruption of the tight junctions between capillary endothelial cells of the BBB and loss of expression of constituent proteins, as well as the recovery of tight junction protein expression, structure, and BBB function by 24 h post-sonication [58]. Concomitantly, BBB permeability to horseradish peroxidase, a large 40 kDa protein with an effective hydrodynamic diameter (d_H) of 6 nm, was increased for 2–4 h after sonication [58]. Subsequent work examining BBB permeability to nanoparticles of various sizes suggests an inverse relationship between the size of an administered compound and the duration of BBB permeability induced by FUS [52]. Specifically, BBB permeability was found to have an approximate half-time to close of 5 h for 1 nm particles, 1.5 h for 4 nm particles, and 1 h for 7 nm particles (Fig. 6.3) [52]. Nonetheless, the extent and duration of BBB opening are also related to mechanical forces experienced during

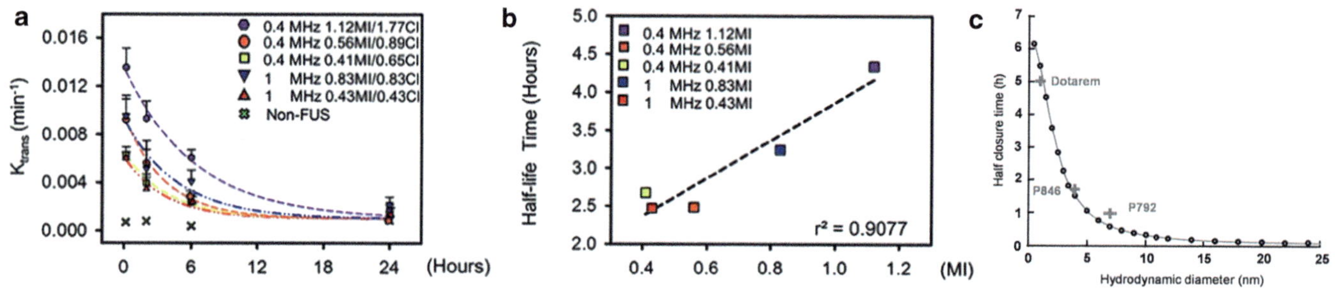

Fig. 6.3 Effect of ultrasound parameters and therapeutic size on BBB opening and drug delivery. Effect of FUS mechanical index ($MI = \frac{\text{power}}{\sqrt{\text{freq}}}$) on the extent of BBB opening and association of hydrodynamic diameter of compounds with brain delivery kinetics after FUS BBB opening. (**a**, **b**) Magnitude of BBB permeability and its longitudinal decay (expressed as half-life in **b**) as a function MI. Increasing MI is associated with greater initial permeability and a longer duration of BBB opening [59]. (**c**) Apparent half-life of BBB opening using tracers of varying hydrodynamic diameter. Larger compounds have a shorter window of brain availability after BBB opening, with quicker decay of permeability [52]. (Reproduced from Meng et al. [15] plots **a** and **b** reproduced from Chu et al. [59] and plot **c** from Marty et al. [52])

sonication, with the mechanical index (power divided by the square root of frequency) most closely associated with these factors [59, 60]. Notably, increased delivery of many larger therapeutics has been reported in preclinical models, including antibodies [61, 62], approximately 150 kDa, $d_H \approx 12$ nm [63, 64], AAV gene therapy vectors about 4000 kDa, $d_H \approx 20$ nm [65, 66], and liposomes ($d_H \approx 240$ nm) [67].

In addition to preclinical evidence of increased drug delivery, there is evidence for improved efficacy of diverse therapeutics in various animal models of human illness [15]. For example, increased delivery of small molecule chemotherapies and associated survival advantages have been demonstrated in many xenograft CNS tumor models [15, 68–70]. Similar drug delivery and survival advantages have been shown in similar models using larger therapeutics, including antibodies [61, 71] and gene therapy vectors [67, 72]. Similarly, increased delivery of antibodies targeting pathogenic proteins has been demonstrated in transgenic animal models of Alzheimer's (AD) and Parkinson's disease (PD) [73–78]. Targeted modulation of neuronal activity has been achieved with acoustically activated nanodroplets, in this case loaded with pentobarbital. The nanodroplets expand to form microbubbles in situ, simultaneously liberating the drug at intensities below those necessary to cause BBB opening [16, 54]. The resulting microbubbles can also serve as sources of cavitation for BBB opening at higher intensities, further enhancing drug delivery at the release site [79]. Thus, the FUS BBB opening provides an ideal platform for enhanced delivery, target engagement, and efficacy on biological endpoints in vivo across a broad range of existing and potential future therapeutics.

Although low-intensity FUS can achieve increased drug delivery and efficacy via physical separation of the tight junction, numerous additional biological effects can be induced, which may augment drug delivery and increase efficacy. As noted above, FUS BBB opening can reduce the expression of clinically relevant multi-drug transporters such as P-gp, which reduce parenchymal delivery of substrates even when the BBB is disrupted [30]. Similarly, FUS increases transcytosis at the BBB, which supports the transport of larger particles across endothelial barriers but is otherwise constitutively repressed at the BBB [15, 58, 80, 81].

Moreover, the potential of FUS to modulate the CNS microenvironment is a fascinating area of research. In animal models, FUS has demonstrated the ability to enhance neuronal uptake of antibodies, autophagy, and microglial phagocytosis. These effects reduce intracellular and extracellular pathogenic protein aggregates, such as tau, alpha-synuclein, and amyloid-beta, opening up new possibilities for therapeutic intervention [74, 76, 82–84]. Understanding the biological effects of FUS is crucial as it can help identify existing therapeutics that can be combined with FUS and guide novel therapeutic strategies optimized to exploit these effects. For instance, while FUS exposure has been shown to cause transient sterile inflammation in numerous studies [85–87], a recent dose-response investigation showed that FUS can achieve BBB opening at intensities lower than levels that trigger parenchymal recruitment of immune cells [88]. Lower intensities of FUS have the potential to enhance the safety of repeated treatments, which could be particularly beneficial in the context of inflammatory illnesses. Such studies could also provide valuable insights into the dosing of FUS cavitation with immunotherapies, especially in treating neuro-oncological illnesses.

Clinical Applications of MR-Guided FUS BBB Opening

Although most existing investigations of FUS BBB opening have been in preclinical settings, many recent clinical trials involving MRgFUS BBB opening have been published in various illnesses affecting the CNS. So far, experience from several small trials primarily in neuro-oncological and neurodegenerative diseases suggests the safety profile of MRgFUS BBB opening is acceptable for single and small numbers of repeated BBB opening events in combination with various therapeutics. In particular, no FUS-related intracranial hemorrhage, seizures, or neurological sequelae have been reported. Nonetheless, preclinical evidence suggests that FUS BBB opening can induce sterile inflammation and potentially recruit leukocytes to the brain parenchyma at higher sonication intensities. These biological effects may have varying positive or negative implications for safety and efficacy in different indications [75, 85, 88].

The first human study of MRgFUS BBB opening was conducted in patients with high-grade gliomas [89]. Subsequently, numerous clinical trials of FUS BBB opening have been initiated, primarily in oncological and neurodegenerative disorders. Increasingly, FUS BBB opening delivers large-molecule biologics, including antibodies and enzyme replacement therapies, in human subjects. Table 6.1 summarizes the FUS devices/modalities, indications, and therapeutics in all active and completed FUS BBB opening trials registered in the NIH Clinical Trials registry. At present, all active and completed trials employ an open-label design.

Early neuro-oncology trials primarily sought to deliver standard-of-care chemotherapies already used for their BBB permeability. More recently, however, therapeutic selection has expanded to include larger biologics that would otherwise have negligible CNS bioavailability and efficacy. For example, in a trial of six cycles of concomitant MRgFUS BBB opening and intravenous infusion of the anti-HER2 antibody trastuzumab (~148 kDa), we demonstrated increased uptake of [^{111}In]-labeled trastuzumab into HER2+ brain metastases after MRgFUS BBB opening relative to infusion without BBB opening (NCT03714243), as well as reduction in tumor volume in some subjects [90]. Recent trials using MRgFUS BBB opening seek to deliver doxorubicin (543 Da), a small molecule chemotherapy with poor BBB permeability [91], to diffuse intrinsic pontine gliomas in pediatric patients (NCT05630209, NCT05615623).

In addition to drug delivery, there is significant interest in the potential to exploit the biological effects of FUS or BBB opening, as well as interactions with drugs. For example, several trials (NCT05370508, NCT04559685, NCT05123534) have combined MRgFUS BBB opening with the ultrasound-sensitive (or "sonosensitizer") 5-aminolevulinic acid (5-ALA), thought to induce ROS production in response to cavitation [92, 93], to activate 5-ALA at the site of drug delivery across the BBB. Similarly, there is great interest in innate immune modulation or stimulation induced by FUS BBB opening [85, 87] to augment endogenous immune responses or the effectiveness of exogenous immunotherapies. For example, a trial of neuronavigated FUS BBB opening in recurrent glioblastoma failed to find an altered immunological response in tumor tissue collected 7 days after BBB opening [88]. However, they were able to replicate this lack of efficacy at similar sonication intensities in rodents and demonstrate that higher-intensity sonications were efficacious in recruiting lymphocytes to the sonication target [88]. Further clinical trials using FUS BBB opening include the delivery of various immune checkpoint inhibitors, including nivolumab, pembrolizumab, balstilimab, and botensilimab, which are currently underway employing both intracranial and transcranial devices (NCT04021420, NCT05864534, NCT05317858). A randomized trial of neoadjuvant and adjuvant pembrolizumab alongside or without MRgFUS BBB opening has been proposed (NCT05879120).

Exploiting immunomodulatory and other biological effects has also been a significant motivator of many trials of FUS BBB opening neurodegenerative disorders. This interest has been driven by preclinical evidence of therapeutic delivery of endogenous antibodies and activation of microglia aiding clearance of pathogenic proteins in animal models of AD [75, 77, 84]. Many early and ongoing clinical trials of FUS BBB opening in AD and other neurodegenerative have sought to target brain pathology while establishing safety data in the absence of drugs (e.g., NCT03671889, NCT03739905, NCT06158789). Encouragingly, results of amyloid PET imaging from early trials suggest good safety and tolerability, as well as some intrinsic potential for amyloid clearance in human patients [94–96]. Additionally, with the approval of aducanumab and lecanemab for AD, a trial employing MRgFUS BBB opening to enhance their delivery is ongoing (NCT05469009). Early results suggest a greater amyloid reduction in targeted brain regions relative to contralateral control regions [97]. Additional trials of MRgFUS BBB opening without the drug in amyotrophic lateral sclerosis and PD further established the safety and tolerability of this intervention across a range of neurodegenerative disorders [78, 98]. In PD, particularly patients with mutations in the gene encoding beta-glucocerebrosidase (GBA-PD), MRgFUS BBB opening has been used to enhance the delivery of a recombinant enzyme replacement therapy (imiglucerase, 55 kDa; NCT04370665, NCT05565443) [99].

In addition to therapeutic indications of MRgFUS, substantial interest and ongoing research is dedicated to diagnostic uses of FUS BBB opening, particularly liquid biopsy [41, 42, 100–102]. Just as FUS BBB opening appears effective at improving the brain penetrance of substances in the systemic circulation, it also seems effective in increasing the release of diverse brain-derived endogenous biomarkers into the systemic circulation [41, 100]. Indeed, significant increases in circulating levels of various brain-derived proteins, including S100β, glial fibrillary acidic protein (GFAP), and cell-free DNA, have been demonstrated in animal mod-

Table 6.1 Active and completed clinical trials of FUS BBB opening

NCT #	Indication	Therapeutic (size)	Enrollment target (*N*)	Location
Intracranial transducer (e.g., SonoCloud)				
NCT04021420	Melanoma brain metastases	Nivolumab (146 kDa)	21	France
NCT05864534	Primary glioblastoma	Balstilimab (143 kDa), Botensilimab (144 kDa), liposomal doxorubicin (d_H ~120–170 nm)	25	USA
NCT04528680	Recurrent glioblastoma	Albumin-bound paclitaxel (~66 kDa) + carboplatin (371 Da)	57	USA
NCT03744026	Recurrent glioblastoma	Carboplatin (371 Da)	38	International, multi-centre
NCT05293197	Malignant pediatric brain tumor	Carboplatin (371 Da)	24	France, multi-centre
NCT02253212	Glioblastoma	Carboplatin (371 Da)	27	France
NCT04614493	Primary glioblastoma	Temozolomide (194 Da)	66	International, multi-centre
NCT03626896	Recurrent glioblastoma	None, proof-of-principle/safety	6	Taiwan
NCT03119961	Alzheimer's disease	None, proof-of-principle/safety	10	France
Transcranial neuronavigated FUS transducer (e.g., NaviFUS and BrainSonix)				
NCT04446416	Recurrent glioblastoma	Bevacizumab (149 kDa)	6	Taiwan
NCT04804709	Progressive diffuse midline glioma	Panobinostat (349 Da)	3	USA
NCT04063514	Low grade gliomas or neurodegenerative dementias	None, proof-of-principle/safety	4	USA
NCT04118764	Alzheimer's disease	None, proof-of-principle/safety	6	USA
Transcranial phased array/MRgFUS (e.g., Exablate)				
NCT05469009	Alzheimer's disease	Aducanumab (~149 kDa) or Lecanemab (~150 kDa)	15	USA
NCT05317858	NSCLC brain metastases	Pembrolizumab (~149 kDa)	20	International, multi-centre
NCT03714243	Breast cancer brain metastases	Trastuzumab (~148 kDa)	10	Canada
NCT04370665	Parkinson's disease	Imiglucerase (55 kDa)	4	Canada
NCT05565443	Parkinson's disease	Imiglucerase (55 kDa)	14	Canada
NCT05630209	Diffuse intrinsic pontine glioma	Doxorubicin (543 Da)	10	USA, multi-centre
NCT05615623	Diffuse intrinsic pontine glioma	Doxorubicin (543 Da)	3	Canada
NCT04440358	Recurrent glioblastoma	Carboplatin (371 Da)	13	International, multi-centre
NCT04417088	Recurrent glioblastoma	Carboplatin (371 Da)	30	USA, multi-centre
NCT04998864	Glioblastoma	Temozolomide (194 Da)	5	International, multi-centre
NCT02343991	High-grade glioma	Temozolomide (194 Da) or liposomal doxorubicin (d_H 120–170 nm)	10	Canada
NCT03551249	Glioblastoma	Temozolomide (194 Da)	20	USA, multi-centre
NCT03616860	Glioblastoma	Temozolomide (194 Da)	20	Canada
NCT03712293	Glioblastoma	Temozolomide (194 Da)	10	Korea
NCT05370508	Recurrent glioblastoma	5-ALA (194 Da), sonodynamic therapy		
NCT04559685	High-grade glioma	5-ALA (194 Da), sonodynamic therapy	30	USA
NCT05123534	Diffuse intrinsic pontine glioma	5-ALA (194 Da), sonodynamic therapy	27	USA, multi-centre
NCT03321487	Amyotrophic lateral sclerosis	None, proof-of-principle/safety	8	Canada
NCT03608553	Parkinson's disease dementia	None, proof-of-principle/safety	10	Spain
NCT03671889	Alzheimer's disease	None, therapeutic	50	USA, multi-centre
NCT03739905	Alzheimer's disease	None, therapeutic	30	Canada
NCT06158789	Alzheimer's disease	None, therapeutic	6	Korea
NCT04526262	Alzheimer's disease	None, proof-of-principle/safety	6	Korea
NCT02986932	Alzheimer's disease	None, proof-of-principle/safety	6	Canada
NCT05383872	Glioblastoma	None, liquid biopsy	57	USA, multi-centre
NCT05733312	Gliomas	None, liquid biopsy	6	USA

All active and completed FUS BBB opening clinical trials registered on ClinicalTrials.gov, arranged by FUS device/modality. Intracranial devices use an implanted transducer for BBB opening at a fixed target, neuronavigated FUS uses a single or small array of transducers positioned via neuronavigation using pre-treatment imaging for targeting, and phased array systems typically employed in MRgFUS BBB opening use select a large subset of a large array of transducers with limited individual maneuverability to produce a small focal convergence of ultrasound energy els and human subjects [41, 100, 103]. Additionally, ddPCR measurements of tumor-derived mutations in glioblastoma patients in genes including IDH1 and TERT suggest enhanced systemic availability of tumor DNA after sonication [41, 102]. Conventional blood-based cfDNA assays intended for liquid biopsy in oncology have demonstrated high sensitivity for ctDNA detection in peripheral tumors with higher cfDNA concentration but much lower sensitivity in glioma patients who also tend to have much lower blood cfDNA concentrations [104]. This is a possible consequence of the BBB preventing cfDNA, often present as a single nucleosome ($d_H \approx$ 6–10 nm) [105, 106] from crossing into the systemic circulation. Thus, FUS BBB opening provides a potential opportunity to improve the sensitivity of existing cfDNA assays in detecting brain tumors. Additionally, there is interest in extending these approaches to liquid biopsy of pathological proteins in neurodegenerative disorders.

Future Directions

Clinical experience with BBB opening with FUS has been promising, and the procedure seems safe and well tolerated. There is evidence supporting the efficacy of FUS in enhancing drug delivery. Nonetheless, concrete evidence of clinical benefit remains to be demonstrated, partly due to the absence of randomized, controlled trials. While existing MRgFUS BBB opening interventions have effectively used existing therapeutic formulations, in most cases, the maximum tolerable systemic exposure limits drug delivery to a target. For example, doxorubicin is a highly effective chemotherapy, but strict limitations are imposed on systemic exposure due to cardiotoxicity. Additionally, most existing drugs used for CNS indications must cross the BBB to some extent by necessity and may have unintended effects in off-target brain regions. With improvements in drug delivery technologies and increasing clinical availability of FUS devices, emerging formulations and therapies optimized for ultrasonic and/or brain delivery are well-positioned to improve both the precision and efficacy of therapeutic delivery to the brain.

At present, the FUS BBB opening for drug delivery relies on the separate administration of both a microbubble ultrasound contrast agent and a therapeutic intended for brain delivery. However, various emerging ultrasound-sensitive drug delivery platforms seek to combine therapeutic payloads with microbubbles to create an all-in-one formulation that can achieve BBB opening while improving focal therapeutic delivery and reducing systemic exposure. For example, microbubble-drug conjugates have been used to deliver both glial-derived neurotrophic factor protein and plasmid gene therapy vectors encoding brain-derived neurotrophic factor in preclinical models, with conjugating microbubbles significantly outperforming the separate formulations [107, 108]. Similarly, solid ultrasound-sensitive drug-loaded perfluorocarbon (PFC) nanodroplets, which can be triggered to convert into traditional PFC microbubbles in situ, have been investigated to deliver many drugs soluble in PFC [17, 109]. Nanodroplets also have the theoretical advantage of better tissue penetration before sonication, which may further augment drug delivery and therapeutic index [17]. Notably, pentobarbital-loaded nanodroplets for focal regional anesthesia have demonstrated the ability to achieve significant effects in behavior assays of motor function and aggression after sonication of the motor cortex and amygdala, respectively [16, 54, 110].

Similarly, an opportunity exists to increase the safety and efficacy of drug delivery via FUS BBB opening by combination with arterial drug delivery at an artery feeding the sonication target. As parenchymal drug delivery is usually proportional to the concentration of the drug in capillaries at the sonication target and often limited by the tolerability of systemic exposure, arterial drug delivery could improve both the therapeutic window and maximal extent of drug delivery achieved by FUS BBB opening. Additionally, the FUS BBB opening provides an opportunity to enhance the spatial specificity of arterial drug delivery. Nonetheless, no published preclinical or clinical studies investigate the therapeutic efficacy of combined arterial drug delivery and FUS BBB opening.

Although MRgFUS allows considerable spatial precision of BBB opening, treatments require substantially more resources than, e.g., traditional drug infusions or neuronavigated FUS. Ideal use cases for MRgFUS BBB opening include delivering disease-modifying therapies with substantial lasting benefits and/or off-target side effects. Many existing BBB-impermeable chemotherapies under active investigation in FUS BBB opening trials present good examples of such treatments [71, 111, 112]. Nonetheless, the rapidly growing repertoire of clinical gene therapies [113, 114] presents an emerging opportunity for precisely delivering brain-targeted, BBB-impermeable vectors for durable therapeutic effects. For example, research on FUS BBB opening for delivery of neuron-specific GDNF gene therapy in animal PD models reveals improvement in histological, biochemical, and behavioral parameters [115, 116]. Significant clinical interest in developing PD gene therapies independent of FUS [117–124] and the pre-existing data supporting the safety of MRgFUS BBB opening and drug delivery in PD [98, 99] make this a strong case for utilizing MRgFUS for controlled BBB penetration.

Similarly, although less extensively investigated, there is great interest in enhancing the delivery of cellular therapies (often genetically modified) using FUS BBB opening. For example, preclinical studies delivering genetically engineered natural killer cells have demonstrated five- to tenfold increased parenchymal abundance and improved survival when combined with simultaneous FUS BBB opening in animal models of various brain tumors [124–126]. Furthermore, given the ability of (relatively) higher intensity FUS BBB opening to recruit lymphocytes into the brain parenchyma in rodents [88], local sterile inflammation, which increases the expression of adhesion proteins and chemoattractants, may also improve the homing of exogenous immune cells to the brain parenchyma.

Conclusion

In summary, FUS and intravascular microbubbles present a compelling approach to achieving focal BBB opening at arbitrary targets in shallow and deep brain structures. Most modern MRgFUS BBB opening trials use a phased array with numerous individually steered ultrasound transducers and fewer receiver transducers. Combining pre-operative CT and MRI imaging, the software can automatically optimize the incident angle, phase, sonication intensity, and subset of active transducers to achieve precise BBB opening throughout a large potential target volume. Sonication of intravascular microbubbles infused or injected during BBB opening produces oscillations (cavitations) and mechanical stress on surrounding vessels, opening tight junctions of brain capillaries. Acoustic feedback from cavitation signals can be used for real-time feedback to tailor ultrasound doses during treatment. Additional biological effects of FUS BBB opening, such as reduced P-gp expression, increased transcytosis, and immunomodulation, may also contribute. Concomitant infusion of various therapeutics has been demonstrated to enhance the delivery of various therapeutics from BBB-impermeable small molecules, biologics, large nanoparticles, and gene therapy vectors. Clinical trials in neuro-oncological and neurodegenerative diseases have provided substantial evidence of safety and tolerability, with early evidence of enhanced drug delivery emerging. Future clinical trials should investigate novel drug delivery platforms optimized for FUS, such as nanodroplets and drug-conjugated microbubbles, and look to emerging gene therapies for promising opportunities for synergistic benefits.

References

1. GBD 2016 Neurology Collaborators. Global, regional, and national burden of neurological disorders, 1990–2016: a systematic analysis for the Global Burden of Disease Study 2016. Lancet Neurol. 2019;18(5):459–80.
2. GBD 2017 US Neurological Disorders Collaborators, Feigin VL, Vos T, Alahdab F, Amit AML, Barnighausen TW, et al. Burden of neurological disorders across the US from 1990–2017: a global burden of disease study. JAMA Neurol. 2021;78(2):165–76.
3. Gooch CL, Pracht E, Borenstein AR. The burden of neurological disease in the United States: a summary report and call to action. Ann Neurol. 2017;81(4):479–84.
4. Wang R, Zhu Y, Liu X, Liao X, He J, Niu L. The clinicopathological features and survival outcomes of patients with different metastatic sites in stage IV breast cancer. BMC Cancer. 2019;19(1):1091.
5. Schor NF, Scott P, Litvina EY, Torborg C, Kim J, Zalutsky R, et al. The NINDS 2021–2026 Strategic Plan: partnership and cross-cutting principles. Cell. 2022;185(9):1445–8.
6. Lindsley CW. New statistics on the cost of new drug development and the trouble with CNS drugs. ACS Chem Neurosci. 2014;5(12):1142.
7. Kesselheim AS, Hwang TJ, Franklin JM. Two decades of new drug development for central nervous system disorders. Nat Rev Drug Discov. 2015;14(12):815–6.
8. Bespalov A, Steckler T, Altevogt B, Koustova E, Skolnick P, Deaver D, et al. Failed trials for central nervous system disorders do not necessarily invalidate preclinical models and drug targets. Nat Rev Drug Discov. 2016;15(7):516.
9. Tsaioun K, Bottlaender M, Mabondzo A, Alzheimer's Drug Discovery Foundation. ADDME—avoiding drug development mistakes early: central nervous system drug discovery perspective. BMC Neurol. 2009;9(Suppl 1):S1.
10. Nance E, Pun SH, Saigal R, Sellers DL. Drug delivery to the central nervous system. Nat Rev Mater. 2022;7(4):314–31.
11. Pardridge WM. Why is the global CNS pharmaceutical market so under-penetrated? Drug Discov Today. 2002;7(1):5–7.
12. Terstappen GC, Meyer AH, Bell RD, Zhang W. Strategies for delivering therapeutics across the blood-brain barrier. Nat Rev Drug Discov. 2021;20(5):362–83.
13. Huang R, Boltze J, Li S. Strategies for improved intra-arterial treatments targeting brain tumors: a systematic review. Front Oncol. 2020;10:1443.
14. Hynynen K, McDannold N, Vykhodtseva N, Jolesz FA. Noninvasive MR imaging-guided focal opening of the blood-brain barrier in rabbits. Radiology. 2001;220(3):640–6.
15. Meng Y, Pople CB, Lea-Banks H, Abrahao A, Davidson B, Suppiah S, et al. Safety and efficacy of focused ultrasound induced blood-brain barrier opening, an integrative review of animal and human studies. J Control Release. 2019;309:25–36.
16. Lea-Banks H, O'Reilly MA, Hamani C, Hynynen K. Localized anesthesia of a specific brain region using ultrasound-responsive barbiturate nanodroplets. Theranostics. 2020;10(6):2849–58.
17. Chowdhury SM, Abou-Elkacem L, Lee T, Dahl J, Lutz AM. Ultrasound and microbubble mediated therapeutic delivery: underlying mechanisms and future outlook. J Control Release. 2020;326:75–90.
18. Banks WA, Reed MJ, Logsdon AF, Rhea EM, Erickson MA. Healthy aging and the blood-brain barrier. Nat Aging. 2021;1(3):243–54.
19. Knox EG, Aburto MR, Clarke G, Cryan JF, O'Driscoll CM. The blood-brain barrier in aging and neurodegeneration. Mol Psychiatry. 2022;27(6):2659–73.
20. Qosa H, Miller DS, Pasinelli P, Trotti D. Regulation of ABC efflux transporters at blood-brain barrier in health and neurological disorders. Brain Res. 2015;1628(Pt B):298–316.
21. Segarra M, Aburto MR, Acker-Palmer A. Blood-brain barrier dynamics to maintain brain homeostasis. Trends Neurosci. 2021;44(5):393–405.
22. Leandro K, Bicker J, Alves G, Falcao A, Fortuna A. ABC transporters in drug-resistant epilepsy: mechanisms of upregulation and therapeutic approaches. Pharmacol Res. 2019;144:357–76.
23. Fletcher JI, Williams RT, Henderson MJ, Norris MD, Haber M. ABC transporters as mediators of drug resistance and contributors to cancer cell biology. Drug Resist Updat. 2016;26:1–9.

24. de Gooijer MC, Kemper EM, Buil LCM, Çitirikkaya CH, Buckle T, Beijnen JH, et al. ATP-binding cassette transporters restrict drug delivery and efficacy against brain tumors even when blood-brain barrier integrity is lost. Cell Rep Med. 2021;2(1):100184.
25. Johnsen KB, Burkhart A, Thomsen LB, Andresen TL, Moos T. Targeting the transferrin receptor for brain drug delivery. Prog Neurobiol. 2019;181:101665.
26. Dong X. Current strategies for brain drug delivery. Theranostics. 2018;8(6):1481–93.
27. Hersh AM, Alomari S, Tyler BM. Crossing the blood-brain barrier: advances in nanoparticle technology for drug delivery in neuro-oncology. Int J Mol Sci. 2022;23(8):4153.
28. Appis AW, Tracy MJ, Feinstein SB. Update on the safety and efficacy of commercial ultrasound contrast agents in cardiac applications. Echo Res Pract. 2015;2(2):R55–62.
29. Ghanouni P, Pauly KB, Elias WJ, Henderson J, Sheehan J, Monteith S, et al. Transcranial MRI-guided focused ultrasound: a review of the technologic and neurologic applications. AJR Am J Roentgenol. 2015;205(1):150–9.
30. Cho H, Lee HY, Han M, Choi JR, Ahn S, Lee T, et al. Localized down-regulation of P-glycoprotein by focused ultrasound and microbubbles induced blood-brain barrier disruption in rat brain. Sci Rep. 2016;6:31201.
31. Meng Y, Hynynen K, Lipsman N. Applications of focused ultrasound in the brain: from thermoablation to drug delivery. Nat Rev Neurol. 2021;17(1):7–22.
32. Meng Y, Jones RM, Davidson B, Huang Y, Pople CB, Surendrakumar S, et al. Technical principles and clinical workflow of transcranial MR-guided focused ultrasound. Stereotact Funct Neurosurg. 2021;99(4):329–42.
33. Sun J, Hynynen K. Focusing of therapeutic ultrasound through a human skull: a numerical study. J Acoust Soc Am. 1998;104(3 Pt 1):1705–15.
34. Sun J, Hynynen K. The potential of transskull ultrasound therapy and surgery using the maximum available skull surface area. J Acoust Soc Am. 1999;105(4):2519–27.
35. Bakay L, Ballantine HT Jr, Hueter TF, Sosa D. Ultrasonically produced changes in the blood-brain barrier. AMA Arch Neurol Psychiatry. 1956;76(5):457–67.
36. Mesiwala AH, Farrell L, Wenzel HJ, Silbergeld DL, Crum LA, Winn HR, et al. High-intensity focused ultrasound selectively disrupts the blood-brain barrier in vivo. Ultrasound Med Biol. 2002;28(3):389–400.
37. O'Reilly MA, Waspe AC, Chopra R, Hynynen K. MRI-guided disruption of the blood-brain barrier using transcranial focused ultrasound in a rat model. J Vis Exp. 2012;61:3555.
38. Huang Y, Meng Y, Pople CB, Bethune A, Jones RM, Abrahao A, et al. Cavitation feedback control of focused ultrasound blood-brain barrier opening for drug delivery in patients with Parkinson's disease. Pharmaceutics. 2022;14(12):2607.
39. Guthkelch AN, Carter LP, Cassady JR, Hynynen KH, Iacono RP, Johnson PC, et al. Treatment of malignant brain tumors with focused ultrasound hyperthermia and radiation: results of a phase I trial. J Neurooncol. 1991;10(3):271–84.
40. Jones RM, Hynynen K. Advances in acoustic monitoring and control of focused ultrasound-mediated increases in blood-brain barrier permeability. Br J Radiol. 2019;92(1096):20180601.
41. Meng Y, Pople CB, Suppiah S, Llinas M, Huang Y, Sahgal A, et al. MR-guided focused ultrasound liquid biopsy enriches circulating biomarkers in patients with brain tumors. Neuro Oncol. 2021;23(10):1789–97.
42. Pacia CP, Yuan J, Yue Y, Xu L, Nazeri A, Desai R, et al. Sonobiopsy for minimally invasive, spatiotemporally-controlled, and sensitive detection of glioblastoma-derived circulating tumor DNA. Theranostics. 2022;12(1):362–78.
43. Meng Y, Pople CB, Lea-Banks H, Hynynen K, Lipsman N, Hamani C. Chapter 10—Focused ultrasound neuromodulation. In: Moro E, Polosan M, Hamani C, editors. International review of neurobiology, vol. 159. Academic; 2021. p. 221–40.
44. Blackmore J, Shrivastava S, Sallet J, Butler CR, Cleveland RO. Ultrasound neuromodulation: a review of results, mechanisms and safety. Ultrasound Med Biol. 2019;45(7):1509–36.
45. Jones RM, McMahon D, Hynynen K. Ultrafast three-dimensional microbubble imaging in vivo predicts tissue damage volume distributions during nonthermal brain ablation. Theranostics. 2020;10(16):7211–30.
46. Franzini A, Moosa S, Prada F, Elias WJ. Ultrasound ablation in neurosurgery: current clinical applications and future perspectives. Neurosurgery. 2020;87(1):1–10.
47. Dubinsky TJ, Khokhlova TD, Khokhlova V, Schade GR. Histotripsy: the next generation of high-intensity focused ultrasound for focal prostate cancer therapy. J Ultrasound Med. 2020;39(6):1057–67.
48. Lu N, Hall TL, Choi D, Gupta D, Daou BJ, Sukovich JR, et al. Transcranial MR-guided histotripsy system. IEEE Trans Ultrason Ferroelectr Freq Control. 2021;68(9):2917–29.
49. Xu Z, Hall TL, Vlaisavljevich E, Lee FT Jr. Histotripsy: the first noninvasive, non-ionizing, non-thermal ablation technique based on ultrasound. Int J Hyperth. 2021;38(1):561–75.
50. Anastasiadis P, Gandhi D, Guo Y, Ahmed AK, Bentzen SM, Arvanitis C, et al. Localized blood-brain barrier opening in infiltrating gliomas with MRI-guided acoustic emissions-controlled focused ultrasound. Proc Natl Acad Sci USA. 2021;118(37):e2103280118.
51. Lipsman N, Meng Y, Bethune AJ, Huang Y, Lam B, Masellis M, et al. Blood-brain barrier opening in Alzheimer's disease using MR-guided focused ultrasound. Nat Commun. 2018;9(1):2336.
52. Marty B, Larrat B, Van Landeghem M, Robic C, Robert P, Port M, et al. Dynamic study of blood-brain barrier closure after its disruption using ultrasound: a quantitative analysis. J Cereb Blood Flow Metab. 2012;32(10):1948–58.
53. Gorick CM, Breza VR, Nowak KM, Cheng VWT, Fisher DG, Debski AC, et al. Applications of focused ultrasound-mediated blood-brain barrier opening. Adv Drug Deliv Rev. 2022;191:114583.
54. Gouveia FV, Lea-Banks H, Aubert I, Lipsman N, Hynynen K, Hamani C. Anesthetic-loaded nanodroplets with focused ultrasound reduces agitation in Alzheimer's mice. Ann Clin Transl Neurol. 2023;10(4):507–19.
55. Chen CC, Sheeran PS, Wu SY, Olumolade OO, Dayton PA, Konofagou EE. Targeted drug delivery with focused ultrasound-induced blood-brain barrier opening using acoustically-activated nanodroplets. J Control Release. 2013;172(3):795–804.
56. Konofagou EE, Tung YS, Choi J, Deffieux T, Baseri B, Vlachos F. Ultrasound-induced blood-brain barrier opening. Curr Pharm Biotechnol. 2012;13(7):1332–45.
57. Hynynen K, McDannold N, Sheikov NA, Jolesz FA, Vykhodtseva N. Local and reversible blood-brain barrier disruption by noninvasive focused ultrasound at frequencies suitable for trans-skull sonications. NeuroImage. 2005;24(1):12–20.
58. Sheikov N, McDannold N, Sharma S, Hynynen K. Effect of focused ultrasound applied with an ultrasound contrast agent on the tight junctional integrity of the brain microvascular endothelium. Ultrasound Med Biol. 2008;34(7):1093–104.
59. Chu PC, Chai WY, Tsai CH, Kang ST, Yeh CK, Liu HL. Focused ultrasound-induced blood-brain barrier opening: association with mechanical index and cavitation index analyzed by dynamic contrast-enhanced magnetic-resonance imaging. Sci Rep. 2016;6:33264.
60. McDannold N, Vykhodtseva N, Hynynen K. Blood-brain barrier disruption induced by focused ultrasound and circulating pre-

formed microbubbles appears to be characterized by the mechanical index. Ultrasound Med Biol. 2008;34(5):834–40.
61. Liu HL, Hsu PH, Lin CY, Huang CW, Chai WY, Chu PC, et al. Focused ultrasound enhances central nervous system delivery of bevacizumab for malignant glioma treatment. Radiology. 2016;281(1):99–108.
62. Kinoshita M, McDannold N, Jolesz FA, Hynynen K. Targeted delivery of antibodies through the blood-brain barrier by MRI-guided focused ultrasound. Biochem Biophys Res Commun. 2006;340(4):1085–90.
63. Sim SL, He T, Tscheliessnig A, Mueller M, Tan RB, Jungbauer A. Protein precipitation by polyethylene glycol: a generalized model based on hydrodynamic radius. J Biotechnol. 2012;157(2):315–9.
64. Al-Ejeh F, Darby JM, Thierry B, Brown MP. A simplified suite of methods to evaluate chelator conjugation of antibodies: effects on hydrodynamic radius and biodistribution. Nucl Med Biol. 2009;36(4):395–402.
65. Wang S, Olumolade OO, Sun T, Samiotaki G, Konofagou EE. Noninvasive, neuron-specific gene therapy can be facilitated by focused ultrasound and recombinant adeno-associated virus. Gene Ther. 2015;22(1):104–10.
66. Hsu PH, Wei KC, Huang CY, Wen CJ, Yen TC, Liu CL, et al. Noninvasive and targeted gene delivery into the brain using microbubble-facilitated focused ultrasound. PLoS One. 2013;8(2):e57682.
67. Zhao G, Huang Q, Wang F, Zhang X, Hu J, Tan Y, et al. Targeted shRNA-loaded liposome complex combined with focused ultrasound for blood brain barrier disruption and suppressing glioma growth. Cancer Lett. 2018;418:147–58.
68. McDannold N, Zhang Y, Supko JG, Power C, Sun T, Peng C, et al. Acoustic feedback enables safe and reliable carboplatin delivery across the blood-brain barrier with a clinical focused ultrasound system and improves survival in a rat glioma model. Theranostics. 2019;9(21):6284–99.
69. Wei KC, Chu PC, Wang HY, Huang CY, Chen PY, Tsai HC, et al. Focused ultrasound-induced blood-brain barrier opening to enhance temozolomide delivery for glioblastoma treatment: a preclinical study. PLoS One. 2013;8(3):e58995.
70. Aryal M, Vykhodtseva N, Zhang YZ, Park J, McDannold N. Multiple treatments with liposomal doxorubicin and ultrasound-induced disruption of blood-tumor and blood-brain barriers improve outcomes in a rat glioma model. J Control Release. 2013;169(1–2):103–11.
71. Park EJ, Zhang YZ, Vykhodtseva N, McDannold N. Ultrasound-mediated blood-brain/blood-tumor barrier disruption improves outcomes with trastuzumab in a breast cancer brain metastasis model. J Control Release. 2012;163(3):277–84.
72. Suzuki R, Namai E, Oda Y, Nishiie N, Otake S, Koshima R, et al. Cancer gene therapy by IL-12 gene delivery using liposomal bubbles and tumoral ultrasound exposure. J Control Release. 2010;142(2):245–50.
73. Karakatsani ME, Blesa J, Konofagou EE. Blood-brain barrier opening with focused ultrasound in experimental models of Parkinson's disease. Mov Disord. 2019;34(9):1252–61.
74. Bajracharya R, Cruz E, Gotz J, Nisbet RM. Ultrasound-mediated delivery of novel tau-specific monoclonal antibody enhances brain uptake but not therapeutic efficacy. J Control Release. 2022;349:634–48.
75. Jordao JF, Thevenot E, Markham-Coultes K, Scarcelli T, Weng YQ, Xhima K, et al. Amyloid-beta plaque reduction, endogenous antibody delivery and glial activation by brain-targeted, transcranial focused ultrasound. Exp Neurol. 2013;248:16–29.
76. Janowicz PW, Leinenga G, Gotz J, Nisbet RM. Ultrasound-mediated blood-brain barrier opening enhances delivery of therapeutically relevant formats of a tau-specific antibody. Sci Rep. 2019;9(1):9255.
77. Jordao JF, Ayala-Grosso CA, Markham K, Huang Y, Chopra R, McLaurin J, et al. Antibodies targeted to the brain with image-guided focused ultrasound reduces amyloid-beta plaque load in the TgCRND8 mouse model of Alzheimer's disease. PLoS One. 2010;5(5):e10549.
78. Abrahao A, Meng Y, Llinas M, Huang Y, Hamani C, Mainprize T, et al. First-in-human trial of blood-brain barrier opening in amyotrophic lateral sclerosis using MR-guided focused ultrasound. Nat Commun. 2019;10(1):4373.
79. Rapoport NY, Kennedy AM, Shea JE, Scaife CL, Nam KH. Controlled and targeted tumor chemotherapy by ultrasound-activated nanoemulsions/microbubbles. J Control Release. 2009;138(3):268–76.
80. Andreone BJ, Chow BW, Tata A, Lacoste B, Ben-Zvi A, Bullock K, et al. Blood-brain barrier permeability is regulated by lipid transport-dependent suppression of caveolae-mediated transcytosis. Neuron. 2017;94(3):581–94.e5.
81. Pandit R, Koh WK, Sullivan RKP, Palliyaguru T, Parton RG, Götz J. Role for caveolin-mediated transcytosis in facilitating transport of large cargoes into the brain via ultrasound. J Control Release. 2020;327:667–75.
82. Zhang H, Sierra C, Kwon N, Karakatsani ME, Jackson-Lewis VR, Przedborski S, et al. Focused-ultrasound mediated anti-alpha-synuclein antibody delivery for the treatment of Parkinson's disease. In: 2018 IEEE International Ultrasonics Symposium (IUS); 2018. p. 22–5.
83. Nisbet RM, Van der Jeugd A, Leinenga G, Evans HT, Janowicz PW, Gotz J. Combined effects of scanning ultrasound and a tau-specific single chain antibody in a tau transgenic mouse model. Brain. 2017;140(5):1220–30.
84. Leinenga G, Gotz J. Scanning ultrasound removes amyloid-beta and restores memory in an Alzheimer's disease mouse model. Sci Transl Med. 2015;7(278):278ra33.
85. Kovacs ZI, Kim S, Jikaria N, Qureshi F, Milo B, Lewis BK, et al. Disrupting the blood-brain barrier by focused ultrasound induces sterile inflammation. Proc Natl Acad Sci USA. 2017;114(1):E75–84.
86. Silburt J, Lipsman N, Aubert I. Disrupting the blood-brain barrier with focused ultrasound: perspectives on inflammation and regeneration. Proc Natl Acad Sci USA. 2017;114(33):E6735–E6.
87. Jung O, Thomas A, Burks SR, Dustin ML, Frank JA, Ferrer M, et al. Neuroinflammation associated with ultrasound-mediated permeabilization of the blood-brain barrier. Trends Neurosci. 2022;45(6):459–70.
88. Chen KT, Chai WY, Lin YJ, Lin CJ, Chen PY, Tsai HC, et al. Neuronavigation-guided focused ultrasound for transcranial blood-brain barrier opening and immunostimulation in brain tumors. Sci Adv. 2021;7(6):eabd0772.
89. Mainprize T, Lipsman N, Huang Y, Meng Y, Bethune A, Ironside S, et al. Blood-brain barrier opening in primary brain tumors with non-invasive MR-guided focused ultrasound: a clinical safety and feasibility study. Sci Rep. 2019;9(1):321.
90. Meng Y, Reilly RM, Pezo RC, Trudeau M, Sahgal A, Singnurkar A, et al. MR-guided focused ultrasound enhances delivery of trastuzumab to Her2-positive brain metastases. Sci Transl Med. 2021;13(615):eabj4011.
91. Park J, Aryal M, Vykhodtseva N, Zhang YZ, McDannold N. Evaluation of permeability, doxorubicin delivery, and drug retention in a rat brain tumor model after ultrasound-induced blood-tumor barrier disruption. J Control Release. 2017;250:77–85.
92. Yamaguchi T, Kitahara S, Kusuda K, Okamoto J, Horise Y, Masamune K, et al. Current landscape of sonodynamic therapy for treating cancer. Cancers (Basel). 2021;13(24):6184.

93. Wu S-K, Santos MA, Marcus SL, Hynynen K. MR-guided focused ultrasound facilitates sonodynamic therapy with 5-aminolevulinic acid in a rat glioma model. Sci Rep. 2019;9(1):10465.
94. Meng Y, Goubran M, Rabin JS, McSweeney M, Ottoy J, Pople CB, et al. Blood-brain barrier opening of the default mode network in Alzheimer's disease with magnetic resonance-guided focused ultrasound. Brain. 2023;146(3):865–72.
95. Rezai AR, Ranjan M, Haut MW, Carpenter J, D'Haese PF, Mehta RI, et al. Focused ultrasound-mediated blood-brain barrier opening in Alzheimer's disease: long-term safety, imaging, and cognitive outcomes. J Neurosurg. 2023;139(1):275–83.
96. D'Haese PF, Ranjan M, Song A, Haut MW, Carpenter J, Dieb G, et al. Beta-amyloid plaque reduction in the hippocampus after focused ultrasound-induced blood-brain barrier opening in Alzheimer's disease. Front Hum Neurosci. 2020;14:593672.
97. Rezai AR, D'Haese PF, Finomore V, Carpenter J, Ranjan M, Wilhelmsen K, et al. Ultrasound blood-brain barrier opening and aducanumab in Alzheimer's disease. N Engl J Med. 2024;390(1):55–62.
98. Gasca-Salas C, Fernandez-Rodriguez B, Pineda-Pardo JA, Rodriguez-Rojas R, Obeso I, Hernandez-Fernandez F, et al. Blood-brain barrier opening with focused ultrasound in Parkinson's disease dementia. Nat Commun. 2021;12(1):779.
99. Meng Y, Pople CB, Huang Y, Jones RM, Ottoy J, Goubran M, et al. Putaminal recombinant glucocerebrosidase delivery with magnetic resonance-guided focused ultrasound in Parkinson's disease: a phase I study. Mov Disord. 2022;37(10):2134–9.
100. Zhu L, Cheng G, Ye D, Nazeri A, Yue Y, Liu W, et al. Focused ultrasound-enabled brain tumor liquid biopsy. Sci Rep. 2018;8(1):6553.
101. Pacia CP, Yuan J, Yue Y, Xu L, Nazeri A, Desai R, et al. Sonobiopsy increases release of circulating tumor DNA for sensitive molecular diagnosis of glioblastoma. J Acoust Soc Am. 2021;150(4_Suppl):A54.
102. Yuan J, Xu L, Chien CY, Yang Y, Yue Y, Fadera S, et al. First-in-human prospective trial of sonobiopsy in high-grade glioma patients using neuronavigation-guided focused ultrasound. NPJ Precis Oncol. 2023;7(1):92.
103. Pacia CP, Zhu L, Yang Y, Yue Y, Nazeri A, Michael Gach H, et al. Feasibility and safety of focused ultrasound-enabled liquid biopsy in the brain of a porcine model. Sci Rep. 2020;10(1):7449.
104. Bettegowda C, Sausen M, Leary RJ, Kinde I, Wang Y, Agrawal N, et al. Detection of circulating tumor DNA in early- and late-stage human malignancies. Sci Transl Med. 2014;6(224):224ra24.
105. Sherwood K, Weimer ET. Characteristics, properties, and potential applications of circulating cell-free DNA in clinical diagnostics: a focus on transplantation. J Immunol Methods. 2018;463:27–38.
106. Banerjee A, Majumder P, Sanyal S, Singh J, Jana K, Das C, et al. The DNA intercalators ethidium bromide and propidium iodide also bind to core histones. FEBS Open Bio. 2014;4:251–9.
107. Wang F, Shi Y, Lu L, Liu L, Cai Y, Zheng H, et al. Targeted delivery of GDNF through the blood-brain barrier by MRI-guided focused ultrasound. PLoS One. 2012;7(12):e52925.
108. Huang Q, Deng J, Wang F, Chen S, Liu Y, Wang Z, et al. Targeted gene delivery to the mouse brain by MRI-guided focused ultrasound-induced blood-brain barrier disruption. Exp Neurol. 2012;233(1):350–6.
109. Lea-Banks H, Hynynen K. Sub-millimetre precision of drug delivery in the brain from ultrasound-triggered nanodroplets. J Control Release. 2021;338:731–41.
110. Lea-Banks H, Meng Y, Wu SK, Belhadjhamida R, Hamani C, Hynynen K. Ultrasound-sensitive nanodroplets achieve targeted neuromodulation. J Control Release. 2021;332:30–9.
111. Kovacs Z, Werner B, Rassi A, Sass JO, Martin-Fiori E, Bernasconi M. Prolonged survival upon ultrasound-enhanced doxorubicin delivery in two syngenic glioblastoma mouse models. J Control Release. 2014;187:74–82.
112. Treat LH, McDannold N, Zhang Y, Vykhodtseva N, Hynynen K. Improved anti-tumor effect of liposomal doxorubicin after targeted blood-brain barrier disruption by MRI-guided focused ultrasound in rat glioma. Ultrasound Med Biol. 2012;38(10):1716–25.
113. Sayed N, Allawadhi P, Khurana A, Singh V, Navik U, Pasumarthi SK, et al. Gene therapy: comprehensive overview and therapeutic applications. Life Sci. 2022;294:120375.
114. Cring MR, Sheffield VC. Gene therapy and gene correction: targets, progress, and challenges for treating human diseases. Gene Ther. 2022;29(1–2):3–12.
115. Lin CY, Hsieh HY, Chen CM, Wu SR, Tsai CH, Huang CY, et al. Non-invasive, neuron-specific gene therapy by focused ultrasound-induced blood-brain barrier opening in Parkinson's disease mouse model. J Control Release. 2016;235:72–81.
116. Mead BP, Kim N, Miller GW, Hodges D, Mastorakos P, Klibanov AL, et al. Novel focused ultrasound gene therapy approach noninvasively restores dopaminergic neuron function in a rat Parkinson's disease model. Nano Lett. 2017;17(6):3533–42.
117. Marras C, Chaudhuri KR, Titova N, Mestre TA. Therapy of Parkinson's disease subtypes. Neurotherapeutics. 2020;17(4):1366–77.
118. Axelsen TM, Woldbye DPD. Gene therapy for Parkinson's disease, an update. J Parkinsons Dis. 2018;8(2):195–215.
119. Christine CW, Richardson RM, Fine EM, Khwaja OS, Liang GS, Meier A, et al. Author response: Safety of AADC gene therapy for moderately advanced Parkinson disease: three-year outcomes from the PD-1101 trial. Neurology. 2022;99(6):259.
120. Christine CW, Richardson RM, Van Laar A, Fine EM, Khwaja OS, Liang GS, et al. Author response: Safety of AADC gene therapy for moderately advanced Parkinson disease: three-year outcomes from the PD-1101 trial. Neurology. 2022;99(6):260–1.
121. Christine CW, Richardson RM, Van Laar AD, Thompson ME, Fine EM, Khwaja OS, et al. Safety of AADC gene therapy for moderately advanced Parkinson disease: three-year outcomes from the PD-1101 trial. Neurology. 2022;98(1):e40–50.
122. Kang UJ, Nakamura K, Zhuang X. Reader response: Safety of AADC gene therapy for moderately advanced Parkinson disease: three-year outcomes from the PD-1101 trial. Neurology. 2022;99(6):258–9.
123. Palma JA. Reader response: Safety of AADC gene therapy for moderately advanced Parkinson disease: three-year outcomes from the PD-1101 trial. Neurology. 2022;99(6):260.
124. Alkins R, Burgess A, Ganguly M, Francia G, Kerbel R, Wels WS, et al. Focused ultrasound delivers targeted immune cells to metastatic brain tumors. Cancer Res. 2013;73(6):1892–9.
125. Alkins R, Burgess A, Kerbel R, Wels WS, Hynynen K. Early treatment of HER2-amplified brain tumors with targeted NK-92 cells and focused ultrasound improves survival. Neuro Oncol. 2016;18(7):974–81.
126. Yang C, Du M, Yan F, Chen Z. Focused ultrasound improves NK-92MI cells infiltration into tumors. Front Pharmacol. 2019;10:326.

7 Intra-arterial Drug Delivery for Brain Tumors

Jake McDermott, Netanel Ben-Shalom, Randy S. D'Amico, and John A. Boockvar

The disease (Glioblastoma Multiforme) is brutal, relentless, unforgiving. We have to remember how they lived, not how they died.

Extracted from the Eulogy to John McCain by Joseph R. Biden (born 1942), American President

Introduction

Intra-arterial (IA) drug delivery is an emerging strategy for treating brain tumors by delivering therapeutic agents directly to the central nervous system (CNS). This approach enables targeted delivery through the tumor's capillary network and the peritumoral vasculature while minimizing systemic toxicity.

Advancements in endovascular catheter technologies have facilitated safe and targeted super-selective intra-arterial cerebral infusions (SSIACI). These advancements, combined with successful IA treatments for other cancers, such as retinoblastoma and hepatocellular carcinoma, have led to renewed interest in IA delivery as a safe and effective strategy for brain tumor treatment [1, 2]. Modern IA delivery overcomes the limitations of traditional drug delivery methods by bypassing the blood-brain barrier (BBB) and by using modern agents with decreased neurotoxicity [3].

IA drug delivery is particularly attractive for treating malignant gliomas, which have limited treatment options and poor survival rates. Current treatments, including surgery, chemotherapy, and radiation, have not provided a cure or significantly improved outcomes [4–7]. The BBB is often blamed for hindering drug delivery to the CNS, and IA delivery with BBB disruption allows direct delivery of effective doses with potentially less toxicity [3, 8].

J. McDermott · N. Ben-Shalom · R. S. D'Amico (✉)
J. A. Boockvar
Lenox Hill Hospital Department of Neurosurgery, Donald and Barbara Zucker School of Medicine at Hofstra/Northwell Health, New York, NY, USA
e-mail: rdamico8@northwell.edu

Despite published successes, interpreting IA delivery outcomes is challenging due to the variability in study designs, protocols, and chemotherapeutic drugs [3]. This chapter examines the preclinical and clinical history of IA delivery and ongoing trials for brain tumor treatment (specifically malignant gliomas). It discusses the challenges and the potential of IA drug delivery.

Brief History

Initial interest in intra-arterial (IA) drug delivery for head and neck cancers and brain cancers, including glioblastoma (GBM), emerged in the 1950s. This interest was sparked when Calvin Klopp accidentally infused nitrogen mustard into a Hodgkin Lymphoma patient's brachial artery [9]. In the 1960s, IA therapy for brain tumors gained momentum as surgeons like Charles Wilson believed it could reduce the systemic toxicities of intravenous (IV) chemotherapies. During his residency at Tulane, Wilson developed a modified Baron food pump to continuously deliver nitrogen mustard chemotherapy through the internal carotid artery to patients with malignant brain tumors [10].

During the 1970s, Stanley Rapaport's work shed light on the role of tight junctions in blood-brain barrier (BBB) permeability and initiated investigations into disrupting the BBB to facilitate drug delivery. Rapaport's group showed that hyperosmolar BBB disruption caused reversible dehydration of endothelial cells and disruption of tight junctions, enabling drugs to cross the BBB [11]. Robert Dedrick's studies on the pharmacokinetics of IA delivery further supported

S. Joshi (ed.), *Arterial Treatment of Neurological Diseases*, https://doi.org/10.1007/978-3-031-80173-0_7

these findings [12]. Building on this knowledge, Neuwelt et al. [13] demonstrated that hyperosmolar BBB disruption increased the concentration of chemotherapies within targeted sites for central nervous system lymphomas.

Advancements in IA delivery continued in the 1990s, but interest declined due to the significant neurotoxicity associated with the drugs under investigation. Unfortunately, this decline occurred just as modern endovascular technology started developing rapidly and novel, safer therapeutic compounds were becoming available, setting the stage for future safe and effective trials of IA therapies for brain tumors [3].

Rationale and Preclinical Support

Intra-arterial (IA) drug delivery offers several advantages compared to standard intravenous (IV) or oral methods. It is based on three critical components: super-selective infusions, BBB disruption, and IA pharmacokinetics.

IA delivery allows for accurate and targeted local delivery of therapeutics by restricting the volume of distribution (Vd) to the targeted pathology and surrounding tissues sharing a vascular supply. Modern endovascular techniques have improved IA treatment for brain tumors, providing effective and minimally invasive options [3, 8].

Various strategies have been identified to enhance IA drug delivery, including methods to increase local extraction, reduce regional blood flow, and improve systemic clearance, Fig. 7.1. Techniques such as transient BBB disruption and flow arrest during infusion have been developed to improve drug delivery, resulting in increased concentrations of chemotherapies within the targeted tissue.

The pharmacokinetics of IA delivery differ from other methods of drug delivery, allowing for more efficient drug perfusion into targeted tissues. This leads to effective regional tissue concentrations with lower total doses, demonstrated in positron emission tomography (PET) measurements showing a significant increase in brain tumor tissue

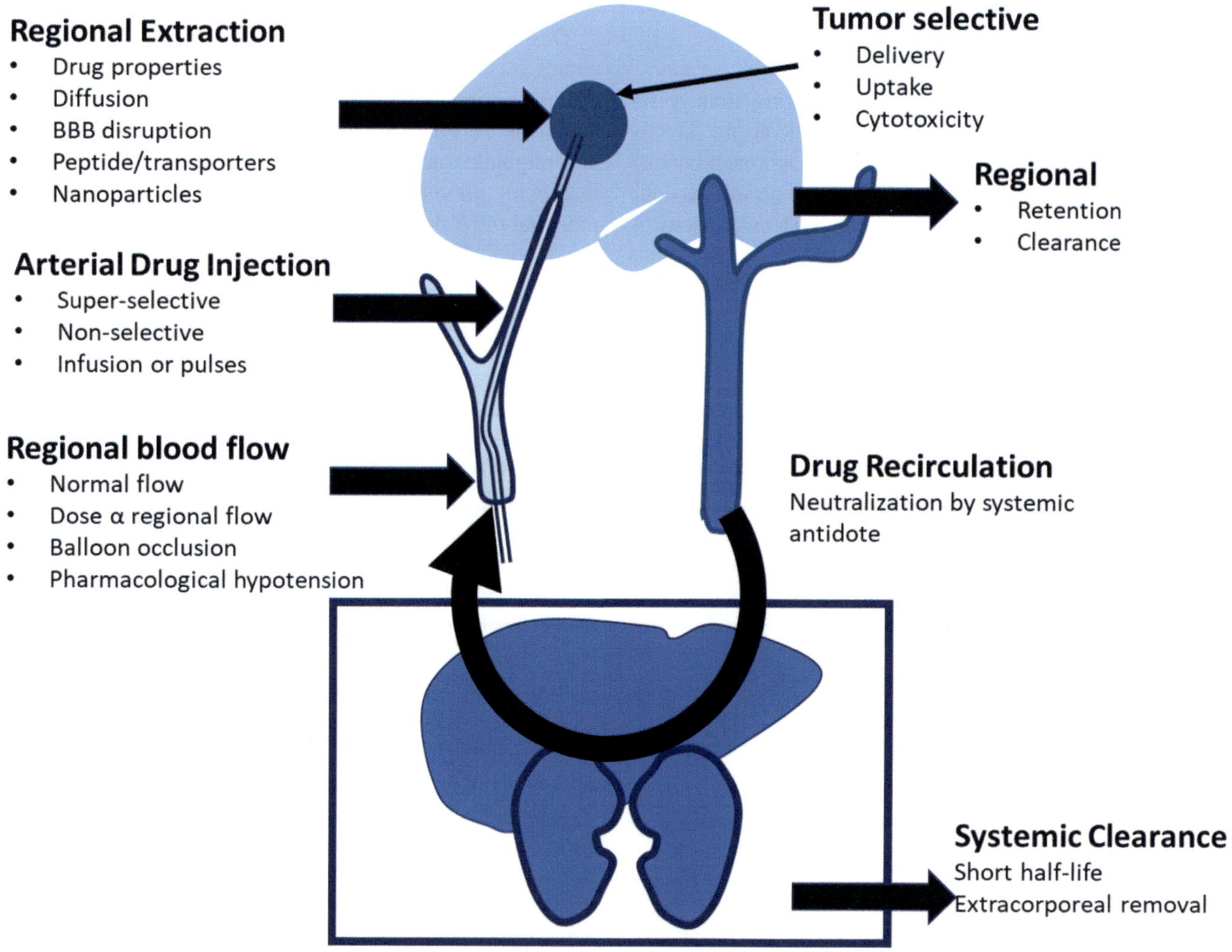

Fig. 7.1 Strategies to improve intraarterial chemotherapy

concentrations with IA compared to IV injections [14]. However, dose advantages depend on several factors, such as method, rate, and infusion duration. Furthermore, successful IA infusion lessens the risk of treatment-related systemic toxicity, permitting multiple treatments with relatively decreased associated treatment-related morbidity [15–20].

Notably, the success of IA chemotherapy in other cancers, such as retinoblastoma, head and neck tumors, and liver cancers, supports its potential efficacy for brain tumor treatment [21–23]. These successes have also contributed to a better understanding of IA delivery and its potential benefits.

Renewed interest in IA drug delivery has led to the development of novel preclinical models to study IA therapy. These models, including xenograft implanted rabbits and in vitro microfluidic "organ-on-a-chip" BBB models, provide valuable insights into the BBB and facilitate a better characterization of IA delivery [24, 25].

BBB Disruption

The blood-brain barrier (BBB) isolates the central nervous system (CNS) from systemic circulation through physical and biochemical barriers. It consists of tight and adherens junctions, efflux pumps, and astrocyte podocytes, which restrict the passage of large molecules [3]. However, this barrier also hinders the delivery of many chemotherapeutic agents to the CNS due to their high molecular weight [13]. Bypassing the BBB is a significant challenge in delivering drugs for brain tumors.

Combining intra-arterial (IA) infusions with BBB disruption expands the possibilities and efficacy of delivering agents to CNS diseases, especially larger therapeutic molecules that the BBB limits. Osmotic disruption is the most commonly used method, involving the infusion of a hypertonic solution like mannitol into targeted cerebral arteries [11, 13, 16, 26, 27]. This creates an osmotic gradient, shrinking endothelial cells and temporarily disrupting tight junctions, increasing BBB permeability. Osmotic disruption can significantly increase the levels of infused chemotherapy [28]. Though variability and unintended neurotoxicity concerns exist, human studies have shown therapeutic benefits and safety when carefully monitored [17, 29–32].

Bradykinin and synthetic analogs have also been used for BBB disruption but with less success than osmotic disruption. These analogs increase permeability in tumor capillaries, but responses and outcomes vary [33, 34]. Additionally, they may not effectively address infiltrating cells within normal brain regions [35, 36].

Emerging techniques like hyperthermia-induced disruption of the peritumoral BBB and magnetic-resonance-guided focused ultrasound (MRgFUS) have also shown promise. During laser interstitial thermal therapy, hyperthermia can induce peak permeability within a few weeks, potentially enhancing IA therapeutic delivery [37]. MRgFUS and recently implantable FUS cranioplasty implants have successfully improved the transport of chemotherapeutic agents and enhanced the uptake of nanoparticles across the BBB for brain tumor and CNS disease treatment [38].

IA Infusion for Brain Tumors

Ongoing clinical trials are listed in Table 7.1. The thrust of clinical research is in the following areas:

IA Bevacizumab for GBM

Bevacizumab, a monoclonal antibody that inhibits vascular endothelial growth factor (VEGF), has shown promising results for recurrent GBM [15, 16, 29, 39]. It binds to VEGF in perivascular spaces where tumor stem cells (TSCs) are known to reside [40, 41]. IA infusion of Bevacizumab after BBB disruption reduces the number of GBM TSCs, offering theoretical benefits to patients with malignant gliomas.

While IV Bevacizumab is effective, it is associated with systemic toxicities [42, 43]. Recent studies have explored IA delivery of Bevacizumab and demonstrated its safety and efficacy alone or combined with chemotherapy. Importantly, Bevacizumab has been shown to increase median progression-free survival (PFS) after a single IA dose. Hence, the question arises whether repeat dosing can improve outcomes [26, 39].

Recent studies of IA Bevacizumab with BBB disruption for newly diagnosed GBM demonstrated significant results. Doses of 15 mg/kg of Bevacizumab at 30, 120, and 210 days post-operatively improved PFS and even OS in a cohort of 23 patients. Median OS was 23.1 months compared to the expected OS of 12–15 months. The treatment-associated toxicities were minimal and well-tolerated by the patients who could complete the regimen. Clinical trials are ongoing for newly diagnosed and recurrent GBM patients [15]. Figures 7.2 and 7.3 show responses to three IA Bevacizumab treatments over several months.

IA Cetuximab for Recurrent GBM

High expression of EGFR in GBM is associated with a poor prognosis. Cetuximab, a recombinant human chimeric antibody, inhibits EGFR and reduces signal transduction. A recent Phase I study explored IA Cetuximab after BBB disruption in recurrent malignant gliomas and determined the maximum tolerated dose (MTD) to be 250 mg/m^2. The study reported potential side effects such as seizures and cerebral edema [26]. Based on these findings, Phase I/II and Phase I trials are currently enrolling to evaluate the effects of IA

Table 7.1 Clinical trials with intraarterial treatment of brain tumors on the National Clinical Trials Registry

NCT number	Title	Interventions	Status
NCT02861898	Super-selective Intra-arterial Repeated Infusion of Cetuximab for the Treatment of Newly Diagnosed Glioblastoma	Intra-arterial Cetuximab. Intra-arterial Mannitol	Recruiting
NCT02800486	Super Selective Intra-arterial Repeated Infusion of Cetuximab (Erbitux) With Reirradiation for Treatment of Relapsed/Refractory GBM, AA, and AOA	Intra-arterial Cetuximab. Intra-arterial Mannitol. Hypo-fractionated reirradiation	Recruiting
NCT02571530	Super-selective Intra-arterial Cerebral Infusion of Trastuzumab for the Treatment of Cerebral Metastases of HER2/Neu Positive Breast Cancer	Intra-arterial Cerebral Infusion of Trastuzumab	Terminated
NCT05773326	Superselective Intra-arterial Cerebral Infusion of Temsirolimus in HGG	Temsirolimus	Recruiting
NCT00983398	Melphalan, Carboplatin, Mannitol, and Sodium Thiosulfate in Treating Patients with Recurrent or Progressive CNS Embryonal or Germ Cell Tumors	Carboplatin, Melphalan, Mannitol, Sodium Thiosulfate: Questionnaire Administration. Quality of Life Assessment	Unknown
NCT05271240	Repeated Superselective Intraarterial Cerebral Infusion (SIACI) of Bevacizumab with Temozolomide and Radiation Compared to Temozolomide and Radiation Alone in Newly Diagnosed GBM	Repeated Superselective Intraarterial Cerebral infusion (SIACI) of Bevacizumab (Avastin) with Temozolomide and Radiation: Temozolomide and Radiation Alone	Recruiting
NCT04994977	Intraarterial Chemotherapy for Newly Diagnosed, Residual, or Recurrent Atypical Choroid Plexus Papilloma and Choroid Plexus Carcinoma Before Second-Look Surgery	Safety of intra-arterial chemotherapy in subjects with ACPP and CPC, measured by the number of serious adverse events that are reported as at least possibly related to the intervention that occurs in subjects on the trial, through study completion, a little over a year for each subject	Recruiting

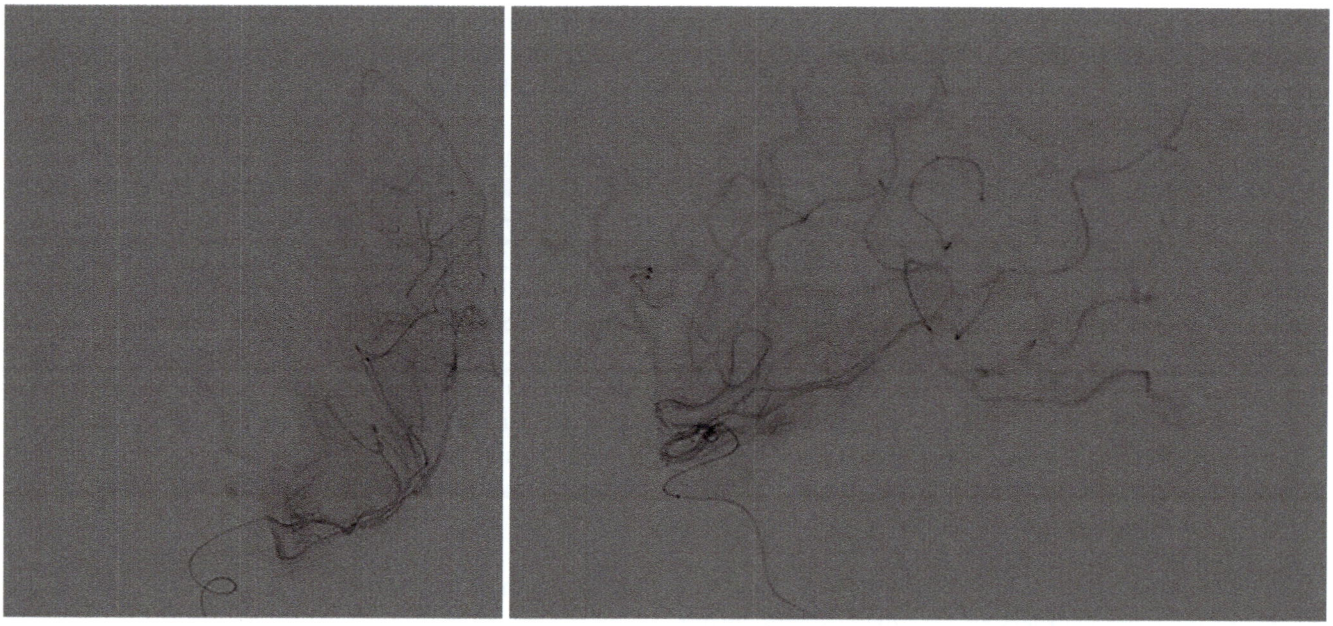

Fig. 7.2 Illustrative case report of IA bevacizumab treatment: A 56-year-old lady was diagnosed with left temporal-opercular Glioblastoma 3.5 years back; the histopathology showed WHO grade IV Glioblastoma, IDH (−) TERT (+), PTEN (+), MGMT (+), KI67 up to 10%. She was treated with Temozolomide for six cycles and 60 Gy of radiation following the first resection. She had her first recurrence after 22 months, for which she was enrolled in a PD1/GITR immunotherapy trial followed by re-resection. She underwent a third surgery (Awake craniotomy) at 24 months follow-up. The imaging at 28 months follow-up showed a recurrent disease for which she was enrolled in the Intra-arterial (IA) Bevacizumab trial. After the first cycle of IA Bevacizumab (at the 29th month), she was stable till the 39th month. Then, follow-up imaging showed recurrence, for which she got a second dose of IA Bevacizumab in the 39th month. Her disease remained stable till the 42nd month when repeat imaging showed progressive disease. She received her third and final dose of IA Avastin in the 42nd month and is pending a follow-up imaging next month. Her KPS is 90 with expressive aphasia, and she was off steroids at her last follow-up in the 42nd month. Angiogram at 42nd month-follow-up for stage 3 IA Bevacizumab infusion showing tumor blush at left MCA territory. The left M1 was micro-catheterized, and 12.5 mL of mannitol (20%) and 45 mL of Bevacizumab were injected

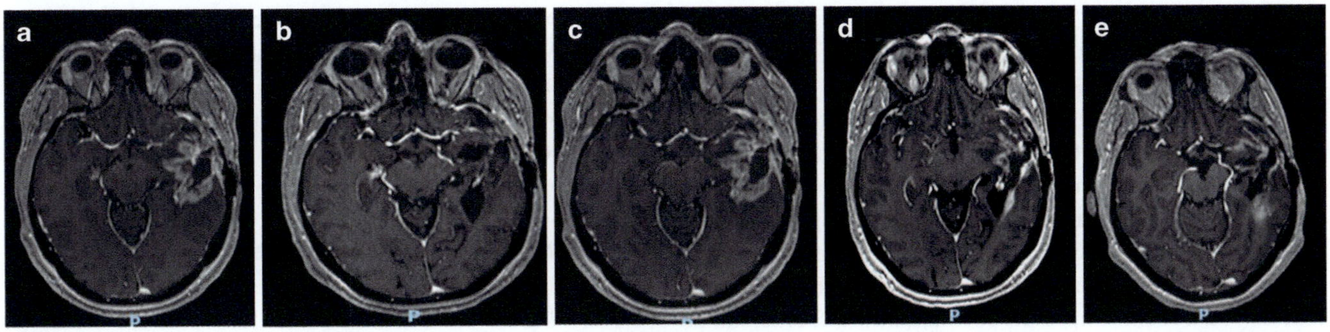

a. MRI (T1-Post contrast) showing recurrent disease at 28 months follow-up (a new enhancing lesion in the resection cavity) which was treated with 1st Dose of IA Bevacizumab →

b. MRI (T1-Post contrast) showing a stable disease at 38 months follow-up →

c. MRI (T1-Post contrast) showing progressive disease at 39 months follow-up (a new enhancing lesion in the resection cavity) which was treated with 2nd Dose of IA Bevacizumab →

d. MRI (T1-Post contrast) showing stable disease at 40 months follow-up →

e. MRI (T1-Post contrast) showing progressive disease at 42 months follow-up which was treated with 3rd Dose of IA Bevacizumab

Fig. 7.3 Illustrative case report of IA bevacizumab treatment: A 56-year-old lady was diagnosed with left temporal-opercular Glioblastoma 3.5 years back; the histopathology showed WHO grade IV Glioblastoma, IDH (−) TERT (+), PTEN (+), MGMT (+), KI67 up to 10%. She was treated with Temozolomide for six cycles and 60 Gy of radiation following the first resection. She had her first recurrence after 22 months, for which she was enrolled in a PD1/GITR immunotherapy trial followed by re-resection. She underwent a third surgery (Awake craniotomy) at 24 months follow-up. The imaging at 28 months follow-up showed a recurrent disease for which she was enrolled in the Intra-arterial (IA) Bevacizumab trial. After the first cycle of IA Bevacizumab (at the 29th month), she was stable till the 39th month. Then, follow-up imaging showed recurrence, for which she got a second dose of IA Bevacizumab in the 39th month. Her disease remained stable till the 42nd month when repeat imaging showed progressive disease. She received her third and final dose of IA Avastin in the 42nd month and is pending a follow-up imaging next month. Her KPS is 90 with expressive aphasia, and she was off steroids at her last follow-up in the 42nd month. MRI images tracking treatment response over 42 months

Cetuximab in recurrent GBM and newly diagnosed EGFR-amplified and overexpressed GBM, respectively [44, 45].

IA Bevacizumab and Cetuximab for Brain Tumors

VEGF receptor overexpression in pediatric ependymoma is linked to a poor prognosis. Combining Bevacizumab and Cetuximab via SSIACI has shown potential benefits in inhibiting both VEGF and EGFR receptors while minimizing systemic toxicities. Rajappa et al. [46] demonstrated tumor regression in a pediatric patient with recurrent posterior fossa ependymoma using superselective balloon-assisted intra-basilar artery infusion of Bevacizumab and Cetuximab. A study assessing this combination for diffuse intrinsic pontine glioma (DIPG) has completed enrollment; results are pending [47].

IA Methotrexate-Based Therapy for Newly Diagnosed Primary CNS Lymphoma

High-dose intra-arterial methotrexate combined with radiotherapy improves responses and prolongs PFS and OS in primary CNS lymphoma patients [48–51]. However, it is associated with a high incidence of delayed neurocognitive toxicity in long-term survivors. Methotrexate has limited BBB permeability, reaching only 5% of plasma levels [52, 53]. In a large study spanning 23 years, intra-carotid or intra-vertebral IA delivery of methotrexate with osmotic BBB disruption showed promising results. The overall tumor response rate was 81.9%, with a 5-year PFS of 31%, a 7-year PFS of 25%, and a median OS of 14 years in low-risk patients. Focal seizures were the most common side effect without long-term consequences [54]. This study suggests that IA methotrexate-based chemotherapy is a safe and effective option for newly diagnosed primary CNS lymphoma, potentially outperforming other treatment regimens.

IA Trastuzamab for Her2/Neu Positive Breast Cancer Cerebral Metastases

Breast cancer is the second leading cause of brain metastases in the USA, driven by the increasing survival of patients with advanced breast cancer. The HER2/neu receptor is a crucial molecular target in aggressive breast cancer. Trastuzumab, a monoclonal antibody, binds to this receptor and inhibits signaling [55].

Recently, an open-label clinical trial assessed the safety and efficacy of intra-arterial Trastuzumab for treating brain metastasis in HER2/neu-positive breast cancer. The trial aimed to determine the maximum tolerated dose (MTD) and evaluate response and overall survival using RECIST criteria. However, recruitment for the trial has been limited, and results are pending [56].

Expanded Uses of IA Drug Delivery

Radiation Necrosis

Radiation exposure to the brain causes microvascular injury and hypoxia, resulting in upregulation of VEGF and increased vascular permeability, leading to vasogenic edema. Some radiation necrosis patients are steroid refractory and experience progressive neurological decline. Bevacizumab inhibits VEGF and improves edema, and IV Bevacizumab has shown durable symptomatic improvement in patients with radiation necrosis but is associated with significant adverse events [57–59].

The ongoing LIBERTI trial assesses the safety and efficacy of a single intra-arterial (IA) injection of low-dose Bevacizumab after BBB disruption for radiation necrosis treatment. IA infusion ensures higher drug delivery, cost-effectiveness, and reduced systemic exposure. IA Bevacizumab may improve steroid requirements, functional status, and quality of life. The trial, with a target enrollment of ten patients, found that eight out of ten patients experienced a mean reduction of radiation necrosis of 74% and were free from recurrence after 12 months. Only one of the ten patients was still steroid-dependent by the end of the trial [60].

IA Delivery of Stem Cells and Nanotherapeutics

Mesenchymal stem cells (MSCs) have shown promise as therapeutics for various nervous system disorders. They have been investigated for traumatic brain injury, multi-system atrophy, and stroke [61–63]. Preclinical studies support using bone marrow-derived human MSCs loaded with delta-24-RGD (BM-hMSC-Delta-24-RGD cells) via SSIACI against gliomas. These loaded MSCs are compatible with different microcatheters and medications used in neuroendovascular therapy. Factors such as catheter diameter, injection velocity, and concurrent use of verapamil or heparin do not affect MSC viability or viral agent anti-glioma activity [64]. This study highlights the potential of endovascular MSC delivery with oncolytic agents for glioma treatment, but further clinical studies are needed.

Yttrium-90

Yttrium-90 (Y-90) microspheres delivered intra-arterially have a distinct advantage over external beam radiation therapy in delivering a higher and more focused dose. Approved in 2021, this treatment has been effective in treating hepatocellular carcinomas and liver metastases, allowing for increased survival in some cases and, in some, providing a bridge to transplant [65]. IA delivery of Y-90 is currently being investigated in an ongoing clinical trial for humans with gliomas. The study investigates the associated toxicities and survival with IA Y-90 for recurrent glioblastoma. Participants are being recruited [66].

IA Delivery of Oncolytic Viruses

DNX-2401 is an oncolytic virus that kills tumor cells through various mechanisms [67–69]. A specific gene deletion enhances its tumor tropism and infectivity [70, 71]. In a Phase I trial, intra-tumoral injection of DNX-2401 in patients with recurrent malignant gliomas reduced tumor size and improved survival in some patients [72]. Based on these results, a Phase I trial is underway to evaluate the intra-arterial delivery of allogeneic bone marrow human MSCs loaded with DNX-2401 for recurrent high-grade gliomas. The trial aims to enroll 36 patients and deliver two doses of BM-hMSCs-DNX-2401 2 weeks apart. Tumor response and survival outcomes will be assessed. The study also includes a dose-escalation phase to determine the maximum tolerated dose, evaluate toxicities, and examine immune responses within the tumor [73].

Challenges of IA Therapy

IA therapy is not without challenges. Most studies have overlooked hydrodynamic factors. Successful IA delivery necessitates rapid drug uptake during its first pass through the tumor's circulation. Understanding the pharmacokinetics of IA delivery requires considering physiological and anatomical factors that affect arterial concentrations, including regional blood flow, injection parameters, endothelial-drug interactions, site-specific pharmacokinetics, and blood-brain barrier (BBB) transit kinetics. These variables depend on the drug and disease; further investigations are needed to characterize them [3, 8].

In particular, "streaming" in IA therapy remains controversial [74]. Streaming occurs when agents infused via IA methods pass through the tissue too quickly, resulting in inadequate tissue penetration and uptake by the targeted lesion. This leads to the uneven distribution of infused agents and has been implicated in treatment failures and neurotoxicity. Several methods have been suggested to mitigate the effects of streaming, such as pulsed injections, injections during diastole, and using catheters with side ports instead of tip exits [75]. Flow arrest using downstream balloon occlusion has also been explored to localize chemotherapy to the tumor region and potentially improve IA delivery. Catheter technologies, including single or double balloon catheters, have been developed to maximize local delivery while minimizing complications [76]. Techniques that allow flow arrest or reductions may be an alternative to increasing IA doses, particularly for tumors with low blood flow, as they can enhance therapeutic effects [77].

The selection of drugs for IA delivery requires careful consideration. Ideal drugs should have reduced local toxicity and manageable systemic complications. Given the biological diversity of brain tumors, and in particular, GBM, applying a single drug to all tumors is unlikely to provide lasting benefits. Ultimately, IA drug selection based on the genotypic and phenotypic characteristics of the tumor will be necessary. Multiple therapies and delivery methods may be required to achieve sustained remission of GBM [3, 8].

Importantly, IA delivery carries unique risks associated with the methodology. These risks include complications related to catheter position and vascular access, local reactions to IA drugs, potential complications such as seizures or neurologic deficits, and systemic toxicities from chemotherapy. Each of these risks should be carefully considered on a case-by-case basis when pursuing IA chemotherapy [3].

Future Directions

Despite renewed interest, intra-arterial (IA) therapy for brain tumors is still in its early stages. Several variables associated with IA therapy require further characterization, considering the rapid advancements in technology and biology. Combining IA drug delivery principles with insights into the molecular characteristics of malignant gliomas and other brain tumors holds great potential. Given the heterogeneity of tumors like GBM, single-agent treatment is unlikely to achieve complete disease control, emphasizing the need for multimodal therapies [8]. Understanding the unique molecular pathogenesis of these tumors is crucial for developing effective IA treatments. With its intermittent and minimally invasive nature, IA drug delivery provides an opportunity to combine therapies targeting different tumor mechanisms and improve long-term outcomes.

Standardization of BBB disruption techniques and a better understanding of BBB kinetics are necessary to facilitate dose standardization for specific agents. Similarly, standardization of endovascular techniques, such as vessel selection and decisions regarding balloon occlusion or flow arrest, needs to be established. Refining these technical aspects will contribute to standardizing IA therapies and their broader application across different CNS pathologies and tumor characteristics.

Hydrodynamic factors in drug delivery and the ultrafast pharmacokinetics of IA drug delivery have been overlooked [8]. Experimental techniques that track tissue drug concentrations can enhance pharmacokinetic models by considering hydrodynamic factors, thus improving the effectiveness and safety of IA delivery. These techniques will expand the range of drugs that can be screened and studied for CNS tumor treatment using IA delivery.

Conclusion

Initial studies of IA drug delivery have shown promising results in a variety of brain tumor types, demonstrating the safety and effectiveness of IA therapy. However, critical aspects of arterial drug delivery need to be addressed in the future. These include refining and standardizing delivery techniques, understanding the complex morphology of GBM, improving drug selection and formulations, and minimizing treatment-related neurological injury. The potential benefits of IA therapy will be better understood with further study.

References

1. Abramson DH, Dunkel IJ, Brodie SE, Kim JW, Gobin YP. A phase I/II study of direct intraarterial (ophthalmic artery) chemotherapy with melphalan for intraocular retinoblastoma. Ophthalmology. 2008;115(8):1398–1404.e1.
2. Lau W, Leung T, Ho S, Chan M, Machin D, Lau J, et al. Adjuvant intra-arterial lipiodol-iodine-131 for resectable hepatocellular carcinoma: a prospective randomized trial. Lancet. 1999;353(9155):797–801.
3. D'Amico RS, Khatri D, Reichman N, Patel NV, Wong T, Fralin SR, et al. Super selective intra-arterial cerebral infusion of modern chemotherapeutics after blood–brain barrier disruption: where are we now, and where we are going. J Neurooncol. 2020;147(2):261–78.
4. Stupp R, Mason WP, van den Bent MJ, Weller M, Fisher B, Taphoorn MJB, et al. Radiotherapy plus concomitant and adjuvant temozolomide for glioblastoma. N Engl J Med. 2005;352(10):987–96.
5. Stern JI, Raizer JJ. Chemotherapy in the treatment of malignant gliomas. Expert Rev Anticancer Ther. 2006;6(5):755–67.
6. Storstein A, Helseth E, Johannesen T, Schellhorn T, Mørk S, Helvoirt R. Høygradige gliomer hos voksne. Tidsskr Den Nor Legeforening. 2011;131(3):238–41.
7. Sanai N, Berger MS. Glioma extent of resection and its impact on patient outcome. Neurosurgery. 2008;62(4):753–66.
8. Joshi S, Ellis JA, Ornstein E, Bruce JN. Intraarterial drug delivery for glioblastoma mutiforme: will the phoenix rise again? J Neurooncol. 2015;124(3):333–43.
9. Klopp CT, Alford TC, Bateman J, Berry GN, Winship T. Fractionated intra-arterial cancer. Chemotherapy with methyl bis amine hydrochloride; a preliminary report. Ann Surg. 1950;132(4):811–32.
10. Wilson CB. Chemotherapy of brain tumors by continuous arterial infusion. Surgery. 1964;55:640–53.
11. Rapoport SI, Hori M, Klatzo I. Reversible osmotic opening of the blood-brain barrier. Science. 1971;173(4001):1026–8.
12. Dedrick RL. Arterial drug infusion: pharmacokinetic problems and pitfalls. JNCI J Natl Cancer Inst. 1988;80(2):84–9.
13. Neuwelt EA, Frenkel EP, Diehl JT, Maravilla KR, Vu LH, Clark WK, et al. Osmotic blood-brain barrier disruption: a new means of increasing chemotherapeutic agent delivery. Trans Am Neurol Assoc. 1979;104:256–60.
14. Tyler JL, Yamamoto YL, Diksic M, Théron J, Villemure JG, Worthington C, et al. Pharmacokinetics of superselective intra-

arterial and intravenous [11C]BCNU evaluated by PET. J Nucl Med. 1986;27(6):775–80.
15. Patel NV, Wong T, Fralin SR, Li M, McKeown A, Gruber D, et al. Repeated superselective intraarterial bevacizumab after blood brain barrier disruption for newly diagnosed glioblastoma: a phase I/II clinical trial. J Neurooncol. 2021;155(2):117–24.
16. Boockvar JA, Tsiouris AJ, Hofstetter CP, Kovanlikaya I, Fralin S, Kesavabhotla K, et al. Safety and maximum tolerated dose of superselective intraarterial cerebral infusion of bevacizumab after osmotic blood-brain barrier disruption for recurrent malignant glioma: clinical article. J Neurosurg. 2011;114(3):624–32.
17. Fortin D, Desjardins A, Benko A, Niyonsega T, Boudrias M. Enhanced chemotherapy delivery by intraarterial infusion and blood-brain barrier disruption in malignant brain tumors: the Sherbrooke experience. Cancer. 2005;103(12):2606–15.
18. Fortin D, Morin PA, Belzile F, Mathieu D, Paré FM. Intra-arterial carboplatin as a salvage strategy in the treatment of recurrent glioblastoma multiforme. J Neurooncol. 2014;119(2):397–403.
19. Jeon JY, Kovanlikaya I, Boockvar JA, Mao X, Shin BK, Burkhardt J, et al. Metabolic response of glioblastoma to superselective intra-arterial cerebral infusion of bevacizumab: a proton MR spectroscopic imaging study. Am J Neuroradiol. 2012;33(11):2095–102.
20. Imbesi F, Marchioni E, Benericetti E, Zappoli F, Galli A, Corato M, et al. A randomized phase III study: comparison between intravenous and intraarterial ACNU administration in newly diagnosed primary glioblastomas. Anticancer Res. 2006;26(1B):553–8.
21. Rashid OM, Sloot S, Zager JS. Regional therapy in metastatic melanoma: an update on minimally invasive intraarterial isolated limb infusion and percutaneous hepatic perfusion. Expert Opin Drug Metab Toxicol. 2014;10(10):1355–64.
22. Stratmann SL. Hepatic artery chemotherapy in the management of colorectal metastases. Bayl Univ Med Cent Proc. 2002;15(4):376–9.
23. Nakasato T, Katoh K, Sone M, Ehara S, Tamakawa Y, Hoshi H, et al. Superselective continuous arterial infusion chemotherapy through the superficial temporal artery for oral cavity tumors. AJNR Am J Neuroradiol. 2000;21(10):1917–22.
24. Park TE, Mustafaoglu N, Herland A, Hasselkus R, Mannix R, FitzGerald EA, et al. Hypoxia-enhanced Blood-Brain Barrier Chip recapitulates human barrier function and shuttling of drugs and antibodies. Nat Commun. 2019;10(1):2621.
25. Sedlakova R, Shivers RR, Del Maestro RF. Ultrastructure of the blood-brain barrier in the rabbit. J Submicrosc Cytol Pathol. 1999;31(1):149–61.
26. Chakraborty S, Filippi CG, Wong T, Ray A, Fralin S, Tsiouris AJ, et al. Superselective intraarterial cerebral infusion of cetuximab after osmotic blood/brain barrier disruption for recurrent malignant glioma: phase I study. J Neurooncol. 2016;128(3):405–15.
27. Doolittle ND, Miner ME, Hall WA, Siegal T, Jerome E, Osztie E, et al. Safety and efficacy of a multicenter study using intraarterial chemotherapy in conjunction with osmotic opening of the blood-brain barrier for the treatment of patients with malignant brain tumors. Cancer. 2000;88(3):637–47.
28. Williams PC, Henner WD, Roman-Goldstein S, Dahlborg SA, Brummett RE, Tableman M, et al. Toxicity and efficacy of carboplatin and etoposide in conjunction with disruption of the blood-brain tumor barrier in the treatment of intracranial neoplasms. Neurosurgery. 1995;37(1):17–27; discussion 27–8.
29. Burkhardt JK, Riina H, Shin BJ, Christos P, Kesavabhotla K, Hofstetter CP, et al. Intra-arterial delivery of bevacizumab after blood-brain barrier disruption for the treatment of recurrent glioblastoma: progression-free survival and overall survival. World Neurosurg. 2012;77(1):130–4.
30. Groothuis DR, Warkne PC, Molnar P, Lapin GD, Mikhael MA. Effect of hyperosmotic blood-brain barrier disruption on transcapillary transport in canine brain tumors. J Neurosurg. 1990;72(3):441–9.
31. Nakagawa H, Groothuis D, Blasberg RG. The effect of graded hypertonic intracarotid infusions on drug delivery to experimental RG-2 gliomas. Neurology. 1984;34(12):1571.
32. Neuwelt EA, Goldman DL, Dahlborg SA, Crossen J, Ramsey F, Roman-Goldstein S, et al. Primary CNS lymphoma treated with osmotic blood-brain barrier disruption: prolonged survival and preservation of cognitive function. J Clin Oncol. 1991;9(9):1580–90.
33. Nomura T, Inamura T, Black KL. Intracarotid infusion of bradykinin selectively increases blood-tumor permeability in 9L and C6 brain tumors. Brain Res. 1994;659(1–2):62–6.
34. Sanovich E, Bartus RT, Friden PM, Dean RL, Le HQ, Brightman MW. Pathway across blood-brain barrier opened by the bradykinin agonist, RMP-7. Brain Res. 1995;705(1–2):125–35.
35. Cloughesy TF, Mochizuki AY, Orpilla JR, Hugo W, Lee AH, Davidson TB, et al. Neoadjuvant anti-PD-1 immunotherapy promotes a survival benefit with intratumoral and systemic immune responses in recurrent glioblastoma. Nat Med. 2019;25(3):477–86.
36. Matsukado K, Inamura T, Nakano S, Fukui M, Bartus RT, Black KL. Enhanced tumor uptake of carboplatin and survival in glioma-bearing rats by intracarotid infusion of bradykinin analog, RMP-7. Neurosurgery. 1996;39(1):125–33; discussion 133–4.
37. Leuthardt EC, Duan C, Kim MJ, Campian JL, Kim AH, Miller-Thomas MM, et al. Hyperthermic laser ablation of recurrent glioblastoma leads to temporary disruption of the peritumoral blood brain barrier. Plos One. 2016;11(2):e0148613.
38. Sonabend AM, Gould A, Amidei C, Ward R, Schmidt KA, Zhang DY, et al. Repeated blood-brain barrier opening with an implantable ultrasound device for delivery of albumin-bound paclitaxel in patients with recurrent glioblastoma: a phase 1 trial. Lancet Oncol. 2023;24(5):509–22.
39. Chakraborty S, Filippi CG, Burkhardt JK, Fralin S, Ray A, Wong T, et al. Durability of single dose intra-arterial bevacizumab after blood/brain barrier disruption for recurrent glioblastoma. J Exp Ther Oncol. 2016;11(4):261–7.
40. Calabrese C, Poppleton H, Kocak M, Hogg TL, Fuller C, Hamner B, et al. A perivascular niche for brain tumor stem cells. Cancer Cell. 2007;11(1):69–82.
41. Müller-Greven G, Carlin CR, Burgett ME, Ahluwalia MS, Lauko A, Nowacki AS, et al. Macropinocytosis of bevacizumab by glioblastoma cells in the perivascular niche affects their survival. Clin Cancer Res. 2017;23(22):7059–71.
42. Lai A, Filka E, McGibbon B, Nghiemphu PL, Graham C, Yong WH, et al. Phase II pilot study of bevacizumab in combination with temozolomide and regional radiation therapy for up-front treatment of patients with newly diagnosed glioblastoma multiforme: interim analysis of safety and tolerability. Int J Radiat Oncol. 2008;71(5):1372–80.
43. Pope WB, Lai A, Nghiemphu P, Mischel P, Cloughesy TF. MRI in patients with high-grade gliomas treated with bevacizumab and chemotherapy. Neurology. 2006;66(8):1258–60.
44. SOM @Hofstra/Northwell JB MD Zucker. Phase II trial of super selective intra-arterial repeated infusion of cetuximab (erbitux) with reirradiation for treatment of relapsed/refractory glioblastoma multiforme, anaplastic astrocytoma, and anaplastic oligoastrocytoma [Internet]. clinicaltrials.gov; 2022 Oct [cited 2023 Jun 14]. Report No.: NCT02800486. https://clinicaltrials.gov/ct2/show/NCT02800486.
45. SOM @Hofstra/Northwell JB MD Zucker. Phase I/II trial of super-selective intra-arterial repeated infusion of cetuximab for the treatment of newly diagnosed glioblastoma [Internet]. clinicaltrials.gov; 2022 Nov [cited 2023 Jun 14]. Report No.: NCT02861898. https://clinicaltrials.gov/ct2/show/NCT02861898.
46. Rajappa P, Krass J, Riina HA, Boockvar JA, Greenfield JP. Super-selective basilar artery infusion of bevacizumab and cetuximab for multiply recurrent pediatric ependymoma. Interv Neuroradiol. 2011;17(4):459–65.

47. McCrea HJ, Ivanidze J, O'Connor A, Hersh EH, Boockvar JA, Gobin YP, et al. Intraarterial delivery of bevacizumab and cetuximab utilizing blood-brain barrier disruption in children with high-grade glioma and diffuse intrinsic pontine glioma: results of a phase I trial. J Neurosurg Pediatr. 2021;28(4):371–9.
48. Abrey LE, DeAngelis LM, Yahalom J. Long-term survival in primary CNS lymphoma. J Clin Oncol. 1998;16(3):859–63.
49. Abrey LE, Yahalom J, DeAngelis LM. Treatment for primary CNS lymphoma: the next step. J Clin Oncol. 2000;18(17):3144–50.
50. Glass J, Gruber ML, Cher L, Hochberg FH. Preirradiation methotrexate chemotherapy of primary central nervous system lymphoma: long-term outcome. J Neurosurg. 1994;81(2):188–95.
51. DeAngelis LM, Yahalom J, Thaler HT, Kher U. Combined modality therapy for primary CNS lymphoma. J Clin Oncol. 1992;10(4):635–43.
52. Muldoon LL, Soussain C, Jahnke K, Johanson C, Siegal T, Smith QR, et al. Chemotherapy delivery issues in central nervous system malignancy: a reality check. J Clin Oncol. 2007;25(16):2295–305.
53. Neuwelt E, Abbott NJ, Abrey L, Banks WA, Blakley B, Davis T, et al. Strategies to advance translational research into brain barriers. Lancet Neurol. 2008;7(1):84–96.
54. Angelov L, Doolittle ND, Kraemer DF, Siegal T, Barnett GH, Peereboom DM, et al. Blood-brain barrier disruption and intra-arterial methotrexate-based therapy for newly diagnosed primary CNS lymphoma: a multi-institutional experience. J Clin Oncol. 2009;27(21):3503–9.
55. Nahta R, Esteva FJ. HER2 therapy: molecular mechanisms of trastuzumab resistance. Breast Cancer Res. 2006;8(6):215.
56. SOM @Hofstra/Northwell JB MD Zucker. Phase 1 trial of super-selective Intra-arterial cerebral infusion of trastuzumab after blood-brain barrier disruption for the treatment of cerebral metastases of HER2/Neu positive breast cancer [Internet]. clinicaltrials.gov; 2021 Oct [cited 2023 Jun 14]. Report No.: NCT02571530. https://clinicaltrials.gov/ct2/show/NCT02571530.
57. Furuse M, Kawabata S, Kuroiwa T, Miyatake SI. Repeated treatments with bevacizumab for recurrent radiation necrosis in patients with malignant brain tumors: a report of 2 cases. J Neurooncol. 2011;102(3):471–5.
58. Levin VA, Bidaut L, Hou P, Kumar AJ, Wefel JS, Bekele BN, et al. Randomized double-blind placebo-controlled trial of bevacizumab therapy for radiation necrosis of the central nervous system. Int J Radiat Oncol. 2011;79(5):1487–95.
59. Zhuang H, Zheng Y, Wang J, Chang JY, Wang X, Yuan Z, et al. Analysis of risk and predictors of brain radiation necrosis after radiosurgery. Oncotarget. 2016;7(7):7773–9.
60. Dashti SR, Kadner RJ, Folley BS, Sheehan JP, Han DY, Kryscio RJ, et al. Single low-dose targeted bevacizumab infusion in adult patients with steroid-refractory radiation necrosis of the brain: a phase II open-label prospective clinical trial. J Neurosurg. 2022;137(6):1676–86.
61. Hasan A, Deeb G, Rahal R, Atwi K, Mondello S, Marei Mady HES, et al. Mesenchymal stem cells in the treatment of traumatic brain injury. Front Neurol. 2017; https://doi.org/10.3389/fneur.2017.00028/full.
62. Jiang Y, Zhu W, Zhu J, Wu L, Xu G, Liu X. Feasibility of delivering mesenchymal stem cells via catheter to the proximal end of the lesion artery in patients with stroke in the territory of the middle cerebral artery. Cell Transplant. 2013;22(12):2291–8.
63. Lee PH, Lee JE, Kim HS, Song SK, Lee HS, Nam HS, et al. A randomized trial of mesenchymal stem cells in multiple system atrophy. Ann Neurol. 2012;72(1):32–40.
64. Srinivasan VM, Gumin J, Camstra KM, Chen SR, Johnson JN, Shimizu Y, et al. Microcatheter delivery of neurotherapeutics: compatibility with mesenchymal stem cells. J Neurosurg. 2020;133(4):1182–90.
65. Murali N, Mouli SK, Riaz A, Lewandowski RJ, Salem R. Extrahepatic applications of yttrium-90 radioembolization. Semin Interv Radiol. 2021;38(4):479–81.
66. Boston Scientific Corporation. FRONTIER: a feasibility study to evaluate the safety of the TheRaSphere GliOblastoma (GBM) device iN PaTIEnts with recurrent GBM [Internet]. clinicaltrials.gov; 2023 May [cited 2023 Jun 14]. Report No.: NCT05303467. https://clinicaltrials.gov/ct2/show/NCT05303467.
67. Kirn D. Replication-selective oncolytic adenoviruses: virotherapy aimed at genetic targets in cancer. Oncogene. 2000;19(56):6660–9.
68. Jiang H, Gomez-Manzano C, Aoki H, Alonso MM, Kondo S, McCormick F, et al. Examination of the therapeutic potential of Delta-24-RGD in brain tumor stem cells: role of autophagic cell death. JNCI J Natl Cancer Inst. 2007;99(18):1410–4.
69. Jiang H, Gomez-Manzano C, Rivera-Molina Y, Lang FF, Conrad CA, Fueyo J. Oncolytic adenovirus research evolution: from cell-cycle checkpoints to immune checkpoints. Curr Opin Virol. 2015;13:33–9.
70. Fueyo J, Gomez-Manzano C, Alemany R, Lee PS, McDonnell TJ, Mitlianga P, et al. A mutant oncolytic adenovirus targeting the Rb pathway produces anti-glioma effect in vivo. Oncogene. 2000;19(1):2–12.
71. Fueyo J, Alemany R, Gomez-Manzano C, Fuller GN, Khan A, Conrad CA, et al. Preclinical characterization of the antiglioma activity of a tropism-enhanced adenovirus targeted to the retinoblastoma pathway. JNCI J Natl Cancer Inst. 2003;95(9):652–60.
72. Lang FF, Conrad C, Gomez-Manzano C, Yung WKA, Sawaya R, Weinberg JS, et al. Phase I study of DNX-2401 (Delta-24-RGD) oncolytic adenovirus: replication and immunotherapeutic effects in recurrent malignant glioma. J Clin Oncol. 2018;36(14):1419–27.
73. M.D. Anderson Cancer Center. Phase I clinical trial of allogeneic bone marrow human mesenchymal stem cells loaded with a tumor selective oncolytic adenovirus, DNX-2401, administered via intra-arterial injection in patients with recurrent high-grade glioma [Internet]. clinicaltrials.gov; 2023 Feb [cited 2023 Jun 14]. Report No.: NCT03896568. https://clinicaltrials.gov/ct2/show/NCT03896568.
74. Agid R, Rubinstein R, Siegal T, Lester H, Bokstein F, Chisin R, et al. Does streaming affect the cerebral distribution of infraophthalmic intracarotid chemotherapy? AJNR Am J Neuroradiol. 2002;23(10):1732–5.
75. Gobin YP, Cloughesy TF, Chow KL, Duckwiler GR, Sayre JW, Milanese K, et al. Intraarterial chemotherapy for brain tumors by using a spatial dose fractionation algorithm and pulsatile delivery. Radiology. 2001;218(3):724–32.
76. Riina HA, Knopman J, Greenfield JP, Fralin S, Gobin YP, Tsiouris AJ, et al. Balloon-assisted superselective intra-arterial cerebral infusion of bevacizumab for malignant brainstem glioma: a technical note. Interv Neuroradiol. 2010;16(1):71–6.
77. Joshi S, Singh-Moon RP, Wang M, Chaudhuri DB, Holcomb M, Straubinger NL, et al. Transient cerebral hypoperfusion assisted intraarterial cationic liposome delivery to brain tissue. J Neurooncol. 2014;118(1):73–82.

The Wada Test: Intraarterial Anesthetics for Localization of Neurological Functions

8

Jeffrey Cole

The human brain, then, is the most complicated organization of matter we know.

Isaac Asimov (1920–1992), Science Fiction Writer

Introduction

The Wada test is an invasive neurovascular procedure that assesses cognitive functioning during temporary anesthesia of a cerebral hemisphere. It is induced by injecting a short-acting anesthetic agent into the internal carotid artery and observing the behavioral response [1]. Commonly mistaken for an acronym, the procedure was named after Juhn A. Wada, MD, who pioneered the technique in the 1940s, initially to better understand the side effects of electroconvulsive therapy for severe psychiatric disorders before the advent of modern neuroleptic and later to help assess language lateralization in patients undergoing neurosurgical intervention for either CNS tumors or, more commonly, for medically refractory epilepsy [2–4].

History

This new advancement was vital at the time because some neurosurgery patients were, unfortunately, exhibiting severe post-operative aphasia, and it became increasingly evident that it was necessary to establish language dominance *pre-operatively*. In years prior, left- or right-handedness was most often used as a proxy for this important distinction. It was believed that most right-handers were left-hemisphere dominant and, conversely, that most left-handers were right-hemisphere dominant. Direct electric cortical stimulation during awake surgeries was the only way to establish cerebral language representation reliably [4]. Gardner injected procaine directly into the cerebral cortex to inactivate suspected language sites as a precursor to this new pharmacological method [5]. Wada later modified the approach, using amobarbital with direct puncture administration into the carotid artery for a more robust hemispheric effect. In the 1950s, he brought this technique into more widespread practice at the Montreal Neurological Institute. Large-scale studies on language lateralization using amobarbital were published in the 1960s and 1970s [6, 7]. In the latter paper, the authors reported on language lateralization as it related to handedness in a large group of patients (n = 262) without clinical evidence of early damage to the left cerebral hemisphere: they found that right-handed people were left dominant in 96% of cases and right dominant in 4% of cases; they also found that left-handed people had left dominance in 70% of cases, bilateral dominance in 15% of cases, and right dominance in 15% of cases.

In addition to the importance of language lateralization, as neurosurgical treatments started to advance in the 1950s, the role of memory and its relation to structural neuroanatomy were not yet fully understood. The infamous case of patient HM is the preeminent example. He underwent bilateral temporal lobe resections for medically refractory epilepsy in 1953 by Dr. William Scoville. Although the surgery cured his seizures, he became densely amnestic, unable to form or retain new memories. Around the same time, neurosurgeon Dr. Wilder Penfield noticed similar detrimental effects in patients undergoing bitemporal resections for severe psychiatric disorders and in patients undergoing unilateral temporal lobe resections in the context of suspected contralateral temporal lobe pathology [8]. It was increasingly apparent that the temporal lobes, especially mesial structures, including the hippocampus, were vital for form-

J. Cole (✉)
Department of Neurology, Columbia University, New York, NY, USA
e-mail: jrc2028@cumc.columbia.edu

S. Joshi (ed.), *Arterial Treatment of Neurological Diseases*, https://doi.org/10.1007/978-3-031-80173-0_8

ing new memories. Importantly, Penfield and some of his contemporaries started considering seizure freedom but concomitant and significant memory impairment as a treatment failure [9, 10]. As with language, it became even more crucial to identify patients at risk for postoperative amnesia before surgery. To address this need, Brenda Milner, Ph.D., further modified the Wada test by including items for memorization during active hemispheric anesthesia. According to Loring et al. [11], the determination for risk of memory decline was based on three main assumptions: (1) unilateral temporal lobe inactivation would not produce a global amnesia effect by itself, (2) amobarbital injected into the carotid artery would cause sufficient functional inactivation of the mesial temporal lobe region in that hemisphere, and (3) contralateral mesial temporal lobe pathology would result in significant memory impairment due to temporary bilateral dysfunction induced by the reversible ipsilateral injection. Landmark studies on Wada memory findings were published in the 1960s and 1970s [12, 13]. The latter paper reported that memory impairment was only present 27 times following 226 separate injections, with memory failure present in 25/110 following injection contralateral to seizure onset and only in 2/116 following ipsilateral injections.

Over time, as more comprehensive epilepsy centers were established around the world in the 1980s and 1990s, the Wada test became the gold standard for assessing both language lateralization and independent hemispheric memory support as part of the presurgical workup for patients who were considering surgery due to the medically refractory nature of their condition.

The Wada Test Protocol

The Wada test is a non-manualized and non-standardized procedure, with varying techniques employed across different epilepsy surgery programs; as such, "Wada testing" refers not to a specific paradigm but rather, to a group of procedures involving the assessment of language and memory functions during temporary anesthesia of a cerebral hemisphere [14]. The following describes the Wada test protocol practiced at Columbia University Irving Medical Center-New York Presbyterian Hospital, and as shown in Fig. 8.1.

The Wada test is considered a same-day outpatient procedure. The patient arrives at the hospital and is brought to the waiting area in the interventional radiology suite. They are dressed with EEG scalp electrodes in a standardized array. The procedure is explained during this time, and baseline language and memory testing are performed. Then, the patient is transferred into the angiography room for preparatory measures. They are lying in a supine position. An area near the groin is shaved and covered with sterile drapes to allow for access to the femoral artery. After injecting local

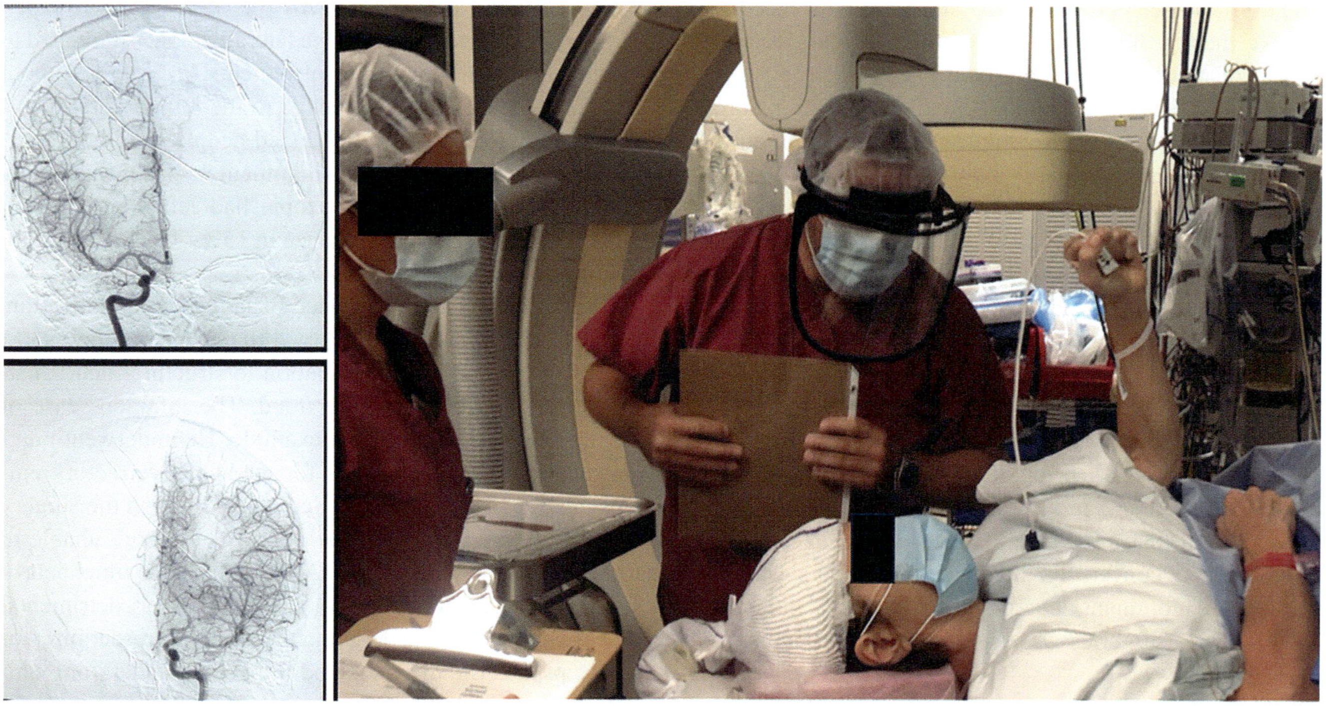

Fig. 8.1 Top left: Angiogram showing intracranial blood vessels with right ICA injection of contrast dye, providing a "roadmap" of where the anesthesia will be perfused. Bottom left: Angiogram showing intracranial blood vessels with left ICA injection of contrast dye provides a similar "roadmap." Right: Patient with right upper extremity hemiplegia and global aphasia following injection of sodium methohexital (Brevital) into the left ICA

anesthetic, the radiologist makes a small puncture incision in the femoral artery, often with Doppler guidance. The radiologist then inserts a wire-guided catheter into the arterial system and manipulates the catheter up and over the aortic arch until it is accurately placed in the internal carotid artery. The side of suspected seizure onset is tested first. The patient must remain still, without moving their head, as there is a risk of arterial dissection or other injury with excessive movements. A cerebral angiogram is performed, using contrast dye, allowing for direct visualization of the intracranial arteries as a "road map" of where the anesthesia will ultimately be perfused. We have used sodium methohexital for years, with doses typically ranging from 4 to 5 mg per injection. When the angiogram is completed, it is time for the actual test to begin. The neuropsychologist and their team enter the room once the radiation is turned off. The examiner needs to stand near the patient's head and ipsilateral to the side of the injection in case the medication causes contralateral hemianopsia. The patient is instructed to raise their arms towards the ceiling and start counting aloud regularly. The radiologist typically injects the medication by hand when the patient reaches number 5. Hemispheric anesthesia is confirmed by ipsilateral EEG slowing and dense contralateral hemiplegia (arm strength 0/5 as tested by a neurologist). The patient is then asked to follow two orally presented commands and to name a series of visually presented pictures and objects, which they have also been instructed to remember. Strength is assessed periodically throughout. Language dominance is inferred when the patient exhibits global aphasia, with an inability to understand or produce words, and, as the medication starts to wear off (arm strength ≥3/5), by the presence of paraphasic errors when trying to speak or repeat phrases. Non-dominance is inferred when the patient can follow commands and accurately name items without paraphasic errors (although dysarthria is sometimes observed). Sodium methohexital is very short-acting, so the testing window is only a few minutes on average; it is essential to note that the radiologist usually withdraws the catheter right away after the desired effects have been obtained to minimize the risk of injury, so there is no option to provide an extra infusion after the initial injection. When the medication is completely worn off (arm strength 5/5 and EEG normalized), there is a 10-min delay before memory assessment for the items presented during the active anesthesia period. Memory is then evaluated by asking the patient if they recall anything spontaneously and, if not, by providing four multiple-choice options (one correct target item, one phonemically related item, one semantically related item, and one unrelated item). After multiple-choice decisions, the patient is asked to rate their subjective confidence, with a score of 3 assigned for "very sure" responses; a score of 2 was assigned for "medium sure" responses, while a score of 1 was assigned for "guessing" responses. Spontaneously recalled items are automatically given a score of 3, and incorrect responses are automatically given 0. Memory scores are then calculated, with ≥67% considered passing for accuracy and ≥2.00 (mean) considered passing for confidence. At this point, the procedure is halfway completed unless the first injection needs to be repeated because of behavioral concerns that raise questions of validity. If not, the radiologist performs the cerebral angiogram on the other side, and the testing portion is repeated with new stimuli. Afterward, the radiologist and the neuropsychologist review the angiogram to determine which vessels were filled and to what extent; the ACA, MCA, PComm, and PCA are assessed, with numerical scores of 3 for maximal filling, 2 for moderate filling, 1 for "flash" filling, and 0 for the absence of filling—this helps with interpretation of the results, especially in cases where the vasculature may be abnormal. The procedure takes less than an hour, and results are available immediately. The patient is later discharged to home after lying down for 6 hours to allow the femoral puncture wound to close effectively and to minimize the risk of hemorrhage.

Wada Experience Narrated by a Patient

A 25-year-old male subject reported his experience during the Wada test as follows:

> *Per the Wada protocol, each side of my brain was put under anesthesia to evaluate each hemisphere's language and memory functions independently.*

Effect of injection of the anesthetic into the dominant hemisphere:

> *When the left side of my brain was being evaluated, the drug was administered just before the neuropsychological portion of the testing began. Once the drug was injected, I quickly felt as if I couldn't speak or understand verbal instructions and couldn't move as I normally would. The right side of my body was extremely weak. A euphoric dazed state occurs, but the key is focusing. I was able to register visual stimuli but unable to produce words to name them. When I was shown the items, I was able to recognize and try to retain the information. During the right hemiplegia, the examiner and I were primarily communicating* via *nonverbal methods (e.g., hand motions, eye contact). As the anesthesia started to wear off, I noticed that my strength was gradually coming back, but I still had some difficulty with my speech, a further indication that this was my language-dominant hemisphere. Within a few minutes, my motor strength and language abilities returned to their normal baseline. After about 10 min, my memory was checked—I was able to recall 1 item spontaneously, as well as recognize the remaining items from multiple-choice options with variable confidence.*

Effect of injection of the anesthetic into the nondominant hemisphere:

> *When the right side of my brain was being evaluated, the drug was again administered just before the neuropsychological portion of the testing began. Once the drug was injected, I was still*

able to speak and follow verbal instructions (e.g., "Point to your nose," "Show me your thumb"), but the left side of my body was extremely weak. I was able to register both verbal and visual stimuli. When I was shown the items, I was able to recognize and try to remember what I had seen. During the left hemiplegia, the examiner and I were able to communicate verbally. As the medication wore off and my strength started to come back, I did not have any trouble with my speech, further verifying that this was not my language-dominant hemisphere. Within a few minutes, my motor strength had returned to normal. After about 10 min, we checked my memory—I could recall four items spontaneously and recognize the remaining items from multiple-choice options with full confidence.

Indications for the Wada Test

Because it is an invasive procedure with inherent risks, the Wada test is used only in certain situations rather than for every epilepsy surgery candidate. Sometimes, it is helpful when there is a question of atypical language dominance or representation such as in individuals who are left-handed or ambidextrous, have an early onset of seizures arising from the left hemisphere, and/or have an early structural lesion in the left hemisphere. It would also be suspected for individuals who do not exhibit post-ictal aphasia following a left-sided seizure, who do exhibit post-ictal aphasia following a right-sided seizure, or who have non-congruent cognitive test findings, including dichotic listening with an apparent left ear advantage [4]. In addition to language, the Wada test is also used when there is a concern for possible memory decline following a proposed surgery involving the mesial temporal structures, such as when there is no imaging evidence of mesial temporal sclerosis or other structural abnormality affecting the hippocampus in question. Similarly, the test can assist when somebody with left temporal lobe seizures performs well on standardized verbal memory tests or poorly on standardized visual memory tests, and vice versa for right temporal lobe seizures. In these situations, measuring the person's memory adequacy (how the hippocampus ipsilateral to the seizure focus functions) is essential to know if the surgeon would remove or ablate a viable structure. It is also necessary to measure the person's memory *reserve* (how the hippocampus contralateral to the seizure focus functions) and whether the "other side" can sufficiently support memory independently.

Potential Complications Associated with the Wada Test

As mentioned earlier, the Wada test is an invasive procedure with inherent risks that must be considered for each patient before proceeding. In one publication [15], a Wada procedure complication was defined as "an unintended adverse and undesirable development in a patient that was clinically significant, requiring medical treatment, additional resource use, or prolonged hospitalization." Unanticipated neurological changes during or immediately after the procedure were found to be procedure-related. However, symptoms associated with the patient's underlying neurological diagnosis (e.g., seizures in people with medically refractory epilepsy) were not considered to be procedure-related. These authors reported on a series of complications in the context of amobarbital use (used exclusively from April 1991 to May 1998, but no longer used at all after July 2004) or methohexital use (used exclusively from August 2004 through June 2013) in a large sample of patients ($n = 431$). In total, 25 patients (5.8% of the total group) experienced an unintended clinical event either during or immediately after the Wada test, including arteriotomy-related hematomas in 13 (3%), seizures in 6 (1.4%), encephalopathy in 3 (0.7%), internal carotid artery vasospasm in 2 (0.5%), injection in the external carotid artery in 1 (0.2%), and status epilepticus in 1 (0.2%). However, only nine patients (2.1% of the total group) had incidents that met the criteria for a *complication* as defined above—this included 0 (0%) of the hematomas and only 2 (0.5%) of the seizures.

A multicenter publication reported complications in 1.09% of patients who underwent Wada testing between 2000 and 2005 [16]. Also, one abstract reported a 1% Wada complication rate, including stroke, femoral neuropathy, left internal artery spasm causing hemiplegia, and temporomandibular joint dislocation [17].

It is perhaps notable that cerebral angiographies alone, without subsequent Wada testing, have been shown to have complications in 0.3–2.63% of patients [18–21].

That said, another significant publication [22] included an extensive series of patients undergoing Wada testing ($n = 677$) with either amobarbital (from 1996 to March 2001) or methohexital (from March 2001 to 2004) and found that as many as 74 (10.9% of the total sample) were affected by complications—this included two distinct complications in 5 of the patients. Complications were described as encephalopathy in 49 patients (7.2%), seizures in 8 patients (1.2%), strokes in 4 patients (0.6%), transient ischemic attacks in 4 patients (0.6%), local hemorrhages at the catheter insertion site in 4 patients (0.6%), carotid artery dissection in 3 patients (0.4%), allergic reaction to contrast dye in 2 patients (0.3%), bleeding from the catheter insertion site in 1 patient (0.1%), and infection in 1 patient (0.1%). They further reported that 14 patients (2% of the total sample) required additional medical workup and treatment due to complications and that lasting deficits with ongoing morbidity for more than 3 months were seen in 4 patients (0.6% of the total sample). They highlighted some significant risk factors for these complications, involving older age for strokes and dissections but younger age for seizures. Moreover, they concluded that amobarbital was more often associated with encephalopathy, whereas methohexital was more often associated with seizures.

The discrepant rates reported in these citations likely reflect different operationalized definitions of a complication, with some sites being more restrictive in assigning this label and other sites perhaps being more liberal in ascribing this classification.

Different Medications Used in the Wada Test

Amobarbital

Historically, amobarbital has been the medication of choice for Wada testing, and its properties are well documented in the literature. However, several alternative drugs have been used in recent years due to its unavailability starting in the early 2000s and restrictions on its use in some countries. These include (but are not limited to) propofol, etomidate, and methohexital. Published research on each of these pharmaceutical agents is reviewed below.

Propofol

Propofol has been increasingly used for Wada testing despite concerns about its broader use, which includes "seizure-like phenomena" [23] and "propofol infusion syndrome" [24]. Propofol's action involves positively modulating the inhibitory function of the neurotransmitter gamma-aminobutyric acid (GABA) through GABA-A receptors.

In a seminal case report, Bazin et al. [25] described the first use of propofol for Wada testing in a 43-year-old ambidextrous man with a brain tumor located in his left temporal-occipital region, in which lateralization of cerebral speech dominance was desired before he underwent a temporal lobectomy. They used a dose of 20 mg injected into the left carotid artery, followed by complete paresis of the right upper extremity after 13 s and total speech arrest for 18 s. The EEG showed slow polymorphic activity over the left frontotemporal area, which decreased in intensity after 6 min; at the same time, motor and speech functions fully recovered, and there was complete amnesia for the entire period. They opted not to inject into the right carotid artery because they obtained the desired results showing left hemisphere language dominance. Notably, there were no significant complications, and the patient only reported the perception of an intense blue light. The authors concluded that the patient's rapid psychomotor recovery and absence of significant adverse effects were "undoubtedly an asset," this initial report led to additional studies using propofol for Wada testing.

In another case report, Silva et al. [26] used propofol for Wada testing in a 26-year-old woman with medically refractory epilepsy. They first injected the left internal carotid artery with a dose of 20 mg, the side of her proposed surgery. The injection resulted in right arm paresis after 11 s and speech arrest for 2 min (followed by another 3 min of mumbling). The EEG showed slow polymorphic activity in the left frontotemporal region, which declined in intensity after 4 min, coinciding with the recovery of motor and speech functions. After a 30-min delay, the right hemisphere was perfused with the same dose in the same fashion. The patient had left arm paresis and inability to speak for 5 min, with arm strength recovering after 6 min. EEG patterns were not included in the report but were presumably similar. The patient described a hot sensation in her head and stated that she wanted to speak but could not do so with the second injection. Memory was assessed after both injections. Results were interpreted as showing bilateral representation for speech and left hemisphere dominance for memory. Once again, given the successful collection of results with no significant adverse effects, the authors concluded that propofol was "good to carry on the Wada test."

Takayama et al. [27] compared patients who underwent bilateral Wada testing with propofol (n = 12, mean dose of 11 mg per injection) with those previously tested with amobarbital (n = 55, mean dose of 104 mg per injection). Diagnostic conditions included epilepsy, brain tumors, and cerebral vascular disease. Contralateral hemiplegia occurred in 22/24 propofol injections and 95/110 amobarbital injections, and retrograde amnesia occurred in 6/22 propofol injections and 26/65 amobarbital injections. Hemispheric dominance for language and memory was successfully evaluated in nearly all propofol patients (12 and 9, respectively), which was similar to rates for the amobarbital patients (52 and 41, respectively). Concerning adverse side effects, 3 of 12 patients in the propofol group exhibited laughing and head/eye version. One of the two patients excluded from statistical analysis (because of left-handedness in one and different doses with left vs. right injections in one) showed face contortion and lacrimation. However, these symptoms did not prevent the patients from completing the Wada test. They further found that the mean recovery time for motor strength was generally longer for amobarbital. In contrast, the mean recovery time of language with the left/dominant injection was typically longer for propofol. The authors concluded that "the Wada test using propofol could replace the traditional Wada test with amobarbital."

In another large retrospective study, Mikuni et al. [28] evaluated 58 patients who underwent Wada testing for presurgical treatment planning between 2001 and 2005, using propofol as the anesthetic agent. The population included people with brain tumors (n = 32), temporal/frontal lobe epilepsy (n = 13), and arteriovenous malformations (n = 13).

They used maximal doses of 15 mg, 10 mg, and 17 mg for these different diagnostic categories, respectively. The authors recorded any adverse reactions and created three distinct classifications: Grade 1 (including eye pain, shivering, face contortion, lacrimation, laughing, and apathy); Grade 2 (including confusion, involuntary movement, and head/eye version); Grade 3 (including increased muscle tone with twitching and rhythmic movements or tonic posturing). Nineteen patients (33% of the total sample) exhibited adverse reactions immediately after propofol administration, including six with Grade 1 symptoms, six with Grade 2 symptoms, and seven with Grade 3 symptoms. However, in most of these patients (with only one exception), the symptoms dissipated within 5 min and were mild enough to continue the testing. Notably, there was no significant difference in memory performance if adverse reactions did or did not occur. Risk factors for any adverse effects included age older than 55. For Grade 3 symptoms, risk factors included age older than 55, diagnosis of AVM, total injection dose >20 mg, and a second injection dose >10 mg. No significant risk factors were specific for Grade 1 or Grade 2 symptoms. In summary, the authors concluded "Despite minor adverse effects of the procedure in a small at-risk population, intracarotid injection of approximately 10 mg propofol for tumors and epilepsy is a reasonably safe method for performance of the Wada test. In contrast, age greater than 55 and a total injection dose greater than 20 mg are important risk factors foretelling potentially severe symptoms."

Mikati et al. [29] compared 25 consecutive patients undergoing Wada testing with propofol with 15 patients previously tested with amobarbital. Pathologies among the groups included mesial temporal/hippocampal sclerosis, tumor, trauma, atrophy, dysgenesis, dysplasia, arteriovenous malformations, hemangioma, infarct, and cyst. The authors found that EEG slowing on the injection side was generally less remarkable for propofol than for amobarbital. Also, the percentage of patients needing more than one dose was significantly higher for propofol (70%) than amobarbital (7%)—this was explained in part by the fact that the propofol group required more extended protocols (because of bilingual testing with multiple parameters), and also that the propofol group protocols were delayed in the start because of side-effects detailed below. One patient, a 28-year-old man with epilepsy, developed an episode of confusion, combativeness, and agitation starting a few seconds after propofol administration, lasting 5 min and subsiding only with diazepam. All patients in the propofol group experienced ipsilateral facial and ocular flushing and discomfort, starting a few seconds after intracarotid injection and lasting about 1–2 min, thereby delaying the onset of testing. Propofol was additionally associated with short-lived chills and tremulousness, with some patients in the amobarbital group also having similar chills. Significantly, side effects in the propofol group did not negatively impact testing, only delaying the start. The protocol was completed for lateralizing speech and memory functions for all patients in both groups. In line with previous researchers, the authors ultimately concluded that "propofol is a reasonable alternative to amobarbital as an anesthetic agent in the Wada test."

Another retrospective analysis of patients undergoing Wada testing between 2004 and 2009 compared the use of amobarbital ($n = 75$) and propofol ($n = 54$) [30]. The patients were under consideration for selective anterior temporal lobectomy for medically refractory epilepsy. The patients underwent unilateral injections ipsilateral to the proposed side of surgery. Statistical analysis showed no significant difference between these medications for pass/fail rates, side effects, or length of hemiplegia. They further stated that there was no significant difference in the number or type of side effects between the groups and that the overall number of side effects in this study was somewhat reduced (total of 29.1% for propofol and 26% for amobarbital) compared to those reported by Mikuni et al. (2005), including zero patients with Grade 3 events for either of the medications [28]. With these findings taken together, they commented that "propofol represents a suitable alternative to amobarbital for use in the Wada test."

Further comparison of bilateral Wada testing for epilepsy with propofol ($n = 29$) versus amobarbital ($n = 18$) was reported by Curot and colleagues [31]. Hemispheric language dominance was successfully identified in 96.5% and 94.4% of the patients, respectively, and hemispheric memory dominance was successfully determined in 72.4% and 77.7% of patients, respectively. There was no significant difference between the groups. The authors also had a particular focus on adverse events that could endanger the patient (hemodynamic and vegetative disorders), create discomfort (pain and dysphoria), or hinder the completion of the test (motor disorders and disturbance of consciousness). They observed adverse events in 65.5% of propofol patients and 44.4% of amobarbital patients, with no statistical difference between the groups. In most cases, these adverse events were mild and short-lived, disappeared before the end of the procedure, and did not interfere with neuropsychological assessment. They further reported that disturbance of consciousness was more intense with amobarbital, that transient euphoria was observed with propofol (3 patients) but not amobarbital, and that ocular symptoms mainly occurred with propofol when it was injected too rapidly (ostensibly making this avoidable with a slower injection). They concluded that "propofol can be used for the Wada test with an efficacy and safety comparable to amobarbital."

In one last publication to be reviewed herein, Mikuni et al. evaluated the effectiveness of intravenous methylprednisolone in reducing the risk of adverse effects during the Wada test [32]. They compared 75 patients who did (study group) and 58 patients who did not (control group) receive this infusion before a standard dose of propofol for testing purposes. The study group included people with brain tumors ($n = 43$), temporal or frontal lobe epilepsy ($n = 18$), and arteriovenous malformations ($n = 14$). In the group receiving antecedent methylprednisolone, nine patients (12%) experienced adverse effects, with all symptoms disappearing within 5 min of propofol injection and not interfering with the test completion. By comparison, 19 patients (33%) experienced adverse effects in the group not receiving antecedent methylprednisolone. Statistical analysis calculated that the study group had a 72% overall risk reduction compared to the control group and a 92% risk reduction for Grade 3 symptoms. There was no significant difference for Grade 1 or Grade 2 symptoms. The authors concluded that intravenous administration of methylprednisolone followed by intracarotid injection of propofol significantly reduces the risk of severe adverse events during Wada testing. The mechanism of action was proposed to improve vascular supply and anti-allergic action, which reduces ischemia-induced cerebral excitability.

Etomidate

Etomidate is yet another medication used in place of amobarbital for Wada testing. However, this drug may have side effects, including myoclonus, tremor, and dystonic posturing in other procedures [33], as well as increased EEG spike activity in patients with epilepsy [34] and epileptiform activity or seizures in people without epilepsy [35]. It is a nonbarbiturate hypnotic agent that produces its effect by acting as a positive allosteric modulator on the gamma-aminobutyric acid (GABA) type A receptor, thus enhancing inhibitory properties.

In a seminal study describing their development of the etomidate speech and memory test (eSAM), Jones-Gotman et al. [36] reported on 16 patients (30 total injections because two only had unilateral testing, eventually reduced to 26 injections because four others were excluded from analysis—13 left hemisphere and 13 right hemispheres) undergoing Wada testing. Nearly all patients had epilepsy, with only one exception involving a right frontal lobe tumor but no epilepsy. The medication was delivered into the internal carotid artery with an initial bolus of 2 mg followed by a steady infusion (3–4 μg/kg/min) to allow for continuous testing without interruption of hemianesthesia. Clinical symptoms—including loss of contralateral upper extremity motor function, changes in speech/language, contralateral facial weakness, and contralateral visual field defects—occurred approximately 40 s after the initial injection. EEG results were examined for 24 of the injections (20 with scalp electrodes and 4 with stereo-depth electrodes); drug-induced changes occurred on average 39 s after injection, with slow waves in the delta range and sometimes theta range, predominantly in the ipsilateral hemisphere (100%) but often in the contralateral frontal region (75%), with dissipation and return to electrophysiological baseline on average 4 min and 13 s after the end of the infusion. Interictal spike activity was also observed with 8 of the injections (33%), including four during scalp EEG recording (3 patients) and four during scalp EEG recording (2 patients). The language was characterized by global aphasia, with 13 tests lasting throughout the infusion, thus indicating language dominance for the injected hemisphere. Memory items were presented on average 3 min and 15 s after injection, and this lasted for just under 2 min, with subsequent yes/no recognition assessed on average 13 min after the initial injection. Memory was considered adequate when 65% or more of the drug-stage objects were recognized. Analyzed injections ipsilateral to the seizure focus resulted in 11 passes and one borderline determination; analyzed injections contralateral to the seizure focus resulted in 4 passes, one borderline determination, and five failures. Two other cases were described separately. Mood changes were evaluated and defined as positive, negative, flat, or labile. When noticeable emotional expression occurred, it was most often positive (nine injections) with lower rates of negative (one injection), flat (one injection), and positive, followed by flat (one injection) and labile (one injection) descriptions. The most notable side-effect involved a shivering-like tremor, most often in the upper extremities for nine patients (12 tests, or 46% of the 26 injections), but this was considered mild in most cases. Overall, based on their experience, the authors concluded that etomidate is a safe alternative to amobarbital for Wada testing "with certain advantages." Specifically, their protocol using continuous infusion was touted as an improvement compared to the traditional procedure because it allowed "all behavioral testing to be completed during full drug effect."

In two case reports, Kowacs et al. also used the etomidate Speech and Memory (eSAM) model for Wada testing [37]. The first patient was a 35-year-old woman who had uncontrolled secondary generalized seizures since age 14 and a 58-year-old female who had refractory epilepsy starting at age 34. In the first instance, injection of etomidate into the right internal carotid artery resulted in "slowing of the EEG tracing on the right hemisphere associated with repetitive rhythmic sharp theta activity" and similar abnormal features with the left-sided injection. In the second patient, injecting etomidate into the left internal carotid artery was followed by "a slowing of the EEG background activity with associated TIRDA activity…on the ipsilateral hemisphere," with comparable findings following the right-sided injection. Language and memory testing was not compromised in either of these studies, despite the presence of irritative EEG activity. Nevertheless, the authors cautioned that "EEG monitoring during the procedure must be encouraged to facilitate the interpretation of the nature of transient cognitive impairment and/or seizure-like phenomena that may eventually occur with the test."

In a later study, Andelman et al. modified the above-described eSAM protocol because they encountered significant side effects [38]. The continuous infusion approach in their first three patients (seizure with secondary generalization in one, prolonged obtundation in one, and severe tremor and myoclonus in all three). They subsequently decided to evaluate the effectiveness of etomidate for Wada testing with only a single bolus injection for an additional 18 patients, with none of them experiencing similar adverse reactions. All 21 patients were candidates for standard anterior temporal lobectomy because they had medically refractory epilepsy (14 with left seizure focus and 7 with right seizure focus), and all had bilateral injections to assess for language dominance and independent hemispheric memory support. They used a dose of 2 mg diluted in 4 cc of saline solution injected into the internal carotid arteries over 60 s. Signs of hemiparesis first started to appear around 40 s after injection, with complete hemiparesis reached by 60 s and lasting for an average of 5 min. Examination of speech function and presentation of memory items was performed for 150–180 s, well within the period of hemiparesis that was continuously checked every 30 s. In their words, "the duration of drug action reliably exceeded the duration of speech testing and presentation of all memory objects in the patients." Using a memory asymmetry calculation, the authors determined that an earlier onset of epilepsy was associated with a higher asymmetry score. In addition, patients with left-hemisphere foci performed more poorly on memory testing than those with right-hemisphere foci. There was no significant difference between these groups in the contralateral memory performance. However, the memory function of the ipsilateral hemisphere in patients with left-hemisphere seizures was significantly lower than that of patients with right-hemisphere seizures. In the absence of meaningful demographic differences between the groups, the different memory performances were thought to be probably due to the effect of the epileptogenic lesion. More importantly, however, this report showed that the modified eSAM procedure, with a single bolus of etomidate, was not only sufficient to complete the necessary testing in the allotted time frame, but it also showed "increased tolerability to etomidate in terms of almost complete eradication of the side-effects displayed with continuous administration by the infusion pump."

Passarelli et al. evaluated 54 prospective patients with medically refractory epilepsy secondary to unilateral mesial temporal sclerosis (MTS), using etomidate for Wada testing during the presurgical workup [39]. The study included bilateral injections into the internal carotid arteries, always starting with the side with MTS (31 left and 23 right). They used an initial bolus of 0.8 mg, which resulted in contralateral hemiplegia in all but one male patient who required an additional bolus of 0.4 mg to achieve this effect. This initial bolus effect lasted 3–8 min (mean 4.8 ± 0.8), with an additional etomidate push necessary in 6 patients (10.7% of the sample) because of partial motor recovery during the procedure. Side effects included tremors in 15 patients (26.8%), dystonia in 11 patients (19.6%), excessive somnolence in 6 patients (10.7%), and a puncture site hematoma in 1 patient (1.9%). However, these problems were mild and transient and did not require procedure interruption. Also, on a positive note, there were no angiographic complications, seizures, or life-threatening issues. Language assessment was possible in all cases, with 52 showing unilateral dominance (50 left and two right) and two patients showing bilateral representation (left > right). Memory evaluation was also achieved in all patients, with memory item presentation lasting from 3.2 to 7 min (mean 4.3 ± 0.96). They calculated scores for memory reserve (performance after injection ipsilateral to the lesion) and memory capacity (performance after injection contralateral to the lesion), as well as a memory asymmetry score (MemCap − MemRes). Four patients (7.4%) failed the memory reserve assessment. There were 16 memory items. There was a significant difference with better memory reserve (12.7 ± 2.5) than memory capacity (10.5 ± 3.5) overall. The authors further noted that 32 of the patients underwent both pre-and post-operative standardized memory testing—analyses showed that there was no significant difference in patients who declined on at least one test when they passed with memory reserve (11/22 or 50%) versus when they had borderline or failing scores with memory reserve (6/10 or 60%), even when patients with left and right MTS were considered separately. When looking at Wada memory asymmetry scores, patients with right MTS who had unfavorable scores were more likely to show declines (4/4 or 100%) than those who had favorable scores (4/9 or 44.4%) on at least one test; this difference was not similarly observed in the left MTS group. Two patients failed the Wada test but underwent surgery. They did not demonstrate a significant global decline or global amnesia afterward. Overall, the authors touted etomidate as a safe and effective alternative medication for Wada testing.

In one final study to be reviewed herein, Banks et al. assessed for awareness of deficits during Wada testing with epilepsy patients who were injected with either amobarbital (n = 32) or etomidate (n = 37) [40]. All of the patients were left-hemisphere language dominant. Testing was conducted over 2 days, with each internal carotid artery injected on the respective days. After standard language and memory testing were completed, and there was a complete return to neurological and cognitive baseline, patients were asked questions regarding their awareness of motor weakness, problems speaking, or difficulty understanding the examiner during anesthesia. Responses were coded into three categories: no awareness, some awareness, or full awareness. Among those in the etomidate group, awareness for the motor deficit was significantly less following right-hemisphere injection (57.5% with no awareness) than it was following left-hemisphere injection (40% with no awareness), with further analysis showing that this difference only reached significance when the seizure focus was in the left hemisphere (e.g., injecting the "good" right side and testing the "bad" left side). Following the left (dominant) hemisphere injection, all patients exhibited speech arrest, and 80% showed some degree of diminished comprehension. Among those with a comprehension deficit, 75% were unaware of this deficit. In comparison, only 10% lacked awareness of their naming impairment, which was true for those with left and right-hemisphere epileptogenic foci. When comparing the two medications, left hemisphere injections included greater awareness of motor weakness with etomidate versus amobarbital (this pattern also approached significance with right hemisphere injections). There was also better awareness of naming deficits with etomidate compared to amobarbital. There was no difference between the medications for awareness of comprehension deficits, which was minimal for all patients. The authors offered some potential explanations for their results. First, when explaining hemispheric differences, they mentioned that von Economo neurons (which have a suggested role in error recognition) are 30% more prevalent in the right versus left cerebral hemisphere in humans, which could impact rates of anosognosia. Second, to explain the difference in medication effects, they noted that both drugs are hypnotics that influence GABAa receptors, but amobarbital has an analgesic effect, whereas etomidate does not. Finally, although not explicitly discussed by the authors in this manner, it could be posited that naming deficits are more akin to Broca's aphasia, which typically involves preserved insight, and comprehension deficits are more akin to Wernicke's aphasia, which is often characterized by impaired insight.

Methohexital

Several studies have been published on the effects of methohexital as a replacement for amobarbital in the Wada test. Methohexital binds to the chloride ionophore site of the gamma-aminobutyric acid (GABA)-A/chloride ionophore receptor complex, thereby enhancing the inhibitory actions of GABA-A in the brain. GABA-A inhibition leads to synaptic inhibition, decreased neuronal excitability, and induction of anesthesia.

Buchtel et al. reported on their observations with methohexital Wada testing in 86 patients (173 procedures), with a more detailed analysis of the behavioral and EEG recovery patterns in 20 patients [41]. The total sample consisted of patients with unilateral temporal lobe epilepsy and MTS (n = 77), parietal lobe epilepsy (n = 1), occipital lobe epilepsy (n = 1), frontal lobe epilepsy (n = 1), orbitofrontal lobe epilepsy (n = 2), temporooccipital lobe epilepsy (n = 2), fronto-parieto-temporal lobe epilepsy (n = 1), and orbitofrontal-anterior temporal-insular epilepsy (n = 1). Their standard procedure generally involved language testing after an initial intracarotid injection of 3 mg, followed by the presentation of memory items after a second intracarotid injection of 2 mg. The latter was given when the patient began to show signs of recovery from the former (e.g., contralateral grip strength ≥2/5 or the beginning of speech production in the dominant hemisphere). Doses varied somewhat depending on the clinical situation at hand. In the cohort, 71 had bilateral hemisphere testing, while 15 had only unilateral hemisphere testing because of complicating variables. Nine patients also underwent super-selective administration into the PCA for more specific memory testing only. With methohexital, the expected neurological changes—hemiplegia, visual field cut, hemineglect with the nondominant injection, and aphasia with the dominant injection—were quickly observed and were "indistinguishable" from the effects of amobarbital that were used by these same examiners in previous years before it became unavailable. When measuring motor outcomes/length of contralateral hemiplegia, the first injection of methohexital (3 mg) lasted for ~90–100 s, and the second injection (2 mg) lasted for ~110–120 s, with a total return to baseline after ~260 s. On rare occasions, a third injection (10 cases) and a fourth injection (1 case) were required due to more rapid recovery. A comparison of the different anesthetics showed that the motor recovery from methohexital (259 ± 63 s) was much faster than that from a standard dose of amobarbital (n = 31, 385 ± 108 s). When measuring EEG outcomes/length of ipsilateral slowing, the combined first and second injections typically showed high amplitude anteriorly predominant delta activity, with a complete return to baseline ~360 s after starting. A brief crossover to the contralateral hemisphere was observed in about half of the cases but quickly dissipated after ~10 s. Notably, there was no activation of interictal epileptiform abnormalities in any of the cases (although it was previously reported that this could be seen with higher doses of 25–50 mg). A comparison of the anesthetics again showed that EEG recovery from methohexital (355 ± 76 s) was more rapid than the same from a standard dose of amobarbital (n = 42, 468 ± 110 s). Based on their experience, the authors stated that "the two anesthetics appear to be equivalent in their ability to determine which hemisphere is dominant for language function and to screen for the risk of amnesia after anterior temporal resection." However, they further commented on several advantages of using methohexital instead of amobarbital. First, patient alertness appeared to be better with methohexital in general. Second, patients' recovery was better after each methohexital injection, allowing for repeat testing within a single session without incremental drowsiness that is often seen with amobarbital. Third, because of more rapid recovery and lack of a cumulative obtundation effect, the lengthy time between amobarbital injections (typically ~45 min) is unnecessary with methohexital, so the entire procedure is much more efficient. It can usually be completed within an hour. On one cautionary note, the authors did emphasize that using methohexital requires keen attention to behavioral changes (grip strength and language) over EEG changes alone (which tend to be faster and less evident with methohexital than amobarbital).

Andelman et al. compared Wada test results between 20 patients [42]. Patients underwent an intracarotid methohexital procedure (IMP) between 2003 and 2005, and 32 patients who had undergone an intracarotid amobarbital procedure (IAP) between 2000 and 2003 in the same medical facility. All patients had medically refractory epilepsy and were candidates for neurological surgery. There were no statistical differences between the groups in age, gender, age at onset of epilepsy, proportion of patients with secondary generalization, proportion of patients with suspected MTS, proportion of patients with anterior cerebral artery cross-flow, or proportion of cerebral language laterality. Each cerebral hemisphere was injected twice in the IMP, first for language function assessment and second for memory function assessment. Language testing included repetition of single words and sentences, comprehension of instructions, and object naming—with speech arrest, disruption of expressive language, and paraphasias during recovery determined to be signs of dominant lateralization. Although this was not the main focus of their paper, the authors noted that "although there was no question about the determination of laterality of cerebral language production in any of our patients, cerebral language comprehension seemed to be bilaterally represented in more patients during methohexital Wada testing than during amobarbital Wada testing." Memory testing involved the presentation of eight physical objects during active anesthesia—with subsequent recognition after full recovery using each target item among two additional foils. Two memory scores were calculated: one for % the items correctly recognized after ipsilateral injection (testing memory in the healthy hemisphere) and one for % correctly recognized after contralateral injection (testing memory in the epileptogenic hemisphere). Wada memory tests were compared with standardized memory tests from paper-and-pencil neuropsychological assessments, including the Rey auditory verbal learning test (RAVLT) and the Rey complex figure (RCF). Statistical analysis revealed no significant difference in contralateral memory support (i.e., memory in the healthy hemisphere) between the methohexital and amobarbital groups. However, there was a substantial difference in ipsilateral memory scores, with the methohexital group showing a higher memory capacity in the hemisphere with the seizure focus. These results were not associated with the laterality of the epileptogenic focus, laterality of language dominance, or any demographic or angiography procedure variables. Moreover, analysis of correlations between ipsilateral Wada memory performance and standardized neuropsychological memory testing showed that the relationship was stronger for patients in the IAP group than the IMP group. The authors had a different conclusion than those of Buchtel et al. [41], specifically that inferred Wada memory support on the side of proposed epilepsy surgery depends on which anesthetic drug is used, and further that stronger correlations with RAVLT or RCF performances might suggest that the degree of adequacy of lateralized memory assessment is possibly higher with the IAP than with the IMP.

Concerning the frequency of seizures during Wada testing, Loddenkemper et al. conducted a retrospective chart review of 761 epilepsy patients [43]. Patients had Wada testing with amobarbital (n = 538, 75–250 mg) or methohexital (n = 222, 3–10 mg) as part of their presurgical workups. Of the 760 patients assessed, 16 (2.1%) had seizures during their Wada test. Three seizures occurred before drug injection (2 before amobarbital and one before methohexital administration, with no significant difference between groups). After the injection of amobarbital, four patients (0.6% of the sample) had a seizure, including one with secondary generalization. The difference in seizure frequency before (2 patients) and after (4 patients) amobarbital injection was insignificant. After methohexital injection, nine patients (4.1% of the sample) had a seizure, including two with secondary generalization. The difference in seizure frequency before (1 patient) and after (9 patients) methohexital injection was statistically significant. The authors concluded that seizures may be more frequent in Wada testing after administration of a barbiturate and, in particular, patients may be more prone to seizures after methohexital injection than amobarbital injection.

In a later study, Loddenkemper et al. again conducted a retrospective chart review of 582 consecutive Wada tests between 1997 and 2003 (amobarbital was used from 1997 to March 2001, and methohexital was used after March 2001) [44]. A total of 1041 injections (left only = 60, right only = 63, and bilateral = 459) were analyzed. Groups tested with amobarbital (n = 449, 75–250 mg) and methohexital (n = 133, 3–10 mg) were compared. Language testing included counting, repetition, spontaneous speech, object naming, and word reading. Memory testing consisted of presenting 9–20 words and objects (number determined by the duration of hemiparesis) during active anesthesia, with recognition using four multiple-choice options 15–30 min after full-strength recovery. With amobarbital, language lateralization in patients with bilateral injections was left in 79.7%, right in 5.9%, bilateral dependent in 13%, and bilateral independent in 1.4%. Memory lateralization was predominantly left in 60.8%, predominantly right in 30.7%, and bilateral in 8.5%. With methohexital, language lateralization in patients with bilateral injections was left in 76%, right in 5.9%, bilateral dependent in 16.3%, and bilateral independent in 1.9%. Memory lateralization was predominantly left in 60.6%, predominantly right in 23.1%, and bilateral in 16.3%. Statistical comparison between the groups showed no significant difference in language or memory lateralization (although bilateral memory was more often seen in the methohexital group compared to the amobarbital group). The length of speech arrest was significantly longer in the amobarbital group, the percentage of retained objects was significantly higher in the methohexital group, and fewer memory items were presented during anesthesia with methohexital compared to anesthesia with amobarbital. The authors concluded that "there seems to be no difference between (the medications) in determining language and memory lateralization." Further, the advantages of using methohexital included shorter recovery times and shorter durations between injections, allowing for more efficient bi-hemispheric testing. One possible downside, however, is a briefer window to present memory items with methohexital owing to its much shorter half-life and the potential risk of seizures described in the previously reviewed study. Nevertheless, this group opted for continued use of methohexital with their future Wada procedures.

An earlier study by Isnard et al. revealed two principal advantages of using methohexital over amobarbital [45]. The first is what they described as "shorter hemispheric narcosis," allowing for the two carotid arteries to be tested in the same session and limiting the risk of drug diffusion to the two hemispheres. The second was the rare occurrence of drowsiness or falling asleep with methohexital, as issues of "vigilance" tend to be more frequent with amobarbital.

Superselective Wada Testing

Standard Wada testing typically involves the injection of amobarbital (or other agents described above) with catheter placement in the internal carotid artery for drug delivery. Carotid injection often results in a general anesthetic effect for the entire cerebral hemisphere, or most of it, which allows for assessment of lateralized dysfunction but obscures evaluation of more localized intra-hemispheric deficits. In some cases, there is even unintended cross-flow to the anterior circulation of the contralateral hemisphere, which can complicate the procedure by causing unwanted obtundation, inattention, and/or disinhibition. In cases where the medical team is interested in a more discrete or focal area within a given hemisphere, it is possible to perform a "super-selective" Wada test, which enables inhibition of an arterial territory supplying a more specific location in the brain, with use of a microcatheter to reach more distal intracranial vessels smaller than 1 mm in diameter.

The selection of the vessel perfused depends on the region or the function of interest. Access to the middle cerebral artery (MCA) territories with superselective infusion would be used to evaluate language functions. With superselective infusion, using this technique, it is possible to perfuse either the anterior language site of the inferior frontal gyrus (near Broca's area) or the posterior language site of the posterior superior temporal gyrus (near Wernicke's area) [46]. They reported on eight cases (three with left dominance and typical language organization, one with left dominance but atypical language organization, two with right dominance and "mirror image" of typical language organization, and two with bilateral dominance and unusual anterior-posterior functional properties). This information can be vital on a case-by-case basis because, in their words, "there is a wide variability in the distribution of language areas in patients with drug-resistant epilepsy."

For assessing memory, the best route would be perfusion of the posterior cerebral artery (PCA) territory because this provides arterial supply to the body and tail of the hippocampus and adjacent mesial temporal structures. It also has the advantage of deactivating this region with minimal effects on language, attention, or motor functions that might otherwise compromise the findings [47]. This group reported on 32 candidates for temporal lobectomy using the super-selective PCA approach. There were no serious complications; all but one of the patients remained alert and cooperative under anesthesia, and 28 showed good contralateral memory support (3 were excluded from surgery because they failed with fewer than 67% of memory items correctly recognized). At the publication, 19 patients had proceeded to surgery, with none showing subsequent global amnesia or significant material-specific memory loss.

Another commonly accessed vessel is the anterior choroidal artery (or the ICA after temporarily blocking the vessel via balloon occlusion distal to the origin of the anterior choroidal artery, AChA), which perfuses several vital structures, including the amygdala and hippocampal head. This modification has some benefits but also one important caveat. Wieser et al. [48] showed that only some patients have their mesial temporal structures supplied by the AChA. Pre-procedure angiographies are therefore important to determine if this region would be irrigated properly for testing purposes.

Fitzsimmons and colleagues described a modified technique in four patients with cerebral arteriovenous malformations who underwent super-selective Wada testing before embolization of the lesions [49]. They used a combination of amobarbital and lidocaine. They found that adding lidocaine detected clinically significant neurological deficits that amobarbital alone did not, likely because they have different pharmacodynamic properties. In short, while amobarbital (and other GABAa agonists) block neuronal functions in the gray matter, lidocaine blocks axonal functions in the white matter. They concluded that using both agents for super-selective Wada testing in patients with cerebral AVMs may improve the sensitivity and predictive value of the test.

Of course, as with any invasive procedure, some potential side effects are associated with the super-selective Wada testing paradigm. According to Hassan et al., these include but are not limited to the following: phantom limb movements, euphoria, agitation or aggression, crying, fear, disinhibition, attentional disturbances, aphasia, motor or somatosensory deficits, cranial nerve palsies, miosis, visual field defects, and ptosis [50]. Possible complications include headaches, nausea, vomiting, thromboembolism, or dissection with subsequent risk of cerebrovascular events. Symptoms would naturally depend on which vessel is being perfused.

Future Directions with Wada and Alternative Techniques

Wada testing can be considered a "disruption technique" because it results in a temporary loss of function (e.g., inability to produce or understand language when the dominant hemisphere is being assessed or failure to remember information when a dysfunctional hippocampus is being tested). Recently, an increasing number of "activation techniques" have been used to measure changes in brain function during language-related tasks, allowing for in vivo or real-time detection of regions presumed to be involved in the task [51]. Functional magnetic resonance imaging (fMRI) is arguably the most widely used method, and it works by showing hemodynamic changes (e.g., increased blood flow to local vasculature) that are presumed to accompany neural activity in that specific location. The benefits of fMRI are as follows: it is non-invasive, can be used repeatedly with minimal time restrictions, and can be used on patients and healthy control subjects with virtually no risks to their health. Furthermore, it provides detailed information about changes in activation across and within the cerebral hemispheres, thus providing valuable information about language lateralization and localization simultaneously. This latter point is important, as it has been shown that language representation is usually not a purely unilateral phenomenon [52].

Research has shown that fMRI has high concordance rates with Wada testing for lateralization purposes [53–56] and reasonable concordance rates for localization purposes with focal electrical stimulation mapping [57–60]. However, these correlations are not perfect, so caution is advised when using this technique for surgical decision-making. Although less publicized to date, there is some evidence that fMRI can also be used as a valid tool for assessing *memory* lateralization in patients with mesial temporal lobe epilepsy [61].

Despite the emerging use of fMRI as an alternative to Wada testing in presurgical evaluations, it also has some notable shortcomings, including the fact that specific functions might be complex to isolate (e.g., language tasks might also activate or "light up" areas associated with auditory processing and sustained attention). It is also assumed that underlying neuropathology has not interfered with normal blood flow or hemodynamic activity in the area(s) of interest. Finally, like the variability seen in Wada testing, there is no uniform or standardized protocol for fMRI studies, so differences in methodologies between centers are bound to yield different results.

Abou-Khalil has described other noninvasive techniques gaining traction in the field, including repetitive transcranial magnetic stimulation (RTMS), event-related brain potentials (ERP), magnetoencephalography (MEG), functional transcranial doppler (fTCD), single photon emission computed tomography (SPECT), positron emission tomography (PET), and near-infrared spectroscopic (NIRS) mapping [62].

Conclusion

In summary, the Wada test is a classic example of intra-arterial drug delivery, and it has been used extensively with good clinical benefits since the 1940s. Furthermore, research has shown that complications related to radiographic techniques and/or medications are rare and manageable. The procedure is a testament to the general safety of anesthetic drug injection when used carefully by highly trained professionals. Newer, less invasive techniques are being employed with increasing frequency, and they hold considerable promise for future research and clinical purposes. However, it can be argued that Wada testing is still the "gold standard" in many centers to determine cerebral language dominance and independently assess memory capacity in each hemisphere. We continue to use Wada testing at Columbia University Irving Medical Center-New York Presbyterian Hospital regularly, and the information it provides is usually vital for surgical planning.

References

1. Wada J, Rasmussen T. Intracarotid injection of sodium amytal for the lateralization of cerebral speech dominance: experimental and clinical observations. J Neurosurg. 1960;17(2):266–82.
2. Wada JA. Youthful season revisited. Brain Cogn. 1997;33(1):7–10.
3. Wada JA. A fateful encounter: sixty years later—reflections on the Wada test. Epilepsia. 2008;49(4):726–7.

4. Loring DW, Meador KJ. History of the Wada test. In: Barr WB, Bieliauskas LA, editors. The Oxford handbook of history of clinical neuropsychology. Oxford: Oxford University Press; 2019.
5. Gardner WJ. Injection of procaine into the brain to locate speech area in left-handed persons. Arch Neurol Psychiatr. 1941;46(6):1035–8.
6. Branch C, Milner B, Rasmussen T. Intracarotid sodium amytal for the lateralization of cerebral speech dominance: observations in 123 patients. J Neurosurg. 1964;21(5):399–405.
7. Rasmussen T, Milner B. The role of early left-brain injury in determining lateralization of cerebral speech functions. Ann N Y Acad Sci. 1977;299:355–69.
8. Penfield W, Milner B. Memory deficit produced by bilateral lesions in the hippocampal zone. AMA Arch Neurol Psychiatry. 1958;79(5):475–97.
9. Penfield W, Jasper H. Epilepsy and the functional anatomy of the human brain. AMA Arch Neurol Psychiatry. 1954;72(5):663–4.
10. Loring DW. History of neuropsychology through epilepsy eyes. Arch Clin Neuropsychol. 2010;25(4):259–73.
11. Loring DW, Meador KJ, Lee GP, King DW. MCG Wada protocol: amobarbital effects and lateralized brain function: the Wada test. In: Amobarbital effects and lateralized brain function: the Wada test. New York: Springer New York; 1992. p. 109–17.
12. Milner B. Study of short-term memory after intracarotid injection of sodium amytal. Trans Am Neurol Assoc. 1962;87:224–6.
13. Milner B. Disorders of learning and memory after temporal lobe lesions in man. Clin Neurosurg. 1972;19:421–46.
14. Cole J, J. HM. Neuropsychology in adult epilepsy surgery. In: Pearson C, Ecklund-Johnson E, Gale S, editors. Neurosurgical neuropsychology: the application of neuropsychology to the practice of neurosurgery: Elsevier; 2019.
15. Beimer NJ, Buchtel HA, Glynn SM. One center's experience with complications during the Wada test. Epilepsia. 2015;56(8):e110–3.
16. Haag A, Knake S, Hamer HM, Boesebeck F, Freitag H, Schulz R, et al. The Wada test in Austrian, Dutch, German, and Swiss epilepsy centers from 2000 to 2005: a review of 1421 procedures. Epilepsy Behav. 2008;13(1):83–9.
17. Macken M, Morris H, editors. Complications of the WADA test. A review of Cleveland Clinic experience. Epilepsia. Philadelphia: Lippincott Williams & Wilkins; 1999.
18. Willinsky RA, Taylor SM, TerBrugge K, Farb RI, Tomlinson G, Montanera W. Neurologic complications of cerebral angiography: prospective analysis of 2,899 procedures and review of the literature. Radiology. 2003;227(2):522–8.
19. Dawkins AA, Evans AL, Wattam J, Romanowski CAJ, Connolly DJA, Hodgson TJ, et al. Complications of cerebral angiography: a prospective analysis of 2,924 consecutive procedures. Neuroradiology. 2007;49(9):753–9.
20. Kaufmann TJ, Huston J, Mandrekar JN, Schleck CD, Thielen KR, Kallmes DF. Complications of diagnostic cerebral angiography: evaluation of 19 826 consecutive patients. Radiology. 2007;243(3):812–9.
21. Fifi JT, Meyers PM, Lavine SD, Cox V, Silverberg L, Mangla S, et al. Complications of modern diagnostic cerebral angiography in an academic medical center. J Vasc Interv Radiol. 2009;20(4):442–7.
22. Loddenkemper T, Morris HH, Möddel G. Complications during the Wada test. Epilepsy Behav. 2008;13(3):551–3.
23. Walder B, Tramèr MR, Seeck M. Seizure-like phenomena and propofol: a systematic review. Neurology. 2002;58(9):1327–32.
24. Kam PC, Cardone D. Propofol infusion syndrome. Anaesthesia. 2007;62(7):690–701.
25. Bazin JE, Picard P, Gabrillargues J, Dordain M. Propofol administered via the carotid artery to achieve a Wada test. Can J Anaesth. 1998;45(7):707–8.
26. Silva TM, Hernández-Fustes OJ, Bueno ML, Varela AM, Machado S. The Wada test with propofol in a patient with epilepsy. Arq Neuropsiquiatr. 2000;58(2a):348–50.
27. Takayama M, Miyamoto S, Ikeda A, Mikuni N, Takahashi JB, Usui K, et al. Intracarotid propofol test for speech and memory dominance in man. Neurology. 2004;63(3):510–5.
28. Mikuni N, Takayama M, Satow T, Yamada S, Hayashi N, Nishida N, et al. Evaluation of adverse effects in intracarotid propofol injection for Wada test. Neurology. 2005;65(11):1813–6.
29. Mikati MA, Naasan G, Tarabay H, El Yamen S, Baydoun A, Comair YG. Intracarotid propofol testing: a comparative study with amobarbital. Epilepsy Behav. 2009;14(3):503–7.
30. Magee JA, Pender NP, Abrahams S, Thornton J, Delanty N, Fortune GM. A comparison of propofol and amobarbital for use in the Wada test. Seizure. 2012;21(5):399–401.
31. Curot J, Denuelle M, Busigny T, Barragan-Jason G, Kany M, Tall P, et al. Bilateral Wada test: amobarbital or propofol? Seizure. 2014;23(2):122–8.
32. Mikuni N, Yokoyama Y, Matsumoto A, Kikuchi T, Yamada S, Hashimoto N, et al. Intravenous methylprednisolone reduces the risk of propofol-induced adverse effects during Wada testing. Neurol Med Chir (Tokyo). 2010;50(8):622–6.
33. Reddy RV, Moorthy SS, Dierdorf SF, Deitch RD Jr, Link L. Excitatory effects and electroencephalographic correlation of etomidate, thiopental, methohexital, and propofol. Anesth Analg. 1993;77(5):1008–11.
34. Ebrahim ZY, DeBoer GE, Luders H, Hahn JF, Lesser RP. Effect of etomidate on the electroencephalogram of patients with epilepsy. Anesth Analg. 1986;65(10):1004–6.
35. Krieger W, Copperman JM, Laxer KD. Seizures with etomidate anesthesia. Anesth Analg. 1985;64(12):1226–7.
36. Jones-Gotman M, Sziklas V, Djordjevic J, Dubeau F, Gotman J, Angle M, et al. Etomidate speech and memory test (eSAM): a new drug and improved intracarotid procedure. Neurology. 2005;65(11):1723–9.
37. Kowacs PA, Mattei TA, Goulart CR, da Rocha SF, Ramina R, Simão CA, et al. Seizure-like activity during etomidate-modified Wada test interfere with the evaluation of cognitive functions? Arq Neuropsiquiatr. 2011;69(5):846–7.
38. Andelman F, Kipervasser S, Maimon S, Fried I, Parmet Y, Neufeld MY. A revised intracarotid etomidate memory (Wada) procedure. Acta Neurol Scand. 2013;127(2):97–102.
39. Passarelli V, Pinto LF, Jorge CL, Puglia P, Adda CC, Wen H-T, et al. The intracarotid etomidate Wada test: a 54-patient series. Epilepsy Behav. 2014;39:73–7.
40. Banks S, Sziklas V, Djordjevic J, Golinski R, Jones-Gotman M. Awareness of deficits during intracarotid anesthetic procedures in epilepsy: comparisons of motor, naming, and comprehension awareness under amobarbital versus under etomidate. Epilepsy Behav. 2010;19(4):591–5.
41. Buchtel HA, Passaro EA, Selwa LM, Deveikis J, Gomez-Hassan D. Sodium Methohexital (Brevital) as an anesthetic in the Wada test. Epilepsia. 2002;43(9):1056–61.
42. Andelman F, Kipervasser S, Reider G II, Fried I, Neufeld MY. Hippocampal memory function as reflected by the intracarotid sodium methohexital Wada test. Epilepsy Behav. 2006;9(4):579–86.
43. Loddenkemper T, Möddel G, Schuele SU, Wyllie E, Morris HH 3rd. Seizures during intracarotid methohexital and amobarbital testing. Epilepsy Behav. 2007;10(1):49–54.
44. Loddenkemper T, Möddel G, Dinner DS, Kim H, Schuele SU, Alexopoulos AV, et al. Language assessment in Wada test: comparison of methohexital and amobarbital. Seizure. 2009;18(9):656–9.
45. Isnard J, Garde P, Fischer C, Duquesnel J, Mauguière F. [Clinical and electroencephalographic manifestations during the Wada test using intracarotid injection of methohexital (Brietal)]. Rev Neurol (Paris). 1994;150(4):266–267.
46. Kakinuma K, Osawa S-I, Hosokawa H, Oyafuso M, Ota S, Kobayashi E, et al. Determination of language areas in patients with

epilepsy using the super-selective Wada test. IBRO Neurosci Rep. 2022;13:156–63.
47. Stabell KE, Bakke SJ, Andresen S, Bjørnæs H, Borchgrevink HM, Due-Tønnessen P, et al. Selective posterior cerebral artery amobarbital test: its role in presurgical memory assessment in temporal lobe epilepsy. Epilepsia. 2004;45(7):817–25.
48. Wieser HG, Müller S, Schiess R, Khan N, Regard M, Landis T, et al. The anterior and posterior selective temporal lobe amobarbital tests: angiographic, clinical, electroencephalographic, PET, SPECT findings, and memory performance. Brain Cogn. 1997;33(1):71–97.
49. Fitzsimmons BF, Marshall RS, Pile-Spellman J, Lazar RM. Neurobehavioral differences in superselective Wada testing with amobarbital versus lidocaine. AJNR Am J Neuroradiol. 2003;24(7):1456–60.
50. Hassan AE, Zacharatos H, Rodriguez GJ, Hanel R. Complications during endovascular provocative testing and bilateral inferior petrosal sinus sampling. In: Khatri R, Rodriguez GJ, Raymond J, Qureshi AI, editors. Complications of neuroendovascular procedures and bailout techniques. Cambridge: Cambridge University Press; 2016. p. 129–47.
51. Cole JR, Hamberger MJ. Language plasticity in epilepsy. In: de Zubicaray GI, Schiller NO, editors. The Oxford handbook of neurolinguistics: Oxford: Oxford University Press; 2019. p. 0.
52. Springer JA, Binder JR, Hammeke TA, Swanson SJ, Frost JA, Bellgowan PS, et al. Language dominance in neurologically normal and epilepsy subjects: a functional MRI study. Brain. 1999;122(11):2033–46.
53. Binder JR, Swanson SJ, Hammeke TA, Morris GL, Mueller WM, Fischer M, et al. Determination of language dominance using functional MRI: a comparison with the Wada test. Neurology. 1996;46(4):978–84.
54. Rutten GJ, van Rijen PC, van Veelen CW, Ramsey NF. Language area localization with three-dimensional functional magnetic resonance imaging matches intrasulcal electrostimulation in Broca's area. Ann Neurol. 1999;46(3):405–8.
55. Woermann FG, Jokeit H, Luerding R, Freitag H, Schulz R, Guertler S, et al. Language lateralization by Wada test and fMRI in 100 patients with epilepsy. Neurology. 2003;61(5):699–701.
56. Benke T, Köylü B, Visani P, Karner E, Brenneis C, Bartha L, et al. Language lateralization in temporal lobe epilepsy: a comparison between fMRI and the Wada test. Epilepsia. 2006;47(8):1308–19.
57. FitzGerald DB, Cosgrove GR, Ronner S, Jiang H, Buchbinder BR, Belliveau JW, et al. Location of language in the cortex: a comparison between functional MR imaging and electrocortical stimulation. AJNR Am J Neuroradiol. 1997;18(8):1529–39.
58. Ruge MI, Victor J, Hosain S, Correa DD, Relkin NR, Tabar V, et al. Concordance between functional magnetic resonance imaging and intraoperative language mapping. Stereotact Funct Neurosurg. 1999;72(2–4):95–102.
59. Carpentier A, Pugh KR, Westerveld M, Studholme C, Skrinjar O, Thompson JL, et al. Functional MRI of language processing: dependence on input modality and temporal lobe epilepsy. Epilepsia. 2001;42(10):1241–54.
60. Pouratian N, Bookheimer SY, Rex DE, Martin NA, Toga AW. Utility of preoperative functional magnetic resonance imaging for identifying language cortices in patients with vascular malformations. J Neurosurg. 2002;97(1):21–32.
61. Golby AJ, Poldrack RA, Illes J, Chen D, Desmond JE, Gabrieli JD. Memory lateralization in medial temporal lobe epilepsy assessed by functional MRI. Epilepsia. 2002;43(8):855–63.
62. Abou-Khalil B. An update on determination of language dominance in screening for epilepsy surgery: the Wada test and newer noninvasive alternatives. Epilepsia. 2007;48(3):442–55.

9 Neuroendovascular Therapies for Acute Ischemic Stroke

Arthur Wang and Philip M. Meyers

There are other things to fear…for example, apoplexy, that lightning bolt which strikes you down without destroying you, yet after which all is finished.

From the Count of Monte Cristo by Alexander Dumas (1802–1870), French Novelist and Playwright

Introduction

Acute ischemic strokes present a heavy health burden on the US population. It is estimated that ischemic strokes affect approximately 795,000 patients in the USA annually [1, 2]. Approximately 30% of these ischemic strokes are large vessel occlusions (LVO) involving the middle cerebral artery or internal carotid artery [3]. In 1995, the National Institute of Neurological Disorders and Stroke (NINDS) group demonstrated the efficacy of intravenous recombinant tissue plasminogen activator (IV-tPA), and a few years later, significant trials were published investigating the efficacy and safety of endovascular stroke therapy [2]. Initially, vessel revascularization rates, as shown in these trials, were low and associated with poor clinical outcomes. However, improvements in device technology and more efficient stroke triage paved the way for the rise of endovascular stroke intervention. Endovascular therapy is the standard of care for patients presenting with LVOs. This chapter discusses the clinical and technical aspects of endovascular stroke therapy and the changing paradigms for selecting endovascular therapy for patients.

Development of Endovascular Stroke Therapy

In 1995, the NINDS group demonstrated that stroke patients given IV-tPA within 3 h of symptom onset had better functional outcomes at 3 and 12 months compared with the placebo group [2]. In 2013, three significant trials (IMS III, SYNTHESIS Expansion, MR RESCUE) cast doubt on the efficacy of endovascular stroke therapy compared to IV-tPA [4–6]. However, there were significant limitations to these trials. Notably, the lack of neuroimaging to confirm a large vessel occlusion, the use of early-generation endovascular technology (intra-arterial thrombolysis, Merci retriever, etc.), and poor stroke triage with long hospital delays were responsible for the lack of benefit seen between endovascular therapy and IV-tPA. However, later trials in 2015–2016 (MR CLEAN, ESCAPE, EXTEND-IA, SWIFT PRIME, REVASCAT, THRACE) investigating the efficacy of more modern endovascular devices (stent retrievers) have each demonstrated the superiority of endovascular therapy over medical management for patients with LVOs [4–8]. These trials highlight three significant modifications that were responsible for the successful application of endovascular stroke therapy:

- More efficient stroke triage and thus shorter time from symptom onset to groin puncture
- Use of newer generation endovascular devices and thus higher recanalization rates
- Use of noninvasive neuroimaging to select patients with LVOs

Stroke Imaging

The purpose of neuroimaging in the evaluation of acute ischemic stroke patients is three-fold: (1) rule out an intracranial hemorrhage, (2) identify the presence and location of the

A. Wang · P. M. Meyers (✉)
Columbia University, New York, NY, USA

S. Joshi (ed.), *Arterial Treatment of Neurological Diseases*, https://doi.org/10.1007/978-3-031-80173-0_9

arterial occlusion and collateral circulation, and (3) evaluate the ratio of irreversible ischemic core/dead tissue versus at risk salvageable tissue/penumbra.

A non-contrast head computed tomography (CT) is often the first imaging modality to exclude an intracranial hemorrhage. CT can also suggest the possibility of a large vessel occlusion through radiographic signs, such as focal hyperdensity within the occluded intracranial vessel (Fig. 9.1).

Advanced imaging, usually CT angiography (CTA), is used to identify a large vessel occlusion and assess collateral circulation. The CTA can be performed immediately after the non-contrast head CT while the patient is still on the CT scanner.

Several methods are used to estimate the ischemic core, each differing in sensitivity, specificity, and accuracy. Before more advanced imaging software, a rapid and widely available method using the non-contrast CT brain scan alone was the ASPECT (Alberta Stroke Program Early CT Score) Score [9]. While quick to obtain, the ASPECT score is the least sensitive method of estimating the ischemic core. Hypoattenuation changes (completed infarction) in ten hemispheric regions on a non-contrast CT are assessed on a 10-point scale (Fig. 9.2). This scoring system has a substantial prognostic value in acute ischemic stroke patients, as lower scores represent larger infarction. In comparison, higher scores represent more minor strokes (i.e., a score of 10 indicates that the area of completed stroke is small). The Interventional Management of Stroke (IMS) III trial demonstrated that patients with ASPECTS of 8–10 are twice as likely to achieve a clinically favorable outcome as those with a lower score [10]. A score < 6 suggests that a large volume of the brain is irreversibly injured, making endovascular recanalization futile and increasing the risk of hemorrhagic conversion of the infarcted tissue.

The most sensitive and accurate method for defining cerebral ischemia and the ischemic core of an acute infarct is diffusion-weighted magnetic resonance imaging (MRI). MRI is not readily available at all institutions, is time intensive, requires specialized equipment, and often introduces an additional delay in treatment. It is, therefore, frequently not practical to obtain in the decision-making process for ischemic stroke patients. An alternative to non-contrast CT with diffusion-weighted MRI is CT-perfusion imaging. By identifying mismatched areas of abnormal cerebral blood flow (CBF) and cerebral blood volume (CBV) relative to the size of the ischemic region, perfusion imaging can delineate the infarcted core from the surrounding ischemic cerebral penumbra (i.e., brain parenchyma salvageable if reperfusion can be rapidly achieved) (Fig. 9.3). A patient who is an ideal candidate for endovascular therapy has a small ischemic core (permanently damaged or infarcted) and large penumbra (reversibly damaged but salvageable) (Fig. 9.4). It has been shown that patients with a sizeable infarcted core exceeding 70 cm^3 are at risk for reperfusion hemorrhage after vessel revascularization. However, outcomes after reperfusion of large cerebral infarctions remain controversial.

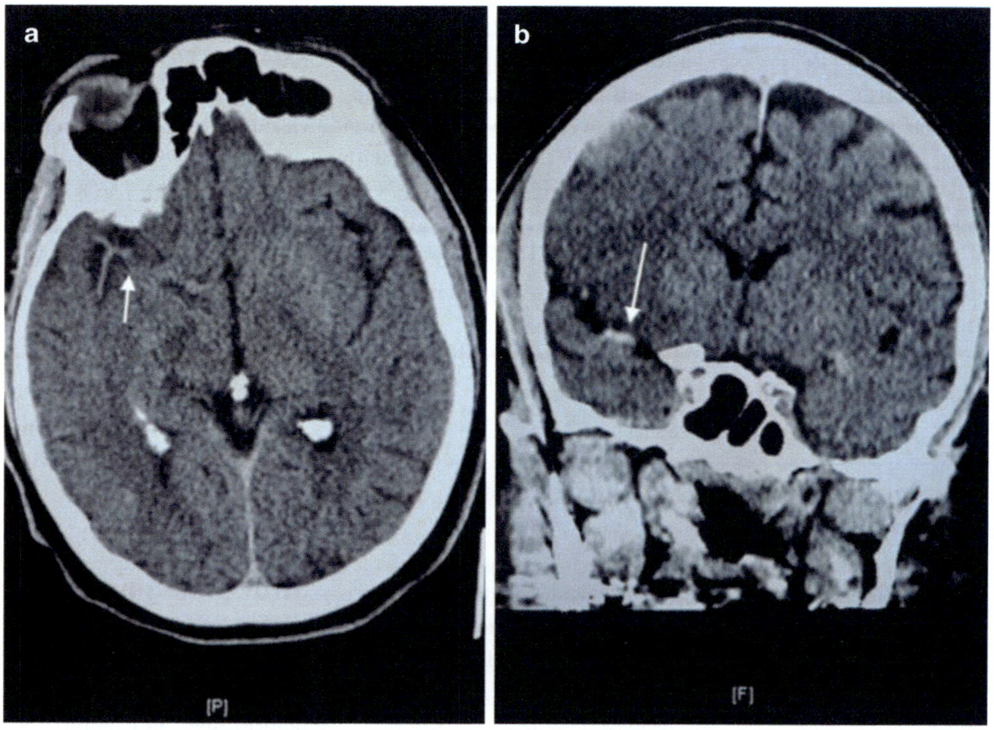

Fig. 9.1 Axial (**a**) and coronal (**b**) reconstruction of non-contrast CT head demonstrating a focal hyperdensity along the right middle cerebral artery "dense" MCA sign

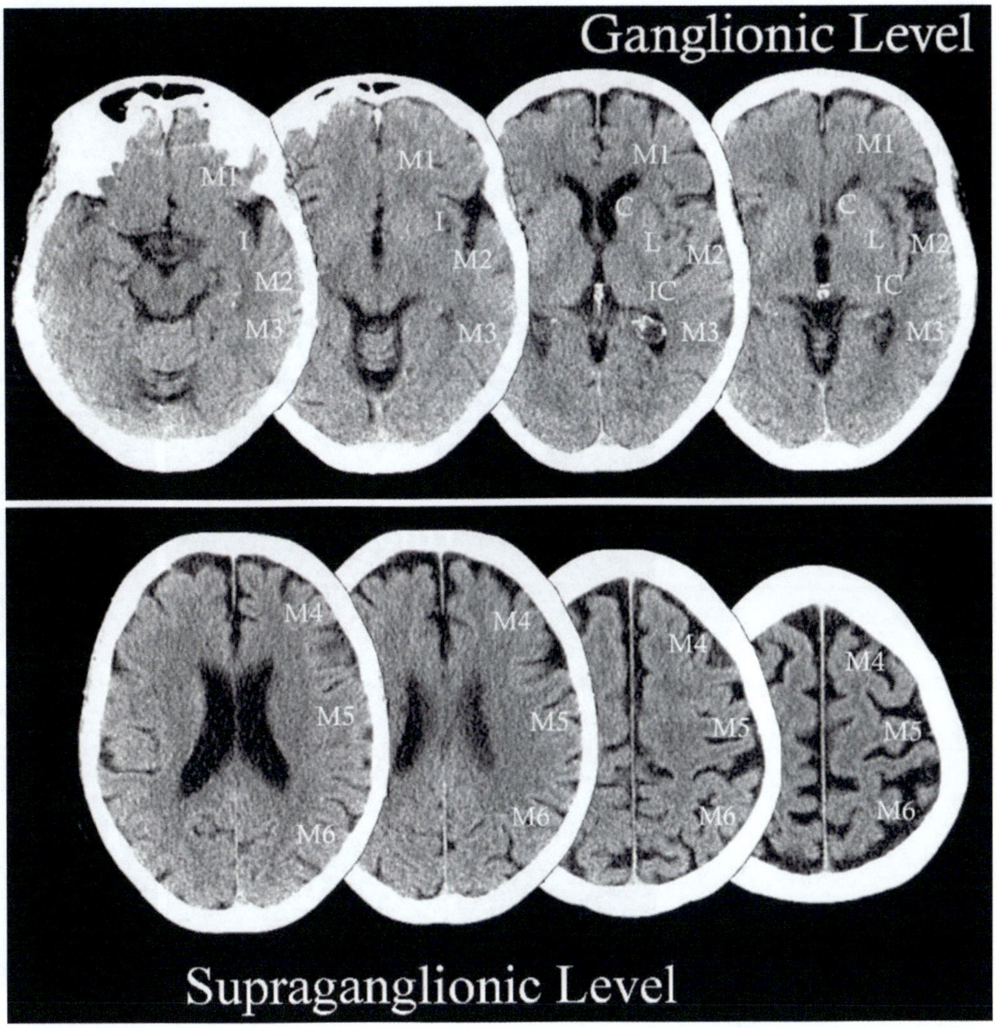

Fig. 9.2 Alberta Stroke Program Early CT Score (ASPECTS). National Institute of Health Stroke Scale (NIHSS)

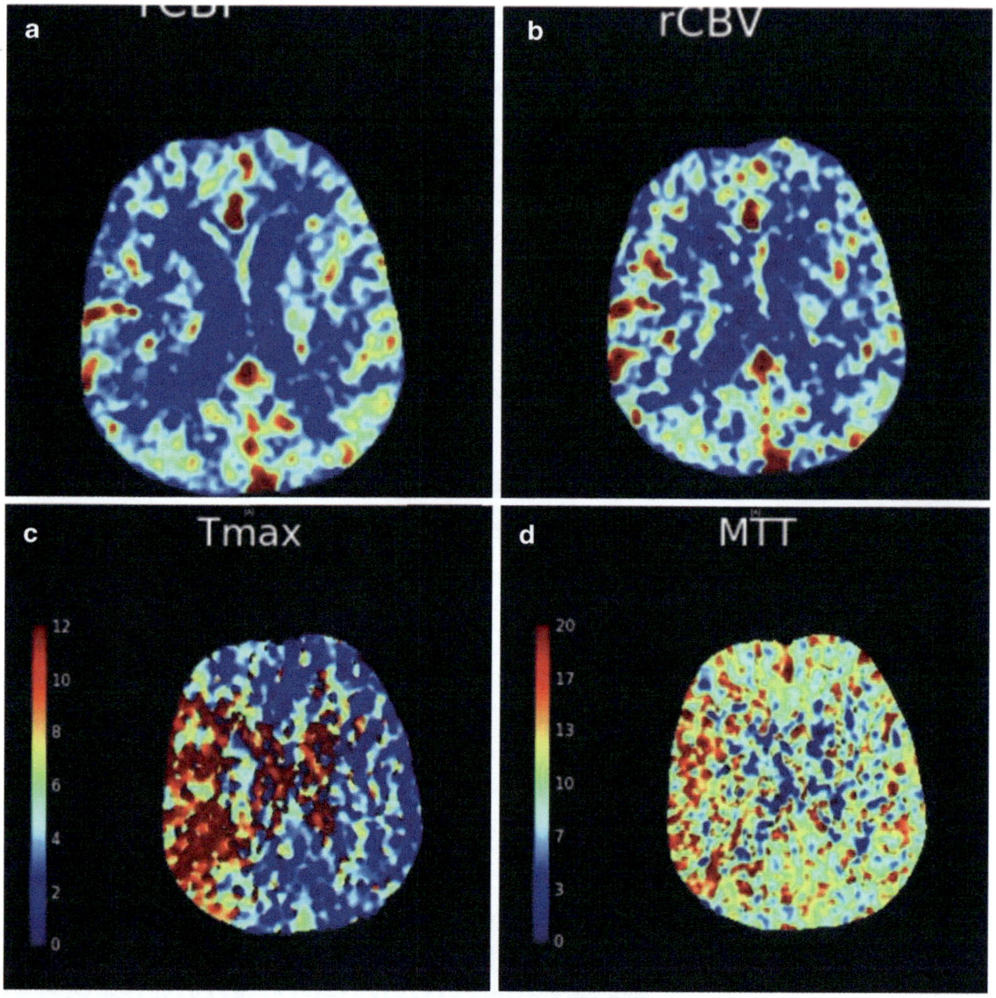

Fig. 9.3 CT Perfusion parameters of cerebral blood flow (**a**), cerebral blood volume (**b**), time-to-maximum (**c**), and mean transit time (**d**)

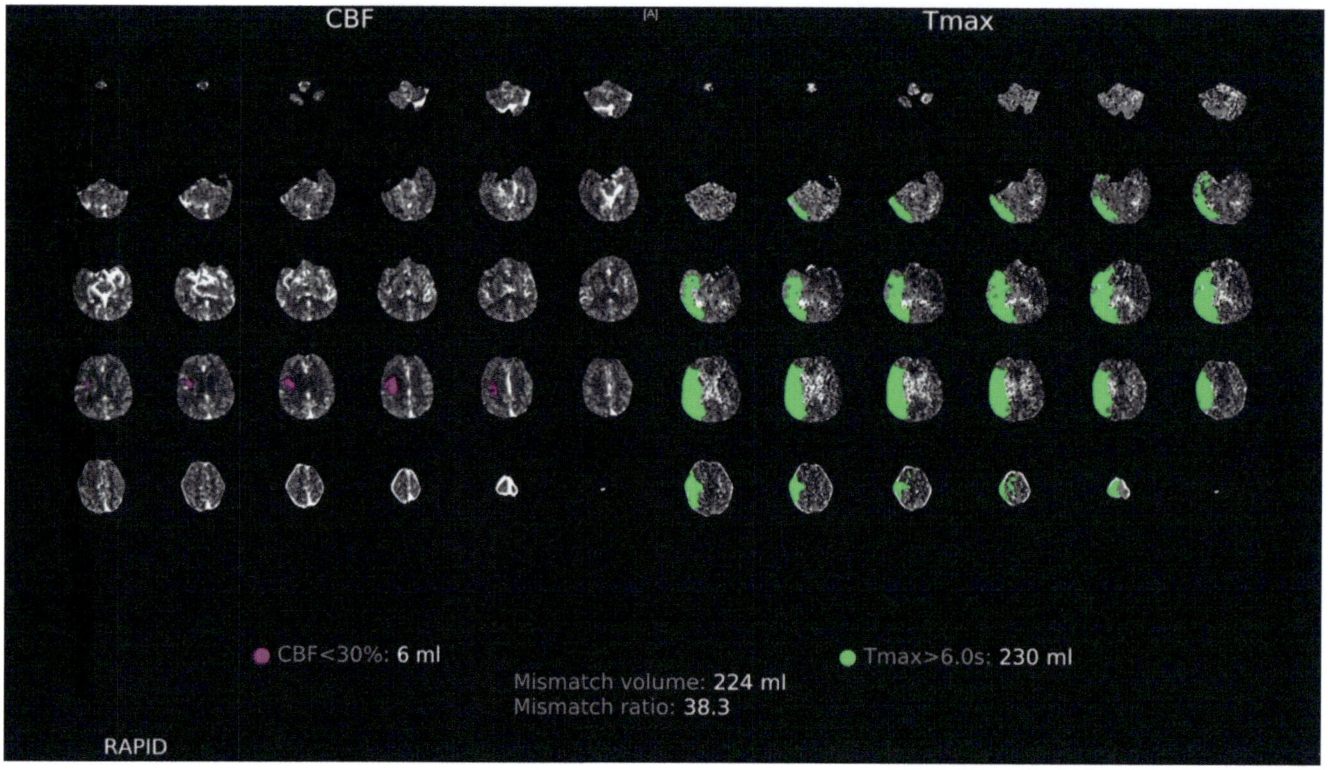

Fig. 9.4 Automated quantified mismatch ratio and volume

Importance of the Penumbra

The ischemic brain tissue supplied by the occluded intracranial vessel is usually a mixture of infarcted brain and penumbra/at-risk tissue (Fig. 9.5). The viability of the penumbra is affected by (1) collateral blood flow and (2) blood pressure. Adequate collateral circulation allows more time for at-risk tissue (penumbra) to remain salvageable and thus for a longer time window until effective reperfusion by endovascular intervention. In an acute ischemic stroke, prominent collateral blood supply to the ischemic area is a predictor of improved clinical outcome. This may be apparent on cross-sectional imaging and sometimes but not reliably, even on catheter angiography.

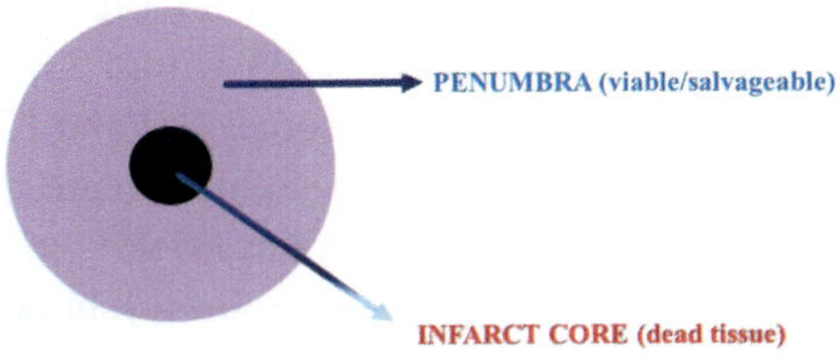

Fig. 9.5 Schematic representation of the relationship between core infarction and penumbral tissue volume

Blood pressure management is a critical factor in ensuring the viability of the penumbra. The 2018 American Heart Association/American Stroke Association Guidelines recommend that blood pressure should be kept at or below 185/110 mmHg before endovascular therapy and reperfusion if no IV t-PA was given (Recommendation II, level of evidence B; for explanation, see legend of Table 9.1) [11]. The limits were initially established to ensure the safety of IV t-PA administration as blood pressure lower than this level protects against an excess risk of intracranial hemorrhage. Until vessel recanalization and reperfusion, higher blood pressure promotes collateral blood flow and maintains penumbral perfusion. Although initially derived from early retrospective data, the lowest acceptable systolic blood pressure value has long been considered 140 mmHg. After reperfusion, blood pressure control appears essential to minimize the risk of reperfusion hemorrhage. The target systolic blood pressure value after reperfusion is below 140 mmHg.

Table 9.1 Randomized control trials: DAWN and DEFUSE-3

	DAWN	DEFUSE 3
Selection criteria		
Last known regular (h)	6–24	6–16
Age (years)	>18	18–90
NIHSS	>10	>6
Infarct volume (mL)	51	70
Results		
Rate of mRS ≥ 2 or functional independence at 90 days: EVT vs. medical management	49% vs. 13% (posterior probability of superiority >0.999)	44.6% vs. 16.7% ($p < 0.001$)

NIHSS NIH Stroke Scale (measure of stroke severity), *mRS* Modified Rankin Scale (measure—from 0 to 6—of neurological outcome, where 0 is return to baseline and 2 is disability but able to self-care, equivalent to functional independence, and 6 is death), *EVT* Endovascular thrombectomy

Time and Changing Paradigm for Stroke Therapy

Two published randomized controlled trials, DAWN and DEFUSE 3, selectively extended the time window to effective endovascular therapy (Table 9.1) [12, 13]. Both studies require confirming the presence of a penumbra in their algorithm to proceed with endovascular treatment. Thus, they introduce a significant paradigm shift from decision-making based on time to decision-making based on imaging according to the amount of salvageable tissue.

DAWN

The DAWN trial was a multi-center stroke trial that evaluated thrombectomy 6–24 h after stroke when there was a mismatch between deficit and infarct volume. It used DWI or CTP Assessment with clinical assessment of stroke deficits in the triage of wake-up and late-presenting strokes. Patients with more significant deficits than infarcts on imaging were randomized to medical treatment or thrombectomy using Trevo (Stryker Neurovascular, Fremont, CA), one of two brands of stent-retrievers [12]. When a difference existed between the severity of clinical presentation and infarct volume, it suggested that a large penumbra causing neuronal dysfunction and deficits existed that was salvageable. In patients with a mismatch between clinical deficit and infarct volume on MRI, clinical outcome (modified Rankin score/mRS) at 90 days was significantly better in the endovascular therapy group than the medical therapy group, even when treated up to 24 h after the last known normal. In conjunction with the data from DEFUSE 3, the FDA approved the expansion of the indications for stroke thrombectomy beyond the initial 6-h window of opportunity.

DEFUSE 3

The DEFUSE 3 trial (Thrombectomy for Stroke at 6–16 h with Selection by Perfusion Imaging) provided additional evidence for endovascular therapy benefits beyond the standard 6-h window [13]. Similar to the DAWN trial, the trial evaluated revascularization of stroke patients with a salvageable penumbra. Patients with LVO up to 16 h from the last-known normal were randomized to EVT or medical therapy based on imaging. The selection criteria included an ischemic core <70 mL, a ratio of volume of penumbra to infarct volume ≥ 1.8, and an absolute volume of penumbra ≥15 mL on MRI with DWI or CT with perfusion imaging. Patients undergoing endovascular treatment had significantly improved 90-day clinical outcomes and functional independence compared to the medical therapy group.

Therapeutics

Intravenous Fibrinolysis

IV-tPA is approved for recanalization in patients presenting with ischemic stroke when presenting within 4.5 h of symptom onset [2, 6]. IV-tPA is given in a total dose of 0.9 mg/kg, as a 10% bolus over 1 min and the rest over 1 h. The NINDS group showed stroke patients given tPA within 3 h of symptom onset had better functional outcomes at 3 and 12 months compared to the placebo group [2]. Symptomatic intracerebral hemorrhage occurred more in the IV-tPA group compared with the placebo group (6.4% vs. 0.6%), but there was no difference in mortality at 3 months or 12 months [2]. The evidence suggests that all patients eligible for IV-tPA should be treated with IV-tPA and taken for endovascular treatment as soon as possible. Table 9.2 shows the inclusion and exclusion criteria for the administration of IV-tPA.

Table 9.2 Inclusion and exclusion criteria for intravenous tissue plasminogen activator

Inclusion criteria
NIHSS ≥4
Symptom onset <4.5 h, with exception of basilary artery occlusion
Age >18 years
Exclusion criteria
Severe head trauma within the past 3 months
Suspicion of subarachnoid hemorrhage
Arterial puncture at non-compressible locations in the past 7 days
Intracranial hemorrhage within the past 6 months
Intracranial arteriovenous malformation or aneurysm
Cerebral or spinal surgery within the past 4 weeks
Uncontrolled hypertions (SBP > 185 mmHg and/or DBP > 110 mmHg)
Serious bleeding event within the past 3 weeks or hemorrhagic diathesis
Childbirth in the past 10 days or the third trimester of the pregnancy
Thrombocytopenia < 100,000
Administration of heparin in the last 48 h and aPTT over the normal range
Therapy by anti-vitamin K and INR > 1.7
Administration of direct thrombin inhibitors or activated factor X inhibitors with significant abnormality of aPTT, INR, thrombocytopenia, and relevant tests of activated factor X activity
Hypoglycemia < 2.7 mmol/L
Early ischemic changes in >1/3 of the MCA territory on CT head

NIHSS National Institute of Health Stroke Scale, *SBP* Systolic blood pressure, *DBP* Diastolic blood pressure, *aPTT* Partial thromboplastin time, *INR* International normalized ratio, *MCA* Middle cerebral artery, *CT* Computed tomography

Mechanical Revascularization

Endovascular mechanical thrombectomy is the standard of care for patients with large vessel occlusion. A large vessel occlusion is considered the intracranial carotid artery (ICA) or M1 segment of the MCA and basilar artery. Five randomized controlled trials (MR CLEAN, ESCAPE, EXTEND-IA, SWIFT PRIME, REVASCAT, THRACE) demonstrated the safety and efficacy of mechanical thrombectomy. In each trial, functional outcomes were substantially improved in patients with large vessel occlusions treated with mechanical thrombectomy. This benefit was seen across multiple subgroups (patients >80 years of age and those with severe strokes as indicated by NIHSS <20). In part, the clinical benefit of mechanical thrombectomy was determined by selection criteria. Only 4.4% of all patients suffered symptomatic intracerebral hemorrhage (sICH), which is lower than some trials evaluating intravenous fibrinolysis.

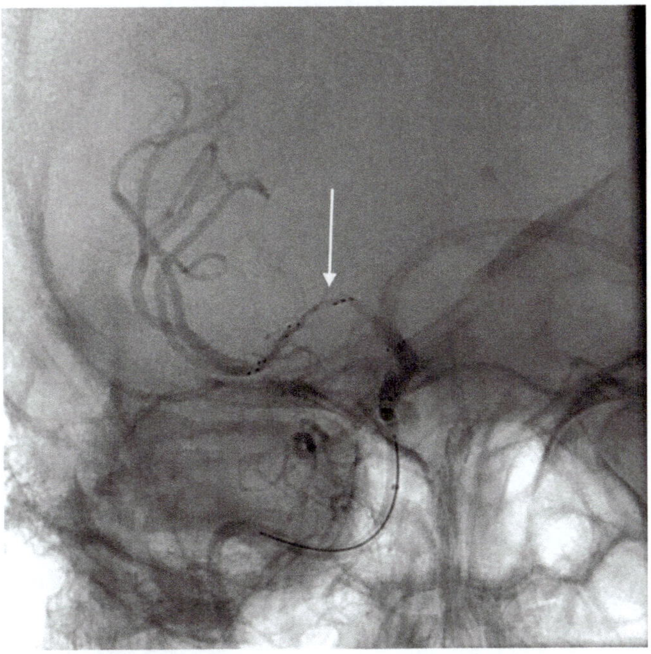

Fig. 9.6 Unsubtracted angiographic projection demonstrating the interstices of the stent-retriever

Stent-Retriever

While the clinical benefit of mechanical thrombectomy over best medical therapy alone is demonstrated, there continues to be ongoing debate regarding the optimal first-line thrombectomy strategy. The most commonly used device in the pivotal randomized control trials was the stent retriever, and as a result, it was felt to be the first-line device for MT. Stent retrievers or "stentrievers" are retrievable stents deployed across the focal occlusion in the intracranial vessel and used to capture and remove the clot (Figs. 9.6 and 9.7). Many trials have shown retrievers have increased recanalization rates and, thus, clinical outcomes compared to first-generation devices (SWIFT PRIME and TREVO 2 trials). When the original five pivotal RCT trials were conducted, each trial utilized stentrievers as the first-line devices for endovascular mechanical thrombectomy [14]. At the time, the two stentrievers that were approved by the US Food and Drug Administration (FDA) were the Trevo ProVue stentriever (Stryker, Kalamazoo, MI, USA) and the Solitaire FR stentriever (ev3/Covidien, Irvine, CA, USA). The two devices came in an array of sizes and lengths to match the diameter of the vessel occlusion. Stentrievers have undergone many iterations over the years. Each medical device company has its latest generation of mechanical thrombectomy devices to optimize clot retrieval while minimizing fragmentation and embolization. The procedure starts with a common transfemoral or trans-radial approach, followed by a guide catheter placed in the artery proximal to the occlusion, usually the cervical internal carotid artery. Using X-ray fluoroscopy, a picture of the occlusion site is taken. Using the digital "roadmap," an intermediate catheter and a microcatheter are advanced to the occlusion site. The microcatheter is advanced across the occlusive thrombus, and the stentriever is then inserted into the microcatheter and unsheathed across the occlusion. As the stent-retriever device expands, it presses the clot against the vessel wall and incorporates the clot within the interstices of the stent (Fig. 9.8). The stentriever,

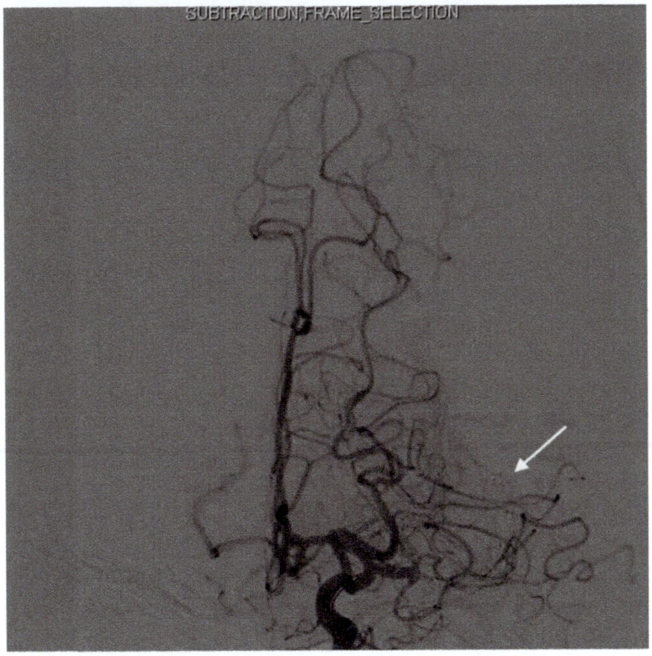

Fig. 9.7 Digitally subtracted angiographic projection of the deployment of the stent-retriever

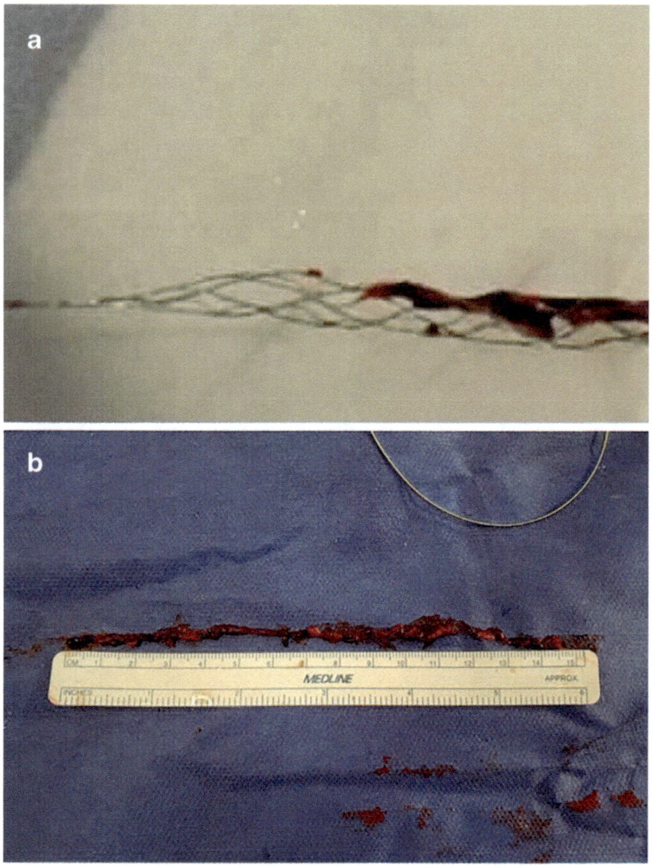

Fig. 9.8 Solitaire stent-retriever with thrombus embedded within the stent after retrieval from the middle cerebral artery

microcatheter, and clot are withdrawn as a single unit into the guide catheter under constant aspiration with a large syringe or aspiration pump. A control angiogram determines if the occlusion is resolved and removed. This process restores cerebral blood flow. If not successful, then the process can be repeated several times.

Suction Aspiration

Direct aspiration (DA) is another technique employed in treating large vessel occlusion [15]. Aspiration may be combined with a stent retriever as described or as a stand-alone method for thrombectomy. This technique involves using a large-bore aspiration catheter guided to the proximal end of the thrombus and then put under negative pressure (by vacuum pump or syringe) to produce suction on the thrombus. The clot is thus trapped at the tip of the catheter, and the goal is to remove the thrombus as a single unit with the aspiration catheter (Fig. 9.9).

In 2014, the ADAPT technique, "a direct aspiration first-pass technique," emerged, utilizing the new generation of large bore aspiration catheters to recanalize vessels [16, 17].

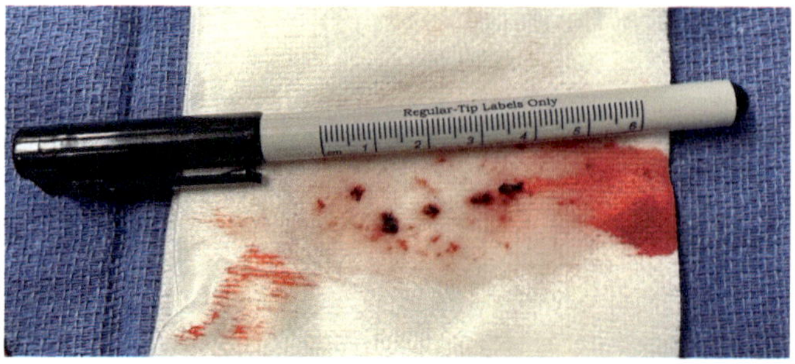

Fig. 9.9 An intravascular thrombus was removed using an aspiration catheter using a direct aspiration technique

This technique utilizes aspiration as the first approach to revascularize the occluded vessel. If this strategy fails, the aspiration catheter is used with a stent retriever to obtain revascularization. The new generation of aspiration catheters have larger lumens to produce more local flow arrest and suction power while being flexible enough to reach the occlusion site. A guide catheter is positioned into the extracranial proximal cervical internal carotid or vertebral artery in the direct aspiration technique. Using a smaller microcatheter and microwire, the aspiration catheter is navigated intracranially to the proximal end of the clot, then the microcatheter and microwire are removed. Once in position, the aspiration catheter is connected to a syringe or a negative vacuum pump and allowed to engage the clot over several minutes (the duration necessary is not well established). The catheter's engagement with the thrombus is confirmed when there is no backflow through the suction tubing. The thrombus is then either aspirated through the catheter or remains at the catheter tip and withdrawn with the aspiration tubing as a unit. If this method is unsuccessful after a few attempts, a stent retriever would be utilized, resulting in a more efficient and cost-effective revascularization strategy.

Over the past several years, some studies have demonstrated that aspiration alone can result in faster reperfusion, higher rates of successful reperfusion, lower rates of major complications (vessel wall damage and distal emboli), and cost-effectiveness compared to stent-retrievers [18, 19]. DA has been used in isolation or in combination with a stent-retriever. Different methods, including Solumbra (Solitaire (Medtronic Neurovascular, Irvine, SA) and Penumbra combination) , ARTS (Aspiration (catheter)-(stent) Retriever Technique for Stroke), and SAVE (Stent retriever Assisted Vacuum-locked Extraction), have described this technique using some different equipment in the literature [20–22].

There are two major randomized controlled trials comparing ADAPT to stent-retrievers. ASTER (Contact Aspiration vs. Stent Retriever for Successful Revascularization) and COMPASS (Aspiration Thrombectomy vs Stent Retriever Thrombectomy as First-Line Approach for Large Vessel Occlusion) showed that direct aspiration is not inferior to stent-retriever thrombectomy [18, 19]. Over the years, data from these studies shows aspiration results in:

- Faster reperfusion times
- Higher rates of successful first-pass reperfusion (Thrombolysis in Cerebral Infraction (TICI) Scale Score 2b or higher)
- Lower rates of significant complications (distal emboli, vessel wall injury)
- Superior cost-effectiveness

Angioplasty and Stent Revascularization

The removal of an intravascular thrombus can reveal an underlying stenosis of the vessel. Stenosis is often secondary to underlying atherosclerotic disease with plaque formation. In Asian populations, for example, atherosclerotic disease is the most common cause of acute ischemic stroke. The stenosis caused by atherosclerotic disease can be flow-limiting and re-occlude the vessel within minutes of revascularization. Alternatively, the atheroma can ulcerate, exposing thrombogenic tissue. Balloon angioplasty and stenting of the intracranial artery is a rescue procedure to re-establish blood flow when stenosis or recurrent thrombosis prevents ongoing patency. While off-label in the setting of an acute ischemic stroke, balloon angioplasty and stenting have been investigated for the treatment of symptomatic intracranial atherosclerotic disease. The SAMMPRIS trial investigated stent angioplasty with the Wingspan device (Stryker, Fremont, CA) plus medical therapy versus aggressive medical therapy alone for the treatment of severe (>70% stenosis) intracranial atherosclerosis (Fig. 9.10) [23]. Unfortunately, the trial failed to demonstrate the superiority of the treatment arm with more adverse outcomes, including periprocedural stroke, hemorrhage, and death rate compared with the medical arm. Analysis of the results showed weaknesses in the methodology of the trial and a subsequent trial, the WEAVE (Wingspan Stent System Post Market Surveillance) trial using the same Wingspan stent was conducted, demonstrating lower than expected adverse outcomes in the treatment arm compared with the medical arm [24]. A total of 97.4% (148 out of 152 patients) did not suffer any adverse outcome 72 h post-procedure. The study demonstrated a low periprocedural

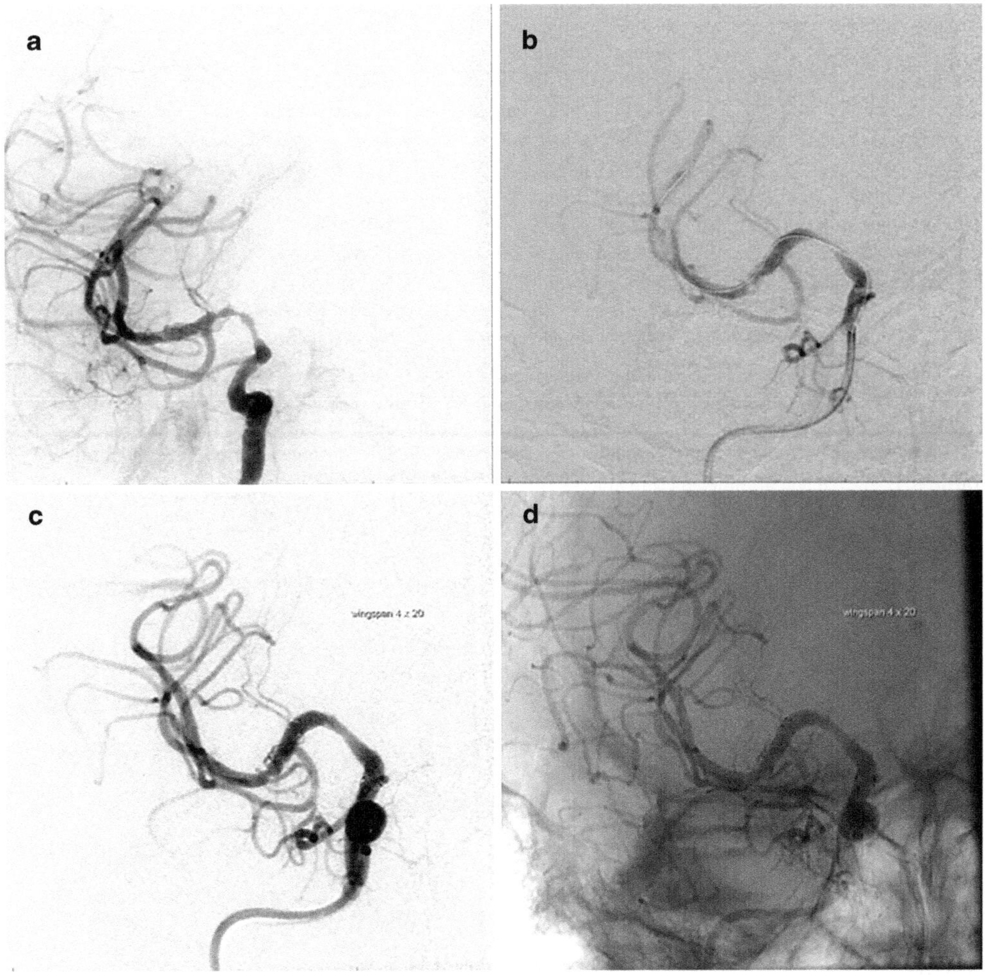

Fig. 9.10 AP angiographic projections demonstrating intracranial atherosclerosis (**a**) with deployment of Wingspan intracranial stent (**b**–**d**)

complication rate and good safety profile when experienced neurointerventionalists perform the procedure in a subacute time frame under careful, proper patient selection.

Effect of Anesthesia on Clinical Outcome

Stroke literature suggested that clinical outcomes from mechanical thrombectomy were better for patients under conscious sedation (CS) than those under general anesthesia (GA) [14]. For this reason, recent guidelines indicated that it might be reasonable to favor conscious sedation over general anesthesia during endovascular therapy for acute ischemic stroke. This recommendation was based on a meta-analysis and subgroup analysis of the Multicenter Randomized Clinical Trial of Endovascular Treatment for Acute Ischemic Stroke in the Netherlands trial (MR CLEAN).

Concerns regarding the use of general anesthesia during endovascular procedures in stroke patients were the increased delay from symptom onset to procedure initiation and potential cerebral hypoperfusion as a result of blood pressure fluctuation during GA. Potential advantages of CS included more rapid initiation of endovascular therapy, the ability to perform neurological exams periprocedural, and fewer blood pressure fluctuations.

Three randomized control trials have been published comparing general anesthesia to sedation in endovascular therapy [25–27]. All showed that GA did not result in poor outcomes compared with CS. Prior data came from small retrospective anesthesia studies that did not specify hemodynamic parameters and anesthetic agents/protocols used. Table 9.3 summarizes these three studies' pertinent design and primary/secondary outcome measures. In all three trials, GA did not result in worse outcomes after endovascular thrombectomy than CS when strict blood pressure was maintained, and hyperventilation was avoided. Table 9.4 lists the advantages and disadvantages of the effects of anesthetic techniques on clinical outcomes in endovascular therapy in these trials.

Table 9.3 Randomized control trials of general anesthesia vs sedation in endovascular mechanical thrombectomy

TRIAL name—*Journal*—Year	**SIESTA—*JAMA*—2016**	**AnSTROKE—*STROKE*—2017**	**GOLIATH—*JAMA NEUROL*—2018**
Country	Germany	Sweden	Denmark
Anesthesia involvement	No Neurointensivists	Yes	Yes
Primary outcome	NIHSS at 24-h	mRS 0–2 at 3 months	Infarct volume
Secondary outcome	mRS 0–2 at 3 months	Infarct volume	mRS 0–2 at 3 months
# of patients GA/sedation	73/77	45/45	65/63
Drugs	Remi/Prop only	GA: Remi/Prop/Sevo vs Sed: Remi only	GA: Prop/Alfenta/Sux Sed: Prop/Fent
Target systolic BP in mmHg	**140–160**	**140–180**	**Minimum 140 or MAP min. 70**
Conversion to GA %	14.3%	15.6%	6.3%
Advantage of GA?	Shorter procedure by 18 min	Not stated	Reperfusion rate higher
Conclusions	At 24 h, **no difference** At 3 months, GA is better	**No difference**	**GA not worse**

NIHSS NIH Stroke Scale (measure of stroke severity), *mRS* Modified Rankin Scale (measure—from 0 to 6—of neurological outcome, where 0 is return to baseline and 2 is disability but able to self-care, equivalent to functional independence, and 6 is death), *GA* General Anesthesia, *Sed.* sedation, *Alfenta.* Alfentanil, *Fent.* Fentanyl, *Prop.* Propofol, *Remi* Remifentanil, *Sux.* Succinylcholine, *Sevo.* Sevoflurane, *Min.* minimum

Table 9.4 Proposed/documented effects of anesthetic technique on outcome in endovascular mechanical thrombectomy

General anesthesia *PRO*	**Sedation *CON***
Immobility: shorter procedure time (SIESTA), better reperfusion rates (GOLIATH), decreased risk of vessel injury, less radiation and dye	Patient motion (SIESTA)
Airway protection	Conversion to general anesthesia 6–15% (SIESTA, AnSTROKE, GOLIATH), risky?
General anesthesia *CON*	**Sedation *PRO***
BP variability, hypotension	+/−
Low $EtCO_2$	No
Time to EVT delay (SIESTA)	Time to EVT start again (10 min)
Increased rate of VAP (SIESTA)	No

VAP ventilator-associated pneumonia, *EVT* endovascular therapy

SIESTA

The Sedation vs. Intubation for Endovascular Stroke Treatment (SIESTA), published in 2016, determined whether conscious sedation was superior to general anesthesia in terms of clinical outcomes after thrombectomy [25]. SIESTA prospectively revealed that there was no difference in post-EVT NIH stroke scale score between patients receiving GA (with Propofol and Remifentanil) and those patients receiving CS (using the same drugs), with strict blood pressure targets and normoventilation at 24-h follow-up. The 3-month follow-up revealed that more patients in the GA group achieved functional independence (modified Rankin Score, mRS 0–2). Overall, the investigators concluded that conscious sedation did not improve the functional outcome compared with general anesthesia.

AnSTROKE

In the Anesthesia During Stroke (AnSTROKE) RCT, 3-month clinical outcome after EVT for anterior circulation LVO was compared in patients receiving CS vs. GA [26]. Patients in the GA group were induced with Propofol and Remifentanil and maintained with Sevoflurane and Remifentanil. Remifentanil infusion was used for CS. Normoventilation was confirmed in both groups. Systolic blood pressure between 140 and 180 mmHg was strictly maintained in both groups. Significantly more patients (98%) in the GA group required vasoactive drugs ($p = 0.007$). No difference in neurological outcome as measured by mRS was evident at 3 months. The importance of strict blood pressure control and avoidance of hypotension was again highlighted in AnSTROKE.

GOLIATH

SIESTA and AnSTROKE showed different results at the 3-month follow-up. The General or Local Anesthesia in Intra Arterial Therapy (GOLIATH) trial promised more clarity [27]. In GOLIATH, general anesthesia with Propofol/Alfentanil/Succinylcholine was compared to sedation with Propofol/Fentanyl. Patients were randomized to GA or CS. The primary endpoint was infarct growth (mL) as demonstrated on MRI diffusion-weighted imaging, which was obtained 48–72 h after symptom onset. There was no statistically significant difference in final infarct volume between the GA and CS patients despite significantly more patients in the GA group suffering a drop in mean arterial pressure greater than 20% from baseline.

Despite evidence from these three randomized control trials, a meta-analysis of data sets from the initial 2015 seven strongly positive randomized trials of endovascular therapy vs medical therapy by the HERMES collaborators studying the effects of GA on clinical outcome showed poorer outcomes in the GA group compared to the non-GA group [28]. Using an odds ratio analysis, the meta-analysis found that for every 100 patients treated under GA, 18 patients would have worse functional outcomes (mRS) compared to the non-GA group.

These differences between the meta-analysis and randomized control trials can be attributed to two reasons. First, in the randomized control trials, patients included in randomization were suitable candidates for either technique, as unconscious, agitated, and vomiting patients were excluded. The anesthetic agents used in the GA and CS groups were standardized, and hemodynamic and ventilation parameters were strictly controlled. In contrast, the meta-analysis from the HERMES collaborators had significant variations in anesthetic agents between the GA and non-GA groups. In addition, local practice and patient variables (level of consciousness, agitation, vomiting) dictated patient selection, and presumably, blood pressure management was not controlled. The HERMES meta-analysis did not specifically evaluate these elements of anesthetic management. Second, there was a delay in reperfusion in the GA group compared to the non-GA group in the meta-analysis, which was not seen in the three RCTs. In the three randomized control trials, the average delay in starting the intervention was <10 min for anesthetic induction. Such a rapid process is challenging to reproduce in most hospitals.

Radiographic Outcomes

The grading scale used to assess angiographic success after endovascular thrombectomy is the modified Thrombolysis in Cerebral Infarction (mTICI) scale. The goal of endovascular revascularization is a goal mTICI 2b or 3 (mTICI 2b requires reperfusion ≥50% or more of the threatened tissue as judged by capillary blush seen on digital subtraction angiography while mTICI 3 is complete revascularization. This result has been correlated with improved patient clinical outcomes following stroke thrombectomy [29]. Some authors have argued for adding another category, TICI 2c, which is near-complete reperfusion but substantially better than the 50% required by TICI 2b [30].

Post-intervention Care

All post-intervention thrombectomy patients require admission to the critical care unit with close monitoring of systolic blood pressure. Although there is little data, avoiding hypertension after endovascular recanalization theoretically limits reperfusion injury. Following acute ischemic stroke, many patients experience dysautoregulation of cerebral blood pressure [31]. CT head imaging within 24 h is a widely accepted standard to evaluate intracranial hemorrhage, and MR imaging is used to assess infarct changes.

Stroke patients require varying degrees of physical therapy and rehabilitation after hospital discharge. Patients who undergo intensive rehabilitative therapies may show improved outcomes at 90 days, but trial results are equivocal. A comprehensive approach, including nurses, physical therapists, and social workers, must facilitate discharge to a skilled nursing facility or inpatient rehabilitation.

Future Directions

The adage "time is brain" denotes the urgency of interventions for ischemic stroke. Endovascular interventions are the fastest route for clot extraction and prevention of neurological injuries. Their effectiveness has been well-established for almost a decade. On the one hand, this raises logistical issues of effectively intervening in the shortest time frame. On the other hand, it opens up new avenues for basic and translational research. The logistics of emergent clot extraction are extensive and complex and require public education, the expansion of hospital outreach programs, assessment of suspected stroke during transport, the creation of emergency hospital protocols, availability of adequate workforce, and setup of stroke intervention facilities with necessary imaging resources close to the emergency room, among others. Thus, many tertiary care centers have now established rapid response stroke teams whose personnel are simultaneously activated when as soon as a potential stroke case is identified. The in-hospital stroke response time will likely improve with advances in telemedicine, artificial intelligence-assisted electronic health data review and treatment planning, and remote robotic interventions.

However, endovascular stroke interventions also create avenues for basic and translational endovascular research. The restoration of cerebral perfusion coincides with the onset of reperfusion injuries. The presence of a catheter perfusing the region of injury at the time of its initiation creates novel therapeutic opportunities. The ability of interventions to instantaneously achieve therapeutic concentrations is matched only by direct injections. However, unlike direct injection, drug diffusion is not a constraint, as arterial injections deliver drugs through a capillary network. Improved arterial drug delivery and better tissue imaging could minimize complications of intraarterial thrombolysis, particularly when the embolic clot is located distally. It could open avenues for newer neuroprotective carrier drug conjugates and the delivery of stem cells or their incubation media to prevent and mitigate neural injury.

Conclusion

Acute ischemic strokes carry a significant risk of morbidity and mortality in the United States and throughout the world. The utilization of Comprehensive Stroke Centers with new-generation endovascular devices has improved patient clinical outcomes by improving recanalization rates, decreasing time to intervention, and reducing complications. Patient outcomes will continue to improve with a focus on improving the efficiency of interhospital transfers and other ways of reducing the time of onset to treatment, such as the advent of the mobile stroke unit. Future research could address the treatment of distal vascular occlusion, managing delayed cases, pharmacological neuroprotection, and neuronal salvage. Arterial pharmacology could help improve stroke outcomes in the future.

References

1. Go AS, Mozaffarian D, Roger VL, Benjamin EJ, Berry JD, Blaha MJ, et al. Heart disease and stroke statistics—2014 update. Circulation. 2014;129(3):e28–e292.
2. National Institute of Neurological Disorders and Stroke rt-PA Stroke Study Group. Tissue plasminogen activator for acute ischemic stroke. N Engl J Med. 1995;333(24):1581–7.
3. Smith WS, Lev MH, English JD, Camargo EC, Chou M, Johnston SC, et al. Significance of large vessel intracranial occlusion causing acute ischemic stroke and TIA. Stroke. 2009;40(12):3834–40.
4. Berkhemer OA, Fransen PS, Beumer D, van den Berg LA, Lingsma HF, Yoo AJ, et al. A randomized trial of intraarterial treatment for acute ischemic stroke. N Engl J Med. 2015;372(1):11–20.
5. Campbell BC, Mitchell PJ, Kleinig TJ, Dewey HM, Churilov L, Yassi N, et al. Endovascular therapy for ischemic stroke with perfusion-imaging selection. N Engl J Med. 2015;372(11):1009–18.
6. Goyal M, Demchuk AM, Menon BK, Eesa M, Rempel JL, Thornton J, et al. Randomized assessment of rapid endovascular treatment of ischemic stroke. N Engl J Med. 2015;372(11):1019–30.
7. Jovin Tudor G, Chamorro A, Cobo E, de Miquel MA, Molina Carlos A, Rovira A, et al. Thrombectomy within 8 hours after symptom onset in ischemic stroke. N Engl J Med. 2015;372(24):2296–306.
8. Saver JL, Goyal M, Bonafe A, Diener HC, Levy EI, Pereira VM, et al. Stent-retriever thrombectomy after intravenous t-PA vs. t-PA alone in stroke. N Engl J Med. 2015;372(24):2285–95.
9. Barber PA, Demchuk AM, Zhang J, Buchan AM. Validity and reliability of a quantitative computed tomography score in predicting outcome of hyperacute stroke before thrombolytic therapy. ASPECTS Study Group. Alberta Stroke Programme Early CT Score. Lancet. 2000;355(9216):1670–4.
10. Al-Ali F, Elias JJ, Tomsick TA, Liebeskind DS, Broderick JP. Relative influence of capillary index score, revascularization, and time on stroke outcomes from the Interventional Management of Stroke III Trial. Stroke. 2015;46(6):1590–4.
11. Powers WJ, Rabinstein AA, Ackerson T, Adeoye OM, Bambakidis NC, Becker K, et al. 2018 guidelines for the early management of patients with acute ischemic stroke: a guideline for healthcare professionals from the American Heart Association/American Stroke Association. Stroke. 2018;49(3):e46–99.
12. Nogueira RG, Jadhav AP, Haussen DC, Bonafe A, Budzik RF, Bhuva P, et al. Thrombectomy 6 to 24 hours after stroke with a mismatch between deficit and infarct. N Engl J Med. 2018;378(1):11–21.

13. Albers GW, Marks MP, Kemp S, Christensen S, Tsai JP, Ortega-Gutierrez S, et al. Thrombectomy for stroke at 6 to 16 hours with selection by perfusion imaging. N Engl J Med. 2018;378(8):708–18.
14. Powers WJ, Derdeyn CP, Biller J, Coffey CS, Hoh BL, Jauch EC, et al. 2015 American Heart Association/American Stroke Association focused update of the 2013 guidelines for the early management of patients with acute ischemic stroke regarding endovascular treatment: a guideline for healthcare professionals from the American Heart Association/American Stroke Association. Stroke. 2015;46(10):3020–35.
15. Boisseau W, Escalard S, Fahed R, Lapergue B, Smajda S, Maier B, et al. Direct aspiration stroke thrombectomy: a comprehensive review. J Neurointerv Surg. 2020;12:1099.
16. Turk AS, Frei D, Fiorella D, Mocco J, Baxter B, Siddiqui A, et al. ADAPT FAST study: a direct aspiration first pass technique for acute stroke thrombectomy. J Neurointerv Surg. 2014;6(4):260–4.
17. Hu YC, Stiefel MF. Force and aspiration analysis of the ADAPT technique in acute ischemic stroke treatment. J Neurointerv Surg. 2016;8(3):244–6.
18. Lapergue B, Blanc R, Gory B, Labreuche J, Duhamel A, Marnat G, et al. Effect of endovascular contact aspiration vs stent retriever on revascularization in patients with acute ischemic stroke and large vessel occlusion: the ASTER randomized clinical trial. JAMA. 2017;318(5):443–52.
19. Turk AS 3rd, Siddiqui A, Fifi JT, De Leacy RA, Fiorella DJ, Gu E, et al. Aspiration thrombectomy versus stent retriever thrombectomy as first-line approach for large vessel occlusion (COMPASS): a multicentre, randomised, open label, blinded outcome, non-inferiority trial. Lancet. 2019;393(10175):998–1008.
20. Humphries W, Hoit D, Doss VT, Elijovich L, Frei D, Loy D, et al. Distal aspiration with retrievable stent assisted thrombectomy for the treatment of acute ischemic stroke. J Neurointerv Surg. 2015;7(2):90–4.
21. Massari F, Henninger N, Lozano JD, Patel A, Kuhn AL, Howk M, et al. ARTS (aspiration-retriever technique for stroke): initial clinical experience. Interv Neuroradiol. 2016;22(3):325–32.
22. Maus V, Behme D, Kabbasch C, Borggrefe J, Tsogkas I, Nikoubashman O, et al. Maximizing first-pass complete reperfusion with SAVE. Clin Neuroradiol. 2018;28(3):327–38.
23. Chimowitz MI, Lynn MJ, Derdeyn CP, Turan TN, Fiorella D, Lane BF, et al. Stenting versus aggressive medical therapy for intracranial arterial stenosis. N Engl J Med. 2011;365(11):993–1003.
24. Alexander MJ, Zauner A, Chaloupka JC, Baxter B, Callison RC, Gupta R, et al. WEAVE trial: final results in 152 on-label patients. Stroke. 2019;50(4):889–94.
25. Schönenberger S, Uhlmann L, Hacke W, Schieber S, Mundiyanapurath S, Purrucker JC, et al. Effect of conscious sedation vs general anesthesia on early neurological improvement among patients with ischemic stroke undergoing endovascular thrombectomy: a randomized clinical trial. JAMA. 2016;316(19):1986–96.
26. Löwhagen Hendén P, Rentzos A, Karlsson J-E, Rosengren L, Leiram B, Sundeman H, et al. General anesthesia versus conscious sedation for endovascular treatment of acute ischemic stroke. Stroke. 2017;48(6):1601–7.
27. Simonsen CZ, Yoo AJ, Sørensen LH, Juul N, Johnsen SP, Andersen G, et al. Effect of general anesthesia and conscious sedation during endovascular therapy on infarct growth and clinical outcomes in acute ischemic stroke: a randomized clinical trial. JAMA Neurol. 2018;75(4):470–7.
28. Campbell BCV, van Zwam WH, Goyal M, Menon BK, Dippel DWJ, Demchuk AM, et al. Effect of general anaesthesia on functional outcome in patients with anterior circulation ischaemic stroke having endovascular thrombectomy versus standard care: a meta-analysis of individual patient data. Lancet Neurol. 2018;17(1):47–53.
29. Zaidat OO, Yoo AJ, Khatri P, Tomsick TA, von Kummer R, Saver JL, et al. Recommendations on angiographic revascularization grading standards for acute ischemic stroke: a consensus statement. Stroke. 2013;44(9):2650–63.
30. LeCouffe NE, Kappelhof M, Treurniet KM, Lingsma HF, Zhang G, Van Den Wijngaard IR, et al. 2B, 2C, or 3: what should be the angiographic target for endovascular treatment in ischemic stroke? Stroke. 2020;51(6):1790–6.
31. Bath PM, Song L, Silva GS, Mistry E, Petersen N, Tsivgoulis G, et al. Blood pressure management for ischemic stroke in the first 24 hours. Stroke. 2022;53(4):1074–84.

Intraarterial Vasodilator Treatment for Cerebral Vasospasm After SAH: Where Are We and Where Do We Go?

10

Jonathan Sisti, Grace Russo, Colin Sperring, and Srini Cherukuri

When persons in good health are suddenly seized with pains in the head, and straightway are laid down speechless, and breathe with stertor, they die in 7 days.

Hippocrates (450–380 BCE), Greek Physician and Philosopher

Introduction

Cerebral vasospasm is the narrowing of the lumen of an intracranial artery either due to contraction of the smooth muscle within the wall or from morphological changes along the vessel's endothelial surface, which typically happens in response to vascular injury and is commonly seen in a delayed fashion following aneurysmal subarachnoid hemorrhage (aSAH). [1] Cerebral blood vessels' small caliber and inability to dilate or respond physiologically during vasospasm results in decreased cerebral blood flow and oxygen delivery. The decrease, if severe, leads to ischemia and cerebral infarction, called delayed cerebral ischemia (DCI). DCI presents as a focal deficit or a reduction of two points on the Glasgow Coma Scale without another attributable clinical cause. Although angiographic cerebral vasospasm occurs in 70% of aSAH, only 30% will develop DCI. While early on, DCI was traditionally thought to be secondary to vasospasm, our current understanding suggests it is more complex and multifactorial. Early brain injury from aneurysmal rupture can result in immediate global ischemic brain injury secondary to acutely increased intracranial cerebral pressure and decreased blood flow, blood-brain barrier breakdown, brain edema, inflammation, and initiation of apoptosis [2–6]. Additional factors that may also contribute include cortical spreading depression, microcirculatory dysfunction, loss of autoregulation, delayed cellular apoptosis, and microthrombosis [7, 8]. Nevertheless, vasospasm is still believed to be the most significant cause of DCI [9].

J. Sisti (✉) · G. Russo · C. Sperring · S. Cherukuri
Columbia University, New York, NY, USA
e-mail: Jas2269@cumc.columbia.edu

Vasospasm typically occurs between 4 and 14 days after aneurysmal rupture, with a peak around 7–8 days, though reports of hyperacute vasospasm are also known to occur [10, 11]. Figure 10.1 illustrates the clinical course of aneurysmal SAH. There are typically two patterns of infarction distribution that are seen: cortical infarcts in the distribution of arteries close to the initial bleed site, occurring in 50% of DCI patients, and multifocal bilateral subcortical infarcts remote from the bleed site, occurring in approximately 40% of patients with DCI. Risk factors for vasospasm include increased volume of subarachnoid blood, hyperglycemia, hypertension, age less than 50 years, smoking history, proximity of the bleed site to large intracranial blood vessels, and presenting clinical condition, which in the setting of subarachnoid hemorrhage is often referred to using the Hunt and Hess Classification as well as the Glasgow Coma Scale [12–15]. It is still unclear if there is a difference in the incidence of vasospasm when considering surgery versus endovascular treatments. Several radiologic grading scales exist, most commonly the Fischer and Claassen scales, which categorize the amount and distribution of subarachnoid blood and are used to predict the likelihood of the development of vasospasm.

High morbidity and mortality are associated with aSAH, though these decrease over time [16]. While initially, case-fatality rates were as high as 50%, this has declined to approximately 30% from 1988 to 2010 [17, 18]. Nevertheless, in patients who can survive the initial bleed and go on to have a procedure to secure the aneurysm from further rebleeding, which is the leading cause of early mortality until obliteration of the aneurysm can be achieved [19], much of the subsequent morbidity is caused by vasospasm and delayed cerebral ischemia, with 30% of survivors never

S. Joshi (ed.), *Arterial Treatment of Neurological Diseases*, https://doi.org/10.1007/978-3-031-80173-0_10

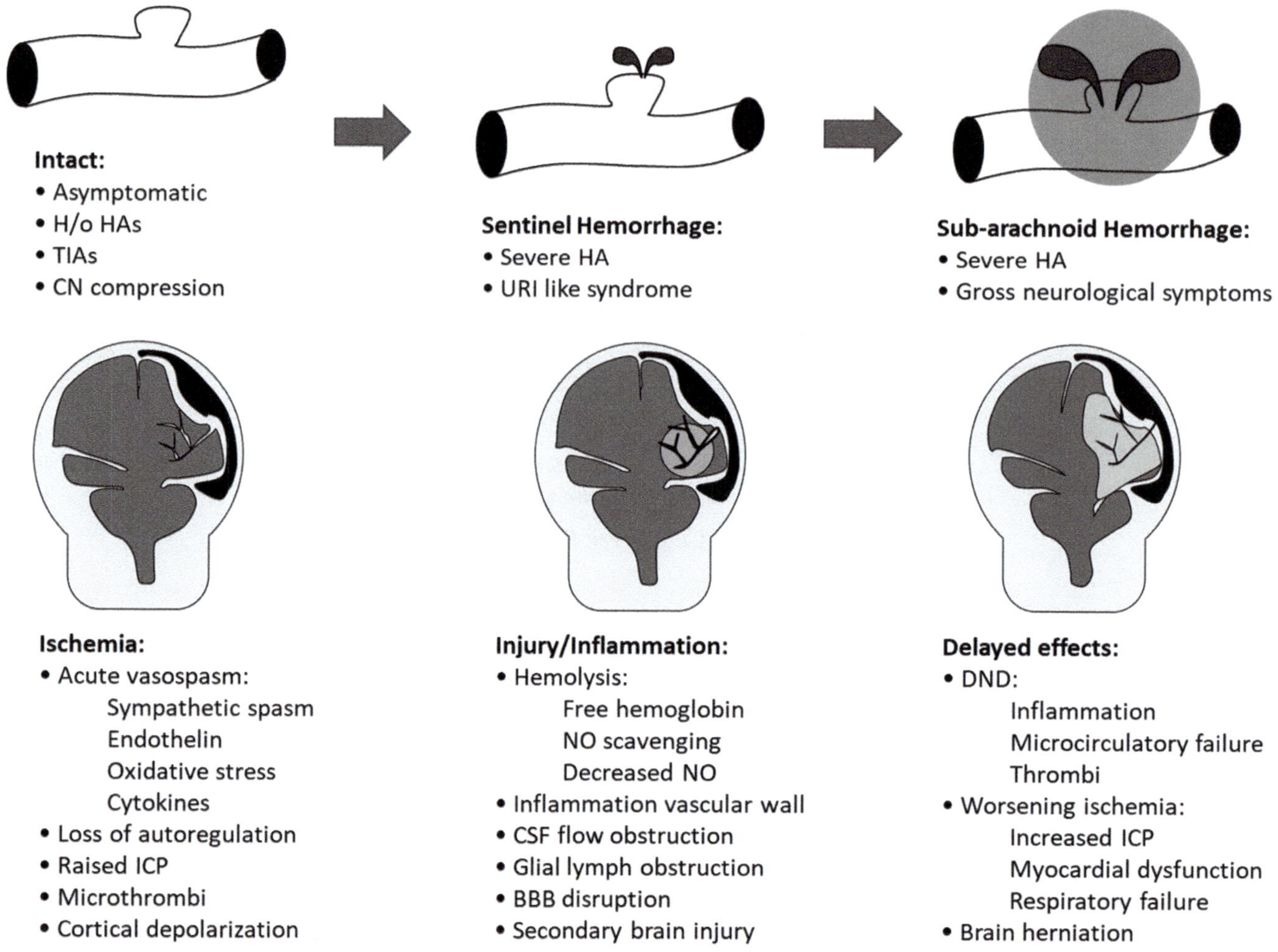

Fig. 10.1 Pathology and symptomatology of aneurysmal rupture and subarachnoid hemorrhage

regaining complete independence and 69% reporting a reduction in quality of life [20, 21]. The risk of poor outcomes following subarachnoid hemorrhage is four times greater if the patient develops cerebral vasospasm and strongly increases with secondary brain insults [15]. It is still unclear, however, how the treatment of vasospasm, especially by endovascular intervention, which carries procedural risk, ultimately affects patient outcomes, though there may be possible benefits in specific subgroups of subarachnoid hemorrhage patients [22]. Intraarterial verapamil treatment is widely used in treating vasospasm following aSAH. However, its impact on survival remains to be proven in randomized control trials. This chapter reviews the pathology of cerebral vasospasm, elaborates on the current treatments, both chemical and mechanical, and discusses their limitations and the future development of arterial vasodilator interventions.

Pathophysiology

The pathophysiology of delayed cerebral ischemia is complex (Fig. 10.2) and incompletely understood. Multiple interacting factors are at play following the initial insult of aneurysmal rupture, including necrosis, inflammation, augmented coagulation, endothelial dysfunction, cortical spreading depression, and blood in subarachnoid spaces; all of which have been hypothesized to play a role in cerebral vasospasm [7]. Although angiographic evidence of cerebral vasospasm is as high as 70%, this is only symptomatic in 20–30% of patients, with a positive predictive value for DCI of 67% [9, 23]. There are conflicting reports regarding the clinical significance of vasospasm, with some claiming that only severe luminal narrowing of at least 50% progresses to DCI [24]. Others suggest a more robust correlation, report-

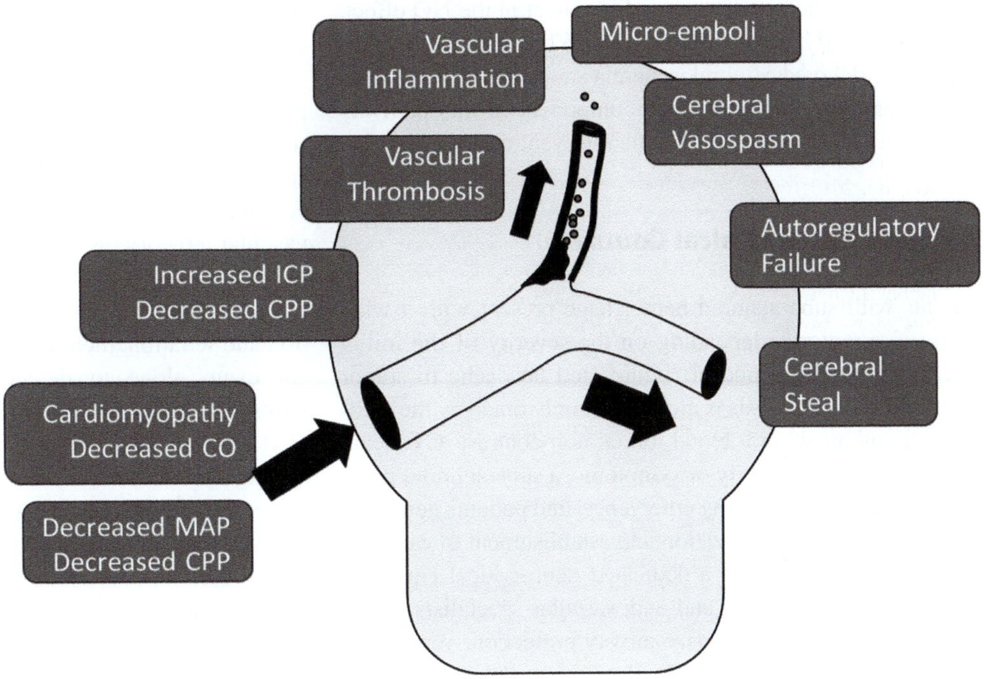

Fig. 10.2 Microvascular and systemic mechanisms of aneurysmal sub-arachnoid hemorrhage affecting tissue perfusion

ing that among patients with no or mild angiographic vasospasm, 3% still developed delayed infarcts [25, 26]. It is possible, however, that the wide range of patient outcomes is related to the choice of investigational treatments and subsequent systemic effects, for example, precipitation of, DCI through their effect on lowering cerebral perfusion pressure. Minimizing systemic side effects provides the rationale for intra-arterial drug delivery for vasospasm treatment, yet, unlike oral nimodipine, the investigational use of intraarterial drugs is not supported by compelling class I evidence in reducing DCI and improving the outcome [27–29].

Any reduction in oxygen delivery relative to metabolic demand can result in ischemia. However, in aSAH, codependent factors influence both the tissue metabolic need and blood supply. Focusing on the former, we see that even within the first 24–48 h after aSAH, early brain injury from global cerebral ischemia and increased intracranial pressure cause a significant increase in inflammation through cytokines known to correlate with changes in blood flow velocity, such as an increase in IL-1beta and IL-6 in both CSF and plasma [30]. There is also an increase in sympathetic tone, often referred to as a "catecholamine surge," that may result from ischemic injury to the hypothalamus and compression to the brain stem following the initial aneurysmal rupture [31]. Additionally, global cerebral ischemia and hypoxia are thought to contribute to endothelial injury, blood-brain barrier distribution, and upregulation of the endothelin-1 pathway [32–34]. Endothelin-1 is a potent endogenous vasoconstrictor produced in endothelial cells and stimulated following ischemia [33]. While the exact mechanism of endothelin-1 and its role in the development of cerebral vasospasm is unknown, it has been demonstrated that plasma concentrations correlate with delayed cerebral ischemia and inhibition of this pathway through receptor antagonism reduces vasospasm [32].

There is a relationship between the amount of subarachnoid blood appreciated on CT as described by the Fischer Scale and cerebral vasospasm [35]. Blood degradation products and oxyhemoglobin, which peak in primate CSF 7 days after SAH and correlate temporally with the typical onset of vasospasm, have been demonstrated to induce cerebral vasoconstriction [36, 37]. While the entire mechanism is not fully understood, several experiments support this model. For example, hematoma evacuation prevented vasospasm in primates [38], and purified oxyhemoglobin-induced vasoconstriction in canine cerebral arteries [39]. Oxyhemoglobin has been shown to increase several vasoconstrictors, such as PGE_2 and superoxide, through its oxidation into methhemoglobin and endothelin-1 while simultaneously inhibiting endothelial-dependent relaxation and decreasing vasodilators, such as PGI_2 and nitric oxide, a critical endothelium-derived mediator of vascular muscle tension [7, 40]. Nitric oxide production and bioavailability further decrease as a result of multiple cascading effects of subarachnoid hemorrhage, including increases in endogenous nitric oxide synthase inhibitors such as asymmetric dimethylarginine, decreases in expression of endothelial and neuronal-specific NOS isoforms, NOS enzyme damage from oxidation due to hemoglobin metabolism and local inflammation, and the presence of superoxide resulting in the "NOS uncoupling" phenomenon whereby there is a disconnect in the NO effect, availability, and homeostasis [32, 41]. While the mechanisms underlying delayed cerebral ischemia and cerebral vasospasm are undoubtedly complex, each component in this pathway presents a potential for therapeutic intervention.

Symptoms and Clinical Course

Patients with subarachnoid hemorrhage present with a wide range of symptoms depending on the severity of the initial bleed, ranging from nuchal rigidity and headache to stupor and coma. The diagnosis is most commonly made by the presence of subarachnoid blood on a non-contrast CT scan. Regardless of the severity of symptoms, a subarachnoid hemorrhage is a life-threatening emergency, and patients generally require immediate stabilization and establishment of care in a high-volume center with a dedicated neurocritical care unit and experienced surgical and endovascular specialists. Early stabilization should emphasize airway protection, ventilatory and hemodynamic support, blood pressure and seizure control, and prompt treatment of increased intracranial pressure. The patient's presenting neurologic status and the severity of the initial hemorrhage are the strongest predictors of outcome, with several grading systems used to efficiently convey such information, such as the Hunt and Hess Scale [42].

Once stabilization of the patient is achieved, the next goal is the prevention of rebleeding of the aneurysm with either endovascular coiling or surgical clipping. Until this goal can be accomplished, several steps should be made to decrease the risk of rebleeding, including antihypertensive therapy, with a goal of systolic blood pressure <160 mmHg, discontinuation of all antithrombotic agents and their appropriate reversal, seizure prophylaxis, pain control, bed rest, the use of stool softeners, and general avoidance of any aggravating care [43]. Additionally, to prevent the complications of cerebral ischemia, aggressive antihypertensive therapy should be avoided to maintain a cerebral perfusion pressure (CPP), which is equal to the mean arterial pressure (MAP) subtracted by the intracranial pressure (ICP), of at least 70 mmHg [44], as well as initiation of maintenance fluids with boluses as needed for euvolemia, and oral nimodipine, 60 mg every 4 h, given as a standard of care for 21 days. Increased intracranial pressure, as evidenced by enlarged ventricles on CT or in a patient with a poor neurologic exam, low level of attention, and inability to follow verbal commands, should receive an external ventricular drain with care not to precipitously drain CSF and acutely drop ICP, which could result in transmural pressure across the aneurysm rupture site, with risk of rebleeding [43].

Aneurysm location is found with vessel imaging through a CT angiogram of the head and neck or on digital subtraction angiography. Treatment consists of aneurysm obliteration using endovascular coiling procedures or through a craniotomy for clip ligation, and this is ideally performed within 24–48 h of rupture. Once the aneurysm is secured, the patient is transferred to a dedicated neurocritical care unit for further management, typically for the duration of the vasospasm window, which can last 2–3 weeks. The symptoms of cerebral vasospasm can be highly variable and depend on the vascular territory involved and the presenting neurologic status of the patient, which may be confounding. Patients with a higher Hunt and Hess grade may require prolonged intubation and sedation, meaning a clinician cannot rely on a physical exam alone to detect the development of cerebral vasospasm. Conversely, in lower-grade patients who remain alert and conversant, the symptoms of cerebral vasospasm are highly variable and unreliable, ranging from asymptomatic to mild headache, decreased attention, sleepiness, abulia, drift, hemiplegia, and cranial neuropathy. Fortunately, in the modern era, many tools are at our disposal to assist in detecting and treating occult cerebral vasospasm.

Diagnostic Investigation

Monitoring for vasospasm in aSAH patients is critical for avoiding DCI. Transcranial Doppler (TCD) is a widely used, low-cost, non-invasive method to measure cerebral vasospasm after aSAH, and daily TCDs are critical for the early identification of vasospasm for at-risk patients. The use and effectiveness of TCD may depend on the operator's experience. TCD detects vasospasm in the Circle of Willis and the internal carotid artery. It is most sensitive to vasospasm in the proximal middle cerebral artery (MCA) and internal carotid artery (ICA). At the same time, it is unreliable at detecting vasospasm in the anterior cerebral artery and arteries of the posterior circulation [10, 45]. Mean velocities <120 cm/s are considered low and carry a high negative predictive value for vasospasm, while mean velocities >180 cm/s are deemed high and carry a high positive predictive value [46]. The Lindegaard ratio (LR) is a calculated ratio specific to the vasospasm of the MCA. It is calculated by dividing the mean MCA velocity by the mean extracranial ipsilateral ICA velocity. To normalize, it is necessary to see if increased velocities are primarily intracranial as opposed to systemic, with an LR > 3 suggestive of vasospasm of the MCA. Single TCD readings alone provide little clinical value; thus, serial examinations are recommended. Elevations in TCD trend require further evaluation for symptomatic vasospasm, including diagnostic cerebral angiogram (DSA), CT angiogram (CTA), and MR angiogram (MRA).

DSA remains the gold standard for diagnosing vasospasm and should be included in managing all patients with symptomatic vasospasm. Specifically, DSA is the most sensitive in detecting medium- and large-vessel spasms. DSA not only provides diagnostic quality but also provides the opportunity to provide potential therapy. CTA has become an increasingly popular modality for assessing these patients. CTA detects suspected symptomatic vasospasm with high sensitivity and specificity [47, 48]. However, CTA may overestimate the magnitude, and thus, it is best to combine it with CT perfusion to assess hypoperfusion [49]. Patients with poor perfusion on CT are 23 times more likely to have DCI than those without appreciable perfusion deficits [50]. Furthermore, CT perfusion has been shown to detect DCI early enough that it is still reversible. Time-of-flight (TOF) MRA provides a non-invasive, contrast-free alternative to DSA and CTA [51]. Previous studies have shown that TOF MRA offers sufficient sensitivity for vasospasm of the ACA but fails to detect vasospasm of the ICA and MCA. Ultimately, it was determined to be inferior to DSA [52]. Comparing MRA to CTA, MRA is superior when visualizing vasculature surrounding platinum coils. However, visualization using MRA is limited when surrounding nitinol stents [53]. MRA requires significant patient cooperation, primarily due to long study times, and images are susceptible to T1-related artifacts, including clips, air after surgery, blood in the arachnoid space, high concentrations of fat, or other high T1-signal tissue [51]. Additionally, the direction of flow has an effect on MRA signal while turbulent flow may falsely create images of narrowed vessels, overestimating the presence of vasospasm [53, 54].

Treatment Options

Aggressive management of aSAH patients with vasospasm is crucial for preventing associated secondary neurological injury. Optimizing cerebral perfusion pressure (CPP) ensures adequate oxygen delivery to meet the brain's changing metabolic demands. Maintenance of CPP > 70 mmHg has been shown to reduce hypoxia and metabolic strain while improving outcomes [55]. Dating back to Kosnik and Hunt in 1976, induction of hypertension has been the most common method of augmenting CPP and resolving neurological deficits for these patients [56]. Following this finding, aggressive volume administration was routinely accepted. Soon, the term "triple-H therapy" was coined, where providers seemingly reversed DCI with the induction of hypertension, hypervolemia, and hemodilution [57, 58]. However, hemodilution decreases oxygen-carrying capacity. Recent trials demonstrate that hypervolemia does not improve outcomes and may increase complications in aSAH patients [57, 58]. Studies have shown that increased mean arterial pressure (MAP) improves brain perfusion. However, randomized clinical trials have failed to demonstrate evidence that induction of hypertension improves outcomes in DCI and have only shown that it may lead to severe complications [59, 60].

Since 1983, nimodipine, a calcium channel blocker (CCB), remains the only pharmacological agent shown to reduce the risk of DCI and improve outcomes in aSAH patients [28]. Notably, despite FDA approval, intravenous (IV) nimodipine has not been shown to reduce the incidence of vasospasm [28, 61, 62]. All aSAH patients should receive nimodipine for the 21 days following their aSAH, regardless of the presence or absence of a neurological deficit [43, 44].

Since the introduction of nimodipine, other vasoactive agents have been introduced and evaluated. In 1993, a randomized controlled trial demonstrated a decreased incidence of DCI when giving aSAH patients high doses of IV nicardipine. However, they failed to show any long-term benefit among these patients [63]. Clazosentan is an inhibitor of Endothelin-1 (ET-1), a potent vasoconstrictor. Increased levels of ET-1 have been reported in the CSF of aSAH vasospasm patients, and increased levels correlate with symptoms of ischemia [33, 64]. Together, this spurred therapeutic interest. However, similar to nicardipine, the IV Clazosentan trials showed reduced rates of vasospasm but failed to demonstrate decreased rates of DCI or improved outcomes [65–67]. IV Nitroglycerin therapy has also been proposed, given that NO levels are known to decrease in the setting of aSAH [68, 69]. It is widely known that NO increases levels of 3, 5-cyclic guanosine monophosphate (cGMP), which leads to the relaxation of smooth muscle cells, vasodilation, and increased CBF [35, 70]. However, the associated pronounced hypotension, even more significant than hypotension following IV nimodipine, and loss of CPP have made IV nitroglycerin inappropriate for clinical use [7]. In a retrospective study, IV milrinone, a phosphodiesterase 3 (PD3) inhibitor, was safe and effective for patients with vasospasm and refractory DCI [71]. More rigorous prospectively evaluated data is required.

Endovascular therapies, including IA dilators and transluminal balloon angioplasty (TBA), have emerged as exciting therapies to treat vasospasm and DCI refractory to medical management. An approach to understanding the multimodality approach to investigate IA vasodilators is shown in Fig. 10.3. IA vasodilators and TBA options are effective for refractory vasospasm [73]. Mechanical vasodilation via TBA improves CBF by disrupting the luminal smooth muscle cells and extracellular matrix. TBA benefits include improved clinical outcomes, angiographic vasospasm, decreased incidence of infarction in treated regions, and low complication rates [74–78]. Risk of complications following TBA alone is considerably less than the risk of complications after pharmacologic IA vasodilation alone [77]. Importantly, prophylactic TBA for aSAH patients has shown no improvement [79]. Normal to supranormal vessel diameter goals for TBA decrease rates of recurrent vasospasm compared to subnormal diameter goals, while balloon compliance does not affect recurrence rates [80, 81]. Self-expandable retrievable stents have been proposed as a method of TBA that would lead to

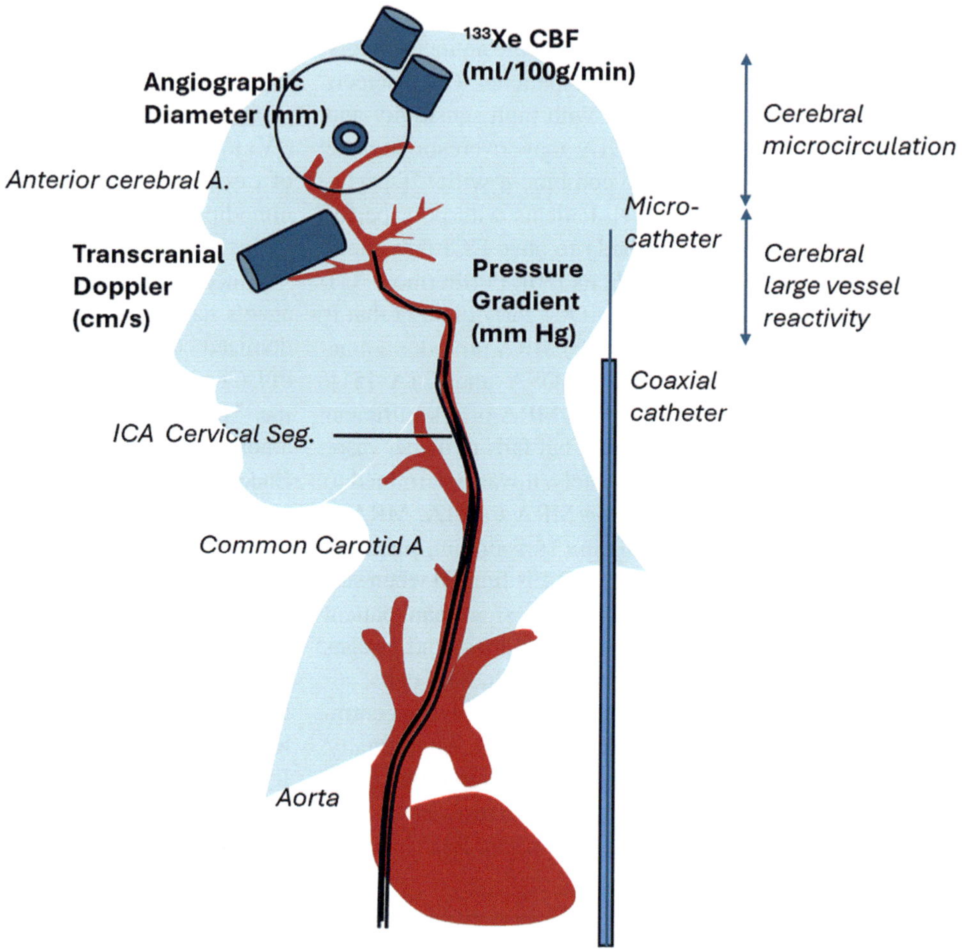

Fig. 10.3 Schematic representation of parameters available to assess pharmacological effects of intraarterial vasodilators with multimodality measurements during cerebral angiography, see Joshi Anesthesiology 2004 [72]

longer durations of vasodilation. These stents are safe and effective, but further studies are required [82]. TBA is limited to large vessels; therefore, a combination therapy of TBA and pharmacologic IA vasodilation has been proposed as rescue therapy for both small and large vessel spasms [83]. IA vasodilators allow targeted treatment of spastic small arteries while avoiding artery rupture from overdilation [21]. CCBs are the preferred IA therapy, and milrinone has also been employed [79, 84]. Specific benefits and pharmacokinetics of IA vasodilators will be discussed in later sections.

Another potential target is that of the immune system and inflammation. Circulating lymphocytes have been shown to invade cerebral arteries in aSAH. The breakdown of the blood-brain barrier (BBB) in aSAH allows immune cells to traffic into CSF and attach to arterial walls [85–88]. Further, monocytes within the CSF have been shown to release ET-1, a potent vasoconstrictor [89]. Follow-up studies have shown that increases in IL-1B, IL-6, and TNF, pro-inflammatory cytokines, in aSAH, and shifts in cytokine concentrations correlate with changes to the velocity of CBF [30, 90]. Given the relationship between SAH and the immune system, anti-inflammatory therapy has been proposed to manage vasospasm and DCI. Traditionally used to treat heart failure, Levosimendan, a calcium channel sensitizer with anti-inflammatory properties, has reduced vasospasm in aSAH patients [91]. Milk fat globule epidermal growth factor 8 (MFG-E8), an anti-inflammatory glycoprotein, promotes phagocytosis of apoptotic cells. It decreases pro-inflammatory signaling in SAH with improved neurologic outcomes in a brain injury rat model [92]. Given the complex interplay between endothelial cells, blood products, and immune cells in aSAH, combination therapy targeting different cell populations may be necessary to improve patient outcomes.

Stellate Ganglion Block (SGB) is another potentially promising alternative to treating anterior and posterior circulation vasospasm [93–95]. The tone of brain vasculature is maintained by noradrenergic sympathetic nerves traveling along the ipsilateral carotid artery and originating from the cervical sympathetic ganglion [96–98]. These vessels constrict in response to sympathetic input and relax when that input is interrupted. Sympathectomy prevents noradrenergic sympathetic vasoconstriction [95]. Many studies have shown decreased flow velocity, increased perfusion, and improved outcomes with SGB [94, 95, 99]. Further, SGB is a bedside procedure with low complication rates [93]. SGB is a valuable adjunct therapy to manage patients with symptomatic vasospasm. BLOCK-CVS, an RCT (NCT04691271), is currently underway to truly understand the effects and safety of SGB for aSAH management [100].

As mentioned previously, the incidence of vasospasm has been directly associated with the presence of blood products in the subarachnoid space [36]. Intentional clearance of blood products, decreasing the rate of hemolysis and spasm, has been proposed as a potential method to reduce the risk of vasospasm and improve outcomes [101, 102]. Clearance of bloody CSF allows for clear circulation of CSF to flush the subarachnoid space. Continuous CSF drainage, typically via external ventricular drain (EVD) or lumbar drain (LD), prevents the rise in ICP in aSAH patients [103–105]. CSF drainage improved clinical outcomes, reduced incidence of symptomatic vasospasm, and reduced rates of DCI. Interestingly, continuous CSF drainage was shown not to affect the prevention of hydrocephalus. LD led to fewer complications and improved mRS scores compared to EVD [103, 106]. One benefit of LD is removing blood products from the intrathecal space, a large CSF cistern [104]. Well-designed RCTs are required to compare differences in LD versus EVD for aSAH.

Intraarterial Treatment:

Vasodilator Drugs

Among the diverse vasodilatory agents, papaverine was among the first agents explored for DCI intra-arterial (IA) treatment. Despite evidence of improved local cerebral blood flow, intra-arterial papaverine (IAP) has largely fallen out of favor due to numerous limitations. Most notably, IAP induces a short-lived response, often necessitating multiple endovascular treatments [107]. IAP has also been associated with elevated ICP, local neurotoxicity, and hypotension [78]. Today, the most common IA agents include verapamil, nicardipine, nimodipine, and milrinone. These agents have become first-line IA therapies given their favorable side effect profile and sustained vasodilatory response compared to papaverine. While no RCT has compared the clinical efficacy of these agents, recent small retrospective studies have begun to provide nuance. One study found that nimodipine could generate a consistent local increase in angiographic vessel diameter. However, this angiographic improvement did not translate consistently to better clinical outcomes [108]. Furthermore, long-term continuous IA nimodipine has been associated with increased cardiac, infectious, and gastrointestinal side effects [79]. It is noteworthy that prolonged and continuous IA nimodipine is reserved as a rescue therapy option for severe refractory DCI. As such, the side effects are likely secondary to the higher-than-normal doses of nimodipine needed for otherwise refractory cases. A more recent prospective study of 43 patients found that IA nimodipine was associated with significant angiographic and clinical recovery without significant complications when adhering to standard endovascular practice [109]. Additionally, another prospective trial found IA milrinone usage associated with improved local vessel patency, improved clinical outcomes, and limited side effects [110]. Interestingly, while rescue IA milrinone has been associated with various adverse side effects, one study found higher-dose IA milrinone to be a viable rescue therapy for patients with DCI refractory to multiple endovascular interventions. It is worth noting that this trial included just six patients who met the criteria for refractory cerebral vasospasm [111]. A larger randomized control trial is needed to elucidate which first-line agents are suitable for higher-dose rescue therapy for refractory DCI. IA verapamil, has been reported in several retrospective studies. However, the results have been mixed [112–115]. In angiographically normal vessels of AVM patients, IA, verapamil decrease both proximal and distal vascular resistance [72, 116]. IA injections were safe and effective in treating vasospasm in one study but did not increase angiographic diameter in another [112, 113]. They are limited by transient effect times and limited effect on more proximal vasculature [114, 115]. Interestingly, IA verapamil significantly improved bilateral perfusion when given as a continuous infusion in anterior and posterior circulations in a patient with severe hypoperfusion [114]. A more extensive retrospective study demonstrated complete radiographic resolution of vasospasm in almost all 12 patients treated with continuous IA verapamil [115]. Continuous IA nimodipine has also been tested. However, data is limited, and results are equivalent to an injection control [117]. Future studies of treatment duration and dosing of IA vasodilators are critical for improving outcomes.

Beyond the promise of single-drug IA therapies, multi-drug IA regimens have recently emerged as potentially superior therapies for DCI. One study found that Nicardipine-Verapamil was associated with improved vessel diameter, improved modified Rankin Scale (mRS) at discharge, and mRS at 90-day follow-up compared to IA nicardipine or verapamil alone [118]. Similarly, another study found that a combination of verapamil and nimodipine improves vessel diameter and mRS at discharge compared to the drugs used independently [119]. However, various combinations of multi-drug IA therapy are not universally beneficial. Studies on a combination of magnesium-nicardipine and nicardipine-milrinone have demonstrated no clinical improvement over using the two drugs alone [120, 121]. Exploring drug combinations to treat vasospasm can improve the outcome and help us better understand the pathological mechanisms.

As a brief note, other IA drug therapies have been explored as a treatment for DCI. These drugs include amrinone, fasudil, dantrolene, magnesium, and nitroglycerine. Overall, studies on these drugs are typically older and have limited enrollment [121–124]. As such, the role of these drugs has been primarily relegated to second-line usage for institutions without access to first-line IA therapies.

Despite the successes of some intra-arterial vasodilatory therapies, concentrations of drugs within the vessel during these procedures are mainly unknown. Several pre-clinical studies have explored the dose-dependent effects of IA nimodipine [125, 126], but there is still an inadequate clinical translation. Understanding in vivo drug concentrations is limited by obvious ethical concerns as intra-arterial sampling carries high risk. However, mathematical models explicitly focusing on intra-arterial delivery of nimodipine suggest that a maximal concentration of 85% is reached relatively quickly compared to IV administration [127]. Further, arterial concentrations of nimodipine were found to be effectively independent of infusion rate, almost entirely dependent on blood flow from the ICA, allowing for shorter infusion durations [127]. While these experiments were theoretical, there is promise in better understanding the pharmacokinetics of intraarterial drug delivery through more sophisticated and advanced modalities such as optical methods.

Monitoring Response of IA Vasodilator Treatment

Serial monitoring is critical for identifying treatment responses and the need for further intervention. Monitoring options for vasospasm are diverse, including physiologic studies, radiologic studies, and clinical examinations. The neurologic exam is the gold standard for detecting symptomatic vasospasm in aSAH patients. It is low-cost, quick, and non-invasive. However, the exam is limited by the examiner's skills and may provide little value for those patients sedated or unconscious. The exact modalities used to diagnose vasospasm in early aSAH can also be used to monitor responses to treatment. As mentioned previously, TCD is another low-cost, non-invasive method to monitor and assess response to intra-arterial therapies via changes in CBF velocity [43]. Similarly, angiography, the best test to determine vessel narrowing, can be repeated serially to assess changes after treatment. Figure 10.4 shows the response to 20 mg of intraarterial verapamil in a patient with cerebral vasospasm. A correlation between intracranial pressure (ICP) and vasospasm has been established for some time. High ICP correlates with prolonged and diffuse vasospasm in aSAH patients. EVD is typically used for ICP measurements, with parenchymal monitoring less frequently used [128]. In addition to these modalities, multiple emerging monitoring methods are under investigation. Cerebral microdialysis (CMD) provides metabolic information from a cellular level. The probe mimics a capillary blood vessel, a semipermeable membranous structure located in the extracellular space to collect molecules by diffusion [129]. Location, determined by CT imaging, is crucial as CMD data is local. Changes to concentrations of glucose and its metabolites, like lactate and pyruvate, may convey conditions of hypoxia or metabolic dysfunction [130]. Ultimately, the pathophysiology is not sufficiently clear. Still, changes to metabolism at the cellular level may be informative in understanding vasospasm in arteries that are too small to be evaluated by angiography. CMD is

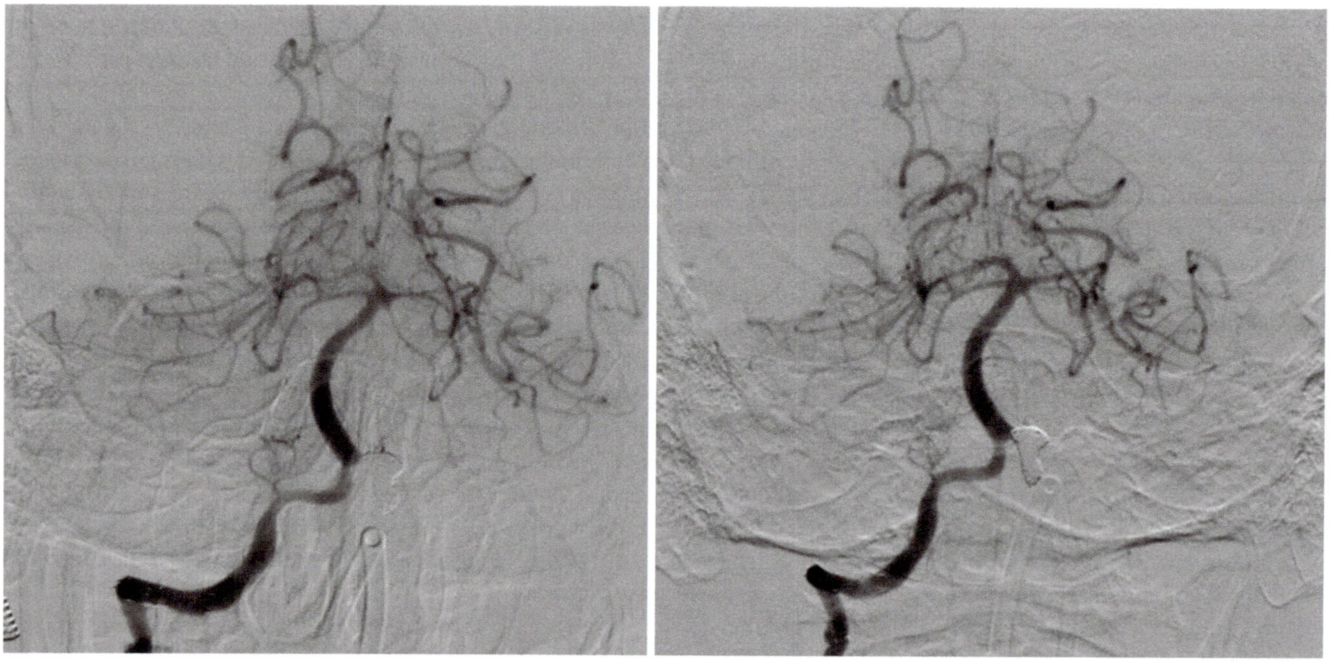

Fig. 10.4 Effect of vasodilator therapy on posterior circulation vasospasm (pre-administration on the left panel, post-administration on the right panel). Twenty milligrams of verapamil was injected into the right vertebral artery over 20 min, with significant improvement in vessel caliber

often part of "multimodal monitoring" (MMM), which typically includes measurements of CIP, CPP, CBF, brain tissue oxygen tension ($PbtO_2$), and electrographic monitoring. Like CMD, monitoring $PbtO_2$ may assess tissue changes where typical modalities, like ICP, would fail. During measurement, oxygen diffuses into a Clark-type invasive probe, and changes in oxygen concentration are translated into electric current, which is quantified [131]. However, tissue hypoxia may occur without increased ICP and is associated with poor outcomes [132, 133]. Thus, monitoring and potentially treating subtle changes in $PbtO_2$ may be course-altering. In combination, $PbtO_2$ and CMD were shown to detect both hypoxia and metabolic derangement when CPP and ICP monitoring failed to do so [134]. Further, in a small study, MMM successfully quantified the efficacy of rescue IA angioplasty via oxygenation and cellular metabolism [135]. However, further studies are still required to better understand how to assess and act on such data. Of multimodal neuromonitoring devices are invasive and risk injury. Meanwhile, near-infrared spectroscopy (NIRS) assesses blood oxygenation non-invasively by measuring the near-infrared light absorption of oxy and deoxyhemoglobin. NIRS measures arterial, venous, and capillary hemoglobin in all tissue within its field by sending near-infrared light at the scalp through the skull. This data calculates oxygen saturation and cerebral hypoxia [131, 136]. NIRS is limited by changes in hemoglobin concentrations, the thickness of the skull, and tissue depth. Data regarding NIRS is equivocal. Some studies have suggested that it is potentially more sensitive than TCDs for measuring changes in oxygenation and can be used to detect changes in oxygenation after IV dobutamine [137]. Others have found that NIRS is limited as a screening tool for vasospam and infraction after SAH [138]. Since NIRS is non-invasive and can be continually monitored at the bedside, it may be worth including in future studies.

Complications of IA Vasodilator Treatment:

Endovascular management of diffuse cerebral vasospasm following aSAH involves intraarterial infusion of vasodilatory drugs and balloon angioplasty, and lacks large-scale randomized clinical trial data. Hence its efficacy remains unknown [45]. These interventions can be associated with significant peri and post-procedural complications. As such, the current expert recommendation is to reserve these treatments for patients with clinically significant vasospasm rather than prophylactically treating patients with angiographic and/or radiographic evidence of vasospasm [45]. This, of course, can be challenging. Many patients with high-grade aSAH have impaired consciousness, hence a poor baseline neurologic exam. Subsequently, clinicians often depend on multi-modal data points, including close trending of neurologic exam, transcranial dopplers, and CT or MR perfusion studies, to inform clinical decision-making regarding the pursuit of endovascular treatment of cerebral vasospasm in patients who are not adequately responding to maximal medical therapy. While further large-scale randomized trials are needed, recent meta-analyses support using IA vasodilators which lead to an angiographic response with good neurological outcome, when the treatment is guided by TCD [21, 139]. The decision to pursue endovascular management of vasospasm should depend on a multidisciplinary review and in-depth risk-benefit analysis, which requires a thorough understanding of peri- and post-procedural complications. Figure 10.5 illustrates the potential complications of intraarterial vasodilator treatment.

Increased ICP

Among patients with cerebral vasospasm in the setting of aneurysmal subarachnoid hemorrhage, IA vasodilators have been reported to result in increased ICP. Of the IA vasodilators, papaverine appears to have the most adverse effect on intracranial pressure. It has been shown to cause increased ICP, independent of systemic blood pressure changes, with a dose-dependent and rate-dependent relationship [140, 141]. One series from the University of Cincinnati showed that of 50 patients treated with IA papaverine, 21 cases needed to be prematurely terminated due to high ICP, and 5 patients died due to intractably high ICP [142, 143].

Calcium channel blockers have also been shown to increase ICP. However, current evidence supports that this is usually a transient effect. Badjatia et al. studied the impact of IA nicardipine in a cohort of 18 patients undergoing endovascular therapy for cerebral vasospasm, treating 44 vessels. In this cohort, ICP was transiently elevated in five patients and persistently in one [144]. The investigators were vigilant about intra-operative ICP monitoring during IA infusion of nicardipine, adjusting the ventriculostomy drains to lower ICP in any patient demonstrating >20 mmHg increase in ICP during the infusion [144]. The patient with persistently elevated ICP, despite drain adjustment, was found to have an intracranial hemorrhage along the tract of the ventriculostomy drain that was placed during the procedure [144]. Therefore, it felt less likely to be a sustained reaction to the drug itself. Current literature supports that IA verapamil may have a dose-dependent effect on ICP. Multiple studies have demonstrated the safety profile of low-dose IA verapamil infusion (mean of 2.5–22 mg/procedure), with no significant changes in hemodynamics or ICP observed [112, 113, 145]. However, in a study conducted by Stuart et al., patients who received a high-dose IA Verapamil infusion (median dose 23 mg, range 15–55 mg) were found to have an 8% decrease in central perfusion pressure and a 30% increase in ICP. The latter remained elevated until post-procedure hour 3 and returned to baseline pressure 8 h after treatment [145, 146].

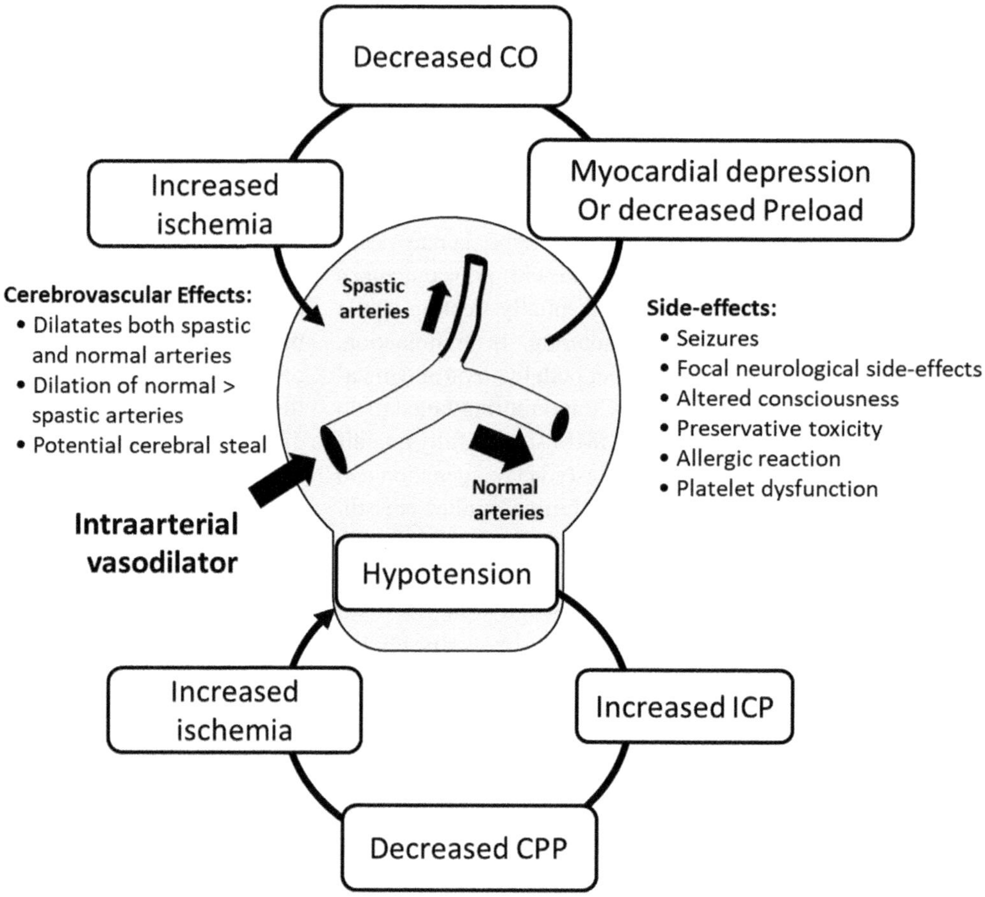

Fig. 10.5 Deleterious effects of intraarterial vasodilator therapy

Given this, close ICP monitoring during the IA vasodilator treatment and immediate post-procedure period is essential to detect and respond to dynamic changes in patients' intracranial pressure.

Seizure

Overall, seizures precipitated by IA infusion of vasodilators are rare [141]. However, IA Papaverine and Verapamil have been associated with ictal events. In one study, papaverine was shown to be a direct proconvulsant in a rat model [147, 148]. There are only a handful of case reports of papaverine-induced seizures in the literature. While never explicitly tested, the proposed mechanism of its pro-epileptogenic effect is thought to be related to the drug interaction with the metabolically challenged neuronal tissue that results after aneurysmal SAH [147]. Mao et al. found that among the 449 high-dose IA verapamil treatments administered in their cohort, 2.9% (13 treatments) resulted in seizures, all of which were successfully treated with intravenous lorazepam without the progression to status epilepticus [145]. While some studies have reported an increased incidence of seizures in IA verapamil dosing over 10 mg, it remains uncertain whether this is directly related to increased dosing or whether it is secondary to the rate of re-perfusion of previously ischemic brain tissue [145, 149]. There are no case reports of intractable seizures secondary to IA vasodilatory therapy or permanent neurologic sequelae resulting from iatrogenic seizure activity.

Neurological deficits

Papaverine is the drug most implicated in causing neurologic deficits during the treatment of medically refractory cerebral vasospasm, which is why it is no longer routinely used in current practice among most centers in the United States. Mathias et al. found that in 36 patients treated with IA papaverine, 6 (16.7%) experienced transient neurologic deficits, including mydriasis, hemiparesis, and respiratory arrest [150]. Papaverine-induced mydriasis can often be mistaken for a cerebral herniation syndrome but usually occurs when the microcatheter tip is proximal to the ophthalmic artery [151]. Transient respiratory depression is associated with papaverine infusion into the posterior circulation, affecting the medullary cardiac and respiratory centers [151]. Additionally, more than 0.3% papaverine concentrations have been associated with microcrystal formation, which theoretically could embolize and result in a neurologic deficit. However, this has not yet been validated in vivo [147, 151]. Papaverine has also been linked to the paradoxical worsening of vasospasm and has been reported to have a direct neurotoxic effect on neuronal gray matter [150, 152, 153].

Some centers are investigating high doses of IA Verapamil in patients with medically refractory, severe vasospasm. In a small case series, prolonged infusion of extra high dose verapamil (mean 220.8 ± 142.2 mg/procedure) successfully reversed angiographic vasospasm in 58.3% of patients while preventing new ischemic insults in 75% [115, 145]. However, prolonged infusion times proposed the theoretical risk of catheter-associated thromboembolic complications during the procedure, although none were reported in this series [145].

Systemic Effects

While rare, multiple treatments of high-dose IA verapamil have been associated with bradycardia and sustained hypotension despite maximal vasopressor support [145]. Rapid infusion of verapamil is more likely to result in hypotension and bradycardia, and this effect can last several hours after the treatment [146, 154]. Papaverine has dose-dependent systemic cardiovascular effects. High doses, rapid administration, and infusion into multiple vascular territories have been shown to cause hemodynamically significant hypotension [143, 147, 150]. Additionally, papaverine is associated with severe thrombocytopenia following IA infusion, the exact mechanism of which is unknown [147, 155]. Milrinone is an agent under active investigation for treating delayed cerebral ischemia secondary to vasospasm. Given its efficacy in the cardiac literature, it is proposed to benefit cerebral vasospasm by directly reducing vascular tone [156]. The subsequent hypotension that results from IA administration of milrinone often requires vasopressor support; however, across various case series, no adverse effects were reported from the subsequent use of vasopressors [71, 156, 157]. Despite promising case studies, no randomized clinical trial, including milrinone, exists; therefore, evidence to support its routine use is currently lacking [21].

Balloon Angioplasty

Transluminal balloon angioplasty (TBA) was first reported as a treatment for SAH in a cohort of 33 patients with subsequent dilation of 105 major cerebral arteries [158]. No randomized clinical control trials have compared pharmacologic vasodilation to TBA in treating delayed cerebral ischemia secondary to cerebral vasospasm after SAH. However, in the recent neurocritical care consensus review of retrospective studies, one method or drug did not show clear superiority over the other, except papaverine, due to its association with neurotoxicity [8, 159].

Two balloon technologies have been utilized for intracranial vasospasm: (1) with the more compliant balloon for intracranial use, (2) coronary balloons adapted for intracranial use [152]. The adapted coronary balloon membrane is a double-lumen, relatively stiff shaft composed of polyethylene or nylon that allows for balloon inflation in one channel and the passage of a guidewire in the other. The balloon is shorter, allowing for improved maneuverability and less vessel tension upon inflation [152]. The specifically designed intracranial balloons consist of a more pliable, single-lumen silicone/elastomer membrane [152]. The balloon is more extended and better adapted for long-segment spastic arteries [152]. The transfemoral approach is most commonly utilized, and intracranial arteries are catheterized, with reliance on a digital roadmap for balloon manipulation over the superimposed, selected vessels [143]. Patients are usually placed under generalized anesthesia to minimize patient movement. The complication of vessel rupture is enhanced due to heparization to a clotting time of two to three times their baseline. The activated clotting time generally exceeds 300 s to reduce thromboembolic risk unless contraindicated [143]. During anesthesia induction, blood pressure must be carefully maintained to prevent a drop in cerebral perfusion pressure during the procedure [143]. The catheter lumen is tapered distal to the balloon, allowing injected contrast to expand the balloon directly [152]. Care must be taken to avoid the guidewire retracting into the catheter lumen once intravascularly placed to avoid contrast and blood retraction, which could lead to poor balloon opacification, unintentional overinflation, and/or difficulty in balloon deflation [152]. Once the location is confirmed, the balloon is inflated with an exquisitely calibrated 1 mL syringe that allows for adjustments in inflation to the 0.01 mL range, and the balloon diameter is calibrated to the volume of injection rather than an insufflation pressure [152]. Once the balloon conforms to the vessel lumen, subsequent inflation must be stopped, given the risk of inadvertent overinflation and vessel rupture. The optimal injection includes a 50/50 mixture of saline and 300 mg/mL of contrast, as higher contrast concentrations may lead to poor deflation [152].

TBA's clinical efficacy is variable and likely dependent on the intervention's timing. Angiographic improvement is notable, reaching 80–100% in most large-scale case series. However, the clinical improvement is less robust, with a broader range of 30–80% in these series [43, 76, 78, 143, 160, 161]. Other studies support that patients taken for TBA within 2 h of neurologic decline have better clinical outcomes than those for which TBA is delayed more significantly than 2 h [154, 159]. This was best illustrated by Rosenwasser et al., who showed that patients treated with TBA within 2 h demonstrated 90% angiographic improvement and 70% clinical improvement, compared to patients treated after 2 h, who had similar angiographic improvement (88%) but significantly decreased clinical improvement (40%) [152, 160]. Additionally, the incidence of infarcts in vessels treated with TBA) is significantly lower compared to those that were not [21, 76]. Recurrence of endovascular retreatment for refractory vasospasm has also been shown to be significantly lower in vessels treated with TBA alone compared to IA vasodilator therapy alone [21, 78].

The disruption of smooth muscle cells, extracellular matrix, and basement membranes of the cells lining the vessel wall endothelium is thought to contribute to the efficacy of TBA as it results in prolonged patency following mechanical dilation, the subsequent increase in cerebral blood flow, and overall resistance to further vasospasm [152]. However, these mechanisms can lead to significant intra-procedural complications. The principal risks associated with this procedure are vessel rupture, dissection, and thromboembolism. Of these, vessel rupture is the most feared, and this typically occurs when the balloon diameter size and vessel wall are discordant. In cases of severe vasospasm, this risk increases due to limited opacification of distal vessels and, subsequently, the increased risk of catheter misplacement [152]. Given the mechanical nature of the intervention and the risk of vessel rupture, TBA is typically reserved for treating larger, proximal vessels. Typical locations include the vertebral artery, basilar artery, supraclinoid internal carotid artery, and the M1 segment of the middle cerebral artery [152]. The exceptions are the proximal ACA and PCA arteries, which inexplicably have a greater risk of vascular injury than the other proximal arteries of the Circle of Willis [154]. Shearing forces generated by manipulating an inflated balloon can result in arterial dissection and subsequent thrombus, pseudoaneurysm, or critical stenosis; therefore, great care must be taken to ensure complete deflation of the balloon before any catheter manipulation [152]. Patients who have suffered SAH are in an inherent hypercoagulable state, leading to an increased risk of thrombus formation around the catheter or balloon, significantly reduced with systemic heparinization [152]. Procedural complications are rare, with some centers estimating a 1% complication rate per ballooned vessel [143].

Given the reported success rate of TBA), mainly when implemented early, prophylactic TBA became a natural point of investigation. In a phase II-multicenter randomized trial investigating prophylactic treatment in patients with Fisher Grade III SAH, no significant difference was found in the primary outcome on the Glasgow Outcome Score. However, there was a trend towards fewer patients who received prophylactic treatment developing delayed cerebral ischemia or requiring eventual therapeutic TBA [161]. However, when balanced with the risk of complications during the procedure, the most recent consensus from the American Stroke Association is that prophylactic TBA is not recommended for treating patients with SAH (Class III, Level B evidence) [43].

Stent Placement

Stenting is another endovascular treatment option for managing delayed cerebral ischemia, and both retrievable and intracranial stents have been utilized. A significant advantage of stent retrievers over TBA is their ability to be deployed in smaller caliber branches of the main cerebral arteries. This ability allows for the vasodilation of more extended segment, distal, vasospastic vessels, which in keeping with Poiseuille's law (volume flow rate is directly proportional to the fourth power of the radius of the vessel), allows for an increase in flow rate to spastic vessels. The unsheathing and resheathing technique for retrievable stents minimizes endothelial damage to the vessels, thereby reducing the risk of precipitating vasospasm [162]. Relatively short deployment times (20 min or less) have been shown to have good treatment response, but the deployment time for maximal effectiveness remains uncertain [162].

One center observed, incidentally, the benefit of intracranial stents for DCI. During aneurysm coiling, instrumentation of the parent vessel affected by vasospasm became further compromised during the intervention. IA vasodilator therapy was ineffective, but stenting the parent vessels restored the blood flow. Following stenting, Khanafer et al. observed decreased vasospasm with perfusion improvement in distal territories supplied by the stented vessels [163]. To follow up on this incidental result, they selected four cases of DCI refractory to chemical and mechanical treatments for endovascular stenting: two cases with one stent placed at M1–M2 Junction, the third with two stents placed in the ipsilateral MCA and ACA, and the fourth had four stents placed, two on each side. There was one transient thrombo-occlusive event during stent placement; otherwise, none of the patients who underwent stenting experienced DCI of the stented vessel territories, suggesting that endovascular stenting may be an acceptable treatment option in refractory vasospasm although requires the use of dual antiplatelet drugs [163].

A significant advantage of stents over TBA is that as opposed to reliance on the proceduralist's mechanical inflation of the balloon, the outward force of the stent is balanced by the inherent centripetal force of the vessel wall, allowing for optimal compliance with significantly lower risk of mechanical vessel rupture [162]. An additional advantage includes the ability to inject IA Vasodilators during the deployment of the stent retriever, allowing for chemical vasodilation of the most distal branches not amenable to mechanical intervention [162]. One study supports that patients treated with stent retrieval before IA vasodilators showed significant vasodilation and significantly reduced development of radiographic or clinical vasospasm compared to patients treated with IA vasodilators before stent retrieval [163, 164]. Drug-eluting stents (DES) for treating

DCI are under investigation. In one in vitro study, laser-cut and polymer-coated stents were designed to be loaded with varying concentrations of verapamil and to elute the drug when vasospasm occurs after SAH [165]. Further in vivo and in vitro studies are needed to determine whether DES may be an effective prophylactic and/or treatment option for DCI.

Clot Retrieval

The strongest predictor of cerebral vasospasm is the number of clots in the subarachnoid space on initial head CT after aneurysmal subarachnoid hemorrhage [166]. This is because the blood degradation products from the subarachnoid clots trigger the cascade responsible for driving cerebral vasospasm [166]. Aggressive surgical clot removal within 24 h of aneurysmal clipping has decreased the probability of developing postoperative symptomatic cerebral vasospasm [167]. Given this, it was hypothesized that an early open surgical approach to aneurysmal SAH may hold an advantage over the endovascular approach in terms of delayed cerebral ischemia and the risk of developing chronic hydrocephalus, given the ability to evacuate the cerebral cisterns of blood clots in the open, as opposed to endovascular, approach. However, one study conducted by Andreas et al. found no significant difference in the rate of development of chronic hydrocephalus in patients treated with early surgical vs. early endovascular approach, with the additional, insignificant trend towards lower rates of shunt dependency in patients treated with an early endovascular approach [168].

Outcome

Regarding outcomes following aSAH, several hallmark randomized clinical trials have been conducted. In 1989, Pickard et al. demonstrated in a randomized, double-blinded, placebo-control trial that oral nimodipine 60 mg four times daily reduces cerebral infarction and improves functional outcomes in patients who have suffered SAH [28]. In 2005, the Lancet published the results of the International Subarachnoid Aneurysm Trial (ISAT), which compared the one-year outcomes of patients with ruptured intracranial aneurysms allocated to surgical clipping versus endovascular coiling and showed that patients who underwent endovascular coiling were more likely to have one-year independent survival compared to the surgical group, with a total survival benefit that continues for at least 7 years. While the risk of late rebleeding was low, it was more commonly seen in the endovascular group [169]. However, the data regarding DCI is much more limited. One randomized clinical trial (RCT) investigated prophylactic TBA use within 96 h of aSAH compared to no intervention. While there was a trend towards improved outcomes and decreased likelihood of subsequent angioplasty, this was countered by three deaths due to arterial rupture in the intervention group, leading to the current American Heart Association/American Stroke Association recommendation against prophylactic TBA (Class III, Level B evidence) [45, 161]. Regarding systemic delivery of drugs used to improve outcomes following SAH, 1 meta-analysis of 14 randomized controlled trials involving 4235 patients concluded that while angiographic vasospasm was significantly reduced following drug administration, clinical outcomes remained unchanged [26]. Notably, no large-scale RCTs are investigating the IA delivery of drugs for treating DCI, including nicardipine, nimodipine, verapamil, and milrinone, commonly used in clinical [8]. The efficacy of IA delivery of these drugs is primarily reported in a smaller scale, largely uncontrolled, retrospective studies, with no clear delineation or superiority of one agent over the other, apart from the reported neurotoxicity associated with papaverine [8]. A 2011 neurocritical care consensus recommended endovascular treatment with IA vasodilators and angioplasty when medical management was ineffective [8, 45]. However, the timing of endovascular intervention for DCI is also unclear. The most recent 2023 neurocritical care consensus stated insufficient evidence to recommend the optimal trigger (change in neurologic exam plus finding on neuroimaging vs. change in neurologic exam alone) for endovascular management of DCI [170]. The Intra Arterial Vasospasm Trial (iVAST), a prospective multicenter RCT, is underway and in phase 4. This trial will compare the IA delivery of nicardipine to verapamil to a combination delivery of nicardipine, verapamil, and nitroglycerin in patients ages 18–80 years old with ruptured intracranial aneurysm who experience symptomatic or asymptomatic (defined as greater than 50% stenosis on DSA performed in centers who do routine DSA 7 days post aneurysm treatment) vasospasm within 3–21 days post-intervention. Pregnant patients, patients with Hunt and Hess Grade 5 aSAH, and patients who receive IA treatment in all three arterial territories are currently excluded. Preliminary results have not yet been published, and study recruitment is estimated to be completed by December 2024. While there is no arm without IA treatment, this will be a valuable study to compare the two IA agents frequently used in current practice to a novel combination therapy approach.

Limitations of Current IA Treatments

IA vasodilator therapy can be associated with many complications, including increased ICP, neurological deficits, and disruption of the BBB, all potentially limiting optimal outcomes for patients with vasospasm. In addition, the endo-

Table 10.1 Clinical trials with "cerebral vasospasm" + "arterial" interventions on the national clinical trial registry

NCT number	Study title	Study status	Condition and intervention
NCT01996436	The Intra-arterial Vasospasm Trial	Recruiting	Cerebral vasospasm Nicardipine/Verapamil/ Nicardipine + Verapamil + Nitroglycerin
NCT01400360	Invasive Diagnostic and Therapeutic Management of Cerebral Vasospasm After Aneurysmatic Subarachnoid Hemorrhage	Unknown	Cerebral vasospasm after subarachnoid hemorrhage. Transluminal balloon angioplasty, IA vasodilators
NCT04649398	Cerebral Nimodipine Concentrations Following Oral, Intra-venous, and Intra-arterial Administration	Recruiting	SAH, delayed cerebral ischemia, vasospasm, cerebral IV or IA Nimodipine
NCT05150002	Cervical Spinal Cord Stimulation in Patients with Cerebral Vasospasm After Subarachnoid Hemorrhage	Recruiting	SAH, delayed cerebral ischemia, vasospasm, cerebral DEVICE: Spinal cord stimulation Spinal cord stimulation, others
NCT05268445	Chemical and Mechanical Angioplasty for Vasospasm (SAVEBRAIN)	Completed	Chemical and mechanical angioplasty
NCT02907879	Contrast Enhanced Ultrasound Imaging for Cerebral Perfusion Measurement in Cerebral Vasospasm After SAH	Terminated	Subarachnoid hemorrhage: IA
NCT06134583	Superior Cervical Sympathetic Block Versus Stellate Ganglion Block in Post-traumatic Subarachnoid Hemorrhage	Not recruiting	Post-traumatic subarachnoid hemorrhage
NCT01613235	Induced Hypertension for Treatment of Delayed Cerebral Ischemia After Aneurysmal Subarachnoid Hemorrhage	Terminated	Cerebral Ischemia, subarachnoid hemorrhage

vascular technology itself may be limited and must be updated to improve outcomes in patients with vasospasm after aSAH. Although improvements to microcatheter navigation have made it easier to approach previously challenging neurovascular locations, some distal areas of vasospasm remain difficult to catheterize selectively. Microcatheter navigation is a significant concern when proximal spasm limits navigability and delivery of IA drugs to an affected region because of impaired flow. IA vasodilator therapy is also not indicated when the vascular narrowing is refractory to endovascular treatment [171]. Further studies are required to understand better the underlying pathophysiologic mechanisms of cerebral vasospasm in specific patient subpopulations and provide insight into why we see different responses.

Reliable assessment tools also limit IA vasodilator therapy. The benefits of treatment are unclear in unconscious patients due to the lack of a detailed neurological exam [172]. Multimodal monitoring may provide some semblance of treatment response, but improvement in focal deficits remains the gold standard. Further, the relationship between arterial vasodilation and clinical improvement is still unclear. Patients who improve clinically after IA vasodilator therapy do not necessarily have corresponding improved vasodilation on angiography [173]. A better assessment of drug delivery and effect is needed. Many emerging optical technologies, such as diffuse reflectance spectroscopy, multispectral and hyperspectral imaging, spatial frequency, domain imaging, confocal microscopy and spectroscopy, and optical coherence tomography, are potential avenues of further research [174].

Lastly, the length of vasodilatory action remains poorly understood. As mentioned previously, CCBs are increasingly used to treat vasospasm. Still, among these options, the duration of effect may be variable, mainly due to the quick transit time of intraarterially infused medications. In a rabbit model, nimodipine and nicardipine were demonstrated to provide more prolonged effects than verapamil [175]. However, no drug provided an effect longer than 2 h. By 3 h, arteries returned to their vasospastic states. Therefore, future studies should be dedicated to either improving the duration of effect for these CCBs or finding better alternatives in drug choice or delivery. Table 10.1 lists the ongoing clinical trials for cerebral vasospasm documented on the National Clinical Trial Registry.

Future Directions

Improving IA vasodilation for vasospasm after aSAH may involve several strategies to understand its mechanisms, enhance its effectiveness and delivery, assess outcomes, and minimize potential complications. Animal models have long been used to study the acute effects of vasospasm, in which mice are sacrificed and their brains fixed for histological analysis [176–178]. However, this only provides insight into the acute effects of vasospasm and its treatment and thus prevents any long-term study about the potential benefits of therapies. Other methods, such as rodent DSA, may avoid animal sacrifice, but its use is severely limited, given the toxicity of contrast to these animals. Similarly, MRA has its own set of hurdles. It is time-consuming and expensive, and the anesthesia requirement creates histopathological artifacts [179]. There are currently no ideal methods to study the long-term effects of vasospasm or its treatment in animal models. Two-photon imaging involving a cranial window may be a viable option, however, where vasculature diameter and oxygenation could be studied.

Identifying the correct patients and monitoring their responses to treatment may also improve in the future. Early prophylactic chemical IA therapy has not been studied. However, given the success of prophylactic mechanical IA therapy, early chemical therapy could also have a preventive role. In a recent RCT, aSAH patients received either prophylactic chemical treatment or angioplasty with symptomatic DCI [161]. Outcomes were similar, but those patients who received early angioplasty were less likely to receive rescue angioplasty. Similar thinking may be appropriate for chemical IA therapy. Prophylaxis is not without complications. Four of 85 patients (4.7%) died from perforation in the intervention arm [161]. However, more studies are needed to determine the optimal timing for IA drug delivery and whether the earlier intervention has a significant clinical benefit.

Traditional monitoring methods with vasospasm have had equivocal clinical relevance when used to assess responses to IA therapies [172, 173]. As mentioned previously, several conventional methods and emerging modalities are used to monitor vasospasm and its response to treatment. Traditional methods, such as physical exams and TCDs, lack sensitivity. Meanwhile, while emerging clinical modalities like $PbtO_2$ monitoring and CMD provide highly granular data, there is little guidance on how to act on their measurements appropriately. Investigators continue to search for the following measurement tools in preclinical studies. Haptoglobin levels in the CSF have been suggested as a marker of imminent vasospasm, given its role as a hemoglobin binder [180]. Free hemoglobin can lead to increased reactive oxygen species (ROS), which may disrupt normal NO and cause both macro- and microvessel dysfunction [181]. Thus, serial measurement of haptoglobin and potential IA haptoglobin therapy may provide new diagnostic and therapeutic insights. Clinical biomarkers have been identified in limited patient cohorts, including the sphingosine-1-phosphate receptor for mRNA, miR-3117-3p, D-dimer, and soluble receptors for advanced glycation end products [181–183]. More expansive clinical studies with better prognostic markers are required.

Patient outcomes may also be improved by focusing on how we deliver drugs to the brain. Improving drug delivery of IA vasodilators requires optimizing existing administration techniques and exploring novel approaches. As mentioned previously, balloon angioplasty can be highly effective but carries the risk of complications. Meanwhile, IA drug delivery provides the added benefit of distal penetration but places patients at independent risk who are drug dependent. A novel hybrid approach combines the advantages of both mechanical and chemical angioplasty, aimed at treating patients who would not usually be able to withstand standard doses of vasodilators or whose anatomy is not suitable for balloon angioplasty [184]. This method involves maneuvering and inflating a balloon catheter immediately proximal to the spasm and then delivering pressure boluses. This approach was trialed on five patients who were refractory to standard of care. All procedures were successful, with vasospasm improved and no complications [184]. Improvements to intraoperative imaging may also refine catheter placement. As previously discussed, advancements in real-time angiographic imaging or optical techniques would allow for more accurate catheter placement and drug delivery and improved assessment of the degree of vasospasm and potential drug choice.

While catheter-based delivery has been the conventional mode of delivery, other groups have explored more novel approaches. Verapamil eluting stents have been shown to deliver verapamil intra-arterially over a prolonged period. However, follow-up animal studies are required to understand whether this technology is feasible [165]. Drug-coated stents have been used to treat intracranial stenosis and may be a helpful addition to the retrievable stents used to treat DCI [168]. Additionally, new devices such as the Comaneci (Rapid Medical, Yokneam, Israel), an approved device for temporary coil embolization, have also shown some promise in the off-label treatment of cerebral vasospasm through operator-controlled variable mechanical dilation with the theoretical benefits of higher radial forces compared to stent retrievers, no implantable hardware without a need for dual antiplatelet therapy as seen in traditional stents, and continued antegrade flow when compared to balloon catheters [185].

Since the initial IA studies, catheter design and technology improvements have allowed for increasingly selective targeting when delivering IA therapies. Specialized microcatheters and microwires are advanced to the small vasospastic arteries where intra-arterial vasodilators can be delivered precisely to distal vessels. These "super-selective" infusions facilitate safer and more effective vasospasm targeting [186–188]. As catheter and wire technology improves, surgeons can target more distal spastic arteries, allowing for safer and more effective treatment.

Conclusions

Vasospasm and DCI following aSAH carry considerable risk of severe morbidity and mortality. For those dealing with aSAH, there is a risk of significant morbidity quadruples if they develop cerebral vasospasm [15]. Despite these known risks, there is no consensus on intraarterial treatment for vasospasm or DCI. Given the complex pathophysiology—including bleeding necrosis, inflammation, procoagulation, and endothelial dysfunction—a multimodal approach must be developed [7]. This paradigm may include diagnostic tools, such as TCDs, DSA, CTA, and MRA. It should be coupled with the combination of both chemical and balloon angioplasty. IA delivery of CCB and multi-drug regiments has shown the most promise, but novel, targeted dilators must be trialed to improve outcomes [115, 118, 119]. Anti-inflammatory therapies should continue to be explored, given the immense role of the immune system in vasospasm [91, 92]. Despite promising results, IA vasodilators are not without complication, and identifying the correct patients and clinical indication is crucial for avoiding the unnecessary risks of both the medication and the procedure itself [145, 146, 150, 161]. These complications, along with poor assessment tools and an incomplete understanding of the underlying pathophysiology of delayed cerebral ischemia, limit the utilization of IA vasodilator therapy. However, clinicians and scientists continue to explore and improve this promising modality by trialing new delivery methods, devices, and patient monitoring. Although maturing, IA vasodilator therapy promises improved outcomes for a highly morbid condition. Protocolized approaches employing a wide range of aggressive diagnostic and therapeutic options are required to improve outcomes beyond small-scale trials.

References

1. Wilkins RH. Cerebral vasospasm. Crit Rev Neurobiol. 1990;6(1):51–77.
2. Bederson JB, Connolly ES Jr, Batjer HH, Dacey RG, Dion JE, Diringer MN, et al. Guidelines for the management of aneurysmal subarachnoid hemorrhage: a statement for healthcare professionals from a special writing group of the Stroke Council, American Heart Association. Stroke. 2009;40(3):994–1025.
3. Cahill J, Calvert JW, Zhang JH. Mechanisms of early brain injury after subarachnoid hemorrhage. J Cereb Blood Flow Metab. 2006;26(11):1341–53.
4. Cahill J, Zhang JH. Subarachnoid hemorrhage: is it time for a new direction? Stroke. 2009;40(3 Suppl):S86–7.
5. Ostrowski RP, Colohan AR, Zhang JH. Mechanisms of hyperbaric oxygen-induced neuroprotection in a rat model of subarachnoid hemorrhage. J Cereb Blood Flow Metab. 2005;25(5):554–71.
6. Voldby B, Enevoldsen EM. Intracranial pressure changes following aneurysm rupture. Part 3: recurrent hemorrhage. J Neurosurg. 1982;56(6):784–9.
7. Budohoski KP, Guilfoyle M, Helmy A, Huuskonen T, Czosnyka M, Kirollos R, et al. The pathophysiology and treatment of delayed cerebral ischaemia following subarachnoid haemorrhage. J Neurol Neurosurg Psychiatry. 2014;85(12):1343–53.
8. Macdonald RL. Delayed neurological deterioration after subarachnoid haemorrhage. Nat Rev Neurol. 2014;10(1):44–58.
9. Rabinstein AA, Friedman JA, Weigand SD, McClelland RL, Fulgham JR, Manno EM, et al. Predictors of cerebral infarction in aneurysmal subarachnoid hemorrhage. Stroke. 2004;35(8):1862–6.
10. Suarez JI. Diagnosis and management of subarachnoid hemorrhage. Continuum (Minneap Minn). 2015;21(5 Neurocritical Care):1263–87.
11. Wilkins RH. Aneurysm rupture during angiography: does acute vasospasm occur? Surg Neurol. 1976;5(5):299–303.
12. Charpentier C, Audibert G, Guillemin F, Civit T, Ducrocq X, Bracard S, et al. Multivariate analysis of predictors of cerebral vasospasm occurrence after aneurysmal subarachnoid hemorrhage. Stroke. 1999;30(7):1402–8.
13. Fisher CM, Kistler JP, Davis JM. Relation of cerebral vasospasm to subarachnoid hemorrhage visualized by computerized tomographic scanning. Neurosurgery. 1980;6(1):1–9.
14. Hop JW, Rinkel GJ, Algra A, van Gijn J. Initial loss of consciousness and risk of delayed cerebral ischemia after aneurysmal subarachnoid hemorrhage. Stroke. 1999;30(11):2268–71.
15. Inagawa T, Yahara K, Ohbayashi N. Risk factors associated with cerebral vasospasm following aneurysmal subarachnoid hemorrhage. Neurol Med Chir (Tokyo). 2014;54(6):465–73.
16. van Gijn J, Kerr RS, Rinkel GJ. Subarachnoid haemorrhage. Lancet. 2007;369(9558):306–18.
17. Hop JW, Rinkel GJ, Algra A, van Gijn J. Case-fatality rates and functional outcome after subarachnoid hemorrhage: a systematic review. Stroke. 1997;28(3):660–4.
18. Mackey J, Khoury JC, Alwell K, Moomaw CJ, Kissela BM, Flaherty ML, et al. Stable incidence but declining case-fatality rates of subarachnoid hemorrhage in a population. Neurology. 2016;87(21):2192–7.
19. Naidech AM, Janjua N, Kreiter KT, Ostapkovich ND, Fitzsimmons BF, Parra A, et al. Predictors and impact of aneurysm rebleeding after subarachnoid hemorrhage. Arch Neurol. 2005;62(3):410–6.
20. Hop JW, Rinkel GJ, Algra A, van Gijn J. Quality of life in patients and partners after aneurysmal subarachnoid hemorrhage. Stroke. 1998;29(4):798–804.
21. Li K, Barras CD, Chandra RV, Kok HK, Maingard JT, Carter NS, et al. A review of the management of cerebral vasospasm after aneurysmal subarachnoid hemorrhage. World Neurosurg. 2019;126:513–27.
22. Vatter H, Guresir E, Konig R, Durner G, Kalff R, Schuss P, et al. Invasive diagnostic and therapeutic management of cerebral vasospasm after aneurysmal subarachnoid hemorrhage (IMCVS)-a phase 2 randomized controlled trial. J Clin Med. 2022;11(20):6197.
23. Dehdashti AR, Mermillod B, Rufenacht DA, Reverdin A, de Tribolet N. Does treatment modality of intracranial ruptured aneurysms influence the incidence of cerebral vasospasm and clinical outcome? Cerebrovasc Dis. 2004;17(1):53–60.
24. Dankbaar JW, Rijsdijk M, van der Schaaf IC, Velthuis BK, Wermer MJ, Rinkel GJ. Relationship between vasospasm, cerebral perfusion, and delayed cerebral ischemia after aneurysmal subarachnoid hemorrhage. Neuroradiology. 2009;51(12):813–9.
25. Crowley RW, Medel R, Dumont AS, Ilodigwe D, Kassell NF, Mayer SA, et al. Angiographic vasospasm is strongly correlated with cerebral infarction after subarachnoid hemorrhage. Stroke. 2011;42(4):919–23.
26. Etminan N, Vergouwen MD, Ilodigwe D, Macdonald RL. Effect of pharmaceutical treatment on vasospasm, delayed cerebral ischemia, and clinical outcome in patients with aneurysmal subarachnoid hemorrhage: a systematic review and meta-analysis. J Cereb Blood Flow Metab. 2011;31(6):1443–51.
27. Petruk KC, West M, Mohr G, Weir BK, Benoit BG, Gentili F, et al. Nimodipine treatment in poor-grade aneurysm patients. Results of a multicenter double-blind placebo-controlled trial. J Neurosurg. 1988;68(4):505–17.

28. Pickard JD, Murray GD, Illingworth R, Shaw MD, Teasdale GM, Foy PM, et al. Effect of oral nimodipine on cerebral infarction and outcome after subarachnoid haemorrhage: British aneurysm nimodipine trial. BMJ. 1989;298(6674):636–42.
29. Rinkel GJ, Feigin VL, Algra A, van den Bergh WM, Vermeulen M, van Gijn J. Calcium antagonists for aneurysmal subarachnoid haemorrhage. Cochrane Database Syst Rev. 2005;(1):CD000277.
30. Fassbender K, Hodapp B, Rossol S, Bertsch T, Schmeck J, Schutt S, et al. Inflammatory cytokines in subarachnoid haemorrhage: association with abnormal blood flow velocities in basal cerebral arteries. J Neurol Neurosurg Psychiatry. 2001;70(4):534–7.
31. Fedina L, Pasztor E, Kocsis B, Berta Z. Activity of peripheral sympathetic efferent nerves in experimental subarachnoid haemorrhage. Part II: observations during the "early vasospasm" period. Acta Neurochir (Wien). 1986;80(1–2):42–6.
32. Dodd WS, Laurent D, Dumont AS, Hasan DM, Jabbour PM, Starke RM, et al. Pathophysiology of delayed cerebral ischemia after subarachnoid hemorrhage: a review. J Am Heart Assoc. 2021;10(15):e021845.
33. Juvela S. Plasma endothelin concentrations after aneurysmal subarachnoid hemorrhage. J Neurosurg. 2000;92(3):390–400.
34. Peeyush Kumar T, McBride DW, Dash PK, Matsumura K, Rubi A, Blackburn SL. Endothelial cell dysfunction and injury in subarachnoid hemorrhage. Mol Neurobiol. 2019;56(3):1992–2006.
35. Griffith TM, Edwards DH, Lewis MJ, Newby AC, Henderson AH. The nature of endothelium-derived vascular relaxant factor. Nature. 1984;308(5960):645–7.
36. Pluta RM, Afshar JK, Boock RJ, Oldfield EH. Temporal changes in perivascular concentrations of oxyhemoglobin, deoxyhemoglobin, and methemoglobin after subarachnoid hemorrhage. J Neurosurg. 1998;88(3):557–61.
37. Toda N. Mechanisms of contracting action of oxyhemoglobin in isolated monkey and dog cerebral arteries. Am J Physiol. 1990;258(1 Pt 2):H57–63.
38. Handa Y, Weir BK, Nosko M, Mosewich R, Tsuji T, Grace M. The effect of timing of clot removal on chronic vasospasm in a primate model. J Neurosurg. 1987;67(4):558–64.
39. Aoki T, Takenaka K, Suzuki S, Kassell NF, Sagher O, Lee KS. The role of hemolysate in the facilitation of oxyhemoglobin-induced contraction in rabbit basilar arteries. J Neurosurg. 1994;81(2):261–6.
40. Kim-Shapiro DB, Schechter AN, Gladwin MT. Unraveling the reactions of nitric oxide, nitrite, and hemoglobin in physiology and therapeutics. Arterioscler Thromb Vasc Biol. 2006;26(4):697–705.
41. Sabri M, Ai J, Knight B, Tariq A, Jeon H, Shang X, et al. Uncoupling of endothelial nitric oxide synthase after experimental subarachnoid hemorrhage. J Cereb Blood Flow Metab. 2011;31(1):190–9.
42. Hunt WE, Hess RM. Surgical risk as related to time of intervention in the repair of intracranial aneurysms. J Neurosurg. 1968;28(1):14–20.
43. Connolly ES Jr, Rabinstein AA, Carhuapoma JR, Derdeyn CP, Dion J, Higashida RT, et al. Guidelines for the management of aneurysmal subarachnoid hemorrhage: a guideline for healthcare professionals from the American Heart Association/American Stroke Association. Stroke. 2012;43(6):1711–37.
44. Diringer MN, Bleck TP, Claude Hemphill J 3rd, Menon D, Shutter L, Vespa P, et al. Critical care management of patients following aneurysmal subarachnoid hemorrhage: recommendations from the Neurocritical Care Society's Multidisciplinary Consensus Conference. Neurocrit Care. 2011;15(2):211–40.
45. Chou SH. Subarachnoid hemorrhage. Continuum (Minneap Minn). 2021;27(5):1201–45.
46. Geraghty JR, Testai FD. Delayed cerebral ischemia after subarachnoid hemorrhage: beyond vasospasm and towards a multifactorial pathophysiology. Curr Atheroscler Rep. 2017;19(12):50.
47. Yoon DY, Choi CS, Kim KH, Cho BM. Multidetector-row CT angiography of cerebral vasospasm after aneurysmal subarachnoid hemorrhage: comparison of volume-rendered images and digital subtraction angiography. AJNR Am J Neuroradiol. 2006;27(2):370–7.
48. Chaudhary SR, Ko N, Dillon WP, Yu MB, Liu S, Criqui GI, et al. Prospective evaluation of multidetector-row CT angiography for the diagnosis of vasospasm following subarachnoid hemorrhage: a comparison with digital subtraction angiography. Cerebrovasc Dis. 2008;25(1–2):144–50.
49. Osgood ML. Aneurysmal subarachnoid hemorrhage: review of the pathophysiology and management strategies. Curr Neurol Neurosci Rep. 2021;21(9):50.
50. Mir DI, Gupta A, Dunning A, Puchi L, Robinson CL, Epstein HA, et al. CT perfusion for detection of delayed cerebral ischemia in aneurysmal subarachnoid hemorrhage: a systematic review and meta-analysis. AJNR Am J Neuroradiol. 2014;35(5):866–71.
51. Carlson AP, Yonas H. Radiographic assessment of vasospasm after aneurysmal subarachnoid hemorrhage: the physiological perspective. Neurol Res. 2009;31(6):593–604.
52. Grandin CB, Cosnard G, Hammer F, Duprez TP, Stroobandt G, Mathurin P. Vasospasm after subarachnoid hemorrhage: diagnosis with MR angiography. AJNR Am J Neuroradiol. 2000;21(9):1611–7.
53. Mills JN, Mehta V, Russin J, Amar AP, Rajamohan A, Mack WJ. Advanced imaging modalities in the detection of cerebral vasospasm. Neurol Res Int. 2013;2013:415960.
54. Oelerich M, Lentschig MG, Zunker P, Reimer P, Rummeny EJ, Schuierer G. Intracranial vascular stenosis and occlusion: comparison of 3D time-of-flight and 3D phase-contrast MR angiography. Neuroradiology. 1998;40(9):567–73.
55. Dreier JP, Woitzik J, Fabricius M, Bhatia R, Major S, Drenckhahn C, et al. Delayed ischaemic neurological deficits after subarachnoid haemorrhage are associated with clusters of spreading depolarizations. Brain. 2006;129(Pt 12):3224–37.
56. Kosnik EJ, Hunt WE. Postoperative hypertension in the management of patients with intracranial arterial aneurysms. J Neurosurg. 1976;45(2):148–54.
57. Egge A, Waterloo K, Sjoholm H, Solberg T, Ingebrigtsen T, Romner B. Prophylactic hyperdynamic postoperative fluid therapy after aneurysmal subarachnoid hemorrhage: a clinical, prospective, randomized, controlled study. Neurosurgery. 2001;49(3):593–605; discussion -6.
58. Lennihan L, Mayer SA, Fink ME, Beckford A, Paik MC, Zhang H, et al. Effect of hypervolemic therapy on cerebral blood flow after subarachnoid hemorrhage: a randomized controlled trial. Stroke. 2000;31(2):383–91.
59. Gathier CS, van den Bergh WM, van der Jagt M, Verweij BH, Dankbaar JW, Muller MC, et al. Induced hypertension for delayed cerebral ischemia after aneurysmal subarachnoid hemorrhage: a randomized clinical trial. Stroke. 2018;49(1):76–83.
60. Rajajee V, Pandey AS, Williamson CA. Subarachnoid hemorrhage and therapy formerly known as "triple-H"—new directions. World Neurosurg. 2019;127:500–1.
61. Allen GS, Ahn HS, Preziosi TJ, Battye R, Boone SC, Boone SC, et al. Cerebral arterial spasm—a controlled trial of nimodipine in patients with subarachnoid hemorrhage. N Engl J Med. 1983;308(11):619–24.
62. Norbeck JS, Weinert C, Cardea JM, Lenz ER. [Social support. Commentaries]. Kango Kenkyu. 1987;20(4):370–379.
63. Haley EC Jr, Kassell NF, Torner JC. A randomized controlled trial of high-dose intravenous nicardipine in aneurysmal subarach-

noid hemorrhage. A report of the Cooperative Aneurysm Study. J Neurosurg. 1993;78(4):537–47.
64. Seifert V, Loffler BM, Zimmermann M, Roux S, Stolke D. Endothelin concentrations in patients with aneurysmal subarachnoid hemorrhage. Correlation with cerebral vasospasm, delayed ischemic neurological deficits, and volume of hematoma. J Neurosurg. 1995;82(1):55–62.
65. Macdonald RL, Higashida RT, Keller E, Mayer SA, Molyneux A, Raabe A, et al. Clazosentan, an endothelin receptor antagonist, in patients with aneurysmal subarachnoid haemorrhage undergoing surgical clipping: a randomised, double-blind, placebo-controlled phase 3 trial (CONSCIOUS-2). Lancet Neurol. 2011;10(7):618–25.
66. Macdonald RL, Higashida RT, Keller E, Mayer SA, Molyneux A, Raabe A, et al. Randomized trial of clazosentan in patients with aneurysmal subarachnoid hemorrhage undergoing endovascular coiling. Stroke. 2012;43(6):1463–9.
67. Macdonald RL, Kassell NF, Mayer S, Ruefenacht D, Schmiedek P, Weidauer S, et al. Clazosentan to overcome neurological ischemia and infarction occurring after subarachnoid hemorrhage (CONSCIOUS-1): randomized, double-blind, placebo-controlled phase 2 dose-finding trial. Stroke. 2008;39(11):3015–21.
68. Khaldi A, Zauner A, Reinert M, Woodward JJ, Bullock MR. Measurement of nitric oxide and brain tissue oxygen tension in patients after severe subarachnoid hemorrhage. Neurosurgery. 2001;49(1):33–8; discussion 8–40.
69. Sehba FA, Schwartz AY, Chereshnev I, Bederson JB. Acute decrease in cerebral nitric oxide levels after subarachnoid hemorrhage. J Cereb Blood Flow Metab. 2000;20(3):604–11.
70. Furchgott RF, Zawadzki JV. The obligatory role of endothelial cells in the relaxation of arterial smooth muscle by acetylcholine. Nature. 1980;288(5789):373–6.
71. Abulhasan YB, Ortiz Jimenez J, Teitelbaum J, Simoneau G, Angle MR. Milrinone for refractory cerebral vasospasm with delayed cerebral ischemia. J Neurosurg. 2020;134(3):971–82.
72. Joshi S, Meyers PM, Pile-Spellman J, Wang M, Sahlein DH. Intracarotid verapamil decreases both proximal and distal human cerebrovascular resistance. Anesthesiology. 2004;100(4):774–81.
73. Boulouis G, Labeyrie MA, Raymond J, Rodriguez-Regent C, Lukaszewicz AC, Bresson D, et al. Treatment of cerebral vasospasm following aneurysmal subarachnoid haemorrhage: a systematic review and meta-analysis. Eur Radiol. 2017;27(8):3333–42.
74. Andereggen L, Beck J, Z'Graggen WJ, Schroth G, Andres RH, Murek M, et al. Feasibility and safety of repeat instant endovascular interventions in patients with refractory cerebral vasospasms. AJNR Am J Neuroradiol. 2017;38(3):561–7.
75. McGuinness B, Gandhi D. Endovascular management of cerebral vasospasm. Neurosurg Clin N Am. 2010;21(2):281–90.
76. Pierot L, Aggour M, Moret J. Vasospasm after aneurysmal subarachnoid hemorrhage: recent advances in endovascular management. Curr Opin Crit Care. 2010;16(2):110–6.
77. Rowland MJ, Hadjipavlou G, Kelly M, Westbrook J, Pattinson KT. Delayed cerebral ischaemia after subarachnoid haemorrhage: looking beyond vasospasm. Br J Anaesth. 2012;109(3):315–29.
78. Stiefel MF, Spiotta AM, Udoetuk JD, Maloney-Wilensky E, Weigele JB, Hurst RW, et al. Intra-arterial papaverine used to treat cerebral vasospasm reduces brain oxygen. Neurocrit Care. 2006;4(2):113–8.
79. Kieninger M, Flessa J, Lindenberg N, Bele S, Redel A, Schneiker A, et al. Side effects of long-term continuous intra-arterial nimodipine infusion in patients with severe refractory cerebral vasospasm after subarachnoid hemorrhage. Neurocrit Care. 2018;28(1):65–76.
80. Abruzzo T, Moran C, Blackham KA, Eskey CJ, Lev R, Meyers P, et al. Invasive interventional management of post-hemorrhagic cerebral vasospasm in patients with aneurysmal subarachnoid hemorrhage. J Neurointerv Surg. 2012;4(3):169–77.
81. Hoh BL, Ogilvy CS. Endovascular treatment of cerebral vasospasm: transluminal balloon angioplasty, intra-arterial papaverine, and intra-arterial nicardipine. Neurosurg Clin N Am. 2005;16(3):501–16, vi.
82. Lopez-Rueda A, Vargas A, Pinana C, Chirife O, Werner M, Aja L, et al. Angioplasty with a retrievable stent to treat vasospasm secondary to subarachnoid hemorrhage due to an aneurysm: a multicenter study of safety and efficacy. Radiologia (Engl Ed). 2022;64(2):103–9.
83. Pandey AS, Elias AE, Chaudhary N, Thompson BG, Gemmete JJ. Endovascular treatment of cerebral vasospasm: vasodilators and angioplasty. Neuroimaging Clin N Am. 2013;23(4):593–604.
84. Lannes M, Zeiler F, Guichon C, Teitelbaum J. The use of Milrinone in patients with delayed cerebral ischemia following subarachnoid hemorrhage: a systematic review. Can J Neurol Sci. 2017;44(2):152–60.
85. Doczi T. The pathogenetic and prognostic significance of blood-brain barrier damage at the acute stage of aneurysmal subarachnoid haemorrhage. Clinical and experimental studies. Acta Neurochir (Wien). 1985;77(3–4):110–32.
86. Doczi T, Joo F, Adam G, Bozoky B, Szerdahelyi P. Blood-brain barrier damage during the acute stage of subarachnoid hemorrhage, as exemplified by a new animal model. Neurosurgery. 1986;18(6):733–9.
87. Doczi T, Joo F, Sonkodi S, Adam G. Increased vulnerability of the blood-brain barrier to experimental subarachnoid hemorrhage in spontaneously hypertensive rats. Stroke. 1986;17(3):498–501.
88. Pradilla G, Chaichana KL, Hoang S, Huang J, Tamargo RJ. Inflammation and cerebral vasospasm after subarachnoid hemorrhage. Neurosurg Clin N Am. 2010;21(2):365–79.
89. Fassbender K, Hodapp B, Rossol S, Bertsch T, Schmeck J, Schutt S, et al. Endothelin-1 in subarachnoid hemorrhage: an acute-phase reactant produced by cerebrospinal fluid leukocytes. Stroke. 2000;31(12):2971–5.
90. Sriram S, Cutler C, Azab M, Reddy R, Peart R, Lucke-Wold B. Neuroinflammation and subarachnoid hemorrhage: a revised look at the literature. Clin Res Commun. 2022;5(3):14.
91. Wanderer S, Andereggen L, Mrosek J, Kashefiolasl S, Schubert GA, Marbacher S, et al. Levosimendan as a therapeutic strategy to prevent neuroinflammation after aneurysmal subarachnoid hemorrhage? J Neurointerv Surg. 2022;14(4):408–12.
92. Xiao Y, Li G, Chen Y, Zuo Y, Rashid K, He T, et al. Milk fat globule-epidermal growth Factor-8 pretreatment attenuates apoptosis and inflammation via the integrin-beta3 pathway after surgical brain injury in rats. Front Neurol. 2018;9:96.
93. Bindra A, Prabhakar H, Singh GP. Stellate ganglion block for relieving vasospasms after coil embolization of basilar tip aneurysms. J Neurosurg Anesthesiol. 2011;23(4):379.
94. Prabhakar H, Jain V, Rath GP, Bithal PK, Dash HH. Stellate ganglion block as alternative to intrathecal papaverine in relieving vasospasm due to subarachnoid hemorrhage. Anesth Analg. 2007;104(5):1311–2.
95. Treggiari MM, Romand JA, Martin JB, Reverdin A, Rufenacht DA, de Tribolet N. Cervical sympathetic block to reverse delayed ischemic neurological deficits after aneurysmal subarachnoid hemorrhage. Stroke. 2003;34(4):961–7.
96. Tuor UI. Local distribution of the effects of sympathetic stimulation on cerebral blood flow in the rat. Brain Res. 1990;529(1–2):224–31.
97. Kurth CD, Wagerle LC, Delivoria-Papadopoulos M. Sympathetic regulation of cerebral blood flow during seizures in newborn lambs. Am J Physiol. 1988;255(3 Pt 2):H563–8.

98. Edvinsson L. Neurogenic mechanisms in the cerebrovascular bed. Autonomic nerves, amine receptors and their effects on cerebral blood flow. Acta Physiol Scand Suppl. 1975;427:1–35.
99. Jain V, Rath GP, Dash HH, Bithal PK, Chouhan RS, Suri A. Stellate ganglion block for treatment of cerebral vasospasm in patients with aneurysmal subarachnoid hemorrhage—A preliminary study. J Anaesthesiol Clin Pharmacol. 2011;27(4):516–21.
100. Jing L, Wu Y, Liang F, Jian M, Bai Y, Wang Y, et al. Effect of early stellate ganglion block in cerebral vasospasm after aneurysmal subarachnoid hemorrhage (BLOCK-CVS): study protocol for a randomized controlled trial. Trials. 2022;23(1):922.
101. Hirashima Y, Kurimoto M, Hayashi N, Umemura K, Hori E, Origasa H, et al. Duration of cerebrospinal fluid drainage in patients with aneurysmal subarachnoid hemorrhage for prevention of symptomatic vasospasm and late hydrocephalus. Neurol Med Chir (Tokyo). 2005;45(4):177–82; discussion 82–3.
102. Hoekema D, Schmidt RH, Ross I. Lumbar drainage for subarachnoid hemorrhage: technical considerations and safety analysis. Neurocrit Care. 2007;7(1):3–9.
103. Qian C, Yu X, Chen J, Gu C, Wang L, Chen G, et al. Effect of the drainage of cerebrospinal fluid in patients with aneurismal subarachnoid hemorrhage: a meta-analysis. Medicine (Baltimore). 2016;95(41):e5140.
104. Borkar SA, Singh M, Kale SS, Suri A, Chandra PS, Kumar R, et al. Spinal cerebrospinal fluid drainage for prevention of vasospasm in aneurysmal subarachnoid hemorrhage: a prospective, randomized controlled study. Asian J Neurosurg. 2018;13(2):238–46.
105. Al-Tamimi YZ, Bhargava D, Feltbower RG, Hall G, Goddard AJ, Quinn AC, et al. Lumbar drainage of cerebrospinal fluid after aneurysmal subarachnoid hemorrhage: a prospective, randomized, controlled trial (LUMAS). Stroke. 2012;43(3):677–82.
106. Hulou MM, Essibayi MA, Benet A, Lawton MT. Lumbar drainage after aneurysmal subarachnoid hemorrhage: a systematic review and meta-analysis. World Neurosurg. 2022;166:261–7.e9.
107. Daou BJ, Koduri S, Thompson BG, Chaudhary N, Pandey AS. Clinical and experimental aspects of aneurysmal subarachnoid hemorrhage. CNS Neurosci Ther. 2019;25(10):1096–112.
108. Bashir A, Andresen M, Bartek J Jr, Cortsen M, Eskesen V, Wagner A. Intra-arterial nimodipine for cerebral vasospasm after subarachnoid haemorrhage: influence on clinical course and predictors of clinical outcome. Neuroradiol J. 2016;29(1):72–81.
109. Jain S, Sinha AK, Goyal S. Evaluation of intra-arterial Nimodipine therapy in post-subarachnoid hemorrhage refractory cerebral vasospasm. Cardiol Cardiovasc Med. 2022;6(4):383–9.
110. Fraticelli AT, Cholley BP, Losser MR, Saint Maurice JP, Payen D. Milrinone for the treatment of cerebral vasospasm after aneurysmal subarachnoid hemorrhage. Stroke. 2008;39(3):893–8.
111. Duman E, Karakoc F, Pinar HU, Dogan R, Firat A, Yildirim E. Higher dose intra-arterial milrinone and intra-arterial combined milrinone-nimodipine infusion as a rescue therapy for refractory cerebral vasospasm. Interv Neuroradiol. 2017;23(6):636–43.
112. Feng L, Fitzsimmons BF, Young WL, Berman MF, Lin E, Aagaard BD, et al. Intraarterially administered verapamil as adjunct therapy for cerebral vasospasm: safety and 2-year experience. AJNR Am J Neuroradiol. 2002;23(8):1284–90.
113. Mazumdar A, Rivet DJ, Derdeyn CP, Cross DT 3rd, Moran CJ. Effect of intraarterial verapamil on the diameter of vasospastic intracranial arteries in patients with cerebral vasospasm. Neurosurg Focus. 2006;21(3):E15.
114. Barbosa S, Jorge N, Silva ML, Maia I, Dias C, Pereira E, et al. Treatment of cerebral vasospasm with continuous intra-arterial nimodipine: a case report. Cureus. 2022;14(10):e30507.
115. Albanese E, Russo A, Quiroga M, Willis RN Jr, Mericle RA, Ulm AJ. Ultrahigh-dose intraarterial infusion of verapamil through an indwelling microcatheter for medically refractory severe vasospasm: initial experience. Clinical article. J Neurosurg. 2010;113(4):913–22.
116. Joshi S, Young WL, Pile-Spellman J, Fogarty-Mack P, Sciacca RR, Hacein-Bey L, et al. Intra-arterial nitrovasodilators do not increase cerebral blood flow in angiographically normal territories of arteriovenous malformation patients. Stroke. 1997;28(6):1115–22.
117. Musahl C, Henkes H, Vajda Z, Coburger J, Hopf N. Continuous local intra-arterial nimodipine administration in severe symptomatic vasospasm after subarachnoid hemorrhage. Neurosurgery. 2011;68(6):1541–7; discussion 7.
118. Chen PR, Bulsara K, Lopez-Rivera V, Sheriff FG, Sanzgiri A, Sheth S, et al. Use of single versus multiple vasodilator agents in the treatment of cerebral vasospasm: is more better than less? Acta Neurochir (Wien). 2021;163(1):161–8.
119. Woodford H, Taylor M, Eftekhar B, Waugh R, Chaganti J. Dual intra-arterial vasodilators in the management of post-aneurysmal subarachnoid haemorrhage vasospasm. Interdiscip Neurosurg. 2022;27:101442.
120. Daftari Besheli L, Tan CO, Bell DL, Hirsch JA, Gupta R. Temporal evolution of vasospasm and clinical outcome after intra-arterial vasodilator therapy in patients with aneurysmal subarachnoid hemorrhage. PLoS One. 2017;12(3):e0174676.
121. Shah QA, Memon MZ, Suri MF, Rodriguez GJ, Kozak OS, Taylor RA, et al. Super-selective intra-arterial magnesium sulfate in combination with nicardipine for the treatment of cerebral vasospasm in patients with subarachnoid hemorrhage. Neurocrit Care. 2009;11(2):190–8.
122. Gatto LAM, Gallo BHD, Koppe GL, Demartini Z. Chemical angioplasty with nitroglycerin for vasospasm after subarachnoid hemorrhage: case series and review. Arq Bras Neurocir. 2022;41(1):e58–69.
123. Ortiz M, Nunna RS, Ravipati K, Tran A, Qureshi AI, Siddiq F. The role of parenteral dantrolene in the contemporary management of cerebral vasospasm in aneurysmal subarachnoid hemorrhage: a systematic review. World Neurosurg. 2022;161:e602–e7.
124. Yoshida K, Watanabe H, Nakamura S. Intraarterial injection of amrinone for vasospasm induced by subarachnoid hemorrhage. AJNR Am J Neuroradiol. 1997;18(3):492–6.
125. Seker F, Hesser J, Neumaier-Probst E, Groden C, Brockmann MA, Schubert R, et al. Dose-response relationship of locally applied nimodipine in an ex vivo model of cerebral vasospasm. Neuroradiology. 2013;55(1):71–6.
126. Firat MM, Gelebek V, Orer HS, Belen D, Firat AK, Balkanci F. Selective intraarterial nimodipine treatment in an experimental subarachnoid hemorrhage model. AJNR Am J Neuroradiol. 2005;26(6):1357–62.
127. Seker F, Hesser J, Brockmann MA, Neumaier-Probst E, Groden C, Schubert R, et al. Pharmacokinetic modeling of intra-arterial nimodipine therapy for subarachnoid hemorrhage-related cerebral vasospasm. Clin Neuroradiol. 2017;27(2):199–203.
128. Alotaibi NM, Wang JZ, Pasarikovski CR, Guha D, Al-Mufti F, Mamdani M, et al. Management of raised intracranial pressure in aneurysmal subarachnoid hemorrhage: time for a consensus? Neurosurg Focus. 2017;43(5):E13.
129. Oddo M, Hutchinson PJ. Understanding and monitoring brain injury: the role of cerebral microdialysis. Intensive Care Med. 2018;44(11):1945–8.
130. Helbok R, Kofler M, Schiefecker AJ, Gaasch M, Rass V, Pfausler B, et al. Clinical use of cerebral microdialysis in patients with aneurysmal subarachnoid hemorrhage-state of the art. Front Neurol. 2017;8:565.
131. Sandsmark DK, Kumar MA, Park S, Levine JM. Multimodal monitoring in subarachnoid hemorrhage. Stroke. 2012;43(5):1440–5.
132. Stiefel MF, Spiotta A, Gracias VH, Garuffe AM, Guillamondegui O, Maloney-Wilensky E, et al. Reduced mortality rate in patients

with severe traumatic brain injury treated with brain tissue oxygen monitoring. J Neurosurg. 2005;103(5):805–11.
133. De Georgia MA. Brain tissue oxygen monitoring in neurocritical care. J Intensive Care Med. 2015;30(8):473–83.
134. Chen HI, Stiefel MF, Oddo M, Milby AH, Maloney-Wilensky E, Frangos S, et al. Detection of cerebral compromise with multimodality monitoring in patients with subarachnoid hemorrhage. Neurosurgery. 2011;69(1):53–63; discussion.
135. Albanna W, Weiss M, Muller M, Brockmann MA, Rieg A, Conzen C, et al. Endovascular rescue therapies for refractory vasospasm after subarachnoid hemorrhage: a prospective evaluation study using multimodal, continuous event neuromonitoring. Neurosurgery. 2017;80(6):942–9.
136. Highton D, Elwell C, Smith M. Noninvasive cerebral oximetry: is there light at the end of the tunnel? Curr Opin Anaesthesiol. 2010;23(5):576–81.
137. Zweifel C, Castellani G, Czosnyka M, Helmy A, Manktelow A, Carrera E, et al. Noninvasive monitoring of cerebrovascular reactivity with near infrared spectroscopy in head-injured patients. J Neurotrauma. 2010;27(11):1951–8.
138. Naidech AM, Bendok BR, Ault ML, Bleck TP. Monitoring with the Somanetics INVOS 5100C after aneurysmal subarachnoid hemorrhage. Neurocrit Care. 2008;9(3):326–31.
139. Venkatraman A, Khawaja AM, Gupta S, Hardas S, Deveikis JP, Harrigan MR, et al. Intra-arterial vasodilators for vasospasm following aneurysmal subarachnoid hemorrhage: a meta-analysis. J Neurointerv Surg. 2018;10(4):380–7.
140. Cross DT 3rd, Moran CJ, Angtuaco EE, Milburn JM, Diringer MN, Dacey RG Jr. Intracranial pressure monitoring during intra-arterial papaverine infusion for cerebral vasospasm. AJNR Am J Neuroradiol. 1998;19(7):1319–23.
141. Westhout FD, Nwagwu CI. Intra-arterial verapamil-induced seizures: case report and review of the literature. Surg Neurol. 2007;67(5):483–6; discussion 6.
142. Andaluz N, Tomsick TA, Tew JM Jr, van Loveren HR, Yeh HS, Zuccarello M. Indications for endovascular therapy for refractory vasospasm after aneurysmal subarachnoid hemorrhage: experience at the University of Cincinnati. Surg Neurol. 2002;58(2):131–8; discussion 8.
143. Zwienenberg-Lee M, Hartman J, Rudisill N, Muizelaar JP. Endovascular management of cerebral vasospasm. Neurosurgery. 2006;59(5 Suppl 3):S139–47; discussion S3–13.
144. Badjatia N, Topcuoglu MA, Pryor JC, Rabinov JD, Ogilvy CS, Carter BS, et al. Preliminary experience with intra-arterial nicardipine as a treatment for cerebral vasospasm. AJNR Am J Neuroradiol. 2004;25(5):819–26.
145. Mao G, Gigliotti MJ, Esplin N, Sexton K. The clinical impact and safety profile of high-dose intra-arterial verapamil treatment for cerebral vasospasm following aneurysmal subarachnoid hemorrhage. Clin Neurol Neurosurg. 2021;202:106546.
146. Stuart RM, Helbok R, Kurtz P, Schmidt M, Fernandez L, Lee K, et al. High-dose intra-arterial verapamil for the treatment of cerebral vasospasm after subarachnoid hemorrhage: prolonged effects on hemodynamic parameters and brain metabolism. Neurosurgery. 2011;68(2):337–45; discussion 45.
147. Carhuapoma JR, Qureshi AI, Tamargo RJ, Mathis JM, Hanley DF. Intra-arterial papaverine-induced seizures: case report and review of the literature. Surg Neurol. 2001;56(3):159–63.
148. Ramzan I. Proconvulsant effect of papaverine on theophylline-induced seizures in rats. Clin Exp Pharmacol Physiol. 1989;16(5):425–7.
149. Rahme R, Abruzzo TA, Zuccarello M, Ringer A. Intra-arterial veramil-induced seizures: drug toxicity or rapid reperfusion? Can J Neurol Sci. 2012;39(4):550–2.
150. Mathis JM, Jensen ME, Dion JE. Technical considerations on intra-arterial papaverine hydrochloride for cerebral vasospasm. Neuroradiology. 1997;39(2):90–8.
151. Liu JK, Couldwell WT. Intra-arterial papaverine infusions for the treatment of cerebral vasospasm induced by aneurysmal subarachnoid hemorrhage. Neurocrit Care. 2005;2(2):124–32.
152. Eddleman CS, Hurley MC, Naidech AM, Batjer HH, Bendok BR. Endovascular options in the treatment of delayed ischemic neurological deficits due to cerebral vasospasm. Neurosurg Focus. 2009;26(3):E6.
153. Smith WS, Dowd CF, Johnston SC, Ko NU, DeArmond SJ, Dillon WP, et al. Neurotoxicity of intra-arterial papaverine preserved with chlorobutanol used for the treatment of cerebral vasospasm after aneurysmal subarachnoid hemorrhage. Stroke. 2004;35(11):2518–22.
154. Koenig MA. Management of delayed cerebral ischemia after subarachnoid hemorrhage. Continuum (Minneap Minn). 2012;18(3):579–97.
155. Miller JA, Cross DT, Moran CJ, Dacey RG Jr, McFarland JG, Diringer MN. Severe thrombocytopenia following intraarterial papaverine administration for treatment of vasospasm. J Neurosurg. 1995;83(3):435–7.
156. Bernier TD, Schontz MJ, Izzy S, Chung DY, Nelson SE, Leslie-Mazwi TM, et al. Treatment of subarachnoid hemorrhage-associated delayed cerebral ischemia with milrinone: a review and proposal. J Neurosurg Anesthesiol. 2021;33(3):195–202.
157. Arakawa Y, Kikuta K, Hojo M, Goto Y, Ishii A, Yamagata S. Milrinone for the treatment of cerebral vasospasm after subarachnoid hemorrhage: report of seven cases. Neurosurgery. 2001;48(4):723–8; discussion 8–30.
158. Zubkov YN, Nikiforov BM, Shustin VA. Balloon catheter technique for dilatation of constricted cerebral arteries after aneurysmal SAH. Acta Neurochir (Wien). 1984;70(1–2):65–79.
159. Kimball MM, Velat GJ, Hoh BL, Participants in the International Multi-Disciplinary Consensus Conference on the Critical Care Management of Subarachnoid Hemorrhage. Critical care guidelines on the endovascular management of cerebral vasospasm. Neurocrit Care. 2011;15(2):336–41.
160. Rosenwasser RH, Armonda RA, Thomas JE, Benitez RP, Gannon PM, Harrop J. Therapeutic modalities for the management of cerebral vasospasm: timing of endovascular options. Neurosurgery. 1999;44(5):975–9; discussion 979–80.
161. Zwienenberg-Lee M, Hartman J, Rudisill N, Madden LK, Smith K, Eskridge J, et al. Effect of prophylactic transluminal balloon angioplasty on cerebral vasospasm and outcome in patients with Fisher grade III subarachnoid hemorrhage: results of a phase II multicenter, randomized, clinical trial. Stroke. 2008;39(6):1759–65.
162. Bhogal P, Loh Y, Brouwer P, Andersson T, Soderman M. Treatment of cerebral vasospasm with self-expandable retrievable stents: proof of concept. J Neurointerv Surg. 2017;9(1):52–9.
163. Khanafer A, Cimpoca A, Bhogal P, Bazner H, Ganslandt O, Henkes H. Intracranial stenting as a bail-out option for posthemorrhagic cerebral vasospasm: a single-center experience with long-term follow-up. BMC Neurol. 2022;22(1):351.
164. Kwon HJ, Lim JW, Koh HS, Park B, Choi SW, Kim SH, et al. Stent-retriever angioplasty for recurrent post-subarachnoid hemorrhagic vasospasm—A single center experience with long-term follow-up. Clin Neuroradiol. 2019;29(4):751–61.
165. Bhambri P, Sarvi A, Wong JH, Sundararaj U, Mitha AP. Verapamil eluting stents as a possible treatment for vasospasm after subarachnoid hemorrhage. J Neurointerv Surg. 2017;9(9):875–9.
166. Ota N, Matsukawa H, Kamiyama H, Tsuboi T, Noda K, Hashimoto A, et al. Preventing cerebral vasospasm after aneurysmal sub-

arachnoid hemorrhage with aggressive cisternal clot removal and nicardipine. World Neurosurg. 2017;107:630–40.
167. Mizukami M, Kawase T, Usami T, Tazawa T. Prevention of vasospasm by early operation with removal of subarachnoid blood. Neurosurgery. 1982;10(3):301–7.
168. Gruber P, Singh S, Andereggen L, Berberat J, Remonda L. Drug-coated balloons for the treatment of symptomatic intracranial high-grade stenosis: a review of the current rationale. Front Neurol. 2021;12:692208.
169. Molyneux AJ, Kerr RS, Yu LM, Clarke M, Sneade M, Yarnold JA, et al. International subarachnoid aneurysm trial (ISAT) of neurosurgical clipping versus endovascular coiling in 2143 patients with ruptured intracranial aneurysms: a randomised comparison of effects on survival, dependency, seizures, rebleeding, subgroups, and aneurysm occlusion. Lancet. 2005;366(9488):809–17.
170. Treggiari MM, Rabinstein AA, Busl KM, Caylor MM, Citerio G, Deem S, et al. Guidelines for the neurocritical care management of aneurysmal subarachnoid hemorrhage. Neurocrit Care. 2023;39:1.
171. Kassell NF, Helm G, Simmons N, Phillips CD, Cail WS. Treatment of cerebral vasospasm with intra-arterial papaverine. J Neurosurg. 1992;77(6):848–52.
172. Hejcl A, Cihlar F, Smolka V, Vachata P, Bartos R, Prochazka J, et al. Chemical angioplasty with spasmolytics for vasospasm after subarachnoid hemorrhage. Acta Neurochir (Wien). 2017;159(4):713–20.
173. Biondi A, Ricciardi GK, Puybasset L, Abdennour L, Longo M, Chiras J, et al. Intra-arterial nimodipine for the treatment of symptomatic cerebral vasospasm after aneurysmal subarachnoid hemorrhage: preliminary results. AJNR Am J Neuroradiol. 2004;25(6):1067–76.
174. Joshi S, Ellis JA, Emala CW. Revisiting intra-arterial drug delivery for treating brain diseases or is it "deja-vu, all over again"? J Neuroanaesth Crit Care. 2014;1(2):108–15.
175. Lim J, Cho YD, Kwon HJ, Byoun SH, Koh HS, Park B, et al. Duration of vasodilatory action after intra-arterial infusions of calcium channel blockers in animal model of cerebral vasospasm. Neurocrit Care. 2021;34(3):867–75.
176. Raslan F, Albert-Weissenberger C, Westermaier T, Saker S, Kleinschnitz C, Lee JY. A modified double injection model of cisterna magna for the study of delayed cerebral vasospasm following subarachnoid hemorrhage in rats. Exp Transl Stroke Med. 2012;4(1):23.
177. Altay T, Smithason S, Volokh N, Rasmussen PA, Ransohoff RM, Provencio JJ. A novel method for subarachnoid hemorrhage to induce vasospasm in mice. J Neurosci Methods. 2009;183(2):136–40.
178. Parra A, McGirt MJ, Sheng H, Laskowitz DT, Pearlstein RD, Warner DS. Mouse model of subarachnoid hemorrhage associated cerebral vasospasm: methodological analysis. Neurol Res. 2002;24(5):510–6.
179. van den Bergh WM, Schepers J, Veldhuis WB, Nicolay K, Tulleken CA, Rinkel GJ. Magnetic resonance imaging in experimental subarachnoid haemorrhage. Acta Neurochir (Wien). 2005;147(9):977–83; discussion 83.
180. Hugelshofer M, Buzzi RM, Schaer CA, Richter H, Akeret K, Anagnostakou V, et al. Haptoglobin administration into the subarachnoid space prevents hemoglobin-induced cerebral vasospasm. J Clin Invest. 2019;129(12):5219–35.
181. Chan AY, Choi EH, Yuki I, Suzuki S, Golshani K, Chen JW, et al. Cerebral vasospasm after subarachnoid hemorrhage: developing treatments. Brain Hemorrhages. 2021;2(1):15–23.
182. Pulcrano-Nicolas AS, Jacquens A, Proust C, Clarencon F, Perret C, Shotar E, et al. Whole blood levels of S1PR4 mRNA associated with cerebral vasospasm after aneurysmal subarachnoid hemorrhage. J Neurosurg. 2019;1-5:1837.
183. Pulcrano-Nicolas AS, Proust C, Clarencon F, Jacquens A, Perret C, Roux M, et al. Whole-blood miRNA sequencing profiling for vasospasm in patients with aneurysmal subarachnoid hemorrhage. Stroke. 2018;49(9):2220–3.
184. Walker M, Erdoes MP, Stricker CG, Bothell J, Kelly CM, Levitt MR. Hybrid microcatheter angioplasty for refractory cerebral vasospasm. J Cerebrovasc Endovasc Neurosurg. 2021;23(2):159–68.
185. Badger CA, Jankowitz BT, Shaikh HA. Treatment of cerebral vasospasm secondary to subarachnoid hemorrhage utilizing the Comaneci device. Interv Neuroradiol. 2020;26(5):582–5.
186. Klopp CT, Alford TC, Bateman J, Berry GN, Winship T. Fractionated intra-arterial cancer; chemotherapy with methyl bis amine hydrochloride; a preliminary report. Ann Surg. 1950;132(4):811–32.
187. Wilson CB. Chemotherapy of brain tumors by continuous arterial infusion. Surgery. 1964;55:640–53.
188. Rapoport SI, Hori M, Klatzo I. Reversible osmotic opening of the blood-brain barrier. Science. 1971;173(4001):1026–8.

11 Lessons from Intra-arterial Chemotherapy for Retinoblastoma

Kyle Zappi, Gary Kocharian, Jasmine H. Francis, David H. Abramson, and Y. Pierre Gobin

Excellence is never an accident. It is always the result of high intention, sincere effort, and intelligent execution; it represents the wise choice of many alternatives—choice, not chance, determines your destiny.

Aristotle (384–322 BCE), Greek Philosopher and Polymath

Introduction

Retinoblastoma (RB) is a common ocular malignancy of childhood, typically diagnosed at a median age of 18 months. Intraarterial chemotherapy of retinoblastoma is a widely accepted application of arterial drug delivery. Even though endovascular interventions in pediatric patients can be technically challenging due to the small size of vessels, the RB treatment has succeeded with a salvage rate of 66–95%. The primary reasons for the success of RB treatment have been the ability to deliver it selectively to the tumor that is principally perfused by the ophthalmic artery, inject the drug as pulses, safely employ blood flow control when needed, and the availability of potent therapeutic agents. This chapter describes the state of RB treatment and what can be applied to treating other neurological diseases.

K. Zappi
Department of Neurological Surgery, Weil Cornell Medicine, New York, NY, USA

G. Kocharian
Department of Neurological Surgery, Weil Cornell Medicine, New York, NY, USA

Division of Interventional Neuroradiology, Weill Cornell Medicine, New York Presbyterian Hospital, New York, NY, USA,

J. H. Francis · D. H. Abramson
Department of Ophthalmic Oncology, Memorial Sloan Kettering Cancer Center, New York, NY, USA,

Y. P. Gobin (✉)
Division of Interventional Neuroradiology, Weill Cornell Medicine, New York Presbyterian Hospital, New York, NY, USA,
e-mail: yvg2001@med.cornell.edu

Retinoblastoma

Retinoblastoma (RB) is a malignancy of the retinal tissues. It is the most common primary ocular malignancy in childhood and comprises approximately 4% of childhood cancers [1]. RB has an incidence of 1 in every 15,000–20,000 live births [2, 3], and in the United States, approximately 300 patients are diagnosed with RB yearly [1]. RB frequently occurs in younger children with a median age of diagnosis of 18 months [2, 4]. Seventy-five percent of children have only one eye affected; 15% of unilateral cases have germline RB1 mutations, most commonly not inherited from a parent. All cases of bilateral and multifocal unilateral RB are germline [2]. The germline form of RB represents approximately 55% of the cases, with the remaining 45% being sporadic [5]. There are rare cases of retinoblastoma that are wildtype *RB1* and instead are driven by N-myc amplification.

RB is of unique significance in the field of genetic oncology. In the early 1970s, it was hypothesized that RB is caused by two (or more) mutational events [6], which was confirmed more than a decade later when it became the first cancer tumor suppressor gene identified and cloned [2]. This revealed that the loss or mutations of both alleles of the retinoblastoma gene (RB1) are required to develop the disease, and this can be somatic or associated with germline RB abnormalities. Germline RB has a penetrance rate of more than 90% [1], necessitating the importance of screening in patients with a familial history of RB [4].

Retinoblastoma usually presents with signs, not symptoms. The most common clinical manifestations of RB include leukocoria, the characteristic "white reflex" seen upon direct illu-

S. Joshi (ed.), *Arterial Treatment of Neurological Diseases*, https://doi.org/10.1007/978-3-031-80173-0_11

mination of the pupil, strabismus, hypopyon, hyphema, enlargement of the orbit, and iris rubeosis or neovascularization of the iris. Proptosis and exophthalmos may occur in later disease progression and typically signify extraocular infiltration [2, 7]. Metastasis of Rb can occur through direct extension through the wall of the eye (common worldwide but rare in the USA) and extension into the optic nerve with CNS or hematogenous spread. Patient survival rates are 99%, and RB is usually curable if treated up to 6 months after initial symptom onset. Delays in diagnosis are associated with a worse prognosis [1].

Historical Treatment of Retinoblastoma

Enucleation has been the most common treatment for advanced RB, especially for tumors that are large with vitreous seeding. Enucleation is an effective strategy, and for most of the twentieth century in the USA, it was the primary way unilateral and some bilateral patients were managed. Still, enucleation is associated with a 3.9% rate of metastatic spread and an overall survival of 98% [8, 9]. In 1903, the first eye with RB was treated by Hilgartner with radiation without the need for enucleation. RB was discovered to be an extremely radiosensitive tumor, ushering in the use of external beam radiotherapy (EBRT) [10, 11] Carl Kupfer 1953 successfully treated RB using nitrogen mustard [12]. During the 1990s, systemic chemotherapy replaced EBRT due to the latter affecting orbitofacial growth and long-term visual deficits secondary to radiation retinopathy [7, 13], cosmetic deformity, cataracts, radiation retinopathy, and vitreous hemorrhage occurs in most patients receiving EBRT [14–16]. Most notably, EBRT also increased the risk of mortality from a second neoplasm by inducing additional somatic mutations in the RB1 gene, which has caused more deaths than primary RB, particularly in patients with hereditary forms of the disease [1, 17].

By the late 1990s, systemic chemotherapy with carboplatin, vincristine, and etoposide replaced external beam irradiation for most tumors. While systemic chemotherapy is quite efficacious in reducing tumor volume, averaging over 50% decrease in volume after three sessions, it cannot cure RB alone. Systemic chemotherapy is often paired with local therapies discussed previously to achieve a cure in small tumors without diffuse vitreous and subretinal seeds [18]. Also, many patients initially managed with systemic chemotherapy require EBRT), compounding the visual deficits associated with both therapies [19]. Systemic chemotherapy is also associated with numerous adverse effects, including nausea and vomiting, hair loss, gastrointestinal toxicity with dehydration, and myelosuppression [20]. Carboplatin is associated with hearing impairment in almost a quarter of patients. For patients receiving chemotherapy in the first 6 months of life, the incidence has been reported as high as 33% within 5 years of treatment [7, 21]. Moreover, secondary acute myelocytic anemia has been reported. A recent review emphasized that systemic chemotherapy is associated with a 140× increased chance of developing secondary leukemia [22, 23].

To avoid the adverse effects of systemic chemotherapy, periocular injection of carboplatin has been utilized. This delivers ten times the chemotherapy concentration to the tumor with a fraction of the systemic dose [24]. Many patients who failed systemic carboplatin had significant clinical responses to periocular carboplatin [25]. However, while avoiding the adverse effects of systemic chemotherapy, periocular inflammation, orbital fat necrosis with fibrosis, optic atrophy, ocular motility changes, pseudopreseptal cellulitis, and visual deficits, including blindness, have been reported [25–28]. Tumors were rarely cured with this therapy [29]. Thus, RB cure may be achieved if chemotherapy is delivered directly to the tumor at a high enough dose while circumventing the local toxicity associated with periocular administration.

Advent of Intra-arterial Chemotherapy

There have been multiple subsequent novel approaches for the local delivery of chemotherapy that have been developed and trialed in human and animal models, including in fibrin sealants [30], episcleral implants [31], miniature catheters [26], and iontophoresis systems [32] with poor to mixed results. In 1954, Reese et al. published the initial results of their experimental procedure involving direct arterial administration of the alkylating agent trimethylene melamine via carotid artery puncture for RB. They reported encouraging results in hundreds of patients [11]. In 1993, a team in Japan led by Kaneko and Mohri enhanced intra-arterial chemotherapy (IAC) by indirect ophthalmic artery access, achieving a local chemotherapy concentration up to 100 times greater than systemic therapy [33]. This technique involved the selective ophthalmic arterial infusion (SOAI) of melphalan by passing a catheter from the femoral artery into the carotid artery. The catheter is advanced past the ophthalmic artery, and a balloon in the catheter is insufflated, occluding the carotid artery distal to the ophthalmic artery. Melphalan is then infused from the catheter, which is directed into the ophthalmic artery. Melphalan was chosen based on the high response in cultured human RB cells and short half-life, which limits systemic toxicity. They reported treating 187 patients with RB using SOAI, with a technical success) rate of 97.51% and no significant complications. They concluded that SOAI using balloon occlusion combined with thermotherapy was safe and efficacious, but almost all their patients also received external beam irradiation and intravitreal chemotherapy [33, 34].

Inspired by the Japanese team, Abramson, Gobin et al. began using selective chemotherapy by direct ophthalmic artery catheterization in 2006 [35]. This technique involved the direct cannulation of the ophthalmic artery with a microcatheter under fluoroscopic guidance [36]. This allowed melphalan to be administered directly into the blood supply of the eye and orbit while keeping systemic concentrations well below the levels that cause toxicity. They initially reported salvaging seven eyes destined to be enucleated with minimal systemic side effects or local toxicity [37]. In 2010, they reported that this technique could be adapted as a tandem bilateral therapy during one session of general anesthesia to treat advanced bilateral disease [38]. There were also no significant systemic adverse effects, given that patients received twice the dose for bilateral disease. Interestingly, the electroretinogram (ERG) improved in half of the eyes in this study [38]. The only recurring side effect was periocular erythema, noted in 16% of patients receiving IAC and spontaneously resolved within 3 months following IAC completion [39].

In 2010, Gobin et al. expanded the indications of IAC to be used as a primary treatment for RB and conducted a prospective study of 78 patients [40]. The drug dosage was based on age, an approximation for eye size, and angioanatomy of the ophthalmic artery and its branches, which is better predictive of ocular toxicity than that of body weight or body surface area. The authors calculated Kaplan-Meier estimates of ocular event-free survival rates at 2 years to be 70.0% for all eyes, 81.7% for eyes that received IAC as primary treatment, and 58.4% for eyes that had previous treatment failure with intravenous chemotherapy and or external beam radiation therapy [40]. The modest survival benefits seen in the early data were further surpassed by improved outcomes with IAC globally.

Global Outcomes Data

IAC for RB has multiple benefits for patients' quality of life. It is a minimally invasive ambulatory procedure requiring no port, hospitalizations, or transfusions, and up to one-third of patients have improved retinal function (ERG) [36]. Ocular survival at institutions that have adopted IAC has increased substantially [35, 41]. A meta-analysis of IAC for RB by Yousef et al. reported an overall globe salvage rate of 66%, with 74% for first-line IAC, 86% for A-C IIRC tumors, and 57% for D-E IIRC tumors [42, 43]. However, a subsequent meta-analysis by Ravindran et al. reported a globe salvage rate of 35% in D-E IIRC tumors [44]. Both studies cited a heterogeneity of reported outcomes due to a lack of sufficient follow-up data. Some institutions adopting IAC as first-line treatment for RB have reported ocular survival rates of up to 95% [41, 45]. Ocular survival is improving at large IAC) centers. Abramson et al. reported an increase in ocular survival of almost 30% over 8 years of using the technique, citing the learning curve and improved combinations of chemotherapeutic agents as reasons for improved outcomes [45]. Ravindran et al. reported an enucleation rate of 11.8%. In some centers, the enucleation rate has now dropped to 5% because, in contrast to systemic chemotherapy, IAC is usually curative [35, 41, 45].

The successful delivery rate for IAC has been reported to be 90% or more. It is only expected to improve with innovations in microcatheter delivery systems and technical proficiency due to surgeon experience [44]. An early hesitation in using IAC for RB originated from concern that while increasing ocular survival, the salvage of these eyes would coincide with an increase in the metastatic spread of RB. A meta-analysis by Runnels et al., which analyzed 24 studies and 1757 eyes, found a metastasis rate of 2.6% [46]. This is close to the 2.7% found by Cao et al., who correspondingly identified no significant difference between the rate of RB metastatic spread with IAC and IVC [47]. Moreover, a 2017 worldwide retrospective review of 1139 patients over 10 years determined that the risk of death due to RB metastases in children treated with IAC as primary or secondary therapy was <1% [48]. Still, deciding to enucleate depends on weighing the risks associated with advanced disease and the cosmetic and functional deficits associated with removing the eye. Enucleation should be strongly considered in eyes with rubeotic glaucoma, buphthalmos, and anterior chamber involvement [44].

IAC has a good risk profile with low rates of ischemic complications [49]. Jenkins et al. recorded ocular complications in the 757 cases reviewed in their meta-analysis, with the most common being retinal detachment (19.3%), vitreous hemorrhage (18.1%), and dysmotility (6.5%) [42]. Ravindran et al. reported additional complications such as cataracts (24%), retinal or choroidal ischemia (13.1%), and chorioretinal atrophy (6.4%). More clinically significant, however, are vascular complications such as ophthalmic artery vasospasm, which has been reported to occur in 8% of patients [42]. The exact pathophysiology of ophthalmic artery vasospasm in IAC is unknown but likely secondary to the arterial endothelium's physical or chemical irritation [50]. Common systemic complications include neutropenia (5.9%), bronchospasm (5.8%), and fever (4.1%) [42]. Another reported complication is SIADH, most likely due to pituitary insufficiency secondary to bilateral balloon insufflation and drug infusion into the cavernous segment of the internal carotid arteries [7]. Less serious reported adverse effects included periorbital edema, erythema, ciliary madarosis, and blepharoptosis [39, 50]. In our experience, the rate of successful IAC delivery is as high as 99.5%, with successful super-selective catheterization approaching 90% in recent years and catheterization-related complications as low as 0.6–1.1% [7].

While historically randomized control trials (RCT) in RB are limited, a 2023 RCT aimed to assess the efficacy and safety of IAC compared with intravenous chemotherapy in treating RB. The study included patients with new-onset unilateral group D or E retinoblastoma without high-risk clinical factors. The patients were randomly assigned to receive either IAC or intravenous chemotherapy. The primary outcome measured was the 2-year progression-free globe salvage rate. The study's findings showed that IAC had a 2-year progression-free globe salvage rate of 53%, while intravenous chemotherapy had a rate of 27%. Myelosuppression, a side effect of chemotherapy, was less common in the intra-arterial chemotherapy group. Two patients in the intra-arterial chemotherapy group experienced ophthalmic artery occlusion, and 13 patients had ophthalmic artery stenosis [51].

Technical Notes and Anatomical Variants

The procedure is performed collaboratively by a neurointerventionist working closely with an ocular oncologist, pediatric oncologist, and anesthesiologist. Table 11.1 summarizes the global trends in IA RB treatment. The IA chemotherapy procedures are conducted under general anesthesia with endotracheal intubation. We recommend using a nasal decongestant such as 0.05% oxymetazoline hydrochloride to vasoconstrict the nasal mucosa and placing topical neosynephrine on the forehead in the distribution of the supratrochlear artery, thereby minimizing chemotherapy flow into the nose, lid, lashes, and glabella. The arterial access site is most commonly the femoral artery. Alternatively, the left or right side, but the radial artery, can be used in older children. The patient is positioned in a way that provides the best access to the femoral artery, with the leg extended and slightly rotated outward.

Once femoral access is achieved, a standard heparin dose of 60–80 U/kg is administered, achieving a PT two to three times higher than baseline. A straight microcatheter, such as the Marathon microcatheter (Medtronic, Mineola, NY) or the Magic 1.5 microcatheter (Balt, Montmorency, France), is inserted over the microwire and is advanced to reach the ophthalmic artery (OA). Conducting the procedure with a well-trained pediatric anesthesia team is essential since OA catheterization can induce a cardio-respiratory reflex, resulting in bronchospasm and de-saturation. This is treated successfully with an IV injection of epinephrine. Once the microcatheter is correctly positioned at the ostium of the OA using a "puff-pull back" technique [7], selective angiography is performed to visualize the arterial anatomy supplying the orbit and the tumor (Fig. 11.1) [51]. Each chemotherapeutic agent is diluted in a 10 mL solution in normal saline for Carboplatin and Melphalan and a 3 mL solution in normal saline for Topotecan. Each drug is injected separately in a pulsatile fashion at a rate and force consistent with the stability of the catheter position at the OA ostium (usually a 0.2 cc pulse every 4–5 s). Each drug is usually injected over 10 min, with fluoroscopic contrast runs mid-injection and post-injection to confirm adequate anterograde flow and absence of reflux into the ICA. The total injection time for three drugs usually ranges from 25 to 30 min. Following a repeat angiogram to rule out any thromboembolic events, the microcatheter and wire are removed. Hemostasis is achieved with manual compression at the puncture site. The patient is closely monitored in the post-anesthesia recovery unit for 5 h, with close neurovascular checks at the puncture site/extremity, before being discharged home. Regular follow-up appointments with complete blood counts are scheduled to assess the treatment's effectiveness and monitor potential side effects 7–10 days postoperatively. Three IAC sessions are usually performed at four-week intervals, but additional treatments may be required depending on the response of the tumor [36, 53].

The dosage and choice of chemotherapy drugs are determined based on the patient's age, tumor characteristics, and

Table 11.1 Summary of global trends

Authors	Year	Eyes treated	Approach	Medication	Results	Complications	Reference
Yamane	2004	610	ICA Balloon	Melphalan	97.51% technical success	None	[33]
Abramson	2008	9	OA	Melphalan	7/9 salvaged	Conjunctival and lid edema [3]	[37]
Brodie	2009	9	OA	Melphalan, Carboplatin	100% retinal preservation	Retinal detachment [4]	[36]
Abramson	2010	8	Bilateral OA	Melphalan, Topotecan	8/8 salvaged	None	[38]
Abramson	2010	28	OA	Melphalan, Topotecan, Carboplatin	27/28 salvaged	None	[40]
Gobin	2011	95	OA	Melphalan	98.5% technical success	None	[35]
Abramson	2015	156	OA	Melphalan, Topotecan, Carboplatin	92.7% salvaged	None	[45]
Abramson	2017	1139	OA	Melphalan, Topotecan, Carboplatin	<1% metastatic deaths	N/A	[48]
Munier	2017	25	OA/ECA	Melphalan	25/25	None	[41]
Shields	2020	341	OA	Melphalan, Topotecan	76% salvage	Retina ischemia (1%), choroidal ischemia (1%)	[50]
Abruzzo	2021	21	OA	Melphalan	N/A	N/A	[52]

OA Ophthalmic Artery, *ECA* External Carotid Artery

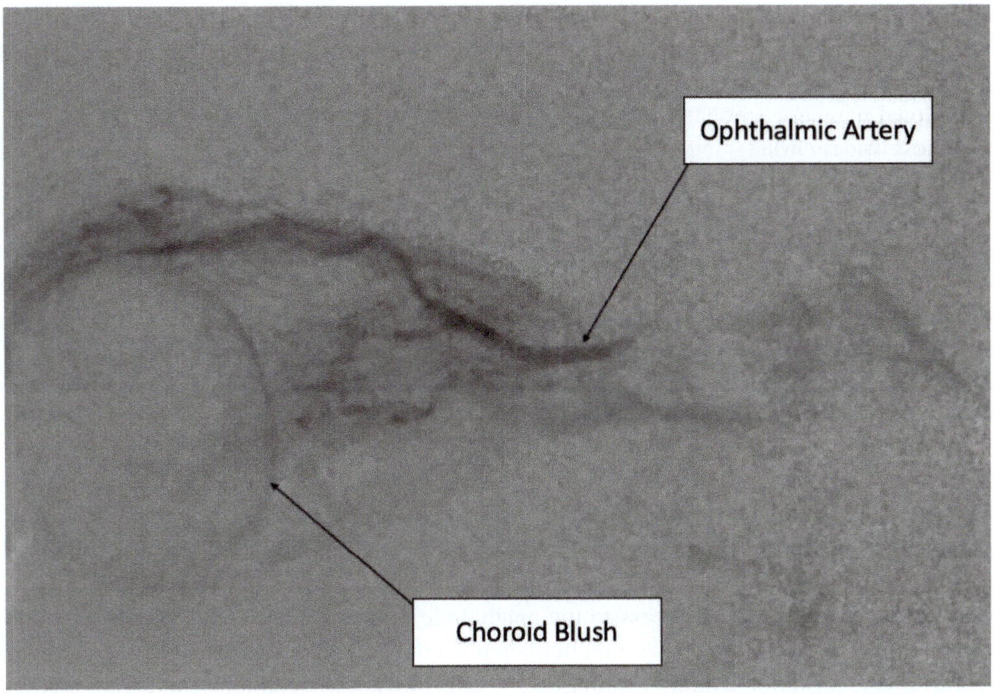

Fig. 11.1 Ophthalmic artery injection with associated choroid blush following direct access (adapted from Carnevale et al. Intra-arterial chemotherapy for Retinoblastoma, JNIS 2023)

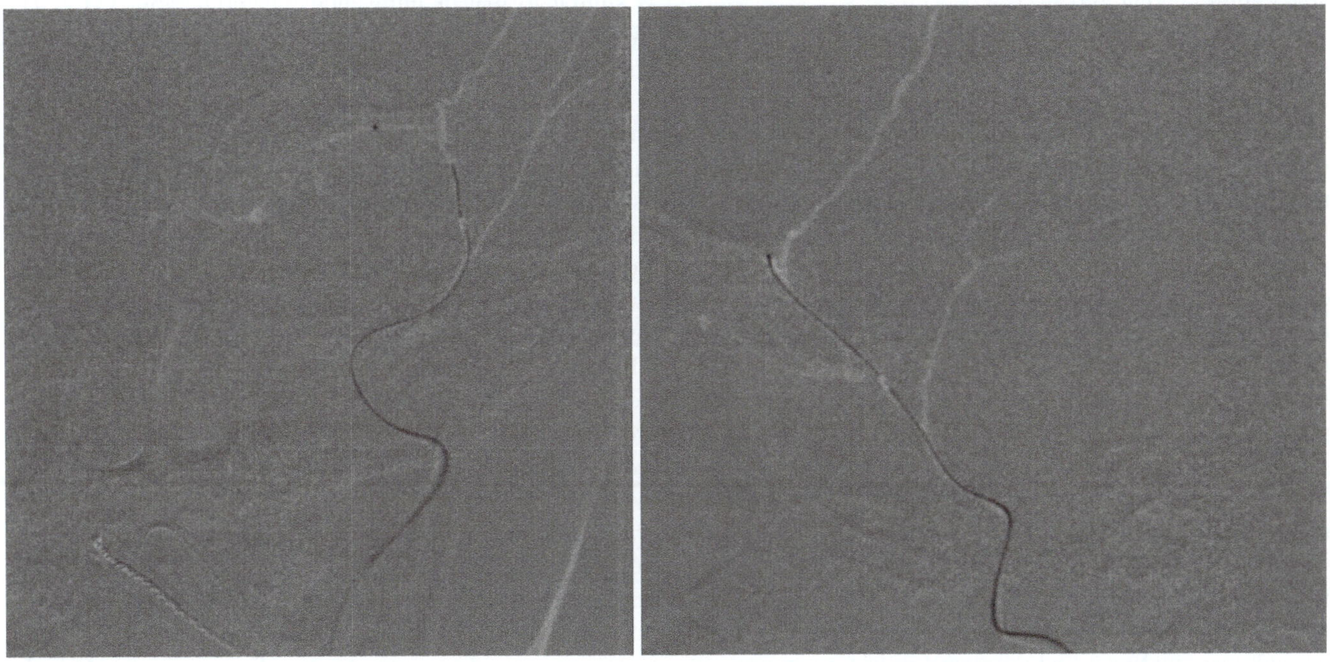

Fig. 11.2 MMA approach to the OA (adapted from Carnevale et al. Intra-arterial chemotherapy for Retinoblastoma, JNIS 2023)

response to previous treatments. The three most used chemotherapeutic agents are melphalan, topotecan hydrochloride, and carboplatin. Continuous intraoperative monitoring is essential to ensure the chemotherapy is effectively delivered. The dose of melphalan ranges from 3 to 7.5 mg, the dose of topotecan hydrochloride ranges from 0.5 to 2 mg, and the dose of carboplatin ranges from 15 to 50 mg [36, 53, 54].

When catheterizing the ophthalmic artery is challenging due to factors such as its small size, vasospasm, or anatomical variations in branching, alternative approaches come into play. In approximately 7% of cases, catheterization is redirected through the middle meningeal artery, a branch of the external carotid artery's internal maxillary artery (Fig. 11.2) [54, 55]. The distal branches of the internal maxillary artery,

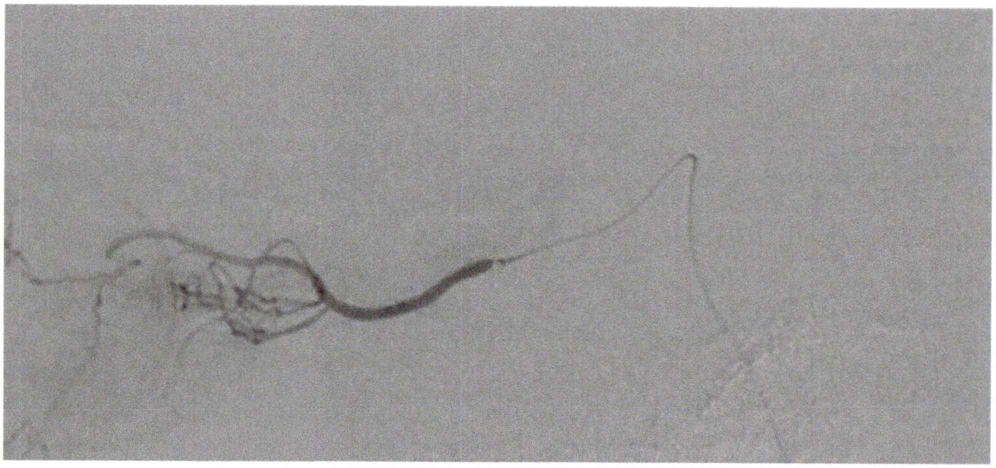

Fig. 11.3 Posterior communicating artery approach to the OA (adapted from Carnevale et al. Intra-arterial chemotherapy for Retinoblastoma, JNIS 2023)

such as the sphenopalatine artery, may anastomose with the ophthalmic artery and can also be used to access the blood supply to the orbit. Finally, access to the ophthalmic artery can be achieved through the posterior circulation via the vertebral artery, posterior communicating artery, and moving retrograde down the ICA until reaching the ophthalmic artery (Fig. 11.3) [7, 53].

The "Japanese technique" is a valuable alternative in scenarios where traditional catheterization proves difficult. This technique involves employing a micro balloon catheter to achieve temporary occlusion of the internal carotid artery right above the origin of the ophthalmic artery. By inflating the balloon, local delivery of chemotherapy to the OA is facilitated, preventing the unintended dispersion of chemotherapeutic drugs into the anterior, middle, and posterior cerebral arteries. The procedure entails diluting the chemotherapeutic drugs in 6 cc of normal saline and administering them rapidly over 4 min. Following drug delivery, the balloon is deflated to mitigate the risk of cerebral ischemic complications [36, 53].

Future Directions

IAC has significantly improved patient outcomes in the treatment of RB. Early trials have reported a substantial increase in ocular survival rates and decreased need for enucleation. The globe salvage rate with IAC varies between 66 and 95%, with some centers reporting enucleation rates as low as 5%. The adoption of IAC has had a profound impact on patient's quality of life, as it is a minimally invasive ambulatory procedure that does not require hospitalization or transfusions. Additionally, up to one-third of patients have improved ERGs after treatment with IAC. The success of IAC has been attributed to its ability to deliver a high concentration of chemotherapy directly to the tumor while minimizing systemic toxicity. This localized delivery of chemotherapy allows for effective tumor control and reduces the need for additional treatments like external beam radiotherapy (EBRT) or enucleation. Despite initial concerns about the risk of metastatic spread with IAC, studies have shown that the metastatic rate is similar to that of intravenous chemotherapy (IVC). The overall risk of death due to RB metastases in children treated with IAC is less than 1%. However, the decision to enucleate is still based on individual factors, such as advanced disease and the associated cosmetic and functional deficits. While there are potential complications associated with IAC, such as retinal detachment, vitreous hemorrhage, and vascular complications like ophthalmic artery vasospasm and occlusion, the risk profile of IAC is generally favorable. Systemic complications, such as neutropenia and bronchospasm, are less frequent with IAC compared to systemic chemotherapy. Clinical trials related to retinoblastoma and its arterial treatments registered on the National Clinical Trials Registry are listed in Table 11.2, and they show the likely evolution of technology in the next several years.

The utilization of IAC for the treatment of RB faces several limitations, hindering its adoption in many communities, especially in lower-middle-income countries. The primary obstacle is the high cost associated with the procedure and the need for specialized infrastructure, such as a neuro-interventional suite. Another limitation of IAC is the need for proficiency in performing the technique. The procedure requires specialized skills and knowledge, as well as repetition and experience with complex access cases, which all healthcare professionals may not easily acquire, especially given the low incidence of the disease. This limitation further restricts the widespread use of IAC, particularly in regions with limited access to specialized training and expertise.

Table 11.2 Trials related to "retinoblastoma" + "arterial" treatment on the National Clinical Trials Registry

NCT number	Study status	Interventions/observation objective	Age
NCT04342572	Active not recruiting	Melphalan	Children, adult
NCT00901238	Completed	IA chemotherapy	Children, adult
NCT04564521	Recruiting	Response to IV Nitroglycerin during IA chemotherapy	Children
NCT00906113	Unknown	IA melphalan	Children
NCT03935074	Completed	IA melphalan	Children
NCT01293539	Terminated	IA Melphalan	Children, adult
NCT00857519	Completed	Melphalan, Carboplatin	Children, adult
NCT04451304	Unknown	Observation of hemodynamic response to IA chemotherapy	Children, adult
NCT03267459	Recruiting	Dynamic contrast-enhanced MRI	C Children, adult
NCT01393769	Terminated	Melphalan	Children
NCT04455139	Terminated	Topotecan Melphalan	Children
NCT01466855	Terminated	IA Topotecan infusion	Children
NCT03559894	Unknown	Transthoracic echocardiography during IA chemotherapy	Children
NCT05028270	Unknown	Superselective balloon-assisted delivery	Children, adult
NCT02097134	Completed	Melphalan	Children, adult
NCT01151748	Withdrawn	IA chemotherapy	Children, adult
NCT02764398	Completed	Observation of hemodynamic response to IA chemotherapy	Children
NCT02116959	Terminated	Melphalan, Carboplatin, Etoposide, Vincristine	Children, adult
NCT04681417	Recruiting	Melphalan, Melphalan + Topotecan, etoposide, carboplatin, and vincristine, OR local treatment without IV chemotherapy. Thermotherapy (local treatment), Cryotherapy (local treatment), Iodine-125 plaques (local treatment), Intravitreal Melphalan	Children
NCT03662776	Enrolling by invitation	Behavioral	Children
NCT01558960	Terminated	Intravitreal Melphalan	Children, adult
NCT04700514	Recruiting	Dexmedetomidine	Children
NCT03866460	Active not recruiting	Distortion product otoacoustic emission measurement (DPOAE)	Children, adult
NCT04903678	Recruiting	Melphalan	Children, adult
NCT02955524	Withdrawn	Tetracaine 0.5%, Lidocaine hydrochloride ophthalmic gel 3.5%	Children, adult
NCT03450590	Completed	Observation of heart rate variability in response to IA chemotherapy	Children, adult
NCT03439397	Unknown	Balloon occlusion, SOAI	Children
NCT02866136	Active not recruiting	Carboplatin, Melphalan, carboplatin, vincristine, Carboplatin + (chemo-thermo-therapy) Local treatment: Laser ablation, cryo-application, ^{125}I-radioactive plaques intravitreal Melphalan	Children

Lessons for Treating Other Neurological Diseases

Intraarterial chemotherapy for RB can avoid mutilating surgery and, in some cases, preserve and even improve vision. Its clinical role is well established, and many centers offer the treatment. As a pediatric tumor, treated often in infancy, it poses technical challenges in selectively delivering the drug to the target site. The question arises: What can be learned from RB treatment that is relevant to treating brain diseases? Compared to IA treatment of brain tumors, there are several advantages to using IA treatment for RB. RB is typically localized within the orbit. A single artery perfuses the malignancy. The host tissue, the retina, is more ischemia-tolerant than the brain. The consequences of injury are usually non-fatal. Hence, in theory, IA treatment of RB will be more likely to be effective than brain tumors. However, both tumors could benefit from the delivery of drugs with super-selective pulsatile injections, particularly when the delivery is assisted by balloon occlusion to localize the drug in the ophthalmic artery. Thus, drug delivery techniques in RB treatment could serve as a paradigm for arterial chemotherapy of brain tumors once the obstacle of the blood-brain barrier is overcome.

Could RB treatment guide the selection of chemotherapy for treating brain tumors? Interestingly, melphalan, a potent non-cell cycle-selective rapidly acting alkylating agent, has been introduced as a single drug for RB treatment [35]. In experimental animals, melphalan has been proven effective for glioma treatment in prolonging survival [56]. However, it has not yet been evaluated clinically. This could be due to the potential risk of white matter injury by lipid-soluble alkylating agents. One of the fundamental challenges in translating RB chemotherapy to GBM is brain tissue's much larger size with far greater structural diversity, infiltrative nature and vascular complexity [57]. Lipid-soluble compounds that penetrate the blood-brain barriers could be trapped in the white matter. An alternate strategy using tumor-selective cell-penetrating peptide-conjugated melphalan has been proposed to treat brain tumors [58].

Conclusion

Intraarterial chemotherapy has revolutionized the management of unilateral and bilateral retinoblastoma, saving more eyes and vision with fewer side effects than all prior approaches for advanced intraocular disease. As the providers become more experienced at performing IAC, the technical success rates are expected to rise, further enhancing its effectiveness. The IAC approach represents a significant advancement in RB treatment, offering a path toward safer and more successful patient treatments and improving the quality of care and outcomes at these centers. While there are host tissue-related differences between the eye and the brain, angiographic techniques and drugs (such as melphalan) developed for RB treatment could inform the development of arterial therapies for brain tumors.

References

1. Abramson DH. Retinoblastoma in the 20th century: past success and future challenges the Weisenfeld lecture. Invest Ophthalmol Vis Sci. 2005;46(8):2683–91.
2. Aerts I, Lumbroso-Le Rouic L, Gauthier-Villars M, Brisse H, Doz F, Desjardins L. Retinoblastoma. Orphanet J Rare Dis. 2006;1:31.
3. Abramson DH, Schefler AC. Update on retinoblastoma. Retina. 2004;24(6):828–48.
4. Baud O, Cormier-Daire V, Lyonnet S, Desjardins L, Turleau C, Doz F. Dysmorphic phenotype and neurological impairment in 22 retinoblastoma patients with constitutional cytogenetic 13q deletion. Clin Genet. 1999;55(6):478–82.
5. Friend SH, Bernards R, Rogelj S, Weinberg RA, Rapaport JM, Albert DM, et al. A human DNA segment with properties of the gene that predisposes to retinoblastoma and osteosarcoma. Nature. 1986;323(6089):643–6.
6. Knudson AG Jr. Mutation and cancer: statistical study of retinoblastoma. Proc Natl Acad Sci U S A. 1971;68(4):820–3.
7. Kocharian G, Gobin YP, Kharas N, Knopman J, Francis JH, Abramson DH. Advancements in super-selective catheterization and drug selection for intra-arterial chemotherapy for retinoblastoma: a 15-year evolution. J Neurointerv Surg. 2024;16(4):398–404.
8. Chantada GL, Dunkel IJ, Antoneli CB, de Davila MT, Arias V, Beaverson K, et al. Risk factors for extraocular relapse following enucleation after failure of chemoreduction in retinoblastoma. Pediatr Blood Cancer. 2007;49(3):256–60.
9. Lu JE, Francis JH, Dunkel IJ, Shields CL, Yu MD, Berry JL, et al. Metastases and death rates after primary enucleation of unilateral retinoblastoma in the USA 2007-2017. Br J Ophthalmol. 2019;103(9):1272–7.
10. Cassady JR, Sagerman RH, Tretter P, Ellsworth RM. Radiation therapy in retinoblastoma. An analysis of 230 cases. Radiology. 1969;93(2):405–9.
11. Reese AB, Hyman GA, Merriam GR Jr, Forrest AW, Kligerman MM. Treatment of retinoblastoma by radiation and triethylenemelamine. AMA Arch Ophthalmol. 1954;53(4):505–13.
12. Kupfer C. Retinoblastoma treated with intravenous nitrogen mustard. Am J Ophthalmol. 1953;36(12):1721–3.
13. Aerts I, Pacquement H, Doz F, Mosseri V, Desjardins L, Sastre X, et al. Outcome of second malignancies after retinoblastoma: a retrospective analysis of 25 patients treated at the Institut curie. Eur J Cancer. 2004;40(10):1522–9.
14. Scott IU, Murray TG, Feuer WJ, Van Quill K, Markoe AM, Ling S, et al. External beam radiotherapy in retinoblastoma: tumor control and comparison of 2 techniques. Arch Ophthalmol. 1999;117(6):766–70.
15. Pradhan DG, Sandridge AL, Mullaney P, Abboud E, Karcioglu ZA, Kandil A, et al. Radiation therapy for retinoblastoma: a retrospective review of 120 patients. Int J Radiat Oncol Biol Phys. 1997;39(1):3–13.
16. Abramson DH, Beaverson KL, Chang ST, Dunkel IJ, McCormick B. Outcome following initial external beam radiotherapy in patients with Reese-Ellsworth group Vb retinoblastoma. Arch Ophthalmol. 2004;122(9):1316–23.
17. Eng C, Li FP, Abramson DH, Ellsworth RM, Wong FL, Goldman MB, et al. Mortality from second tumors among long-term survivors of retinoblastoma. J Natl Cancer Inst. 1993;85(14):1121–8.
18. De Potter P. Current treatment of retinoblastoma. Curr Opin Ophthalmol. 2002;13(5):331–6.
19. Chan MP, Hungerford JL, Kingston JE, Plowman PN. Salvage external beam radiotherapy after failed primary chemotherapy for bilateral retinoblastoma: rate of eye and vision preservation. Br J Ophthalmol. 2009;93(7):891–4.
20. Benz MS, Scott IU, Murray TG, Kramer D, Toledano S. Complications of systemic chemotherapy as treatment of retinoblastoma. Arch Ophthalmol. 2000;118(4):572–5.
21. Toral-Martinnon R, Collado-Corona MA, Mora-Magana I, Leal-Leal C, Gutierrez-Castrellon P, Gonzalez-de Leo S. [Evaluation of cisplatin ototoxicity by the audiometric curve in retinoblastoma]. Cir Cir. 2006;74(2):79–82.
22. Gombos DS, Hungerford J, Abramson DH, Kingston J, Chantada G, Dunkel IJ, et al. Secondary acute myelogenous leukemia in patients with retinoblastoma: is chemotherapy a factor? Ophthalmology. 2007;114(7):1378–83.
23. Villanueva G, Sampor C, Moreno F, Alderete D, Moresco A, Pinto N, et al. Subsequent malignant neoplasms in the pediatric age in retinoblastoma survivors in Argentina. Pediatr Blood Cancer. 2022;69(8):e29710.
24. Tsui JY, Dalgard C, Van Quill KR, Lee L, Grossniklaus HE, Edelhauser HF, et al. Subconjunctival topotecan in fibrin sealant in the treatment of transgenic murine retinoblastoma. Invest Ophthalmol Vis Sci. 2008;49(2):490–6.
25. Abramson DH, Frank CM, Dunkel IJ. A phase I/II study of subconjunctival carboplatin for intraocular retinoblastoma. Ophthalmology. 1999;106(10):1947–50.
26. Schmack I, Hubbard GB, Kang SJ, Aaberg TM Jr, Grossniklaus HE. Ischemic necrosis and atrophy of the optic nerve after periocular carboplatin injection for intraocular retinoblastoma. Am J Ophthalmol. 2006;142(2):310–5.
27. Mulvihill A, Budning A, Jay V, Vandenhoven C, Heon E, Gallie BL, et al. Ocular motility changes after subtenon carboplatin chemotherapy for retinoblastoma. Arch Ophthalmol. 2003;121(8):1120–4.

28. Kiratli H, Kocabeyoglu S, Bilgic S. Severe pseudo-preseptal cellulitis following sub-tenon's carboplatin injection for intraocular retinoblastoma. J AAPOS. 2007;11(4):404–5.
29. Marr BP, Dunkel IJ, Linker A, Abramson DH. Periocular carboplatin for retinoblastoma: long-term report (12 years) on efficacy and toxicity. Br J Ophthalmol. 2012;96(6):881–3.
30. Martin NE, Kim JW, Abramson DH. Fibrin sealant for retinoblastoma: where are we? J Ocul Pharmacol Ther. 2008;24(5):433–8.
31. Carcaboso AM, Chiappetta DA, Opezzo JA, Hocht C, Fandino AC, Croxatto JO, et al. Episcleral implants for topotecan delivery to the posterior segment of the eye. Invest Ophthalmol Vis Sci. 2010;51(4):2126–34.
32. Hayden BC, Jockovich ME, Murray TG, Voigt M, Milne P, Kralinger M, et al. Pharmacokinetics of systemic versus focal carboplatin chemotherapy in the rabbit eye: possible implication in the treatment of retinoblastoma. Invest Ophthalmol Vis Sci. 2004;45(10):3644–9.
33. Yamane T, Kaneko A, Mohri M. The technique of ophthalmic arterial infusion therapy for patients with intraocular retinoblastoma. Int J Clin Oncol. 2004;9(2):69–73.
34. Schaiquevich P, Buitrago E, Taich P, Torbidoni A, Ceciliano A, Fandino A, et al. Pharmacokinetic analysis of melphalan after superselective ophthalmic artery infusion in preclinical models and retinoblastoma patients. Invest Ophthalmol Vis Sci. 2012;53(7):4205–12.
35. Gobin YP, Dunkel IJ, Marr BP, Brodie SE, Abramson DH. Intra-arterial chemotherapy for the management of retinoblastoma: four-year experience. Arch Ophthalmol. 2011;129(6):732–7.
36. Brodie SE, Pierre Gobin Y, Dunkel IJ, Kim JW, Abramson DH. Persistence of retinal function after selective ophthalmic artery chemotherapy infusion for retinoblastoma. Doc Ophthalmol. 2009;119(1):13–22.
37. Abramson DH, Dunkel IJ, Brodie SE, Kim JW, Gobin YP. A phase I/II study of direct intraarterial (ophthalmic artery) chemotherapy with melphalan for intraocular retinoblastoma initial results. Ophthalmology. 2008;115(8):1398–404, 1404 e1.
38. Abramson DH, Dunkel IJ, Brodie SE, Marr B, Gobin YP. Bilateral superselective ophthalmic artery chemotherapy for bilateral retinoblastoma: tandem therapy. Arch Ophthalmol. 2010;128(3):370–2.
39. Marr B, Gobin PY, Dunkel IJ, Brodie SE, Abramson DH. Spontaneously resolving periocular erythema and ciliary madarosis following intra-arterial chemotherapy for retinoblastoma. Middle East Afr J Ophthalmol. 2010;17(3):207–9.
40. Abramson DH, Dunkel IJ, Brodie SE, Marr B, Gobin YP. Superselective ophthalmic artery chemotherapy as primary treatment for retinoblastoma (chemosurgery). Ophthalmology. 2010;117(8):1623–9.
41. Munier FL, Mosimann P, Puccinelli F, Gaillard MC, Stathopoulos C, Houghton S, et al. First-line intra-arterial versus intravenous chemotherapy in unilateral sporadic group D retinoblastoma: evidence of better visual outcomes, ocular survival and shorter time to success with intra-arterial delivery from retrospective review of 20 years of treatment. Br J Ophthalmol. 2017;101(8):1086–93.
42. Jenkins R, Lemire C, Altamirano-Lamarque F, Orbach DB, Vanderveen D, Shah AS, et al. Complications of intra-arterial chemotherapy (IAC) for retinoblastoma: an updated, comprehensive review: American Academy of Ophthalmology; 2023 [updated August 24, 2023]. https://www.aao.org/education/disease-review/complications-of-intra-arterial-chemotherapy-iac-r.
43. Yousef YA, Soliman SE, Astudillo PPP, Durairaj P, Dimaras H, Chan HSL, et al. Intra-arterial chemotherapy for retinoblastoma: a systematic review. JAMA Ophthalmol. 2016;134(5):584–91.
44. Ravindran K, Dalvin LA, Pulido JS, Brinjikji W. Intra-arterial chemotherapy for retinoblastoma: an updated systematic review and meta-analysis. J Neurointerv Surg. 2019;11(12):1266–72.
45. Abramson DH, Fabius AW, Issa R, Francis JH, Marr BP, Dunkel IJ, et al. Advanced unilateral retinoblastoma: the impact of ophthalmic artery chemosurgery on enucleation rate and patient survival at MSKCC. PLoS One. 2015;10(12):e0145436.
46. Runnels J, Acosta G, Rose A, Haynes M, Nikolaidis D, Wong A, et al. The role for intra-arterial chemotherapy for refractory retinoblastoma: a systematic review. Clin Transl Oncol. 2021;23(10):2066–77.
47. Chen Q, Zhang B, Dong Y, Mo X, Zhang L, Huang W, et al. Comparison between intravenous chemotherapy and intra-arterial chemotherapy for retinoblastoma: a meta-analysis. BMC Cancer. 2018;18(1):486.
48. Abramson DH, Shields CL, Jabbour P, Teixeira LF, Fonseca JRF, Marques MCP, et al. Metastatic deaths in retinoblastoma patients treated with intraarterial chemotherapy (ophthalmic artery chemosurgery) worldwide. Int J Retina Vitreous. 2017;3:40.
49. Shields CL, Dockery PW, Yaghy A, Duffner ER, Levin HJ, Taylor OS, et al. Intra-arterial chemotherapy for retinoblastoma in 341 consecutive eyes (1,292 infusions): comparative analysis of outcomes based on patient age, race, and sex. J AAPOS. 2021;25(3):150.e1–9.
50. Shields CL, Bianciotto CG, Jabbour P, Griffin GC, Ramasubramanian A, Rosenwasser R, et al. Intra-arterial chemotherapy for retinoblastoma: report no. 2, treatment complications. Arch Ophthalmol. 2011;129(11):1407–15.
51. Wen X, Fan J, Jin M, Jiang H, Li J, Han M, et al. Intravenous versus super-selected intra-arterial chemotherapy in children with advanced unilateral retinoblastoma: an open-label, multicentre, randomised trial. Lancet Child Adolesc Health. 2023;7(9):613–20.
52. Abruzzo T, Abraham K, Karani KB, Geller JI, Vadivelu S, Racadio JM, et al. Correlation of technical and adjunctive factors with quantitative tumor reduction in children undergoing selective ophthalmic artery infusion chemotherapy for retinoblastoma. AJNR Am J Neuroradiol. 2021;42(2):354–61.
53. Manjandavida FP, Stathopoulos C, Zhang J, Honavar SG, Shields CL. Intra-arterial chemotherapy in retinoblastoma—A paradigm change. Indian J Ophthalmol. 2019;67(6):740–54.
54. Klufas MA, Gobin YP, Marr B, Brodie SE, Dunkel IJ, Abramson DH. Intra-arterial chemotherapy as a treatment for intraocular retinoblastoma: alternatives to direct ophthalmic artery catheterization. AJNR Am J Neuroradiol. 2012;33(8):1608–14.
55. Carnevale JA, Goldberg J, Kocharian G, Rivera M, Giantini Larsen A, Garton A, et al. Intra-arterial chemotherapy for retinoblastoma. J Neurointerv Surg. 2023;15(3):303–4.
56. Kurpad SN, Friedman HS, Archer GE, McLendon RE, Petros WM, Fuchs HE, et al. Intraarterial administration of melphalan for treatment of intracranial human glioma xenografts in athymic rats. Cancer Res. 1995;55(17):3803–9.
57. Mahaley MS Jr, Whaley RA, Blue M, Bertsch L. Central neurotoxicity following intracarotid BCNU chemotherapy for malignant gliomas. J Neurooncol. 1986;3(4):297–314.
58. Joshi S, Cooke JRN, Ellis JA, Emala CW, Bruce JN. Targeting brain tumors by intra-arterial delivery of cell-penetrating peptides: a novel approach for primary and metastatic brain malignancy. J Neurooncol. 2017;135(3):497–506.

12 Developing Arterial Drugs: Lessons from the Hepatic Artery and Other Arterial Injections

Asad Baig, T Clark Gamblin, Ricardo J. Bello, and Shailendra Joshi

No problem can withstand the assault of sustained thinking.

M. de Voltaire (1694–1778), French Philosopher, Historian, and Satirist

Introduction

Interventional radiology has advanced rapidly in the last three decades. Most of the focus has been on developing catheters, endovascular devices, and imaging technology, but less on developing pharmaceuticals that can be delivered through arteries. In recent years, imaging devices amounted to $25 billion in annual global sales, while endovascular devices (catheters/stents) amounted to an additional $5.2 billion. The global market will increase by 5% annually over the next decade [1]. Most neurological treatments with IA injections consist of off-label use of intravenous drugs. These drugs are not specifically designed to be retained by the target site after arterial injections. Models show that the advantage of IA injections will significantly diminish unless the drugs are retained in the tissue during their first pass through the regional circulation [2–6]. In contrast to treating neurological diseases, arterial drug delivery is an accepted treatment for liver cancers. A wide range of drugs, drug formulations, and delivery methods have been developed in the last two decades. Today, arterial infusion methods are used for destruction of early-stage liver cancers, as a bridge to surgery or transplant, or as treatment of choice for advanced malignancy. Despite considerable differences in the host organ, the success of hepatic artery infusion therapy provides a road map for the development of arterial drugs for treating neurological diseases. The current strategy to improve IA delivery is often based on safely injecting intravenous drug formulations to benefit from the high regional first-pass drug concentrations. Little emphasis is placed on selecting and developing drug formulations that are rapidly taken up during their first pass through arterial irrigation. HAI success shows the role drug selection and drug formulations can play in improving outcomes of arterial treatments.

One of the fundamental problems with arterial injection is that the biomechanics of such injections are often overlooked. A problem of arterial drug delivery is that at low infusion rates, it is difficult to ensure even distribution of the drugs due to streaming [7]. Streaming can be minimized by pulsed delivery. However, pulsatile drug injection results in their rapid transit through arterial irrigation, which is challenging to investigate and optimize [8, 9]. Flow arrest (FA) arterial drug delivery radically changes the pharmacokinetic paradigm by delivering pure drugs to the target site. It physically restricts delivery to non-target sites and, within the target site, avoids contact with blood cells, serum proteins, and circulating enzymes. Flow-arrest arterial delivery could significantly enhance the effectiveness of neural tissue targeting approaches that have been developed for direct tissue or intravenous injections. The first-pass pharmacokinetics of drugs after arterial injections is highly complex and is affected by many factors listed in Table 12.1. A problem in investigating the first-pass kinetics of IA delivery is to assess tissue drug concentrations within a sub-second timeframe after IA injections. Conventional pharmacokinetic methods of tissue biopsy with chemical analysis or PET studies are not readily feasible. Chapters 19 and 20 discuss how the

A. Baig
Columbia University, New York, NY, USA

T. C. Gamblin · R. J. Bello
Medical College of Wisconsin, Milwaukee, WI, USA

S. Joshi (✉)
Department of Anesthesiology, Columbia University Irving Medical Center, New York, NY, USA
e-mail: sj121@cumc.columbia.edu

S. Joshi (ed.), *Arterial Treatment of Neurological Diseases*, https://doi.org/10.1007/978-3-031-80173-0_12

Table 12.1 Factors affecting first-pass concentrations of the drug after IA injection

Factor	Parameter	Anticipated effects
Tissue condition	Site of infusion	Distal infusions result in greater streaming compared to proximal infusions
	Blood flow volume/time	The higher the background flows, the greater the streaming
	Vascular dead space	Affects dilution and transit time
Injection	Type of catheter	Endon vs. side port affects streaming
	Volume of injection	Determines dilution and streaming
	Injection concentration	Determines peak concentration, uptake, regional toxicity
	Injection frequency	Uptake and maintenance of tissue concentrations
	Flow velocity	Determines streaming
	Bolus transit time	Determines uptake and clearance
	Diastolic injection	It enhances drug and blood mixing and decreases streaming
Nature of drug	Protein binding	Free drug concentration
	Vascular penetration	Delivery to tissue compartment
	Vascular clearance	Metabolism by blood cells, serum enzymes, and endothelium
Compartmental characteristics	The volume of distribution (Vd)	The capacity of regional tissue for the drug
	Regional clearance	Metabolism in the regional site
	Tissue diffusion	Rate of saturation of regional compartment
	Tissue retention	Efflux rate from the tissue compartment
Recirculating drug concentrations	Cardiac output	Determine systemic delivery and concentrations
	Systemic clearance	Determines recirculating concentrations

optical method can provide a rapid, site-specific, tissue-invasive, repeated assessment of tissue drug concentrations that are safe, cost-effective, and quickly undertaken in conventional wet labs. Such an approach combined with post-mortem imaging can help to understand and optimize the first-pass kinetics of IA drug delivery.

This chapter briefly discusses how drugs have been developed for hepatic artery chemotherapy. It primarily discusses arterial drug delivery to the liver. The chapter summarizes other experiences, such as developing radiocontrast agents and accidental arterial drug injections, that also provide clues to arterial drug development. This chapter aims to identify drug properties that can help develop arterial drugs and enhance the effectiveness and safety of arterial delivery.

The Need to Develop Drugs Specifically for Intraarterial Injections

Conventional drug design relies on the pharmacokinetic properties of compounds, such as protein binding and lipid solubility, that result in preferential uptake by the target organ. However, if a drug is directly delivered to the site by IA injections, the emphasis on these characteristics becomes somewhat redundant. The most significant pharmacokinetic characteristic of IA delivery of a drug or a formulation is its rapid uptake during its first pass through the tissue and its sustained retention afterward [2]. The uptake should preferably be limited to the pathology [4]. Classical preclinical drug development does not select compounds for IA use or assess them for their IA efficacy. Other than for HAI and angiographic contrast, compounds are seldom specifically optimized for IA injections. Consequently, most arterial treatments are based on the off-label use of intravenous drug formulations.

Before embarking on a discussion on drug development, it should be noted that arterial drug delivery carries inherent risks. Arterial drugs often challenge the fundamental tenant of medicine of avoiding harm. Arterial drug injections carry the risk of vascular injury and thrombotic and hemorrhagic complications. The overall risk of cerebral angiography is about 1.3%, an inherent risk with arterial interventions even without drug delivery [10]. Therefore, the benefits of IA drug delivery must outweigh the risks of the standard treatment. For example, faced with a relentless and fatal outcome of brain tumors, the hazards of arterial chemotherapy infusion are justified [11]. Chapters 17 and 18 discuss that better angiographic techniques and catheters can further reduce procedural risks. Modern arterial chemotherapy emerged from an accidental IA injection of nitrogen mustard in the brachial artery, causing a significant local injury [12]. However, the injury was reversible and could be justified in the context of a poor outcome with standard cancer treatment. Within a decade, IA nitrogen mustards were being evaluated for many cancers despite the potential hazards of such treatments. Perhaps arterial drug delivery should be considered "pharmacological tissue surgery," and the risk-benefit analysis should be similar to any surgical procedure.

An ideal IA drug or drug formulation should be regionally safe and ensure maximum regional uptake and adequate retention of drugs to achieve the desired therapeutic effect. In the absence of direct experimental data to guide the development of arterial drugs, the desired properties of arterial drugs can be gleaned from the review of the following literature:

- Desirable properties of arterial drugs based on conceptual models
- Hazardous drug characteristics that led to harm after accidental arterial drug injections
- Characteristics of angiographic contrast agents

Table 12.2 Host organ characteristics impacting drug delivery

	Liver	Brain
Host organ	1500 g	1350 g
Organ function	Diffusely distributed	Local and highly specialized
Ischemia/injury tolerance	Yes	No
Tumor cell drug uptake	Yes	Limited by BBB
Regeneration	Yes	No
Blood flow characteristics		
Blood flow	100 mL/100 g/min	50 mL/100 g/min
	Hepatic A 25 mL/100 g/min	Carotid A: 350 mL/min/artery
	Portal V 75 mL/100 g/min	Vertebral A: 150 mL/min/artery
Organ perfusion	Communicating: portal system	Non-communicating end arteries
Tumor blood flow	Hepatic artery	From multiple arteries
Tumor-blood barrier	None	Yes, often requires disruption
Therapeutic implications		
Particle embolization	Possible	No
Organ-specific uptake	Yes, with 5FU	None yet
IA treatment options	Chemotherapy	Chemo ineffective
	Radioactive particles	
	Embolic entities	
Long-term infusion over weeks	Possible	Not practical: stroke risk
IA Rx impact	Significant, clinically accepted	Unproven, experimental

- Strategies available to enhance first-pass uptake of the drugs
- Drugs developed for hepatic artery chemo- and radiation therapy

Perhaps the safest prolonged use of arterial drugs has been for HAI, where infusions are carried over weeks through implantable pumps [13, 14]. HAI drugs are selected based on their first-pass extraction, systemic clearance, and potential local complications. There is also extensive pharmacokinetic data with these drugs from preclinical and clinical studies. Even though the liver is a unique organ in relation to its blood flow, ischemia tolerance, and regenerative capacity, drugs used for HAI infusions are relevant to rationalize drug development for other applications, Table 12.2.

Desirable Properties of Arterial Drugs Based on Computational Models

Several researchers developed the basic model of IA drug delivery in the 1970s and 1980s [3–6]. The models revealed that IA drug delivery is effective when there is low regional blood flow, high regional extraction, and high systemic clearance. Based on these models, an ideal arterial drug should have:

- Rapid uptake by the target site
- Drug retention at the target site
- Minimal metabolism at the target site, to achieve the desired effect
- Rapid clearance from systemic circulation
- Ability to selectively target pathological cells within the arterial irrigation

A classic drug with high first-pass extraction is Floxuridine (FUDR). The liver extracts about 95% of the drug on its first pass after IA infusion [15]. Based on the computational modeling, floxuridine is a prototype of an ideal drug for arterial infusion for treating liver malignancy [16]. At the same time, there is also highly selective tumor uptake that is 15-fold greater than the normal cells. FURD is also suited for arterial injections because it has a circulating half-life of about 16 min. Therefore, whatever drug reaches systemic circulation will be rapidly cleared. Randomized studies have shown an increase in survival for patients with liver metastases from colorectal cancer treated with a combination of FUDR via HAI and systemic chemotherapy compared to systemic chemotherapy alone [17, 18]. HAI chemotherapy has proven effective even after failure to respond to systemic therapy. Similarly, 90% of patients with inoperable IDH1/2-mutated-cholangiocarcinoma survived 2 years after treatment with IA floxuridine and systemic chemotherapy [19].

Impact of Flow Arrest on Arterial Drug Delivery

The effectiveness of arterial drug delivery is radically altered when the drug is injected during complete or nearly complete cessation of blood flow [20]. Under these conditions, the drug bolus completely displaces the blood in the vascular dead space. Thus, the drug is delivered to the target site without blood cells or protein exposure. The FA-IA technique delivers tissue-targeting molecules to reach the targeting site in pristine conditions without any attenuation by blood components. The FA-IA delivery method can significantly augment the benefits of tissue-targeting technologies [21–24].

The effectiveness of carrier, receptor, adsorptive uptake, other tissue-targeting molecules, and nanoparticles could be significantly enhanced without dilution or non-specific attenuation by blood.

The bolus injection of drugs during flow arrest offers the following advantages:

- Precisely controls drug distribution
- Avoids variation in tissue concentrations due to streaming
- Avoid dilution with blood to achieve high concentrations
- Increases transit time through the capillary network to augment tissue uptake
- Avoids the uptake and metabolism of drugs by blood cells
- Avoids opsonization by serum proteins
- Minimize non-specific binding to proteins and blood cells to protect targeting mechanisms such as surface charge, ligands, receptor-antibodies, and carriers
- Decrease hemodynamic stress to improve ligand-receptor binding
- Could overcome interstitial pressure within tumors to achieve better tumor penetration

Flow arrest drug delivery can be achieved by administering bolus injections of adenosine or by balloon occlusion. It has been used for treating neurological diseases. Pile-Spellman et al. used high-dose adenosine boluses for embolic occlusion of high-flow cerebral arterio-venous malformations with methacrylate [25, 26]. Riina et al. demonstrated the feasibility of balloon occlusion in delivering mannitol and bevacizumab [27, 28]. The technique has been used in treating pediatric pontine tumors [29]. Chapter 20 describes how cationic particles and peptides can target experimental brain tumors in vivo using the FA-IA technique. Malignant and apoptotic cells have overexpression of anionic lipids such as phosphatidyl serine. Cationic cell-penetrating peptide, a trans-activator of transcription (TAT), can cross the blood-brain/tumor barrier and is selectively taken up by cancer cells. FA-IA delivery of TAT and similar peptides could be effective carriers for therapeutic compounds to treat cancers, stroke, and neurodegenerative diseases [24].

Balloon-occluding catheters have been used to treat retinoblastomas to direct drug delivery to the ophthalmic artery [30–35]. Similarly, balloon occlusion has been used to treat hepatic malignancy. Both femoral and radial approaches have been used for this purpose [36–38]. Chemotherapeutic agents can also be dissolved in lipiodol or delivered as drug-eluting beads, thereby occluding feeding arteries to decrease blood flow. Such embolization delays regional clearance and create a depot to extend the delivery of chemotherapeutic agents [39]. The advantages of balloon occlusion are (1) minimizing reflux into the hepatic artery to prevent non-target delivery, (2) alter the blood flow pattern by decreasing the pressure gradient between the distal hepatic artery and the portal circulation, thus localizing the drugs to the tumor, and (3) decrease the interstitial pressure in the tumor to achieve more uniform tumor drug delivery [38, 39]. However, balloon occlusion delivery could result in greater hepatotoxicity; hence, it is recommended that pressure measurements guide flow occlusion [40].

Learning from Accidental Arterial Drug Injections

To develop safe formulations of drugs for arterial injections, one can get some guidance by reviewing accidental or iatrogenic complications [41, 42]. Table 12.3 summarizes the accidental and iatrogenic complications of arterial drug injections described in Chap. 16. These complications can range from transient pain to those resulting in significant tissue destruction.

What can be deduced from iatrogenic complications of arterial drug injections [42] is the following:

- Some compounds are inherently tissue-toxic due to their pharmacological properties. Chemotherapeutic drugs, certain antibotics, vasoconstrictors, preservatives, and solvents are an example.
- Regional tissue injury can occur with water and lipid-soluble drugs.
- Water-soluble drugs are generally safer than lipid-soluble drugs.

Table 12.3 Consequences of accidental iatrogenic arterial injections

No injury-after discontinuation	Propofol, midazolam, dopamine infusion, neostigmine and glycopyrrolate, neostigmine and atropine, Demerol, aminocaproic acid, rocuronium and fentanyl, dexmedetomidine, succinylcholine
No injury with minimal treatment	Atracurium, small doses of pentothal
No permanent injury with Rx	Azlocillin, ephedrine, nitrogen mustard
Chronic pain, motor/sensory loss	Diazepam, clindamycin
Severe injury despite Rx (tissue necrosis, contractures, gangrene, need for amputation)	Diazepam, penicillin, pentazocine, paracetamol/benzyl alcohol, benzylpenicillin, amiodarone, diclofenac/benzyl alcohol, thiopental, crushed prescription opioids, barbiturates
Fatal	Phenytoin (progressive gangrene)

- Drugs can form crystals, leading to injury. Drugs like papaverine and mannitol could crystallize during IA use. The illicit use of crushed tablets that contain methylcellulose is a known cause of embolic injury.
- Complications can be due to the total dose, concentrations, hyperosmolarity, and pH.
- Preservatives in intravenous drugs injected arterially can cause tissue injury, such as:
  - Benzyl alcohol (0.8–2%) can cause tissue necrosis.
  - Chlorobutanol has been suspected of being a cause of neurotoxicity.

Learning from Formulations of Radiocontrast Agents

Radiocontrast agents require the optimization of compounds that are opaque to X-rays. As described in the chapter on the historical review of IA drug delivery, these contrast agents contain iodine. Iodine-containing compounds inherently carry the risk of allergic reactions, nephropathy, and thyroid dysfunction [43]. Many other contrast-related complications are due to their physical properties and due to the expansion of blood volume. Despite potential complications, these compounds are the most frequently used IA drugs. Millions of angiograms are safely done each year. Contrast injections can help determine the safe osmolarity, viscosity, and tonicity parameters that could be used to develop arterial drugs. Compared to intravenous injections, complications with a given contrast agent are worse when injected intraarterially.

Complications during the use of contrast agents include:

- Major complications [44, 45]:
  - Allergic reactions: Anaphylaxis and anaphylactoid reactions
  - Nephrotoxicity
  - Cardiovascular side effects:
    - Vascular loading
    - Bradycardia
    - Pulmonary hypertension
    - Hypotension
  - Preservative toxicity: EDTA/citrate-induced hypocalcemia:
    - Arrhythmias
    - Hypotension
  - Endothelial injury/activation: Vascular thrombosis
  - Increased Blood-Brain Barrier (BBB) permeability and neurological complications
- Minor Complications:
  - Pain on injection and, if extravasated, pain due to resulting tissue injury
  - Flushing and warmth on injection
  - Metallic taste, nausea, dizziness, and vomiting

The formulation of contrast agents and their development over time is an example of the evolution of arterial drugs for a specific application. By manipulating their chemical composition, osmolality, tonicity, and viscosity, modern contrast agents are considerably safer than their predecessors [46]. Though they still pose clinical hazards, the complications are manageable within the guidelines for safe use [47].

Methods to Enhance First-Pass Extraction of Drugs

Rapid uptake must occur during the initial pass through the regional circulation for IA drugs to be effective. However, drug uptake might be restricted by blood-tissue barriers. A classic example of this is the BBB. Some techniques developed for penetrating the BBB could be used for arterial drug delivery Fig. 12.1. These include:

- *Small molecule therapy:*
- The presence of BBB barriers restricts the free diffusion of compounds [48]. This free diffusion probably occurs through the aqueous pores. Free diffusion of compounds is essentially determined by the following [49]:
  - Molecular weights: The diffusion of molecules weighing 300 Daltons (Da) is a hundred times greater than those weighing 450 Da. Generally, molecules under 400 Daltons can easily penetrate the BBB.
  - Molecular size: The molecular area/volume is likely more critical than molecular weight. Compounds with molecular area >100 sq. Å impede diffusion, whereas those under 50 sq. Å can cross the BBB.
  - Ability to form hydrogen bonds: Drugs that can form more than ten hydrogen bonds poorly penetrate the BBB, while those forming <5 hydrogen bonds can do so easily.
  - Molecular flexibility: Drugs that permit rotation of the molecules can diffuse easier across the BBB than rigid ones.

  Recent cancer treatments target cell signaling pathways with large (≈140 kDa) antibodies or smaller molecules (<400 Da). However, only 2% of the small molecules developed for cancer treatment can cross the BBB yet are less effective in treating brain cancers. Temozolomide (mol wt. 192 Da) can easily penetrate the BBB, and the CSF concentrations are 30% of those of the arterial blood. IA temozolomide can improve drug delivery with or without BBB disruption, but the outcome has yet to be improved with IA delivery in clinical trials [28].

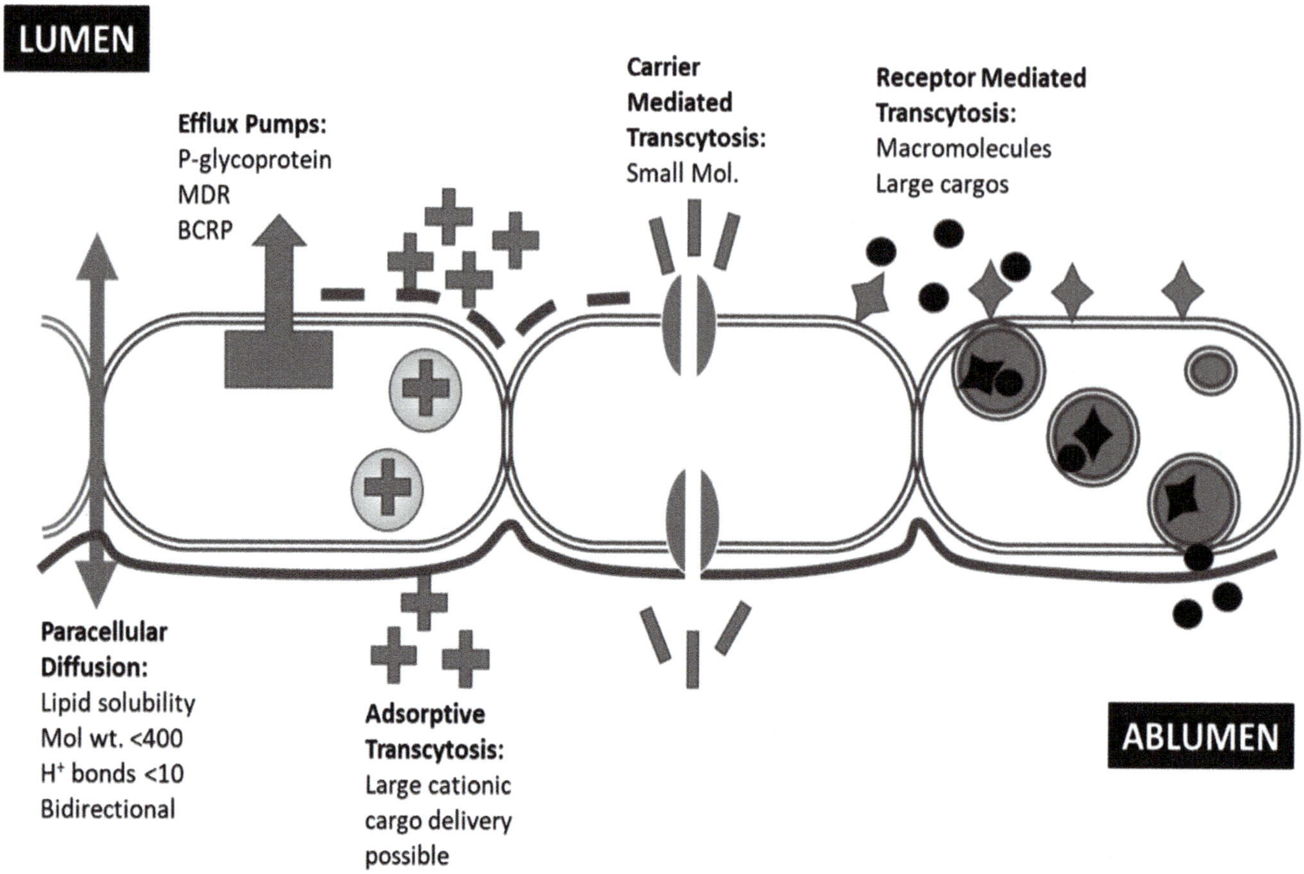

Fig. 12.1 Drug transport mechanisms across the blood-brain barrier

- *Increased lipid solubility:* The drug's lipid solubility is determined by the extent of hydrogen bonding. For drugs to cross the BBB, they should form less than eight hydrogen bonds [48]. The number of hydrogen bonds can be decreased by adding functional groups.
  - For example, in the case of morphine, if two hydroxyl groups are acetylated to form heroin, The BBB permeability increases 10× [48, 50]
  - Nitrogen mustards represent some of the most potent lipid-soluble compounds in cancer treatment. The problem with increased lipid solubility with bolus injection is that tissue concentration may not be sustained. Unless the drug is trapped in the tissue, it will also be cleared rapidly once the arterial concentration declines [2]. Furthermore, small lipid-soluble molecules are often extruded by the p-glycoprotein transport.
  - Another problem is the retention of lipid-soluble compounds by white matter with higher lipid content and lower blood flow. Such drug retention could explain the white matter injuries seen with IA nitrogen mustard treatments [51]

  Thus, increasing lipid solubility is an effective way to improve drug delivery, but it also poses several challenges. FA-IA delivery can enhance the deposition of lipid-soluble drugs sevenfold compared to an IA infusion and 24-fold greater than an IV infusion [20]. Thus, lipid-soluble compounds might need careful dose adjustments, particularly with flow arrest.
- *Concurrent disruption of the blood-brain barrier:* Many drugs other than those used as anesthetics and those used for treating psychiatric illnesses do not cross the blood-brain and blood-tumor barrier. IA mannitol has been used to disrupt the barrier and enhance drug delivery during its first pass through the cerebral circulation [52, 53]. Mannitol is also a vasodilator, increasing blood flow. It has the potential to improve the delivery of the recirculating drug [54]. However, IA mannitol has reported neurological complications, and the degree of disruption can vary considerably. An alternative strategy to mannitol, such as focused ultrasound, has emerged. The disruption can be enhanced using microbubbles; ultrasound could also release the drug from nanoparticles. However, the technology remains experimental. Super-selective delivery into a smaller region could also enhance mannitol safety. FA-IA bevacizumab with concurrent BBB disruption is safe in GBM patients [27].
- *Carrier-mediated drug uptake:* FA-IA delivery permits the delivery of high drug concentrations locally to the tar-

get site. Carrier assisted drug delivery with FA-IA technique can greatly augment tissue-selective delivery as it delivers pure drug conjugates to the target site as demonstrated by videomicroscopy [20]. Drugs with similar structural properties mimicking the natural substrate of the carrier can be selectively delivered to the target site. Carriers can be expressed on non-target cells; therefore, target selectivity is somewhat attenuated when the drugs are injected intravenously. FA-IA delivery could enhance carriers' effectiveness by selectively delivering them to the target site. A companion chapter discusses carrier transport in detail, and some of the major carriers that can transport drugs across the BBB are listed in Table 12.4. Of all carrier systems, neutral amino acid transporter (LAT1, Fig. 12.2) is one of the most widely used carrier systems for drug delivery, and it is overexpressed in many cancer cell lines [55]

LAT1 is primarily expressed in the basolateral surface of the cell membrane. It is coupled with CD98 on the cell surface. It is often difficult to demonstrate by immunohistochemistry. However, mRNA and protein expression studies show expression in several tissues, such as the cortex, retina, esophagus, testis, bone marrow, and placenta. Besides L-phenylalanine, LAT1 transports leucine, isoleucine, methionine, tryptophan, valine, and tyrosine. LAT 1 is widely expressed in many cancer cell lines. It offers an attractive cancer-targeting strategy. Inhibition of LAT1 can deny cancer cells essential amino acids and inhibit cell growth. LAT1 is a very efficient transporter for delivering drugs and nanoparticles. The topic of

Table 12.4 Carriers across the blood-brain barriers that could enhance arterial drug delivery[a]

Carrier	Transport rate	Concentration (pMol/mg)	Km (μM)	Vmax (nmol/min/g)	Prototypic carrier	Substrate and drugs transported
Large neutral amino acid	3000	0.43 ± 0.09	26 ± 6	22 ± 4	LAT1	L-phenylalanine: Melphalan, L-dopa, gabapentin, paraquat
Monocarboxylic acid	2700	2.3 ± 0.8	1800 ± 600	91 ± 35	MCT1	L-lactic acid: Salicylate, valproic acid, simvastatin
Glucose	600	139 ± 46	11,000 ± 1400	1420 ± 140	GLUT1	D-glucose: Glycoconjugates Glyconanoparticles
Basic amino acid	270	1.1 ± 0.2	40 ± 24	5 ± 3	CAT1	L-arginine, histidine, lysine, pyrrolysine, ornithine
Purine nucleoside	–	<0.14	25 ± 3	0.75 ± 0.08	CNT2	Adenosine, uridine, inosine, guanidine: floxuridine, fluoropyrimidine, zidovudine, ribavirin

[a] See reviews by Pardridge and Zhang [48, 55]. Transport rate across BBB: molecules/s

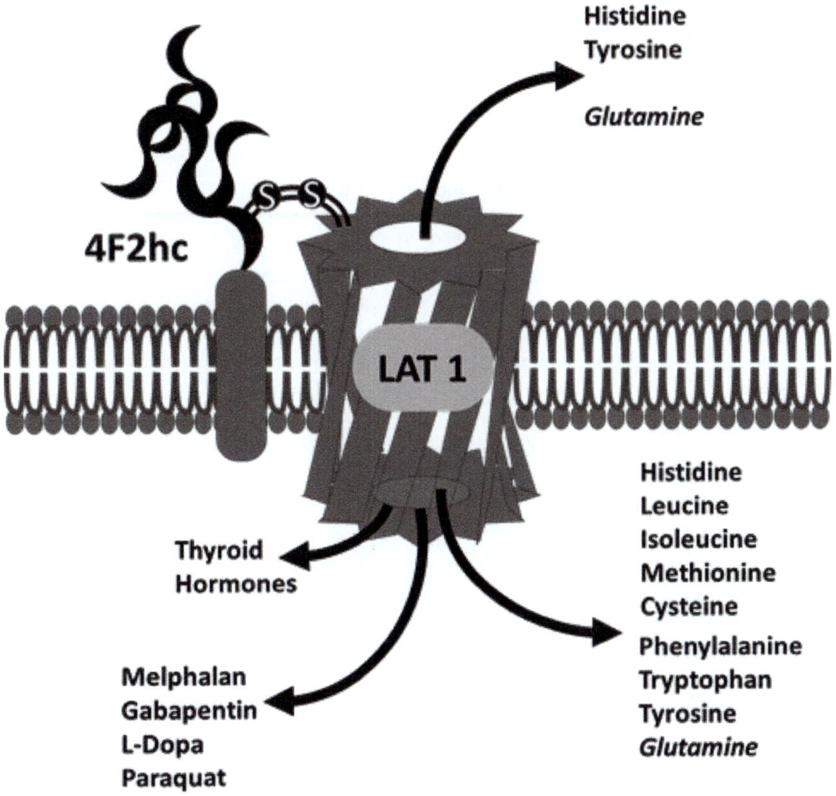

Fig. 12.2 L-Type of Amino Acid Transporter -1

Amino Acid Transporters for Drug Delivery was reviewed by Zhang et al and that of LAT-1 by Puris et al. in 2020 and summary is presented in Table 12.5 [55, 87].

The main concerns with carrier-based drug delivery are the lack of target cell specificity, substrate specificity, and competition with endogenous substrates. There are also problems with demonstrating the efficacy of delivery. Carrier-mediated drug delivery is effective for small molecules. Macromolecules and nanoparticle carriers help localize the target site, but internalization may require another mechanism. The limitation of carrier-mediated transport is due to competition with the natural substrates in circulation that can be overcome by FA-IA delivery. When FA-IA delivers pure drug to the target site, the first-pass contact with blood proteins and circulating substrates can be avoided.

- *Receptor-mediated drug uptake:* Receptor-mediated transcytosis delivers macromolecules and large nanoparticles across endothelial cells [89, 90]. These include receptors for insulin, transferrin, lipoproteins, KS5, and rabies virus capsular proteins. See the recent comprehensive review on Brain Drug Delivery by Pardridge [48]. Table 12.6 summarizes key receptor-mediated drug delivery mechanisms.

- *Adsorptive transcytosis:* Adsorption mechanisms can facilitate drug development through the cationization of proteins or by employing cell-penetrating peptides capable of binding the endoluminal surface of endothelial cells. These molecules then follow transcytosis pathways, transporting small molecules and proteins across the BBB. See the review by Herve et al. and summarized from the publication in Table 12.7 [88]

- *Embolic carrier-assisted chemotherapy:* Although the arterial delivery of embolic materials for treating neurological diseases carries the risk of stroke, embolic materials are used clinically to reduce tumor blood flow before surgery [130], ablate arteriovenous malformations [131] and during treatment of certain brain aneurysms [132, 133]. It is conceivable that embolic modalities could be

Table 12.5 LAT1 conjugated compounds for potential arterial drug delivery applications[a]

Strategy	Representative compounds		Proposed clinical use	References
Natural substrate	l-phenylalanine, leucine, isoleucine, valine, Tryptophan, methionine, tyrosine		Depletion/ inhibits cancer growth	[56, 57]
Prodrugs and drugs	Chemotherapeutic	Melphalan	Several cancers	[58]
	Antiepileptic	Gabapentin	N/A	[59–61]
	Parkinson's Ds	L-DOPA	N/A	[59, 62–64]
LAT1 inhibitor	Non-selective substrate	BCH	Epidermoid carcinoma, C6 glioma and osteosarcoma	[65]
	Binds to LAT1	Compounds 5/17	Cervical cancer	[66, 67]
	Inhibition of recombinant LAT1	Compounds 28/46/36	proteoliposomes	[68]
	LAT1 blocker	JPH203	Brain, Colorectal cancers, thyroid, solid tumors, leukemias	[66]
	LAT1 competitive inhibitor	SKN103	Pancreatic and squamous Ca	[69]
	Antibody	mAbLAT1	Epithelial and glandular malignancies	[70]
Substrate drug conjugates	Methionine-Au-Np	Doxorubicin	Liver, lung, breast Ca	[71]
	Threonine	Gemcitabine-threonine amide (GCB) converted to CBG-triphosphate	Pancreatic ovarian, bladder, small cell lung cancer, GBM	[72]
	Efflux inhibitor probenicid	Amino acid-probenecid conjugate	Breast cancer	[73]
Liposomes and nanoparticles	L-DOPA	WP1066	Glioma	[74]
	L- and D-DOPA	Multibranched AuNP	Breast Ca	[75]
	Glutamate	Docetaxel liposomes	GBM	[76]
	Glutamate	Paclitaxel Nanocarrier	Breast and cervical cancer	[77]
	L-Methionine	Ligand affinity	In-silico	[78]
Sensitizers	Tyrosine	Fluorescein-5-meleimide	Cervical cancer imaging	[79]
PET ligand	Tyrosine	18F-Fluoroethyl-L-tyrosine	GBM	[80, 81]
	Methionine	11C-Methionine	GBM	[82, 83, 160]
	DOPA	18F DOPA	GBM	[84]
Boron neutron capture	Phenylalanine	P-boronophenylalanine	GBM and Pancreatic Ca cells	[85, 86]

[a] See reviews by Zhang et al., Puris et al., and Halfliger et al. [55, 66, 87]

Table 12.6 Receptor-mediated transcytosis with potential for arterial drug delivery applications

Receptor	Characteristic	References
Insulin	Insulin has half-life is 10 min, and carries risk of hypoglycemia Treatment of Alzheimer's disease; mucopolysaccharidosis	[91–93]
Insulin receptor antibodies and insulin -like growth factors I/II	Effective in rats with IA delivery and for cancer targeting	[91, 93–96]
Transferrin	Transferrin delivery is ineffective due to naturally high circulating levels Anti-transferrin receptor antibody effective for drug delivery Treatment of Alzheimer's disease, glycogen storage disease, stroke	[97–101]
Lipoproteins	Examples include ApoE, ApoB, and Aingopep-2 mediated For gene delivery, liposomal guidance, and conjugated chemotherapy	[102–106]
Leptin	Delivery of leptin conjugate by intranasal route effective in mice	[107]
Amyloid beta protein I-40, I-42	Effective in vivo delivery	[108–110]
FC5	Fragment of the heavy domain of antibody to endothelial cells targets. Stable, lightweight, accumulate in the brain	[111–113]
Rabies virus glycoprotein	Target nicotinic acetylcholine receptors. Effective siRNA delivery possible	[114–118]

Table 12.7 Adsorptive mediated transcytosis mechanisms with potential arterial drug delivery applications

Cationic entity	Mechanism	In-vivo/model	References
Protamine	Not known	Rat: IA injection	[119]
Histone	Not known	Rat: IA injection	[120]
Avidin	Not known	In-vitro	[121]
Agglutinin: Wheat Germ	Not known	Rat: IV or intraventricular/sub-arachnoid	[122]
Agglutinin: Ricin 1	Not known	In-vitro	[123]
Cationic albumin	Not known	Rat: IA injection	[124, 125]
Cationic antibodies	Not known	Rat: IA injection	[124–126]
Cationic antibody fragments	Caveolae mediated	Rat: IA injection	[127]
TAT	Direct penetration likely in high concentrations	Rat: IA injection	[24]
Syn B	Caveolae-independent	Rat: IA injection	[128, 129]

developed for treating certain CNS malignancies. In the case of the liver, a wide range of embolic agents with various particle sizes and properties have been developed. The rationale for embolization for liver cancer is the following:

- Decrease blood flow, causing tumor ischemia and necrosis.
- Selectively deliver chemotherapeutic agents to the tumor site.
- Sustained local release of chemotherapeutic agents.
- Due to the trapping of the drug in the liver, there is less systemic exposure to the drug.
- Embolic material might increase local absorption and biological effectiveness of drugs.

Therefore, to get maximum benefits from embolic treatments, the operational goal of such interventions is to densely pack the hepatic arterial branches with particles without overspilling into the systemic circulation. A variety of embolic materials have been developed for treating liver malignancy. These include:

- *Bland embolic material*: The objective of bland particles that do not contain chemotherapeutic drugs is to cause ischemic necrosis of the tumor. Although tumors can have large arteriovenous fistulae, typical vessels feeding the tumors are in the 25–75 μm range. Thus, particles 40–150 μm are needed to occlude these vessels, while larger particles, 500–750 μm, might be needed to occlude a fistula [39]
- *Lipiodol (ethiodized oil)* is a radiocontrast agent for imaging hepatic neoplasm with IA injections. The particle size of lipiodol can range from 100 to 300 nm. Conventional trans-arterial chemoembolization uses chemotherapy agents mixed with lipiodol (cTACE). This contrast agent can be used only with adequate biliary drainage. It carries the risk of pulmonary and cerebral embolization. It can lead to allergic reactions and can potentially injure the liver. Lipiodol is somewhat structurally unstable, and although it can reach distal branches, new structurally flexible embolic agents have greater reach [134]
- *Cellulose embolization*: Drugs delivered through ethyl cellulose particles were used for TACE to occlude the vessels and deliver chemotherapeutic drugs and sclerosing agents.

- *Drug-eluting beads* (DEBs): DEBs are made of superabsorbent polymers loaded with chemotherapeutic drugs. DEBs vary in size from 100 to 700 μm. Smaller DEBs (100–300 μm) might be more effective than the larger ones. Drugs can diffuse from the DEBs to a distance of 600 μm in the adjacent tissue. DEBs can be covalently bound to iodine to enhance their X-ray imaging. The superiority of cTACE over DEB-TACE is contested. Both improve patient survival [135–137]
- *Transarterial radioembolization (TARE)*: Yttrium-90 is a beta emitter with a half-life of about 64–65 h. Its radiation penetrates a mean of 2.4 mm (range 2–11 mm) of the tissue. Thus, it is well-suited for intravascular brachytherapy and is the most widely used isotope. TARE is indicated for intermediate-stage hepatocellular carcinoma [138–140]
- The two formulations used for ^{90}Y-TARE include:

  Glass beads containing 90Y have a specific activity of about 2500 Bq.

  Resins have ^{90}Y bonded to the surface and have a specific activity of 50–400 Bq.

  TARE can be used for either (1) radiation lobectomy, in which the treated lobe of the liver atrophies and there is compensatory hypertrophy of the other lobe, (2) radiation segmentectomy, when two or more liver segments are treated, and (3) modified radiation lobectomy combines high-dose radiation treatment of the tumor segment while a low-dose treatment is given to the entire lobe [139]

The complications of TARE have decreased over time. Local complications more frequent with metastatic disease include perihepatic/pleural effusion, biliary necrosis/biloma, and hepatic abscess. Complications from non-target site irradiations have significantly decreased due to proper patient selection, better imaging, personalized dosing, and particle delivery. Nontarget site complications include radiation injuries to the gut, gall bladder, pancreases and lungs [139]

The Importance of First-Pass Pharmacokinetics

Intra-arterial delivery of chemotherapy via hepatic artery infusion pump has been clinically accepted and widely used in the past 20 years to treat selected patients with advanced hepatobiliary cancers. Another cancer that is routinely treated with IA drugs is retinoblastoma. However, as a larger organ, the liver poses very different challenges. Both these organs have relative vascular isolation. In the case of retinoblastoma, the ophthalmic artery perfuses the tumor, enabling relatively selective drug delivery. In the case of the liver, the perfusion of the organ is exceedingly complex and the catheter location has to be carefully optimized as shown in Fig. 12.3. The hepatic artery and the portal vein perfuse the liver. These two systems autoregulate to maintain a constant blood flow. The two systems also demonstrate reciprocal

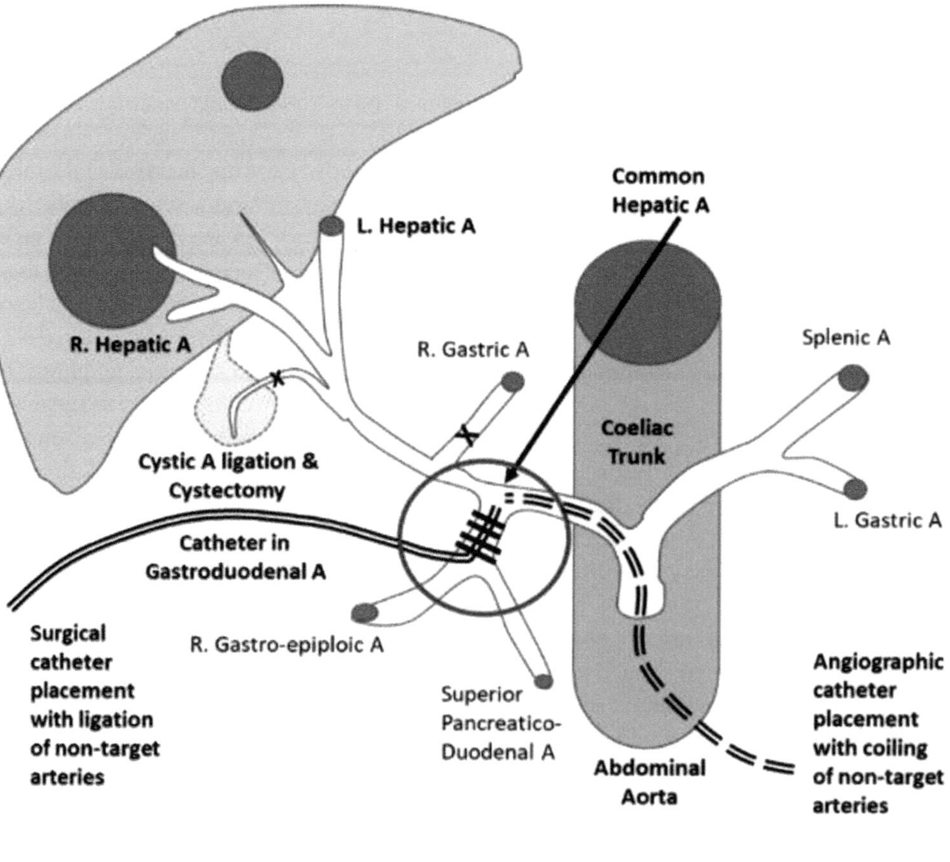

Fig. 12.3 Vascular access and optimization for hepatic artery infusion

flows. Hepatic artery blood flow increases when portal pressure declines. The hepatic artery carries oxygenated blood. However, the portal vein carries partially deoxygenated blood. Because metastatic lesions in the liver are primarily perfused via the hepatic artery, infusion of FRDU into the hepatic artery preferentially targets hepatic tumors over normal liver parenchyma. Beyond that, there are a few other similarities in treating these two malignancies. Retinoblastoma affects a relatively small region of the body compared to the large size of the liver. Thus, relatively greater amounts of drug relative to the tumor mass can be delivered while avoiding systemic toxicity. That is not the case with a large organ such as the liver. Due to its large size, despite significant differences, hepatic artery infusion provides valuable lessons for developing drugs for arterial treatment of neurological diseases.

Table 12.2 compares the challenges of treating liver and brain cancers with IA drug delivery. The favorable characteristics of the host tissue in the case of liver cancers include a sizeable functional reserve, ischemia and injury tolerance, and regenerative capacity. However, there are also significant challenges for example, in advanced stages of liver cancer, the disease is multifocal, requiring perfusion of the entire organ, which poses technical challenges. Superselective injections are highly desirable for arterial drug delivery may not be possible with advanced liver disease. However, the hepatic artery selectively perfuses the malignant tumors and could help to target them. Although the variable origin of the hepatic artery requires technical expertise. One of the essential precautions taken with HAI is improving vascular isolation by embolizing or ligating atrial branches of the coeliac trunk and irrigating non-target tissues. The isolation from these arteries, Fig. 12.3, restricts chemotherapy selectively to tumors, minimizing the risks of complications related to the gallbladder and gut.

About 20% of the patients have atypical arterial anatomy, which can lead to complications and treatment failures. Catheter dislodgement, arterial thrombosis, catheter thrombosis, arterial dissection, bleeding, and stenosis have been reported during HAI therapy. However, surgical experience, drug selection, improved catheters, improved implantable pumps, and minimally invasive surgical techniques have reduced those risks.

Models of arterial drug delivery [2, 4] reveal that IA drug delivery is most effective when there is:

- Low regional blood flow
- High regional extraction without conversion to inactive metabolites
- High total body clearance

All three of these conditions are met during HAI. The first is low regional blood flow. For example, while the total hepatic blood flow is about 1200 mL/min, the hepatic artery only provides a fourth of the blood flow or about 300 mL/min. Since the drug is infused into the proper hepatic artery, it has a considerably higher impact on drug delivery than infusion in the portal vein. Furthermore, there is evidence that the blood supply to metastatic lesions in the liver primarily comes from the hepatic artery, unlike normal liver parenchyma. This explains why experimental tumor models have shown that hepatic artery infusion is 15× more effective than portal vein infusion, and randomized studies have failed to show a response in patients treated with portal vein infusion. About 20–40% of patients respond to hepatic artery infusion, can rise to 80–90% in the first year when combined with systemic therapy [16]. Also, compared to an infusion in the carotid artery, where a similar blood volume infuses about 400 g of brain tissue, the hepatic artery is more efficient as it perfuses a larger volume of tissue, about 1500 g. Thus, hepatic artery perfusion/gm tissue is much less than the brain. Second is the capability of the liver to extract the drugs. For example, floxuridine has 95% hepatic extraction, meaning only 5% of the drug reaches systemic circulation. The third is the rapid clearance of the drugs. Several drugs in Table 12.8 have elimination half-lives of a few minutes. It is estimated that IA infusion of floxuridine is 400 times more effective than IV infusion.

Several studies have demonstrated the benefits of HAI treatment over IV therapy. However, HAI yields the best

Table 12.8 Pharmacokinetic parameters of drugs used for hepatic artery infusion (HAI) therapy

Drug	Mol wt.	First pass extraction	Elimination half-life	Vd	Protein binding	Clearance	Comment
Floxuridine	246	95%	16 min	N/A	N/A	>200 L/h	Prodrug
5 Fluorouracil	130	80%	10–20 min[a]	N/A	8–12%	>200 L/h	90% excreted in the urine in 1 h
Doxorubicin	543	80%	20–48 h	1400 L	75%	30 L/h	
Epirubicin	543	60%	1.5–30 h	1800 L	77%	70 L/h	
Cisplatin	300	25%	20–30 min	20 L	90% Pt	26 L/h	Irreversible protein binding
Oxaliplatin	397	50%	16.8 h	–	90% Pt	25 L/h	Irreversible protein binding
Gemcitabine	263	55–90%[a]	32–94 min	86 L	10%	140 L/h	

[a] Dose-dependent. All values calculated for a 72 kg person with 1.72 m^2 BSA

results when combined with systemic treatment. The emergence of tyrosine kinase and checkpoint inhibitors as first— and second-line concurrent therapies seems to improve outcomes further [141, 142].

Pharmacodynamic Considerations

In addition to the pharmacokinetic considerations, there are pharmacodynamic ones. Drug or drug cargo should be selected based on therapeutic objective, their desired onset of action and duration of effect, their required frequency of administration, and whether long-term infusion is possible. In the case of cancer treatment, effective drugs will have a relatively early onset of effect, their concentration-time cytotoxicity should be low, and they should not cause treatment failure due to cell cycle specificity. Furthermore, the total dose required for these drugs to have a practical cytotoxic effect should be accompanied by no more than an acceptable level of local toxicity and a low likelihood of causing systemic toxicity. Given higher concentration in target tissues and lower potential for systemic toxicity if the drug's systemic clearance is truly rapid, it might be possible to achieve the goal of near total cell kill. However, as drugs are developed, fractional kill goals may achievable with lower doses or shorter treatments.

Additional Concerns with Arterial Drugs:

Other factors that can enhance the pharmacokinetics of IA drugs include monitoring drug delivery, avoiding formulations where the active ingredient is mixed with harmful preservatives in the IA setting, and systemic measures conducted concurrently with IA drug administration to enhance its effects.

- *Monitoring IA drug delivery:*
  - Defining the angioarchitecture of the target site. As is the case for HAI, ligation of side branches of the target arterial system can enhance the delivery of IA into the target tissue and mitigate toxicity to other tissues [18, 141].
  - Placement of catheters under imaging guidance. Reducing the risk of catheter malposition improves outcomes for patients undergoing IA treatment. Intraoperative direct visualization or imaging guidance can confirm adequate catheter placement for IA drug delivery.
  - Testing for drug distribution after IA delivery during surgery or afterward. Several testing modalities have been proposed for IA drug delivery technology. These include:

    Angiography at the catheter placement can confirm positioning.

    Dye injections- such as fluorescein under a Woods lamp, methylene blue, or, more recently, indocyanine green administration, can be performed intraoperatively to confirm drug delivery to the adequate tissue bed.

    PET imaging- follow-up when needed, verifying target tissue delivery prior to chemotherapy.
  - In-vivo monitoring of drug delivery: Multifunctional carrier systems: With large drug carriers, developing dual-function carrier molecules that can carry tracers and therapeutic compounds might be possible. Dual-function gold carriers, that are potentially radiologically and optically traceable, have been tagged with optical dyes and ligands to increase target selectivity [75]. In conjunction with nanocarriers tailored to malignant cell microenvironment, monitorable nanotherapeutics would be highly relevant to arterial delivery [143].
- *Selection of solvents and preservatives:*
  - Avoidance of toxic preservatives. This involves the toxic capacity of the preservatives in question and their specific risk of harm in the IA setting [144]. Avoid benzyl alcohol, given the significant risk in retrospective studies of severe target tissue injury [41, 42, 145]
  - Perfluorocarbons. Data suggest that these lipophilic molecules can improve pharmacokinetics by being used for drug delivery [146]
- *Concurrent measures to enhance arterial drug delivery:*
  - Options to reduce blood flow: several measures are available to reduce blood flow and improve IA drug delivery: balloon occlusion of target arterial system [27], facilitating flow arrest and drug delivery in ideal conditions, inducing a cardiac pause with adenosine [25, 26], adding IA vasoconstrictors [4], hyperventilating the patient [147] or inducing deep anesthesia [148] to improve delivery to brain tumors.
  - Measures to induce chemo-sensitization: Hyperthermia can enhance drug penetration and increase chemosensitivity [149]
  - Efflux transport inhibitors: Lipid-soluble compounds delivered to cells and rendered ineffective by efflux transporters. These efflux proteins eliminate drugs from the cells, leading to treatment resistance to antibiotics and chemotherapeutic drugs. To overcome treatment resistance, verapamil, a p-gap inhibitor, has been administered with chemotherapeutic drugs. IA verapamil is widely used to treat vasospasm. IA verapamil offers a method to overcome treatment resistance due to efflux protein inhibition [150]
  - Systemic rescue: in the case of drugs with suboptimal systemic clearance and known systemic toxicity for

which there is a known antidote [151]. Furthermore, IA drugs with complementary systemic chemotherapy may improve drug tolerance and treatment outcomes [19]
- Enhanced clearance: Systemic clearance can be facilitated with either extracorporeal removal of the drug [152, 153] or changes in the acid-base balance to favor excretion, such as forced alkaline diuresis although it could potentiate nephrotoxicity [154, 155]
- Arterial radioembolization is useful when inadequate arterial access or microcirculatory failure prevents the direct delivery of chemotherapeutic drugs to the tumor target.

Current Limitations and Future Developments of Arterial Drugs

Maximizing Arterial Drug Delivery

The widely accepted advance in drug delivery via the hepatic artery contrasts with the general failure to develop applications of arterial drugs to treat neurological diseases. The fundamental difference lies in host tissue characteristics. In the case of HAI, occlusion of the artery is well tolerated, while even transient interruption of blood flow carries the risk of stroke, yet flow arrest is for short periods and is often used clinically during endovascular and neurosurgical procedures. The challenge in developing the application of arterial drugs for treating neurological diseases is to optimize drug delivery within short periods of flow arrests that do not risk neurological injuries. Drug formulations must be optimized for rapid uptake and sustained retention to avail the benefits of arterial drug delivery. As reviewed in this chapter, many transport systems have been developed for brain and tumor-selective drug intake. At the same time, arterial drugs pose certain unavoidable risks. Those risks have to be balanced with the benefits of such treatments.

This review makes the case that for maximum benefits of arterial treatments, it is necessary to optimize blood flow distribution to target pathology selectively and, when possible, safely use FA-IA delivery. While many technologies to target neuropathologies have been developed, they have seldom been tested during flow arrest. The advantages of FA-IA delivery include:

- Superselective pharmacological interventions: Superselective delivery can change the risk-benefit of arterial treatment. Selectivity of delivery, for example, could bring radio embolic agents into play whose risks would otherwise be hard to justify. These embolic approaches could be used for local radiation treatments.
- Better control of drug distribution to regional arterial irrigation guided by imaging.
- With effective first-pass uptake, IA drug delivery would instantly achieve therapeutic concentrations at the target site, decreasing the required doses and the time needed to treat effectively.
- Substantial dose reduction may affect the choice of chemotherapy, favoring more potent drugs that are not cell-cycle specific, such as melphalan.
- Reduced contact with blood and circulating proteins enhances the target selectivity of homing strategies. Improved arterial drug delivery could be a force multiplier for tumor targeting strategies.
- The targeted nature of IA drugs could permit the administration of several drugs to the target site while avoiding systemic pharmacokinetic and pharmacodynamic interactions.
- The development and drug formulations based on first-pass extraction through the cerebral circulation will decrease systemic toxicity, as illustrated by the evolution of HAI.
- In addition, systemic side effects can be further decreased by neutralizing the drug with an antidote, removing the recirculating drug by extracorporeal hemoperfusion, or employing drugs with exceedingly short half-lives. While extracorporeal removal has been used in the past, it is highly intrusive and carries the risk of multiple vascular cannulation and embolic injury. Developing drugs with high first-pass extraction circumvents the need for such adjuvant procedures.

Concerns, Problems, and Limitations of Arterial Drugs

- Local toxicity or injury for central nervous system indications. The potential risk of stroke must be balanced against the chances of surviving a fatal disease (brain tumor) or impending neurological morbidity. As described above, local toxicity may be minimized with concurrent measures; however, all intra-arterial interventions will carry the risk of complications related to IA access.
- IA drugs require exceedingly rapid uptake with sufficient retention in the target site or having the desired duration of effect, limiting the currently available drug options for IA administration.
- It may be challenging to achieve all the desired therapeutic effects within the short time permitted by most IA interventions for neurological purposes, which last a few minutes and seldom more than an hour. For example, chemotherapy for brain tumors could be achieved swiftly, while treatment of stroke-reperfusion injury may take hours.
- Additional risks of IA drugs include long-term drug safety of catheterization, embolic complications, catheter migration, vascular injury, and closed-system drug deliv-

ery problems that must be addressed if more prolonged infusions are used.

Given these risks and benefits with currently available options for IA drug administration, the clinical indications for IA drugs are presently limited. However, current options do not lack scientific evidence to support their use or safety, which has been available for decades.

Current Clinically Accepted Applications of Arterial Drugs

- The most widely used arterial drugs are radiocontrast agents, which have become exceedingly safe, permitting millions of angiographic procedures worldwide each year.
- Cancer treatments: IA drugs have been established as a treatment for hepatobiliary malignant disease via hepatic artery infusion and for retinoblastoma with super-selective ophthalmic artery infusion.
- IA vasodilators have been developed to treat vasospasm, mainly in the central nervous system, though this may also be translated to other subspecialties.
- IA thrombolytics are often used in vascular surgery to treat peripheral artery disease with acute critical limb ischemia and were used for treating stroke. Mechanical thrombectomy, with or without stenting, has superseded the use of arterial thrombolytics for embolic stroke due to rapid recanalization and less risk of hemorrhagic conversion.
- Neurological: Besides BBB disruption, treating vasospasm, certain brain tumors, and intraarterial thrombolysis for stroke, intra-arterial delivery is used to occlude tumor vessels and embolize vascular malformations.
- Additionally, intra-arterial delivery of anesthetics permits Wada testing before resection of ablation of brain tumors and epilepsy.

Optimized IA delivery systems and drugs developed explicitly for IA administration can potentially advance the treatment of cancer, stroke, neurodegenerative diseases, and vascular diseases. For brain cancer, the benefits of IA delivery for glioblastoma treatment are still unproven [149, 156]. FA-arterial delivery may not require disruption of BBB due to the ability to target malignant tissues. Improved IA drug delivery might present the opportunity for "pharmacologic surgery" as an alternative to conventional oncologic resection, as in the case of retinoblastoma. In the case of stroke, IA drug delivery allows time-dependent multidrug interventions, which, if carefully selected, minimize systemic interactions of these drugs. Similarly, treating neurodegenerative diseases may be improved using IA antiapoptotic drugs, delivery of growth factors, stem cells, and gene vectors. Various chapters in this book have discussed some of these emerging applications.

Conclusion

In conclusion, arterial drug delivery is substantially more complicated than intravenous drug injections. The first attempts at intravenous anesthetics began in 1660 when Robert Boyle and Christopher Wren injected tincture of opium in dogs to produce sleep [157]. However, intravenous drugs were not routinely used until the mid-twentieth century. Jose Goyanes demonstrated the first arterial drug delivery in 1908 [158, 159]. Technologies needed for safe arterial delivery, such as imaging, catheters, and anticoagulation protocols, are still developing. Thus, the arterial approach is still in its infancy relative to intravenous injections. Even in this early stage of technology development, the impact of arterial treatments is evident in the treatment of liver cancers, where arterial drug delivery has a well-established role. The success of hepatic artery infusions is due to a wide range of drugs and drug formulations developed for clinical use. Based on HAI and other sources of information, we can arrive at desirable properties of arterial drugs:

- The drug must have significant first-pass extraction.
- It should have high systemic clearance and a small volume of distribution.
- It should be tissue nontoxic across a wide range of concentrations.
- It should be preferably water-soluble to avoid potentially tissue-toxic solvents.
- It should be retained for sufficient time and concentration for the desired therapeutic effect.
- It should be pH neutral, isotonic, and iso-osmotic.
- It should be stable, not precipitate, and contain no toxic preservative.

The challenges in treating neurological diseases are far more daunting than those in treating liver diseases due to the complex nature of the tissue and the devastating impact of any injury. These challenges are further enhanced by the rapid transit of the drugs through the cerebral circulation. In the case of the liver, arterial blood flow can be arrested for a sustained period, and embolic material can provide depots of drugs to treat tumors. That is not the case for neurological diseases where cessation of blood flow beyond 3–5 min could result in stroke. Thus, investigating and optimizing the first-pass uptake of the drug will be essential to treat neurological diseases. Conversely, a compelling argument can be made that if drug and drug formulations are not optimized for arterial delivery, the potential of arterial drugs in treating neurological diseases will remain untapped.

References

1. Anonymous. Interventional radiology market—by product (MRI systems, CT scanners, ultrasound imaging systems, angiography systems), by application (Cardiology, Oncology, Urology, Gastroenterology, Obstetrics, Gynecology), by end-use & forecast, 2022–2030. 2022. https://www.gminsights.com/industry-analysis/interventional-radiology-market.
2. Cooke JN, Ellis JA, Hossain S, Nguyen J, Bruce JN, Joshi S. Computational pharmacokinetic rationale for intra-arterial delivery to the brain. Drug Deliv Transl Res. 2016;6(5):622–9.
3. Dedrick RL. Interspecies scaling of regional drug delivery. J Pharm Sci. 1986;75(11):1047–52.
4. Dedrick RL. Arterial drug infusion: pharmacokinetic problems and pitfalls. J Natl Cancer Inst. 1988;80(2):84–9.
5. Eckman WW, Patlak CS, Fenstermacher JD. A critical evaluation of the principles governing the advantages of intra-arterial infusions. J Pharmacokinet Biopharm. 1974;2(3):257–85.
6. Fenstermacher J, Gazendam J. Intra-arterial infusions of drugs and hyperosmotic solutions as ways of enhancing CNS chemotherapy. Cancer Treat Rep. 1981;65(Suppl 2):27–37.
7. Lutz RJ, Dedrick RL, Boretos JW, Oldfield EH, Blacklock JB, Doppman JL. Mixing studies during intracarotid artery infusions in an in vitro model. J Neurosurg. 1986;64(2):277–83.
8. Saris SC, Blasberg RG, Carson RE, deVroom HL, Lutz R, Dedrick RL, et al. Intravascular streaming during carotid artery infusions. Demonstration in humans and reduction using diastole-phased pulsatile administration. J Neurosurg. 1991;74(5):763–72.
9. Saris SC, Shook DR, Blasberg RG, Dedrick RL, Doppman JL, Bankiewicz KS, et al. Carotid artery mixing with diastole-phased pulsed drug infusion. J Neurosurg. 1987;67(5):721–5.
10. Willinsky RA, Taylor SM, TerBrugge K, Farb RI, Tomlinson G, Montanera W. Neurologic complications of cerebral angiography: prospective analysis of 2,899 procedures and review of the literature. Radiology. 2003;227(2):522–8.
11. Liang J, Lv X, Lu C, Ye X, Chen X, Fu J, et al. Prognostic factors of patients with gliomas—an analysis on 335 patients with glioblastoma and other forms of gliomas. BMC Cancer. 2020;20(1):35.
12. Klopp CT, Alford TC, Bateman J, Berry GN, Winship T. Fractionated intra-arterial cancer; chemotherapy with methyl bis amine hydrochloride; a preliminary report. Ann Surg. 1950;132(4):811–32.
13. Anteby R, Kemeny NE, Kingham TP, D'Angelica MI, Wei AC, Balachandran VP, et al. Getting chemotherapy directly to the liver: the historical evolution of hepatic artery chemotherapy. J Am Coll Surg. 2021;232(3):332–8.
14. Napier KJ, Lidsky ME, James OG, Wildman-Tobriner B. Hepatic arterial infusion pumps: what the radiologist needs to know. Radiographics. 2021;41(3):895–908.
15. Laface C, Laforgia M, Molinari P, Ugenti I, Gadaleta CD, Porta C, et al. Hepatic arterial infusion of chemotherapy for advanced hepatobiliary cancers: state of the art. Cancers (Basel). 2021;13(12):3091.
16. Power DG, Kemeny NE. The role of floxuridine in metastatic liver disease. Mol Cancer Ther. 2009;8(5):1015–25.
17. Buisman FE, Filipe WF, Galjart B, Grunhagen DJ, Homs MYV, Moelker A, et al. Adjuvant intra-arterial chemotherapy for patients with resected colorectal liver metastases: a systematic review and meta-analysis. HPB (Oxford). 2022;24(3):299–308.
18. Doussot A, Kemeny NE, D'Angelica MI. Hepatic arterial infusional chemotherapy in the management of colorectal cancer liver metastases. Hepat Oncol. 2015;2(3):275–90.
19. Cercek A, Boerner T, Tan BR, Chou JF, Gonen M, Boucher TM, et al. Assessment of hepatic arterial infusion of floxuridine in combination with systemic gemcitabine and oxaliplatin in patients with unresectable intrahepatic cholangiocarcinoma: a phase 2 clinical trial. JAMA Oncol. 2020;6(1):60–7.
20. Joshi S, Wang M, Etu JJ, Suckow RF, Cooper TB, Feinmark SJ, et al. Transient cerebral hypoperfusion enhances intraarterial carmustine deposition into brain tissue. J Neurooncol. 2008;86(2):123–32.
21. Nguyen J, Cooke JRN, Ellis JA, Deci M, Emala CW, Bruce JN, et al. Cationizable lipid micelles as vehicles for intraarterial glioma treatment. J Neurooncol. 2016;128(1):21–8.
22. Nguyen J, Hossain SS, Cooke JRN, Ellis JA, Deci MB, Emala CW, et al. Flow arrest intra-arterial delivery of small TAT-decorated and neutral micelles to gliomas. J Neurooncol. 2017;133(1):77–85.
23. Joshi S, Singh-Moon RP, Ellis JA, Chaudhuri DB, Wang M, Reif R, et al. Cerebral hypoperfusion-assisted intra-arterial deposition of liposomes in normal and glioma-bearing rats. Neurosurgery. 2015;76(1):92–100.
24. Joshi S, Cooke JRN, Ellis JA, Emala CW, Bruce JN. Targeting brain tumors by intra-arterial delivery of cell-penetrating peptides: a novel approach for primary and metastatic brain malignancy. J Neurooncol. 2017;135(3):497–506.
25. Pile-Spellman J, Young WL, Joshi S, Duong H, Vang MC, Hartmann A, et al. Adenosine-induced cardiac pause for endovascular embolization of cerebral arteriovenous malformations: technical case report. Neurosurgery. 1999;44(4):881–6; discussion 6–7.
26. Hashimoto T, Young WL, Aagaard BD, Joshi S, Ostapkovich ND, Pile-Spellman J. Adenosine-induced ventricular asystole to induce transient profound systemic hypotension in patients undergoing endovascular therapy. Dose-response characteristics. Anesthesiology. 2000;93(4):998–1001.
27. Riina HA, Knopman J, Greenfield JP, Fralin S, Gobin YP, Tsiouris AJ, et al. Balloon-assisted superselective intra-arterial cerebral infusion of bevacizumab for malignant brainstem glioma. A technical note. Interv Neuroradiol. 2010;16(1):71–6.
28. Burkhardt JK, Riina HA, Shin BJ, Moliterno JA, Hofstetter CP, Boockvar JA. Intra-arterial chemotherapy for malignant gliomas: a critical analysis. Interv Neuroradiol. 2011;17(3):286–95.
29. McCrea HJ, Ivanidze J, O'Connor A, Hersh EH, Boockvar JA, Gobin YP, et al. Intraarterial delivery of bevacizumab and cetuximab utilizing blood-brain barrier disruption in children with high-grade glioma and diffuse intrinsic pontine glioma: results of a phase I trial. J Neurosurg Pediatr. 2021;28(4):371–9.
30. Maddy K, Luther E, Walker A, Hackett A, Lu V, Starke R. Algorithm for evaluating ophthalmic artery pseudo-occlusion during intra-arterial chemotherapy for retinoblastoma. Interv Neuroradiol. 2023:15910199231169843.
31. Marasligiller SA, Williams BK, Vadivelu S, Correa ZM, Abruzzo TA, Nicola MD, et al. Ocular survival after intra-arterial chemotherapy for retinoblastoma improves with accrual of experience and programmatic evolution. Pediatr Blood Cancer. 2023;70(2):e30071.
32. Pham CT, Blanc R, Lumbroso-Le Rouic L, Pistocchi S, Bartolini B, Piotin M. Access to the ophthalmic artery by retrograde approach through the posterior communicating artery for intra-arterial chemotherapy of retinoblastoma. Neuroradiology. 2012;54(8):845–8.
33. Quinn C, Tummala R, Anderson J, Dahlheimer T, Nascene D, Jagadeesan B. Effectiveness of alternative routes of intra-arterial chemotherapy administration for retinoblastoma: potential for response and complications. Interv Neuroradiol. 2019;25(5):556–61.
34. Stenzel E, Goricke S, Temming P, Biewald E, Zulow S, Gobel J, et al. Feasibility of intra-arterial chemotherapy for retinoblastoma: experiences in a large single center cohort study. Neuroradiology. 2019;61(3):351–7.
35. Yamane T, Kaneko A, Mohri M. The technique of ophthalmic arterial infusion therapy for patients with intraocular retinoblastoma. Int J Clin Oncol. 2004;9(2):69–73.

36. Koganemaru M, Abe T, Anai H, Tanaka N, Nonoshita M, Iwamoto R, et al. A newly developed double lumen microballoon catheter with a side hole: initial experience of intraarterial infusion chemotherapy and/or embolization. Jpn J Radiol. 2012;30(10):870–4.
37. Minami Y, Minami T, Chishina H, Arizumi T, Takita M, Kitai S, et al. Balloon-occluded transcatheter arterial chemoembolization for hepatocellular carcinoma: a single-center experience. Oncology. 2015;89(Suppl 2):27–32.
38. Goldman DT, Singh M, Patel RS, Nowakowski FS, Bishay V, Ranade M, et al. Balloon-occluded transarterial chemoembolization for the treatment of hepatocellular carcinoma: a single-center US preliminary experience. J Vasc Interv Radiol. 2019;30(3):342–6.
39. Devcic Z, Toskich BB. Embolic locoregional therapy for the treatment of hepatocellular carcinoma. Endovasc Today. 2020;19(4):54–9.
40. Irie T, Kuramochi M, Takahashi N. Dense accumulation of lipiodol emulsion in hepatocellular carcinoma nodule during selective balloon-occluded transarterial chemoembolization: measurement of balloon-occluded arterial stump pressure. Cardiovasc Intervent Radiol. 2013;36(3):706–13.
41. Sen S, Chini EN, Brown MJ. Complications after unintentional intra-arterial injection of drugs: risks, outcomes, and management strategies. Mayo Clin Proc. 2005;80(6):783–95.
42. Lokoff A, Maynes JT. The incidence, significance, and management of accidental intra-arterial injection: a narrative review. Can J Anaesth. 2019;66(5):576–92.
43. Pasternak JJ, Williamson EE. Clinical pharmacology, uses, and adverse reactions of iodinated contrast agents: a primer for the non-radiologist. Mayo Clin Proc. 2012;87(4):390–402.
44. Andreucci M, Solomon R, Tasanarong A. Side effects of radiographic contrast media: pathogenesis, risk factors, and prevention. Biomed Res Int. 2014;2014:741018.
45. Currie GM. Pharmacology, part 5: CT and MRI contrast media. J Nucl Med Technol. 2019;47(3):189–202.
46. Singh J, Daftary A. Iodinated contrast media reactions. J Nucl Med Technol. 2008;36:69–74.
47. Thomsen HS. Guidelines for contrast media from the European Society of Urogenital Radiology. AJR Am J Roentgenol. 2003;181(6):1463–71.
48. Pardridge WM. A historical review of brain drug delivery. Pharmaceutics. 2022;14(6):1283.
49. Pardridge WM. Drug transport across the blood-brain barrier. J Cereb Blood Flow Metab. 2012;32(11):1959–72.
50. Oldendorf WH, Hyman S, Braun L, Oldendorf SZ. Blood-brain barrier: penetration of morphine, codeine, heroin, and methadone after carotid injection. Science. 1972;178(4064):984–6.
51. Rosenblum MK, Delattre JY, Walker RW, Shapiro WR. Fatal necrotizing encephalopathy complicating treatment of malignant gliomas with intra-arterial BCNU and irradiation: a pathological study. J Neurooncol. 1989;7(3):269–81.
52. Uluc K, Ambady P, McIntyre MK, Tabb JP, Kersch CN, Nerison CS, et al. Safety of intra-arterial chemotherapy with or without osmotic blood-brain barrier disruption for the treatment of patients with brain tumors. Neurooncol Adv. 2022;4(1):vdac104.
53. Neuwelt E, Ambady P, Muldoon L, McConnell H, Doolittle N. Outwitting the blood-brain barrier. Oncology (Williston Park). 2016;30(11):963, 966–7.
54. Joshi S, Singh-Moon R, Wang M, Bruce JN, Bigio IJ, Mayevsky A. Real-time hemodynamic response and mitochondrial function changes with intracarotid mannitol injection. Brain Res. 2014;1549:42–51.
55. Zhang L, Sui C, Yang W, Luo Q. Amino acid transporters: emerging roles in drug delivery for tumor-targeting. Asian J Pharm Sci. 2020;15:192–206.
56. Kanai Y. Amino acid transporter LAT1 (SLC7A5) as a molecular target for cancer diagnosis and therapeutics. Pharmacol Ther. 2022;230:107964.
57. Yan R, Li Y, Muller J, Zhang Y, Singer S, Xia L, et al. Mechanism of substrate transport and inhibition of the human LAT1-4F2hc amino acid transporter. Cell Discov. 2021;7(1):16.
58. Matharu J, Oki J, Worthen DR, Smith QR, Crooks PA. Regiospecific and conformationally restrained analogs of melphalan and DL-2-NAM-7 and their affinities for the large neutral amino acid transporter (system LAT1) of the blood-brain barrier. Bioorg Med Chem Lett. 2010;20(12):3688–91.
59. Karkkainen J, Laitinen T, Markowicz-Piasecka M, Montaser A, Lehtonen M, Rautio J, et al. Molecular characteristics supporting l-type amino acid transporter 1 (LAT1)-mediated translocation. Bioorg Chem. 2021;112:104921.
60. Lu X. The role of large neutral amino acid transporter (LAT1) in cancer. Curr Cancer Drug Targets. 2019;19(11):863–76.
61. Dickens D, Webb SD, Antonyuk S, Giannoudis A, Owen A, Radisch S, et al. Transport of gabapentin by LAT1 (SLC7A5). Biochem Pharmacol. 2013;85(11):1672–83.
62. Singh N, Ecker GF. Insights into the structure, function, and ligand discovery of the large neutral amino acid transporter 1, LAT1. Int J Mol Sci. 2018;19(5):1278.
63. Peura L, Malmioja K, Huttunen K, Leppanen J, Hamalainen M, Forsberg MM, et al. Design, synthesis and brain uptake of LAT1-targeted amino acid prodrugs of dopamine. Pharm Res. 2013;30(10):2523–37.
64. Kageyama T, Nakamura M, Matsuo A, Yamasaki Y, Takakura Y, Hashida M, et al. The 4F2hc/LAT1 complex transports L-DOPA across the blood-brain barrier. Brain Res. 2000;879(1–2):115–21.
65. Kim CS, Cho SH, Chun HS, Lee SY, Endou H, Kanai Y, et al. BCH, an inhibitor of system L amino acid transporters, induces apoptosis in cancer cells. Biol Pharm Bull. 2008;31(6):1096–100.
66. Hafliger P, Charles RP. The L-type amino acid transporter LAT1-an emerging target in cancer. Int J Mol Sci. 2019;20(10):2428.
67. Napolitano L, Scalise M, Koyioni M, Koutentis P, Catto M, Eberini I, et al. Potent inhibitors of human LAT1 (SLC7A5) transporter based on dithiazole and dithiazine compounds for development of anticancer drugs. Biochem Pharmacol. 2017;143:39–52.
68. Singh N, Scalise M, Galluccio M, Wieder M, Seidel T, Langer T, et al. Discovery of potent inhibitors for the large neutral amino acid transporter 1 (LAT1) by structure-based methods. Int J Mol Sci. 2018;20(1)
69. Kongpracha P, Nagamori S, Wiriyasermkul P, Tanaka Y, Kaneda K, Okuda S, et al. Structure-activity relationship of a novel series of inhibitors for cancer type transporter L-type amino acid transporter 1 (LAT1). J Pharmacol Sci. 2017;133(2):96–102.
70. Ueda S, Hayashi H, Miyamoto T, Abe S, Hirai K, Matsukura K, et al. Anti-tumor effects of mAb against L-type amino acid transporter 1 (LAT1) bound to human and monkey LAT1 with dual avidity modes. Cancer Sci. 2019;110(2):674–85.
71. Chen H, Li B, Ren X, Li S, Ma Y, Cui S, et al. Multifunctional near-infrared-emitting nano-conjugates based on gold clusters for tumor imaging and therapy. Biomaterials. 2012;33(33):8461–76.
72. Hong S, Fang Z, Jung HY, Yoon JH, Hong SS, Maeng HJ. Synthesis of gemcitabine-threonine amide prodrug effective on pancreatic cancer cells with improved pharmacokinetic properties. Molecules. 2018;23(10):2608.
73. Huttunen J, Gynther M, Huttunen KM. Targeted efflux transporter inhibitors—A solution to improve poor cellular accumulation of anti-cancer agents. Int J Pharm. 2018;550(1–2):278–89.
74. Bhunia S, Vangala V, Bhattacharya D, Ravuri HG, Kuncha M, Chakravarty S, et al. Large amino acid transporter 1 selective liposomes of l-DOPA functionalized Amphiphile for combating glioblastoma. Mol Pharm. 2017;14(11):3834–47.

75. Ong ZY, Chen S, Nabavi E, Regoutz A, Payne DJ, Elson DS, et al. Multibranched gold nanoparticles with intrinsic LAT-1 targeting capabilities for selective photothermal therapy of breast cancer. ACS Appl Mater Interfaces. 2017;9(45):39259–70.
76. Li L, Di X, Zhang S, Kan Q, Liu H, Lu T, et al. Large amino acid transporter 1 mediated glutamate modified docetaxel-loaded liposomes for glioma targeting. Colloids Surf B Biointerfaces. 2016;141:260–7.
77. Li L, Di X, Wu M, Sun Z, Zhong L, Wang Y, et al. Targeting tumor highly-expressed LAT1 transporter with amino acid-modified nanoparticles: toward a novel active targeting strategy in breast cancer therapy. Nanomedicine. 2017;13(3):987–98.
78. Waddad AY, Ramharack P, Soliman MES, Govender T. Grafted hyaluronic acid N-acetyl-l-methionine for targeting of LAT1 receptor: in-silico, synthesis and microscale thermophoresis studies. Int J Biol Macromol. 2019;125:767–77.
79. Matsuura M, Ohshima M, Hiruta Y, Nishimura T, Nagase K, Kanazawa H. LAT1-targeting thermoresponsive fluorescent polymer probes for cancer cell imaging. Int J Mol Sci. 2018;19(6):1646.
80. Manzarbeitia-Arroba B, Hodolic M, Pichler R, Osipova O, Soriano-Castrejon AM, Garcia-Vicente AM. (18)F-Fluoroethyl-L tyrosine positron emission tomography radiomics in the differentiation of treatment-related changes from disease progression in patients with glioblastoma. Cancers (Basel). 2023;16(1):195.
81. Krys D, Mattingly S, Glubrecht D, Wuest M, Wuest F. PET imaging of L-type amino acid transporter (LAT1) and Cystine-glutamate antiporter (x(c)(−)) with [(18)F]FDOPA and [(18)F]FSPG in breast cancer models. Mol Imaging Biol. 2020;22(6):1562–71.
82. Ohmura K, Kumagai N, Kumagai M, Ikegame Y, Shinoda J, Yano H, et al. Combining methionine-PET and MRI fluid-attenuated inversion-recovery mismatch to determine glioma molecular subtype. J Neuroimaging. 2023;33(4):652–60.
83. Takenaka S, Asano Y, Shinoda J, Nomura Y, Yonezawa S, Miwa K, et al. Comparison of (11)C-methionine, (11)C-choline, and (18)F-fluorodeoxyglucose-PET for distinguishing glioma recurrence from radiation necrosis. Neurol Med Chir (Tokyo). 2014;54(4):280–9.
84. Youland RS, Kitange GJ, Peterson TE, Pafundi DH, Ramiscal JA, Pokorny JL, et al. The role of LAT1 in (18)F-DOPA uptake in malignant gliomas. J Neurooncol. 2013;111(1):11–8.
85. Kondo N, Hikida M, Nakada M, Sakurai Y, Hirata E, Takeno S, et al. Glioma stem-like cells can be targeted in boron neutron capture therapy with boronophenylalanine. Cancers (Basel). 2020;12(10):3040.
86. Wang S, Zhang Z, Miao L, Zhang J, Tang F, Teng M, et al. Construction of targeted (10)B delivery agents and their uptake in gastric and pancreatic cancer cells. Front Oncol. 2023;13:1105472.
87. Puris E, Gynther M, Auriola S, Huttunen KM. L-type amino acid transporter 1 as a target for drug delivery. Pharm Res. 2020;37(5):88.
88. Herve F, Ghinea N, Scherrmann JM. CNS delivery via adsorptive transcytosis. AAPS J. 2008;10(3):455–72.
89. Xiao G, Gan LS. Receptor-mediated endocytosis and brain delivery of therapeutic biologics. Int J Cell Biol. 2013;2013:703545.
90. Rennick JJ, Johnston APR, Parton RG. Key principles and methods for studying the endocytosis of biological and nanoparticle therapeutics. Nat Nanotechnol. 2021;16(3):266–76.
91. Pardridge WM, Kang YS, Buciak JL, Yang J. Human insulin receptor monoclonal antibody undergoes high affinity binding to human brain capillaries in vitro and rapid transcytosis through the blood-brain barrier in vivo in the primate. Pharm Res. 1995;12(6):807–16.
92. Pardridge WM. Transport of insulin-related peptides and glucose across the blood-brain barrier. Ann N Y Acad Sci. 1993;692:126–37.
93. Pardridge WM. Kinetics of blood-brain barrier transport of monoclonal antibodies targeting the insulin receptor and the transferrin receptor. Pharmaceuticals (Basel). 2021;15(1):3.
94. Reinhardt RR, Bondy CA. Insulin-like growth factors cross the blood-brain barrier. Endocrinology. 1994;135(5):1753–61.
95. Brahmkhatri VP, Prasanna C, Atreya HS. Insulin-like growth factor system in cancer: novel targeted therapies. Biomed Res Int. 2015;2015:538019.
96. Rosenzweig SA, Atreya HS. Defining the pathway to insulin-like growth factor system targeting in cancer. Biochem Pharmacol. 2010;80(8):1115–24.
97. Descamps L, Dehouck MP, Torpier G, Cecchelli R. Receptor-mediated transcytosis of transferrin through blood-brain barrier endothelial cells. Am J Phys. 1996;270(4 Pt 2):H1149–58.
98. Broadwell RD, Baker-Cairns BJ, Friden PM, Oliver C, Villegas JC. Transcytosis of protein through the mammalian cerebral epithelium and endothelium. III. Receptor-mediated transcytosis through the blood-brain barrier of blood-borne transferrin and antibody against the transferrin receptor. Exp Neurol. 1996;142(1):47–65.
99. Tashima T. Brain cancer chemotherapy through a delivery system across the blood-brain barrier into the brain based on receptor-mediated transcytosis using monoclonal antibody conjugates. Biomedicines. 2022;10(7):1597.
100. Cerletti A, Drewe J, Fricker G, Eberle AN, Huwyler J. Endocytosis and transcytosis of an immunoliposome-based brain drug delivery system. J Drug Target. 2000;8(6):435–46.
101. Choudhury H, Pandey M, Chin PX, Phang YL, Cheah JY, Ooi SC, et al. Transferrin receptors-targeting nanocarriers for efficient targeted delivery and transcytosis of drugs into the brain tumors: a review of recent advancements and emerging trends. Drug Deliv Transl Res. 2018;8(5):1545–63.
102. Dehouck B, Fenart L, Dehouck MP, Pierce A, Torpier G, Cecchelli R. A new function for the LDL receptor: transcytosis of LDL across the blood-brain barrier. J Cell Biol. 1997;138(4):877–89.
103. Molino Y, David M, Varini K, Jabes F, Gaudin N, Fortoul A, et al. Use of LDL receptor-targeting peptide vectors for in vitro and in vivo cargo transport across the blood-brain barrier. FASEB J. 2017;31(5):1807–27.
104. Nikanjam M, Gibbs AR, Hunt CA, Budinger TF, Forte TM. Synthetic nano-LDL with paclitaxel oleate as a targeted drug delivery vehicle for glioblastoma multiforme. J Control Release. 2007;124(3):163–71.
105. Pawar S, Koneru T, McCord E, Tatiparti K, Sau S, Iyer AK. LDL receptors and their role in targeted therapy for glioma: a review. Drug Discov Today. 2021;26(5):1212–25.
106. Pinzon-Daza M, Garzon R, Couraud P, Romero I, Weksler B, Ghigo D, et al. The association of statins plus LDL receptor-targeted liposome-encapsulated doxorubicin increases in vitro drug delivery across blood-brain barrier cells. Br J Pharmacol. 2012;167(7):1431–47.
107. Yuan D, Yi X, Zhao Y, Poon CD, Bullock KM, Hansen KM, et al. Intranasal delivery of N-terminal modified leptin-pluronic conjugate for treatment of obesity. J Control Release. 2017;263:172–84.
108. Shibata M, Yamada S, Kumar SR, Calero M, Bading J, Frangione B, et al. Clearance of Alzheimer's amyloid-ss(1-40) peptide from brain by LDL receptor-related protein-1 at the blood-brain barrier. J Clin Invest. 2000;106(12):1489–99.
109. Merino-Zamorano C, Fernandez-de Retana S, Montanola A, Batlle A, Saint-Pol J, Mysiorek C, et al. Modulation of amyloid-beta1-40 transport by ApoA1 and ApoJ across an in vitro model of the blood-brain barrier. J Alzheimers Dis. 2016;53(2):677–91.
110. Poduslo JF, Curran GL, Sanyal B, Selkoe DJ. Receptor-mediated transport of human amyloid beta-protein 1-40 and 1-42 at the blood-brain barrier. Neurobiol Dis. 1999;6(3):190–9.

111. Abulrob A, Sprong H, Van Bergen en Henegouwen P, Stanimirovic D. The blood-brain barrier transmigrating single domain antibody: mechanisms of transport and antigenic epitopes in human brain endothelial cells. J Neurochem. 2005;95(4):1201–14.
112. Thom G, Hatcher J, Hearn A, Paterson J, Rodrigo N, Beljean A, et al. Isolation of blood-brain barrier-crossing antibodies from a phage display library by competitive elution and their ability to penetrate the central nervous system. MAbs. 2018;10(2):304–14.
113. Webster CI, Caram-Salas N, Haqqani AS, Thom G, Brown L, Rennie K, et al. Brain penetration, target engagement, and disposition of the blood-brain barrier-crossing bispecific antibody antagonist of metabotropic glutamate receptor type 1. FASEB J. 2016;30(5):1927–40.
114. Dos Santos RB, Arora S, Kanekiyo T, Singh J. Efficient neuronal targeting and transfection using RVG and transferrin-conjugated liposomes. Brain Res. 2020;1734:146738.
115. Gao Y, Wang ZY, Zhang J, Zhang Y, Huo H, Wang T, et al. RVG-peptide-linked trimethylated chitosan for delivery of siRNA to the brain. Biomacromolecules. 2014;15(3):1010–8.
116. Ji F, Xu L, Long K, Zhang F, Zhang M, Lu X, et al. Rabies virus glycoprotein 29 (RVG29) promotes CAR-T immunotherapy for glioma. Transl Res. 2023;259:1–12.
117. Kim SS, Ye C, Kumar P, Chiu I, Subramanya S, Wu H, et al. Targeted delivery of siRNA to macrophages for anti-inflammatory treatment. Mol Ther. 2010;18(5):993–1001.
118. You L, Wang J, Liu T, Zhang Y, Han X, Wang T, et al. Targeted brain delivery of rabies virus glycoprotein 29-modified deferoxamine-loaded nanoparticles reverses functional deficits in parkinsonian mice. ACS Nano. 2018;12(5):4123–39.
119. Pardridge WM, Buciak JL, Kang YS, Boado RJ. Protamine-mediated transport of albumin into brain and other organs of the rat. Binding and endocytosis of protamine-albumin complex by microvascular endothelium. J Clin Invest. 1993;92(5):2224–9.
120. Pardridge WM, Triguero D, Buciak J. Transport of histone through the blood-brain barrier. J Pharmacol Exp Ther. 1989;251(3):821–6.
121. Pardridge WM, Boado RJ. Enhanced cellular uptake of biotinylated antisense oligonucleotide or peptide mediated by avidin, a cationic protein. FEBS Lett. 1991;288(1–2):30–2.
122. Villegas JC, Broadwell RD. Transcytosis of protein through the mammalian cerebral epithelium and endothelium. II. Adsorptive transcytosis of WGA-HRP and the blood-brain and brain-blood barriers. J Neurocytol. 1993;22(2):67–80.
123. Raub TJ, Audus KL. Adsorptive endocytosis and membrane recycling by cultured primary bovine brain microvessel endothelial cell monolayers. J Cell Sci. 1990;97(Pt 1):127–38.
124. Bickel U, Yoshikawa T, Pardridge WM. Delivery of peptides and proteins through the blood-brain barrier. Adv Drug Deliv Rev. 2001;46(1–3):247–79.
125. Pardridge WM, Triguero D, Buciak J, Yang J. Evaluation of cationized rat albumin as a potential blood-brain barrier drug transport vector. J Pharmacol Exp Ther. 1990;255(2):893–9.
126. Bickel U. Antibody delivery through the blood-brain barrier. Adv Drug Deliv Rev. 1995;15(1–3):53–72.
127. Girod J, Fenart L, Regina A, Dehouck MP, Hong G, Scherrmann JM, et al. Transport of cationized anti-tetanus Fab'2 fragments across an in vitro blood-brain barrier model: involvement of the transcytosis pathway. J Neurochem. 1999;73(5):2002–8.
128. Rousselle C, Smirnova M, Clair P, Lefauconnier JM, Chavanieu A, Calas B, et al. Enhanced delivery of doxorubicin into the brain via a peptide-vector-mediated strategy: saturation kinetics and specificity. J Pharmacol Exp Ther. 2001;296(1):124–31.
129. Drin G, Cottin S, Blanc E, Rees AR, Temsamani J. Studies on the internalization mechanism of cationic cell-penetrating peptides. J Biol Chem. 2003;278(33):31192–201.
130. Schartz D, Furst T, Ellens N, Kohli GS, Rahmani R, Akkipeddi SMK, et al. Preoperative embolization of meningiomas facilitates reduced surgical complications and improved clinical outcomes: a meta-analysis of matched cohort studies. Clin Neuroradiol. 2023;33(3):755–62.
131. Alfter M, Albina-Palmarola P, Cimpoca A, Diaz-Peregrino R, Jans P, Ganslandt O, et al. Multi-stage treatment for Spetzler-Martin grades III, IV, and V arteriovenous malformations: preoperative embolization and microsurgical resection in a consecutive series of 250 patients. J Clin Med. 2023;12(18):5990.
132. Yoshikawa MH, Rabelo NN, Telles JPM, Pipek LZ, Barbosa GB, Barbato NC, et al. Temporary arterial occlusion (TAO) as independent prognostic factor in unruptured aneurysm surgery: a cohort study. J Clin Neurosci. 2022;99:78–81.
133. Yoshikawa MH, Rabelo NN, Telles JPM, Pipek LZ, Barbosa GB, Barbato NC, et al. Role of temporary arterial occlusion in subarachnoid hemorrhage outcomes: a prospective cohort study. Acta Cir Bras. 2023;38:e387923.
134. Wang D, Rao W. Bench-to-bedside development of multifunctional flexible embolic agents. Theranostics. 2023;13(7):2114–39.
135. Facciorusso A. Drug-eluting beads transarterial chemoembolization for hepatocellular carcinoma: current state of the art. World J Gastroenterol. 2018;24(2):161–9.
136. Padia SA, Shivaram G, Bastawrous S, Bhargava P, Vo NJ, Vaidya S, et al. Safety and efficacy of drug-eluting bead chemoembolization for hepatocellular carcinoma: comparison of small-versus medium-size particles. J Vasc Interv Radiol. 2013;24(3):301–6.
137. Prajapati HJ, Xing M, Spivey JR, Hanish SI, El-Rayes BF, Kauh JS, et al. Survival, efficacy, and safety of small versus large doxorubicin drug-eluting beads TACE chemoembolization in patients with unresectable HCC. AJR Am J Roentgenol. 2014;203(6):W706–14.
138. Keane G, Lam M, de Jong H. Beyond the MAA-Y90 paradigm: the evolution of radioembolization dosimetry approaches and scout particles. Semin Intervent Radiol. 2021;38(5):542–53.
139. Miller FH, Lopes Vendrami C, Gabr A, Horowitz JM, Kelahan LC, Riaz A, et al. Evolution of radioembolization in treatment of hepatocellular carcinoma: a pictorial review. Radiographics. 2021;41(6):1802–18.
140. Saini A, Wallace A, Alzubaidi S, Knuttinen MG, Naidu S, Sheth R, et al. History and evolution of Yttrium-90 radioembolization for hepatocellular carcinoma. J Clin Med. 2019;8(1):55.
141. Massani M, Bonariol L, Stecca T. Hepatic arterial infusion chemotherapy for unresectable intrahepatic cholangiocarcinoma, a comprehensive review. J Clin Med. 2021;10(12):2552.
142. Yan L, Lin J, Ke K, Wu Z, Huang J, Huang N, et al. A meta-analysis comparing hepatic arterial infusion chemotherapy and sorafenib for advanced hepatocellular carcinoma. Transl Cancer Res. 2022;11(1):99–112.
143. Yang S, Cai C, Wang H, Ma X, Shao A, Sheng J, et al. Drug delivery strategy in hepatocellular carcinoma therapy. Cell Commun Signal. 2022;20(1):26.
144. Anonymous. Top ten additive commonly used in parentral products 2024. https://mycoscience.com/top-ten-additives-commonly-used-in-parenteral-products/#:~:text=Benzyl%20alcohol%2C%20phenol%2C%20and%20parabens,used%20preservative%20in%20vaccine%20products.
145. Nair B. Final report on the safety assessment of benzyl alcohol, benzoic acid, and sodium benzoate. Int J Toxicol. 2001;20(Suppl 3):23–50.
146. Kakaei N, Amirian R, Azadi M, Mohammadi G, Izadi Z. Perfluorocarbons: a perspective of theranostic applications and challenges. Front Bioeng Biotechnol. 2023;11:1115254.
147. Claassen J, Thijssen DHJ, Panerai RB, Faraci FM. Regulation of cerebral blood flow in humans: physiology and clinical implications of autoregulation. Physiol Rev. 2021;101(4):1487–559.
148. Slupe AM, Kirsch JR. Effects of anesthesia on cerebral blood flow, metabolism, and neuroprotection. J Cereb Blood Flow Metab. 2018;38(12):2192–208.

149. Crezee J, Franken NAP, Oei AL. Hyperthermia-based anti-cancer treatments. Cancers (Basel). 2021;13(6):1240.
150. Summers MA, Moore JL, McAuley JW. Use of verapamil as a potential P-glycoprotein inhibitor in a patient with refractory epilepsy. Ann Pharmacother. 2004;38(10):1631–4.
151. Neuwelt EA, Brummett RE, Doolittle ND, Muldoon LL, Kroll RA, Pagel MA, et al. First evidence of otoprotection against carboplatin-induced hearing loss with a two-compartment system in patients with central nervous system malignancy using sodium thiosulfate. J Pharmacol Exp Ther. 1998;286(1): 77–84.
152. Dedrick RL, Oldfield EH, Collins JM. Arterial drug infusion with extracorporeal removal. I. Theoretic basis with particular reference to the brain. Cancer Treat Rep. 1984;68(2):373–80.
153. Oldfield EH, Dedrick RL, Chatterji DC, Yeager RL, Girton ME, Kornblith PL, et al. Arterial drug infusion with extracorporeal removal. II. Internal carotid carmustine in the rhesus monkey. Cancer Treat Rep. 1985;69(3):293–303.
154. Ries F. Nephrotoxicity of chemotherapy. Eur J Cancer Clin Oncol. 1988;24(6):951–3.
155. Ries F, Klastersky J. Nephrotoxicity induced by cancer chemotherapy with special emphasis on cisplatin toxicity. Am J Kidney Dis. 1986;8(5):368–79.
156. Pinkiewicz M, Pinkiewicz M, Walecki J, Zawadzki M. A systematic review on intra-arterial cerebral infusions of chemotherapeutics in the treatment of glioblastoma multiforme: the state-of-the-art. Front Oncol. 2022;12:950167.
157. Dagnino J. Wren, Boyle, and the origins of intravenous injections and the Royal Society of London. Anesthesiology. 2009;111(4):923–4; author reply 4.
158. Vaca Miguel JM, Granda Juesas J, Garcia Camarero EJ, Alaejos Estebanez A, Llorente de la Fuente A, Tamayo Gomez E. [Intra-arterial regional anesthesia]. Rev Esp Anestesiol Reanim. 1990;37(6):356–359.
159. Die-Goyanes A, Die-Trill J. [Jose Goyanes. Surgeon and humanist]. Cir Esp. 2008;83(1):8–11.
160. Roesler R, Dini SA, Isolan GR. Neuroinflammation and immunoregulation in glioblastoma and brain metastases: recent developments in imaging approaches. Clin Exp Immunol. 2021;206(3):314–24.

Hepatic Arterial Infusion Therapy: Strategies for Safe Long-term Arterial Infusions

13

Grey Leonard, Sreenivasa Chandana, Asad Beg, and Perry Shen

Is life worth living? It all depends on the liver.

William James (1842–1910), American Philosopher and Psychologist

Introduction

This chapter discusses the current status of hepatic arterial infusion (HAI) pumps, including the physiologic rationale, technical insertion techniques (including open and robotic approaches), a brief overview of applications in oncology, and strategies to enable long-term arterial infusion. Long-term chemotherapy has also been used to treat head and neck cancers and locally invasive breast cancers. Due to the potential risk of stroke, its use in treating neurological diseases has hitherto been limited. However, with advances in catheter technology, anticoagulation, and novel antiplatelet therapies, there could be future applications of long-term infusion for treating neurological diseases. Finally, this chapter assesses the challenges in developing prolonged arterial delivery for neurological diseases.

Anatomic Rationale

The liver is a unique organ due to its particular blood supply and metabolic functions. HAI therapy uses these features to maximize cytotoxic chemotherapy delivered to tumor cells while sparing normal hepatic parenchyma. Metastatic lesions to the liver derive more than 80% of their blood supply from the hepatic arterial circulation, whereas normal liver parenchyma is supplied primarily by the portal system [1]. Given this arrangement, HAI therapy achieves a high concentration of chemotherapy in the liver while sparing the systemic circulation due to the liver's first-pass metabolism [2]. Anatomically, the catheter is typically inserted via the gastroduodenal artery (GDA), allowing flow into the right and left hepatic arteries (Fig. 13.1). In a recent autopsy study, the origin of the hepatic arteries followed the standard anatomy 72% of the time, while in 28%, there were variant origins, such as replaced right and left hepatic arteries [3]. The potential for these aberrations must be considered during pump insertion to minimize the risk of malperfusion, defined as inadequate drug delivery or escape of drug outside the boundaries of the liver.

G. Leonard · P. Shen (✉)
Atrium Health Wake Forest Baptist, Section Surgical Oncology, Winston-Salem, NC, USA
e-mail: pshen@wakehealth.edu

S. Chandana
The Cancer and Hematology Centers, Grand Rapids, MI, USA

A. Beg
Division of Interventional Radiology, Columbia University, New York, NY, USA

S. Joshi (ed.), *Arterial Treatment of Neurological Diseases*, https://doi.org/10.1007/978-3-031-80173-0_13

Fig. 13.1 Position of the hepatic artery infusion catheter

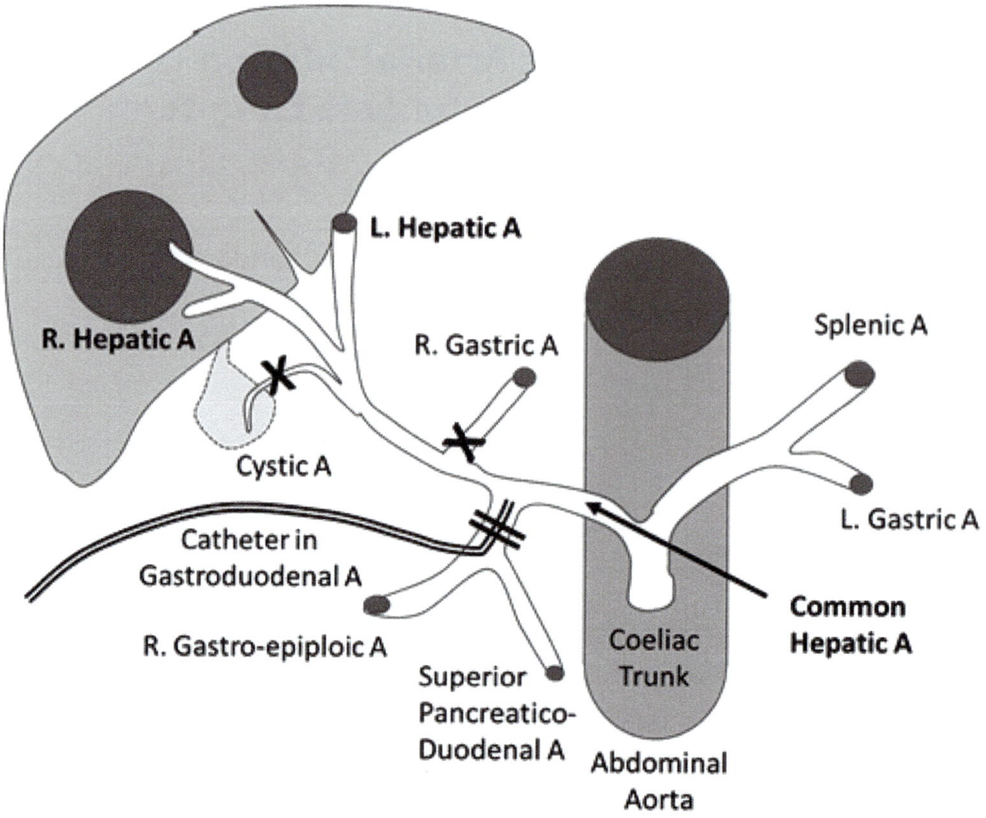

Open and Robotic Approaches

Most HAI pumps are inserted using an open approach, whereby the optimal incision is typically dictated by the necessity of other procedures (colon and/or liver resection vs. ablation). A cholecystectomy is standard as the cystic artery generally is downstream from the catheter insertion, and the gallbladder is at risk for cholecystitis due to regional drug exposure. The common hepatic artery (CHA) and the proper hepatic artery (PHA) junction are defined for catheter placement and the relationship with the GDA. The GDA must be skeletonized to an adequate length for the catheter to be secured with the tip abutting the junction of the GDA and the CHA. Furthermore, the GDA should be exposed circumferentially from its origin at the CHA to the superior border of the pancreas as progression distally increases the likelihood of branches supplying the duodenum [4]. Skeletonizing the PHA for approximately 2 cm is recommended to prevent extrahepatic perfusion of the stomach or duodenum, which can lead to GI ulceration (Fig. 13.1). The pump pocket is made, and the device is secured within the subcutaneous fat. Once the catheter is securely in place, hepatic perfusion is confirmed with an injection of methylene blue via the hepatic pump catheter.

Minimally invasive approaches (MIS) to HAI catheter placement have advanced to the robotic platform. The robotic procedure mimics an open approach with the typical modifications of this platform. After insufflation and port placement, the CHA, GDA, and PHA are skeletonized as above. A silk suture is used to ligate the GDA distally, and two additional sutures are placed proximally in preparation for catheter insertion. Robotic vascular clamps are then placed on the CHA and PHA. A vein pick and 11-blade are inserted through the ports, and a transverse arteriotomy is made. The vein pick is used to insert the catheter, which is then secured with a suture. The clamps are removed, and a methylene blue test is performed to assess for malperfusion. This approach enjoys the general advantages of MIS surgery compared to open procedures, such as smaller incisions and better pain control. In a retrospective comparison by Qadan et al. in 2017, between robotic, open, and laparoscopic HAI pump placement approaches, there was a trend toward a shorter length of stay where concomitant resections were omitted, four for robotic vs. 5 days for open and laparoscopic ($p = 0.09$), respectively [5]. Additionally, there was a lower conversion rate for the robotic approach compared to laparoscopic (17% vs. 67%, $p < 0.01$) and a similar overall complication rate between the three approaches. While this was at a single institution between two surgeons, these results will likely become more generalizable as the HAI pump and robotic experience increase.

HAI Therapy for Liver Malignancy

HAI for Colorectal Liver Metastasis

HAI therapy for CRLM is not a new treatment option. One early and notable study (1999) looking at two-year overall survival (OS) and progression-free survival (PFS) showed a benefit to pump-infuse floxuridine (FUDR) with systemic 5-fluorouracil (5-FU) and leucovorin (LV) over the same systemic therapy alone [6]. Median overall survival was 68.4 months with HAI vs. 58.8 months in the systemic therapy alone group. Critics have since stated the differential benefits of the HAI therapy in this study were likely due to outdated chemotherapy in the systemic arm. Since then, the combination of chemotherapy with 5-FU, leucovorin, and possibly oxaliplatin (FOLFOX) and/or irinotecan (FOLFIRI) has become more common in CRLM. Table 13.1 contains a compilation of commonly used systemic chemotherapy regimens with suggested doses in conjunction with HAI pump FUDR therapy in various cancers. Given this criticism, researchers began examining HAI therapy in combination with modern systemic therapy. Kemeny et al. 2001, in a phase I trial, studied a combination of HAI Pump FUDR and intravenous irinotecan [7]. They concluded that irinotecan's maximum tolerated dose (MTD) was 100 mg/m^2 3 weeks on, while the FUDR was 016 mg/kg daily. The median time to progression was 8.1 months, and the median OS was 20 months [7].

Progressing to combination HAI therapy with platinum-based chemotherapy, Kemeny et al., in 2005 [8], studied two different oxaliplatin-based systemic chemotherapy regimens to FUDR-based HAI therapy. In one group of 21 patients, a combination of oxaliplatin and Irinotecan was studied as dose escalation of each drug. In another group of 15 patients, a fixed dose of oxaliplatin (100 mg/m^2) with an escalating dose of infusion of 5 FU/LV. The MTD for Oxaliplatin was 100 mg/m^2, Irinotecan 150 mg/m^2, given every 2 weeks, and FUDR 0.12 mg/kg × 30 mL divided by pump flow rate. The MTD for LV was 400 mg/m^2, and 5-FU was 1400 mg/m^2 by continuous infusion over 48 h. Seven out of 21 patients in the Oxaliplatin and Irinotecan group were able to undergo liver surgery, and 2 had complete pathological responses. The median OS was 36 and 22 months in the two groups. In a phase I trial in 2009, Kemeny et al. [9] demonstrated the safety of the combination of HAI with FUDR in addition to FOLFOX systemic therapy in 49 CRLM patients treated with Oxaliplatin and Irinotecan in combination with HAI FUDR. The median OS for treatment-naive patients was 50.8 months, while it was 35 months in previously treated patients.

The most common toxicities included diarrhea, neutropenia, and neurotoxicity, and the authors noted that attenuated systemic therapy doses with HAI were both safe and effective. The authors found that 92% of patients had at least a partial response, and 47% achieved enough of a response to go on to resection. Again, in 2009, Kemeny et al. provided further evidence of the safety and efficacy of HAI with modern systemic therapy in a Phase-I clinical trial of HAI FUDR combined with FOLFOX [10]. The oxaliplatin dose was escalated from 85 to 100 mg/m^2, and the 5-FU 48-h continuous infusion doses were increased from 1000 to 2000 mg/m^2. The LV dose was fixed at 400 mg/m^2). MTD was determined to be oxaliplatin at 85 mg/m^2 and 5-FU by continuous infusion at 2000 g/m^2 with LV at 400 mg/m^2. Dose-limiting toxicities include diarrhea and hyperbilirubinemia.

Keeping up with modern chemotherapy regimens, Kemeny and colleagues studied the addition of bevacizumab to systemic therapy with HAI in 2011. A randomized phase II trial was conducted with HAI FUDR and systemic therapy (FOLFOX or FOLFIRI) with or without bevacizumab [11]. There was no statistical significance in 4-year RFS (46% vs. 37%) or OS (85% vs. 81%) between the groups. Interestingly, there was a significant difference in the biliary stenosis with increased bilirubin >3 mg/dL noted (0/38 versus 5/35

Table 13.1 Commonly used chemotherapy regimens with HAI pump therapy

HAI pump FUDR dosing—0.12 to 0.14 mg/kg (divided by the pump flow rate) in combination with 25 mg of dexamethasone, 30,000 units of heparin, and normal saline. It will flow continuously for 14 days. On day 15, residual will be removed from the pump, followed by injection of heparinized saline (30,000 units of heparin in 30 mL of normal saline) on days 15–28	
CRLM regimens	
(a)	FOLFOX—5-FU 2000 mg/m^2 CIV for 46 h, Leucovorin 400 mg/m^2 IVP, Oxaliplatin 85 mg/m^2 over 2–3 h
(b)	FOLFIRI—5-FU 2000 mg/m^2 CIV for 46 h, Leucovorin 400 mg/m^2 IVP, Irinotecan 150 mg/m^2 over 1.5 h
(c)	Oxaliplatin/Irinotecan—Oxaliplatin IV 85 mg/m^2 over 2–3 h, Irinotecan 150 mg/m^2 over 1.5 h
(d)	FOLFIRI and Panitumumab—5-FU 2000 mg/m^2 CIV for 46 h, Leucovorin 400 mg/m^2 IVP, Irinotecan 150 mg/m^2 over 1.5 h, and Panitumumab IV 6 mg/m^2 over 0.5–1 h
Cholangiocarcinoma regimens	
(a)	Gemcitabine/Cisplatin—Gemcitabine IV 800 mg/m^2 over 30 months, Cisplatin 25 mg/m^2 over 1–2 h, 1 L NS mixed with KCL and MgSO4 over 2–3 h as prehydration on days 1 and 8 of 21-day cycle
(b)	Gemcitabine/Oxaliplatin—Gemcitabine IV 800 mg/m^2 over 30 months, and oxaliplatin 85 mg/m^2 IV over 2–3 h every 14 days

Each cycle is 28 days. FUDR is given on days 1–14, while systemic chemotherapy is given on days 1 and 15 of the 28-day cycle
5-FU 5 Fluoro Uracil, *NS* normal saline, *CIV* Continuous IV, *KCL* Potassium Chloride, MgSO4 Magnesium Chloride

patients, $p = 0.02$, *No Bevacizumab* vs. *Bevacizumab arms*). The nonefficacy of bevacizumab in the setting was confirmed in a phase II study by D'Angelica and colleagues in 2015 [12]. The addition of bevacizumab did not improve conversion rates or survival and had an unacceptable rate of biliary complications. Given these data, the addition of bevacizumab is not recommended with HAI therapy.

In a long-term follow-up study by Pak and colleagues in 2018 in unresectable CRLM patients, the conversion rate with HAI with systemic therapy (excluding bevacizumab) was 52% [13]. Furthermore, conversion to resection was the only factor associated with increased disease-free or overall survival. The authors noted that after a median follow-up of 86 months, 14% of patients had no evidence of disease. As such, combination HAI therapy likely has benefits in modern systemic chemotherapy and carries a significant potential for cure. Verheij and colleagues found a 55% conversion rate in initially unresectable tumors [14]. A long-term follow-up study by Kemeny's group in 2016 for resectable disease from four prospective trials shows increasing long-term survival with HAI and systemic therapy [15]. Notably, the 5-year OS before 2003 was 56%, whereas after, in the modern chemotherapy era, it rose to 78%. These data suggest that modern systemic therapy with HAI is safe and increasingly more effective. To further clarify the role of HAI therapy in unresectable CRLM, the EA2222 (PUMP trial, NCT05863195) is being conducted as a large, randomized phase III trial, which will randomize patients with unresectable CRLM in a 2:1 fashion to combined treatment with HAI FUDR and systemic therapy or systemic therapy alone.

Additional comparison studies have been conducted, examining the potential superiority of HAI with systemic therapy compared to systemic therapy alone. Goéré et al. studied resected patients receiving adjuvant HAI therapy compared to modern systemic therapy [16]. The 3-year OS was longer in the HAI group (75% vs. 62%, $p = 0.17$), in addition to longer 3-year DFS (33% vs. 5%). In a long-term database study by Groot Koerkamp et al. examining patients with CRLM with complete resection, systemic therapy was only compared with HAI plus systemic treatment, divided into modern vs. premodern chemotherapy [17]. This study demonstrated a significant survival advantage with HAI therapy with a median OS of 67 vs. 44 months. When comparing modern chemotherapy only, the survival advantage persisted, 67 vs. 47 months ($p < 0.01$). The patients were matched using seven known and independent prognostic factors. In the matched comparison, HAI therapy was associated with a hazard ratio (HR) for OS of 0.67 (95% CI 0.59–0.76). The benefits of HAI therapy, compared to systemic treatment only, were more pronounced in subgroups of patients with node-negative cancer and those with a low clinical risk score (0–2). The clinical risk score was composed of the following five elements from Fong et al., where one point is assigned for each factor: node-positive disease, identification of metastasis to the liver in <12 months (synchronous), >1 hepatic metastatic lesion, largest hepatic metastasis >5 cm and CEA > 200 ng/mL [18]. A recent systematic review and meta-analysis published by Buisman et al. comparing HAI vs. no HAI (+/− systemic therapy) in resected CRLM patients in the adjuvant setting found a pooled HR of 0.77 (95% CI 0.64–0.93) in favor of HAI therapy [19]. This study included 15 studies and 3584 patients and found significant benefits when HAI was combined with systemic therapy and when a subcutaneous pump was used instead of a percutaneous approach.

Advances in technology may be available to identify patients with a greater or lesser probability of benefitting from HAI therapy for CRLM. Next-generation genetic sequencing can detect particular genetic alterations associated with various outcomes [20]. Datta et al. examined genomic profiles related to conversion to resection in CRLM patients who were initially unresectable and received HAI and systemic therapy [21]. This study had a 40% conversion to a resection rate (commensurate with studies above [9, 13]), a median OS of 66 months, and a 5-year OS of 51%. Mutations in SOX9 and BRAF were associated with a higher conversion rate, while BRAF, RAS-pathway mutations, and the combination RAS/RAF-TP53 were associated with worse overall survival. Narayan et al. examined CRLM patients who received HAI and/or systemic therapy and recurred [22]. There was a 58% recurrence rate. Increased recurrence rates were associated with alteration in KRAS and the RAS/RAF pathways. Again, the combination RAS/RAF-TP53, on multivariate analysis, was associated with increased recurrence rates (HR 2.14, 95% CI 1.38–3.31). These data demonstrate conceptually the potential use of genetic sequencing for prognosis in CRLM patients and may indicate targeted therapeutics. Furthermore, genetic data may contribute to clinical decision-making and patient selection for HAI therapy.

In summary, Tables 13.2 and 13.3 list the outcomes of significant studies of HAI in treating CRLM. HAI therapy studies have advanced with the growing repertoire of systemic chemotherapy for CRLM and show great promise in unresectable disease, primarily because of the increased likelihood of conversion to resection. With resectable disease, the long-term survival with HAI may be superior to systemic therapy alone.

HAI Therapy for Intrahepatic Cholangiocarcinoma

In addition to CRLM, HAI therapy has applications for intrahepatic cholangiocarcinoma, a disease associated with a one

Table 13.2 Outcomes of HAI therapy in CRLM

Study	Disease	Year	Comparison	Outcomes	Results	Reference
Kemeny et al.	Resected	1999	HAI + Systemic vs. Systemic	2-year OS	86% vs. 72% ($p = 0.03$)	[6]
Goéré et al.	Resected	2013	HAI + Systemic vs. Systemic	3-year OS	75% vs. 62% ($p = 0.17$)	[16]
Kemeny et al.	Resected	2016	HAI + Systemic (modern)	5-year OS	78%	[15]
Groot Koerkamp et al.	Resected	2017	HAI + Systemic vs. Systemic	Median OS	67 vs. 44 months ($p = <0.01$)	[17]
Buisman et al.	Resected	2022	HAI ± Systemic vs. ± Systemic	Hazard ratio	0.77 (95% CI 0.64–0.93)	[19]
Kemeny et al.	Unresectable	2009	HAI + Systemic	Conversion to resection	47%	[9]
Pak et al.	Unresectable	2017	HAI + Systemic	Conversion to resection	52%	[13]

Table 13.3 Outcomes in therapies for intrahepatic cholangiocarcinoma

Study	Disease	Year	Comparison	Outcomes	Results	Reference
Valle et al.	Unresectable biliary tract	2010	Gem + Cis vs. Gem	Median OS	11.7 vs. 8.0 months ($p < 0.01$)	[23]
TOPAZ-1	Unresectable biliary tract	2022	Gem + Cis + Durvalumab vs. Gem + Cis	2-year OS	24.9 vs. 10.4% ($p = 0.02$)	[24]
Cercek et al.	Unresectable ICC	2020	HAI + Gem + Oxaliplatin	6-month PFS	80%	[25]
Franssen et al.	Unresectable ICC	2022	HAI vs. Gem + Cis	Median OS	27.7 vs. 11.7 months ($p < 0.01$)	[26]

and 5-year OS rate of 30% and 18%, respectively, irrespective of resectability [27]. The median OS for unresectable tumors has been estimated at 11 months [25]. Traditional chemotherapy for unresectable and metastatic biliary tract cancer (including extrahepatic cholangiocarcinoma and gallbladder adenocarcinoma) has been a combination of gemcitabine and cisplatin with a median OS of 11.7 months [23]. This was an improvement of gemcitabine alone (median OS 8.7 months).

Recently, the TOPAZ-1 trial showed mild superiority over the gemcitabine–cisplatin combination for biliary tract cancer with the addition of durvalumab [24]. Early results demonstrated a 24-month OS of 25% in the durvalumab group vs. 10% for the gemcitabine–cisplatin group. While this new drug combination is promising, it highlights the low bar for success in a dismal disease.

With experience in HAI therapy, the Memorial Sloan Kettering and Washington University groups combined in a phase II clinic trial examining the addition of HAI therapy to gemcitabine and oxaliplatin [25]. In the combined HAI arm, the median OS was 25 months. This trial included unresectable ICC with the inclusion of resectable regional lymph nodes. Distant metastatic disease was excluded. These results warrant further investigation, which is currently being conducted in a multicenter, randomized phase II clinical trial of HAI therapy plus Gemcitabine/Oxaliplatin for unresectable ICC (NCT04891289). However, in a recent retrospective analysis involving a total of 266 patients with liver-confined unresectable ICC, it was shown that the addition of HAI FUDR to systemic gemcitabine and cisplatin improved OS compared to chemotherapy alone (27.7 vs. 11.7 months). The 3-year OS was 34.1% vs. 1.8% [26].

In summary, intrahepatic cholangiocarcinoma is a devastating disease with few treatment options. HAI with systemic therapy presents an exciting, potent, novel tool for treating ICC patients.

HAI Pump Care

The availability of implantable pumps enables the patient to receive continuous chemotherapy outside the hospital. The basic design of the pump is shown in Fig. 13.2. Using implantable pumps for HAI creates a closed drug delivery system. An implantable pump allows activities such as swimming, which are impossible with an external infusion device. Once the pump is implanted, the patient recovers until their safe discharge from the hospital. Typically, the pump is tested by a nuclear medicine study that injects Technetium-99m macro-aggregated albumin into the pump and observes its distribution. Liver-only perfusion clears the pump for use. At this stage, care for the patient predominantly becomes the purview of the medical oncologist, with pump therapy beginning around 2–4 weeks post implant. The patient's body heat powers the pump delivery, so the pump has no internal energy source or moving parts. The pump is typically refilled every 2 weeks, alternating between floxuridine and heparinized saline with concomitant laboratory liver function tests. Depending on the primary tumor type, these pump cycles are typically coordinated with additional systemic chemother-

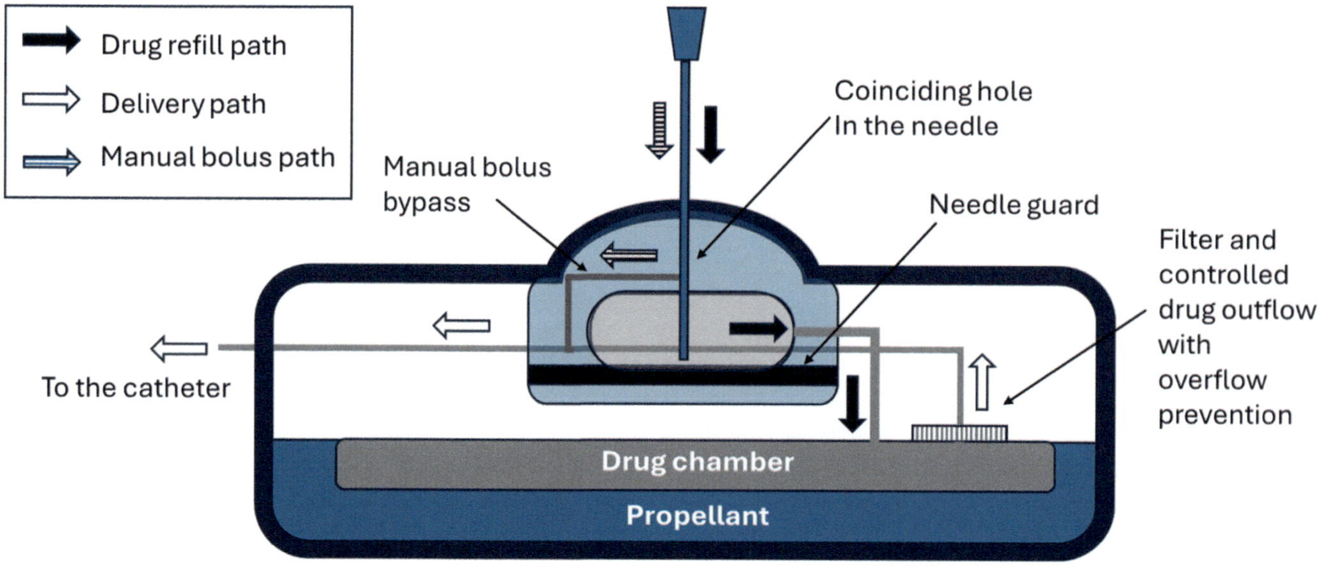

Fig. 13.2 Schematic diagram showing the construction of a hepatic artery infusion pump

apy. Patients do not receive systemic anticoagulation or regular imaging to confirm continued accurate pump catheter position. While pumps may be removed after therapy, they also may be left in place indefinitely and maintained should future use become necessary.

HAI Pump Chemotherapy

Several agents were used as HAI Pump chemotherapies. These include 5-fluorouracil (5-FU), floxuridine (FUDR), oxaliplatin, mitomycin C, dexamethasone, and leucovorin. FUDR, a prodrug of 5-FU, is the agent most commonly used for HAI pump chemotherapy. FUDR, the deoxyribonucleoside derivative of 5-FU, is a pyrimidine antimetabolite and works through the inhibition of thymidylate synthase. FUDR's principal mechanism of action is through 5 fluoro-2′-deoxyuridine-5′ monophosphate (FdUMP). It has a short half-life, and up to 95% of the drug is extracted in the liver, which decreases systemic toxicity. Consequently, the addition of HAI to a systemic intravenous chemotherapy regimen typically does not result in additional systemic side effects [28]. Some of the side effects of HAI pump chemotherapies include biliary toxicity, leading to elevated liver enzymes, and GI toxicities, which include diarrhea, gastric ulceration, and rarely pancreatitis. FUDR is instilled for a 14-day infusion with heparin and normal saline or glycerol to prevent catheter clotting. A randomized phase II study showed that the addition of Dexamethasone to FUDR was effective in avoiding biliary toxicity [29]. Doses of FUDR will be determined based on the patient's weight, liver enzyme trends, and individualized flow rate calculation.

HAI Complications and Management

Complications are not uncommon after HAI pump placement. Allen et al. reviewed a single institution's experience with 544 pump placements [30]. Pump complications occurred in 22%. Patients are monitored for signs of pump pocket infections, such as fevers, erythema, pus, and leukocytosis. Infections may require antibiotics, surgical washout, and or pump removal. Arterial complications were most common and included arterial thrombosis, malperfusion such as extrahepatic and incomplete hepatic perfusion, and hemorrhage. Notably, no arterial thromboses occurred after 1995. Factors associated with pump complications included the pump model, non-GDA cannulation, earlier era of insertion, and <25 cases performed previously by the primary surgeon. Extrahepatic perfusion (EHP) may occur due to variant anatomy or missed ligation of vessels. This error is mitigated by the recommended technical steps for catheter placement described earlier in this chapter. EHP may be discovered by nuclear medicine scintigraphy despite a normal liver-only intraoperative distribution of the methylene blue dye [31]. Sofoclueus et al. reported that 9% (43 of 475) of HAI patients had identifiable EHP on postoperative scintigraphy [32]. The typical management of EHP) is salvage percutaneous arterial embolization of the feeding vessel. Only 7% (32 of 475) of this study had angiographic abnormalities. Eight of the 32 had either arterial thrombosis or catheter erosion, which rendered EHP unsalvageable. Of the remaining 24 patients, 88% achieved technically successful embolization. As such, EHP is rare but identifiable by scintigraphy and best managed by salvage percutaneous embolization.

Catheter thrombosis is an occlusive complication that may occur after pump placement. This is typically discovered as difficulty with pump infusion. To determine the cause, a fluoroscopic pump study may be performed to rule out malposition or kinking. If a catheter thrombosis is discovered, management depends upon the timing. Early thrombosis may be managed with gentle heparin flushing. Late thrombosis due to fibrin sheath formation requires tissue plasminogen activator(tPA) injection. However, this should not be performed if the clot extends into the arterial lumen due to the risk of pseudoaneurysm formation. These procedures are typically performed in the interventional radiology suite.

Arterial complications may occur during pump placement. First among these are arterial dissections, where the intimal layer of the arterial wall forms a false channel disconnected from the anatomical lumen. Catheters inserted into this space will not properly perfuse the liver and are typically noticed after injecting methylene blue into the pump. Here, the blue dye may accumulate in the lumen or perfuse on one or the other side of the liver. If discovered intraoperatively, attempts may be made at reinsertion. Unfortunately, this problem may often be unrecoverable, highlighting the importance of proper arteriotomy and insertion of vein pick [33].

Pseudoaneurysm may also occur due to erosion of the catheter tip through the arterial wall. CT scans may show layering blood products around the insertion site and problems with pump flow [34]. Should the hematoma become loosened, a potential life-threatening hemorrhage may occur. This problem is typically managed by passing a stent across the CHA to the PHA, excluding the GHA [30].

Patient factors may contribute to arterial complications as well. In addition to the malperfusion caused by variant branches discussed above, the GDA itself may be too short for proper cannulation. In severe celiac artery stenosis, blood flood to the liver may originate predominantly from the SMA through GDA in a retrograde fashion, in which case using the GDA would be prohibitive. There are alternative cannulation sites [30] and options for venous conduits [35], particularly from the greater saphenous vein with a low complication rate.

The biliary system is at risk for complications from HAI pump placement, given the dependence on arterial blood supply [6]. Abnormal liver function tests detect complications related to the biliary system and may require dexamethasone infusion [34]. In one study, biliary sclerosis occurred in 5.5% of patients who underwent pump placement. Still, this finding had no material impact on long-term patient survival if salvage procedures such as stenting or drainage were utilized [36].

Alternative Arterial Liver Therapies

Table 13.4 lists the clinical trials with HAI on the National Clinical Trials Registry, many of which hope to advance the efficacy and safety of such treatments. HAI therapy must be considered within the context of other intra-arterial therapeutics (IAT) of unresectable hepatic tumors, including transarterial chemoembolization (TACE) and transarterial radioembolization (TARE). HAI pump therapy has extrinsic advantages such as ease of administration over repeated cycles and reliable access to the arterial system. In contrast, TACE and TARE do not require surgery or pump management. There is a lack of data directly comparing IAT therapies for ICC and CRLM, likely due to patient heterogeneity and variance in specific treatment methods (type of chemotherapy and embolization, radiation dose). Wright et al. compared surgical treatment ($n = 57$) vs. IAT (TACE $n = 41$, HAI $n = 16$) for multifocal ICC and found no advantage in the surgical group [37]. While OS remained poor, HAI therapy recorded the highest median OS of 39 months vs. 20 for surgery and 15 for TACE. In a multivariate analysis, HAI had an HR of 0.29 (95% CI 0.13–0.65) compared with surgery, where TACE had an HR of 0.73 (95% CI 0.43–1.25). Noting the high morbidity of surgery, the authors highlighted the potential role and benefit of HAI therapy, albeit in the setting of a retrospective review with small numbers of patients. In unresectable CRLM, TACE is considered an adjunct therapy to systemic chemotherapy. Gruber-Rouh et al. analyzed data from 564 patients with CRLM who received TACE. There was a median of 6 sessions per patient with varied chemotherapy agents [38]. There was a median overall survival of 14.3 months. For TARE, NCCN guidelines recommended its usage in unresectable, liver-dominant, or liver-limited, chemotherapy-resistant patients [39]. In a combined analysis of the SIRFLOX and FOXFIRE trials, comparing systemic FOLFOX therapy for unresectable CRLM vs. FOLFOX and selective internal radiotherapy (SIRT) to liver found a median OS of 23 months in the systemic alone group vs. 25 months in the systemic plus SIRT group [40]. This difference was not statistically significant, and the authors concluded that using SIRT up-front could not be recommended, and patients should be carefully selected for its use. Of the three IAT therapies, only HAI has shown possible advantages in OS when given in conjunction with standard systemic therapy.

Table 13.4 Ongoing trials involving intra-arterial hepatic therapy for malignancy

NCT trial number	Status	Location	Therapy	Rationale
NCT05698459	Recruiting	China	Biological: OH2 injection; Transcatheter	Phase I: Advanced HCC
NCT04837885	Recruiting	France	177Lu-DOTATATE; HAI pump	Phase II; Hepatic neuroendocrine tumor
NCT04701281	Recruiting	Australia	Oxaliplatin + Capecitabine; Transcatheter	Phase I/II; CRLM
NCT04601428	Recruiting	Taiwan	Biological: CSR02-Tab-TF; Transcathete	Phase I: HCC
NCT05053555	Recruiting	USA, MDA	High dose-rate brachytherapy	Phase NA: Unresectable liver malignancies
NCT01214343	Recruiting	Japan	Sorafenib systemic; Cisplatin + 5-FU; HAI pump	Phase III: HCC
NCT02885753	Recruiting	France	LV5FU2 ± Irinotecan	Phase III: CRLM
NCT04003792	Recruiting	Israel	Systemic FOLFIRI + Bevacizumab; Oxaliplatin HAI pump	Phase II: CRLM
NCT04898504	Recruiting	Norway	HAI Floxuridine + second-line chemotherapy vs. Liver transplant	Phase II: CRLM
NCT04595266	Recruiting	Spain	LIFEPEARLS® + TACE	Phase II: CRLM
NCT03727633	Recruiting	France	Idarubicin/Lipiodol; Transcatheter	Phase II: HCC
NCT05103020	Recruiting	Korea	Oxaliplatin—HAI pump; systemic FOLFIRI	Phase II: CRLM
NCT04544098	Active, not recruiting	USA, MSK	177Lu-DOTATATE; HAI pump	Phase I: Hepatic neuroendocrine tumor
NCT02174549	Active, not recruiting	USA, Stanford	Tirapazamine; Transcatheter	Phase I/II: hepatic neuroendocrine tumor
NCT03028311	Active, not recruiting	USA, MDA	Y-90	Phase I: Primary or metastatic liver cancer
NCT02856126	Unknown	China	HAI chemotherapy + Sorafenib vs. TACE + Sorafenib	Phase III: HCC
NCT03687853	Unknown	China	HAI chemotherapy	Phase NA; PDAC liver metastasis prophylaxis
NCT00027768	Unknown	Singapore	Radioactive iodine; Transcatheter	Phase III: HCC
NCT00183885	Unknown	USA, USC	Cisplatin + Mitomycin-C; HAI Pump	Phase II: HCC
NCT04552093	Unknown	Netherlands	Floxuridine HAI pump + systemic FOLFOX/ FOLFIRI	Phase II/III; CRLM
NCT03469479	Unknown	China	Neoadjuvant TACE	Phase III: Resectable HCC

NCT04764409 Is a prospective observational study of complications of transcatheter therapy—excluded from the table
NCT04796025 Excluded as it is a new systemic therapy with TACE for HCC; no HA infusion
NCT03107416 Excluded given therapy is a diuretic in combination with TACE
NCT03326375 Excluded given just comparison of SBRT to TACE
NCT04069468 Excluded—Observational
NCT04903548 Excluded—Observational

Implication for Neurological Diseases

Long-term catheter placement has played an essential role in treating liver cancer. The liver's regenerative capacity and the desire to decrease blood flow by embolization during HAI run contrary to treating neurological diseases. Although long-term catheter placements have been used for treating cerebral sinus thrombosis [41], there are few other applications for treating brain cancer, vasospasm, and stroke. Long-term chemotherapy infusions over days effectively treat extracranial tumors [42]. However, prolonged infusions are currently impractical for arterial chemotherapy of brain tumors that require multiple single treatment sessions over several weeks [43]. During the treatment of cerebral vasospasm, arterial vasodilator infusions are administered daily over several days. During venous sinus thrombosis, thrombolytic infusion lasts several hours. Chapter 23 proposes stroke interventions that will require long-term catheter placement. Thus, developing technology for long-term catheter placement in the cerebral circulation has several applications. The key component in this advance will require improvements in catheter technology, bedside technology to detect displacement of catheters, infusion pumps, anticoagulation, and antiplatelet drugs. Safe long-term infusions can offer new avenues to treat neurological diseases.

Some other techniques of HAI could be applied to brain tumor treatments. These include the need to alter arterial networks by ligating arteries delivering to nontarget sites, selecting drugs taken by the target tissue, altering blood flow to enhance tumor uptake, and perhaps developing emboli materials used for TACE and TARE that selectively target tumors. While embolic materials carry the risk of stroke, modern superselective catheters could selectively embolize pathology [44–46]. Techniques developed for treating high-flow vascular lesions could be applied to treating brain tumors [47]. These include transient flow arrest with adenosine that can target embolic material highly selectively to even very high-flow lesions [48]. Could these embolic materials be used to deliver radioisotopes or chemotherapy for brain tumor treatments remains to be investigated. Selective embolization of brain tumors is an aspect of HAI that could be applied to brain tumor treatment.

Another significant lesson of HAI for brain tumor treatment is to develop compounds and carriers with high first-pass uptake, significant regional extraction, and sustained retention. Clinical reports have already established the safety of superselective delivery with concurrent flow modulation to brain tumors. The future treatment of brain tumors and other neurological diseases will require the development of compounds with site-specific uptake and sustained retention. To the contrary, there is also cautionary evidence of potential complications of long-term catheter placements. Impacted catheters during cerebral angiography pose embolic and infective risks [49]. Considering all the risks of long-term cerebral arterial catheterization, the prudent strategy in the near term—until safe long-term cerebral catheterization is possible—is the development of efficacious tumor-selective drugs that are rapidly extracted and sufficiently retained might be the more prudent strategy [50].

Conclusion

In conclusion, HAI therapy takes advantage of nature by delivering concentrated chemotherapy to arterially dependent liver tumors. Indications are not limited to but broadly include CRLM and ICC. Pumps with similar outcomes may be placed as an open procedure or using a surgical robot. For CRLM and ICC, pump therapy may be a valuable adjunct to modern systemic therapy in selected patients, requiring multidisciplinary support from surgeons, medical oncologists, interventional radiologists, and nuclear medicine physicians. A summary of studies for CRLM and ICC is given in Tables 13.2 and 13.3. HAI is likely superior to other IATs for CRLM and ICC, such as TACE and TARE. The complexity and multidisciplinary nature of pump placement is best optimized in high-volume centers, though pump placement may become more common as expertise grows and is disseminated. Careful patient selection is mandatory based on disease status and anatomy. Complications may occur intraoperatively and/or postoperatively, including malperfusion, dissection, pseudoaneurysm/erosion, biliary sclerosis, pump pocket seroma, and/or infection. Most of these complications may be salvaged with careful and prompt observation and care. Given the growing expertise and care coordination, HAI therapy remains a promising therapeutic option in the oncologic armamentarium for primary and secondary hepatic malignancies. Some of the advances in HAI might be relevant to treating neurological diseases. Still, the inherent risk of stroke and the need to manipulate blood flow pose significant hurdles to long-term arterial infusions in neurological patients.

References

1. Breedis C, Young G. The blood supply of neoplasms in the liver. Am J Pathol. 1954;30(5):969–77.
2. Collins JM. Pharmacologic rationale for regional drug delivery. J Clin Oncol. 1984;2(5):498–504.
3. Garg S, Kumar KH, Sahni D, Yadav TD, Aggarwal A, Gupta T. Anatomy of the hepatic arteries and their extrahepatic branches in the human liver: a cadaveric study. Ann Anat. 2020;227:151409.
4. Perez DR, Kemeny NE, Brown KT, Gewirtz AN, Paty PB, Jarnagin WR, et al. Angiographic identification of extrahepatic perfusion after hepatic arterial pump placement: implications for surgical prevention. HPB (Oxford). 2014;16(8):744–8.
5. Qadan M, D'Angelica MI, Kemeny NE, Cercek A, Kingham TP. Robotic hepatic arterial infusion pump placement. HPB (Oxford). 2017;19(5):429–35.
6. Kemeny N, Huang Y, Cohen AM, Shi W, Conti JA, Brennan MF, et al. Hepatic arterial infusion of chemotherapy after resection of hepatic metastases from colorectal cancer. N Engl J Med. 1999;341(27):2039–48.
7. Kemeny N, Gonen M, Sullivan D, Schwartz L, Benedetti F, Saltz L, et al. Phase I study of hepatic arterial infusion of floxuridine and dexamethasone with systemic irinotecan for unresectable hepatic metastases from colorectal cancer. J Clin Oncol. 2001;19(10):2687–95.
8. Kemeny N, Jarnagin W, Paty P, Gonen M, Schwartz L, Morse M, et al. Phase I trial of systemic oxaliplatin combination chemotherapy with hepatic arterial infusion in patients with unresectable liver metastases from colorectal cancer. J Clin Oncol. 2005;23(22):4888–96.
9. Kemeny NE, Melendez FD, Capanu M, Paty PB, Fong Y, Schwartz LH, et al. Conversion to resectability using hepatic artery infusion plus systemic chemotherapy for the treatment of unresectable liver metastases from colorectal carcinoma. J Clin Oncol. 2009;27(21):3465–71.
10. Kemeny N, Capanu M, D'Angelica M, Jarnagin W, Haviland D, Dematteo R, et al. Phase I trial of adjuvant hepatic arterial infusion (HAI) with floxuridine (FUDR) and dexamethasone plus systemic oxaliplatin, 5-fluorouracil and leucovorin in patients with resected liver metastases from colorectal cancer. Ann Oncol. 2009;20(7):1236–41.
11. Kemeny NE, Jarnagin WR, Capanu M, Fong Y, Gewirtz AN, Dematteo RP, et al. Randomized phase II trial of adjuvant hepatic arterial infusion and systemic chemotherapy with or without bevacizumab in patients with resected hepatic metastases from colorectal cancer. J Clin Oncol. 2011;29(7):884–9.
12. D'Angelica MI, Correa-Gallego C, Paty PB, Cercek A, Gewirtz AN, Chou JF, et al. Phase II trial of hepatic artery infusional and systemic chemotherapy for patients with unresectable hepatic metastases from colorectal cancer: conversion to resection and long-term outcomes. Ann Surg. 2015;261(2):353–60.
13. Pak LM, Kemeny NE, Capanu M, Chou JF, Boucher T, Cercek A, et al. Prospective phase II trial of combination hepatic artery infu-

sion and systemic chemotherapy for unresectable colorectal liver metastases: long term results and curative potential. J Surg Oncol. 2018;117(4):634–43.
14. Verheij FS, Kuhlmann KFD, Silliman DR, Soares KC, Kingham TP, Balachandran VP, et al. Combined hepatic arterial infusion pump and systemic chemotherapy in the modern era for chemotherapy-naive patients with unresectable colorectal liver metastases. Ann Surg Oncol. 2023;30(13):7950–9.
15. Kemeny NE, Chou JF, Boucher TM, Capanu M, DeMatteo RP, Jarnagin WR, et al. Updated long-term survival for patients with metastatic colorectal cancer treated with liver resection followed by hepatic arterial infusion and systemic chemotherapy. J Surg Oncol. 2016;113(5):477–84.
16. Goéré D, Benhaim L, Bonnet S, Malka D, Faron M, Elias D, et al. Adjuvant chemotherapy after resection of colorectal liver metastases in patients at high risk of hepatic recurrence: a comparative study between hepatic arterial infusion of oxaliplatin and modern systemic chemotherapy. Ann Surg. 2013;257(1):114–20.
17. Groot Koerkamp B, Sadot E, Kemeny NE, Gonen M, Leal JN, Allen PJ, et al. Perioperative hepatic arterial infusion pump chemotherapy is associated with longer survival after resection of colorectal liver metastases: a propensity score analysis. J Clin Oncol. 2017;35(17):1938–44.
18. Fong Y, Fortner J, Sun RL, Brennan MF, Blumgart LH. Clinical score for predicting recurrence after hepatic resection for metastatic colorectal cancer: analysis of 1001 consecutive cases. Ann Surg. 1999;230(3):309–18; discussion 18–21.
19. Buisman FE, Filipe WF, Galjart B, Grunhagen DJ, Homs MYV, Moelker A, et al. Adjuvant intra-arterial chemotherapy for patients with resected colorectal liver metastases: a systematic review and meta-analysis. HPB (Oxford). 2022;24(3):299–308.
20. Cheng DT, Mitchell TN, Zehir A, Shah RH, Benayed R, Syed A, et al. Memorial Sloan Kettering-integrated mutation profiling of actionable cancer targets (MSK-IMPACT): a hybridization capture-based next-generation sequencing clinical assay for solid tumor molecular oncology. J Mol Diagn. 2015;17(3):251–64.
21. Datta J, Narayan RR, Goldman DA, Chatila WK, Gonen M, Strong J, et al. Distinct genomic profiles are associated with conversion to resection and survival in patients with initially unresectable colorectal liver metastases treated with systemic and hepatic artery chemotherapy. Ann Surg. 2022;276(5):e474–e82.
22. Narayan RR, Datta J, Goldman DA, Aveson VG, Walch HS, Sanchez-Vega F, et al. Genomic predictors of recurrence patterns after complete resection of colorectal liver metastases and adjuvant hepatic artery infusion chemotherapy. Ann Surg Oncol. 2022;29(12):7579–88.
23. Valle J, Wasan H, Palmer DH, Cunningham D, Anthoney A, Maraveyas A, et al. Cisplatin plus gemcitabine versus gemcitabine for biliary tract cancer. N Engl J Med. 2010;362(14):1273–81.
24. Oh DY, Lee KH, Lee DW, Yoon J, Kim TY, Bang JH, et al. Gemcitabine and cisplatin plus durvalumab with or without tremelimumab in chemotherapy-naive patients with advanced biliary tract cancer: an open-label, single-centre, phase 2 study. Lancet Gastroenterol Hepatol. 2022;7(6):522–32.
25. Cercek A, Boerner T, Tan BR, Chou JF, Gonen M, Boucher TM, et al. Assessment of hepatic arterial infusion of floxuridine in combination with systemic gemcitabine and oxaliplatin in patients with unresectable intrahepatic cholangiocarcinoma: a phase 2 clinical trial. JAMA Oncol. 2020;6(1):60–7.
26. Franssen S, Holster J, Jolissaint JS, Soares KC, Nooijen L, Klümpen HJ, et al. A patient-level comparison of systemic chemotherapy and hepatic arterial infusion pump chemotherapy for unresectable intrahepatic cholangiocarcinoma. HPB (Oxford) [Internet]. 2022;24:S459–S60 pp. https://www.hpbonline.org/article/S1365-182X(22)01124-8/fulltext.
27. El-Diwany R, Pawlik TM, Ejaz A. Intrahepatic cholangiocarcinoma. Surg Oncol Clin N Am. 2019;28(4):587–99.
28. Ensminger WD, Gyves JW. Clinical pharmacology of hepatic arterial chemotherapy. Semin Oncol. 1983;10(2):176–82.
29. Kemeny N, Seiter K, Niedzwiecki D, Chapman D, Sigurdson E, Cohen A, et al. A randomized trial of intrahepatic infusion of fluorodeoxyuridine with dexamethasone versus fluorodeoxyuridine alone in the treatment of metastatic colorectal cancer. Cancer. 1992;69(2):327–34.
30. Allen PJ, Nissan A, Picon AI, Kemeny N, Dudrick P, Ben-Porat L, et al. Technical complications and durability of hepatic artery infusion pumps for unresectable colorectal liver metastases: an institutional experience of 544 consecutive cases. J Am Coll Surg. 2005;201(1):57–65.
31. Callahan MK, Kemeny NE. Implanted hepatic arterial infusion pumps. Cancer J. 2010;16(2):142–9.
32. Sofocleous CT, Schubert J, Kemeny N, Covey AM, Brody LA, Getrajdman GI, et al. Arterial embolization for salvage of hepatic artery infusion pumps. J Vasc Interv Radiol. 2006;17(5):801–6.
33. Sharib JM, Creasy JM, Wildman-Tobriner B, Kim C, Uronis H, Hsu SD, et al. Hepatic artery infusion pumps: a surgical toolkit for intraoperative decision-making and management of hepatic artery infusion-specific complications. Ann Surg. 2022;276(6):943–56.
34. Napier KJ, Lidsky ME, James OG, Wildman-Tobriner B. Hepatic arterial infusion pumps: what the radiologist needs to know. Radiographics. 2021;41(3):895–908.
35. Yezhelyev M, Osgood M, Egnatashvili V, Lumsden A, Staley CA, Kooby DA. Saphenous vein graft conduits for insertion of hepatic arterial infusion pumps in patients with abnormal hepatic arterial anatomy. J Surg Oncol. 2008;97(1):85–9.
36. Ito K, Ito H, Kemeny NE, Gonen M, Allen PJ, Paty PB, et al. Biliary sclerosis after hepatic arterial infusion pump chemotherapy for patients with colorectal cancer liver metastasis: incidence, clinical features, and risk factors. Ann Surg Oncol. 2012;19(5):1609–17.
37. Wright GP, Perkins S, Jones H, Zureikat AH, Marsh JW, Holtzman MP, et al. Surgical resection does not improve survival in multifocal intrahepatic cholangiocarcinoma: a comparison of surgical resection with intra-arterial therapies. Ann Surg Oncol. 2018;25(1):83–90.
38. Gruber-Rouh T, Naguib NN, Eichler K, Ackermann H, Zangos S, Trojan J, et al. Transarterial chemoembolization of unresectable systemic chemotherapy-refractory liver metastases from colorectal cancer: long-term results over a 10-year period. Int J Cancer. 2014;134(5):1225–31.
39. Benson AB, Venook AP, Al-Hawary MM, Arain MA, Chen YJ, Ciombor KK, et al. Colon cancer, version 2.2021, NCCN clinical practice guidelines in oncology. J Natl Compr Cancer Netw. 2021;19(3):329–59.
40. Wasan HS, Gibbs P, Sharma NK, Taieb J, Heinemann V, Ricke J, et al. First-line selective internal radiotherapy plus chemotherapy versus chemotherapy alone in patients with liver metastases from colorectal cancer (FOXFIRE, SIRFLOX, and FOXFIRE-Global): a combined analysis of three multicentre, randomised, phase 3 trials. Lancet Oncol. 2017;18(9):1159–71.
41. Waugh J, Plumb P, Rollins N, Dowling MM. Prolonged direct catheter thrombolysis of cerebral venous sinus thrombosis in children: a case series. J Child Neurol. 2012;27(3):337–45.
42. Ii N, Fuwa N, Toyomasu Y, Takada A, Nomura M, Kawamura T, et al. A novel external carotid arterial sheath system for intra-arterial infusion chemotherapy of head and neck cancer. Cardiovasc Intervent Radiol. 2017;40(7):1099–104.
43. Patel NV, Wong T, Fralin SR, Li M, McKeown A, Gruber D, et al. Repeated superselective intraarterial bevacizumab after blood brain barrier disruption for newly diagnosed glioblastoma: a phase I/II clinical trial. J Neurooncol. 2021;155(2):117–24.
44. Riina HA, Burkhardt JK, Santillan A, Bassani L, Patsalides A, Boockvar JA. Short-term clinico-radiographic response to super-selective intra-arterial cerebral infusion of bevacizumab for the treatment of vestibular schwannomas in neurofibromatosis type 2. Interv Neuroradiol. 2012;18(2):127–32.

45. Riina HA, Fraser JF, Fralin S, Knopman J, Scheff RJ, Boockvar JA. Superselective intraarterial cerebral infusion of bevacizumab: a revival of interventional neuro-oncology for malignant glioma. J Exp Ther Oncol. 2009;8(2):145–50.
46. Riina HA, Knopman J, Greenfield JP, Fralin S, Gobin YP, Tsiouris AJ, et al. Balloon-assisted superselective intra-arterial cerebral infusion of bevacizumab for malignant brainstem glioma. A technical note. Interv Neuroradiol. 2010;16(1):71–6.
47. Pile-Spellman J, Young WL, Joshi S, Duong H, Vang MC, Hartmann A, et al. Adenosine-induced cardiac pause for endovascular embolization of cerebral arteriovenous malformations: technical case report. Neurosurgery. 1999;44(4):881–6; discussion 6–7.
48. Hashimoto T, Young WL, Aagaard BD, Joshi S, Ostapkovich ND, Pile-Spellman J. Adenosine-induced ventricular asystole to induce transient profound systemic hypotension in patients undergoing endovascular therapy. Dose-response characteristics. Anesthesiology. 2000;93(4):998–1001.
49. Mirdamadi A, Mirdamadi N. A case of recurrent osteomyelitis due to retained micro-catheter after cerebral angiography. IDCases. 2024;36:e02005.
50. Cooke JN, Ellis JA, Hossain S, Nguyen J, Bruce JN, Joshi S. Computational pharmacokinetic rationale for intra-arterial delivery to the brain. Drug Deliv Transl Res. 2016;6(5):622–9.

Intra-arterial Gene Delivery for Neurodegenerative Diseases

14

Jonathan M. Fischell

Medicine is not only a science; it is also an art. It does not consist of compounding pills and plasters; it deals with the very processes of life, which must be understood before they may be guided.

Paracelsus (1493–1541), Swiss Physician

Introduction

In the past 20 years, incredible advances have been made in modern medicine, allowing for the discovery and implementation of countless treatments for diseases previously considered untreatable. The fields of oncology and autoimmunity have seen a large proportion of these improvements due to a better understanding of the molecular mechanisms underlying these diseases and the use of monoclonal antibodies to target these mechanisms specifically. While treatments for neurologic diseases often lag behind their systemic counterparts, the field of neurology has also seen substantial growth—intra-arterial (IA) therapy for ischemic stroke, effective disease modifying therapies (DMTs) for neuro-immunologic diseases such as multiple sclerosis and myasthenia gravis, neurosurgical treatments for refractory epilepsy, calcitonin gene-related peptide (CGRP) antagonists for migraine, deep brain stimulation (DBS) for a variety of neurologic conditions (including but not limited to movement disorders), and gene therapy for spinal muscular atrophy (SMA) are just a few of the critical advances in neurology in the past decade. Despite these advances, and those in neurology, there are almost no approved DMTs for neurodegenerative diseases (NDDs), with the exception being the new monoclonal antibodies, Aducanumab and Lecanemab, for Alzheimer's disease (AD) [1]. Despite their approval, the meaningful clinical effectiveness of these medications remains a source of significant debate. NDDs include but are not limited to AD, Parkinson's disease (PD), amyotrophic lateral sclerosis (ALS), Huntington's disease (HD), frontotemporal lobar degeneration (FTLD), spinocerebellar ataxias (SCAs), lysosomal storage disease (LSDs), prion diseases, and many more and represent a vast proportion of neurologic illnesses in patients today. Many are extremely common, all are life-altering diagnoses with high morbidity to patients and families, all are ultimately fatal, and none have approved and effective DMTs. It is safe to say there is a hugely unmet need for effective DMTs for NDDs.

Many scientists and clinicians worldwide are working together to improve treatments for NDDs. While a wide variety of strategies are being investigated to treat NDDs, genetic therapy offers immense hope. The major challenge for clinical translation of gene therapies for NDDs is efficient and targeted delivery. How do we get genetic therapy to the intracellular compartment, typically of the neurons, where it can exert its therapeutic effect? How do we minimize off-target deliveries, which can be harmful or potentially fatal? In this chapter, we will (1) discuss the pathogenesis of NDDs, the rationale for using gene therapies as DMTs for NDDs and types of genetic therapy; (2) review methods for gene therapy delivery to the brain, including vectors, capsid engineering, and non-IA routes; (3) evaluate the potential benefits and limitations of IA delivery of gene therapy vectors and review preclinical investigations of this strategy for brain gene therapy; and finally (4) thoroughly review physical methods for disrupting the BBB to allow the passage of gene therapy vectors efficiently to the brain with a focus on how these methods could be combined with IA route for maximum effectiveness.

J. M. Fischell (✉)
Department of Neurology, University of Maryland School of Medicine, Baltimore, MD, USA
e-mail: jonathan.fischell@som.umaryland.edu

S. Joshi (ed.), *Arterial Treatment of Neurological Diseases*, https://doi.org/10.1007/978-3-031-80173-0_14

Pathogenesis of NDDs and Rationale for the Use of Genetic Therapy for Disease Modification

The fundamental feature of most neurodegenerative diseases (NDDs) is the toxic accumulation of misfolded protein aggregates [2–4], which are termed "proteinopathies." As the needs of a cell are dynamic, it must constantly create new proteins to maintain or alter cellular functions or to replace old or dysfunctional proteins. All healthy cells exist in a balanced state of protein creation and removal, known as proteostasis [2]. To achieve proteostasis, in the face of constantly evolving protein needs, cells have adopted various mechanisms for removing unwanted proteins [2–5]. Degradation of proteins is typically accomplished by digestion via the proteasome or by autophagocytosis, forming lysosomes [2, 6]. Once in lysosomes, proteins can either be degraded by lysosomal proteases or expelled into the extracellular matrix via exocytosis, where extracellular proteases degrade them [6]. While a healthy cell can keep its protein burden manageable, in NDDs, its proteostatic capabilities are overwhelmed for several reasons. Often, there is a genetic basis for the enhanced proteostatic stress [6], either predisposing a cellular protein to aggregation or impairing cellular machinery for handling proteostatic stress [4]. As dysfunctional or misfolded proteins increase, they often form less soluble toxic aggregates that alter transcription, intracellular signaling, or cell sequestering to impair cell functions. Ultimately, this forward feedback loop results in cellular death [5]. In many NDDs, all cells share a genetic background predisposing to proteostatic stress. As the cells are exposed to other environmental oxidative or inflammatory stressors [2], more and more cells become afflicted and die. Furthermore, in many cases, including but likely not limited to Prion disease and Parkinson's disease [2], pathological proteins are also transmitted through the extracellular space, cell to cell, in an infectious-like manner [4]. As time passes, more cells are destroyed, and since neurons do not regenerate, neurologic function worsens as the brain deteriorates [2–5, 7–12]. Identifying the definitive pathogenic target is often necessary to develop a DMT for any disorder. Targeting more proximal steps in the pathogenesis of a disorder is also more likely to be successful than targeting downstream consequences. Targeting noncausative proteins, which may result from an underlying problem rather than the problem itself, could lead to ineffective therapeutics. Thus, by identifying and targeting the causative proteins, we can hope to develop therapeutics with the most clinical effect.

Proteinopathies can be divided by underlying pathogenesis, specifically, those caused by a mutation in a single gene vs. those with complex pathogenesis, which are generally polygenic risks with environmental triggers. Single-gene proteinopathies typically result from gain-of-function mutations in proteins, predisposing them to form pathogenic aggregates (e.g., Huntington's disease) [13] or loss-of-function mutations in proteins critical to maintaining proteostasis (e.g., LSDs) [14]. Proteinopathies with complex pathogenesis are not attributable to a single gene mutation; however, in most cases, they are attributable to a single (or small number of) pathogenic protein (Fig. 14.1). For example, sporadic PD is a heterogeneous condition with several alleles that confer increased risk [15]. The single unifying pathologic factor for most forms of sporadic PD is the pathologic accumulation of α-synuclein aggregates [16]. Although similar to PD, many proteinopathies cause the toxic accumulation of just one or two pathogenic proteins in sporadic PD. Just as the abnormal gene in single disorders serves as a high-yield target for genetic manipulation, pathogenic proteins in complex proteinopathies are also logical targets with the highest chance of yielding effective disease modification. Following this thought process, the next question becomes: "What type of therapeutic intervention allows for the specific modification of a single intracellular protein?". The answer is genetic therapy.

Overview of Genetic Therapy for NDDs

Genetic (gene) therapy is the introduction of nucleic acids, capable of modifying protein expression, into target cells to "correct" a disease phenotype [11]. Genetic therapies can be introduced in vivo or ex vivo. In vivo*, gene therapy requires delivering a gene therapy platform directly to* the patient. To do this safely, careful consideration of the delivery method is needed to reduce the risk of adverse effects of the therapeutic. Ex vivo gene therapy involves harvesting effector cells from a patient, introducing a genetic modification in vitro, *and* then transplanting those cells back into the patient [17]. Examples of ex vivo gene therapy being used in the clinic are chimeric antigen T-cell (CAR-T) therapies for the treatment of various malignancies [18] and genetic diseases [17]. The benefit of ex vivo gene therapy is that it directly delivers a therapeutic to target cells in a controlled environment. This eliminates two significant risks and challenges faced by in vivo gene therapy—delivery of the gene therapy platform to off-target cells and immune activation by a gene therapy vector when introduced directly into the patient. Unfortunately, this method cannot be used to treat NDDs because harvest and reimplantation of neurons in the brain is

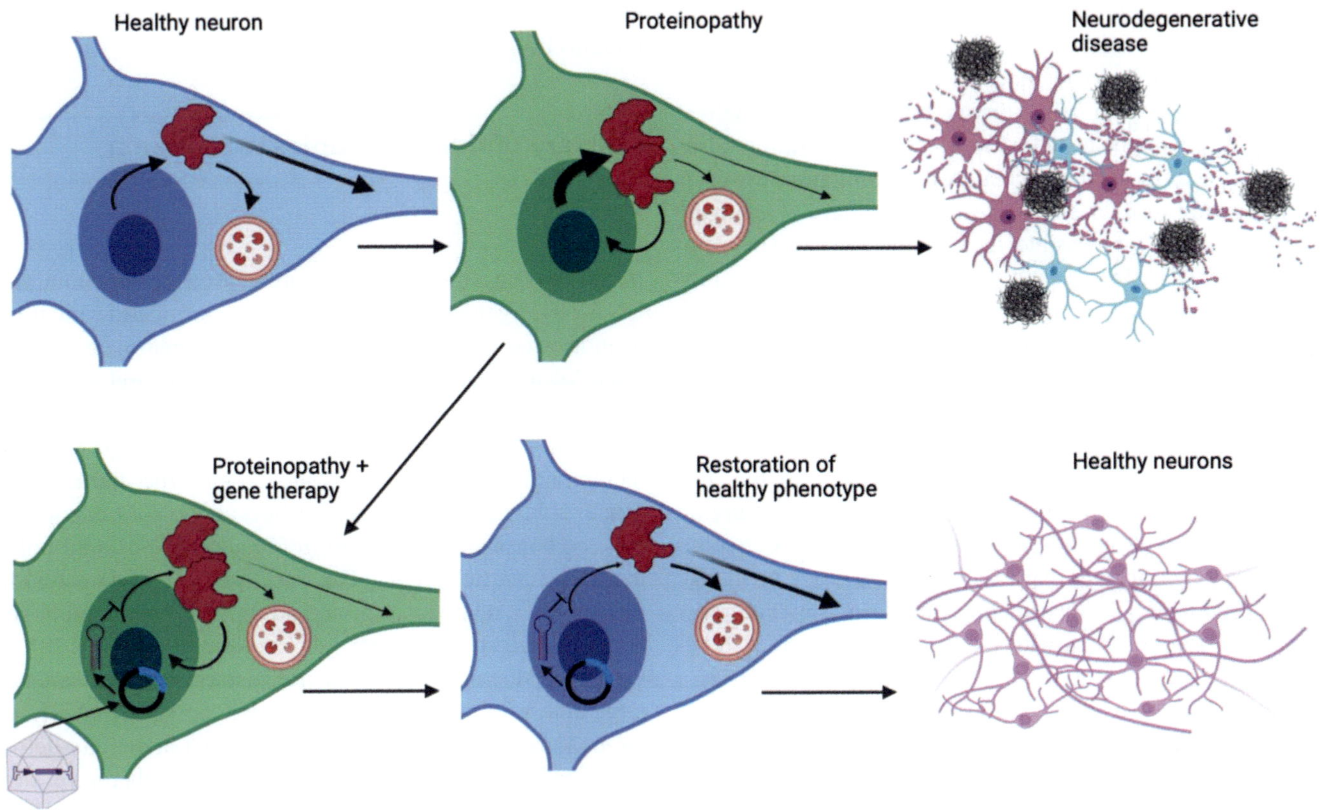

Fig. 14.1 Genetic therapy for neurodegenerative proteinopathies. In healthy neurons, proteins exist in a steady state of production, performing essential functions and then being degraded. In the case of proteinopathies, proteostatic homeostasis is disturbed, which is related to an inefficient genetic background and environmental trigger that leads to the formation of insoluble protein aggregates. These aggregates build up, modify translation, or sequester useful forms of the protein such that it cannot perform its critical function, ultimately leading to repent protein buildup and cell death. Gene therapy offers a means to modify this process directly. For example, an AAV can deliver a plasmid encoding a short hairpin RNA (shRNA), which decreases expression of the pathogenic protein, reducing the formation of toxic aggregates and ultimately restoring a healthy neuronal phenotype (*Created with* www.biorender.com)

impossible. Therefore, this chapter focuses on strategies for improving the safety and effectiveness of in vivo gene delivery to the brain.

In a broad sense, genetic therapy includes RNA-based therapeutics, such as antisense oligonucleotides (ASOs) and DNA-based therapeutics. At present, most clinical trials investigating genetic therapies for NDDs are ASOs. ASOs are short (16–21 bases), synthetic, single strands of RNA that can selectively modify mRNA [19]. In most cases, these therapies are designed to decrease (knockdown) protein production by targeting a specific mRNA for degradation via an RNA-induced silences complex (RISC) [19]. However, ASOs can also be used as splice modifiers, such as in the landmark genetic therapy, nusinersen (Spinraza) for SMA [20]. There are many clinical trials of ASOs under investigation for NDDs involving the CNS, including PD, HD, progressive supranuclear palsy (PSP), ALS, and FTD (*clinicaltrials.gov*). While ASOs do not cross the blood–brain barrier (BBB), they can be delivered intrathecally. ASOs can cross into the intracellular compartment of cells, and therefore, they do not require a vector for delivery, reducing the risk of vector-associated immunotoxicity. This said, there are several significant downsides to RNA-based gene therapy with ASOs. First, unlike DNA, which can remain stable for years or even a lifetime in a target cell after delivery, therapeutic RNA molecules are degraded over weeks to months, requiring recurrent infusions to maintain therapeutic effectiveness [21]. Second, owing to their simplicity, ASOs are not targetable to a specific tissue or cell type but rather enter whichever cells are most convenient. Most ASOs are being delivered intrathecally (IT) at the lumbar spine 4 and 5 (L4-L5 IT-L) level and are expected to travel up the thecal space to the brain. While this method may be sufficient for diseases involving the spinal cord or peripheral nerves, the proportion of ASOs that reach the brain is unknown but is likely very low. This may pose a significant problem in trials investigating ASOs for diseases of the brain. To combat this, one could conceive of using more targeted delivery methods such as intracisternal (ICM) or IA delivery with BBB disruption (BBBD) to deliver ASOs. However, the need for recurrent administration raises concerns with these approaches. A final limitation of ASOs is that owing to their simple design, they have a relatively restricted range of possible therapeutic effects. This contrasts with DNA-based gene therapies, which can theoretically utilize any existing protein.

DNA-based gene therapy (Fig. 14.1) often delivers DNA as an extra-chromosomal (episomal) plasmid. However, some vectors facilitate the insertion of the therapeutic DNA sequence directly into the host's chromosome. The benefit of episomal plasmids is that, by not inserting into the host genome, they do not risk insertional mutagenesis (disruption of host gene expression by the inserted DNA) and are considered a generally safer approach. However, one challenge with introducing DNA as an episomal plasmid is that transgenes are not replicated with the rest of the genome; therefore, DNA can be lost when cells turn over. This raises a problem when considering gene therapy for systemic diseases; however, it is not a problem in nondividing cells such as neurons. For this reason, vectors that introduce genes as episomal plasmids are preferable for gene therapy for NDDs of the CNS. Once the therapeutic DNA is introduced to the nucleus, host cells will express the transgene using its machinery and produce a new protein. This protein will be produced as long as the plasmid (or inserted DNA sequence) persists, which will be for the cell's life without extrinsic factors such as an immune response to the transgene [22]. This can mean life-long therapeutic effectiveness with a single dose, not requiring readministration. This strategy is especially desirable for gene therapy for NDDs of the CNS both because neurons are an ideal cell type for the maintenance of episomal plasmids and because delivering therapeutics to the brain often requires more risky or invasive means. Thus, readministration should be avoided. Onasemnogene abeparvovec (Zolgensma) is the first-ever approved DNA-based, single-dose gene therapy for a neurologic disease (SMA) [23–25]. Patients with SMA type 1, as were treated in the initial study, typically do not live past the age of 2–3 years. Yet, at the five-year extension study of these patients, all were alive, and many could even walk [26]. Both feats were unheard of for patients with SMA type 1 before this landmark medication. This example highlights the revolutionary potential of DNA-based gene therapy when harnessed appropriately.

Despite the high potential of DNA-based gene therapies for treating neurologic diseases, no therapies for NDDs involving the brain are currently approved, and very few are even under investigation in clinical trials. While multiple factors make DNA-based gene therapy for NDDs challenging, most would agree that the most significant challenge remains drug delivery.

Delivery of Gene Therapies to the Brain

Vectors

In most NDDs, the target cells are neurons in the brain. All DNA-based gene therapies require a vector to allow the therapeutic gene to enter the intracellular compartment of neurons. Vectors can be nonviral or viral. Nonviral strategies generally involve placing the transgene of interest inside a nonpolar nanomaterial, which can pass through the cell membrane, depositing its contents into the intracellular space. Nonviral vectors include liposomes, gold nanoparticles, carbon nanotubes, solid-lipid nanoparticles, and polymeric nanoparticles [27]. The benefit of nonviral vectors is that they are relatively simple and typically nonimmunogenetic, though some vectors still exert direct toxicity [28]. A significant downside with nonviral vectors is that they are not targetable to a specific organ or cell type. The inability to target particular cells generally means that nonvirally delivered genes may enter any cell they contact; therefore, off-target delivery is high, especially when the infusion site is a considerable distance from the target site. Furthermore, a nanoparticle's chemical and physical properties influence its pharmacokinetics, and some nanoparticles have been demonstrated to distribute throughout the brain even after IT-L infusion [28].

Unlike nonviral vectors, viruses have evolved over hundreds of millions of years to deliver a foreign gene to the intracellular compartment of cells. With viral vectors, a transgene is placed within the capsid of a virus instead of the viral genome, including genes for replication of the virus. The most frequently used viral vectors for gene therapy delivery to the nervous system are adeno-associated viruses (AAVs) [25, 29–34]. AAVs are much less immunogenic than most other viral vectors. They exist in many different natural serotypes, each with different tissue tropism, and they can be easily engineered to modify tropism further [35–39]. Some naturally occurring serotypes of AAV, such as AAV9 and AAVrh10 [34, 40], are even able to cross the BBB, though they do this highly inefficiently compared to engineered vectors [35–37]. The major downside to AAVs is their small size, which can be a significant limitation when a large transgene is required [25]. It is possible to work around limitations by removing unnecessary genetic elements and creating compact but efficacious versions of transgenes [41].

Viral capsids enter the intracellular space of cells using receptors that mediate internalization, and, in many cases, these receptors remain unknown. The presence of specific receptors on the viral capsid can allow cell or tissue-specific tropism. Furthermore, viral capsids are made of easily modifiable that further enhance the vector's tropism. The downside to viral vectors is that all viruses risk immunogenicity (though some viruses more than others). Immunogenicity with viral vectors poses a significant safety risk, and over the years, patients have died from immune-mediated adverse effects from viral gene therapies. AAVs, for example, are known to cause acute liver failure and thrombotic microangiopathy at high systemic doses [42] and neurotoxicity, including but not limited to dorsal root ganglion (DRG) toxicity, at high doses within the CNS [43–46]. For this reason, it is critical to maximally exploit the advantages of viral vectors, namely cell/tissue-specific tropism and modifiable tropism, to improve delivery efficiency and safety.

One difficulty with modifying viruses for enhanced delivery properties is that cell-specific receptors for internalization remain unknown. To combat that, groups have developed strategies termed directed evolution, which involves the evolution of viral capsids to enhance internalization without requiring prior knowledge of the underlying biological properties. The general concept of directed evolution involves the generation of a library of millions or billions of variants of viral capsids, then injecting all viruses into a host organism, finally harvesting the target tissue, and using next-generation sequencing to identify variants that reached the target in the greatest proportion [35–38]. The first iteration of AAV capsid evolution selected vectors in mice using a Cre-lox system called CREATE [36]. This endeavor yielded AAV-PHP.B, which has been demonstrated to drastically enhance BBB transduction compared to its parent vector, AAV9 [36]. While the AAV-PHP.B is highly effective in the specific strain of mice in which it was evolved, its properties did not translate to NHPs or even certain other strains of mice, highlighting that capsid evolution only has a high degree of certainty of effectiveness in the species in which it was screened [47–49]. The same group recently published a new paper where a similar capsid evolution process was performed in marmosets, yielding a novel variant, AAV.CAP-Mac [50]. This variant was then tested on Rhesus Macaques and was found to improve brain transduction by nine-fold and reduce liver transduction by roughly 30% compared to AAV9 [50]. While it is promising that this vector was identified to be effective in NHPs and that its effectiveness was not limited to marmosets in which it was screened, it remains to be seen if its properties will apply to humans. A potential strategy to evolve viruses with a greater likelihood of properties that translate to humans would be to evolve viruses in human cells in vitro [21], for example, in an organoid model of the human BBB. After this, variants were screened for a second time in NHPs to ensure they were effective in vivo [21].

Non-IA Delivery Routes

The delivery route is a powerful tool to modulate delivery efficiency without modifying the vector. The delivery efficiency can be conceptualized simply as the ratio of vectors delivered to target cells vs. off-target cells. It is well established that the route markedly alters the biodistribution of a therapeutic agent; therefore, the route should be viewed as an opportunity to improve on-target delivery further. To create the most efficient gene therapy delivery system, one must optimize both intrinsic factors of the therapy, such as the vector or capsid, and extrinsic factors, such as the delivery route. Various delivery routes have been used, or conceived of, for delivering gene therapy to the brain. These routes include IV, IT (which can be further broken down by location in the neuroaxis), intranasal (IN), IA, or direct intracranial (dIC). Historically, dIC has been the most widely employed delivery route in human studies as it is easily validated in animal models, does not need to take the BBB into account, and can reliably achieve a high therapeutic concentration at a specific site, thus limiting off-target delivery. Despite these factors, dIC is a poor delivery route for gene therapy for NDDs as it only allows localized delivery, and neurodegeneration is known to be a global process (though specific brain structures are affected earlier than others, depending on the disease). dIC is also invasive, requiring craniotomy and a needle track through brain parenchyma, exposing the brain to direct damage or secondary damage from surgical complications such as infection or hemorrhage [42, 51].

On the other hand, IV delivery is also frequently used in human gene therapy trials. The IV route is noninvasive and global, which is an advantage for treating NDDs. However, it does not specifically target the brain, and the therapeutic agent has to penetrate the BBB. These limitations explain why only a tiny fraction of infused vectors are found in the brain after IV delivery while ~1000× more are found in the liver [48, 52–55]. The problem means exceptionally high doses are necessary to achieve meaningful concentrations in the brain using standard gene therapy vectors such as AAV9. While engineered capsids drastically enhanced BBB crossing may lessen this problem, none have been validated with this property in humans. Additionally, even if engineered vectors with enhanced BBB crossing in humans did exist, the IV route would theoretically be suboptimal compared to the IA route as vectors still travel throughout the body before reaching the brain, allowing plenty of opportunities for them to get sequestered in other organs such as the liver (Fig. 14.2). Given these limitations, it is not surprising that most severe adverse events and deaths with gene therapies have been with high doses infused intravenously [56]. Despite the significant flaws with dIC and IV delivery, almost every clinical trial of gene therapies for NDDs involving the brain has used

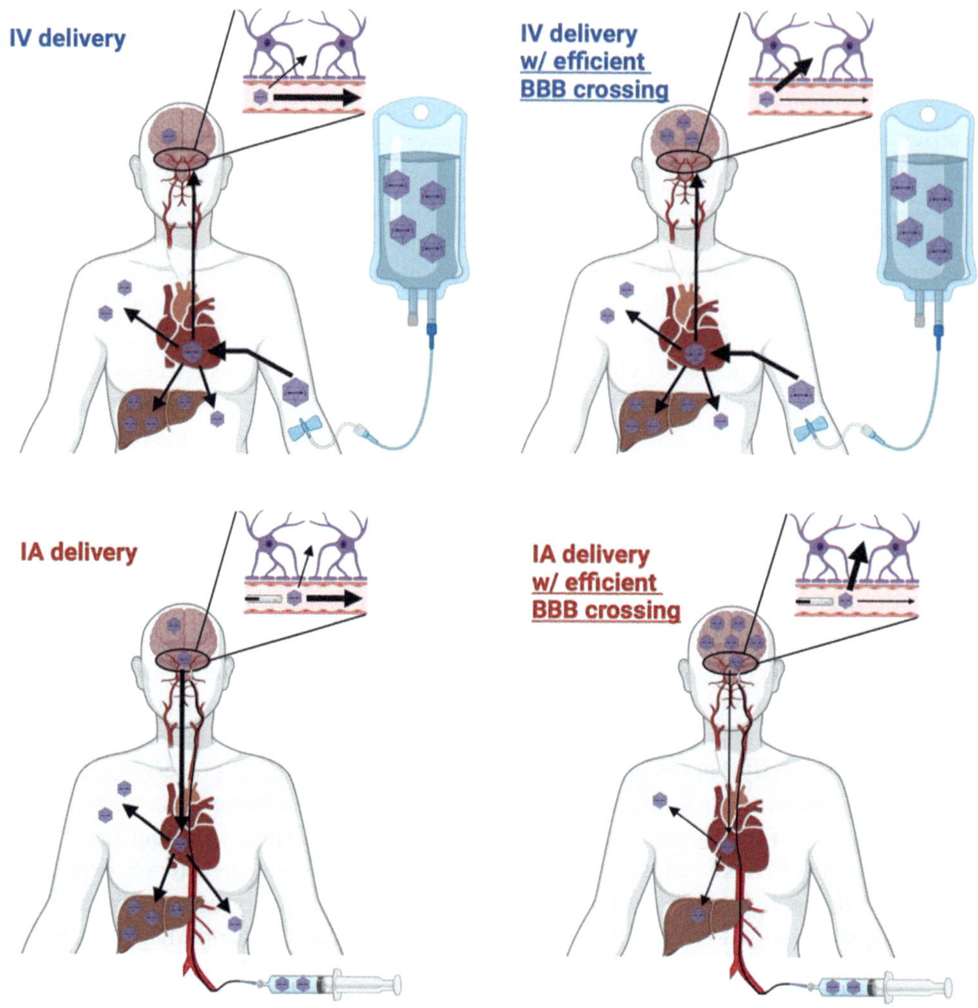

Fig. 14.2 Intravascular delivery of gene therapies to the brain. IV delivery neither targets gene therapy vectors to the brain nor intrinsically allows their passage to the brain through the BBB. This results in highly inefficient delivery where most vectors are delivered to off-target peripheral tissues, and almost no vectors are delivered to target cells in the brain. Combining IV delivery with methods such as capsid engineering for enhanced BBB transduction or physical methods of BBBD, such as IA mannitol or focused ultrasound, can enhance the number of vectors delivered to the brain. However, because the delivery route does not direct vectors to the brain, many vectors will still be delivered to off-target organs before even reaching the brain. IA delivery directs vectors to the brain, potentially reducing off-target delivery. However, without efficient BBB crossing, most vectors will not enter the brain on the first pass, and the IA route will provide little or no benefit compared to IV delivery. The combination of IA delivery and methods for efficient BBB transduction produces a synergistic effect where a large portion of vectors can enter the brain on the first pass, increasing on-target and reducing off-target delivery (*Created with* www.biorender.com)

these routes. Consequently, gene therapies for brain diseases have earned a reputation for being ineffective and/or dangerous. It is imperative that more advanced delivery routes, which maximize safety and efficiency, are developed to realize the goal of translating gene therapies to the clinic for the treatment of NDDs.

More advanced delivery methods include IT, IN, and IA. IT routes are in the early stages of investigation but show merit for the global delivery of gene therapy vectors across the BBB. IT can be divided into IT-L, intracisternal (ICM), and intracerebroventricular (ICV). The IT-L route is the least invasive IT delivery route, but it is limited by the long-distance therapeutics that must travel to reach the brain. This increases the number of vectors delivered to the spinal cord rather than the brain. Additionally, therapeutics in the CSF are constantly lost to the bloodstream [28, 57]. It stands to reason that the greater the distance a vector needs to travel, the more the proportion will be lost to systemic circulation. Consequently, some studies find minimal brain delivery with the IT-L route in NHP models [28, 58], others suggest that it could be effective [57, 59].

The intracisternal route (ICM) involves infusing vectors into the CSF at the level of the cisterna magna rather than the lumbar spinal cord. In doing so, vectors are released closer to the brain parenchyma, logically increasing brain delivery. The ICM route is effective in most animal models [57, 59–67]. That said, several concerns remain with ICM delivery. Most notably, this route requires the placement of a needle near the medulla, damage to which results in high morbidity and potentially death. Also, ICM delivery is not commonly used in a clinical setting, and few interventionalists are trained to use it, thereby limiting widespread translatability. To mitigate these limitations, thecal space is accessed at L4-L5, and a temporary catheter (or microcatheter) is advanced to the level of the cisterna magna to release the vectors [28, 68]. This method allows biodistribution similar to the ICM route but with the safety of the IT-L route. However, this approach is less efficient than the ICV route for brain delivery [28].

Although CSF flow dynamics are complex and nonunidirectional [57], CSF typically flows inferiorly from the cisterna magna down toward the spinal cord [69], rather than superiorly toward the brain. This causes problems for infratentorial delivery routes, including ICM. The ICV route is effective for brain gene therapy [28, 57, 59, 62, 70–72]. Though effective, like dIC delivery, ICV delivery requires a craniotomy and needle insertion through healthy brain tissue to reach its target. For this reason, it carries the risks of infection and hemorrhage, and therefore, despite its high efficiency, it is generally avoided.

Last, briefly, the IN route releases gene therapy vectors as a nasal spray, which then diffuses into nasal blood vessels and can be up taken into the brain [73]. Although this route releases vectors closer to the brain than a typical intravenous injection, it may not substantially improve IV delivery unless vectors can be rapidly translocated across the BBB before entering the systemic circulation. Combining IN delivery with focused ultrasound (FUS) to disrupt the BBB can lead to highly efficient gene delivery in mice [74]. Though few studies have employed this delivery method in the past 10 years, it may be worth reassessing it with novel BBB disruption methods such as FUS.

IA Route for Gene Therapy Delivery to the Brain

Overview, Benefits, and Limitations

The IA route is minimally invasive, where therapeutics are delivered directly to the brain through the arterial system, thereby reducing systemic absorption. IA delivery can range from global to regional super-selective, depending on which artery is infused. To achieve global delivery, with a consistent amount throughout the brain, all four vessels perfusing the brain are injected—the bilateral internal carotid arteries and the bilateral vertebral arteries. Super-selective delivery can be achieved by infusing a distal blood vessel, allowing only the small region supplied by that blood vessel to achieve high vector concentrations [75]. This method can reduce the total dose and further limit systemic toxicity. In the case of NDDs, it is often advisable to perform global gene therapy. This is because, as stated previously, most NDDs cause neurodegeneration throughout the brain, even if a specific region or pathway is affected earlier in the disease course. For example, PD preferentially damages dopaminergic neurons in the substantia nigra resulting in the motor symptoms. However, there are also several nonmotor manifestations of PD—autonomic dysfunction, sleep disorders, sensory symptoms, neuropsychiatric symptoms, and dementia [76]. These nonmotor symptoms can be just as problematic for many patients as the motor symptoms, which are not improved by DBS or levodopa. A similar logic applies to most NDDs involving the brain, such as AD, HD, and others. Therefore, global gene therapy is optimal for most NDDs to prevent global brain degeneration later in the disease course, even if patients are not manifesting global cerebral dysfunction at the time of treatment. Alternatively, super-selective gene therapy may be a fantastic tool for certain diseases, such as neurologic malignancies [75, 77–80], focal epilepsy, and stroke [81, 82].

Despite great potential, IA delivery is one of the least explored delivery routes for gene therapy to the brain (Fig. 14.2). IA delivery provides several advantages while targeting the brain: (1) It allows targeted delivery to the brain before the other organs. (2) It uses the brain's extensive capillary network, depositing the vectors close to the target cells. (3) IA procedure is safe, minimally invasive, and routinely performed for the diagnosis and treatment of ischemic stroke and aneurysms. (4) The IA route can also be used with osmotic BBB disruption with IA mannitol, as discussed elsewhere in the book. There are several limitations to this delivery strategy. The IA route relies on the "first pass effect" to improve efficiency. After IA infusion, gene therapy vectors have a single opportunity to enter the brain before continuing to systemic circulation. If only a small fraction of the vectors can enter the brain on the first pass, IA delivery over IV will have little or no benefit. For this reason, IA delivery should be combined with physical BBBD methods. Alternatively, engineered AAVs can drastically enhance BBB transduction in humans in the future (Fig. 14.2). Secondly, while minimally invasive, IA procedures carry more risks than IV. These include groin site or (rarely) retroperitoneal hematoma, arterial wall injury, and embolic strokes [83] (though these strokes are typically punctate and asymptomatic). Despite these risks, DNA-based gene therapies should not require readministration, and the minor risks of a single IA procedure are likely to be outweighed by the benefit of reducing potentially life-threatening immunotoxicity.

IA Gene Therapy in Preclinical Models

Unfortunately, very few preclinical studies have investigated IA delivery of gene therapies to the brain. Preclinical investigations of IA are uncommon because they are technically demanding in small animals compared to other delivery methods. This is ironic because the IA route is straightforward and highly utilized in hospitals. This section will review the studies on gene therapy delivery via the IA route and emphasize points that can be gleaned from each.

Foley et al. delivered AAVrh10 via intracarotid infusion and BBBD using a mouse model using IA mannitol [84]. Mannitol is a highly hydrophilic molecule that opens the BBB when infused at high concentrations IA by "pulling" water out of endothelial cells, causing them to shrink; this temporarily disrupts the integrity of tight junctions and allows for the passage of therapeutics through the BBB to the brain parenchyma. This method of BBBD will be discussed in greater detail in section "Strategies for BBB Opening". In the study by Foley, they first compared different volumes and flow rates of mannitol using magnetic resonance imaging (MRI) with contrast to assess the patency of the BBB. In their study, increasing the total volume of mannitol increased the distribution of BBB opening while modifying the flow rate had no effect. They found that a volume of 750 μL of 25% mannitol was necessary for global BBBD. Pretreated with IA mannitol increased vector delivery compared to saline control. They then compared IA delivery of AAVrh.10 to IV and IA with IA mannitol and found that IA delivery significantly increased brain delivery compared to IV. They also quantified delivery to multiple other tissues. They found a slight decrease in muscle delivery with IA but no significant difference in off-target delivery, including the liver. Unfortunately, they observed a much greater number of mice died in the high-dose mannitol group compared to the lower-dose groups, emphasizing that IA mannitol may be unsafe, at least using their protocol and parameters in mice.

Janson et al. compared IA with IA mannitol to ICV with IA mannitol to deliver AAV5 in mice [85]. AAV5 is a natural serotype that cannot naturally cross the BBB. They found that ICV with IA mannitol delivery led to superior brain delivery compared to IA with IA mannitol as measured by immunofluorescence and IDUA activity assays. They also found that a portion of the IA delivered AAVs in the liver, suggesting that vectors were not efficiently taken up during the first pass with their method. A fundamental limitation of this paper is that they did not use MRI with contrast to confirm that their mannitol protocol sufficiently opened the BBB. Further, they only injected 14 μL/g (about 280 μL) of 25% mannitol, which is far less than the dose that Foley et al. found necessary for BBB opening. With this significant limitation, it isn't easy to draw meaningful conclusions about IA vs. ICV delivery other than reinforcing the necessity of effective mitigation of the BBB for IA delivery to provide any value.

Morabito et al. evaluated IA (intracarotid) to IV delivery of AAV-PHP.B in mice [52]. It is worth noting that evaluating the delivery routes was a small part of this larger paper. However, the remainder of the paper is out of the scope of this chapter. AAV-PHP.B is an engineered vector with enhanced BBB crossing [36]. It was created using directed evolution and screened in C57 mice. For this reason, it has been determined that the BBB crossing potential of AAV-PHP.B does not translate to NHPs or even other strains of mice [48, 49]. However, it is highly effective at BBB crossing in C57 mice used in this study. They found comparable GFP expression with both routes. However, the IA route resulted in an approximately five-fold reduction in off-target delivery to the liver, heart, and muscle. This paper highlights the value of IA delivery in reducing nontarget delivery to systemic organs when an effective method of BBB penetration is concurrently used.

Yoon et al. used the IA (intracarotid) route with AAVhu.32 to deliver the alpha-mannosidase (MANB) gene in cats [55]. AAVhu.32 is a naturally occurring vector that can cross the BBB like AAV9, though not nearly as efficiently as engineered vectors. In their first analysis, they found that AAVhu.32 resulted in approximately four-fold higher GFP expression after IV delivery compared to AAV9 and about two-fold greater than AAVrh.8. They then delivered their AAVhu.32-MANB vector via the IA route in a cat model of alpha-mannosidosis. Their therapy significantly increased MANB activity throughout the brain, which was greater in the brain than in the liver, kidney, heart, and spleen. They did not compare this route to other routes. This therapy reversed the behavioral and pathological phenotype of alpha-mannosidosis in their cat model.

Liguore et al. compared IA, IV, ICV, and ICM delivery of AAV-PHP.B in C57 mice and IA vs. ICM delivery in NHPs [54]. In mice, all four routes had comparable delivery efficiency throughout the brain, suggesting that intravascular delivery methods with adequate BBB penetration can be just as effective as IT methods. In NHPs, they found that ICM delivery was markedly more efficient than IA delivery. This is likely because the enhanced BBB transduction of AAV-PHP.B is not conserved in NHPs; thus, this vector would not be able to take advantage of the first pass effect. It remains unexplored if IA delivery, an effective means of crossing the BBB, can be as efficient as ICM or other IT routes in NHPs (or humans).

A key theme among these studies is the importance of highly efficient BBB crossing to derive benefit from the IA route. Two of the four studies comparing the IA route to other routes in preclinical models demonstrated its benefits. Foley et al. found greater brain delivery with IA injection with IA mannitol compared to IV in mice, and Morabito et al. found a five-fold reduction in off-target delivery compared to IV. Although neither Janson et al. nor Liguore et al. found the IA route inferior to IT delivery, the BBB was likely not adequately bypassed in either study. It, therefore, remains unclear if IA delivery *with* efficient BBB crossing can be as (or more) efficient than ICV or ICM routes in NHPs or humans. If this were the case, the IA route would be preferred, given the simplicity of performing IA infusions in a clinical setting and the lower risks associated with the procedure. Future investigations should compare the IA route *with highly efficient BBB crossing* to ICM and ICV delivery in NHPs, after which translation to human patients should be strongly considered.

Strategies for BBB Opening

As demonstrated in the previous section, the benefit of IA delivery is contingent upon the efficient crossing of the BBB. While naturally occurring AAVs such as AAV9 can cross the BBB, they do so inefficiently and cannot be relied upon to improve delivery efficiency using the IA route. Strategies to enhance the crossing of the BBB can be divided into methods that modify the vector to enhance crossing through an intact BBB or methods that aim to open the BBB to allow vectors to go unhindered. Previously, we discussed capsid engineering to discover novel AAV variants with enhanced ability to cross the BBB in mice and NHPs. While this method may yield variants with properties confirmed to be effective in humans, this is not yet the case. Strategies to open the BBB, such as IA mannitol and focused ultrasound (FUS), are alternative approaches to tackling the problem of the BBB (Fig. 14.3). Both methods have been demonstrated to be safe and effective at opening the BBB and enhancing the delivery of therapeutics (which are typically unable to cross the BBB) in human patients.

Osmotic BBBD with IA Mannitol

Mannitol, a sugar alcohol, is a highly hydrophilic molecule. It is regularly used intravenously in clinical practice to treat cerebral edema and reduce intracranial pressure [86]. IA delivery allows much higher local concentrations of mannitol for a shorter duration. Instead of pulling water from the brain parenchyma, like IV delivery, IA delivery pulls water from the endothelial cells that line the BBB. This causes them to shrink, placing physical strain on the tight junctions between cells, ultimately causing them to dissociate [21]. This opens holes in the BBB, allowing molecules typically incapable of crossing the BBB to do so with high efficiency (Fig. 14.3). Over hours, the tight junctions re-form, reconstituting the intact BBB [21].

One group has developed a reliable protocol for opening the BBB using IA mannitol in mice, allowing for the study of its utility in this preclinical model [87–89]. Using real-time MRI, these authors could identify the optimal infusion rate of mannitol to disrupt the BBB in each mouse globally [87–91]. They have also developed methods for quantifying delivery efficiency in vivo using bioluminescence imaging [90], intravital microscopy [87], or by radiolabeling and using positron emission tomography (PET) scanning [92]. In doing so, they have quantitatively demonstrated that IA delivery with IA mannitol for BBBD can be used to enhance the delivery of monoclonal antibodies [87, 92], and stem cells [90] to the brain. As discussed, IA delivery with IA mannitol has also been shown to enhance the delivery of AAVs [84]. However, this study's methodology did not allow for a precise BBB opening and resulted in considerable toxicity. It would be interesting to investigate AAVs for gene therapy delivery using more advanced BBBD techniques.

Thus far, IA delivery with IA mannitol for BBBD in human patients has only been investigated for delivering antineoplastic agents for treating CNS malignancies. Although it has yet to be used for delivering gene therapies in humans, much can be inferred from the neuro-oncology literature. Osmotic disruption of the BBB was first described by a pioneering paper by Rapoport et al. in 1971 [93]. Ten years later, in 1981, Neuwelt et al. published the first paper using IA mannitol to disrupt the BBB in human patients with malignant brain tumors. Over the next two decades, few studies expanded upon this work, mainly because endovascular technology was insufficient for more widespread clinical translation [75].

Interest in IA delivery with IA mannitol resurfaced in the 1990s, and Doolittle et al. published a large multicenter study of patients receiving IA chemotherapy with IA mannitol in the year 2000 [94]. In this study, the authors performed repeated treatments (up to 2 days per week) of IA chemotherapy, mainly with BBBD with IA mannitol, in a cohort of 221 patients. The number of treatments with BBBD totaled 2204 with BBBD and 260 without. Doolittle et al. pretreated patients with an anticonvulsant to reduce the risk of seizures and atropine immediately before mannitol to reduce the risk of bradycardia [94]. Potentially treatment-related adverse events included 4/221 (1.8%) patients with intracranial herniation (possibly due to asymmetric cerebral edema from BBBD); 11/221 (5.0%) with asymptomatic intimal tears; 7/221 (3.2%) with cardiac arrhythmia (potentially related to bradycardia or atropine); 3/221 (1.4%) had strokes; and none were reported to have seizures despite this known potential side effect [94]. The 30-day morality was proportionally lower in the group receiving IA chemotherapy with BBBD compared to those without [94]. This study was not designed to compare the efficacy of IA delivery with BBBD to standard IV chemotherapy. However, it did strongly support the safety of using IA mannitol for BBBD, even 20+ years ago. Since then, several smaller studies have pub-

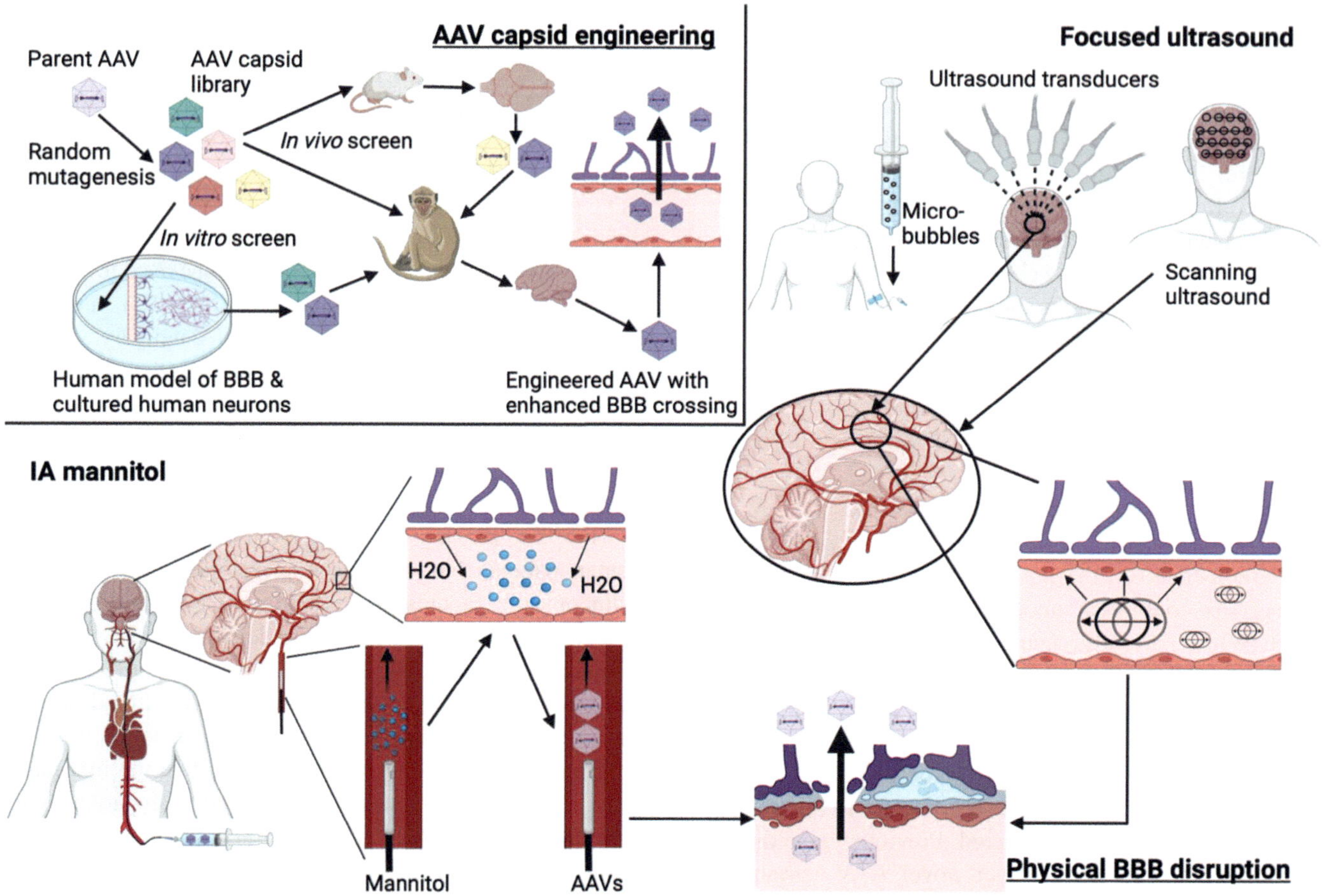

Fig. 14.3 Strategies for enhancing BBB transduction of AAVs or other gene therapies for delivery to the brain. Strategies for delivering AAVs to the brain can be divided into AAV capsid engineering and physical BBB disruption. AAV capsid engineering involves creating a vast library of AAV variants using random mutagenesis and then screening those variants in models. The delivery of viruses into the vasculature requires vectors to cross the BBB to reach the brain. This is typically performed in vivo, in mice or NHPs, but could be performed in vitro to maximize the likelihood of generating properties that work in humans. In the case of in vitro screening, a second step of in vivo screening in NHPs should be performed to ensure vector viability in a living model. Vectors are harvested from target tissues (brains of organisms or cultured neurons) and then sequenced to identify the most effective variants. Successful variants can be identified with novel properties that allow them to cross the BBB without disruption (*Created with* www.biorender.com)

lished IA delivery with IA mannitol for the delivery of chemotherapeutics and monoclonal antibodies for various neurologic malignancies [95–100]. Though complications varied between studies, all concluded that IA delivery with IA mannitol was safe overall. None of these studies compared IA with IA mannitol to standard IV therapy; thus, its effectiveness for treating CNS malignancies remains unclear.

One challenge faced by earlier studies investigating IA delivery with IA mannitol is confirming, in real-time, that the BBB was effectively disrupted. One strategy for doing this is to use an MRI with IV contrast shortly after mannitol infusion [101]. While effective, this strategy requires transporting patients to an adjacent MRI suite, which may be logistically challenging intraoperatively. Alternatively, one group demonstrated the effectiveness of direct current electroencephalogram (DC-EEG) in identifying BBB openings [100]. They found that BBB opening with IA mannitol creates a large negative-voltage deflection over the territory infused, allowing for precise identification of BBB opening in real-time in the operating room. This method could provide an effective means for confirming BBB opening and allow interventionalists to minimize the amount of mannitol used on an individual patient basis, theoretically reducing the risk of side effects.

Although the studies above support the safety of IA delivery with IA mannitol, it is certainly not without risks. Each study took significant precautions to facilitate the safest possible therapy. Potential complications of BBBD with IA mannitol include seizures, bradycardia, cerebral edema, and stroke [94, 99]. The risk of cerebral edema with IA mannitol is thought to be proportional to the volume of BBBD [99]. Of the studies investigating IA delivery with IA mannitol above, three performed super-selective delivery [96–98]. The remaining studies limited their treatment to the vascular distribution of a single large artery (internal carotid or vertebral) [94, 99, 100]. This challenge raises a critical concern with adopting IA delivery with IA mannitol for gene therapy for NDDs, where global delivery throughout the brain is desired. That said, multivessel therapy has yet to be tried; thus, it remains unclear if it will lead to harm. Additionally, as Doolittle et al. demonstrated, repeated administrations separated by time are safe and feasible [94].

Thus, one could perform three separate treatments (right carotid, left carotid, and dominant vertebral artery) over days, weeks, or months. This strategy may, however, be limited by the development of anti-AAV-neutralizing antibodies (nABs) or increasing the risk of immune-mediated toxicity with successive treatments. The following steps for investigating IA delivery with IA mannitol should include confirming its effectiveness for AAV delivery in an NHP model and developing protocols for BBBD in humans.

Focused Ultrasound

The underlying principle of FUS is the convergence of a multitude of ultrasound waves into a small volume. FUS devices can either use a single concave transducer or a phased array of smaller transducers [102]. MRI guidance is used to target a specific area within the brain. Focused ultrasound transfers its energy precisely to the target tissue where the beam converges. When ultrasound waves are released continuously, the target tissue is rapidly heated, producing a focal lesion termed high-intensity FUS. This lesioning method is approved as a minimally invasive alternative to DBS for treating essential tremors and is under clinical investigation for PD [102, 103]. FUS can also be used in a pulsatile fashion, allowing the energy to dissipate between pulses. Rather than heating tissue and producing a lesion, pulsatile FUS (pFUS) delivers repeated energy pulses to the target zone. Patients are pretreated with an IV infusion of microbubbles. The bubbles circulate throughout the body, including in arterial vasculature of the brain where pFUS is applied. The energy from the ultrasound waves causes the gas-filled microbubbles to compress and expand in a process called cavitation [104]. Stable cavitation of microbubbles induces oscillation causing them to physically collide with endothelial cells lining the BBB, which disrupts tight junctions and produces a transient opening of the BBB (Fig. 14.3) [104, 105]. Like BBBD with IA mannitol, BBB opening lasts several hours, allowing large molecules, including (but not limited to) gene therapy vectors, to pass through before tight junctions reform and the BBB is reconstituted. Because this chapter focuses exclusively on the delivery of therapeutics to the brain rather than tissue ablation, for the remainder of the section, it will be presumed that all FUS discussed is pFUS.

MRI-guided FUS (MRgFUS) has yet to be used to deliver gene therapies to the brain in humans, several studies have confirmed its safety and effectiveness for opening the BBB in small phase one clinical trials for ALS [106], PD [107–109], and AD [110]. Additionally, one group has used it to enhance the delivery of the enzyme glucocerebrosidase in patients with PD [108]. While this small study did not demonstrate any clinical benefit, it required multiple repeated treatments, unlike a glucocerebrosidase gene therapy, which would be a single dose. Yet, it is the first to our knowledge to use MRgFUS to deliver a therapeutic for the treatment of an NDD. MRgFUS has been proven safe in most studies, with no severe adverse events. However, it is noteworthy that it necessitates a stereotactic frame (which must be drilled into the scalp of patients), and most patients report headaches related to the procedure. Although this does not constitute a series risk, most patients would likely agree that minimizing recurrent procedures would be ideal.

Many studies have demonstrated that MRgFUS efficiently delivers otherwise impermeable AAVs across the BBB for gene therapy in mice and rats [74, 111–116]. Most studies use the IV route to deliver AAV with FUS. FUS allows several AAV serotypes (not just those with innate BBB crossing potential) to penetrate the BBB. However, it does not direct the AAVs to the brain; the vast majority are delivered to peripheral organs such as the liver [111, 114–116]. One interesting study compared the IV + FUS to IN + FUS and found that the IN route allowed approximately 40× greater brain transduction with the same dose [74]. This is likely a demonstration of the "first pass" effect and should apply to IA delivery. The combination of IA delivery with FUS has yet to be described (to our knowledge). Further, the anatomy of the nasal passage and brain in a mouse is situated to allow effective delivery throughout the brain with the IN route. However, in humans, IN delivery would likely result in an uneven distribution favoring anterior and inferior structures. This study suggests the value of the first pass effect when coupled with highly efficient BBB crossing, but in humans, the IA route may be superior to the IN route for achieving this effect. Another mouse study compared IV delivery of AAV9 and AAV PHP.B, each with MRgFUS [113]. They found AAV9 concentrated only in sonicated regions, while PHP.B seemingly ignored the BBBD with FUS and distributed evenly throughout the brain. This finding confirms that physical BBB opening does not benefit engineered vectors, which can already cross the BBB efficiently.

A final preclinical study highlighted in this section investigated AAV delivery with FUS in NHPs, providing several valuable insights [109]. This study treated six NHPs with MRI-guided pulsatile FUS, termed low-intensity focused ultrasound (LIFU). They first used FUS to create multiple, small volume, distinct regions of BBB opening, confirming patency of the BBB with contrast T1 MRI. Next, they delivered an AAV-PHP.eB vector containing a GFP transgene intravenously and found ~20–50× increased expression in sonicated regions compared to nonsonicated controls in the NHPs treated with small volume LIFU. They then modified their protocol to target multiple areas in the same region (the putamen), reducing the predefined spacing between lesions from 2 to 1 mm. This produced a much larger, homogenous region of BBBD—subsequent IV delivery of AAV-PHP.eB containing GFP led to a ~20–50× enhancement of GFP expression in sonicated regions in 2/3 NHPs. The third NHP, which had pre-existing anti-AAV nABs, had virtually no GFP expression with or without sonication. This finding highlights the major impediment of pre-existing nABs with AAV gene therapy delivered IV. Though it has never been tested, IA delivery may allow successful gene therapy despite nABs. AAVs would not need to travel through the systemic circulation to be exposed to nABs before reaching the target. It is noteworthy that AAV-PHP.eB does not demonstrate increased BBB transduction in NHPs. Thus, the parent AAV9 vector was used in the study. Posttreatment MRI was performed 30 days after the FUS and viral delivery. It confirmed that the BBB functions recovered, and no hemorrhages or lesions were associated with the procedure. NHPs clinically tolerated the procedure, assuring the safety of the method.

The most significant challenge faced when considering implementing FUS as a tool for enhancing the delivery of gene therapies to the brain for NDDs is its focality. Although the authors described above were able to produce a larger volume of BBB opening, this still only targeted the unilateral putamen, which would be insufficient for treating most NDDs that impact neurons globally. One potential strategy to combat this is scanning ultrasound (SUS), which a group in Australia has pioneered [117–124]. This group has developed a method where the focus of the ultrasound waves moves in a "zigzag" pattern across the brain in mice [122]. Their work suggests that this is sufficient to open the BBB globally throughout the brain. However, they do not use the typical T1 MRI with contrast to confirm the region of BBB opening, nor have they used this method combined with gene therapy vectors to demonstrate widespread enhancement of gene delivery. They have shown that this method enhances the clearance of amyloid and tau from the brain in mouse models of AD. They have also demonstrated that this method enhances brain delivery of monoclonal antibodies [120]. Overall, SUS holds great potential for enhancing the global delivery of gene therapy vectors to the brain to treat NDDs.

One potential risk associated with BBBD with FUS is an inflammatory response. However, there is mixed data to support this. Microglial and T-cell activation in mice has been reported in focal regions treated with AAV9 and FUS. However, a diffuse microglial and T-cell activation with AAV-PHP.B was also observed, which did not correspond to the sonicated region [113]. This suggests the inflammatory response was to the AAV vector rather than FUS-mediated BBBD. Two other reports in mice did not find any evidence of microglial activation [112, 115]. NHPs showed no evidence of microglial activation in sonicated regions after AAV delivery [109]. On the other hand, SUS consistently led to microglial and immune system activation throughout the brain, though no clinical deficits were noted in the mice [117, 119, 121, 123]. Unlike the broader BBB opening with SUS, the targeted BBB opening with FUS seems unlikely to lead to significant immune system activation. Still, the clinical implications of this resulting inflammation with SUS remain unclear.

FUS offers an additional tool to be considered for delivering gene therapies to the brain for NDDs. It raises several concerns that need to be addressed before it can be effectively used for gene delivery. First, with IV delivery, FUS does not minimize the amount of vectors reaching the liver and other peripheral organs. This puts the patients at risk of systemic immune-mediated toxicity and/or exposing vectors to nABs. Hazards of off-target delivery could be mitigated with IA delivery, allowing the brain to see much higher concentrations of vectors on the first pass, fully taking advantage of the open BBB. Unfortunately, the combination of these two methods has not been tried, likely because IA mannitol is a much simpler solution if the arterial circulation is to be accessed anyway. Secondly, as stated before, the lack of a global BBB opening severely limits its utility for treating NDDs. SUS is promising but is still in the early stages of the investigation; further investigation of SUS for delivering AAVs and translation to NHPs and, ultimately, humans may be valuable.

Summary, Limitations, and Recommendations

This chapter reviewed the existing body of literature, presented hypotheses, and suggested future directions for investigation for IA delivery of gene therapies for the treatment of NDDs involving the brain. Because gene therapy is far from the only therapeutic under investigation for the treatment of NDDs, especially those with complex pathogenesis, it was felt to be necessary to fully explain the rationale for its value in the first section. In short, most NDDs can be attributed to a single gene or single protein. One of the potential reasons for the failure of therapeutics for NDDs is that they do not specifically target the underlying problem in the correct location. The problem in proteinopathies is the toxic accumulation of proteins, which occurs intracellularly. Neither targeting downstream consequences of that toxic accumulation nor utilizing extracellular therapies is likely to be highly effective. Gene therapy can solve both problems, and DNA-based gene therapies should allow for life-long correction with a single treatment.

Gene therapies, however, do not yet exist in clinical practice for diseases primarily involving the brain, mainly because of the delivery challenge. Thus far, most clinical trials have used dIC or IV delivery, neither suited for global gene therapies for NDDs. More advanced delivery methods are necessary to improve gene therapy's safety and feasibility for NDDs involving the brain. IT delivery provides a potential solution to this challenge; however, IT-L delivery is likely too far from the brain to allow highly efficient gene transfer, and ICV is very invasive. ICM delivery has considerable potential, though the CSF flow dynamics may not be as well suited as the vasculature for evenly distributing vectors throughout the brain. It also carries risks of neurotoxicity, including DRG toxicity; it is not well established in clinical practice, and accessing the thecal space immediately adjacent to the medulla may not be ideal. IA delivery provides a compelling alternative to all these routes as it directs vectors to the brain, is minimally invasive, and is well established in clinical practice. Unfortunately, IA delivery of gene therapies has rarely been done, even in preclinical models. The most significant hurdle to IA gene delivery is the efficient penetration of BBB. If vectors cannot cross the BBB during their first pass through the cerebral circulation, the benefits of IA delivery will be limited and no different than IV injections.

There are three major strategies under investigation for enhancing BBB crossing of gene therapy vectors (Fig. 14.3): (1) AAV capsid engineering using directed evolution to enhance BBB transduction, (2) IA delivery with IA mannitol, and (3) FUS/SUS. All these strategies show significant promise, but none have been developed to the degree that they are ready for human translation, as summarized in Table 14.1. Future directions should focus on improving and implementing these strategies with IA delivery. Most AAV capsid engineering has been done using a mouse model for screening, but this is highly unlikely to translate to humans. While recent work has progressed to using NHPs, which is more likely to succeed, there are no guarantees. Perhaps we should step back and evolve AAVs in vitro, in human cells, before screening in NHPs. IA delivery with IA mannitol may be the most developed of the three potential solutions to the BBB as it has been widely utilized in human patients. The major limitation with this method, at this time, is that it has only been used to open the BBB in a single vascular distribution in humans, which would not allow global delivery, which is needed for treating NDDs. Further investigation should center around developing protocols for safely and globally opening the BBB in humans using this strategy. If this is not safe to do in a single pass, one may consider splitting this therapy into two or three separate instances over several days. Separating instances over weeks or months may be safer. Still, it may lead to problems with the immune system, which could significantly limit therapeutic efficacy or increase the risk of adverse effects. Finally, FUS is an effective strategy for opening the BBB. However, it is too localized in its current iteration to be useful for most NDDs. SUS may be a good alternative, but it has only been used in mice. Further validation of this strategy and translation to NHPs and humans will be necessary if this method for BBBD is to be used for gene therapy for NDDs. Additionally,

Table 14.1 Current landscape of methods for enhancing intravascular gene therapy delivery to the brain validated in preclinical models and humans

	Mouse	NHP	Human
IA + AAV no BBBD	(−)	(−)	0
IV + engineered AAV with enhanced BBBD	(++)	(+)	0
IA + engineered AAV with enhanced BBBD	(+)	0	0
IA + IA Mannitol	(++)	0	(+ Safe)
IA + IA Mannitol + AAV	(+)	0	0
IV + FUS	(++)	(+)	(+ Safe)
IV + FUS + AAV	(++)	(+)	0
IV + FUS + engineered AAV with enhanced BBBD	(−)	0	0
IV + SUS	(+)	0	0
IV + SUS + AAV	0	0	0
IA + FUS or SUS	0	0	0
IA + FUS or SUS + AAV	0	0	0

The table indicates the strength of evidence from the current body literature supporting each method. Key: (−) evidence demonstrates no benefit, (+) weak evidence in support of benefit, (++) strong evidence in support of benefit, (+ Safe) evidence in support of safety but not necessarily benefit, 0 has never been studied to our knowledge

BBBD Blood–brain barrier disruption

current strategies using FUS have mainly used the IV route and, therefore, are still plagued by very high off-target systemic delivery, risking toxicity. IA delivery with SUS may be effective; however, if IA delivery is to be performed anyway, it is far simpler to use IA mannitol to disrupt the BBB.

Conclusions

Overall, the IA delivery route has a large amount of untapped potential for providing the means to efficiently deliver gene therapies to the brain for the treatment of NDDs. This chapter provided an outline explaining the rationale for gene therapy for NDDs, the challenges associated with delivery, the current landscape of preclinical and clinical research investigating IA delivery, and high-value strategies that may be relevant to this pursuit. Though this method has significant theoretical value, it is in its early stages of investigation. Much research must validate this route and translate it to a clinical setting. We are on the cusp of breakthroughs for treating a broad range of neurologic disorders, including NDDs with gene therapies, and we must develop the tools necessary to allow safe delivery for their broad translation. The IA route *with efficient BBB crossing* may be the critical step in advancing gene therapies for NDDs, allowing for the translation of many DMTs for these disorders. Though much research remains to be done, the benefit of developing a safe and effective strategy for delivering gene therapies to the brain is hugely worthwhile. We hope that investigators will use this chapter as a guide to push this field forward so that, someday, we may live in a world where NDDs are no longer untreatable and ultimately fatal.

References

1. van Dyck C, Aisen S, Bateman R, Chen C, Gee M, Kanekiyo M, et al. Lecanemab in early Alzheimer's disease. N Engl J Med. 2023;388(1):9.
2. Sweeney P, Park H, Baumann M, Dunlop J, Frydman J, Kopito R, et al. Protein misfolding in neurodegenerative diseases: implications and strategies. Transl Neurodegener. 2017;6(1):1–13.
3. Kovacs GG. Molecular pathological classification of neurodegenerative diseases: turning towards precision medicine. Int J Mol Sci. 2016;17(2):189.
4. Kovacs GG. Molecular pathology of neurodegenerative diseases: principles and practice. J Clin Pathol. 2019;72(11):725–35.
5. Gorman AM. Neuronal cell death in neurodegenerative diseases: recurring themes around protein handling: apoptosis review series. J Cell Mol Med. 2008;12(6A):2263–80.
6. Lakhani CM, Tierney BT, Manrai AK, Yang J, Visscher PM, Patel CJ. 乳鼠心肌提取 HHS public access. Physiol Behav. 2019;176(3):139–148.
7. Pearce MM. Prion-like transmission of pathogenic protein aggregates in genetic models of neurodegenerative disease. Curr Opin Genet Dev [Internet]. 2017;44:149–155. https://doi.org/10.1016/j.gde.2017.03.011.
8. Larson MH, Gilbert LA, Wang X, Lim WA, Weissman JS, Qi LS. CRISPR interference (CRISPRi) for sequence-specific control of gene expression. Nat Protoc. 2013;8(11):2180–96.
9. Maeder ML, Gersbach CA. Genome-editing technologies for gene and cell therapy. Mol Ther. 2016;24(3):430–46.
10. Yang S, Chang R, Yang H, Zhao T, Hong Y, Kong HE. CRISPR/Cas9- mediated therapeutic effects in Huntington's disease mice. 2017.
11. Ingusci S, Verlengia G, Soukupova M, Zucchini S, Simonato M. Gene therapy tools for brain diseases. Front Pharmacol [Internet]. 2019;10:724. https://www.frontiersin.org/article/10.3389/fphar.2019.00724/full.
12. Agustín-Pavón C, Isalan M. Synthetic biology and therapeutic strategies for the degenerating brain: synthetic biology approaches can transform classical cell and gene therapies, to provide new cures for neurodegenerative diseases. Bioessays. 2014;36(10):979–90.
13. Wild EJ, Tabrizi S. Therapies targeting DNA and RNA in Huntington's disease. Lancet Neurol. 2018;16(10):837–47.
14. Filocamo M, Morrone A. Lysosomal storage disorders: molecular basis and laboratory testing. Hum Genomics. 2011;5(3):156–69.
15. Blauwendraat C, Heilbron K, Vallerga CL, Bandres-Ciga S, von Coelln R, Pihlstrøm L, et al. Parkinson's disease age at onset genome-wide association study: defining heritability, genetic loci, and α-synuclein mechanisms. Mov Disord. 2019;34:866–75.
16. Srinivasan E, Chandrasekhar G, Chandrasekar P, Anbarasu K, Vickram AS, Karunakaran R, et al. Alpha-Synuclein aggregation in Parkinson's disease. Front Med. 2021;8:736978.
17. Abraham AA, Tisdale JF. Gene therapy for sickle cell disease: moving from the bench to the bedside. Blood [Internet]. 2021;138(11):932–941. https://doi.org/10.1182/blood.2019003776.
18. June CH, Sadelain M. Chimeric antigen receptor therapy. N Engl J Med. 2018;379(1):64–73.
19. Drahansky M, Paridah M, Moradbak A, Mohamed A, Owolabi F, Taiwo AW, Asniza M, et al. Antisense oligonucleotides, a novel developing targeting therapy. Intech [Internet]. 2016;i(tourism):13. https://www.intechopen.com/books/advanced-biometric-technologies/liveness-detection-in-biometrics.
20. Yin W, Rogge M. Targeting RNA: a transformative therapeutic strategy. Clin Transl Sci. 2019;12(2):98–112.
21. Fischell JM, Fishman PS. A multifaceted approach to optimizing AAV delivery to the brain for the treatment of neurodegenerative diseases. Front Neurosci. 2021;15:747726.
22. Lufino MMP, Edser PAH, Wade-Martins R. Advances in high-capacity extrachromosomal vector technology: episomal maintenance, vector delivery, and transgene expression. Mol Ther [Internet]. 2008;16(9):1525–1538. https://doi.org/10.1038/mt.2008.156.
23. Keeler AM, Flotte TR. Recombinant adeno-associated virus gene therapy in light of Luxturna (and Zolgensma and Glybera): where are we, and how did we get here? Annu Rev Virol. 2019;6(1):601–21.
24. Hoy SM. Onasemnogene abeparvovec: first global approval. Drugs [Internet]. 2019;79(11):1255–1262. https://doi.org/10.1007/s40265-019-01162-5.
25. Hudry E, Vandenberghe LH. Therapeutic AAV gene transfer to the nervous system: a clinical reality. Neuron [Internet]. 2019;101(5):839–862. https://doi.org/10.1016/j.neuron.2019.02.017.
26. Mendell JR, Al-zaidy SA, Lehman KJ, Mccolly M, Lowes LP, Alfano LN, et al. Five-year extension results of the phase 1 START trial of onasemnogene abeparvovec in spinal muscular atrophy. JAMA Neurol. 2021;43205(7):834–41.

27. Ediriweera GR, Chen L, Yerbury JJ, Thurecht KJ, Vine KL. Non-viral vector-mediated gene therapy for ALS: challenges and future perspectives. Mol Pharm. 2021;18(6):2142–60.
28. Bey K, Deniaud J, Dubreil L, Joussemet B, Cristini J, Ciron C, et al. Intra-CSF AAV9 and AAVrh10 administration in nonhuman primates: promising routes and vectors for which neurological diseases? Mol Ther Methods Clin Dev [Internet]. 2020;17:771–784. https://doi.org/10.1016/j.omtm.2020.04.001.
29. DiMattia MA, Nam H-J, Van Vliet K, Mitchell M, Bennett A, Gurda BL, et al. Structural insight into the unique properties of adeno-associated virus serotype 9. J Virol. 2012;86(12):6947–58.
30. Lykken EA, Shyng C, Edwards RJ, Rozenberg A, Gray SJ. Recent progress and considerations for AAV gene therapies targeting the central nervous system. J Neurodev Disord. 2018;10(1):1–10.
31. Snyder BR, Gray SJ, Quach ET, Huang JW, Leung CH, Samulski RJ, et al. Comparison of adeno-associated viral vector serotypes for spinal cord and motor neuron gene delivery. Hum Gene Ther. 2011;22(9):1129–35.
32. Zincarelli C, Soltys S, Rengo G, Rabinowitz JE. Analysis of AAV serotypes 1-9 mediated gene expression and tropism in mice after systemic injection. Mol Ther. 2008;16:1073.
33. Hocquemiller M, Giersch L, Audrain M, Parker S, Cartier N. Adeno-associated virus-based gene therapy for CNS diseases. Hum Gene Ther. 2016;27(7):478–96.
34. Saraiva J, Nobre RJ, Pereira de Almeida L. Gene therapy for the CNS using AAVs: the impact of systemic delivery by AAV9. J Control Release [Internet]. 2016;241:94–109. https://doi.org/10.1016/j.jconrel.2016.09.011.
35. Büning H, Srivastava A. Capsid modifications for targeting and improving the efficacy of AAV vectors. Mol Ther Methods Clin Dev [Internet]. 2019;12:248–265. https://doi.org/10.1016/j.omtm.2019.01.008.
36. Deverman BE, Pravdo PL, Simpson BP, Kumar SR, Chan KY, Banerjee A, et al. Cre-dependent selection yields AAV variants for widespread gene transfer to the adult brain. Nat Biotechnol [Internet]. 2016;34(2):204–209. http://www.ncbi.nlm.nih.gov/pubmed/26829320, http://www.pubmedcentral.nih.gov/articlerender.fcgi?artid=PMC5088052.
37. Chan KY, Jang MJ, Yoo BB, Greenbaum A, Ravi N, Wu W-L, et al. Engineered AAVs for efficient noninvasive gene delivery to the central and peripheral nervous system. Nat Neurosci. 2017;20:1172–9.
38. Hanlon KS, Meltzer JC, Buzhdygan T, Cheng MJ, Sena-Esteves M, Bennett RE, et al. Selection of an efficient AAV vector for robust CNS transgene expression. Mol Ther Methods Clin Dev [Internet]. 2019;15:320–332. https://doi.org/10.1016/j.omtm.2019.10.007.
39. Pulicherla N, Shen S, Yadav S, Debbink K, Govindasamy L, Agbandje-Mckenna M, et al. Engineering liver-detargeted AAV9 vectors for cardiac and musculoskeletal gene transfer. Mol Ther [Internet]. 2011;19(6):1070–1078. https://doi.org/10.1038/mt.2011.22/nature06264.
40. Tanguy Y, Biferi MG, Besse A, Astord S, Cohen-Tannoudji M, Marais T, et al. Systemic AAVrh10 provides higher transgene expression than AAV9 in the brain and the spinal cord of neonatal mice. Front Mol Neurosci. 2015;8:36.
41. Lau CH, Ho JWT, Lo PK, Tin C. Targeted transgene activation in the brain tissue by systemic delivery of engineered AAV1 expressing CRISPRa. Mol Ther Nucleic Acids [Internet]. 2019;16:637–649. https://doi.org/10.1016/j.omtn.2019.04.015.
42. Flotte TR, Gessler DJ. Gene therapy for rare neurological disorders. Clin Pharmacol Ther. 2022;111(4):743–57.
43. Hordeaux J, Hinderer C, Goode T, Katz N, Buza EL, Bell P, et al. Toxicology study of intra-cisterna magna adeno-associated virus 9 expressing human alpha-L-Iduronidase in rhesus macaques. Mol Ther Methods Clin Dev [Internet]. 2018;10:79–88. https://doi.org/10.1016/j.omtm.2018.06.003.
44. Hinderer C, Katz N, Buza EL, Dyer C, Goode T, Bell P, et al. Severe toxicity in nonhuman primates and piglets following high-dose intravenous administration of an adeno-associated virus vector expressing human SMN. Hum Gene Ther [Internet]. 2018;29(3):285–298. http://www.liebertpub.com/doi/10.1089/hum.2018.015.
45. Perez BA, Shutterly A, Chan YK, Byrne BJ, Corti M. Management of neuroinflammatory responses to AAV-mediated gene therapies for neurodegenerative diseases. Brain Sci. 2020;10(2):119.
46. Samaranch L, Sebastian WS, Kells AP, Salegio EA, Heller G, Bringas JR, et al. AAV9-mediated expression of a non-self protein in nonhuman primate central nervous system triggers widespread neuroinflammation driven by antigen-presenting cell transduction. Mol Ther [Internet]. 2014;22(2):329–337. https://doi.org/10.1038/mt.2013.266.
47. Hordeaux J, Yuan Y, Clark PM, Wang Q, Martino RA, Sims JJ, et al. The GPI-linked protein LY6A drives AAV-PHP.B transport across the blood-brain barrier. Mol Ther [Internet]. 2019;27(5):912–921. https://doi.org/10.1016/j.ymthe.2019.02.013.
48. Hordeaux J, Wang Q, Katz N, Buza EL, Bell P, Wilson JM. The neurotropic properties of AAV-PHP.B are limited to C57BL/6J mice. Mol Ther. 2018;26(3):664–8.
49. Matsuzaki Y, Konno A, Mochizuki R, Shinohara Y, Nitta K, Okada Y, et al. Intravenous administration of the adeno-associated virus-PHP.B capsid fails to upregulate transduction efficiency in the marmoset brain. Neurosci Lett [Internet]. 2018;665:182–188. https://doi.org/10.1016/j.neulet.2017.11.049.
50. Chuapoco MR, Flytzanis NC, Goeden N, Octeau JC, Roxas KM, Chan KY, et al. Adeno-associated viral vectors for functional intravenous gene transfer throughout the non-human primate brain. Nat Nanotechnol. 2023;18:1241.
51. Fugate JE. Complications of neurosurgery. Continuum (Minneap Minn). 2015;21(5):1425–44.
52. Morabito G, Giannelli SG, Ordazzo G, Bido S, Castoldi V, Indrigo M, et al. AAV-PHP.B-mediated global-scale expression in the mouse nervous system enables GBA1 gene therapy for wide protection from synucleinopathy. Mol Ther [Internet]. 2017;25(12):2727–2742. https://doi.org/10.1016/j.ymthe.2017.08.004.
53. Lim JA, Yi H, Gao F, Raben N, Kishnani PS, Sun B. Intravenous injection of an AAV-PHP.B vector encoding human acid α-glucosidase rescues both muscle and CNS defects in murine Pompe disease. Mol Ther Methods Clin Dev [Internet]. 2019;12:233–245. https://doi.org/10.1016/j.omtm.2019.01.006.
54. Liguore WA, Domire JS, Button D, Wang Y, Dufour BD, Srinivasan S, et al. AAV-PHP.B administration results in a differential pattern of CNS biodistribution in non-human primates compared with mice. Mol Ther [Internet]. 2019;27(11):2018–2037. https://doi.org/10.1016/j.ymthe.2019.07.017.
55. Yoon SY, Hunter JE, Chawla S, Clarke DL, Molony C, O'Donnell PA, et al. Global CNS correction in a large brain model of human alpha-mannosidosis by intravascular gene therapy. Brain. 2020;143(7):2058–72.
56. High-dose AAV gene therapy deaths. Nat Biotechnol. 2020;38:910.
57. Fowler M, Cotter J, Knight BE, Sevick-muraca EM, Sandberg DI, Sirianni RW. Intrathecal drug delivery in the era of nanomedicine. Adv Drug Deliv Rev. 2020;165–166:77–95.
58. Ohno K, Samaranch L, Hadaczek P, Bringas JR, Allen PC, Sudhakar V, et al. Kinetics and MR-based monitoring of AAV9 vector delivery into cerebrospinal fluid of nonhuman primates. Mol Ther Methods Clin Dev. 2019;13:47.
59. Hinderer C, Bell P, Katz N, Vite CH, Louboutin JP, Bote E, et al. Evaluation of intrathecal routes of administration for adeno-associated viral vectors in large animals. Hum Gene Ther. 2018;29(1):15–24.

60. Bucher T, Dubreil L, Colle MA, Maquigneau M, Deniaud J, Ledevin M, et al. Intracisternal delivery of AAV9 results in oligodendrocyte and motor neuron transduction in the whole central nervous system of cats. Gene Ther. 2014;21(5):522–8.
61. Bey K, Ciron C, Dubreil L, Deniaud J, Ledevin M, Cristini J, et al. Efficient CNS targeting in adult mice by intrathecal infusion of single-stranded AAV9-GFP for gene therapy of neurological disorders. Gene Ther. 2017;24(5):325–32.
62. Rosenberg JB, Kaplitt MG, De BP, Chen A, Flagiello T, Salami C, et al. AAVrh.10-mediated APOE2 central nervous system gene therapy for APOE4-associated Alzheimer's disease. Hum Gene Ther Clin Dev. 2018;29(1):24–47.
63. Matsuzaki Y, Konno A, Mukai R, Honda F, Hirato M, Yoshimoto Y, et al. Transduction profile of the marmoset central nervous system using adeno-associated virus serotype 9 vectors. Mol Neurobiol. 2017;54(3):1745–58.
64. Kondratov O, Kondratova L, Mandel RJ, Coleman K, Savage MA, Gray-Edwards HL, et al. A comprehensive study of a 29-capsid AAV library in a non-human primate central nervous system. Mol Ther [Internet]. 2021;29(9):2806–2820. https://doi.org/10.1016/j.ymthe.2021.07.010.
65. Chatterjee D, Marmion DJ, McBride JL, Manfredsson FP, Butler D, Messer A, et al. Enhanced CNS transduction from AAV.PHP.eB infusion into the cisterna magna of older adult rats compared to AAV9. Gene Ther [Internet]. 2022;29:390. https://doi.org/10.1038/s41434-021-00244-y.
66. Chatterjee D, Marmion DJ, McBride JL, Manfredsson FP, Butler D, Messer A, et al. Enhanced CNS transduction from AAV.PHP.eB infusion into the cisterna magna of older adult rats compared to AAV9. Gene Ther. 2022;29(6):390–7.
67. Kurokawa Y, Osaka H, Kouga T, Jimbo E, Muramatsu K, Nakamura S, et al. Gene therapy in a mouse model of Niemann-pick disease type C1. Hum Gene Ther. 2021;32(11–12):589–98.
68. Taghian T, Marosfoi MG, Puri AS, Cataltepe OI, King RM, Diffie EB, et al. A safe and reliable technique for CNS delivery of AAV vectors in the cisterna magna. Mol Ther. 2020;28(2):411–21.
69. Johanson CE, Duncan JA, Stopa EG, Baird A. Enhanced prospects for drug delivery and brain targeting by the choroid plexus-CSF route. Pharm Res. 2005;22(7):1011–37.
70. Belur LR, Romero M, Lee J, Podetz-Pedersen KM, Nan Z, Riedl MS, et al. Comparative effectiveness of intracerebroventricular, intrathecal, and intranasal routes of AAV9 vector administration for genetic therapy of neurologic disease in murine mucopolysaccharidosis type I. Front Mol Neurosci. 2021;14:618360.
71. Meyer K, Ferraiuolo L, Schmelzer L, Braun L, McGovern V, Likhite S, et al. Improving single injection CSF delivery of AAV9-mediated gene therapy for SMA: a dose-response study in mice and nonhuman primates. Mol Ther. 2015;23(3):477–87.
72. Shababi M, Villalón E, Kaifer KA, DeMarco V, Lorson CL. A direct comparison of IV and ICV delivery methods for gene replacement therapy in a mouse model of SMARD1. Mol Ther Methods Clin Dev [Internet]. 2018;10:348–360. https://doi.org/10.1016/j.omtm.2018.08.005.
73. Dhas N, Mehta T, Sharma S, Garkal A, Yadav D, Hariharan K. Intranasal gene therapy for the treatment of neurological disorders [Internet]. In: Direct nose-to-brain drug delivery. Elsevier; 2021. 351–387 p. https://doi.org/10.1016/B978-0-12-822522-6.00017-5.
74. Ye D, Yuan J, Yang Y, Yue Y, Hu Z, Fadera S, et al. Incisionless targeted adeno-associated viral vector delivery to the brain by focused ultrasound-mediated intranasal administration. EBioMedicine [Internet]. 2022;84:104277. https://doi.org/10.1016/j.ebiom.2022.104277.
75. Amico RSD, Khatri D, Reichman N, Patel NV, Wong T, Fralin SR, et al. Super selective intra-arterial cerebral infusion of modern chemotherapeutics after blood—brain barrier disruption: where are we now, and where we are going. J Neurooncol [Internet]. 2020;147(2):261–278. https://doi.org/10.1007/s11060-020-03435-6.
76. Jankovic J. Parkinson's disease: clinical features and diagnosis. J Neurol Neurosurg Psychiatry. 2008;79(4):368–76.
77. Patel NV, Wong T, Fralin SR, Li M, Mckeown A, Gruber D. Repeated superselective intraarterial bevacizumab after blood brain barrier disruption for newly diagnosed glioblastoma: a phase I/II clinical trial. J Neurooncol [Internet]. 2021;155:117. https://doi.org/10.1007/s11060-021-03851-2.
78. Joshi S, Ellis JA, Ornstein E, Bruce JN. Intraarterial drug delivery for glioblastoma mutiforme: will the phoenix rise again? J Neurooncol. 2015;124(3):333–43.
79. Burkhard J-K, Riina H, Shin BJ, Christos P, Kesavabhotla K, Hofstetter CP, et al. Intra-arterial delivery of bevacizumab after blood-brain barrier disruption for the treatment of recurrent glioblastoma: progression-free survival and overall survival. Word Neurosurg. 2012;71(2):233–6.
80. Rechberger JS, Brown CA, Thiele F, Power EA, David J. Superselective intra-arterial cerebral infusion to improve brain tumor drug delivery. Ther Deliv. 2022;13:1–4.
81. Spiliopoulos S, Festas G, Reppas L, Brountzos E. Intra-arterial administration of cell-based biological agents for ischemic stroke therapy [Internet]. vol. 19, Expert opinion on biological therapy. Taylor & Francis; 2019. 249–259 p. https://doi.org/10.1080/14712598.2019.1566454.
82. Link TW, Santillan A, Patsalides A. Intra-arterial neuroprotective therapy as an adjunct to endovascular intervention in acute ischemic stroke: a review of the literature and future directions. Interv Neuroradiol. 2020;26(4):405–15.
83. Davis MC, Deveikis JP, Harrigan MR. Clinical presentation, imaging, and management of complications due to neurointerventional procedures. Semin Intervent Radiol. 2015;32(2):98–107.
84. Foley CP, Rubin DG, Santillan A, Sondhi D, Dyke JP, Crystal RG, et al. Intra-arterial delivery of AAV vectors to the mouse brain after mannitol mediated blood brain barrier disruption. PLoS One. 2014;32(7):736–40.
85. Janson CG, Romanova LG, Leone P, Nan Z, Belur L, Scott McIvor R, et al. Comparison of endovascular and intraventricular gene therapy with adeno-associated virus-α-L-iduronidase for hurler disease. Neurosurgery [Internet]. 2014;74(1):99–111. https://doi.org/10.1038/s41598-021-85820-3.
86. Koenig MA. Cerebral edema and elevated intracranial pressure. Continuum (Minneap Minn). 2018;24(6):1588–602.
87. Chu C, Jablonska A, Lesniak WG, Thomas AM, Lan X, Linville RM, et al. Optimization of osmotic blood-brain barrier opening to enable intravital microscopy studies on drug delivery in mouse cortex. J Control Release [Internet]. 2020;317:312–321. https://doi.org/10.1016/j.jconrel.2019.11.019.
88. Chu C, Liu G, Janowski M, Bulte JWM, Li S, Pearl M, et al. Real-time MRI guidance for reproducible hyperosmolar opening of the blood-brain barrier in mice. Front Neurol. 2018;9:921.
89. Chu C, Jablonska A, Gao Y, Lan X, Lesniak WG, Liu G, et al. Hyperosmolar blood–brain barrier opening using intra-arterial injection of hyperosmotic mannitol in mice under real-time MRI guidance. Nat Protoc. 2023;17(1):76–94.
90. Walczak P, Wojtkiewicz J, Nowakowski A, Habich A, Holak P, Xu J, et al. Real-time MRI for precise and predictable intra-arterial stem cell delivery to the central nervous system. J Cereb Blood Flow Metab. 2017;37(7):2346–58.
91. Janowski M, Walczak P, Pearl MS. Predicting and optimizing the territory of blood-brain barrier opening by superselective intra-arterial cerebral infusion under dynamic susceptibility contrast MRI guidance. J Cereb Blood Flow Metab. 2016;36(3):569–75.
92. Lesniak WG, Chu C, Jablonska A, Du Y, Pomper MG, Walczak P, et al. A distinct advantage to intraarterial delivery of 89Zr-bevacizumab in PET imaging of mice with and with-

out osmotic opening of the blood–brain barrier. J Nucl Med. 2019;60(5):617–22.
93. Rapoport SI, Hori M, Klatzo I. Reversible osmotic opening of the blood-brain barrier. Science. 1971;173(4001):1026–8.
94. Doolittle ND, Miner ME, Hall WA, Siegal T, Hanson EJ, Osztie E, et al. Safety and efficacy of a multicenter study using intraarterial chemotherapy in conjunction with osmotic opening of the blood-brain barrier for the treatment of patients with malignant brain tumors. Cancer. 2000;88(3):637–47.
95. Hall WA, Doolittle ND, Daman M, Bruns PK, Muldoon L, Fortin D, et al. Osmotic blood–brain barrier disruption chemotherapy for diffuse pontine gliomas. J Neurooncol. 2006;77:279–84.
96. Boockvar JA, Hofstetter AJTCP, Kovanlikaya II, Fralin S, Kesavabhotla K, Seedial SM, et al. Safety and maximum tolerated dose of superselective intraarterial cerebral infusion of bevacizumab after osmotic blood-brain barrier disruption for recurrent malignant glioma. J Neurosurg [Internet]. 2011;114(3):624–632. https://www.ncbi.nlm.nih.gov/pmc/articles/PMC3624763/pdf/nihms412728.pdf.
97. Burkhardt J-K, Riina H, Shin BJ, Christos P, Kesavabhotla K, Hofstetter CP, et al. Intra-arterial delivery of bevacizumab after blood-brain barrier disruption for the treatment of recurrent glioblastoma: progression-free survival and overall survival. World Neurosurg. 2012;77(1):130–4.
98. Chakraborty S, Filippi CG, Wong T, Demopoulos A, Mccrea HJ, Bodhinayake I. Superselective intraarterial cerebral infusion of cetuximab after osmotic blood / brain barrier disruption for recurrent malignant glioma: phase I study. J Neurooncol. 2016;128(3):405–15.
99. Morin C, Vanderweyen D. Management of primary central nervous system lymphoma using intra-arterial chemotherapy with osmotic blood-brain barrier disruption: retrospective analysis of the Sherbrooke cohort. Front Oncol. 2021;10:543648.
100. Kiviniemi V, Korhonen V, Kortelainen J, Rytky S, Siniluoto T. Real-time monitoring of human blood-brain barrier disruption. PLoS One. 2017;12(3):1–16.
101. Zawadzki M, Walecki J, Kostkiewicz B, Kostyra K, Pearl MS, Solaiyappan M, et al. Real-time MRI guidance for intra-arterial drug delivery in a patient with a brain tumor: technical note. BMJ Case Rep. 2019;12(1):10–3.
102. Fishman PS, Frenkel V. Treatment of movement disorders with focused ultrasound. J Cent Nerv Syst Dis [Internet]. 2017;9:1179573517705670. http://www.ncbi.nlm.nih.gov/pubmed/28615985, http://www.pubmedcentral.nih.gov/articlerender.fcgi?artid=PMC5462491.
103. Fishman PS, Frenkel V. Focused ultrasound: an emerging therapeutic modality for neurologic disease. Neurotherapeutics. 2017;14(2):393–404.
104. Fan CH, Lin CY, Liu HL, Yeh CK. Ultrasound targeted CNS gene delivery for Parkinson's disease treatment. J Control Release [Internet]. 2017;261:246–262. https://doi.org/10.1016/j.jconrel.2017.07.004.
105. Fishman PS, Fischell JM. Focused ultrasound mediated opening of the blood-brain barrier for neurodegenerative diseases. Front Neurol. 2021;12:749047.
106. Wijesooriya et al.pdf.
107. Gasca-Salas C, Fernández-Rodríguez B, Pineda-Pardo JA, Rodríguez-Rojas R, Obeso I, Hernández-Fernández F, et al. Blood-brain barrier opening with focused ultrasound in Parkinson's disease dementia. Nat Commun [Internet]. 2021;12(1):1–7. https://doi.org/10.1038/s41467-021-21022-9.
108. Meng Y, Pople CB, Huang Y, Jones RM, Ottoy J, Goubran M, et al. Putaminal recombinant glucocerebrosidase delivery with magnetic resonance—guided focused ultrasound in Parkinson's disease: a phase I study methods. Mov Disord. 2022;37(10):2134–44.
109. Blesa J, Pineda-pardo JA, Inoue K, Gasca-salas C, Balzano T, Del Rey NLG, et al. BBB opening with focused ultrasound in nonhuman primates and Parkinson's disease patients: targeted AAV vector delivery and PET imaging. Sci Adv. 2023;9:eadf4888.
110. Mehta RI, Carpenter JS, Mehta RI, Haut MW, Ranjan M, Najib U, et al. Blood-brain barrier opening with MRI-guided focused ultrasound elicits meningeal venous permeability in humans with early Alzheimer disease. Radiology. 2021;298(3):654.
111. Wang S, Olumolade OO, Sun T, Samiotaki G, Konofagou EE. Noninvasive, neuron-specific gene therapy can be facilitated by focused ultrasound and recombinant adeno-associated virus. Gene Ther [Internet]. 2015;22(1):104–110. https://doi.org/10.1038/gt.2014.91.
112. Xhima K, Nabbouh F, Hynynen K, Aubert I, Tandon A. Noninvasive delivery of an α-synuclein gene silencing vector with magnetic resonance–guided focused ultrasound. Mov Disord. 2018;33(10):1567–79.
113. Kofoed RH, Heinen S, Silburt J, Dubey S, Dibia CL, Maes M, et al. Transgene distribution and immune response after ultrasound delivery of rAAV9 and PHP.B to the brain in a mouse model of amyloidosis. Mol Ther Methods Clin Dev [Internet]. 2021;23:390–405. 10.1016/j.omtm.2021.10.001.
114. Alonso A, Reinz E, Leuchs B, Kleinschmidt J, Fatar M, Geers B, et al. Focal delivery of AAV2/1-transgenes into the rat brain by localized ultrasound-induced BBB opening. Mol Ther Nucleic Acids. 2013;2:e73.
115. Stavarache MA, Petersen N, Jurgens EM, Milstein ER, Rosenfeld ZB, Ballon DJ, et al. Safe and stable noninvasive focal gene delivery to the mammalian brain following focused ultrasound. J Neurosurg. 2019;130(3):989–98.
116. Hahn R, Lilian C, Noseworthy K, Xhima K, Vacaresse N, Hynynen K, et al. Efficacy of gene delivery to the brain using AAV and ultrasound depends on serotypes and brain areas. J Control Release [Internet]. 2022;351:667–680. https://doi.org/10.1016/j.jconrel.2022.09.048.
117. Leinenga G, Götz J. Scanning ultrasound removes amyloid- b and restores memory in an Alzheimer's disease mouse model. Sci Transl Med. 2015;7(278):1–12.
118. Nisbet RM, Van Der Jeugd A, Leinenga G, Evans HT, Janowicz PW, Götz J. Combined effects of scanning ultrasound and a tau-specific single chain antibody in a tau transgenic mouse model. Brain. 2017;140(5):1220–30.
119. Leinenga G, Götz J. Safety and efficacy of scanning ultrasound treatment of aged APP23 mice. Front Neurosci. 2018;12:55.
120. Kofoed RH, Noseworthy K, Wu K, Sivadas S, Stanek L, Elmer B, et al. The engineered AAV2-HBKO promotes non-invasive gene delivery to large brain regions beyond ultrasound targeted sites. Mol Ther Methods Clin Dev [Internet]. 2019;27:167–184. https://doi.org/10.1016/j.omtm.2022.09.011.
121. Leinenga G, Koh WK, Götz J. A comparative study of the effects of Aducanumab and scanning ultrasound on amyloid plaques and behavior in the APP23 mouse model of Alzheimer disease. Alzheimers Res Ther. 2021;4:1–14.
122. Götz J, Richter-stretton G, Cruz E. Therapeutic ultrasound as a treatment modality for physiological and pathological ageing including Alzheimer's disease. Pharmaceutics. 2021;13:1002.
123. Nisbet RM, Bajracharya R, Cruz E, Jürgen G. Ultrasound-mediated delivery of novel tau-specific monoclonal antibody enhances brain uptake but not therapeutic efficacy. J Control Release. 2022;349:634–48.
124. Batts AJ, Ji R, Noel RL, Kline-Schoder AR, Bae S, Kwon N, et al. Using a novel rapid alternating steering angles pulse sequence to evaluate the impact of theranostic ultrasound-mediated ultra-short pulse length on blood-brain barrier opening volume and closure, cavitation mapping, drug delivery feasibility, and safety. Theranostics. 2023;13(3):1180.

15 Intra-arterial Delivery of Stem Cells: Their Role in Stroke Treatment

Alexander Ramos and Shailendra Joshi

Stem cell research can revolutionize medicine, more than anything since antibiotics.

Ronald Reagan (1911–2004), American President

Introduction

The potential application of stem cells for treating brain diseases offers hope for treating ailments that have hitherto been considered incurable. The neural tissue cannot generally regenerate in postnatal life. Stem cell therapy is, therefore, uniquely relevant to treating neurological diseases. Significant strides have been made in the last decade in understanding stem cells' biology and tapping their therapeutic potential. Recent advances in genetic engineering have the potential to enhance stem cell technology in the future. However, effective delivery of stem cells remains a significant hurdle. In most cases, for stem cell treatment to be effective, it requires delivering a sufficient number of viable cells to the therapeutic niche where they can integrate and function effectively. Although, some benefits of stem cells can be obtained from nonviable cells, and the supernatant of stem cell cultures, the secretome. When delivered intravenously, 95% of mesenchymal stem cells are trapped in the lungs, and only <5% reach the target tissues [1]. The challenge in CNS stem cell delivery is compounded by the presence of the blood–brain barrier. Stem cell delivery to nervous tissue can be achieved by direct intraparenchymal injections, intranasal injections, intrathecal injections, or arterial injections. For maximum therapeutic benefit, targeted delivery of stem cells to the therapeutic niche with minimal exposure to other tissues is necessary. Delivery to nontarget tissues could result in inflammatory and immune responses such as, in the lungs.

Effective locoregional delivery is imperative for the success of stem cell treatment. Of the four possible methods of locoregional delivery to the brain mentioned above, arterial drug delivery offers the greatest site flexibility, tissue reach, speed of intervention, and ease of repeat dosing. Entrapment rates with arterial delivery can be further improved with stem cell selection, the inclusion of adhesion molecules, and MRI-assisted image guided delivery [1, 2]. Arterial delivery of stem cells is highly relevant to stroke treatment where the catheter for delivery might be in place during reperfusion after endovascular interventions. This chapter introduces stem cells, the role of arterial delivery and the potential and challenges in intraarterial stem cell delivery for neurological diseases and stroke treatments.

A. Ramos
Columbia University, New York, NY, USA

S. Joshi (✉)
Department of Anesthesiology, Columbia University Irving Medical Center, New York, NY, USA
e-mail: sj121@cumc.columbia.edu

S. Joshi (ed.), *Arterial Treatment of Neurological Diseases*, https://doi.org/10.1007/978-3-031-80173-0_15

Stem Cell Basics

Stem Cell Terminology

Before discussing stem cells, it is imperative to introduce some of the key terms frequently used in the field.

- Stem cells have two basic properties: unlimited "self-renewing" and "differentiating capabilities." The third property is less recognized as "functional reconstitution" [3].
  - Self-renewing: The ability to generate daughter cells identical to the initiator cell.
  - Differentiating capabilities: Commitment to a cell lineage or a terminal transition to a specific phenotype with morphological and functional characteristics.
  - Functional reconstitution: Ability to function as the native tissue.
- Potency is the capacity to differentiate into other cell types [4].
- Plasticity refers to the ability to differentiate adult cells and assume new phenotypic identities [5].
- Embryonic stem cells: These are obtained from the inner cell mass of the blastocyst, typically a 3- to 5-day-old embryo, and can develop into any cell type. They can be embryonic (from the three germ layers) or extraembryonic (from the placenta and supporting structures) [6].
- Totipotent: These cells can develop into any of the three primary germ layers and extra-embryonic layers [7].
- There are multitudes of embryonic stem cells. They can be pluripotent (multilineage: all adult cell types) or multipotent: At least two cell types from the single lineage (adult cell types, e.g., bone marrow that gives rise to various blood cells) (Fig. 15.1).
- Gastrulation is the process of transforming the zygote into a recognizable outline of an organism [8, 9]. This results in the formation of the three germ layers: endodermal, which includes "many" internal organs; mesodermal, which includes muscle and blood cells; and ectodermal, which includes skin and neurons. Some investigators consider the neural crest cells to be the fourth germ layer [10].
- Progenitor cells: These are similar to embryonic stem cells in that they are self-renewing and can differentiate. However, they are more lineage-restricted than the parent cell with less capacity to proliferate compared to stem cells; for example, neural progenitor cells are derived from embryonic stem cells and can self-renew, but they only generate neural lineage cells.

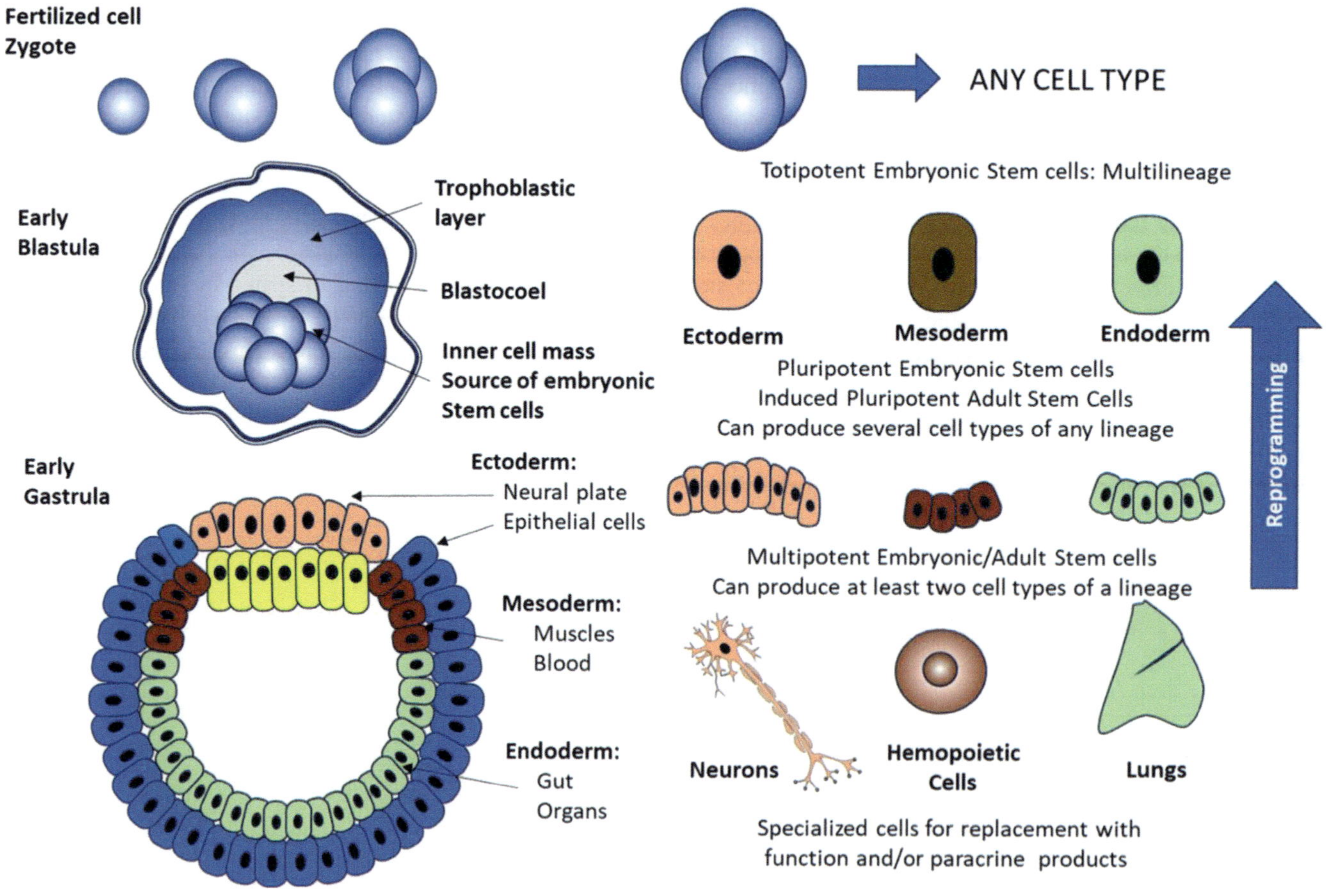

Fig. 15.1 The early development of the embryo and the types of stem cells

- Stemness is the capacity of the cell to self-renew and differentiate into other cell types to replace healthy cells but could also lead to malignancy [11].
- Niche is he anatomical and functional environment of the stem cell.
- Stem cells are found in many organs in adults, such as:
  - Bone marrow: mesenchymal and hematopoietic stem cells
  - Dental pulp
  - Heart and liver
  - Skin
  - Brain: subventricular zone of lateral ventricle and subgranular zone of the hippocampus

Sources of Stem Cells

- Embryonic stem cells can be obtained at the blastocyst stage of embryo development from the inner cell mass totipotent cells (Fig. 15.1).
- Human pluripotent stem cells (hPSC) can be obtained from bone marrow, umbilical cord stroma, cord blood, adipose tissue, and several other organs.
- Progenitor neural stem cells are found in the brain, spinal cord, and the hypothalamus.
- Induced Pluripotent stem cells are prepared by reprogramming and transforming adult cells.
- Stem cells can be autografts (from self as a source), allografts (from the same species), or xenografts (from another species).
- Sources of stem cells which are clinically accessible, include bone marrow, umbilical cord blood, adipose tissue, and dental pulp.

Characteristics of Stem Cells

Table 15.1 summarizes and extends on the major types of stem cells and their sources, surface markers, and advantages and disadvantages, as reviewed by Harting [3].

Table 15.1 Stem cell features relevant for arterial delivery applications of stem cells

Cell type	Characteristic	Source	Advantage	Disadvantage
Adult stem cells: Bone marrow-derived				
Mesenchymal stromal cells (MSCs) [12, 13]	Plastic adherence Surface markers include CD 73, CD105, CD90, CD11b, CD34, CD45 lack CD13, 31 and SSEA-1 MHC I (+) II (−)	Bone marrow, blood, adipose tissue, umbilical cord, spleen	Easy to harvest Immune privileged, Less ethical controversy	Tumorigenesis possible; weak potency, larger cell sizes, greater risk of embolic complications
Multipotent adult progenitor cells (MAPCs) [14]	Plastic adherence. Surface markers CD 13, 31, SSEA-1 Lack MHC I and II, CD 3, 11b, 19, 34, 44	Bone marrow, muscle, and brain	Greater potency: In-vitro diversify in any of the three germ layer cells	Difficult harvesting, cultured
Hematopoietic stem cells (HSCs): Pluripotent hematopoietic stem cells, long- and short-term reconstituting cells (LTRC and STRC) [15]	Surface markers: CD34 and CD90 positive while Lin, CD38 and CD45 negative	Bone marrow Umbilical cord blood, mobilized peripheral blood, fetal liver	Most investigated cells. They can differentiate to myeloid and lymphoid blood cells	Enlarged HSCs may loose potency
Mononuclear cells: Mixture of MSCs, HSCs, and nonstem/progenitor cells [16, 17]	Variable immunotype; Surface marker increase with age: CD11a, CD11b, CD43, and CD45 in rodents	Bone marrow	Rapidly harvested and processed from bone marrow in adequate numbers for self-treatment	Inconsistent results, embolization risk with arterial delivery
Nervous system-derived cell population				
Neural progenitor cell (NPCs) [18, 19]	Surface marker: CD133 Nestin, SOX2, others	Although found in adults are derived from embryonic stem cells	Develop into diverse neural cells, including functional neurons	Harvesting from adults can limit use. Must derive and expand from ESCs
Human ESC-derived NPCs [20]	Express ESC markers such as OCT4, TRA 1–81, SOX 2, and NANOG	Human-derived embryonic stem cells. Conversion from somatic cells possible.	Readily differentiate into dopaminergic neurons and astrocytes	Ethical issues with embryonic research.
Neural crest stem cells [21]	Positive for CD9 and CD29, P75 receptor	Neural tube, sciatic nerve, and intestine	Multipotent cells differentiate into several subtypes	Embryonic harvest limits use but can be derived from adult cells.

(continued)

Table 15.1 (continued)

Cell type	Characteristic	Source	Advantage	Disadvantage
Other niche-derived stem cells				
Umbilical cord blood and umbilical cord matrix stroma stem/progenitor cells [22]	Exceedingly heterogeneous cells, CD34 expressed in 1–3% cells	1 mL of cord blood contains: 8000 erythroid progenitor cells; 12,000–24,000 myeloid progenitor cells; 1000–10,000 multipotent progenitor cells		Carry autologous disease or premalignant condition; longer graft time that BMSC
Embryonic stem cells (ESC) [23]	Stage-specific embryonic antigen (SSEA) 3 and 4, TRA-1-60 and 81, and Alkaline phosphatase positive	Blastocyst stage of the zygote	Stable developmental potential. Differentiate into several cell types	Ethical issues with embryonic research. Ectopic tissue development: ESCs have malignant potential
Induced pluripotent stem cells (iPSC)				
iPSC [24]	TRA-1-60, TRA-1-81, SSEA-4	Variety of adult cells of humans and rodents when introduced to transcription factors	Personalized source, Differentiate into several cell types, Gene edited	Potential oncogenesis

Stem Cells Relevant for Neurological Applications

Embryonic Stem Cells (ESCs)

ESCs can proliferate indefinitely while retaining their potency to develop into any of the three embryonic germ layers. Due to their ability to proliferate, they pose a risk of tumorigenesis. These totipotent cells are derived from the inner cell mass of the early mammalian embryos. Being derived from embryos, their use raises ethical concerns if used for clinical research. For most clinical uses, the ESCs are transformed into specified precursor cells. ESCs have been used to treat Parkinson's disease in experimental animals, including primates. They are effective in models of Amyotrophic lateral sclerosis and multiple sclerosis. Due to ethical concerns, ESCs have been largely replaced by induced pluripotent stem cells, iPSCs.

Induced Pluripotent Stem Cells (iPSCs)

Ethical concerns raised by embryonic stem cells can be circumvented by reprogramming adult somatic cells to divide and differentiate like ESCs. This transformation is achieved by introduction of four transcription factors: octamer binding transcription factor 4 (OCT4), myelocytomatosis (MYC), Kruppel-like factor-4 (KLF4), and SRY-related high mobility BOX protein (SOX-2). There are several applications of iPSCs for providing cell models for various neurological diseases, from Fragile X and Down syndrome to Parkinson's and Alzheimer's diseases. By injecting human iPSCs in mice, a human-mouse chimera can be developed with human neurons and glial cells in the mouse brain. Induced progenitor stem cells can also provide 2-D and 3-D organ models to investigate drug delivery and pharmacological applications. Brain organoids have been developed to better understand development and disease. The challenges in using iPSCs in clinical trials include variability in reprogramming, manufacturing, quality control, and potential for malignant transformation. Some of these challenges may be overcome by delivery of the secretome alone [25]. Studies that have used these cells for better understanding Parkinson's Disease, Huntington's Disease, amyotrophic lateral sclerosis (ALS), and spinal muscular atrophy, underscore their potential in neurological research and clinical applications [26].

Mesenchymal Stem Cells (MSCs)

MSCs occur in many adult tissues and the umbilical cord blood and stroma (Worton's jelly) [22]. These cells characteristically adhere to plastic surfaces. They are large, 5–50 μm in size. MSCs are easy to isolate and process. These cells are found in the bone marrow, umbilical cord/ umbilical cord blood, placenta, amniotic fluid, adipose tissue, dental tissue, salivary gland, synovial fluid, and menstrual blood. Bone marrow, umbilical cord, and adipose tissue are the MSC sources in clinical and experimental settings. The umbilical cord cells have more differentiation potential than the bone marrow or adipose tissue MSCs. MCSs lack HLA-II and are generally immunologically inert. Their abundant availability in various tissues makes their harvesting convenient. Extensive clinical research has been undertaken with the MSCs, and their safety profile is reasonably well established. However, there are still some immunological concerns with these cells [27].

MSCs can replace cells, suppress the inflammatory response, are neuroprotective and antiapoptotic, and promote angiogenesis. They can also serve as therapeutic carriers for drug microcapsules and oncolytic viruses. MSC exosomes may be able to penetrate the BBB.

The safety of MSCs has been demonstrated in several Alzheimer's disease clinical trials. Brody et al. showed improvement in a small phase I trial, which showed lesser cognitive decline and improved inflammatory biomarkers and hippocampal volume with low-dose intravenous MSC treatment [28]. In Parkinson's disease, MSCs can replenish lost cells or provide trophic factors to improve cell health. MSC exomes are also being used to deliver neuroprotective agents. When incubated with the MSC secretome, neural stem cells show better engraftment and differentiation. MSC treatment shows clinical improvement in Parkinson's disease patients. In multiple sclerosis, an inflammatory disease, immunomodulation by MSCs is beneficial. While animal models show the benefits of MSC treatment, clinical trials have arrived at conflicting results with BM-MSCs. Although delivering stem cells in the carcinogenic environment of glioblastoma multiforme seems counterintuitive, the tumor tropism of MSCs has been exploited to deliver conditionally activated oncolytic viruses to tumor cells in Phase I and II clinical trials. The rationale for the use of stem cells in ischemic stroke is that multiple injury pathways related to ischemia, inflammation, apoptosis, angiogenesis, immune response, and neural plasticity determine the outcome, all of which can be altered by stem cells. Animal models reveal that pathological parameters and functional outcomes are improved with MSC treatment. Clinical trials reveal improvements in motor function and infarct dimensions after BM-MSC treatment, but the results are inconsistent. Other MSC clinical trials have shown the safety of the techniques with intravenous delivery, but clinical improvement is inconsistent [27].

Neural Stem Cells (NSC) and Neural Progenitor Cells (NPCs)

NSCs can develop into any cell type in the brain, while NPCs have a more limited differentiation capability. NPCs are derived from embryonic stem cells. Unlike embryonic stem cells, these cells are committed to developing neural tissue such as neurons, astrocytes, or oligodendrocytes. These cells are found in fetal and postnatal life in specific locations in the mammalian brain, such as the subgranular zone of the dentate gyrus and the subventricular zone surrounding the lateral ventricles. While well-characterized in animal models, the relevance of these adult populations in humans remains controversial. The other locations of NPCs in adults include radial glial cells in the cerebellum (Bergmann's glia), retina (Muller's glia), and spinal cord. iPSCs can also be a source of NPCs. The NPCs, when directly injected into the target site, improve functional outcomes in stroke models. The benefits are due to the integration in host tissue and the release of paracrine mediators. NPCs are also derived from human embryonic stem cells and can be transformed into dopaminergic neurons and astrocytes [29].

Bone Marrow Mononuclear Cells (BM-MNCs)

BM-MNCs are cells in the bone marrow with rounded or nonlobulated nuclei lacking cytoplasmic granules with characteristic stem cell properties. These include primitive multipotent stem cells, MSCs, small embryonic-like stem cells, multipotent adult progenitor cells, endothelial progenitor cells, tissue-committed stem cells, and hemangioblasts [17]. These cells are released from the marrow during stress and can be engrafted in many injured tissues. They can integrate with the injured tissue, trigger angiogenesis, and release paracrine factors. These factors are cytoprotective, antiapoptotic, anti-inflammatory, and antifibrosis, and help recruit other stem cells. BM-MNCs are relatively small stem cells (5–12 μm), thus carry a lower risk of embolic vascular occlusion. The size of the cells is an essential determinant of engraftment after coronary injections. In an early SPECT study, arterial injections of autologous 99Tc-labeled BM-MNCs were initially deposited in the brain in chronic stroke settings but, after 24 h, were better seen in other organs. BM-MNC delivery was well tolerated [30].

Method of Tracking Stem Cells

The key to improving stem cell applications is the ability to track their delivery. Tracking stem cells in vivo is necessary to assess their delivery, uptake, redistribution, viability, and functionality. Labeling stem cells with static reporters, such as dyes and quantum dots, poses a challenge as they are diluted in tissues after injection and through cell division. Furthermore, static reporters may not indicate the viability of the cells as they might be phagocytosed, and the signal does not accurately report their loss. Viral transfection techniques overcome this

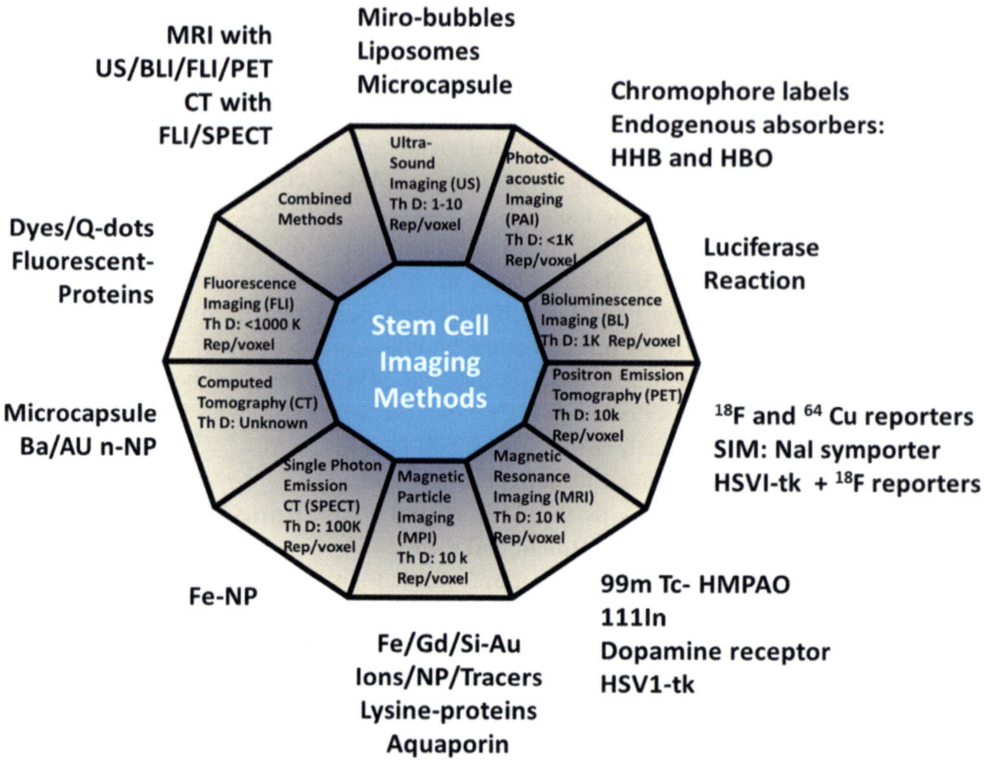

Fig. 15.2 Stem cell imaging modalities and reporters. The sensitivity is determined by the reporter/voxel needed to be detected by the method. THD: Threshold for detection (see Bose RJC et al.)

problem as the reporter genes continue to function in the progeny of the stem cells.

Figure 15.2 lists some techniques for imaging stem cells in vivo. These techniques could be classified as direct or indirect labels.

- **Direct labels** are fixed labels that are engrafted onto the cells. Fixed labels include dyes, quantum dots, radioactive labels, iron oxide labels, and microbubbles. The concentrations of the label decline as the stem cells divide and migrate. Furthermore, the signal would still be recorded as viable cells even if the cell dies and is phagocytosed. Direct labeling is a more straightforward process and helpful in understanding the delivery and uptake of stem cells, but not over more extended periods. The failure to longitudinally monitor the stem cells prevents assessment of their viability and function.
- **Indirect labels**: Indirect labeling involves the injection of a reporter gene for a fluorescent marker, an enzyme for bioluminescence for optical imaging, or an iron transporter for magnetic resonance imaging. The transfection of the stem cells could be temporary by injecting a nanoparticle. If the gene is not replicating, the signal will attenuate due to dilution and cell division. The advantage of introducing a gene into the host cell genome is that it is active in viable cells. However, the signal is conserved as the cell divides. Transfection of cells with viral vectors carries risks of mutagenesis, immune reactions, and side effects. Thus, it is clinically challenging.

Stem Cell Delivery Methods

The delivery of stem cells is substantially different from the delivery of drugs. Stem cells are metabolically active entities. Assuring viability from harvesting to delivery is necessary for cell replacement, although some benefits can be evident from cell-free secretome injections. Unlike drugs, stem cells have tissue tropism and migrate actively to injured or inflamed cells. Their paracrine factors are complex, with limited diffusion beyond the injection site. Although some of the immunomodulatory actions of stem cells can be remotely achieved, the benefits of stem cell treatment significantly improve with local delivery. Delivering stem cells to the target site promptly, effectively, safely, and conveniently has been a hurdle in translational research.

The route of stem cell delivery, listed in Table 15.2, depends on the application. Intravenous injection is the best way to deliver the cells for systemic diseases. However, locoregional delivery is superior to intravenous delivery for

Table 15.2 Routes of stem cell delivery

Route	Rationale	Advantage	Disadvantage	Typical application
Intravenous	Systemic delivery	Simplicity. Immune modulation. It could be helpful for delivery to the lungs, spleen, or liver	Trapping by the lungs, spleen, and liver makes stem cell targeting difficult Inefficient, non-targeted delivery could lead to complications	Widely used for most disease conditions
Topical	Local delivery	Simplicity Requires delivery scaffolds (collagen/synthetic)	The application to surface-exposed pathologies (skin burns or organ surfaces), although effectiveness has been debated	N/A
Direct injection	Local delivery	Excellent cell load deposition, relatively simple	Tissue invasive	Parkinson's disease
Intra-arterial	Local delivery	Acceptable local delivery. It is a ubiquitous method that is applicable across organs	Embolic risk Needs optimization Redistribution to other organs	Ischemic stroke
Inhalation	Local delivery	Simplicity Restricted to trachea bronchial tree and alveoli	Limited to respiratory applications	N/A
Intranasal	Local delivery	Cranial deposition through cranial nerves and perivascular migration Could bypass the blood–brain barrier	Nonspecific site targeting	Multiple sclerosis
Intraventricular	Local delivery		Nonspecific site targeting	Alzheimer's disease

treating focal pathologies, partly because it avoids the cells' sequestration by the lungs, liver, and spleen.

Arterial Delivery of Stem Cells for Non-neurological Diseases

Peripheral Vascular Disease

Stem cell injections are effective in PVD in part due to local release of paracrine factors that promote neovascularization; incorporation of stem cells into the tissue is not the sole benefit [12, 31]. Direct injection into the adjacent muscle, intra-arterial injections, or a combination of both has been used. Direct injections efficiently deliver cells to the muscle surrounding the artery. However, it risks cell loss due to tissue ischemia secondary to vascular insufficiency. On the other hand, arterial injections give the stem cells a ready supply of oxygenated blood. However, regional deposition of stem cells is much less effective than that by direct injection. Stem cell treatments result in symptomatic improvement; whether they reduce the likelihood of amputation is contested. Both direct and arterial injections result in similar benefits.

Acute Kidney Injury (AKI)

AKI is associated with oxidative injuries, inflammation, and fibrosis. These processes lead to the deterioration of kidney functions and can be halted or reversed by stem cells. In animals, intravenous delivery of MSCs ameliorates kidney injury [32, 33]. Several animal studies reveal the beneficial effects of intra-arterial stem cell delivery for AKI. Following 45 min of renal ischemia, renal artery infusion of 10^5 MSCs resulted in better delivery than through the tail vein or the carotid artery. However, higher doses led to more MSC deposition and worsening of injury [34]. Injection of MSCs was most effective if the delivery was concurrent with ischemia compared to pre- and postischemic injury [35]. In clinical trials, the benefits of stem cell treatment in AKI have been inconsistent. Suprarenal arterial infusion of MSCs can prevent the deterioration of renal function after surgery and improve the outcome [36].

Liver Diseases

The cytoprotective, antiapoptotic, antifibrosis, and immunomodulatory paracrine effects of stem cells are beneficial in treating liver damage. Although the liver sequesters stem cells, intravenously delivered cells tend to accumulate more in the lungs and spleen. Intraportal and hepatic arterial injections are superior to intravenous injections for delivering stem cells. A meta-analysis of 23 controlled trials revealed that hepatic artery infusion was superior to intravenous infusion and improved liver function parameters [37].

Diabetes Mellitus

The benefits of stem cell therapy for type 2 diabetes mellitus are due to the improvements in islet cell function and glucose homeostasis rather than the replacement of β cells [38]. These have resulted in a decrease in HbA1C, a reduction in insulin requirements, and an increase in C-reactive protein [39]. Other studies did not observe a decrease in insulin requirements. Evidence suggests that the outcome of arterial infusions is superior to the intravenous delivery of stem cells [40]. The pancreas's remote location favors arterial drug delivery via the dorsal pancreatic artery or through branches of the coeliac trunk. However, animal models using human bone marrow SCs show that the benefits of stem cell transplant may be temporary, lasting 4–45 days, and could result in neoplastic transformation [41].

Cardiac Disease

A variety of stem cell treatments are available for treating myocardial ischemia. These include MNCs, MSCs, cardiac stem cells, and iPSCs from cardiac myocytes. The benefits of treatment can be both from cell integration into tissue and paracrine effects that improve myocardial performance [38]. Although there are many possible routes of stem cell delivery, direct injection of stem cells is thought to be more efficient than intracoronary injection. Balloon occlusion is sometimes used with arterial delivery to enhance local uptake [42]. Direct injection requires surgical exposure and has limited application. Arterial delivery is attractive as radiological interventions are often needed in acute settings. A hybrid technique using microinjections through arterial access was developed to improve regional deposition [13]. The amount of cells delivered with intra-arterial injection is a function of cell size. Larger MNSCs are more efficiently trapped after arterial delivery [43]. The potential risk of arterial delivery of stem cells in the possibility of embolic occlusion of the artery, arrhythmia, and malignant transformation since iPSCs yield the best clinical results.

Neurological Applications of Stem Cells

Derivatives of Stem Cell Research:

- **Cell replacement to restore tissue integrity and function:**
  - Focal cell degeneration: Parkinson's disease
  - Lost/damaged cells: Stroke, TBI and SCI
  - Replacement of abnormal cells: Epilepsy
- **Beneficial paracrine effects:**
  - Proangiogenetic factors benefit stroke, ischemic/hypoxic brain injury
  - Anti-inflammation: SCs modulate T-cell and macrophage function and promote anti-inflammatory cytokines, such as IL-10 and TGF-β, useful in conditions like multiple sclerosis.
  - Antiapoptotic, e.g., neurodegenerative diseases
  - Host cell recruitment
  - Cell proliferation
- **Cytological and organoid research**:
  - Cell studies: Mechanisms of tissue healing, repair, and regeneration
  - Development of 2- to 3-dimensional cytological models
  - Cerebral organoid
  - Human-animal chimera
- **Disease models**: Investigating stem cells from animal disease models, developing potential treatment strategies, and generating induced stem cells from a cohort of patients to investigate a specific disease, e.g., generating motor neurons obtained from patients with ALS as models of disease evolution.
- **Drug testing**: Investigate drug toxicity related to specific cells, tissue, or an individual.
- **Vehicles for drug delivery**: Drug microcapsule-loaded mesenchymal stem cells
- **Cancer treatment**: Delivery of oncolytic viruses to glioma cells
- **Secretome formulation**: Hydrogels, scaffolds, patches, microneedle patch
- **Stem cell exosomes**: Peptides, drugs, gene delivery

Arterial Stem Cell Delivery

Delivery of stem cells by arterial injections has a broad appeal across many organs. While these techniques could be similar in some respects, they must be adapted to meet the tissue needs. For example, arterial stem cell delivery to the liver will significantly differ from that of the brain in terms of cell type and even the manner of injection. In the case of the liver, embolic occlusion might aid the delivery of stem cells, while in the case of the brain, any embolic event could worsen tissue injury. As seen in the above section, there are certain similarities in arterial drug delivery for diseases across various organs. These include:

- Greater ability to target tissue compared to intravenous delivery but less than direct injection.
- Cell size is an essential determinant of the extent of deposition.
- The number of injected cells can determine the outcome.
- Excessive number of cells can adversely affect the outcome.

- Cells can redistribute from the injection site with delayed lung, liver, and spleen localization.
- Labeling stem cells with suitable reporters can help to determine their regional kinetics.
- Benefits of stem cell delivery can be due to their paracrine effects.

Pros and Cons of Arterial Stem Cell Delivery

- Pros

Delivers cells in high concentration to the target site
Avoids dilution by circulating blood volume
Minimizes uptake by lungs, spleen, and liver
More effective than IV delivery
Minimally invasive compared to direct injection
Arterial or angiographic procedures are relatively routine and safe
It can be undertaken concurrently with other arterial interventions
Ubiquitous cross-organ appeal

- Cons

Requires arterial puncture and catheter placement
Carries embolic risk with larger MSCs and greater cell loads
Tissue injury from injection pressure/jet
Entrapment rates can be meager, and only 1–5% of injected cells may be deposited
Redistribution can be rapid with small stem cells

Optimizing Arterial Stem Cell Delivery

Computational models of arterial drug delivery reveal that drug delivery is most effective when there is low regional blood flow, high regional extraction, and high systemic clearance [44]. However, the rules of drug delivery cannot be applied to living stem cells. Unlike drug molecules, stem cells are large and pose embolic risks, which are directly related to their size [13]. Thus, excessive regional deposition with large cells or more significant injected cell numbers could be potentially harmful [45]. Furthermore, clearance, i.e., by nontarget site delivery, could lead to unanticipated development of the stem cells at the nontarget site and malignant transformation [41]. Despite differences, there are similarities. For example, arterial drug delivery can deliver a large number of stem cells to the target site, and judicious flow reduction could improve their retention [42]. Regional extraction could be improved with better monitoring of stem cells by surface labeling to track their location [13]. As with drugs, the blood–brain barrier hinders stem cell delivery; thus, ultrasonic disruption has been used to enhance local deposition [46].

Arterial delivery of drugs and stem cells requires an assessment of local and systemic drug concentrations. Optimizing their delivery, ensuring safety, and fully benefiting from stem cell technology will be challenging without the ability to track stem cells in the body after injection. Several factors affect arterial stem cell delivery to the brain. These include:

Size of Stem Cells:

Brain capillaries are about 5–10 μm in diameter. While RBCs (7 μm) can pass through capillaries, white blood cells (10–25 μm) are restricted in movement. The size of the WBCs is similar to that of stem cells. However, the size of stem cells varies greatly. In general, MNSCs are about 6–12 μm, the NSCs are 10–20 μm, and the BMSCs are 5–50 μm [45]. Thus, based on size alone, MNSCs would pose little embolic risk, NSCs would pose some embolic risk, and BMSCs would pose the most significant risk. Guzman et al. reviewed the reported embolic complications of studies with different stem cells and found the risk to be directly proportional to the size of the cells [47].

Dose of Stem Cells:

Determining optimum arterial drug doses has always been challenging [48]. The challenge is significantly increased in the case of stem cells. Guzman et al. used dose/gram of brain weight to optimize doses across animal models and stem cells. The dose of stem cells impairing blood flow in mice is 7.5×10^5 cells/g, but increased mortality was seen with 12.5×10^5 cells/g of brain weight. In the rats, high doses of MNSCs 150×10^5 cells/g of tissue are well tolerated, while the dose of NSCs associated with embolic complications seems to be 10×10^5 cells/g of tissue. In dogs, microembolic complications occurred with 0.4×10^5 cells/g of brain tissue [47]. Due to the risk of embolic injury, which seems to be cell-related and animal-model dependent, it is prudent to monitor regional blood flow and limit stem cell doses to those that do not decrease flow [45]. One consideration is that intracarotid injections may not perfuse the whole brain due to variations in anatomy, and weight correction should be based on perfused tissue volume [49]. Furthermore, laboratory animals have variations in the carotid anatomy, and correct vascular isolation is necessary to apply weight-based dose corrections [50].

Infusion Rate:

In most angiographic procedures, contrast agents are manually injected as boluses. This ensures sufficient opacification vessel. In clinical angiography, the injection volume varies considerably with the infused vessels. It ranges from 7 to 10 mL/s, 6 to 8 mL/s, and 5 to 8 mL/s for the common carotid artery, internal carotid artery, and vertebral artery, respectively [51]. This volume of injection is more than the blood flow. During clinical angiography, radiologists manually optimize the pressure of injection to achieve the desired image quality. Excessive injection pressure can lead to hemorrhagic complications, as have been reported during arterial chemotherapy and thrombolysis for stroke [52, 53]. Stem cell delivery is likely to be undertaken to the injured tissue; careful determination of infusion rates is needed to avoid hemorrhagic or embolic complications.

Timing of Injection:
The benefits of stem cell treatment are evident in animal ischemic stroke studies. However, these benefits seem to be time-dependent. Several studies have revealed more benefits in the subacute phase. Reperfusion after stroke is associated with the breakdown of the blood–brain barrier and influx of white blood cells between 48 and 72 h after stroke. Injection at this time will be ideally suited for the engraftment of the stem cells. Ischemia and acidosis in the early stages of reperfusion could adversely affect stem cell survival [47]. Other investigators have suggested that stem cells be delivered not concurrently but 24–48 h after reperfusion [45, 54, 55].

Stem Cell-Intrinsic Properties:
Autologous bone marrow and mesenchymal stem cells are the most attractive stem cell populations due to the relative lack of immune response. On the other hand, they have limited and variable ability to integrate into nonnative neural tissues. Neural stem cells can integrate more efficiently in the native brain niche, but directing their differentiation and integration integration can be challenging.

Adjuvant Measures to Improve Arterial Stem Cell Delivery:

- Flow arrest delivery in coronary circulation; however, it poses the risk of increasing ischemic injury in settings of stroke [42].
- BBB disruption [46].
- Optimizing Culture Conditions: Stem cell cultured with nerve growth factors and brain derived neurotropic growth factor increase MSC engraftment rates by about 15–20%, 24 h after TBI [56].
- Ligand Decoration: Enriching NSCs with surface ligands CD49 that could increase adhesion to the vascular endothelium [55].
- Magnetic targeting could improve arterial delivery, as with intraventricular and intravenous stem cell delivery [57].

Clinical Effectiveness of Stem Cell Treatment

Meta-analysis of 16 clinical studies revealed that locoregional delivery, via stereotactic transplant or intracarotid injection, of stem cells is significantly more effective than intravenous delivery [58]. Another meta-analysis of 26 studies, 9 before 2010, revealed that stem cell treatment was well tolerated across various delivery methods and showed a trend toward improving the neurological outcome [59]. A more recent review of clinical trials discussed arterial injection of stem cells and suggested their use in acute stroke but raised concerns about redistribution after arterial injection [60].

While there is no proven long-term benefit of intra-arterial stem cell treatment in controlled and sufficiently powered clinical trials, there is enough evidence to suggest that stem cell treatment holds promise and their delivery is different from conventional drugs. Failure of pharmacological neuroprotection over the last four decades compels us to look elsewhere. As experience grows with thrombectomy, the intervention window will expand based on perfusion parameters. Stem cell therapies12.5 could offer hope to people beyond the thrombectomy time window or those unsuitable for such treatments. One of the biggest hurdles to establishing the benefits of stem cell treatment is the inability to track them in vivo. Combined CT-MRI suites are now available for stroke treatment in some medical centers. Superparamagnetic iron oxide nanoparticles could label the stem cells to monitor their delivery in a CT-MR environment. Another approach to track stem cells is labeling them with ^{111}In SPECT imaging [61]. The signal of such fixed reporters degrades over time due to dilution and cell division. However, these methods can provide initial brain uptake and clearance data, which will be invaluable for optimizing arterial stem cell delivery.

Challenges and Limitations of Arterial Stem Cell Treatments

Some of the challenges in developing stem cell applications are shown in Fig. 15.3. These include:

- Availability of stem cells: The most likely neurological application of intra-arterial stem cells will be stroke treatment. Such treatment is best undertaken over 1–3 days after injury. This gives sufficient time to harvest and process autologous stem cells. The quality of autologous stem cells could be affected by several factors, including age, diabetes, gender, and obesity. Smoking also affects stem cell functions and therapeutic response [62]. MSCs that lack HLAII antigens are considered safe for allogeneic transplants and are, therefore, attractive for urgent care [45].
- Immune rejection: Allogeneic stem cells can trigger an immune reaction, resulting in transplant failure.
- Embolism: The dose and size of stem cells increase the risk of embolism. If used in a CT or MR environment, monitoring blood flow by contrast transit could minimize the risk.
- Tissue engulfment, integration, and functionality:
- Operational:
  - Ethical and regulatory issues are more critical for stem cells derived from fetal tissue but have been partly addressed by reprogramming adult cells.

  - Production of stem cells requires compliance with rigorous FDA guidelines.
  - Delivery methods should be optimized and compared in well-controlled studies.
- Duration of effect: Some data suggest that stem cell treatment benefits might be finite. In an animal model of diabetes, stem cell implants failed after 45 days and could lead to malignant transformation [41]. On the other hand, patients receiving human fetal allografts for treating Parkinson's disease have evidence of functioning grafts several years after transplantation [63]. Thus, the viability and renewability of the cells after delivery will need to be assessed. Careful cell line selection will be required to assure long-term viability.

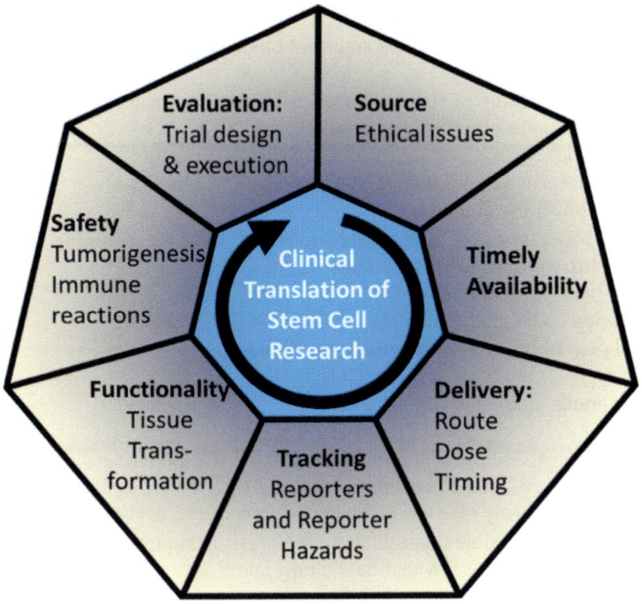

Fig. 15.3 Challenges in developing stem cell applications

Intra-Arterial Stem Cell Delivery Trials

Table 15.3 lists the ongoing stem cell trials for acute ischemic stroke as reported on the National Clinical Trial Registry website.

Future Challenges and Applications

Since antiquity, neurological diseases like apoplexy or traumatic brain and spinal injuries have had the aura of helpless finality. Even recently, after the failure of NXY 059, a Lancet editorial questioned whether research in neuroprotective pharmaceuticals should continue after the failures of hundreds of compounds in clinical trials [64]. While there could be many causes for the failure of over a thousand neuropro-

Table 15.3 Acute ischemic stroke (AIS) trials extracted from the National Clinical Trials website

NCT number Phase	Objective	Status
Intra-arterial delivery		
NCT00761982 Phase 1 and 2	Determine the safety and efficacy of autologous CD34+ subset bone marrow stem cell infusion into **the middle cerebral artery** in acute MCA stroke	Completed
NCT00535197 Phase 1 and 2	Determine the safety and tolerability of an autologous CD34+ subset bone marrow stem cell **infusion into the middle cerebral artery** in patients with acute total or partial anterior circulation syndrome (TACS/PACS)	Completed
NCT00473057 Phase 1	To assess the safety of **arterial** autologous bone marrow transplantation in patients with an ischemic MCA stroke within 90 days from symptoms onset	Completed
NCT04434768 Phase 1	To assess the safety of dual administration of UCMSC **via arterial and intravenous delivery** in human subjects using rigorous recruitment criteria and careful dosing.	Recruiting
Intravenous/intranasal delivery		
NCT03186456 Phase 1	Determine the safety and efficacy of treating acute ischemic stroke patients with human umbilical cord mesenchymal stem cells. via **intravenous** forearm delivery.	Suspended
NCT04047563 Phase 3	Prospective, multicentric, randomized, double-blind, parallel, saline-controlled phase II clinical study to evaluate the efficacy of sovateltide (IRL-1620 or PMZ-1620) with standard supportive care in AIS patients	Completed
NCT05955326 Phase 4	Prospective, multicenter, randomized, double-blind, parallel, phase IV study to evaluate the safety and efficacy of sovateltide (PMZ-1620, IRL-1620) treatment for AIS	Not yet recruiting
NCT04097652 Phase 1	This is a UMC119-06 dose escalation, open-label, single-center study in adults with AIS. UMC119-06 is ex-vivo cultured human umbilical cord tissue-derived mesenchymal stem cell product	Recruiting
NCT06129175 Phase 2 and 3	To assess Barthel index (BI) and modified Rankin Scale (mRS) scores within 1 year of Neuroncell-EX infusion in AIC patients	Recruiting

(continued)

Table 15.3 (continued)

NCT number Phase	Objective	Status
NCT03384433 Phase 1 and 2	To assess the effect of cell-free exosomes derived from mesenchymal stem cells (MSCs) on disability of AIS patients	Unknown
NCT02157896	Assess prognosis in AIS by comparing serum vascular endothelial growth factor (VEGF) and Endostatin (ES) and circulating endothelial progenitor cells (EPCs) in peripheral blood	Completed
NCT05522569	To assess **intravenous** allogeneic human mesenchymal stem cells (Allo-hMSCs) to treat AIS	Not available
NCT01289795	To determine levels of circulating endothelial progenitor cells (cEPC) in AIS	Unknown
NCT03735277 Phase 1	This phase one study investigates the safety and efficacy of **intravenous** allogeneic cord blood hematopoietic progenitor cells (HPC, Cord Blood) with 9 days of AIS	Unknown
NCT01310114 Phase 2	The study's primary objective is to assess the safety and tolerability of Human Placenta-Derived Cells (PDA001) at three different dose levels versus placebo (vehicle control) administered **intravenously** in subjects following ischemic stroke	Terminated
NCT03004976 Phase 2	Determine the efficacy of a single **intravenous** dose of unrelated donor umbilical cord blood (UCB) for improving functional outcomes in patients with AIS over a year	Completed
NCT06138210 Phase 1	This is a multicenter, randomized, double-blinded, placebo-controlled, dose-escalation trial. It aims to evaluate the safety and preliminary efficacy of **intravenous** exosomes derived from human induced pluripotent stem cells (GD-iExo-003) in acute ischemic stroke	Not yet recruiting
NCT04608838 Phase 1 and 2	To evaluate the safety and efficacy of a single **intravenous** administration of JTR-161 (allogeneic stem cell product derived from the dental pulp of healthy adult humans) to patients with AIC	Completed
NCT01501773 Phase:2	To assess the safety, feasibility, and efficacy of **intravenous** autologous bone marrow mononuclear cells (BMMC) in patients with AIS	Completed
NCT02397018 Phase 1	To assess the safety of a single**, intravenous** infusion of banked allogeneic umbilical cord blood within 3–10 days of the AIS. Interview follow-up at 1-, 6-, and 12-month postinfusion and a neurological exam, MRI, and blood tests at 90 days	Completed
NCT04046484 Phase 2	A prospective, multicentric, randomized, double-blind, parallel, saline-controlled phase II clinical study to compare the safety and efficacy of PMZ-1620 (INN: Sovateltide) therapy and standard supportive care in patients with AIS	Completed
NCT05993884 Phase 1	A single-center, randomized, double-blind, placebo-controlled, dose-escalation clinical study to investigate the safety and efficacy of EPCs transplantation in acute ischemic stroke	Not yet recruiting
NCT04093336 Phase 1 and 2	A placebo-controlled, randomized, double-blind study including phase 1 and 2. Phase I study assesses safety assessment, and phase 2 study assesses the effectiveness of **intravenous** human umbilical cord mesenchymal stem cells MSCs in AIS	Recruiting
NCT01678534 **Phase 2**	Phase II clinical trial, pilot, single-center, prospective, randomized, double-blind, placebo-controlled, with sequential inclusion of patients with AIC	Completed
NCT05008588 Phase 1 and 2	To determine the effectiveness of a combination of **intranasal** conditioned medium (CM) with intraparenchymal umbilical cord mesenchymal stem cells (UC-MSCs) transplantation in acute stroke patients to induce neurogenesis	Recruiting
NCT02425670 Phase 2	Primary hypothesis: **Intravenous** injection of bone marrow mononuclear cells (30–500 million) in patients with subacute ischemic stroke results in reduced infarct volume and improved neurological function compared to those without the injection	Completed
NCT00901381 Phase 2	To investigate leucostim (Filgrastim; granulocyte-colony stimulating factor; G-CSF) for AIS	Completed

tective compounds for operational and scientific reasons, we could also have used the wrong tools to address the problem. The neural tissues' lack of regenerative capacity may have led to these failures. The cytoprotective, antiapoptotic, and regenerative capacity of stem cells could address this limitation.

Ischemic stroke, which accounts for almost four-fifths of all strokes, constitutes a significant healthcare burden. Yet, we see the potential of using stem cells to treat acute ischemic stroke. However, in Table 15.3, very few clinical studies have investigated arterial delivery. While not mentioned in the table, many studies have investigated intracoronary stem cell treatments. Stem cell therapy for neurological diseases is far more challenging than those for the heart. Preclinical experiments suggest that, unless the stem cells are carefully selected and delivered in the optimum doses, effectively and at the right time, the treatment will fail and could worsen the injury.

Arterial delivery is considered to be the preferred stem cell delivery method for treating acute ischemic stroke. This is partly due to the recent improvement in stroke outcomes due to early thrombectomy and thrombolysis. However, only a third of the patients who meet treatment criteria benefit from such interventions. Having arterial access to the injury site paves the way for stem cell treatments. Most preclinical studies suggest that such a route of drug delivery could be superior to intravenous infusion.

Furthermore, due to arterial interventions for stroke, there is an urgency for developing stroke units that have combined MR and CT imaging facilities to save the time needed to assess and treat stroke. The problem with such dual units is the coregistration of the images when the patient is moved from one scanner to another. This has led to the design of a combined CT-MRI scanner. The CT-MRI scanner comprises a double doughnut-shaped pair of superconducting 1.5 T magnets (blue) with a multisource interior CT (red) (Fig. 15.4). Thus, CT-MRI images can be obtained in a single scanner without moving the patient [65].

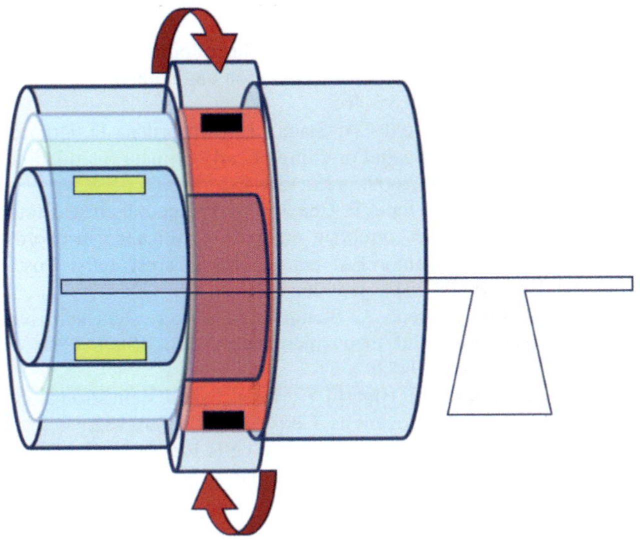

Fig. 15.4 A representation of a combined CT (red) MR (blue) scanner design proposed by Wang et al. [65].

The availability of combined CT-MR images in independent and combined canners also opens avenues for stem cell application, such as by tracking paramagnetically labeled stem cells. Effective deposition of these cells without obstructing the blood flow will be crucial for stroke treatments. The embolic risk is much less with MNSCs; however, these cells are rapidly redistributed and lack potency. Therefore, there is a need to transplant more potent MSCs effectively. Future treatments might not just rely on potent stem cells, but rather an array of stem cell products, as shown in Fig. 15.5. While thrombectomy is very effective in restoring the microcirculation, the microcirculatory flow might take time to recover. In such a situation, using MSCs could be potentially harmful; stem cell secretomes and exosomes might be safe.

The use of stem cell secretome obtained from the culture media with cytoprotective, anti-inflammatory, antiapoptotic, and tissue-tropic properties but with no risk of embolic injury could be used. In the next phase of treatment, stem cell exomes (40–160 nm) with tissue tropism could deliver anti-apoptotic and therapeutic compounds also without embolic risk. Using stem cell secretomes and exomes carries minimal

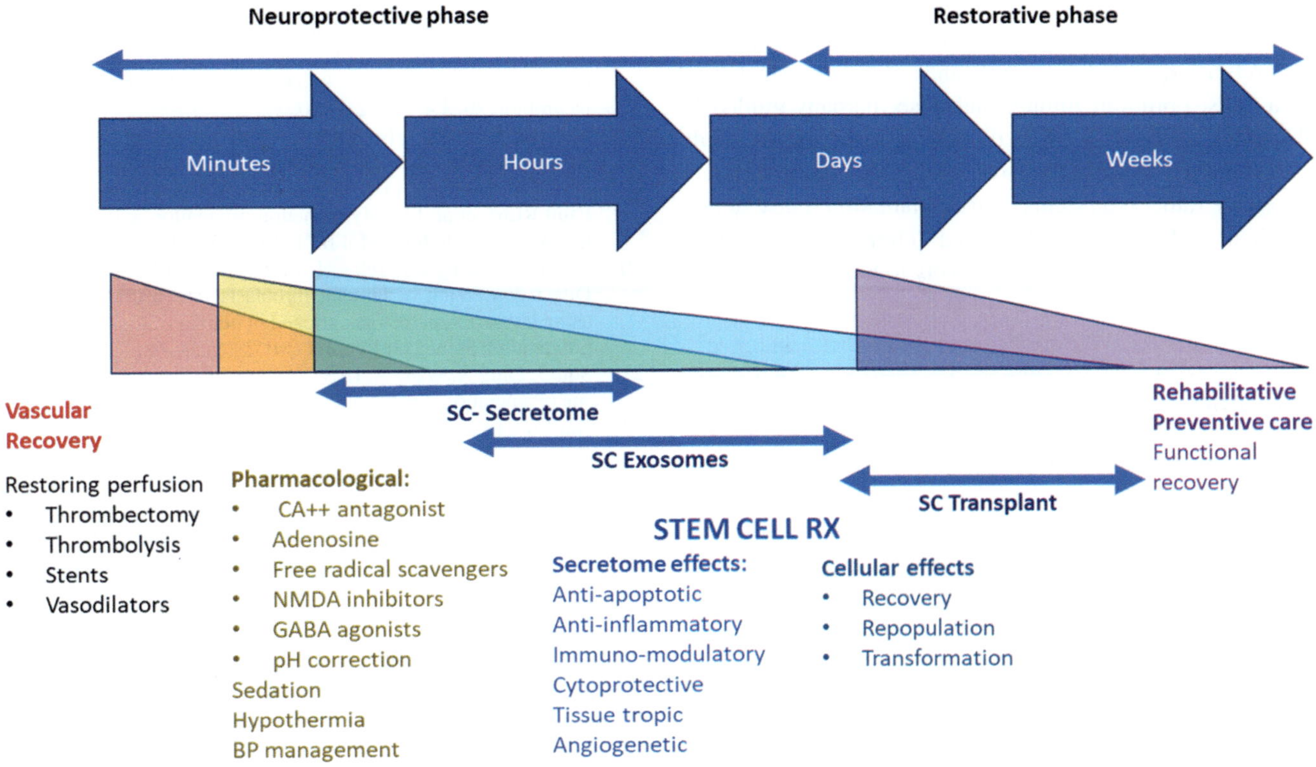

Fig. 15.5 Proposed use of stem cells for stroke acute ischemic stroke treatment

immunological risks and can be stored and ready to use. Pretreatment by these modalities could pave the way for stem cell treatment in 24–48 h when tissue perfusion is better established. Delivering stem cell products could improve engraftment, repopulation, and transformation. Rather than single-shot stem cell delivery, the sequenced use of stem cell products strategically guided by imaging data could offer novel future treatments for ischemic stroke.

Conclusions

This review sought to briefly describe the promises and pitfalls of stem cell therapy. The current approved clinical applications of stem cell therapy are limited to the treatment of hematological disorders. The FDA has not yet approved exosome-based products. There an intense effort to validate the use of stem cell treatment in many aspects of medicine. Considerable resources have been directed to regenerative medicine to develop stem cells, exomes, and secretomes. However, the effective delivery of stem cells is one of the biggest hurdles to technological development. It is likely that stem cell applications for ophthalmology and dentistry, where there is easy access to target sites, will soon be approved. There are many neurological applications of stem cells, but they face far greater delivery hurdles than posed by any other organ. Arterial drug delivery provides easy access to cerebral tissue. In the setting of stroke—where endovascular technology is highly developed—delivering stem cells through arterial injections is particularly attractive. Ongoing research has revealed the significance of proper selection of stem cells, optimum timing, and dose, perhaps guided by blood flow. It could well be that the first successful results with stem cell therapy for stroke will come from stem cell secretome rather than stem cell transplantation. The extent to which arterial delivery will be used to treat other neurological disorders is unclear, but it is likely to be most relevant in treating stroke.

References

1. Prockop DJ. Repair of tissues by adult stem/progenitor cells (MSCs): controversies, myths, and changing paradigms. Mol Ther. 2009;17(6):939–46.
2. Malysz-Cymborska I, Golubczyk D, Kalkowski L, Kwiatkowska J, Zawadzki M, Glodek J, et al. Intra-arterial transplantation of stem cells in large animals as a minimally-invasive strategy for the treatment of disseminated neurodegeneration. Sci Rep. 2021;11(1):6581.
3. Harting MT. Basics of stem and proginator cells. In: Cox CS, editor. Proginator cell therapy for neurological diseases. Stem cell biology and regenerative medicine. New York: Springer; 2011. p. 1–18.
4. Singh VK, Saini A, Kalsan M, Kumar N, Chandra R. Describing the stem cell potency: the various methods of functional assessment and in silico diagnostics. Front Cell Dev Biol. 2016;4:134.
5. Filip S, Mokrý J, English D, Vojácek J. Stem cell plasticity and issues of stem cell therapy. Folia Biol (Praha). 2005;51(6):180–7.
6. Wei Y, Zhang E, Yu L, Ci B, Guo L, Sakurai M, et al. Dissecting embryonic and extra-embryonic lineage crosstalk with stem cell co-culture. bioRxiv. 2023.
7. Ghazimoradi MH, Khalafizadeh A, Babashah S. A critical review on induced totipotent stem cells: types and methods. Stem Cell Res. 2022;63:102857.
8. Arias AM, Marikawa Y, Moris N. Gastruloids: pluripotent stem cell models of mammalian gastrulation and embryo engineering. Dev Biol. 2022;488:35–46.
9. Bergmann S, Penfold CA, Slatery E, Siriwardena D, Drummer C, Clark S, et al. Spatial profiling of early primate gastrulation in utero. Nature. 2022;609(7925):136–43.
10. Le Douarin NM, Dupin E. Chapter 1—The neural crest, a fourth germ layer of the vertebrate embryo: significance in chordate evolution. In: Trainor PA, editor. Neural crest cells. Boston: Academic Press; 2014. p. 3–26.
11. Aponte PM, Caicedo A. Stemness in cancer: stem cells, cancer stem cells, and their microenvironment. Stem Cells Int. 2017;2017(1):5619472.
12. Mohamad Yusoff F, Higashi Y. Mesenchymal stem/stromal cells for therapeutic angiogenesis. Cells. 2023;12(17):2162.
13. Copland IB. Mesenchymal stromal cells for cardiovascular disease. J Cardiovasc Dis Res. 2011;2(1):3–13.
14. Verfaillie CM, Crabbe A. Chapter 28—Multipotent adult progenitor cells. In: Lanza R, Gearhart J, Hogan B, Melton D, Pedersen R, Thomas ED, et al., editors. Essentials of stem cell biology. 2nd ed. San Diego: Academic Press; 2009. p. 233–41.
15. Lengefeld J, Cheng CW, Maretich P, Blair M, Hagen H, McReynolds MR, et al. Cell size is a determinant of stem cell potential during aging. Sci Adv. 2021;7(46):eabk0271.
16. Henry TD, Moyé L, Traverse JH. Consistently inconsistent—Bone marrow mononuclear stem cell therapy following acute myocardial infarction. Circ Res. 2016;119(3):404–6.
17. Nguyen QT, Thanh LN, Hoang VT, Phan TTK, Heke M, Hoang DM. Bone marrow-derived mononuclear cells in the treatment of neurological diseases: knowns and unknowns. Cell Mol Neurobiol. 2023;43(7):3211–50.
18. Martínez-Cerdeño V, Noctor SC. Neural progenitor cell terminology. Front Neuroanat. 2018;12:104.
19. Park TIH, Waldvogel HJ, Montgomery JM, Mee EW, Bergin PS, Faull RLM, et al. Identifying neural progenitor cells in the adult human brain. Methods Mol Biol. 2022;2389:125–54.
20. Hou PS, Chuang CY, Yeh CH, Chiang W, Liu HJ, Lin TN, et al. Direct conversion of human fibroblasts into neural progenitors using transcription factors enriched in human ESC-derived neural progenitors. Stem Cell Reports. 2017;8(1):54–68.
21. Soto J, Ding X, Wang A, Li S. Neural crest-like stem cells for tissue regeneration. Stem Cells Transl Medz. 2021;10(5):681–93.
22. Nagamura-Inoue T, He H. Umbilical cord-derived mesenchymal stem cells: their advantages and potential clinical utility. World J Stem Cells. 2014;6(2):195–202.
23. Zakrzewski W, Dobrzyński M, Szymonowicz M, Rybak Z. Stem cells: past, present, and future. Stem Cell Res Ther. 2019;10(1):68.
24. Shi Y, Inoue H, Wu JC, Yamanaka S. Induced pluripotent stem cell technology: a decade of progress. Nat Rev Drug Discov. 2017;16(2):115–30.
25. Li F, Zhang J, Yi K, Wang H, Wei H, Chan HF, et al. Delivery of stem cell secretome for therapeutic applications. ACS Appl Bio Mater. 2022;5(5):2009–30.
26. Valadez-Barba V, Cota-Coronado A, Hernández-Pérez OR, Lugo-Fabres PH, Padilla-Camberos E, Díaz NF, et al. iPSC for modeling neurodegenerative disorders. Regen Ther. 2020;15:332–9.
27. Musiał-Wysocka A, Kot M, Majka M. The pros and cons of mesenchymal stem cell-based therapies. Cell Transplant. 2019;28(7):801–12.

28. Brody M, Agronin M, Herskowitz BJ, Bookheimer SY, Small GW, Hitchinson B, et al. Results and insights from a phase I clinical trial of Lomecel-B for Alzheimer's disease. Alzheimers Dement. 2023;19(1):261–73.
29. Jeon K, Park K, Jetten AM. Efficient neural differentiation using single-cell culture of human embryonic stem cells. J Vis Exp. 2020;(155).
30. Vasconcelos-dos-Santos A, Rosado-de-Castro PH, Lopes de Souza SA, da Costa SJ, Ramos AB, Rodriguez de Freitas G, et al. Intravenous and intra-arterial administration of bone marrow mononuclear cells after focal cerebral ischemia: is there a difference in biodistribution and efficacy? Stem Cell Res. 2012;9(1):1–8.
31. Huang NF, Stern B, Oropeza BP, Zaitseva TS, Paukshto MV, Zoldan J. Bioengineering cell therapy for treatment of peripheral artery disease. Arterioscler Thromb Vasc Biol. 2024;44(3):e66–81.
32. Wang Y, He J, Pei X, Zhao W. Systematic review and meta-analysis of mesenchymal stem/stromal cells therapy for impaired renal function in small animal models. Nephrology (Carlton). 2013;18(3):201–8.
33. Zhuo W, Liao L, Xu T, Wu W, Yang S, Tan J. Mesenchymal stem cells ameliorate ischemia-reperfusion-induced renal dysfunction by improving the antioxidant/oxidant balance in the ischemic kidney. Urol Int. 2011;86(2):191–6.
34. Cai J, Yu X, Xu R, Fang Y, Qian X, Liu S, et al. Maximum efficacy of mesenchymal stem cells in rat model of renal ischemia-reperfusion injury: renal artery administration with optimal numbers. PLoS One. 2014;9(3):e92347.
35. Jang MJ, You D, Park JY, Kim K, Aum J, Lee C, et al. Hypoxic preconditioned mesenchymal stromal cell therapy in a rat model of renal ischemia-reperfusion injury: development of optimal protocol to potentiate therapeutic efficacy. Int J Stem Cells. 2018;11(2):157–67.
36. Togel FE, Westenfelder C. Kidney protection and regeneration following acute injury: progress through stem cell therapy. Am J Kidney Dis. 2012;60(6):1012–22.
37. Zhao L, Chen S, Shi X, Cao H, Li L. A pooled analysis of mesenchymal stem cell-based therapy for liver disease. Stem Cell Res Ther. 2018;9(1):72.
38. Ng NN, Thakor AS. Locoregional delivery of stem cell-based therapies. Sci Transl Med. 2020;12(547):eaba4564.
39. Hu J, Li C, Wang L, Zhang X, Zhang M, Gao H, et al. Long term effects of the implantation of autologous bone marrow mononuclear cells for type 2 diabetes mellitus. Endocr J. 2012;59(11):1031–9.
40. Sood V, Mittal BR, Bhansali A, Singh B, Khandelwal N, Marwaha N, et al. Biodistribution of 18F-FDG-labeled autologous bone marrow-derived stem cells in patients with type 2 diabetes mellitus: exploring targeted and intravenous routes of delivery. Clin Nucl Med. 2015;40(9):697–700.
41. Tang DQ, Wang Q, Burkhardt BR, Litherland SA, Atkinson MA, Yang LJ. In vitro generation of functional insulin-producing cells from human bone marrow-derived stem cells, but long-term culture running risk of malignant transformation. Am J Stem Cells. 2012;1(2):114–27.
42. Sheng CC, Zhou L, Hao J. Current stem cell delivery methods for myocardial repair. Biomed Res Int. 2013;2013:547902.
43. Campbell NG, Kaneko M, Shintani Y, Narita T, Sawhney V, Coppen SR, et al. Cell size critically determines initial retention of bone marrow mononuclear cells in the heart after intracoronary injection: evidence from a rat model. PLoS One. 2016;11(7):e0158232.
44. Dedrick RL. Arterial drug infusion: pharmacokinetic problems and pitfalls. J Natl Cancer Inst. 1988;80(2):84–9.
45. Watanabe M, Yavagal DR. Intra-arterial delivery of mesenchymal stem cells. Brain Circ. 2016;2(3):114–7.
46. Burgess A, Ayala-Grosso CA, Ganguly M, Jordao JF, Aubert I, Hynynen K. Targeted delivery of neural stem cells to the brain using MRI-guided focused ultrasound to disrupt the blood-brain barrier. PLoS One. 2011;6(11):e27877.
47. Guzman R, Janowski M, Walczak P. Intra-arterial delivery of cell therapies for stroke. Stroke. 2018;49(5):1075–82.
48. Joshi S, Meyers PM, Ornstein E. Intracarotid delivery of drugs: the potential and the pitfalls. Anesthesiology. 2008;109(3):543–64.
49. Lee JS, Hamilton MG, Zabramski JM. Variations in the anatomy of the rabbit cervical carotid artery. Stroke. 1994;25(2):501–3.
50. Joshi S, Wang M, Hartl R. Retinal discoloration test. J Cereb Blood Flow Metab. 2004;24(3):305–8.
51. Yousem DM, Trinh BC. Injection rates for neuroangiography: results of a survey. AJNR Am J Neuroradiol. 2001;22(10):1838–40.
52. Khatri P, Broderick JP, Khoury JC, Carrozzella JA, Tomsick TA, Ims I, et al. Microcatheter contrast injections during intra-arterial thrombolysis may increase intracranial hemorrhage risk. Stroke. 2008;39(12):3283–7.
53. Liang T, Zhang X, Li J, Hua X, Zhao P, Ji X. Intra-arterial chemotherapy as primary treatment for advanced unilateral retinoblastoma in China. Front Med (Lausanne). 2022;9:855661.
54. Shen LH, Li Y, Chen J, Zhang J, Vanguri P, Borneman J, et al. Intracarotid transplantation of bone marrow stromal cells increases axon-myelin remodeling after stroke. Neuroscience. 2006;137(2):393–9.
55. Guzman R, De Los Angeles A, Cheshier S, Choi R, Hoang S, Liauw J, et al. Intracarotid injection of fluorescence activated cell-sorted CD49d-positive neural stem cells improves targeted cell delivery and behavior after stroke in a mouse stroke model. Stroke. 2008;39(4):1300–6.
56. Lu D, Li Y, Wang L, Chen J, Mahmood A, Chopp M. Intraarterial administration of marrow stromal cells in a rat model of traumatic brain injury. J Neurotrauma. 2001;18(8):813–9.
57. Sun C, Zhang AD, Chen HH, Bian J, Liu ZJ. Magnet-targeted delivery of bone marrow-derived mesenchymal stem cells improves therapeutic efficacy following hypoxic-ischemic brain injury. Neural Regen Res. 2021;16(11):2324–9.
58. Chen L, Zhang G, Khan AA, Guo X, Gu Y. Clinical efficacy and meta-analysis of stem cell therapies for patients with brain ischemia. Stem Cells Int. 2016;2016:6129579.
59. Nagpal A, Choy FC, Howell S, Hillier S, Chan F, Hamilton-Bruce MA, et al. Safety and effectiveness of stem cell therapies in early-phase clinical trials in stroke: a systematic review and meta-analysis. Stem Cell Res Ther. 2017;8(1):191.
60. Kawabori M, Shichinohe H, Kuroda S, Houkin K. Clinical trials of stem cell therapy for cerebral ischemic stroke. Int J Mol Sci. 2020;21(19):7380.
61. Yamaguchi S, Yoshida M, Horie N, Satoh K, Fukuda Y, Ishizaka S, et al. Stem cell therapy for acute/subacute ischemic stroke with a focus on intraarterial stem cell transplantation: from basic research to clinical trials. Bioengineering (Basel). 2022;10(1):33.
62. Gholamrezanezhad A, Mirpour S, Bagheri M, Mohamadnejad M, Alimoghaddam K, Abdolahzadeh L, et al. In vivo tracking of 111In-oxine labeled mesenchymal stem cells following infusion in patients with advanced cirrhosis. Nucl Med Biol. 2011;38(7):961–7.
63. Barker RA, Drouin-Ouellet J, Parmar M. Cell-based therapies for Parkinson disease—past insights and future potential. Nat Rev Neurol. 2015;11(9):492–503.
64. Anonymous. Neuroprotection: the end of an era? Lancet. 2006;368(9547):1548.
65. Wang G, Liu F, Liu F, Cao G, Gao H, Vannier MW. Design proposed for a combined MRI/computed-tomography scanner. 2013. https://spie.org/news/4860-design-proposed-for-a-combined-mri-computed-tomography-scanner#_=_.

Complication of Arterial Drug Injections: Treading Cautiously Beyond Primum Non-Nocere

16

Jake Rachiele, Phillip M. Meyers, and Shailendra Joshi

Good decisions come from experience. Experience comes from bad ones.

Mark Twain (1835–1910), American Humorist and Essayist

Introduction

The long-held adage "Primum Non-Nocere," or "first do no harm," has been considered a foundational tenet of medicine for over two millennia [1]. However, its relevance to modern medicine has recently been questioned. Modern medical and surgical interventions can be considered potentially hazardous. Therefore, avoiding harm in contemporary medicine is sometimes challenging, which questions the relevance of this ancient phrase. The proposed replacement phrase is "*Primum Noce Apte*," or "do harm appropriately," which seems more apt [2]. Modern medicine reflects the balance of the benefits and the risks. When the former outweighs the latter, a treatment can be justified. Nowhere is this debate more relevant than with intra-arterial drug delivery. A procedure that certainly carries the risks and has a chequered history of past failures. Consequently, reports of complications due to arterial drug injections exacerbate the bias against arterial drug delivery. In any meaningful review of the subject, one has to acknowledge all the complications of this mode of drug delivery, whether they are procedural or accidental. The net outcome of arterial drug injections is determined by various factors, many of which can be prevented by improved techniques and better drug formulations. Thus, complications of arterial drug injection have to be reviewed with the broadest approach. This chapter will review the complications, their pathogenic mechanisms, underlying patterns, and treatment outcomes of arterial injections collectively. To apply the knowledge to improve arterial drug delivery for neurological interventions.

Accidental arterial injections could be self-administered during substance abuse or iatrogenic in hospital settings. Self-injected complications can be due to vascular injury or are drug-related. Iatrogenic injuries could occur in three circumstances: (a) during the angiographic procedures, such as during thrombolysis for stroke; (b) in the Intensive Care Units (ICUs); and (c) in the operating rooms. In the latter cases, either an intravenous catheter is misplaced, or intravenous drugs are accidentally injected into the arterial line. Arterial chemotherapy evolved after an accidental injection of chemotherapeutic drugs and follow-up investigations [3, 4]. Complications during angiography are the subject of a separate chapter. Although the hazardous circumstances of self-administered accidental arterial injection are unlikely to occur during careful therapeutic injections, there are potential lessons that may be relevant to arterial drug development. These include complication risks that are associated with specific drugs and drug formulations observed after accidental injections. Common to both self-administered and iatrogenic injuries are injuries due to emboli such as air, thrombi, or even drug crystals and particles [5]. Those risks must be assessed relative to the benefits of treatments. Arterial drug delivery should be seen as pharmacological surgery, and the risk/benefit of the procedure has to be individually assessed in each case.

As reviewed extensively by other authors [6, 7], there are many reports of injuries due to accidental self-inflicted arte-

J. Rachiele
University of Miami, Department of Anesthesiology, Miami, FL, USA

P. M. Meyers
Columbia University, New York, NY, USA

S. Joshi (✉)
Department of Anesthesiology, Columbia University Irving Medical Center, New York, NY, USA
e-mail: sj121@cumc.columbia.edu

S. Joshi (ed.), *Arterial Treatment of Neurological Diseases*, https://doi.org/10.1007/978-3-031-80173-0_16

rial injections and how these injuries evolve in a specific pattern [6–9]. The effects range from transient pain and flushing to tissue gangrene, limb loss, and death [10–13]. Some of these injuries have been systemically investigated, and identifying their characteristics could lead to more effective treatment and safer arterial drug formulations [14, 15]. Pharmacokinetic models suggest that arterial injections can instantaneously generate effective tissue site concentrations as a fraction of whole-body dose, thereby minimizing systemic side effects [16, 17]. Generally, that concept has been applied to patients in extremis when conventional drug delivery has failed [18]. Arterial drugs have been used to treat a wide range of neurological diseases, including acute ischemic stroke, vasospasm, and tumors [19]. However, the evidence to support therapeutic applications is often weak or lacking. The lack of proven effectiveness of arterial treatments contrasts with the WADA test, where arterial anesthetic drug injections have been used to localize brain function for the last 70 years [20]. Thus, the failure of arterial drug delivery in treating neurological diseases and the possibility of complications of such injections should not dissuade us from exploring such interventions. On the contrary, it should be used to improve patient selection, delivery techniques, drug selection, and drug formulations. Yet, one must be aware of the potential complications of such interventions upfront and proceed with caution [5]. This chapter seeks to apply what we can learn from the reported complications of iatrogenic and accidental arterial injections, which could help develop safer drugs in the future.

Types of Complications

The complications of arterial drug delivery can be broadly classified as procedural and accidental. Procedural complications are not accidental and are often anticipated. They are relevant to a discussion of arterial drug injections because those risks will be a part of any drug delivery effort and have to be minimized as well. Accidental complications are the unintended injection of drugs into arteries, either iatrogenic or during illicit drug use (Fig. 16.1).

Procedural complications: Arterial drug injections carry inherent risks due to vascular access and the injection process itself. These risks are independent of the pharmacological properties of the drugs being delivered. Drug-related complications can also be due to extravasation of the contrast media that can lead to significant local injury [21]. Some complications are related to the *access site* (groin or wrist), while others are related to the target organ, such as the brain, liver, or heart. Some examples of *access site* complications include groin hematomas, retroperitoneal bleeds, dissection, vascular perforation, aneurysm formation, and nerve injury

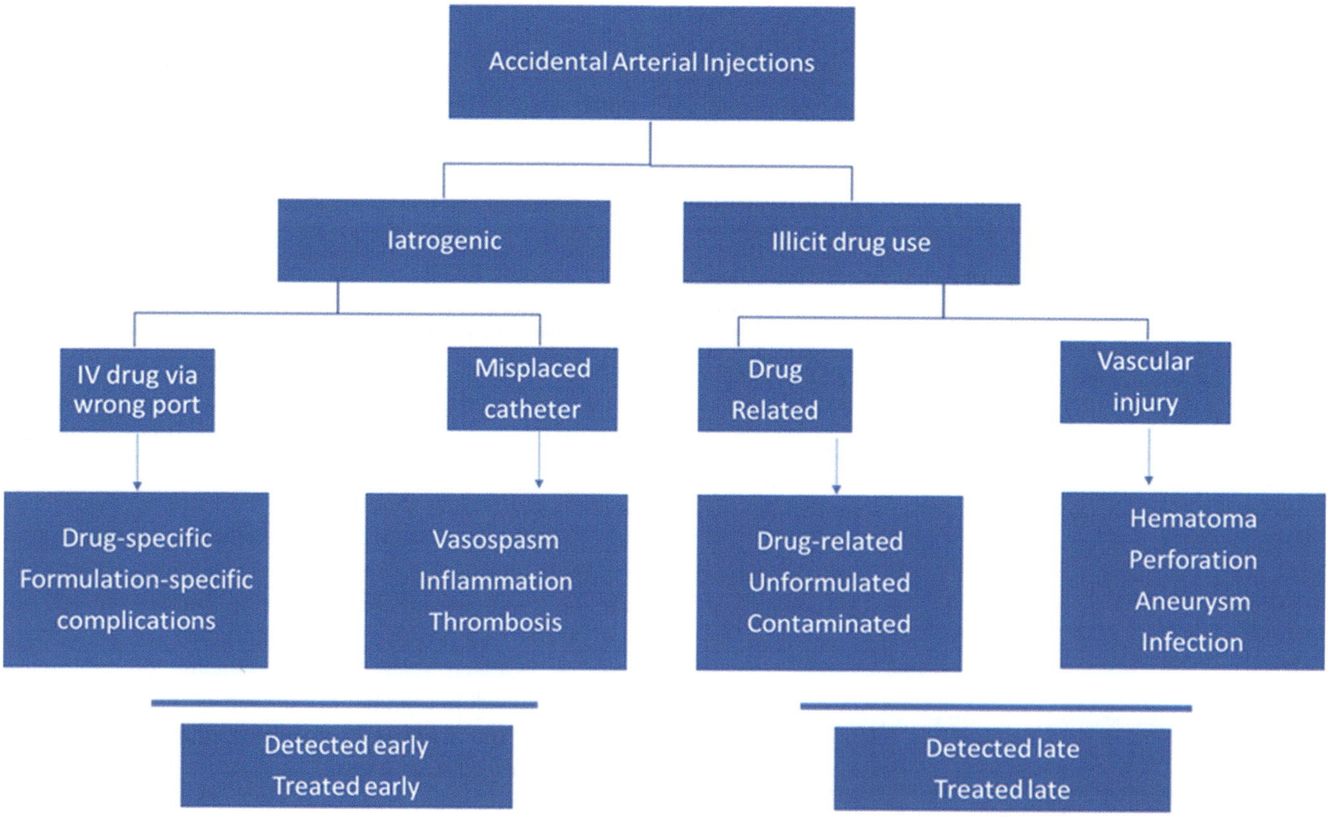

Fig. 16.1 Overview of complications due to accidental arterial injections

Table 16.1 Possible complications of cerebral angiography

Access site complications	Cerebral arterial complications	Systemic complications
Groin hematoma	Vasospasm	Arrhythmias
Retroperitoneal bleed	Dissection	Systemic embolism
Dissection	Perforation	Myocardial infarction
Pseudoaneurysm	Pseudoaneurysm	Allergic reaction
Arteriovenous malformation	Embolism	Infection
Distal thromboembolism	Stroke	Radiation injury
Thrombosis		Contrast renal injury
Trans-radial: 5% occlusion		Death

[5, 22–24]. Also, complications related to air embolism, clots, and debris from endothelial plaques could occur during angiographic procedures and accidental injections. Similarly, angiography could trigger vasospasm that could decrease blood flow. Furthermore, another aspect of procedural risk is that arterial drug delivery may require temporary arrest of blood flow to augment drug delivery [25–28]. Flow arrest methods, such as balloon occlusion, adenosine cardiac pause [29–31], or rapid ventricular pacing [32], are available. The potential ischemic complications of each of these methods must be assessed for the target organ. Complications could be due to the high injection pressure that could lead to hemorrhagic transformation, such as in necrotic tumors or infarcted [32, 33]. Table 16.1 lists the potential complications of arterial drug delivery for treating neurological diseases that could occur irrespective of therapeutic compounds. While the complication rates of cerebral angiography are exceedingly low, any drug delivery procedure has to consider these complications and whether the drugs could enhance such risks [22]. For example, melphalan suppresses platelet function [34]. Could it increase the risk of bleeding into tumors that might have structurally weak vessels and lead to hemorrhages, such as those seen with retinoblastoma treatment? [32] The risks of angiographic procedures can be mitigated by recognizing high-risk populations, adequate hydration, measures to minimize thromboembolic risk, better catheters and guide wire use, and close radiological and clinical patient monitoring during and after the procedure. Further, the mitigation of complications of angiography is discussed in the next chapter.

Iatrogenic complications due to drugs: Excessive concentration of the drugs achieved by arterial injection can be locally toxic to tissues. In addition, when higher doses are used, there can be systemic toxicity as well. In the case of the liver, arterial chemotherapy is associated with chemical hepatitis, sclerosing cholangitis, and biliary toxicity [35]. Thus, low-dose 5FU or chemotherapeutic drug combinations have been developed to minimize hepatotoxicity [36]. Another therapeutic injury associated with arterial chemotherapy of brain tumors is white matter injury after intra-arterial carmustine treatment [37]. White matter has less blood flow and a higher lipid content than gray matter or brain tumors. Therefore, there is a potential trapping of the BCNU and ACNU, which are highly lipid-soluble in the white matter. Retaining these drugs in the white matter could explain the white matter injury after such treatments. Similarly, with stem cell therapy, careful dosing of cells is necessary to prevent embolic injury [38, 39]. Thus, iatrogenic injuries with arterial drugs can occur even during planned procedures and may require careful dose titrations.

Accidental complications can be *iatrogenic,* caused by trained personnel under sterile conditions, or due to *drug misuse* with their illicit use.

Accidental iatrogenic complications typically occur in the critical care units or the ORs when intravenous drugs are accidentally injected into an established arterial line. With the increased use of invasive blood pressure monitoring, there have been several reports of accidental injections into arterial lines. The subject of accidental arterial injection has been extensively reviewed by Sen et al. in 2005 and, more recently, by Lokoff et al. in 2019 [6, 7]. In these reviews, both authors list the reports of accidental arterial drug injections, the manifestations, and treatment outcomes. A summary of their report is presented in Table 16.2. The most significant iatrogenic injuries have occurred after injecting phenytoin [41–43] and promethazine [6, 12, 44]. In the case of phenytoin, progressive gangrene eventually led to the individual's death [42]. In the case of promethazine, there was extensive tissue damage, requiring surgery and resulting in persistent painful disability and significant depression. Arterial injections have been used for deliberate drug delivery in critical situations. There are case reports of intentional arterial injection of atropine [45] and midazolam [46] when intravenous access was not feasible, no complications with drug injections were reported. In the 1950s, arterial access was used for fluid resuscitation during the Korean War, although the practice was later abandoned [47].

Complications during the illicit use of drugs are seen in substance abuse cases who accidentally or deliberately inject drugs into the arteries. These are usually injections of crushed tablets or powders prepared in unsterile conditions [48–52] and contain tablet fragments and physical stabilizers like cellulose, whose emboli can obstruct blood flow [48]. Furthermore, drug abuse can result in severe injury due to the repeated use of these compounds, the desire to conceal, and the delay in seeking help [53, 54].

Table 16.2 Treatment and outcome of accidental arterial injections [6, 7, 40]

Severity	Drugs
No injury-after discontinuation transient effects, no treatment needed	Propofol, midazolam, dopamine infusion, neostigmine and glycopyrrolate, neostigmine and atropine, Demerol, aminocaproic acid, rocuronium and fentanyl, dexmedetomidine, succinylcholine, atropine, sugammadex
No injury with medical treatment (analgesics, anti coagulation, nitroglycerine, hot compresses)	Atracurium, small doses of pentothal, ephedrine
No injury with surgical Rx (blocks, IA thrombolysis)	Azlocillin, chlordiazepoxide
Chronic residue, despite treatment	Diazepam, clindamycin
Severe injury despite intense Rx (blocks, thrombolysis, debridement, amputation)	Diazepam, temazepam, chlordiazepoxide, pentazocine, meperidine, paracetamol/benzyl alcohol, benzylpenicillin, floxacillin, clindamycin, amiodarone, diclofenac/benzyl alcohol, thiopental, secobarbital, methohexital, phenytoin, cocaine, amphetamines
Fatal	Phenytoin

Pathogenesis

- *Regional toxicity of arterial drugs*: *Regional* complications that occur after intentional arterial injections may involve additional mechanisms of injury that are unexplained by systemic pharmacodynamics. These could be due to (a) *Excessive concentrations*: PET studies show that arterial injections can achieve peak tissue concentrations 50× greater than intravenous injections [55]. Predicting the peak regional concentrations after arterial drug injections is challenging due to the interaction between the complex hemodynamic and pharmacokinetic factors [56, 57]. An example of dose-related side effects is propofol injection for the localization of brain functions. During Wada testing, 10 mg of propofol is well tolerated, but a higher dose of 20 mg leads to seizures and transient neurological symptoms [58]. Such small doses of propofol given intravenously are anticonvulsive and usually cause minimal sedation. (b) *Regional toxicity*: Complications may also be due to a tissue-specific injury seen only with regional administration—for example, intra-arterial papaverine treatment for cerebral vasospasm results in neurological side effects [59–61]. These could be due to the neurotoxic effects of papaverine, which are also seen with direct topical application [62–64]. (c) *Pharmacological nonspecificity*: Arterial papaverine also provides an excellent example of a drug with diverse cellular effects, making it difficult to establish causation should a complication occur [61]. Due to neurological complications, verapamil has largely replaced papaverine for intra-arterial treatment of cerebral vasospasm [65]. (d) *Hemodynamic effects*: Side effects of arterial drugs could be due to the hemodynamic effects of the drug. These may result in an excessive rise of ICP with intra-arterial vasodilators or redistribution of blood flow due to cerebral steal [66–68]. (e) *Micro-crystallization* of the drugs can also be a factor in regional injury and is suspected in the case of papaverine [60, 61]. It could also factor in neurological complications seen with intra-arterial mannitol when used to disrupt the blood–brain barrier for treating brain tumors. (f) *Preservative toxicity*: The use of solvent in drugs such as chlorobutanol [63, 69] or methylparaben [70, 71] has also been associated with complications due to neurotoxicity or allergic reactions [72]. The former has been invoked to explain papaverine's toxicity, while the latter may explain pallor after accidental arterial lidocaine injection. (g) *Solvents and lipid solubility*: The presence of benzyl alcohol and greater lipid solubility of the drug increase the likelihood of complications after arterial injections [73–76]. (h) *Effect of tissue perfusion*: Tissue perfusion can affect regional toxicity. For example, accidental drug infusion into the brachial artery can lead to blistering and skin necrosis. Yet, arterial injections of the same dose and concentrations in a high-flow organ such as the kidney are tolerated [3].
- *Complications of accidental iatrogenic injection of drugs*: Although Goyanes developed the arterial drug injection technique in 1908, the complications of accidental arterial injection were first described in 1942 [77]. By the decade's end, several reports emerged regarding the severe complications of accidental arterial injections of anesthetic drugs. Although intravenous drugs were first experimented with in the seventeenth century, they did not find wide application until the emergence of antibiotics and anesthetic drugs in the late 1930s. There is no recent epidemiological data on the incidence of accidental iatrogenic arterial injections. Accidental iatrogenic injections have been historically cited to occur in 1: 3500–1:55,000 of general anesthetics. Yet, there is suspicion that many of such accidents go unreported [6, 7].

The risk factors for accidental arterial injection include the following. *Site of injection*: Antecubital fossa where veins and arteries are nearby or in the forearm/radial groove with high branching radial artery. That could result in unrecognized arterial placement of a venous catheter. In patients with *indwelling arterial* lines with ports arterial and venous ports in close proximity to each otherports resulting in accidental injection into the arterial line. In patients with *impaired consciousness* who cannot respond to pain due to such injections. Patients with *difficult IV access,* such as those who are obese or with obliterated limb venous network due to past repeat injections.

Accidental arterial injections in clinical practice often involve benzodiazepines [48, 78], psychiatric drugs [79], and antibiotics [80–82]. The consequence of such injection can range from mild transient discomfort to limb gangrene, amputation, and even death (Table 16.2). These may require minimal treatment or result in severe disability with crippling physical and psychological effects. Accidental injections reveal that water-soluble drugs are usually well-tolerated. Complications are more likely with poorly water-soluble drugs. In experimental animals, injection of ketamine was safe, but that of diazepam caused injury [83]. Aqueous soluble preparation of acetaminophen was safe, but that with benzyl alcohol caused significant injuries [84].

- *Complications of accidental arterial injection due to misuse of drugs*: Illicit use of drugs poses many additional challenges that are not seen with accidental iatrogenic injections. These injections are often undertaken in unhygienic conditions, using unsterile needles and syringes by untrained individuals. Thus, they carry substantial risks of vascular injury and infection. In addition, the drugs are reconstituted by crushing tablets dissolved in unsterile water. Crushing tablets that often contain binding agents, such as cellulose, predispose to embolic injury [48, 49, 85]. Most cases of accidental arterial injection with illicit drugs involve benzodiazepines, usually in the forearm. Due to the desire to conceal the complications and the repetitive nature of substance abuse, intervention is often delayed, and the consequences are severe [50, 53, 54].

Presentation

Injuries due to accidental arterial injection of drugs usually present with signs and symptoms that tend to appear in a specific sequence (Table 16.3) [6, 7, 86, 87]. Immediately during injection, there is pain, usually accompanied by blanching or unexplained skin flushing. Although arterial pulses are present, capillary perfusion diminishes over the next few hours. Subsequently, edema, ischemia, compartment syndrome, inflammation, and necrosis set in. Prevention and mitigation of accidental or intentional arterial injection injuries require awareness that these injuries can occur despite precautions [86]. Thus, the early detection of accidental injection is of paramount importance.

Table 16.3 Clinical evolution of arterial drug injections

Time	Symptoms and signs	Possible mechanism
Immediately (0–30 min)	Pain during injection Blanching Flushing Numbness possible Weakness possible	Antidromic pain response Norepinephrine release Vasospasm Lipid embolization Microcrystal emboli Osmotic stress
Early (30 min to 4 h)	Pulses palpable Capillary perfusion impaired Nail bed pallor Poor capillary refill	Endothelial injury Inflammation Vasospasm
4–24 h	Skin mottling Venous congestion Numbness Muscle cramps Motor weakness Cold limb	Inflammation Thrombosis
Day 1–2	Increasing pain Tissue edema Loss of motor functions Compartment syndrome	Inflammation Ischemia
Day 2–7	Rhabdomyolysis Contracture	Ischemia Necrosis
Day 7–14	Tissue necrosis Gangrene	Surgical intervention and repair

Mechanism of Tissue Injury

Figure 16.2 illustrates the factors and mechanisms that cause tissue injury after arterial injection. However, most mechanisms ignore the effect of underlying blood flow. Over the last 70 years, many injury reports have occurred after arterial injection into the limbs [88]. Yet, during Wada testing, anesthetic drugs have been safely used when injected into the carotid artery [89–92]. The lack of tissue injury could be due to a high cerebral blood flow of 50 mL/100 g/min compared to the skin's 2–4 mL/100 g/min [93, 94]. Due to the high blood flow, drugs are diluted and buffered during cerebral arterial injections, but there is hardly any dilution with a limb injection. Consequently, the tissue toxic effects of anesthetic drugs are more potentiated with limb injections. Due to low tissue perfusion, factors such as concentration, pH, and lipid solubility play a much more significant role in determining injury severity.

The pathogenic mechanisms of tissue injury after arterial injection include [6, 7, 83]:

- Endothelial injury:
  - Endothelial cell toxicity due to high concentrations of delivered drugs.
  - Osmotic stress with hypertonic drug formulations, such as mannitol and sodium bicarbonate.
  - Injury is associated with lipid-soluble drugs, while most water-soluble drugs seem safe.
  - Drug preservatives such as benzyl alcohol are associated with endothelial cell injury.
- Vasospasm: vasospasm after arterial drug injection associated with injuries is biphasic. An initial vasospastic response is immediate and lasts about 15 min. A second phase of vasospasm begins after 24 h.
  - Arterial wall punctures sometimes cause minimal pain. Thus, excessive or unanticipated pain during any injection should be carefully assessed.
  - Pain with an arterial propofol injection is not associated with tissue injury.
  - Norepinephrine plays a critical role as vasospasm can be enhanced or attenuated after arterial drug injection by pretreatment with norepinephrine agonists and antagonists, respectively.
  - Endothelial injury leads to platelet activation and the loss of endothelium-derived vasodilators, thus predisposing to vasospasm and altered response to circulating vasodilators.
- Tissue ischemia:
  - Precipitation of highly alkaline drugs, such as thiopental, can result in crystallization and microcrystal embolization.
  - Hemolysis of RBC and platelet activation and tissue hypoperfusion leading to thrombus formation
  - Inflammation, edema, and compartment syndrome

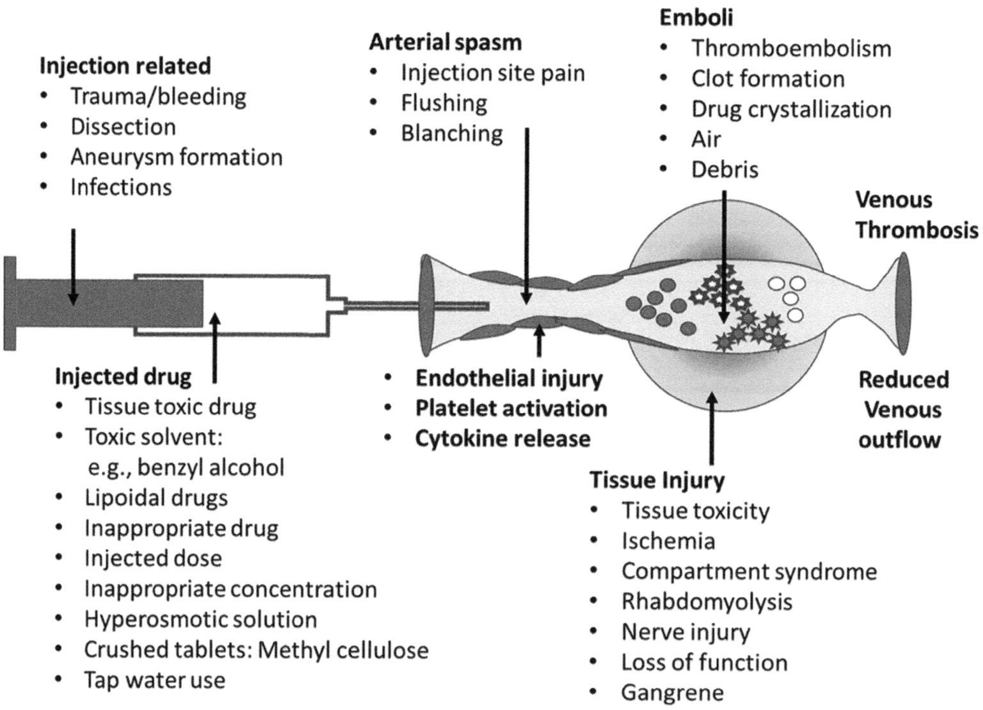

Fig. 16.2 Pathogenic mechanisms of accidental arterial drug injection injuries

Complications of Therapeutic Arterial Interventions

The incidence of complications with arterial administration of drugs in treating neurological disease is listed in Table 16.4. Neurological disease treatment poses many challenges that are not seen with other tissues. Neural tissue is structurally complex. It is exceedingly well perfused. It is vulnerable to ischemic injury. In addition, the blood–brain barrier, which protects it, prevents the uptake of many drugs. The functional impact of any injury to neural tissue can be devastating. Studies cited in the table are representative of the expected complication rates. However, all these studies are retrospective reviews and may underestimate the incidence of the injury because some of these complications are transient and may be. There is also some consideration as to the definition of each complication. For instance, the incidence of encephalopathy in WADA testing was 7.2%, with total complications at 11% [100], while most publications list complication rates of 2% or less.

Two clinical applications of arterial drugs are the treatment of retinoblastoma and advanced primary and secondary liver cancers. The complications for both these treatments are vascular access complications and cytotoxicity of drugs. Hepatic artery chemotherapy can result in inadvertent drug perfusion into the gastric or cystic artery, causing gastritis or gallbladder necrosis. Proper catheterization techniques and cholecystectomy have decreased the likelihood of these complications. Similarly, despite selective ophthalmic artery catheterization, there are extraocular complications of treatment in retinoblastoma. The reported complications of retinoblastoma include pigmentation of the retina (47%), III Cranial Nerve palsy (40%), vitreous hemorrhage (27%), orbital edema (20%), and permanent retinal detachment (7%) [101]. However, with a success rate of 80%, the procedure's risks can be justified as an alternative to surgery. Significant complications arising from chemotherapeutic drugs have also been reported with hepatic artery infusion chemotherapy, which includes liver injury. Yet, hepatic artery chemotherapy is now a well-accepted technique for advanced liver cancer treatments as it significantly improves survival with advanced diseases. In both these cases, efforts are underway to seek safer catheterization techniques and less toxic drug combinations [35, 102].

Table 16.4 Representative studies on complications of specific arterial drug interventions

Osmotic BBB disruption (mannitol) [95]	IA chemotherapy [96]	Wada testing (anesthetic drugs) [97]	Vasospasm (verapamil) [98]	Thrombolysis (rTPA) [99]
17 patients 210 procedures	48 patients 392 procedures	436 patients	189 patients 346 procedures	451 patients
Focal seizures (13%)	Groin hematomas (2.6%)	Hematoma (3%)	Vessel dissection (2%)	Symptomatic ICH (4%)
Vasospasm (9%)	Carotid dissection (0.5%)	Seizures (1.4%)	Cognitive impairment (1.1%)	Intracerebral bleed (0.2); extracranial bleed (0.4%)
Inc. HR with ST seg dep. (4.3%)	Seizures (1.5%)	ICA vasospasm (0.5%)	Vessel perforation (0.5%)	Angioedema (0.4%); anaphylaxis (0.2%)
Generalized seizures (2%)	Transient visual disturbances Hemiparesis (1.8%)	Encephalopathy (0.3%)	Intractably raised ICP (0.5%)	Epistaxis (0.2%) GI bleed (0.2%) Gum bleed (0.2%)
Impaired cognition (7.6%)	Popliteal emboli (0.25%)	Status (0.2%)		
Nausea/Vomiting (11.9%)				
Headache (6%)				
Transient motor deficits (3.8%)				

Management

The prevention of complications due to arterial drug injection begins with the proper scientific rationalization of the treatment, proper drug selection, appropriate formulation, avoidance of known potentiators, safe delivery, close monitoring during and after delivery, and immediate intervention as needed (Fig. 16.3) [86].

These complications are likely when the target site is poorly perfused, such as in limb vessels. Poor perfusion leads to higher injected concentration, increased time for tissue drug uptake, and prolonged clearance from the target site. Furthermore, to enhance safety, drugs have to be suitably formulated for arterial injection; lipid formulation should be carefully assessed, and toxic preservatives avoided. As shown in Table 16.2, a wide range of compounds can be tolerated with a low risk of complications. Although micellar preparations such as propofol cause pain on injection, they are unlikely to cause injury. Robust bench research should precede any use of therapeutic compounds backed by phase I and II studies, which is not the case in many instances. The use of arterial drugs is often clinically justified in extremis when conventional treatments are no longer effective. This is neither a good rationale for the use of arterial drugs nor a fair basis to assess their effectiveness or resulting complications.

Developing screening for drugs and drug formulations specifically for arterial injections is necessary to enhance the safety of such injections. Careful attention should be paid to catheter selection, execution of the delivery method, safety of flow control, safe pulse design, monitoring injection pressure, and technically adept execution of the angiographic procedure. Judicious anticoagulation should be used to avoid thromboembolic complications. All these measures are ignored during accidental injections, and the consequences can be dire.

Managing accidental arterial injection: Accidental arterial injections are not so rare. Almost 30% of the directors were aware of one or more accidental arterial injections in their intensive care units in the UK in the preceding 5 years [86]. The broad approach for treating both iatrogenic and illicit injections is managed similarly. They are mainly based on reversing the anticipated pathogenic mechanisms, as due to the sporadic nature of these events, a randomized control trial is challenging to undertake. Thus, the broad protocols for management have changed little over time [6, 7, 86, 87], and consist of the following:

- In case of iatrogenic accidental infusion, assess the risk and keep the catheter in situ for:
  - Angiography
  - Thrombolysis: intra-arterial thrombolysis with
    - Urokinase
    - Streptokinase
- Initiate anticoagulation with heparin unless otherwise contraindicated
- Pain management
- Limb elevation
- Massage
- Regional nerve block to annul pain and increase blood flow
- Antibiotics as needed
- Hyperbaric oxygen therapy
- Monitor:
  - Clinical: Observe capillary refill, cyanosis, skin temperature, and sensory deficits. If, at 48 h, two or fewer of these symptoms are evident, there is a 90% chance of recovery
  - Doppler
  - Angiography

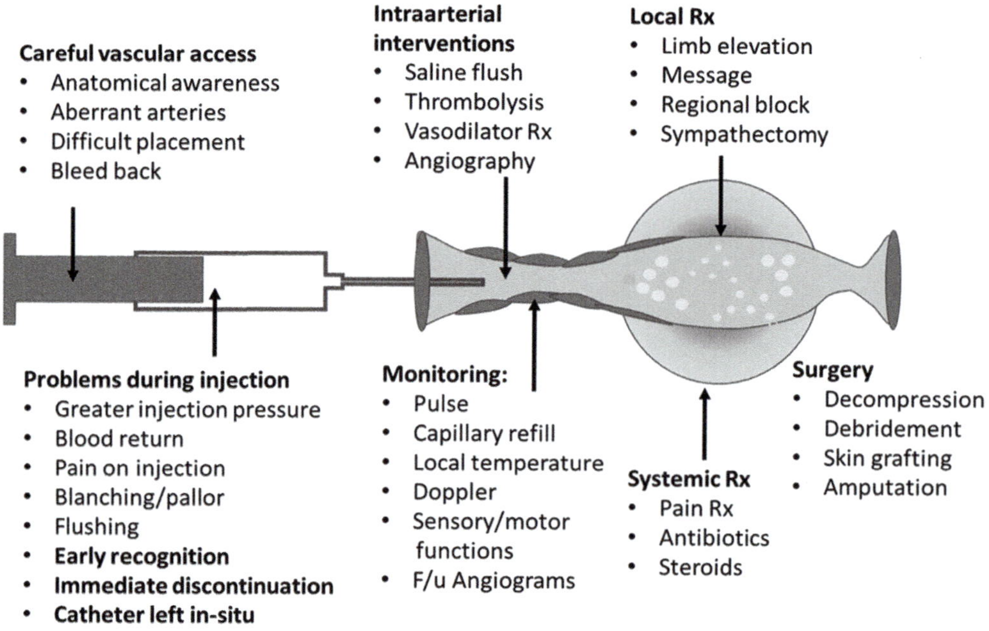

Fig. 16.3 Prevention and treatment of accidental arterial injection injuries

- Sympathectomy, corticosteroids, and vasodilators have not proven to be effective
- Surgical interventions and rehabilitative care as needed

Conclusions

The objective of presenting this chapter is primarily to emphasize the risks of arterial drug delivery. Figure 16.4 illustrates the overall view of measures that could enhance the safety of arterial drug injections. Complications resulting from accidental arterial injections could provide valuable experience to guide safer arterial injections. Arterial chemotherapy developed after an unintentional injection of nitrogen mustard into the brachial artery that caused severe skin reactions. However, those effects were transient and would not exclude using such an approach to treat fatal diseases like cancers. Inherent in any arterial treatment are access-related complications. Acutely, there is the risk of vascular injury, plaque, air, and thromboembolism risk. Chronically, there is the risk of thrombosis, perforation, migration, and aneurysm formation. Thus, arterial drug delivery should be considered as tissue-level pharmacological surgery. A risk-benefit analysis will be needed for treatment on a case-by-case basis. Given the profound impact of neurological diseases, risk avoidance is not an option.

Patient selection for arterial drug treatments will require careful assessment of comorbidities, pathology, and drug interventions. Even, for a given diagnosis detailed imaging and assessment of the angioarchitecture of the pathology will be an additional consideration. The altering the flow pattern, safely disrupting the BBB, and manipulating blood flow will be needed to deliver drugs effectively. The success of delivery will determine the treatment's course and effectiveness. The cumulative risks of arterial drug interventions must be justified before such treatments. Complications of accidental injections illustrate the hazards of such interventions that sometimes occur even in the hands of trained personnel. This chapter reviewed the complications of arterial drug injections. Its strategic objective was to learn from accidental arterial injections that could help formulate drugs for arterial delivery. These drugs should avoid endothelial cell injury. They should preferably be water soluble, without toxic preservatives or solvents, avoid precipitation or crystallization after injection, and be administered in safe concentrations. Arterial drug delivery is a complex problem, yet it is the only way tissue-level medicine can be undertaken relatively safely. Learning from complications of accidental injections may help to develop safer drugs. Drugs that could offer novel treatment of neurological diseases, some of which have hitherto defied conventional medical interventions. *Gratias Tibi Primum Non-Nocere, Salvete Primium Noce Apate!*

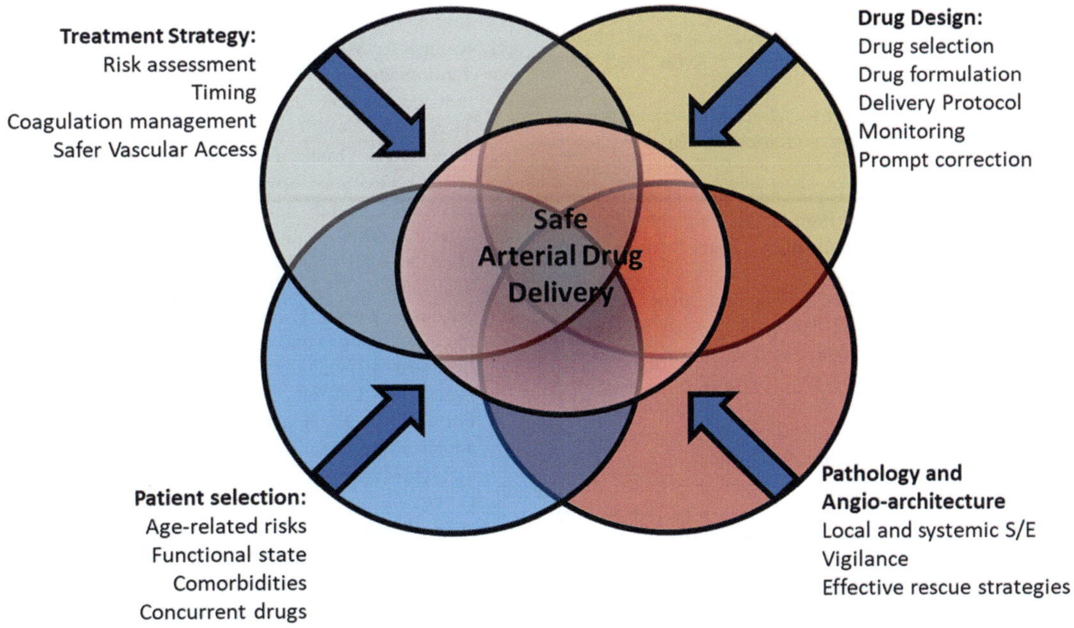

Fig. 16.4 An overview of safe arterial drug delivery

References

1. Smith CM. Origin and uses of primum non nocere—above all, do no harm! J Clin Pharmacol. 2005;45(4):371–7.
2. Bernstein J. Not the last word: Primum non nocere is harmful. Primum noce apte may help. Clin Orthop Relat Res. 2023;481(2):211–3.
3. Klopp CT, Alford TC, Bateman J, Berry GN, Winship T. Fractionated intra-arterial cancer; chemotherapy with methyl bis amine hydrochloride; a preliminary report. Ann Surg. 1950;132(4):811–32.
4. Klopp CT, Alford TC, Bateman J, Berry GN, Winship T. Fractionated intra-arterial cancer; chemotherapy with methyl bis amine hydrochloride; a preliminary report. Trans Meet Am Surg Assoc Am Surg Assoc. 1950;68:490–511.
5. Omeh DJ, Shlofmitz E. Angiography. Florida: StatPearls Publishing; 2023. https://www.ncbi.nlm.nih.gov/books/NBK557477/.
6. Sen S, Chini EN, Brown MJ. Complications after unintentional intra-arterial injection of drugs: risks, outcomes, and management strategies. Mayo Clin Proc. 2005;80(6):783–95.
7. Lokoff A, Maynes JT. The incidence, significance, and management of accidental intra-arterial injection: a narrative review. Can J Anaesth. 2019;66(5):576–92.
8. Stone HH, Donnelly CC. The accidental intraarterial injection of thiopental. Anesthesiology. 1961;22:995–1006.
9. Ellertson DG, Lazarus HM, Auerbach R. Patterns of acute vascular injury after intra-arterial barbiturate injection. Am J Surg. 1973;126(6):813–7.
10. Mazumder JK, Metcalf IR, Holland AJ. Inadvertent intra-arterial injection of thiopentone. Can Anaesth Soc J. 1980;27(4):395–8.
11. Khan ZH, Noorbaksh S. An accidental intra-arterial injection of thiopental on the dorsum of the foot—a case report. Acta Anaesthesiol Taiwan. 2004;42(1):55–8.
12. Mahajan SS, Tandon VR, Sarin R, Roshi, Gupta AK, Kohli A. Digital gangrene induced by inadvertent intra-arterial cocktail injection of anesthetic agents such as pentazocine, promethazine, and atropine: a serious adverse drug experience. Indian J Pharmacol. 2018;50(6):354–7.
13. Malik A, Ikramullah, Khan MG, Ali Shah SM, Ilyas M. Accidental intra arterial injection and limb ischemia. J Ayub Med Coll Abbottabad. 2017;29(2):230–3.
14. MacPherson RD, McLeod LJ, Grove AJ. Intra-arterial thiopentone is directly toxic to vascular endothelium. Br J Anaesth. 1991;67(5):546–52.
15. Hanci V, Ozbilgin S, Ozbal S, Kamaci G, Ates H, Boztas N, et al. Evaluation of the effects of intra-arterial sugammadex and dexmedetomidine: an experimental study. Braz J Anesthesiol. 2016;66(5):456–64.
16. Dedrick RL. Interspecies scaling of regional drug delivery. J Pharm Sci. 1986;75(11):1047–52.
17. Dedrick RL. Arterial drug infusion: pharmacokinetic problems and pitfalls. J Natl Cancer Inst. 1988;80(2):84–9.
18. Ellis JA, Banu M, Hossain SS, Singh-Moon R, Lavine SD, Bruce JN, et al. Reassessing the role of intra-arterial drug delivery for glioblastoma multiforme treatment. J Drug Deliv. 2015;2015:405735.
19. Joshi S, Meyers PM, Ornstein E. Intracarotid delivery of drugs: the potential and the pitfalls. Anesthesiology. 2008;109(3):543–64.
20. Wada JA. A fateful encounter: sixty years later—reflections on the Wada test. Epilepsia. 2008;49(4):726–7.
21. Thomas R, Vermaak L, Price G. Iodinated contrast media extravasation injuries: should osmolality and the pattern of distribution affect management?: a literature review and case report comparison. Eplasty. 2022;22:e23.
22. Fifi JT, Meyers PM, Lavine SD, Cox V, Silverberg L, Mangla S, et al. Complications of modern diagnostic cerebral angiography in an academic medical center. J Vasc Interv Radiol. 2009;20(4):442–7.
23. Al-Hijji MA, Lennon RJ, Gulati R, El Sabbagh A, Park JY, Crusan D, et al. Safety and risk of major complications with diagnostic cardiac catheterization. Circ Cardiovasc Interv. 2019;12(7):e007791.
24. Massani M, Bonariol L, Stecca T. Hepatic arterial infusion chemotherapy for unresectable intrahepatic cholangiocarcinoma, a comprehensive review. J Clin Med. 2021;10(12):2552.
25. Joshi S, Wang M, Etu JJ, Suckow RF, Cooper TB, Feinmark SJ, et al. Transient cerebral hypoperfusion enhances intraarterial carmustine deposition into brain tissue. J Neurooncol. 2008;86(2):123–32.
26. Joshi S, Wang M, Etu JJ, Nishanian EV, Pile-Spellman J. Cerebral blood flow affects dose requirements of intracarotid propofol for electrocerebral silence. Anesthesiology. 2006;104(2):290–8, discussion 5A.
27. Joshi S, Wang M, Etu JJ, Pile-Spellman J. Reducing cerebral blood flow increases the duration of electroencephalographic silence by intracarotid thiopental. Anesth Analg. 2005;101(3):851–8.
28. Riina HA, Burkhardt JK, Santillan A, Bassani L, Patsalides A, Boockvar JA. Short-term clinico-radiographic response to super-selective intra-arterial cerebral infusion of bevacizumab for the treatment of vestibular schwannomas in neurofibromatosis type 2. Interv Neuroradiol. 2012;18(2):127–32.
29. Hashimoto T, Young WL, Aagaard BD, Joshi S, Ostapkovich ND, Pile-Spellman J. Adenosine-induced ventricular asystole to induce transient profound systemic hypotension in patients undergoing endovascular therapy. Dose-response characteristics. Anesthesiology. 2000;93(4):998–1001.
30. Pile-Spellman J, Young WL, Joshi S, Duong H, Vang MC, Hartmann A, et al. Adenosine-induced cardiac pause for endovascular embolization of cerebral arteriovenous malformations: technical case report. Neurosurgery. 1999;44(4):881–6; discussion 6–7.
31. Kahn RA, Moskowitz DM, Marin ML, Hollier LH, Parsons R, Teodorescu V, et al. Safety and efficacy of high-dose adenosine-induced asystole during endovascular AAA repair. J Endovasc Ther. 2000;7(4):292–6.
32. Monroy JE, Orbach DB, VanderVeen D. Complications of intra-arterial chemotherapy for retinoblastoma. Semin Ophthalmol. 2014;29(5–6):429–33.
33. Zhang J, Yang Y, Sun H, Xing Y. Hemorrhagic transformation after cerebral infarction: current concepts and challenges. Ann Transl Med. 2014;2(8):81.
34. Klener P, Kubisz P, Suranova J. Influence of cytotoxic drugs on platelet functions and coagulation in vitro. IV. Melphalan. Thromb Haemost. 1977;37(1):53–61.
35. Laface C, Laforgia M, Molinari P, Ugenti I, Gadaleta CD, Porta C, et al. Hepatic arterial infusion of chemotherapy for advanced hepatobiliary cancers: state of the art. Cancers (Basel). 2021;13(12):3091.
36. Cercek A, Boerner T, Tan BR, Chou JF, Gonen M, Boucher TM, et al. Assessment of hepatic arterial infusion of floxuridine in combination with systemic gemcitabine and oxaliplatin in patients with unresectable intrahepatic cholangiocarcinoma: a phase 2 clinical trial. JAMA Oncol. 2020;6(1):60–7.

37. Rosenblum MK, Delattre J-Y, Walker RW, Shapiro WR. Fatal necrotizing encephalopathy complicating treatment of malignant gliomas with intra-arterial BCNU and irradiation: A pathological study. Journal of Neuro-Oncology. 1989;7(3):269–81.
38. Watanabe M, Yavagal DR. Intra-arterial delivery of mesenchymal stem cells. Brain Circ. 2016;2(3):114–7.
39. Guzman R, Janowski M, Walczak P. Intra-arterial delivery of cell therapies for stroke. Stroke. 2018;49(5):1075–82.
40. McCullum A, Reid D. Management of accidental intra-arterial injections. World Federation of Societies of Anesthesiologists; 2023. https://resources.wfsahq.org/atotw/management-of-accidental-intra-arterial-injections/.
41. Khan ZH, Faghihnassiri S. An accidental intra-arterial injection of phenytoin in a 43-year-old woman. Saudi J Anaesth. 2016;10(3):342–4.
42. McLean CR, Cheng KS, Clifton MA. Fatal case of accidental intra-arterial phenytoin injection. Eur J Vasc Endovasc Surg. 2002;23(4):378–9.
43. Sintenie JB, Tuinebreijer WE, Kreis RW, Breederveld RS. Digital gangrene after accidental intra-arterial injection of phenytoin (epanutin). Eur J Surg. 1992;158(5):315–6.
44. Mostafavi H, Samimi M. Accidental intra-arterial injection of promethazine HCl during general anesthesia: report of a case. Anesthesiology. 1971;35(6):645–6.
45. Fikkers BG, Wuis EW, Wijnen MH, Scheffer GJ. Intraarterial injection of anesthetic drugs. Anesth Analg. 2006;103(3):792–4.
46. Ali MA, Yahya M. Intentional intra-arterial injection of midazolam in a patient with status epilepticus in the intensive care unit. Saudi J Anaesth. 2017;11(4):476–8.
47. Vyskocil JJ, Kruse JA, Wilson RF. Techniques for vascular access when venous entry is impossible. Route depends on urgency and the agent to be administered. J Crit Illn. 1993;8(4):539–45.
48. Détriché G, Goudot G, Khider L, Galloula A, Guillet M, Lillo-Le Louët A, et al. Acute digital ischemia after arterial injection of crushed zolpidem tablets: role of microcrystalline cellulose? A case report. Front Pharmacol. 2020;11:560382.
49. Gramenz P, Roberts D, Schrag L. Intra-arterial self-injection of methadone tablets into the femoral artery. J Emerg Med. 2010;39(3):e125–7.
50. Leifert JA, Bossaller L, Uhl M. Acute ischaemia of the leg following accidental intra-arterial injection of dissolved flunitrazepam tablets. Vasa. 2008;37(4):374–8.
51. Radeleff B, Stampfl U, Sommer CM, Bellemann N, Hyhlik-Duerr A, Weber MA, et al. Successful thrombolysis and spasmolysis of acute leg ischemia after accidental intra-arterial injection of dissolved flunitrazepam tablets. Cardiovasc Intervent Radiol. 2011;34(5):1085–9.
52. Rohm S, Staab H, Schulz H, Richter O, Aust G. Good clinical outcome after accidental intra-arterial injection of flunitrazepam tablets in 16 drug abusers with critical limb ischaemia. Eur J Vasc Endovasc Surg. 2014;47(1):61–7.
53. Cooper JC, Griffiths AB, Jones RB, Raftery AT. Accidental intra-arterial injection in drug addicts. Eur J Vasc Surg. 1992;6(4):430–3.
54. Haj-Yahia S, Rabi I, Adar R. [Ischemic complications of accidental intra-arterial injection in drug addicts]. Harefuah. 1996;131(5–6):178–80.
55. Tyler JL, Yamamoto YL, Diksic M, Theron J, Villemure JG, Worthington C, et al. Pharmacokinetics of superselective intra-arterial and intravenous [11C]BCNU evaluated by PET. J Nucl Med. 1986;27(6):775–80.
56. Hossain SS, Hughes TJ, Decuzzi P. Vascular deposition patterns for nanoparticles in an inflamed patient-specific arterial tree. Biomech Model Mechanobiol. 2014;13(3):585–97.
57. Hossain SS, Zhang Y, Liang X, Hussain F, Ferrari M, Hughes TJ, et al. In silico vascular modeling for personalized nanoparticle delivery. Nanomedicine (Lond). 2013;8(3):343–57.
58. Mikuni N, Takayama M, Satow T, Yamada S, Hayashi N, Nishida N, et al. Evaluation of adverse effects in intracarotid propofol injection for Wada test. Neurology. 2005;65(11):1813–6.
59. Tsukahara T, Yoshimura S, Kazekawa K, Hashimoto N. Intra-arterial papaverine for the treatment of cerebral vasospasm after subarachnoid hemorrhage. J Auton Nerv Syst. 1994;49(Suppl):S163–6.
60. Yoshimura S, Hashimoto N, Goto Y, Sampei K, Tsukahara T, Iihara K. Intraarterial infusion of high-concentration papaverine damages cerebral arteries in rats. AJNR Am J Neuroradiol. 1996;17(10):1891–4.
61. Joshi S, Young WL, Pile-Spellman J. Does papaverine cause endothelial injury in clinically relevant doses? AJNR Am J Neuroradiol. 1997;18(9):1797–800.
62. Kimball MM, Velat GJ, Hoh BL, Participants in the International Multi-Disciplinary Consensus Conference on the Critical Care Management of Subarachnoid Hemorrhage. Critical care guidelines on the endovascular management of cerebral vasospasm. Neurocrit Care. 2011;15(2):336–41.
63. Smith WS, Dowd CF, Johnston SC, Ko NU, DeArmond SJ, Dillon WP, et al. Neurotoxicity of intra-arterial papaverine preserved with chlorobutanol used for the treatment of cerebral vasospasm after aneurysmal subarachnoid hemorrhage. Stroke. 2004;35(11):2518–22.
64. Zhou X, Alambyan V, Ostergard T, Pace J, Kohen M, Manjila S, et al. Prolonged intracisternal Papaverine toxicity: index case description and proposed mechanism of action. World Neurosurg. 2018;109:251–7.
65. Feng L, Fitzsimmons BF, Young WL, Berman MF, Lin E, Aagaard BD, et al. Intraarterially administered verapamil as adjunct therapy for cerebral vasospasm: safety and 2-year experience. AJNR Am J Neuroradiol. 2002;23(8):1284–90.
66. Collins L, Lam L, Kleinig O, Proudman W, Zhang R, Bagster M, et al. Verapamil in the treatment of reversible cerebral vasoconstriction syndrome: a systematic review. J Clin Neurosci. 2023;113:130–41.
67. Yamaki VN, Cavalcanti DD, Figueiredo EG. Delayed ischemic neurologic deficit after aneurysmal subarachnoid hemorrhage. Asian J Neurosurg. 2019;14(3):641–7.
68. Shimamura N, Naraoka M, Matsuda N, Kakuta K, Ohkuma H. Prophylactic intra-arterial injection of vasodilator for asymptomatic vasospasm converts the patient to symptomatic vasospasm due to severe microcirculatory imbalance. Biomed Res Int. 2014;2014:382484.
69. Nordt SP. Chlorobutanol toxicity. Ann Pharmacother. 1996;30(10):1179–80.
70. Hu C, Bai Y, Sun B, Zhou X, Chen L. Exposure to methylparaben at environmentally realistic concentrations significantly impairs neuronal health in adult zebrafish. J Environ Sci (China). 2023;132:134–44.
71. Ninomiya R, Nishijima T, Aoshima M, Sakaguchi H, Tokura Y. Sensory irritation to methylparaben is caused by its low metabolism in the skin. J Dermatol. 2023;50(7):888–94.
72. Bina B, Hersh EV, Hilario M, Alvarez K, McLaughlin B. True allergy to amide local anesthetics: a review and case presentation. Anesth Prog. 2018;65(2):119–23.
73. Takadera T, Ohyashiki T. Benzyl alcohol inhibits N-methyl-D: -aspartate receptor-mediated neurotoxicity and calcium accumulation in cultured rat cortical neurons. J Biomed Sci. 2008;15(6):767–70.

74. Chang YS, Lin CF, Wu CL, Kuo PY, Wu FS, Shieh CC, et al. Mechanisms underlying benzyl alcohol cytotoxicity (triamcinolone acetonide preservative) in human retinal pigment epithelial cells. Invest Ophthalmol Vis Sci. 2011;52(7):4214–22.
75. Chang YS, Wu CL, Tseng SH, Kuo PY, Tseng SY. In vitro benzyl alcohol cytotoxicity: implications for intravitreal use of triamcinolone acetonide. Exp Eye Res. 2008;86(6):942–50.
76. Terrazas P, Salamanca E, Davila M, Manner S, Gimenez A, Sterner AO. SAR:s for the antiparasitic plant metabolite Pulchrol. 1. The benzyl alcohol functionality. Molecules. 2020;25(13):3058.
77. Van der Post C. Report of a Case of Mistaken Injection of Pentothal Sodium Into an Aberrant Ulnar Artery. Anesthesia & Analgesia. 1942;21(3):58–9.
78. Schulz S, Aksü T, Igde A, Hengstmann J. [Acute ischemia of the leg in a drug addict]. Vasa. 2002;31(1):57–61.
79. Heber R, Helmig L. [Gangrene of the hand and forearm following accidental intra-arterial injection of phenothiazines]. Med Welt. 1976;27(42):2026–28.
80. Salama T, Aghoutane EM, Fezzazi RE. [Gangrene of the hand due to accidental intra-arterial injection of floxacilline: about a case]. Pan Afr Med J. 2016;25:221.
81. Schanzer H, Gribetz I, Jacobson JH 2nd. Accidental intra-arterial injection of penicillin G. A preventable catastrophe. JAMA. 1979;242(12):1289–90.
82. Tsoulos NG. Accidental intra-arterial injection of penicillin. JAMA. 1980;243(8):733.
83. Knill RL, Evans D. Pathogenesis of gangrene following intra-arterial injection of drugs: a new hypothesis. Can Anaesth Soc J. 1975;22(6):637–46.
84. Samanta S, Chakraborty N, Samanta S. Accidental intra-arterial injection of paracetamol: different preparations, different results. Eur J Anaesthesiol. 2014;31(4):236–7.
85. Goldberg I, Bahar A, Yosipovitch Z. Gangrene of the upper extremity following intra-arterial injection of drugs. A case report and review of the literature. Clin Orthop Relat Res. 1984(188):223–29.
86. McCallum A, Reid D. Management of accidental intra-arterial injections. World Federation of Societies of Anesthesiologists; 2023. pp. 1–6. https://resources.wfsahq.org/atotw/management-of-accidental-intra-arterial-injections/.
87. Treiman GS, Yellin AE, Weaver FA, Barlow WE, Treiman RL, Gaspar MR. An effective treatment protocol for intraarterial drug injection. J Vasc Surg. 1990;12(4):456–65; discussion 65–6.
88. Prabhu R, Shenoy R, Thinda N, Patel A, Sadhu S. Be careful with an IV line. J Clin Diagn Res. 2014;8(3):166–7.
89. Curot J, Denuelle M, Busigny T, Barragan-Jason G, Kany M, Tall P, et al. Bilateral Wada test: amobarbital or propofol? Seizure. 2014;23(2):122–8.
90. Yamaguchi T, Shojima M, Delashaw JB Jr, Watanabe E. Wada test using secobarbital sodium (Ional) to determine language dominance. Br J Neurosurg. 2011;25(2):203–9.
91. Patel A, Wordell C, Szarlej D. Alternatives to sodium amobarbital in the Wada test. Ann Pharmacother. 2011;45(3):395–401.
92. Buchtel HA, Passaro EA, Selwa LM, Deveikis J, Gomez-Hassan D. Sodium methohexital (brevital) as an anesthetic in the Wada test. Epilepsia. 2002;43(9):1056–61.
93. Harris JP, McLaughlin AF, Quinn RJ, Page S, May J. Skin blood flow measurement with xenon-133 to predict healing of lower extremity amputations. Aust N Z J Surg. 1986;56(5):413–5.
94. Olesen J, Paulson OB, Lassen NA. Regional cerebral blood flow in man determined by the initial slope of the clearance of intra-arterially injected 133Xe. Stroke. 1971;2(6):519–40.
95. Elkassabany NM, Bhatia J, Deogaonkar A, Barnett GH, Lotto M, Maurtua M, et al. Perioperative complications of blood brain barrier disruption under general anesthesia: a retrospective review. J Neurosurg Anesthesiol. 2008;20(1):45–8.
96. Gelman M, Chakeres DW, Newton HB. Brain tumors: complications of cerebral angiography accompanied by intraarterial chemotherapy. Radiology. 1999;213(1):135–40.
97. Beimer NJ, Buchtel HA, Glynn SM. One center's experience with complications during the Wada test. Epilepsia. 2015;56(8):e110–3.
98. Jun P, Ko NU, English JD, Dowd CF, Halbach VV, Higashida RT, et al. Endovascular treatment of medically refractory cerebral vasospasm following aneurysmal subarachnoid hemorrhage. AJNR Am J Neuroradiol. 2010;31(10):1911–6.
99. Han TS, Gulli G, Fry CH, Affley B, Robin J, Fluck D, et al. Adverse consequences of immediate thrombolysis-related complications: a multi-centre registry-based cohort study of acute stroke. J Thromb Thrombolysis. 2022;53(1):218–27.
100. Loddenkemper T, Morris HH, Moddel G. Complications during the Wada test. Epilepsy Behav. 2008;13(3):551–3.
101. Muen WJ, Kingston JE, Robertson F, Brew S, Sagoo MS, Reddy MA. Efficacy and complications of super-selective intra-ophthalmic artery melphalan for the treatment of refractory retinoblastoma. Ophthalmology. 2012;119(3):611–6.
102. Carnevale JA, Goldberg J, Kocharian G, Rivera M, Giantini Larsen A, Garton A, et al. Intra-arterial chemotherapy for retinoblastoma. J Neurointerv Surg. 2023;15(3):303–4.

Enhancing the Safety of Angiographic Procedures for Drug Delivery: An Overview of Safety Precautions in Interventional Neuroradiology Procedures

17

Deborah Boyett, Tala Rawashdeh, and Alexander Ramos

The man who has anticipated the coming of troubles takes away their power when they arrive.

Lucius Annaeus Seneca (4 BCE–65 AD), Roman Philosopher and Playwright

Introduction

Intra-arterial drug delivery represents a pivotal advancement in the targeted treatment of various medical conditions, including cerebral vasospasm, intracranial chemotherapy, and intracranial tumors. Clinicians can achieve higher local drug concentrations by administering therapeutic agents directly into the arterial system while minimizing systemic exposure and associated side effects. However, the success of this approach, which is a testament to the effectiveness of safety protocols and technological innovations, hinges on meticulous attention to these measures that mitigate the inherent risks.

This chapter delves into the safety considerations essential for effective intra-arterial drug delivery. We will explore the historical context and technological progressions that have shaped current practices. We will emphasize the importance of safe arterial access, advanced imaging modalities, and the development of adjuvant pharmaceutical therapeutics to enhance the safety of arterial drug delivery.

History

Interventional neuroradiology utilizes radiological imaging and catheter technology to diagnose and treat vascular diseases in the central nervous system. First described by Dr. Kori in his paper titled "Interventional Neurology: a Subspeciality Whose Time Has Come," the subspecialty has evolved to cover intra-arterial procedures such as carotid angioplasty, intracranial thrombolysis, embolization, and chemotherapy, with continued evolution toward expanding therapies such as intra-arterial drug, gene, and stem-cell delivery [1, 2].

Dr. Jose Goyanes Capdevila undertook arterial drug delivery in 1908. A Spanish vascular surgeon, he envisioned and demonstrated the feasibility of intra-arterial anesthesia, which later formed the basis for the regional application of drugs used to treat neoplastic conditions through arterial and venous vascular catheterization. The first attempts at arterial drug delivery involved experiments on dogs before the discovery of X-rays, catheters, or anticoagulants, all discoveries essential to interventional radiology today. The following year, Goyanes successfully used intra-arterial anesthetics to enable surgery in 72 patients with few treatment failures [1, 2]. The original technique involved applying an Esmarch bandage, elevating the limb, and applying a compressor tube close to the armpit. A calculated quantity of the anesthetic solution is injected subcutaneously into the wrist to locate the radial artery, and catheterization of the artery is achieved—the volume and mass of the area to be anesthetized determine the quantity of the solution [3].

Several disruptive technologies of the last century have rendered interventional neuroradiology safe, enabling the wide use of neuroangiographic procedures. The notable landmarks in the evolution of concepts and techniques of interventional radiology have been reviewed elsewhere in this book. However, certain developments stand out in the context of the safety of such procedures that are enumerated here. In 1927, Dr. Egas Moniz, who later became the Chair of Neurology at the University of Lisbon in Portugal, performed the first cerebral angiogram. His initial

D. Boyett · T. Rawashdeh · A. Ramos (✉)
Columbia University, New York, NY, USA
e-mail: ar4680@cumc.columbia.edu

S. Joshi (ed.), *Arterial Treatment of Neurological Diseases*, https://doi.org/10.1007/978-3-031-80173-0_17

intent was to improve the technique of pneumoencephalography for cerebral imaging. After performing his early studies on human cadavers and dogs, Dr. Moniz began applying his techniques to living patients. Injecting a 70% solution of strontium bromide directly into the carotid arteries led to the death of 1 of his patients secondary to thrombosis of the artery. As a result, Moniz adjusted the contrast media to a more dilute iodide salt, ultimately visualizing the cranial circulation successfully [4].

Dr. Sven-Ivar Seldinger, a radiologist at the Karolinska Institute in Stockholm, introduced percutaneous vascular access in 1953, enhancing its safety. His technique involved puncturing the vessel with a hollow needle, sliding a wire into the vessel through the needle, removing the needle, and then inserting a catheter over the wire. These principles remain the basis of safe endovascular access today [5].

During the 1960s, neurosurgeons mainly performed cerebral angiograms. Mehmed Gazi Yasargil, the "father of microneurosurgery," performed extensive cerebral angiography between the 50s and 60s. In 1965, Per Amundsen, a radiologist at Ulleval Hospital in Norway, was the first to implement the Seldinger technique to catheterize great vessels from the femoral artery, bringing this technique to the United States while serving at the University of California, San Francisco [6].

Endovascular neurosurgery has revolutionized the management of various cerebrovascular conditions, providing minimally invasive alternatives to traditional surgical approaches. While offering numerous benefits, ensuring patient safety remains paramount in this specialized field. Safety in endovascular neurosurgery encompasses a comprehensive understanding of procedural risks, meticulous technique, advanced imaging guidance, and effective complication management. This chapter delves into the critical safety aspects of endovascular neurosurgery, highlighting strategies to minimize risks and optimize patient outcomes.

Preprocedural Assessment and Planning

A thorough preprocedural evaluation is fundamental to ensuring patient safety in endovascular neurosurgery [7]. This assessment includes a detailed medical history review, focusing on comorbidities, medication use, and prior neurosurgical interventions. Advanced imaging studies, such as magnetic resonance imaging (MRI) and computed tomography angiography (CTA), are essential for precise anatomical delineation and lesion characterization.

Assessment of Comorbidities

- *Cardiac function*
  - *Functional status*: The functional capacity of the cardiovascular system plays a crucial role in ensuring adequate cerebral perfusion and overall hemodynamic stability during neuroendovascular procedures. Several factors related to cardiac function must be assessed before initiation of the procedure, including baseline hemodynamic stability, procedural needs, and fluid management considerations (discussed below). Close collaboration between neurointerventionalists, anesthesiologists, and other multidisciplinary team members is essential to assess and optimize cardiac function, minimize procedural risks, and ensure the successful completion of neuroendovascular interventions while prioritizing patient safety.
  - *Hemodynamic instability risk*: Systemic blood pressure, heart rate, and cardiac output are critical for adequate cerebral perfusion during neuroendovascular procedures. Patients with compromised cardiac function, such as those with heart failure or arrhythmias, may be more prone to hemodynamic instability or bradycardic events during catheterization of the great vessels.
  - *Hemorrhagic risk*: Patients with impaired cardiac function may be at increased risk of bleeding complications during neuroendovascular procedures, especially if they are on *anticoagulant* or *antiplatelet therapy*. Cardiac conditions associated with increased bleeding risk include atrial fibrillation, mechanical heart valves, and cardiomyopathies. Close coordination with cardiology colleagues may be necessary to optimize antithrombotic management and minimize bleeding complications in these patients.
  - *Anesthetic considerations*: Patients with compromised cardiac function may have reduced tolerance to sedation or anesthesia, which can pose challenges during neuroendovascular procedures. Careful selection of anesthesia techniques and vigilant hemodynamic monitoring are essential to maintain cardiovascular stability and optimize patient safety throughout the procedure [7, 8].
- *Renal function*
  - *Baseline functions*: Creatinine, a waste product produced by muscles from the breakdown of creatine, is primarily filtered out of the blood by the kidneys and excreted through urine. Serum creatinine levels serve as a vital marker of renal function, with elevated levels indicative of impaired kidney function. Iodinated contrast agents are used for imaging guidance during endovascular procedures, and these contrast agents can exert nephrotoxic effects, particularly in patients with pre-existing renal impairment. The procedural risks and benefits must be carefully weighed, considering the potential for exacerbating renal dysfunction versus the anticipated benefit of the diagnostic or therapeutic procedure. Close monitoring of renal function pre- and

postprocedure is essential in this patient population to promptly identify and manage any decline in renal function [8].

- *Contrast-induced nephropathy (CIN) risk*: Endovascular procedures frequently use iodinated contrast agents for imaging guidance. These contrast agents can exert nephrotoxic effects, particularly in patients with pre-existing renal impairment. Elevated creatinine levels signify reduced renal function and increase the risk of contrast-induced nephropathy. Therefore, patients with elevated baseline creatinine levels are at a heightened risk of renal injury following contrast exposure during endovascular procedures. Close attention to renal function, hydration status, and judicious use of contrast agents are critical in minimizing the risk of CIN in these patients.
- *Fluid management considerations*: Adequate hydration prevents contrast-induced nephropathy. Patients with elevated creatinine levels may have compromised renal function and may require careful fluid management strategies to maintain renal perfusion and minimize the risk of renal injury. Optimizing hydration status before, during, and after endovascular procedures is essential in mitigating the risk of contrast-induced nephropathy.
- *Necessity for contrast-sparing techniques*: In patients with elevated creatinine levels and underlying renal dysfunction, minimizing contrast exposure is paramount to reducing the risk of contrast-induced nephropathy. Endovascular operators may employ various contrast-sparing techniques, such as low contrast volume protocols and intermittent fluoroscopy, whenever feasible. These strategies aim to achieve the necessary procedural goals while limiting the nephrotoxic effects of contrast agents.

- *Hepatic function*
  - *Baseline functions*: The liver is responsible for metabolizing drugs and toxins, synthesizing proteins, and regulating various metabolic processes, making its function critical in the context of endovascular interventions. Hepatic function significantly impacts the safety and outcomes of endovascular procedures through its effects on drug clearance and coagulation status. Careful patient selection, assessment of hepatic function, and periprocedural management are essential in optimizing outcomes in this patient population.
  - *Drug metabolism*: Many medications used during endovascular procedures, such as anticoagulants, antiplatelet agents, and sedatives, are metabolized by the liver. An impaired hepatic function can alter the metabolism and clearance of these medications, leading to altered pharmacokinetics and an increased risk of adverse effects or therapeutic failure. Dosage adjustments or alternative medications may be necessary for patients with hepatic dysfunction to ensure safe and effective pharmacotherapy during the procedure.
  - *Coagulation status*: The liver synthesizes several clotting factors and regulatory proteins essential for maintaining hemostasis. In patients with liver disease, particularly those with advanced cirrhosis, alterations in coagulation parameters, such as prolonged prothrombin time (PT) and reduced levels of clotting factors, may predispose to bleeding complications during endovascular procedures. Close monitoring of coagulation status and judicious use of anticoagulants and hemostatic agents are essential to mitigate the risk of bleeding in patients with hepatic dysfunction.

Procedural Planning and Navigation

Neurological imaging, such as magnetic resonance imaging (MRI) and computed tomography (CT), provides essential anatomical information. Preprocedural imaging helps identify the location and extent of neurovascular pathology, plan optimal access routes, and anticipate potential procedural challenges. By leveraging the strengths of various imaging modalities and advanced techniques, clinicians can optimize treatment strategies, improve procedural outcomes, and enhance patient care in neuroendovascular interventions.

- *Magnetic resonance imaging (MRI)*: MRI is a versatile imaging modality that offers high-resolution, multiplanar imaging of the brain and surrounding vasculature, making it invaluable in preprocedural assessment for neuroendovascular procedures. Key MRI sequences used in this context include:
  - T1-weighted imaging: Provides excellent anatomical detail and visualization of brain structures, aiding in identifying lesions, vascular anatomy, and surrounding structures.
  - T2-weighted imaging: Highlights areas of edema, ischemia, or hemorrhage, aiding in the characterization of neurovascular pathology and guiding treatment planning.
  - Diffusion-weighted imaging (DWI): Sensitive to the motion of water molecules, DWI is highly effective in detecting acute ischemic strokes and assessing tissue viability, helping determine the extent of ischemic injury, and guiding revascularization strategies.
- *Magnetic resonance angiography (MRA, time of flight based)*: This noninvasive procedure visualizes the cerebral vasculature, including arteries and veins, providing information on vascular anatomy, stenosis, or aneurysms.

- *Contrast-enhanced MRA*: This technique utilizes intravenous gadolinium-based contrast agents to enhance vascular visualization. It is beneficial for assessing dynamic vascular pathologies, such as arteriovenous malformations (AVMs) or fistulas.
- *Computed tomography (CT)*: CT imaging is widely utilized in the preprocedural evaluation of neuroendovascular pathology, offering rapid acquisition, excellent spatial resolution, and multiplanar reconstructions. Key CT sequences and techniques include:
  - *Noncontrast CT*: Provides rapid assessment of hemorrhage, ischemia, or mass effect, aiding in the identification and characterization of acute neurological conditions.
  - *CT angiography (CTA)*: This procedure utilizes intravenous contrast agents to visualize the cerebral vasculature, providing detailed information on arterial anatomy, stenosis, or occlusions.
  - *Perfusion CT*: Quantifies cerebral blood flow, volume, and mean transit time, offering valuable insights into tissue perfusion deficits and the extent of ischemic injury. It is advantageous in evaluating acute stroke patients.
- *Digital subtraction angiography (DSA)*: DSA remains the gold standard for vascular imaging in neuroendovascular procedures, offering real-time, high-resolution visualization of the cerebral vasculature. The key strength of DSA is dynamic imaging, which provides real-time visualization of blood flow dynamics, allowing for the assessment of collateral circulation, vascular filling patterns, and the presence of vascular lesions such as aneurysms or arteriovenous malformations.

Procedural Safety Measures

Sterile Technique

Strict adherence to sterile technique is imperative to minimize the risk of procedural site infections. Sterile draping, appropriate hand hygiene/mask utilization, and sterile equipment handling are essential to maintaining a sterile field.

Vascular Access

Careful selection of vascular access sites and meticulous catheter manipulation are crucial to prevent arterial injury, dissection, or perforation. Real-time fluoroscopic and ultrasonographic guidance aids in optimizing catheter placement and minimizing vascular trauma. Selecting the most suitable arterial vascular access site is the first step in ensuring the effectiveness and safety of diagnostic procedures or interventional treatment.

Femoral Access

In the United States, femoral arterial access is the most often used vascular access technique for neurointerventional procedures and cerebral angiography [9]. The artery's size and caliber allow for larger-bore equipment and robust stability of catheter systems. Femoral access is a common source of challenges during angiography and intervention and a frequently overlooked crucial component of the process [10].

- *Anatomic considerations*: The most frequent source of difficulties during catheterization is the location of the arterial puncture site beyond the common femoral artery (CFA). However, significant complications are still infrequent [11]. Understanding the common femoral artery's typical path is essential. As the external iliac artery traverses the pelvic brim at the level of the inguinal ligament, which runs from the pubic tubercle to the anterior superior iliac crest's spine, it becomes the common femoral artery. Following its passage through the femoral sheath, the CFA splits into the profunda femoris and superficial femoral arteries. The femoral nerve is located outside the femoral sheath and lateral to the femoral artery. The femoral artery is located laterally within the femoral sheath, and the femoral vein is located medially. The smallest and most medial compartment contains efferent lymphatic veins and lymph node tissue embedded in a tiny amount of areolar tissue in the femoral canal. The mnemonic "NAVEL" can be used to remember the relative location of this vasculature in the *right* groin.
- *Fluoroscopic guidance*: The inferior edge of the femoral head is observed to be associated with or above the femoral artery bifurcation. Multiple studies have verified the use of fluoroscopic guidance for femoral artery access and have found that the incidence of acquiring CFA access was comparable to anatomic methods [12–14].
  - *Steps*:

    The hemostat's tip is placed at or below the inguinal crease and verified by fluoroscopy to be near the femoral head's inferior border.

    Local anesthetic is administered at the planned site of puncture.

    A hollow-bore needle punctures at a 30–45° angle. With this trajectory, the CFA is punctured at the level of the femoral head.

    A wire is passed into the needle and verified to traverse medially toward the aorta. If it passes laterally, it is withdrawn and course redirected under fluoroscopic guidance.
  - *Advantages*:

    Most operators are familiar with this technique.

    This technique permits rapid access, and the caliber of the CFA provides a large target for puncture.

    It is possible to observe the existence and degree of vascular calcification.

- *Disadvantages*:

  Following local anesthetic infiltration, the location of the skin entrance point may differ from that of the femoral head's inferior border.

  This technique does not visualize the bifurcation and may not be accurate in patients with a high bifurcation (superior to the femoral head midpoint).

  Femoral artery access is associated with a higher risk of bleeding complications compared to radial access, particularly the dreaded retroperitoneal hematoma. The femoral artery is located deep within the groin, making it more susceptible to hematoma formation and access site-related bleeding, particularly in patients with elevated INR levels or those who are on anticoagulant therapy.

  Delayed ambulation: Depending on the closure type, patients may be required to remain on bed rest for an extended period to minimize the risk of bleeding site complications.

- *Ultrasonographic guidance*: Operators have expanded the use of ultrasound-guided venous access to include femoral arterial access. This technique significantly reduced the time needed for access and the rate of vascular access complications in a multicenter prospective randomized single-blinded trial. Though widespread adoption of this approach has been limited, it offers a suitable alternative to fluoroscopy-guided femoral access with minimum training and additional equipment [15].
  - *Steps*:

    The bifurcation is located through imaging the CFA along the long and short axes.

    The ultra-sound is directed toward the bifurcation while imaging it in the short axis.

    The needle is advanced using the dominant hand while the US probe is held in the nondominant hand. The operator may start 1 cm below the US probe depending on the needle trajectory.

    The short-axis view is reviewed for the needle tip tenting vessel.

    The needle is advanced until the tip is visualized in the vessel's lumen, and a blood backflow is observed.

    A guidewire is passed in the usual manner, and additional fluoroscopic guidance may be used to verify the trajectory of the wire.
  - *Advantages*:

    The technique enables the medical professional to identify and avoid arterial calcification, plaque, and a pulsating femoral vein.

    "Side-walling," or punctures to the side and rear walls are prevented.
  - *Disadvantages*:

    Learning curve: Operator training and expertise are necessary to become proficient with visualizing the needle tip. If the ultrasound beam intersects the proximal needle shaft rather than the tip, the depth of the needle tip may be underestimated.

    Visualizing the bifurcation relative to the femoral head is significant, as it determines the effectiveness of arterial compression after the sheath is removed. Additionally, in patients with a high bifurcation, a puncture at the CFA may increase the risk of retroperitoneal hematoma.

Radial Access

Trans-radial access (TRA) is the best-studied alternative access site in neurointervention. It has garnered growing utilization due to its reduced bleeding risk and ease of puncture site closure.

- *Anatomic considerations*: Assessment for collateral circulation in the hand may be performed using Allen's test or the Barbeau test. However, several randomized trials have found that postprocedure symptomatic hand ischemia is almost negligible regardless of the preprocedure collateral testing results.
- *Common techniques*: The diameter of the radial artery may be first assessed and measured by ultrasonography. Various measures to increase the diameter of the radial artery include topical lidocaine and nitroglycerin 30 min before puncture [16], and fluid and light anesthetic administration.
- *Ultrasonographic guidance*: The small caliber of the radial artery necessitates successful puncture at the first attempt to avoid radial artery vasospasm and subsequent inability to access the artery.
  - *Steps*:

    Local anesthetic is administered at the access site to minimize discomfort.

    The radial artery is sufficiently large for puncture and accommodation of the sheath 2–3 cm proximal to the palmar wrist crease.

    As in the femoral artery approach, ultrasonographic visualization of the needle tip is crucial for successful radial artery puncture. The artery may be punctured at a 45° angle using a micro-puncture needle tip. The micro-puncture needle is advanced until arterial blood return is observed.

    A flexible guidewire is passed through the needle and advanced gently to prevent arterial injury or dissection.

    A radial artery sheath is inserted over the guidewire. The radial artery may accommodate 5Fr and 6Fr sheath sizes.

To prevent radial artery vasospasm and occlusion, a radial "cocktail" consisting of unfractionated heparin, verapamil, and/or nitroglycerin is administered intra-arterially [17].

- *Advantages*:

  Lower bleeding risk: Radial access has a significantly lower risk of bleeding complications than femoral access. This is particularly beneficial for patients with elevated INR levels, as it reduces the risk of access site-related bleeding events.

  Reduced hematoma formation: Radial artery access typically results in smaller hematoma formation at the access site than femoral access. This advantage is particularly relevant for patients with coagulopathy or elevated INR levels, as it minimizes the risk of bleeding complications.

  Enhanced patient comfort: Radial access is generally more comfortable for patients than femoral access. The radial artery is located superficially, allowing easier access and reducing the need for deep arterial punctures. This can lead to improved patient satisfaction.

  Faster ambulation: Radial artery access enables quicker ambulation postprocedure than femoral access. Patients can often mobilize sooner and resume normal activities, reducing the length of hospital stay and improving overall patient satisfaction.

- *Disadvantages*:

  Learning curve: Radial artery access requires specialized training and expertise, and healthcare providers transitioning from femoral to radial access may experience a learning curve.

  Limited catheter selection: The smaller caliber of the radial artery may limit the selection of catheters and guidewires for specific procedures.

  Risk of radial artery occlusion: Prolonged use of radial artery access for invasive procedures may increase the risk of radial artery occlusion.

Microcatheter Technique

Microcatheter techniques have significantly enhanced the safety and efficacy of intra-arterial drug delivery by superselectively delivering drugs to the pathology [18]. These improvements focus on precise drug targeting, reducing systemic exposure, and minimizing procedural risks.

- *Superselective catheterization*: Modern microcatheters are designed to navigate intricate vascular pathways and reach target sites with high precision. Superselective catheterization ensures that drugs are delivered directly to the tumor, sparing healthy tissue and reducing systemic side effects. This precision is crucial in minimizing damage to nontarget areas and enhancing the therapeutic efficacy of the treatment.
- *Microcatheter features*:
  - *Flexibility and hydrophilic coating*: Developing more flexible microcatheters allows more straightforward navigation through tortuous vascular pathways. Coating with hydrophilic materials can also reduce friction and facilitate maneuverability through blood vessels, thus improving navigation and positioning accuracy for targeted drug delivery.
  - *Improved biocompatibility*: Biocompatibility can reduce the risk of adverse reactions such as thrombosis or inflammation. These materials are designed to be nonreactive with blood and tissues, ensuring safer long-term use during prolonged procedures.
  - *Dual-lumen capability*: Dual-lumen microcatheters, which have two separate channels, allow for simultaneous delivery of therapeutic agents and embolic materials. This capability is advantageous in chemoembolization procedures, where chemotherapy drugs and embolizing agents are administered together to maximize the therapeutic impact while minimizing systemic toxicity.

Flow Control Methods

- Flow control methods in superselective intra-arterial drug delivery are crucial for maximizing therapeutic efficacy and minimizing systemic exposure. These methods focus on precise targeting, maintaining drug concentration, and preventing nontarget embolization.
  - *Balloon-assisted techniques*: Balloon-tipped microcatheters can temporarily occlude blood flow in the targeted vessel during drug delivery. This balloon-occlusion technique increases the concentration of the therapeutic agent in the tumor area. It also reduces the drug washout rate, enhancing the treatment's effectiveness compared to IV dosing in cerebral diseases [18].
  - *Adenosine-induced transient asystole*: A growing method of partial flow arrest in the treatment of cerebral arteriovenous malformations or high flow fistulas, in which rapid blood flow transit can limit glue delivery's effectiveness and safety. Adenosine, an endogenous purine nucleoside with a half-life of approximately 10 s, is currently indicated for the treatment of supraventricular tachycardia in small doses (10–12 mg) as it slows the conduction time through the atrioventricular (AV) node. In higher doses (up to 64 mg), it can be used to induce high degree AV block, resulting in transient asystole and profound systemic hypotension. This provides a much slower and more controlled glue delivery without significant sequelae in circulatory, neurological, and renal functions [19, 20].

Radiation Safety

Endovascular neurosurgery involves ionizing X-rays for procedural guidance. To ensure patient and operator safety, adherence to radiation safety principles, such as minimizing fluoroscopy time, maximizing distance from the radiation source, and utilizing radiation shielding, is paramount. Fundamental principles and strategies for radiation safety include:

- *Optimization of imaging parameters*: Utilize appropriate imaging protocols and parameters to achieve optimal image quality with the lowest possible radiation dose.
  - Adjust the fluoroscopy settings based on procedural requirements and patient characteristics, such as body weight and habitus, pulse rate, frame rate, and magnification.
  - Use collimation to restrict the radiation field to the area of interest and minimize unnecessary exposure to surrounding tissues.
  - Reduce the patient's distance from the radiation source to minimize scatter radiation and enhance image quality.
- *Minimization of fluoroscopy time*: To minimize fluoroscopy time, optimize procedural techniques, such as rapid catheterization and efficient navigation through vascular anatomy.
  - Use intermittent fluoroscopy instead of continuous fluoroscopy whenever possible to reduce cumulative radiation dose.
  - Employ image acquisition techniques, such as digital subtraction angiography (DSA) and roadmap imaging, to minimize the need for prolonged fluoroscopic guidance.
- *Protective shielding and equipment*:
  - Use lead aprons, thyroid shields, and protective eyewear to shield healthcare providers and staff from scattered radiation.
  - Position protective shielding devices, such as lead drapes and table skirts, to minimize radiation exposure to nonessential areas of the body.
  - Ensure proper maintenance of radiation shielding equipment.
- *Radiation monitoring devices*:
  - Implement radiation monitoring devices, such as dosimeters and radiation badges, to measure and track radiation exposure for healthcare providers and staff.
  - Regularly assess radiation dose levels and review cumulative dose reports to identify individuals at risk of exceeding recommended exposure limits.
  - Regularly review radiation safety protocols and procedures.
- *Education and training*:
  - Provide comprehensive radiation safety training for healthcare providers and staff involved in INR procedures, emphasizing the principles of ALARA (As Low As Reasonably Achievable) and dose optimization.

Management of Anticoagulation

Anticoagulation prevents thromboembolic complications, particularly in patients with pre-existing cardiovascular conditions or undergoing concomitant antithrombotic therapy. Key considerations include:

- *Periprocedural anticoagulation*:
  - Temporary cessation or adjustment of anticoagulant and antiplatelet medications may be necessary to minimize the risk of bleeding complications. This decision should be made in consultation with a multidisciplinary team, considering the patient's underlying condition and procedural risk.
  - Bridging therapy heparin or therapeutic Lovenox may be warranted in high-risk patients.
  - Radial access may be considered to minimize the risk of hematoma formation and retroperitoneal bleeding.
- *Procedural anticoagulation*:
  - Patients may require therapeutic anticoagulation to prevent thrombotic complications during endovascular procedures. Knowing the weight and baseline activated clotting time (ACT) is necessary to titrate anticoagulation agents appropriately.
  - ACT is a point-of-care test that evaluates coagulation's intrinsic pathway and provides real-time anticoagulation status assessment during invasive procedures. ACT measures the time for blood to clot after activating the intrinsic coagulation pathway. The test involves adding an activator (e.g., kaolin, celite) to whole blood to initiate coagulation, followed by monitoring clot formation using a coagulation analyzer. ACT reflects the combined effects of various coagulation factors, platelets, and inhibitors in the intrinsic pathway, providing a global assessment of coagulation function.
  - ACT monitoring is performed regularly throughout the procedure, with initial baseline measurements obtained before initiating anticoagulation therapy.
  - Target ACT ranges may vary depending on the type of procedure, patient weight, and institutional protocols, with higher targets often used for more complex or high-risk interventions.
  - By titrating heparin infusion rates based on ACT measurements, healthcare providers can optimize anticoagulation therapy and minimize the risk of thrombotic and bleeding complications.

- *Anticoagulant reversal agents*: In cases of emergent bleeding or excessive anticoagulation, reversal agents such as protamine sulfate (for heparin) or prothrombin complex concentrate (for vitamin K antagonists) can be administered to restore hemostasis rapidly.
- *Preprocedural activated clotting time (ACT)* monitoring should be used to guide reversal. Close monitoring of coagulation parameters is essential to guide the appropriate use of reversal agents and prevent thrombotic complications.
- *Postprocedural anticoagulation*: During the transition period, close monitoring for signs of bleeding or thrombosis is essential. Gradual reintroduction of anticoagulant therapy, guided by serial laboratory testing and clinical assessment, can minimize the risk of thromboembolic events while ensuring adequate hemostasis.

Arterial Closure Devices

Proper management of access site hemostasis and monitoring for signs of bleeding or hematoma formation are essential components of postprocedural care. Arterial closure devices or manual compression techniques may be utilized to achieve hemostasis effectively.

Arterial closure devices are crucial in mitigating the risk of vascular complications following intra-arterial catheterization. These devices facilitate rapid hemostasis and promote early ambulation, reducing the duration of postprocedural observation and hospital stay. Commonly used arterial closure devices include:

- Suture-based devices: These devices deploy sutures or clips to approximate the arterial puncture site, effectively sealing the vessel. Examples include the Perclose ProGlide™ and MynxControl™ or MynxGrip™ systems.
- Collagen plugs: Collagen-based plugs expand upon contact with blood, forming a mechanical barrier against bleeding. The Angio-Seal™ and Exoseal™ are the most popular collagen plug devices.
- Vascular compression devices: Designed for arterial closure after radial artery access, the TR Band™ is a compression device to achieve hemostasis and maintain radial artery patency. The TR Band™ applies controlled pressure to the radial artery access site, facilitating rapid and effective hemostasis while minimizing the risk of complications. Compared to manual compression techniques, it has been shown to significantly reduce the incidence of access site-related complications, such as bleeding, hematoma formation, and radial artery occlusion (reference).

Complication Management

Close neurological monitoring in the postprocedural period enables early detection of neurological deficits or complications, such as hemorrhage or thromboembolism.

- *Vessel perforation or dissection*: Immediate recognition and intervention are critical if vessel perforation or dissection is suspected.
  - Techniques such as balloon tamponade, stent placement, or coil embolization may be employed to achieve hemostasis and restore vessel integrity.
  - Management of anticoagulation, either immediate reversal in the case of perforation or anticoagulation loading in the case of dissection requiring stenting, is critical to patient safety and optimal outcomes.
- *Radial artery vasospasm*: Patients may experience postprocedural radial artery vasospasm symptoms, including pain and numbness or coolness of the affected hand.
  - Nonpharmacological measures, such as warm compresses and fluids, can alleviate symptoms and encourage arterial vasodilation.
- *Thromboembolic events*: Thromboembolic complications, including clot formation or embolization, pose a significant risk during endovascular procedures.
  - Prompt administration of antithrombotic agents, such as antiplatelet or anticoagulant medications, and mechanical thrombectomy may be necessary to restore vessel patency and prevent ischemic sequelae.
- *Contrast-induced nephropathy*: Contrast-induced nephropathy is a potential complication following the administration of iodinated contrast agents.
  - Adequate hydration, preprocedural renal function assessment, and judicious contrast use can help minimize the risk of renal injury.
- *Pharmaceutical risks*: The pharmacological agents can exacerbate the risks associated with interventional procedures. Therefore, selecting appropriate drugs and developing careful infusion protocols are essential to minimize complications. Although drug selection and infusion protocols are beyond the scope of this chapter, this section outlines the considerations and precautions necessary for safer drug delivery.
  - Drug-induced hypotension and increased intracranial pressure:

    When used to treat cerebral vasospasm, verapamil can induce hypotension and increase intracranial pressure. To prevent these complications, it is critical to have blood pressure support and CSF drainage available during the procedure.

- Management of hyperosmotic agents:
  Hyperosmotic agents, used for disrupting the blood–brain barrier, can cause bradycardia and seizures. Anticipating these potential adverse effects and having protocols in place for their management is vital. This includes continuously monitoring the patient's cardiac and neurological status and being prepared with appropriate interventions to address any complications.
- Dose and duration adjustments for chemotherapy:
  The dose and duration of chemotherapy must be meticulously adjusted based on the specific vessel and organ being perfused [21]. Over- or underdosing can lead to suboptimal treatment outcomes or increased toxicity. Tailoring the chemotherapy regimen to the patient's anatomy and the characteristics of the tumor ensures that the therapeutic effects are maximized while minimizing systemic exposure and adverse effects.

Future Directions

The global angiography market is estimated to be worth $12.7 billion in 2023 and will increase to $23.3 billion by 2033 [22]. While data on the number of cerebral angiograms is not readily available, it is estimated that 4 million coronary angiograms are performed annually in America and Europe [23]. The fact that millions of angiographic procedures are being done each year is a testament to the safety of angiography procedures. It is generally accepted that the complication rate of cerebral angiography is about 3.2%. The notable complications of cerebral angiography are groin hematoma (1.32%) and neurological complications, which occur in about 0.68% and are usually transient. Permanent neurological injuries occur in 0.13%. Thus, despite the procedure's overall safety, there is room to improve [24].

Enabling safe arterial injections during transient flow arrest is at the core of effective arterial drug delivery for neurological diseases. This chapter describes many advances that have made routine angiography safe. However, the focus in the future will be the development of better catheters, anticoagulant and antiplatelet treatment, and adjuvant measures that enable safer flow arrest. Techniques such as hypothermia or deep intravenous anesthesia could be neuroprotective yet decrease the blood flow and increase the safety of transient flow arrest. Future angiographic imaging techniques, whether in an X-ray or MR environment, could help monitor blood flow, drug delivery, and therapeutic effects.

There is certainly room for improvement in arterial drug development. Despite the explosive and spectacular development of endovascular tools, intra-arterial pharmacology has seen few advances in the last two decades. We can cautiously look to innovations in the endovascular treatment of hepatocellular carcinoma for inspiration, including the use of radiopaque microspheres to improve drug localization and reduce systemic side effects and the development of venous filtration systems that enable posttarget chemotherapy filtration to limit systemic exposure [25, 26]. We must not forget the potential for multimodality treatments to outperform historical management. Multiple studies demonstrate that varied combinations of transarterial chemoembolization, transarterial drug-eluting bead delivery, radiofrequency ablation, and systemic therapy can improve overall survival and local tumor control [27, 28]. As with all innovations, rigorous clinical trials and postmarket surveillance are essential to identify potential complications early and refine techniques and protocols. Developing endovascular techniques for safe drug delivery is a critical part of any future arterial treatments of neurological diseases. The field of intra-arterial drug delivery in endovascular surgery has the potential to improve patient outcomes.

Conclusion

Ensuring safety in intra-arterial drug delivery demands a comprehensive and multidisciplinary approach, integrating meticulous preprocedural planning, precise procedural execution, effective complication management, and vigilant postprocedural care. This will involve neurologists, anesthesiologists, and interventionalists. Continued research and innovations in this field promise further advancements in safety and efficacy, solidifying intra-arterial drug delivery as a cornerstone of modern interventional radiology. On the technical front, there will be improvements related to endovascular procedures. There will be further technical improvements from safer arteriotomy, better catheters, improved flow-occluding devices, precise anticoagulation management, and rapid and effective vascular closure. This chapter provided an overview of the vital safety measures integral to intra-arterial drug delivery. Detailed examination of current practices, historical developments, and technological advancements underscores the critical importance of safety in achieving successful therapeutic outcomes. As the field continues to evolve, maintaining a focus on safety will be paramount to leveraging the full potential of intra-arterial drug delivery.

References

1. Vaquero Puerta C, Del Río Sola ML, San Norberto García EM, Brizuela Sanz JA, Ediciones Universidad de V. José Goyanes Capdevila (1876–1964): pionero de la cirugía vascular española. 2017.
2. Kori SH. Interventional neurology: a subspecialty whose time has come. Neurology. 1993;43(11):2395–9.

3. Márquez-Espinós C, Pérez A, Aragón F, Torres LM. Intra-arterial regional anesthesia: a Spanish contribution. Int Congr Ser. 2002;1242:537–40.
4. Artico M, Spoletini M, Fumagalli L, Biagioni F, Ryskalin L, Fornai F, et al. Egas Moniz: 90 years (1927-2017) from cerebral angiography. Front Neuroanat. 2017;11:81.
5. Greitz T. Sven-Ivar Seldinger. AJNR Am J Neuroradiol. 1999;20(6):1180–1.
6. Qureshi AI. Textbook of interventional neurology. Cambridge: Cambridge University Press; 2011.
7. Young WL, Pile-Spellman J. Anesthetic considerations for interventional neuroradiology. Anesthesiology. 1994;80(2):427–56.
8. Joshi S, Young WL. Anesthesia for interventional neuroradiological procedures. In: Scientific proceedings—first national conference of the Indian Society of Neuroanaesthesiology and Critical Care. New Delhi: Department of Anaesthesiology, G.B. Pant Hospital; 1999. p. 149–52.
9. Rao SV, Ou FS, Wang TY, Roe MT, Brindis R, Rumsfeld JS, et al. Trends in the prevalence and outcomes of radial and femoral approaches to percutaneous coronary intervention: a report from the National Cardiovascular Data Registry. JACC Cardiovasc Interv. 2008;1(4):379–86.
10. Babu SC, Piccorelli GO, Shah PM, Stein JH, Clauss RH. Incidence and results of arterial complications among 16,350 patients undergoing cardiac catheterization. J Vasc Surg. 1989;10(2):113–6.
11. Holland B, Applegate R. Femoral vascular access—approaches and available devices. Interv Cardiol Rev. 2012;7:108.
12. Huggins CE, Gillespie MJ, Tan WA, Laundon RC, Costello FM, Darrah SB, et al. A prospective randomized clinical trial of the use of fluoroscopy in obtaining femoral arterial access. J Invasive Cardiol. 2009;21(3):105–9.
13. Jacobi JA, Schussler JM, Johnson KB. Routine femoral head fluoroscopy to reduce complications in coronary catheterization. Proc (Bayl Univ Med Cent). 2009;22(1):7–8.
14. Abu-Fadel MS, Sparling JM, Zacharias SJ, Aston CE, Saucedo JF, Schechter E, et al. Fluoroscopy vs. traditional guided femoral arterial access and the use of closure devices: a randomized controlled trial. Catheter Cardiovasc Interv. 2009;74(4):533–9.
15. Seto AH, Abu-Fadel MS, Sparling JM, Zacharias SJ, Daly TS, Harrison AT, et al. Real-time ultrasound guidance facilitates femoral arterial access and reduces vascular complications: FAUST (Femoral Arterial Access with Ultrasound Trial). JACC Cardiovasc Interv. 2010;3(7):751–8.
16. Beyer AT, Ng R, Singh A, Zimmet J, Shunk K, Yeghiazarians Y, et al. Topical nitroglycerin and lidocaine to dilate the radial artery prior to transradial cardiac catheterization: a randomized, placebo-controlled, double-blind clinical trial: the PRE-DILATE study. Int J Cardiol. 2013;168(3):2575–8.
17. Kwok CS, Rashid M, Fraser D, Nolan J, Mamas M. Intra-arterial vasodilators to prevent radial artery spasm: a systematic review and pooled analysis of clinical studies. Cardiovasc Revasc Med. 2015;16(8):484–90.
18. Riina HA, Knopman J, Greenfield JP, Fralin S, Gobin YP, Tsiouris AJ, et al. Balloon-assisted superselective intra-arterial cerebral infusion of bevacizumab for malignant brainstem glioma. A technical note. Interv Neuroradiol. 2010;16(1):71–6.
19. Pile-Spellman J, Young WL, Joshi S, Duong H, Vang MC, Hartmann A, et al. Adenosine-induced cardiac pause for endovascular embolization of cerebral arteriovenous malformations: technical case report. Neurosurgery. 1999;44(4):881–6; discussion 6–7.
20. Hashimoto T, Young William L, Aagaard Beverly D, Joshi S, Ostapkovich Noeleen D, Pile-Spellman J. Adenosine-induced ventricular asystole to induce transient profound systemic hypotension in patients undergoing endovascular therapy: dose–response characteristics. Anesthesiology. 2000;93(4):998–1001.
21. Gobin YP, Cloughesy TF, Chow KL, Duckwiler GR, Sayre JW, Milanese K, et al. Intraarterial chemotherapy for brain tumors by using a spatial dose fractionation algorithm and pulsatile delivery. Radiology. 2001;218(3):724–32.
22. FMI Inc. Angiography devices market outlook (2023–2033). https://www.futuremarketinsights.com/reports/angiography-devices-market.
23. Beştemir A, Apaydın Z, Kılınç AY. Analysis of coronary angiography and revascularization rates made over 5 years in public institutions in Türkiye. Anatol J Cardiol. 2023;27(9):529–33.
24. Tafelmeier S, Kesseler E, Iancu AM, Nikoubashman O, Wiesmann M. Spectrum of complications and complication rates after diagnostic catheter angiography in neuroradiology. Clin Neuroradiol. 2023;33(3):763–8.
25. Patel AS, Saeed M, Yee EJ, Yang J, Lam GJ, Losey AD, et al. Development and validation of endovascular chemotherapy filter device for removing high-dose doxorubicin: preclinical study. J Med Device. 2014;8(4):0410081–8.
26. Pérez-López A, Martín-Sabroso C, Gómez-Lázaro L, Torres-Suárez AI, Aparicio-Blanco J. Embolization therapy with microspheres for the treatment of liver cancer: state-of-the-art of clinical translation. Acta Biomater. 2022;149:1–15.
27. Liu B, Zhang Y, Chen H, Li W, Tsochatzis E. The combination of transcatheter arterial chemoembolisation (TACE) and thermal ablation versus TACE alone for hepatocellular carcinoma. Cochrane Database Syst Rev. 2022;1(1):CD013345.
28. Chen YC, Huang CW, Li CC, Chang TK, Su WC, Chen PJ, et al. Efficacy of transarterial chemoembolization with drug-eluting beads combined with systemic chemotherapy and targeted therapy in colorectal cancer liver metastasis. World J Surg Oncol. 2023;21(1):378.

18 Evolution of Transvascular Catheter From Material, Construction, and Technological Perspectives

Sean Lynn

The angiographic catheter can be more than a tool for passive means for diagnostic observation; used with imagination, it can become an important surgical instrument.

Charles Theodore Dotter (1920–1985), the Father of Interventional Radiology

Introduction

Interventional therapies are part of the growing trend toward less invasive techniques in modern clinical practice [1–7]. These therapies are obsoleting current surgical procedures and offering hope in areas considered beyond medical treatment a generation ago [8–13]. While interventional therapies were pioneered in the mid-1960s, they are still an evolving and growing area of modern medicine. Interventional medical practitioners are specialists who do minimally invasive procedures instead of surgery or other treatments. The common feature of most interventional therapies is that they are catheter-based [14]. Catheters have been defined as tubular medical devices for insertion into canals, vessels, passageways, or body cavities, usually to permit injection or withdrawal of fluids or to keep a passage open [15]. This chapter will examine the history of these interventional or transvascular catheters from a technology and materials perspective. Understanding some essential steps and concepts that drove the evolution from simple tubing to the ultra-thin, metal-reinforced multilayer composites of today is an insightful journey. It's also a journey poorly documented from the perspective of transvascular catheter technology rather than the clinical perspective.

Today's transvascular catheter technology offers a modular, adaptable platform tailored to meet new or emerging clinical needs. Understanding its technological evolution can open minds and inspire clinicians and designers to ask what is truly possible in this space. The technological developments that made the emergence of transvascular catheterization feasible are discussed alongside the evolution of catheter materials and design and the refinement of clinical practice as various clinical specialties emerged and matured.

S. Lynn (✉)
Teleflex Medical OEM, Annacotty Business Park, Anacotty, Co Limerick, Ireland
e-mail: sean.lynn@teleflex.com

Early Vascular Imaging and Right Heart Catheterization

Medical imaging began in 1895 with Conrad Roentgen's discovery of the X-ray [16, 17]. The development of contrast media allowed physicians to gradually develop skills and techniques in visualizing the vascular system [18]. Carlos Heuser, an Argentine radiologist, is recorded as having performed the first angiogram on a living person in 1919 [19]. Over the next 10 years, firsts in clinical angiography (Brooks) and cerebral angiography (Moniz) were recorded [20]. At this point, contrast media was injected directly into the vascular system using a syringe to facilitate imaging. Developing a practical vascular imaging approach created the initial need for transvascular catheter-based medicine.

In 1929, Werner Forssmann (a medical intern in Berlin) passed a lubricated ureteral catheter into his heart using a venous puncture of his left arm as an access point. His report included a photograph of an X-ray showing the catheter in the heart, and as such, he was the first to document human right heart catheterization [21, 22]. His insightful leap was that there was a better, easier, and safer way of accessing the cardiac chambers than the direct needle-based approaches of the time [23]. Ureteral catheters of the time were radiopaque and made from soft rubber (latex), which had been vulcanized [24, 25]. The flexibility made these catheters appeal to the early innovators in the vascular space, as synthetic

S. Joshi (ed.), *Arterial Treatment of Neurological Diseases*, https://doi.org/10.1007/978-3-031-80173-0_18

polymerization was still in its infancy. The 1930–1940 decade saw the industrial development of today's leading thermoplastics: polystyrene, polyvinylchloride, polyolefins, and polymethyl methacrylate [26].

Cournard and Dickenson Richards systematically catheterized the right side of the heart to measure pulmonary blood flow [27]. Cournand's first paper (1941) while working at Bellevue Hospital refers directly to Forssmann's earlier work [28]. Richards and Cournard applied catheterization to a variety of cardiac conditions, including valvular heart disease, heart failure, and congenital heart disease [29]. Cournard, Richards, and Forssmann were awarded the Nobel Prize in 1956 for their collective contributions to cardiac catheterization [30, 31].

Transvascular Catheter Materials

Cournard's catheters were developed collaboratively with the United States Catheter and Instruments Corporation (USCI) [32]. Norman Jeckel, cofounder of USCI [33], had been granted a patent in 1946 for a novel catheter design described as a braided fabric structure with a PVC varnish applied to it [34]. Jeckel initially worked for American Cystoscope Makers Inc. (ACMI), and early thinking in vascular catheter design was influenced by knowledge acquired at ACMI, which included developing the first woven catheters produced in the USA [35]. The Cournand catheter consisted of an inner framework of fabric covered with polyvinyl chloride with comminuted tin added for radiopacity [24]. This is the earliest description of a composite transvascular catheter.

Intravenous Catheterization

At this point, it is worth examining the technological evolution that led to intravenous catheterization as we know it today. In 1945, Zimmerman [36] and Meyers [37] independently reported using plastic tubing placed into vessels through large caliber introducer needles. Zimmerman used vinylite (polyvinylchloride) and Meyers polyethylene [38]. The needles were withdrawn, leaving the catheter tubing as a pliable channel for intravenous therapy. This approach improved patient comfort compared to a rigid needle and was easier for the medical staff to manage.

In 1950, Massa and associates advanced the needle approach by introducing polyvinylchloride (PVC) tubing attached over a 16 Ga short needle, which was threaded over a 19 Ga needle, which acted as a stylet [39]. When the 19 Ga needle stylet was removed, the plastic tubing, the same size as the access site, reduced the leakage. Massa's experiences working in the cardiac catheterization laboratory at the Mayo Clinic informed the concept. His design reduced leakage at the venous access site, allowed a hub to be attached to the cannula, and was technically more straightforward than the Zimmermann–Myers technique [40]. Massa's invention marked the point where, finally, a catheter was available that could be directly threaded into a vessel after venipuncture with a needle [41]. While the technique was simple, the frequency of phlebitis (inflammation of the vein) developing in the vessel and the tendency toward thrombus (blood clot) formation within the catheter were practical drawbacks [42].

Emergence of Extruded PVC-P

Polyvinyl chloride (PVC) is a rigid material with a glass transition temperature of 80 °C. In biomedical applications such as catheters, it is used in its flexible form, plasticized PVC (PVC-P). Compounding it with plasticizers in concentrations reaching 50% makes it a soft, flexible, and adaptable catheter material. In the 1930s, W.L. Semon, working for BF Goodrich, was granted a patent on using di-2-ethylhexyl phthalate (DEHP) as a plasticizer in PVC [43]. This technological advancement set the scene for PVC-P to become one of the most dominant materials in the transvascular catheter space. The technology to process PVC-P leaned heavily on that used for rubber processing, and PVC-P was first seen commercially as an alternative to natural rubber [44]. As a material, its low cost, inertness, high transparency, ease of sterilization, and strength led to its widespread use in medical applications [45]. PVC-P was found to be used in blood bags, replacing glass as early as 1947 [46]. In the catheter space, it was used for vascular applications such as intravenous infusions [47], and central venous pressure measurements [48]. It was also used for feeding tubes, among other applications [49]. The emergence of thermoplastic elastomers (discussed later) provided more options for catheter designers in later years, but in the 1950s and 1960s, PVC-P was a key intravascular catheter material.

In 2002, the FDA issued a notification regarding the exposure to DEHP-plasticized PVC. As DEHP is not covalently bound within the PVC-DEHP matrix, it can leach from the material into the contacting physiological medium [50]. In more recent studies, DEHP has been labeled as a category-2 toxic compound [51]. This has led to a move away from PVC for many new applications.

The Search for Inert and Biocompatible Materials Such as Polyethylene

By 1947, the synthetic polymer polyethylene became a material of choice for cardiac catheters [31]. From the literature of the time, its adoption across multiple therapy areas was described. Aortography [52, 53], angiography [54, 55], and intravenous catheterization [38, 56] represent its widespread use. Polyethylene offers advantages as a more biocompatible material that is less likely to cause clotting issues in intravenous therapy [57]. It also provided practical advantages in being drawn to reduce its diameter and be shape-set in boiling water [24].

Polyethylene was foundational to the access technique developed by Dr. Sven-Ivar Seldinger in 1952 [58, 59]. He described using a polyethylene catheter tube in his seminal 1953 paper [59]. The technique reduced blood loss, complications, and the potential risks of arterial puncture [60]. Today, catheters are predominantly introduced or access the vasculature using the Seldinger or modified Seldinger technique. All clinicians did not immediately adopt this change, and it took 10 years, particularly the work of Dotter and Gruentzig in the USA [60] and Erik Boijsen in Sweden [61], to make it the accepted access practice for vascular catheterization. Rappaport [62] described coating their polyethylene catheters with silicone oil to reduce thrombosis in 1955.

Search for Silicone Elastomers

Coating catheters with silicone oil to reduce thrombus was a logical step. Jaques [63] and Margulies [64] described how silicone coating on syringes and glassware increased the time required for blood clotting compared to untreated surfaces. In the 1940s, silicones became commercially available after Hyde of Dow Corning demonstrated silicone resins' thermal stability and high electrical resistance. Rochow of General Electric found a direct method to prepare silicones from silicon and methyl chloride [65]. Implant applications were described by Lahey and DeNicola [66], in the late 1940s. Silastic (a portmanteau of silicone and plastic) was trademarked by Dow Corning in 1948. Silicone elastomers' chemical stability and elastic nature benefit many applications, from long-term implantation to a wide range of catheter-based therapies. Stewart in 1961 [67] described silicone catheters' softness and flexibility, tissue inertness, durability, and ease of insertion as critical characteristics. Luessenhop and Velasquez reported the first catheterization of brain vessels was in 1964 using a silicone elastomer-based catheter [68]. Silicone catheters and pump refinements were critical technological advances in hepatic artery infusion chemotherapy [69]. Silicone elastomers were the key construction material in many other therapy areas, including urology [70], parenteral nutrition, and central venous catheters [71].

Development of Fluoropolymers

Medical experimentation with Teflon (PTFE) began in 1949 [72]. It was used for biomedical applications in implants [73, 74] and catheters [75–77]. Teflon was introduced in 1969 for intravenous catheters. Teflon cannulae were easy to slide over the needle and thus easy to thread into veins and were resistant to "peel back" (the tendency of the catheter tip to roll outward when it met resistance) [47]. Teflon FEP (a melt-processable fluoropolymer version of Teflon PTFE) became the dominant fluoropolymer material for this application. Tough and self-lubricating, Teflon was also flexible, nontoxic, and tissue-compatible. It dominated this space until the emergence of a polyurethane alternative in 1983. Polyurethane exhibited a lower incidence of phlebitis than Teflon [78]. Today, polyurethane and Teflon FEP remain the dominant materials used in peripheral intravenous catheters (PIVC).

Teflon or polytetrafluoroethylene (PTFE) has become a critical and widely used material across the broad and complex interventional catheter space. Composite interventional catheters typically comprise a PTFE inner layer wrapped with a fine strand and a metal reinforcement layer covered with a TPE (thermoplastic elastomer) outer layer [79]. As a material, it has found a niche as an inner layer for catheters based on its low friction coefficient and chemical inertness. The outer surface of the PTFE layers is etched with a sodium naphthalene solution to provide a polar surface that can adhere to the conventional polar polymers such as polyamides, polyurethanes, and poly-ether-block-amide copolymers (PEBAs) that are used as catheter outer layers.

Lessons from Intravenous Catheterization:

Peripheral Venous Catheters

Peripheral intravenous catheters (PIVCs) are 6 cm or shorter and suitable for 3–5 days. Longer peripheral catheters (LPCs) can range from 6 to 15 cm in length, and Midline catheters (MCs), which are 15–25 cm long, can be used for 1–4 weeks [80]. Midline catheters extend as far as the axillary vein but do not enter the subclavian vein. All are considered peripheral devices and can only be used to deliver peripherally compatible infusates. While most intravenous fluids, medications, and blood products are peripherally compatible, infusates that are considered vesicants (chemotherapy drugs), irritants, or hyperosmolar (>900 Osm/L) are contraindicated for delivery by PIVC [81]. The limitations of peripheral intravenous catheterization led to the development of central venous catheterization. The need for longer-duration therapies sparked the development of novel materials and catheter techniques as the catheter–body interaction factors were better understood.

Parenteral Nutrition (PN)

Patients who cannot use their gastrointestinal system for feeding are sustained using parenteral nutrition. Central venous hyperalimentation (TPN) or parenteral nutrition was developed by Dudrick, Wilmore, Vars, and Rhoads in the 1960s and provided a route to administer all the necessary nutrients by vein [82]. Through structured experimentation, Dudrick and his associates grasped that introducing the nutrients directly to the superior vena cava via a jugular vein allows them to infuse the hypertonic solutions continuously 24 h a day. The high blood flow at that point of the vasculature diluted the hypertonic infusate to normal osmolarity, and the concentrations of the nutrient components in the blood were observed to be within normal ranges [83]. This meant that the nutrients could be provided in a manner that limited side effects and, with later refinements, could sustain the life of patients who previously had no clinical treatment options.

Silicone rubber or silastic was the primary catheter material used for PN therapy from the late 1960s to the mid-1970s, when the technique was developed and refined through the application. Notable milestones were the introduction by Broviac, a right atrial silastic catheter with a polyester cuff, which was inserted for central venous access and tunneled subcutaneously for long-term placement [84]. Tunneling meant the catheter was located more securely and less prone to infection. However, the small diameter of the catheter meant it often had clotting issues when used for blood sampling or delivery of blood products. Hickman increased the catheter's internal diameter from 0.22 to 0.32 mm (more than doubling the lumen cross-sectional area) and thickened the wall, which allowed it to be used for leukemia patients undergoing bone marrow transplants [85]. Later, Hickman innovations included a dual-lumen version, which allowed separation of PN and then both blood sampling or infusion through the other lumen, and a triple-lumen version, where all mentioned functions were separated. Even today, the Hickman catheter remains an essential therapeutic tool for long-term central vascular access for ambulatory home parenteral nutrition.

Central Venous Catheterization for Oncology

The beginning of peripherally inserted central catheters (PICCs) can be attributed to the pioneering work of Werner Forssmann (mentioned earlier). Central venous catheters enable clinicians to monitor and support the body in stabilizing the circulation during and after surgery. It is used mainly for administration of antibiotics, chemotherapy, fluid resuscitation, and parenteral nutrition. It is also used for hemodialysis and is the preferred choice for vascular access in many short-term therapies.

Short-duration central venous catheters are specialist polyurethane devices of 20–30 cm in length and up to 8 Fr in diameter that are implanted via puncture of a central vein (internal jugular, subclavian, axillary, or femoral), with the tip positioned close to the cavo-atrial junction [86]. There are versions with single or multiple lumens, which are always for continuous use, exclusively in patients admitted to the hospital because of the risks of catheter displacement and infection. Duration of use is generally up to 3 weeks for oncology. Products are impregnated or coated to reduce the risk of infections (i.e., Teleflex Arrowg+ard Blue Plus® CVC or Cook Spectrum® CVC).

PICCs are nontunneled, central catheters inserted through a peripheral vein of the arm. They are 50–60 cm long and made of silicone or second—or third-generation polyurethane. The PICC material (silicone versus polyurethane) can influence the risk of complications since some types of polyurethane may be associated with a higher incidence of thrombosis [87]. The advantage of polyurethane PICCs is that they have more significant flow rates due to thinner walls, which can be advantageous in hematology. That higher flow rate is rarely beneficial in oncology, where pump-driven intravenous infusions are used for chemotherapy. Some studies have suggested that PICCs may be preferable to CVCs because they are associated with fewer mechanical complications at insertion, lower costs (since they are mainly inserted by nurses at the bedside), and a lower infection rate [88, 89]. PICCs can also be left longer than CVCs, with Gallieni suggesting 3–12 months of use [90].

Fluoroscopy for Catheter Visualization for Navigation

Collective technology changes, including the replacement of single-plate angiograms by automatic film cassette changers (1949) [19], rapid film-changing technology [91], and image intensification (1950) [59], allowed sharper imaging with less radiation exposure and contrast media use. Medical imaging became more refined and, therefore, better able to support the requirements of catheter-based procedures.

A literature review shows that lack of radiopacity has emerged as an issue in adopting polyethylene as a vascular catheter material. In 1940, a patent for a radiopaque catheter for urology based on an extrusion process for cellulosic material incorporating bismuth was filed [92]. Various approaches were tried to compensate for polyethylene's lack of radiopacity, including leaving the wire guide within the catheter and injecting contrast media to see it under fluoroscopy [59]. Odman described the first radiopaque polyethylene catheter in 1956, which was achieved by incorporating a heavy metal salt into the polymer matrix [93].

It was becoming increasingly apparent to clinicians that the toxic effects of intervascular contrast agents were dose-related [20, 94, 95]. Hence, clinicians focused on the catheter being radiopaque and more maneuverable. Odman proposed the visualization of each arterial branch of the aorta separately [96]. This required radiopaque catheters with distal shapes that facilitated entry into the particular branch of the aorta to be imaged. Distal shaping of catheters was one simple, practical approach widely described at the time [32, 97]. Other approaches for magnetic guidance by Tillander [98] and the use of a wire and catheter combination by Radner [99] appeared in the literature but did not become the adopted practice.

Early Catheter Design:

A detailed paper by Odman compares the performance of four vascular catheter structures in terms of performance (summarized in Table 18.1) [24]. It provides a good overview of catheter technology at the end of the 1950s. In summary, these catheters had large diameters [32, 100] that allowed low-pressure contrast injection [101]. The clinical risk of high-pressure injection was understood [102, 103]. For example, the placement of a catheter tip in the heart during high-pressure injections could cause arrhythmia or heart wall damage [104, 105]. Standard practice was to inject contrast media only with the catheter tip away from the vessel or heart wall [61].

Tornvall suggested using a metal catheter tip to improve patient safety, occluding the leader with an open-ended catheter [107]. This design, using side holes, allowed injection stability and the use of the Seldinger method. Another alternative was using a closed-tip catheter such as the NIH (National Institute of Health; catheter made by USCI). This catheter, designed for selective angiocardiography, had a thinner wall than the Cournand catheter of the same external gage, greater luminal diameter, a closed tip, and discharges through 4 spirally placed side holes 1–2 cm proximal to the tip (see Fig. 18.1) [108].

Using a closed-ended catheter with side holes allowed safe injection and eliminated recoil [109, 110]. These closed-ended catheters were used in the late 1950s. They were proposed for various procedures, such as investigating severe aorta injury [111] and for assessing cardiac valve function before valve surgery [112]. While they solved the recoil and

Table 18.1 Vascular catheter comparison (late 1950s' technology) [106]

Design	OD mm (Fr)	Wall (mm)	Construction	Shapability
Radiopaque PE Kifa	2.85 (8.5 Fr)	0.6	Polyethylene with heavy metal salt as a radiopacifier	Good
Lehman	3.33 (10 Fr)	0.6	The fabric structure is laminated PVC with powdered tin as a radiopacifier	Poor
Cournard	3.33 (10 Fr)	0.8	The fabric structure is laminated PVC with powdered tin as a radiopacifier	Poor
Ruchelit	3.33 (10 Fr)	Thick wall (above 0.8)	PVC with mercury sulfide as radiopacifier	Poor

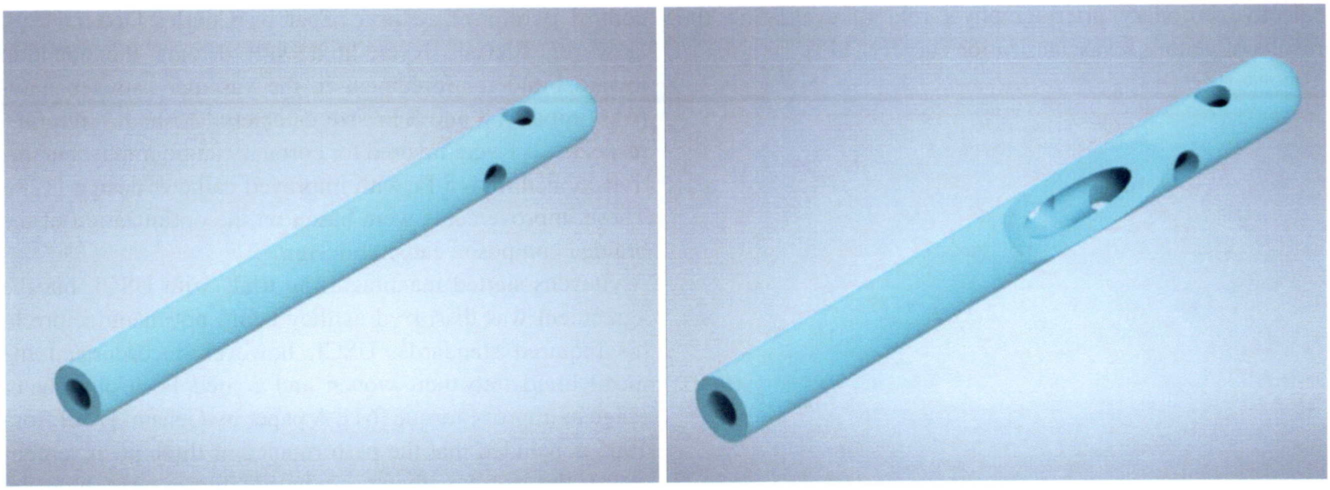

Fig. 18.1 The distal tip of the NIH catheter shows closed-end and distal discharge holes. **Left**: The NIH catheter tip configuration (3.0 mm outer diameter). **Right**: NIH catheter tip with a cut-through, 3.0 mm outer diameter

allowed safer injection, they were not a perfect solution. Issues with perforation of the heart wall and surrounding tissue were noted [108].

The First Selective Coronary Angiogram

In October 1958, at the Cleveland Clinic, Mason Sones, while attempting to complete a left ventricular imaging study, accidentally intubated the ostium of the right coronary artery, thus completing the first selective coronary arteriogram [113]. Up to this point, it was believed that direct injection of contrast media into a coronary artery would cause a heart attack or a potentially fatal misfiring of the heart's central pacemaker [114].

Sones refined the technique and published a study on 1020 patients 3 years later [115]. The Sones catheter (developed with USCI) used the established thin-walled radiopaque woven structure [61]. It was 8 Fr tapering to 5 Fr for the distal 7 cm tip. It had an end hole and four side holes within 1 cm of the tip (see Fig. 18.2) [116]. This composite-based design provided proximal pushability, radiopacity, high burst pressure, and an atraumatic flexible tapered tip section. In biomedical engineering terms, this catheter design is the platform composite intravascular catheter design that served as the technological foundation for a range of specialist catheters that were to be derived from it.

Radiographers of average training could use the Sones catheter to visualize the aorta, left ventricle, and coronary arteries [61]. Selective coronary arteriography clearly showed the choke points of blood flow in the coronary arteries [114]. Sones's technique was later used to identify candidates for revascularization surgery [117]. In 1968, Rene Favaloro (working with Sones) published an article outlining selective coronary arteriography's role in evaluating the results of venous revascularization surgery [118].

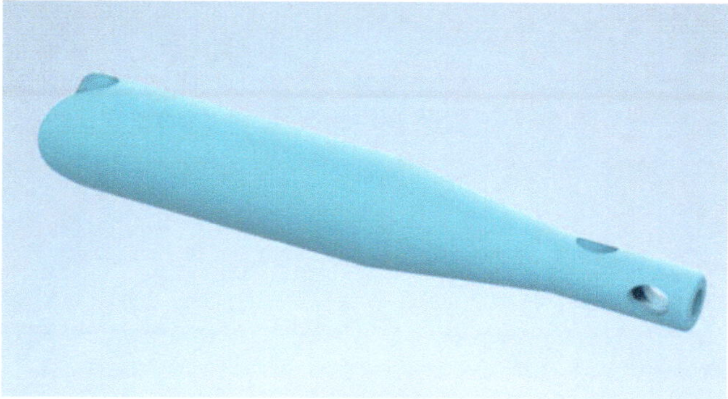

Fig. 18.2 Distal tip of Sones catheter. The four side holes are closer to the tip than the NIH design. The second pair is at 90° to the first. The tip is open rather than closed. The outer diameter tapers from 2.67 to 1.67 mm

In 1962, Ricketts and Abrams [119] described an approach using preformed polyethylene coronary catheters with a Seldinger femoral artery approach. The left and right catheters were shaped differently to use the anatomy to help facilitate placement. Eric Boijsen had been a visiting professor at Stanford in 1962 and worked with Abrams (potentially explaining Abrams's early US advocacy of the Seldinger technique) [120]. This contrasted with Sones's approach, which used a single catheter to catheterize both coronary arteries using the brachial artery cut-down method for vascular access [121].

Amplatz [122] and Judkins [123] independently introduced the transfemoral approach for selective coronary arteriography in 1967. This was simpler and eventually demonstrated to be safer [124], and became widely adopted [122, 125–127]. Part of the explanation for its broad adoption toward the end of the 1960s rather than when it was first described by Ricketts and Abrams was the evolution in catheter technology in the intervening years. Both techniques used preshaped catheters that needed highly torque-able (ideally steel-braided) catheter shafts [128].

Emergence of Steel Braided Composite Catheters

In the early 1960s, Robert Stevens (of Cordis Corporation) developed a prototype metal braided catheter with excellent radiopacity (bismuth subcarbonate milled into the polyurethane before extrusion), torqueability, and high burst pressure [61]. The tip section contained no wire, which improved shape retention and softness. A catheter prototype by Lowell Edwards (Founder of Edwards Lifesciences) built in 1960 consisting of a hollow flexible shaft braided with 12 stainless steel wires that provided reasonable torqueability/ rotary control is referred to in a paper by Charles Dotter [129]. However, Stevens is credited with driving the adaption toward braid reinforcement in the vascular catheter space [61]. Initially, 8 and 7 Fr size catheters (2.7 and 3 mm OD, respectively) were favored for coronary angiography, but this transitioned to 4–5 Fr with improved catheter design [128]. These improvements were based on the optimization of the braided composite catheter design.

Stevens started manufacturing trials with USCI, but the agreement was dissolved as they could not manufacture to his required standards. USCI, however, incorporated the metal braid into their woven and coated Positrol catheter range to improve torque [61]. A paper by Gensini [130] from 1965 concluded that the performance of these positive control ("Positrol") catheters reduced fluoroscopy time by 50–80% and allowed straightforward manipulation of catheters. This simplified selective catheterization of small vessels and allowed tortuosity of the aortic arch to be more readily overcome.

Stevens received a patent on a braided catheter using steel wire in 1969 [131]. Cordis's catheter range, "Ducor," was based on the first commercial thermoplastic elastomer, a polyurethane (Estane) [132, 133]. The innovative Ducor catheter range significantly improved over the available catheters [122, 126, 134]. The metal braided catheter with an inner and outer extruded polymer layer became the standard within the catheter market. Cook developed a similarly structured catheter ("Torcon," a combination of torque and control). This was a steel-braided polyethylene catheter [135], USCI-developed Positrol II, a polyurethane-based version similar to "Ducor" with better tip shape retention than the Positrol I catheter range [61]. Today, all selective angiography catheters are based on the technology that Stevens/Cordis pioneered.

Braid reinforcement has come to dominate the majority of composite interventional catheter designs as it allows designs to be tailored to provide optimal mechanical properties for diverse interventional catheter applications [136]. Carey's review on braided catheters [137] mentions the dearth of literature and resorts to referencing patents. Based on the patents cited, braid reinforcement was used to achieve properties such as high torque, low flexural rigidity, high kink resistance, and high longitudinal compressive strength [137]. Three principal braid patterns, regular diamond and diamond half load, are used, with each pattern providing different torque and kink resistance levels [138].

Roth's article outlines how varying the outer and inner material layers around a standard braid structure can achieve a wide range of vastly different mechanical properties, including torque response [139]. Kucklick has defined torqueability [140] as the ability of a catheter to transmit twisting forces without kinking or absorbing the torsion in the catheter. Today, torqueability is a crucial performance requirement for composite interventional catheters. The FDA recommends that the torque strength of stent delivery systems be measured by methods that lock the distal end and then rotate the proximal end to failure [141]. Braiding enhances the catheter's axial and torsional control, thereby reducing or virtually eliminating the lag associated with the physician's push/pull or rotational input [142].

Importance of Shape and Shape Retention

More than 67% of the mortality risk associated with diagnostic coronary angiography relates to trauma of the left coronary artery. This explains the importance of shape, shape retention, and having an atraumatic catheter tip design. Judkins introduced the transfemoral approach for selective coronary arteriography in 1967. His approach required specific catheter shafts for left and right coronary arteries. Judkins modified catheters using a design approach based on three curves (see Fig. 18.3). This allowed enlarged aorta or unusual anatomy to be treated by catheter shape selection to match the anatomy [123].

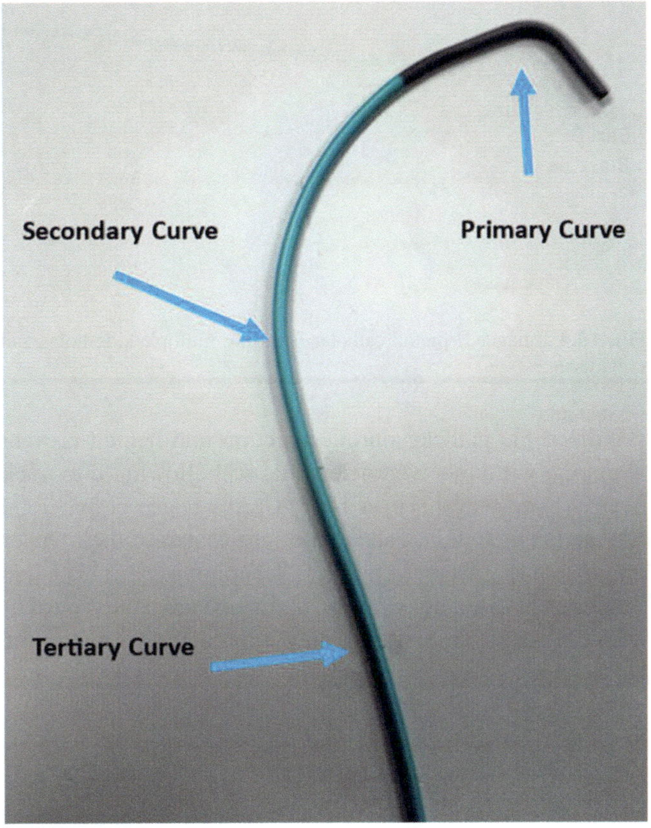

Fig. 18.3 The three-curve catheter design technique developed by Judkins

Judkins achieved his ideal designs through shape and tip modification to the standard Cordis Ducor catheters of the time [61]. The tip was changed from pencil tip to bullet tip to reduce intimal damage; distal 2 cm were reduced from 8 to 5.5 Fr (taper similar to Sones catheter design), and side holes were eliminated to reduce blood clotting risk [123]. The heat shaping and tapering of the catheter were techniques Judkins learned during his time working with Erik Boijsen at the University of Lund in Sweden, and these techniques are described in a coauthored paper [143]. In 1966, the hook-tail catheter was suggested by Boijsen and Judkins as a method of minimizing recoil, thus allowing safer injection while still allowing the use of the Seldinger access technique [31].

Judkins introduced his pigtail catheter, Fig. 18.4, which was based on the hook and tail catheter, in 1968 [19]. It measured aortic and ventricular pressures while permitting contrast injection into the left ventriculogram [125]. It featured an elongated coiled shape with multiple side holes to accommodate rapid injection without the damaging effect of a jet of contrast from the end hole against the endocardium (see Fig. 18.3) [61]. Unlike closed-end catheters, the spiral design

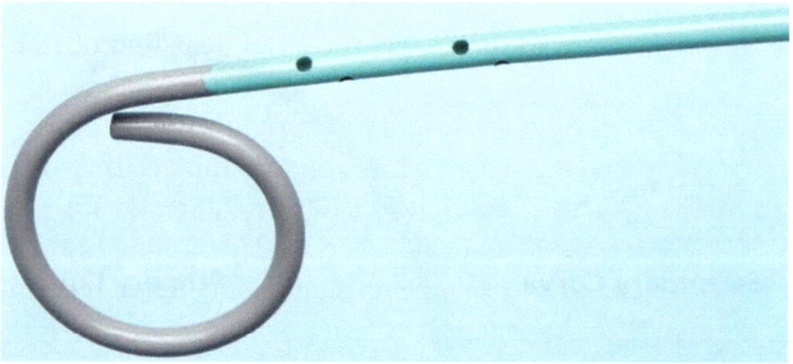

Fig. 18.4 Imager II pigtail catheter featuring multiple side holes and coiled shape

stabilized the catheter during injection and helped prevent whipping within the ventricle while still allowing it to track over a guide wire [27]. In 1968, Cordis began commercial production of Judkins catheter designs as part of their Ducor range [144], Amplatz [122], Schoonmaker [127], and Simmons [145], among others, and made valuable contributions to catheter shaping and approaches for specific anatomy.

From Diagnosis to Therapy; the Emergence of Interventional Medicine

Charles Dotter has been acknowledged as the father of Interventional Radiology [146], and his contribution changed the clinical perspective of catheters to one that recognized their therapeutic and diagnostic value [147]. In 1963, Dotter, examining a patient with an obstruction in the iliac artery, inadvertently pushed the catheter through the site of the obstruction and discovered he had unblocked it [19]. In medical terms, he had completed a transluminal recanalization of an occluded iliac artery while attempting retrograde aortography [60]. He presented his technique and catheter biopsy, flow-guided catheterization, occlusion catheterization, and the rationale of catheter endarterectomy at the Czechoslovak Radiological Congress in Prague in June 1963 [148]. He closed his presentation by asserting that a catheter with some imagination can be turned into a surgical instrument [149].

In January 1964, Charles Dotter and his colleague Melvin Judkins performed the first percutaneous transluminal angioplasty procedure (PTA) [19]. Later, in 1964, they published a paper [150] that detailed the results of 15 procedures in which four of the seven possible amputations were averted [151]. The technique involved advancing a guide wire through the stenosis (blockage) and then advancing the smaller and, subsequently, a larger dilating telescopic Teflon catheter over the guide wire. Introducing large-bore rigid dilators percutaneously and applying large shear forces to atherosclerotic plaque made the technique cumbersome, crude, and risky. In addition, the "snowplow effect" pushed the atheromatous debris aside, which could potentially obstruct the branch vessels adding a risk of clinical complications [19]. Technical refinements, including increased dilator tip tapers and reducing the dilator diameters from 15 and 9 Fr to 12 and 8 Fr, respectively, reduced the risks and complications in using these devices [151].

Improving PTA, the Ability to Apply Radial Shear Force

The following conceptual leap was the application of radial rather than shear force to the atherosclerotic plaque within the vasculature. Dotter describes a device with an expandable section (balloon) at the end of his seminal 1964 paper on PTA [150]. In 1966, Dotter fabricated a woven fiberglass sheath surrounding a simple balloon catheter; however, this reinforced balloon catheter was never used in patients [152]. In Europe, PTA was viewed more seriously than in the USA [153]. Porstmann described the first clinically applicable balloon catheter for PTA in 1973 [151]. Dotter iteratively improved this design and used it to treat iliac artery obstructions in 48 patients [154]. However, thrombus formation meant that these therapies were not adopted [151]. Dotter and Porstmann's approaches did not require strong (noncompliant) balloon material.

Thomas Fogarty developed his embolectomy catheter in 1960 and patented it in 1969 [155]. It had a compliant balloon mounted on a catheter and was the first therapeutic balloon catheter for vascular applications [156]. It was an effective, noninvasive means of removing intravascular clots [157, 158]. The catheter was pushed through the clot. The compliant balloon inflated, occluding the lumen, and the clot was pulled back toward the catheter entry point. However, the compliant balloon used in this catheter configuration did not apply a radial force, so its applicability for PTA was limited. Eberhart Zeitler published 15 papers on PTA and popularized the Dotter coaxial catheter PTA method in Europe [151]. Teflon catheter size was reduced progressively from 12 and 8 Fr to a single 9 Fr dilation catheter tapering to 5 Fr [159, 160]. Side holes were added to Dotter's early design to allow the use of contrast media [19]. Andreas Gruentzig learned coaxial PTA and the European refinements of PTA from Zeitler [114]. He developed his skill with the Dotter method, performing 42 cases between late 1971 and 1974 in Zurich, refining his skills and profoundly understanding the limitations of the technique [114].

On February 12, 1974, Gruentzig demonstrated the balloon-based PTA procedure by treating the stenosis (narrowing) of a patient's superficial femoral artery [161]. Gruentzig solved the balloon issue by using PVC [162]. Polyvinylchloride (PVC) allowed the formation of a semi-compliant balloon. The PVC balloon was mounted onto a diagnostic catheter [163]. Holes were made through the catheter wall in the balloon region to allow inflation. An occlusion stylette was passed through the catheter, blocking the end hole end, thus allowing the balloon to be inflated. This bulky device significantly increased size when the balloon was placed on the catheter [164]. In 1975, Gruentzig developed a coaxial system and successfully used it for peripheral arterial angioplasty [165]. The redesign allowed the central lumen for contrast injection and pressure monitoring and the second lumen (the space between the outer sheath and the inner body) to inflate/deflate the balloon. This catheter design was more flexible and had a lower profile than the earlier single-lumen version [163]. The outer sheath was a PVC tube with a distendable section (balloon) incorporated toward the catheter tip. The inner shaft was still based on a standard angiographic catheter [164].

PTCA for Treating Coronary Arterial Disease

The design platform was refined, improved, and reduced in profile. On September 16, 1977, Andreas Gruentzig performed the first coronary angioplasty in Zurich. A patent filed by Gruentzig and Schneider on November 21, 1977, gives further details of the catheter technology [166]. Supporting patent claims 10–13 refer to the guide catheter construction and a preshaped hose of synthetic fiber fabric formed of polyamide with an outer protective layer of fluoroethylenepropylene (Teflon FEP). Gruentzig published a letter in the Lancet detailing the procedure in five patients [167]. Recognition of the potential of percutaneous revascularization of coronary arteries was immediate. Studies comparing percutaneous to surgical revascularization surgery demonstrated that it was safer, lower cost, and faster recovering as early as 1985 [168–170].

Immediate focus was placed on improving the equipment. In 1978, guiding catheters were 9.4 Fr, solid, stiff Teflon tubes with poor torqueability [163]. However, by 1980, guiding catheters composed of PTFE, woven mesh, and polyurethane were being used [19]. ACS (Advanced Cardiovascular Systems) launched an alternative PTCA system in 1982 [171]. This system was based on the patents that John Simpson had filed [172, 173]. The patents describe a coaxial system that used irradiated modified polyethylene as the guide sheath's outer layer and for key dilation catheter components, including the balloon segment. It also used a nonfixed guide wire compared to the fixed wire of the earlier Gruentzig system. This resulted in a much more maneuverable system [174].

By 1983, guide catheters had reduced to 8 Fr with thinner walls, and balloon inflation pressures had increased from 6 to 12 atmospheres [175]. Between 1977 and 1986, guide catheters, guidewires, and balloon catheter technology were refined, with lower profiles and higher inflation pressures being the key developments [176]. New balloon materials such as PET (polyethylene terephthalate) became available, allowing higher pressures (greater than 20 atmospheres) with thinner walls and lower compliance (stretch) [177]. These advances, particularly in the dilation equipment, were the key determinant in overall procedure success and safety [178]. In the first decade of percutaneous transluminal coronary angioplasty (PTCA), success rates went from 61% to 78% despite treating more complex cases [179].

However, the approach's shortcomings were apparent. These included inadequate dilation, dissection, and late restenosis, which stimulated the development of other techniques [174]. These techniques to remove atherosclerotic plaque included directional, rotation, and extraction atherectomy, laser angioplasty, and coronary stent placement [174, 180]. Despite improved procedural success with rotational atherectomy, restenosis rates increased in patients treated with laser angioplasty (46%) and rotational angioplasty (48%) compared to PTCA (35%) [181]. Atherectomy techniques were extensively used to treat peripheral arterial disease (PAD) [182]. The catheter components of these diverse atherectomy devices are generally reinforced outer sheaths, usually PTFE-lined, with good pushability and torque transmission [183–185].

Early Coronary Stenting and the Emergence of Drug Eluting Stents (DES)

Coronary stents were developed to overcome the issues with POBA (plain old balloon angioplasty) by scaffolding the balloon-dilated artery, sealing the dissection flaps, and preventing late recoil. The Wall Stent (Schneider Inc.) was Sigwart's first stent implanted in a human coronary artery. The technical challenges in using its delivery system limited its clinical utility until its withdrawal from the market in 1991 [186].

The FDA approved the Gianturco-Roubin stent (a coil-based design) to treat acute vessel closure following balloon angioplasty in early 1993 [187]. The coil stent structure was wrapped tightly around a compliant polyethylene dilation balloon catheter for deployment using a standard 8 Fr guide sheath. The Palmaz-Schatz stent was the second FDA-approved coronary stent in 1994 [188]. The 15 mm balloon-expandable, stainless-steel stent was the first slotted tube stent design. The slotted tube designs increased the surface coverage of the stented lesion and applied more radial force [189]. Several flexible stent designs were developed, with the balloon-expanded slotted tube approach dominating [190]. Higher incidences of stent thrombosis (thrombotic occlusion of a stent) and restenosis (gradual narrowing of the inner lumen of a stent) with WALLSTENT and the Gianturco-

Roubin stent meant they gradually faded from the market [191].

Clinical evidence (European BENESTENT and US STRESS trials) demonstrated that the Palmaz-Shatz stent significantly reduced restenosis rates compared to balloon-based PTCA. Longer-term studies revealed rates of in-stent restenosis as high as 20–30% [192]. It was concluded that the presence of the stent promotes restenosis by causing the proliferation of vascular smooth muscle cells. To reduce this neointimal hyperplasia, antiproliferative drugs were coated onto the metal scaffolds, and this began the generation of drug-eluting stents (DES) [193]. The first generation of DES used antiproliferative agents based on paclitaxel and sirolimus analogs. The Cypher (sirolimus-eluting stent) and the Taxus (paclitaxel-eluting stent) were the first devices approved by the FDA. In long-term trials, concerns emerged regarding their safety due to very late thrombotic events, which were associated with a high rate of death and myocardial infarction.

During this time, stent materials went from stainless steel to cobalt-chromium and platinum-chromium steels, making stent struts thinner (from 150 to 75 μm). Trials confirmed thinner struts resulted in lower rates of restenosis [194]. The second-generation DESs were designed using these thinner strut stents as their platform. They are more refined and have a rapid drug elution profile. They also employed new biocompatible polymer coatings and less toxic antiproliferative drugs [195]. In 2001, Ulrich Speck and his team proposed and tested the concept of a drug-coated balloon (DCB) [196]. DCBs offer a means for sustained antirestenotic therapy without the drawbacks of a permanent implant being placed in the vasculature. It's an approved therapy for stent restenosis (ISR) and in small coronary vessels in Europe [197]. The treatment was thought to reduce the risk of a late inflammatory response due to the lack of foreign material and thrombogenicity. However, evidence emerged showing the efficacy of DCB-only for treating de novo lesions in large coronary arteries (greater than 3 mm).

Polymer Materials

Biological Response to Interventional Catheters

The availability of synthetic polymer materials in the late 1920s made the creative concepts of medical device pioneers more feasible [198]. Table 18.2 summarizes the early material experimentation of pioneers in the search for optimal vascular catheter materials. Materials such as Nylon (Polyamide), Dacron (Polyester), Orlon (Polyacrylonitrile), Ivalon (Polyvinyl alcohol), and Teflon (Polytetrafluoroethylene) were evaluated as potential vascular graft replacement materials in the late 1950s [199].

For those developing early implantable devices (between 1950 and 1980), it became increasingly apparent that the best biological performance was obtained from materials that were the least reactive chemically [200]. Materials were selected or developed as understanding grew for implant applications because they were nontoxic, nonimmunogenic, nonthrombogenic, noncarcinogenic, and nonirritant. This thinking has been applied to materials for vascular catheters (admittedly with recognition for the shorter duration of use and the level of blood and tissue contact) through ISO 10993 guidelines [201].

In April 1987, the FDA issued General Program Memorandum G87-1 "Tripartite Biocompatibility Guidance [206]. This was built on ANSI and ASTM standards [207]. It allowed all manufacturers to select appropriate tests to evaluate adverse biological responses to medical devices. In 1992, ISO 10993 was released. In 1995, the FDA mandated compliance with ISO 10993 for all submissions [206]. ISO 10993 contains two tables and a flow chart, allowing manufacturers to determine testing requirements principally based on duration of use and type of blood contact [208]. Before 1987, catheter manufacturers relied on USP Class VI certification to determine which materials were likely suitable for catheter applications [208]. It is now accepted that biocompatibil-

Table 18.2 Materials used in vascular catheters in the early years

Rubber latex	Rubber	Forssmann [24]	1927
PVC dispersion	Thermoplastic	Cournand [24]	Early 1940s
Polyethylene	Thermoplastic	Pierce [53]	1951
Radiopaque polyethylene	Thermoplastic	Odman [24]	1953
PTFE (Teflon)	Intractable thermoplastic	Gensini [202], Nordenström [76], Barr [203]	1960–1963
Silastic	Silicone rubber	Stewart [67], Dickson [204], McKissock [205]	1956–1960

ity is a complex characteristic of a system and not a specific material characteristic [209].

Experimentation between the mid-1950s and late 1960s marked a significant period in developing a clearer understanding of the ideal properties of vascular catheter tubing. Materials should be nonthrombogenic and not induce an inflammatory response in the endothelium layer of the vasculature [210]. Literature of the time showed awareness of the damage stiff catheters could cause to the vasculature [211–213]. Soft elastomeric materials were difficult to advance due to their poor pushability. Interventional catheters require a high degree of column strength to enable a clinician to transmit sufficient force through the tube for the distal tip to advance deep within the vasculature around tortuous vessels and across calcifications or lesions. Column strength is vital in deploying interventional devices and relates directly to catheter pushability. Today, composite catheter designs using complex reinforcement technologies and specific polymers allow sophisticated catheters to be produced with the desired column strength in various catheter sections [138]. The distal section can have lower column strength, allowing improved tracking and the proximal end can be optimized for high column strength, maximizing catheter pushability. Achieving the ideal properties of vascular catheters required the development of a new class of polymer materials: thermoplastic elastomers.

Polymer Materials for Interventional Catheter Applications

The first thermoplastic elastomer was polyester-based urethane (TPU), commercialized by BF Goodrich under the trade name Estane® [133]. The patent was granted on January 27, 1959 [214]. Estane® was used in "Ducor" (the first commercial metal wire braided catheter), which Cordis commercialized. Polyester-based polyurethanes proved susceptible to hydrolytic degradation within the body (in implant applications) [215]. This urgent need spurred the development of other materials for implant applications, with work on heart valves, artificial hearts, and vascular grafts, all of which require more biocompatible and degradation-resistant materials [216–218]. Considering the short period inside the body, this would have had little consequence for many vascular catheter applications but was important in the development of catheters that spent longer periods inside the body (i.e., central venous catheters). Generally more biocompatible and degradation resistant materials have less issue with thrombus formation and related complications within the vascular system.

Polyether urethanes, initially in solvent-based versions such as Biomer and Avothane, were introduced next [215] Pellethane®, introduced by Upjohn company in 1971 [219], was melt processable and had a lower cost than earlier polyether-based urethanes [220]. By the mid-1970s, a family of grades, "the Pellethane 2363 series," aimed at the biomedical market, was released. Failure of polyether-based polyurethanes (Pellethane 2363 80A) from oxidative degradation due to metal ion degradation (MIO) and induced environmental stress cracking (ESC) were noted in pacemaker lead failures in the early 1980s [221, 222]. Dow restricted using the Pellethane 2363 range to short-term implants in 1992 [220]. The term "short-term implant" is a device classification composed of interventional catheter-type therapies.

In 1979, an aliphatic polyurethane (Tecoflex®) from Thermedics exhibited improved resistance to yellowing and UV degradation compared to earlier polyurethane grades [223]. Thermedics later commercialized polycarbonate-based polyurethanes Carbothane® with increased alcohol resistance [224]. Catheters that are placed in the body for periods of up to 30 days (central venous catheters (CVCs) and peripheral infusion central catheters (PICCs)) are used with locking solutions often containing alcohol to maintain their effectiveness [225]. These third-generation carbonate-based urethanes, with their improved alcohol resistance, dominate central venous catheter (CVC) and other short-term implant-type applications [224, 226]. Thermoplastic carbonate urethane (TPCU) technology provides the basis of the very soft polyurethanes and polyurethane blends available as Chronoflex® AR or Chronoflex® AL [227]. These ultra-soft polyurethanes are used in the distal end of catheter shafts for various percutaneous neurovascular applications [228]. Extremely soft distal catheter materials are required due to the delicacy of the cerebral vasculature and the clinical need for highly kink-resistant yet trackable catheters for new therapies [229]. A review article listing construction details of guiding catheters for neurovascular use lists polyurethane and Polyblend® as distal tip materials [230]. Other materials, such as the Neusoft™ range from PolyOne®, allow materials of Shore A hardness as low as 42A to be used [231].

Polyamide fiber was used in USCI) woven-type construction, which Norman Jeckel patented and described in several papers in the early 1960s [24, 232]. The literature of the early 1960s also describes polyamide tubing as a stiffer alternative to polyethylene [233, 234]. With the commercialization of polyamide (Nylon) 11 and 12 and their derivatives, an alternative to polyurethane for vascular catheters emerged. Production of Polyamide 11 was started in 1949 [235]. Organico commercialized Polyamide 11 in France in 1955.

Today, Arkema (a descendant of Organico) produces Polyamide 11 in France and the USA as "Rilsan BESNO" [236]. Polyamide 12 was first commercialized in 1959 [237] and has similar mechanical and thermal properties to Polyamide 11. Both materials were used in catheter applications before polyether-block-amide (PEBA) materials emerged. Medical-grade Polyamide 11 (Rilsan BESNO® MED) and 12 (Rilsamid ASNO® MED and Vistamed L21 Care®) have been explicitly introduced for catheters in the last decade and are used where high mechanical performance is required. Polyamide 11 and 12 grades find applications in noncompliant balloons, proximal ends of guide catheters, and delivery systems [210, 238].

Plasticized versions of Polyamide 11, such as "BESNO P40," were developed to provide flexible tubing options for industrial applications in the early 1970s. These grades featured Butyl-Benzene-sulfonamide as the plasticizer [239]. These plasticized materials provided an option for creating more flexible materials before the availability of polyamide-based thermoplastic elastomers. Throughout the 1970s, ATO Chemie focused on developing nonplasticized flexible polyamide-based polymers [240]. As an expert in Polyamide 11 and 12 technologies, ATO Chemie knew the limitations and drawbacks of plasticizer technology. Technically, the first polyamide elastomer was produced by Huls AG (Now Degussa AG) in Germany in 1977 under the trade name Vestamid E [241]. In 1980, ATO Chemie (Now Arkema) received a patent for the technology to produce poly-ether-ester-amide block copolymers [242]. This material, PEBAX®, was launched commercially in 1981 [240]. Altering the structure and molecular weight of the polyamide and polyether segments in PEBAX® modifies mechanical properties [243]. Over the next decade, the PEBAX® durometer range was widened to provide options for various catheter applications. Pebax in SA (sans additive) grades became available in the early 1990s with USP Class VI testing certification [241].

Their processability, mechanical properties, and biocompatibility have made PEBA attractive for medical device applications [244]. With the selective use of grades, PEBA can meet the requirements of most interventional catheter applications, making it the most commonly used interventional catheter material [245]. Applications include diagnostic catheters, guiding catheters, microcatheters, and delivery systems [244, 246]. The emergence of medical-grade thermoplastic elastomers with low durometer values that are chemically and thermally compatible allows almost infinite customization of catheter properties. These materials can be combined in longitudinal sections along the outside surface of a composite catheter to tailor the stiffness to fit the requirements of any area of the vasculature (very low durometer materials are key for the flexibility and trackability required for many neurovascular catheter applications).

Thrombogenicity was a grave concern in the early evolution of interventional catheter-based therapies [247–249]. Due to changes in the polymers used, the smaller diameters of catheters today relative to vessel size, the smooth nature of the inner and outer surfaces, and the increased use of flushing and ancillary medicines, thrombogenicity is now a minor concern for short-term catheter interventions [250].

Polymer Materials: Catheter Coating

Coatings, particularly hydrophilic coatings, have improved catheter performance regarding thrombogenicity [250]. The first attempts at providing low-friction surfaces for catheters involved the application of nonpermanent coatings such as silicone oil, olive oil, or glycerin and the use of conventional low-friction polymers such as fluoroplastics, silicone, and polyethylene [251]. Amplatz and others demonstrated heparin bound to the surface of a catheter as an insoluble precipitate effectively reduced thrombus formation [252]. Later work on silicone and PTFE coatings showed limited effectiveness in reducing thrombus formation in vivo [253, 254]. To reduce friction between the device and the vasculature, a selection of hydrophilic polymers, including polyvinylpyrrolidone (PVP), polyacrylic acid, polyethylene oxide (PEO), and polysaccharides, were used [81]. The first vascular hydrophilic coated devices were guidewires placed on the market by Terumo in the mid-1980s [255]. Terumo applied that coating to catheters in the early 1990s. It improved catheter tracking and control and was less traumatic to the vasculature [256].

Trackability describes the ability of a catheter to follow over a guide wire through a tortuous vessel. Several factors influence trackability, including catheter outer diameter and length, column strength, and the frictional resistance between the guide wire and catheter and the outer catheter surface and the vessel wall [257]. The hydrophilic coating reduces the frictional resistance with the vasculature and improves trackability. Hydrophobic liners (discussed further on) minimize frictional resistance of the inner catheter surface. Kenny regarded trackability as the main feature that guided catheter development [258].

The hydrophilic coating has widened the capabilities of interventional device designers by providing new opportunities to achieve performance requirements. Larger diameter and longer devices can be inserted through the vasculature for the same or lower force for a smaller or shorter device [259]. Reductions in insertion force, patient discomfort [260, 261], and improvements in trackability, control [261], and decreased thrombogenicity [262] improved catheter performance. Furthermore, hydrophilic coatings, such as antimicrobial and drug-eluting, enhanced their safety and applications [259].

Polymers for the Construction of Ultra-Thin Layers and Complex Structures

Both PTFE and HDPE are hydrophobic materials [210]. A hydrophobic surface repels water with a static contact angle above 90° [263]. Both materials are regularly used as inner lining layers of interventional catheters to provide an excellent sliding movement on the guide wire and reduce the friction required to deliver various implants through the catheter [210]. Hydrophobic inner layers offer an alternative route to a low-friction surface where a tightly packed implant is delivered. Hydrophilic coatings would require fluid activation and could create emboli through shearing the coating under the radial force applied by an implant being advanced through the inner bore of a catheter delivery system. There is considerable concern and focus on emboli generated from catheter coatings in interventional therapies [81, 264]. Increasingly complex catheter property demands from areas such as ischemic stroke treatment, structural heart, and lower profile delivery systems have pushed the development and adoption of alternative materials and catheter fabrication techniques [229, 265, 266].

Polyimide has found application as an inner (liner) layer for thin wall composite catheters and in applications where high strength and low profile are required [267]. Polyimides exhibit high stiffness, tensile properties, and a very high melt point [268]. The first commercial polyimide was prepared using a two step method by Endrey [269]. This material was patented by Du Pont under the trade name Kapton [270]. Polyimide is applied using a thermally cured solution coating process [267, 271]. The coating process allows material deposition to very exact dimensions in ultra-thin layers. Polyimide is also available in composite form with PEBA, polyamide, or polyurethane outer layers [272, 273]. PTFE solution coating can be carried out using similar processing technology [274, 275]. Both polyimide and film-cast PTFE allow complex metal-reinforced composites to be manufactured in ultra-thin walls [271]. These ultra-thin-walled composite catheters are vital to advancing catheter techniques in neurovascular therapies [229, 276, 277].

Guiding Catheters and Introducer Sheaths: Facilitating Therapies

By 1985, guiding catheters had evolved to a design based on a PTFE liner, a braid layer with an outer layer of polyurethane or polyethylene [278]. In 1985, Van Tassel demonstrated that a soft tip section significantly reduced vascular trauma with coronary catheterization [279]. Guide catheter manufacturers adopted this approach [163]. By this point, radiopaque markers such as tantalum or platinum rings were being incorporated into the distal end of the catheter shafts [278].

Studies have shown that smaller guide catheter sizes correlate with fewer clinical complications [280–282]. Most coronary interventions use 6 or 7 Fr guide catheters today [283]. Modern guide catheters of 6 Fr (2 mm outside diameter) have typical wall thicknesses of 0.12 mm [27]. This thin wall incorporates a Teflon liner, metal, or plastic braid to transmit torque and provide stiffness for backup support and a smooth outer layer to resist thrombus formation [27]. Outer layers are typically multidurometer sections of thermoplastic elastomer (PEBA or polyurethane-based). Outer materials are selected to provide the right balance between support and flexibility [283]. The technology developed for PTCA was foundational to the development of guide catheters for various therapeutic areas (neurology, stenting, atherectomy, etc.).

With the development of closed-end catheters, the need for catheter sheaths grew due to the increased use of catheter manometers, bioptomes (heart biopsy sampling devices), and flow meters [284]. These devices could not be introduced over a wire (Seldinger technique). The first vascular access or "Desilets-Hoffman" sheath was described in 1965 [285]. These sheaths simplified placing specialized catheters within the vasculature. Closed-end catheters with side holes were less likely to suffer recoil during injection, higher pressures could be used, and the likelihood of perforation of the myocardium was reduced. This first vascular access sheath was constructed from Mylar (oriented polyethylene terephthalate (PET)) purchased from a drinking straw company. A 0.002 in. thick Mylar tubing was glued to a steel cannula, which acted as a proximal hub and anchor for the sheath [286]. In a later 1966 paper [287], Desilets describes how Teflon (PTFE) showed promise for venous studies but could not be made thin enough for access use. Cook Inc. started commercial production of the Desilets-Hoffman sheath in 1965. Later, in 1969, improvement in Teflon extrusion techniques allowed a thin-walled Teflon tube to replace the Mylar in the sheath introducer [288]. Early versions required a catheter closely matched in size to the sheath's inner diameter to avoid excessive bleeding during use [286].

Minimizing Blood Loss: Hemostasis Valves

In 1974, the ability to downsize catheter size while minimizing blood loss was described [289]. Attaching a Tuohy-Borst adaptor to the sheath allowed an almost bloodless interchange of varying diameter and nontapered catheters [286]. Cordis introduced the first sheath introducers with hemostasis valves designed to minimize blood loss during an angioplasty procedure in the mid-1970s [290]. The 1977 patent assigned to Robert Stevens describes using a dual gasket system in a housing [291]. The use of these devices for left heart catheterization was described in 1979 [292, 293]. Vascular access site sheaths allow catheter exchange with minimal blood loss [128]. The development of the vascular access sheath was a foundation stone in the emergence of complex catheter-based therapies, in which multiple catheters are used throughout the procedure. It also allowed more complex interventions to be contemplated.

Further Refinement: Kink Resistance

Coil-reinforced silicone tubing for drainage was described in a 1971 patent [294]. Descriptions of coil reinforcement for fluid flow [295] and intravenous feeding followed [296] and a patent issued to Kocak [297]. This patent describes a process for creating a valved introducer with a sheath body based on a solution-coated spirally coiled spring. It claimed flexible tubing with both kink and crush resistance. Arrow International (Teleflex) introduced the Super Arrow Flex product line in 1993 [298]. The patent describes an extremely thin, flat metal coil surrounded externally by a plastic coating [299]. Cook Medical's coil-reinforced sheath patent from 1995 [300] describes a flat spirally wound coiled catheter with a PTFE liner and a polyamide outer layer. This technology became the platform for the Cook Flexor range of access sheaths [288]. Guiding sheaths are similar to reinforced introducer sheaths with longer lengths and shaped tips [301]. They facilitate the passage of a smaller catheter or endovascular device through a tortuous path to a treatment location [302]. A relatively flexible PEBA-type polymer surrounds the coiled reinforcement compared to the stiffer materials used in guiding catheters. The technologies used for guiding sheaths would later be used in delivery systems for emerging EVAR, TEVAR, and TAVI therapies.

Today, coil reinforcement is recognized as improving kink performance, minimizing ovalization of the inner lumen, and maximizing hoop strength in interventional catheters [303]. Variable pitch coiling has been used in vascular graft delivery systems to achieve different properties on both ends of the delivery system [304]. A tight pitch at the distal end minimizes ovalization, thus minimizing graft deployment forces. A wider pitch in the proximal end maximizes column strength. Generally, in very complex demanding applications, coil reinforcement is often used distally for kink resistance and trackability, and braid is used in the proximal end and for most of the catheter length for pushability and tensile strength [142]. The Sofia distal access catheter used in neurovascular applications is an example [230].

Neurovascular Catheters: Challenge of Delicate Anatomy

Catheter-based procedure development in neurointerventional radiology lags behind that of other interventional fields. The tortuosity, narrowness, delicacy of intracranial arteries, and the presence of the carotid siphon are obstacles to intracranial navigation [305]. Since the field's inception, intracranial access through the skull base and around the ophthalmic genu has been challenging for endovascular neurosurgeons [306]. Figure 18.5 outlines the vasculature relevant to neurovascular procedures and the complex vascular geometry the catheters must navigate during neurosurgical procedures.

The first microcatheterization of brain vessels was reported in 1964 [68]. This involved a silastic (silicone) catheter introduced through the carotid artery. Later, the POD, a magnetically directed microcatheter [307], Debrun's coaxial catheter [308], and Hieshima flow-directed polyethylene microcatheter [309] marked the stages in the progression of neurovascular microcatheter technology.

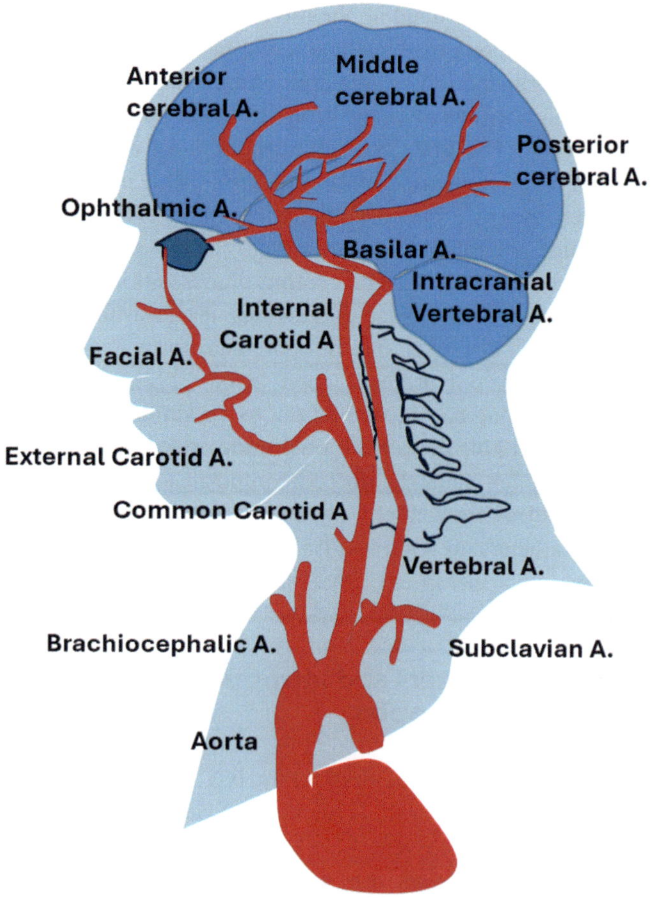

Fig. 18.5 Schematic anatomy for catheter-based neurovascular therapies

In 1986, Target Therapeutics introduced the tracker microcatheter [310]. Construction details of the catheter are described in a patent granted in 1988 [311]. This 3.2 Fr unreinforced catheter had a stiff proximal section made from rigid materials (polypropylene or high-density polyethylene) with a short flexible distal section made from low stiffness low-density polyethylene. The catheter fitted closely over a steerable guide wire with a deformable tip to negotiate vascular bends [305]. This innovation allowed the possibility of direct catheterization of cerebral aneurysms for the first time. The tracker catheter's flexibility enabled access for treatment but required extensive manipulation for placement [306]. Fastracker, a next-generation version, was a hydrographically coated Polyether urethane microcatheter (Tracker was silicone coated) [262]. Reduction in friction from hydrographic coating allowed easier manipulation for catheter placement.

Endovascular therapies for intracranial aneurysms emerged in the 1990s with the advent of the Guglielmi detachable coil system [312]. This therapy demonstrated efficacy in trials against the accepted open surgical procedure of neurosurgical clipping [313, 314]. The tracker catheter was used to deliver endovascular coils, but the inner lumen was easily scored, and the absence of reinforcement resulted in kinking [306]. In the mid-1990s, the microcatheter design evolved to meet the challenges of providing trackable catheters that were pushable, and more resistant to kinking and ovalization [306, 315–317]. As PTFE-lined microcatheters became the accepted design platform, other innovations were introduced, mainly in distal tip flexibility. These included platinum micro coils, braid structures with spiral reinforcement in the distal section, and even softer distal catheter materials [306]. Catheters were also downsized to facilitate the miniaturization of aneurysm coil technology [318]. These innovations were driven by the need to reduce kinking and improve usability and workability to facilitate catheter placement for aneurysm coil placement [306].

The guide catheter provides the stability of microcatheters and is fundamental to successful and safe endovascular interventions [319]. The neuron guide catheter was explicitly designed for neurovascular procedures [306]. This guide catheter has a variable stiffness profile that allows higher positioning in the anatomy than earlier catheter designs (see Fig. 18.6), providing additional microcatheter support [320].

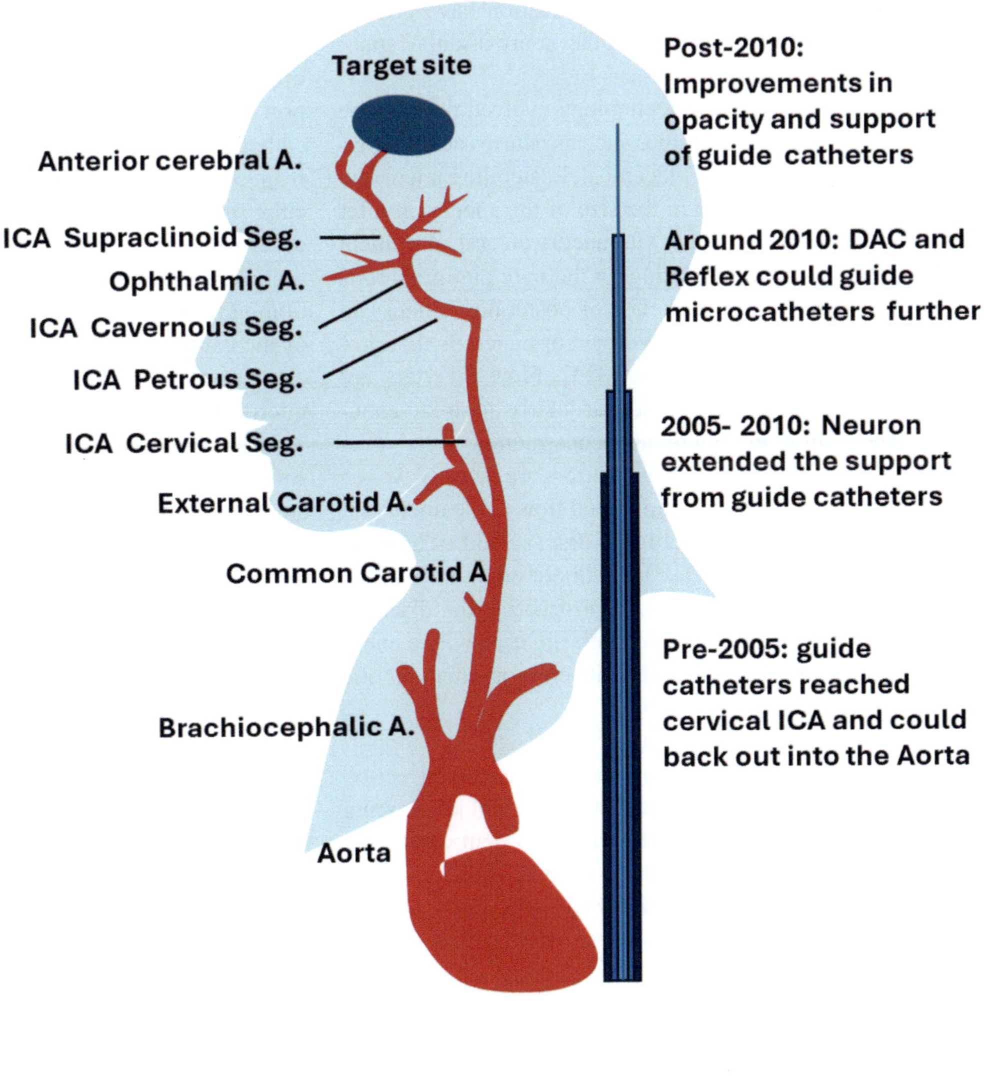

Fig. 18.6 The evolution of neurovascular guiding catheters

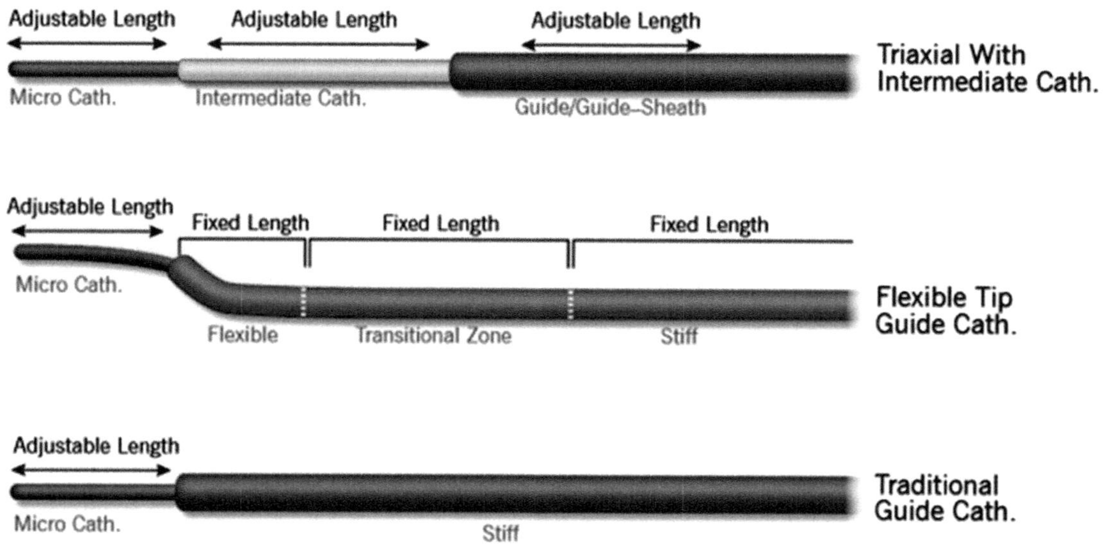

Fig. 18.7 Evolution of catheter navigation of approaches [321]

The Neuron could be positioned around the right angles in the vascular anatomy at the skull base [276]. Improvements in microcatheter technology and the development of neurovascular-specific guide catheters (see Fig. 18.7 middle image) that can achieve intracranial position have created complication-free distal access in the neurovascular space [276].

Guide and microcatheter technology evolved to meet the needs of neurovascular therapies such as neurovascular angiography and aneurysm coil placement. Postcoiling aneurysm recanalization (an increase in the size of the aneurysm after therapy) remains a challenge with aneurysm coil placement [322]. Coatings promote clotting on the bare platinum coils are used to reduce the occurrence of postcoiling aneurysm recanalization. These include hydrogel or materials that promote an inflammatory response [323]. Flow diverters are stent-like devices deployed endovascularly to treat aneurysms. They allow endoluminal reconstruction rather than endovascular filling [324]. Flow diverters are densely woven wire-based devices that interrupt blood flow at the aneurysm neck to increase blood stagnation in the sac and trigger the thrombosis-based healing cascade without embolic material [306]. They treat aneurysms by reconstructing the diseased parent artery [312, 325]. Flow diverters are used where aneurysms have wide necks, and filling with coils or other embolic materials is not viable.

There has been a shift in the design of catheter support systems for flow diversion from the classic biaxial set-up (Guide catheter and microcatheter) with cervical positioning of guide catheters to a more robust triaxial system with intracranial positioning of intermediate support catheters [312, 326]. Using an intermediate catheter (see Fig. 18.7), this triaxial catheter approach has become standard across a range of neurovascular therapies, mainly where tortuosity is a concern, i.e., deployment of aneurysm coils and thrombectomy [106, 327, 328]. Intermediate catheters (such as Concentric Medical's (Now Stryker's) Outreach DAC catheter or Reflex from Reverse Medical (now Navien Medtronic)) are highly trackable catheters with very thin walls that can track further up the vasculature (over a microcatheter) and provide support for a range of neurovascular therapies [329, 330]. These catheters continue to evolve and are structurally different from the guide catheters (even those modified for neurovascular use) and the microcatheters. These catheters have been described as having nitinol spiral reinforcement in the distal section with many distinct stiffness zones gradually transitioning from very soft to more rigid toward the proximal end of the catheter [326]. This minimizes the amount of microcatheter exposed unsupported and acts as a fulcrum for microcatheter withdrawal (see Fig. 18.7 (top of the image)). This is important as microcatheter distal sections become softer and microcatheter profiles reduce. Intermediate catheters also provide another option for the aspiration of clots, representing an advancement in neurovascular thrombectomy technology [328, 331].

Steerable and Deflectable Catheters; Catheter Positioning for Targeted Therapy

In 1951, Tillander reported using a steerable magnetic catheter based on a single copper coil that articulated a steel-tipped catheter [98]. The size and power consumption to navigate the catheter tip were shown to be impractical [332]. Using a Niobium-Titanium (NbTi) filament wound superconducting coil improved the guiding ability of this conceptual approach while reducing its power consumption [333]. This technology, combined with improvements in imaging, led to the MNS (Magnetic Navigation System) Telstar [334]. This system was superseded by a second-generation Niobe system that's silent, more reliable, and responsive [335]. This technology has been used successfully in catheter ablation procedures to treat atrial fibrillation [336, 337] and percutaneous coronary intervention [338].

The first commercial controllable tip deflector for interventional catheters was the USCI) Muller tip deflecting system [61]. This system evolved from the guide wire, and the literature describes its use in angiography and chemotherapy in 1968 and 1970, respectively [339, 340]. Grollman describes how the system worked; a 0.035 in. tip deflecting wire was placed in the system and introduced through the catheter, allowing selective catheterization of each coronary artery as this wire was deflected [341]. Muller's patent outlines how manipulating an inner tension wire resulted in the straightening or curvature of the distal tip [342].

Barchilon achieved the placement of the deflection mechanism inside the catheter wall rather than within the catheter lumen. His 1969 patent outlines a design with deflection cables buried in the catheter wall with 360° single-location deflection. This was key as it allowed an unobstructed inner lumen that had the potential to be used for implant or device delivery [343]. Bentov received a patent (1971) for a four-direction steerable catheter used in the bronchial tree and gastrointestinal tract [344]. Both designs were too large for vascular applications at the time. Mechanical actuation based on cable or tendon steering describes the most significant and commercially available styles of steering catheters used in cardiology (the principal market for steerable catheters) [345]. A schematic representation of a four-directional braided catheter profile is shown in Fig. 18.8c.

Steerable catheters for vascular applications are generally mechanically actuated thin wall composite sheaths [346]. These catheters rely on a tendon-based continuum system where the actuation tendons are terminated at the catheter tip [347]. Flexible polymers, braided or coiled reinforcement can be layered to obtain the different characteristics in different directions [345]. Varying the lengths of outer material sections can also tailor the catheter shaft's deflection properties. Steering limitations arise from the interaction between catheter components, tortuous vasculature, and the dynamic environment [346]. The tendons are tracked through steering lumens, generally Polyimide, PTFE, or a thin-walled composite construction. These steering channels minimize frictional force and run through the catheter walls or may protrude very slightly into the inner lumen of the catheter, as shown in Fig. 18.8b.

The most straightforward steering system for a mechanically actuated catheter consists of one spring-like construction with one or two steering cables fixed at the tip generally to a steering band, providing a one degree of freedom tip deflection in one or two directions in a single plane (see Fig. 18.8a) [345]. As outlined earlier, omnidirectional or four-directional steering gives two degrees of freedom, with the catheter tip able to move in two planes perpendicular to each other. This is achieved with four tendons and a single steering band. Omni-directional steering simplifies catheter manipulation for a physician as the catheter does not need to be rotated [346]. Theoretically, two steering bands can be added to a single catheter assembly to create multiple-segment actuation (Fig. 18.9). A catheter of this type could create multiplanar movements inside the heart or other structures [345]. A patent for second-generation delivery system for a mitral valve clip is an example of a delivery system using this design approach [348].

Using two distinct catheter shafts, a coaxial steerable catheter technique can achieve the above outcome [335]. In the coaxial technique, an outer sheath with two deflection cables at 180° to each other is used to create a stable plat-

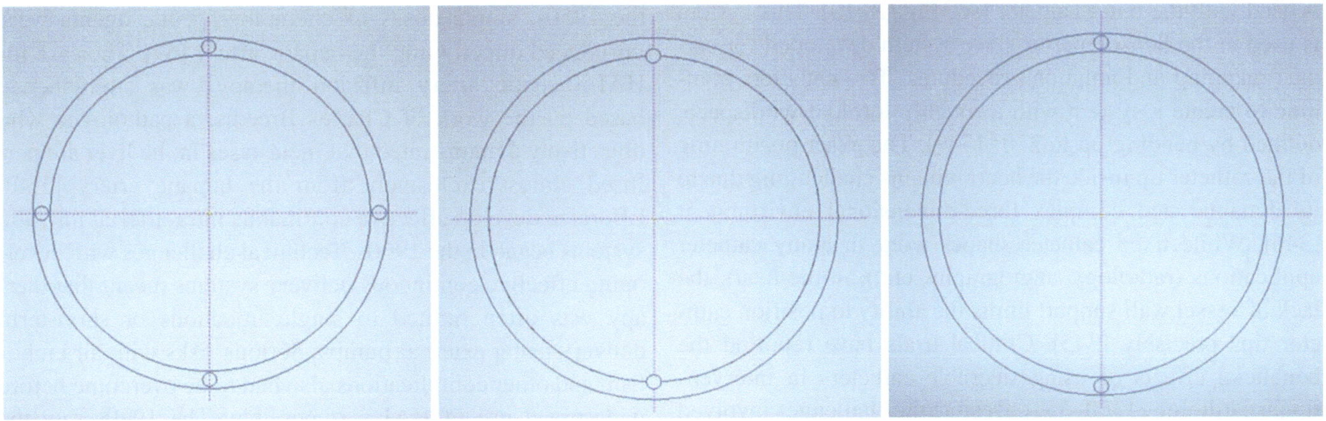

Fig. 18.8 Cross-sections of various steering approaches. **Left**: Dual steering channels. **Middle**: Dual steering channels protruding into the internal lumen. **Right**: Four steering channels in the catheter wall

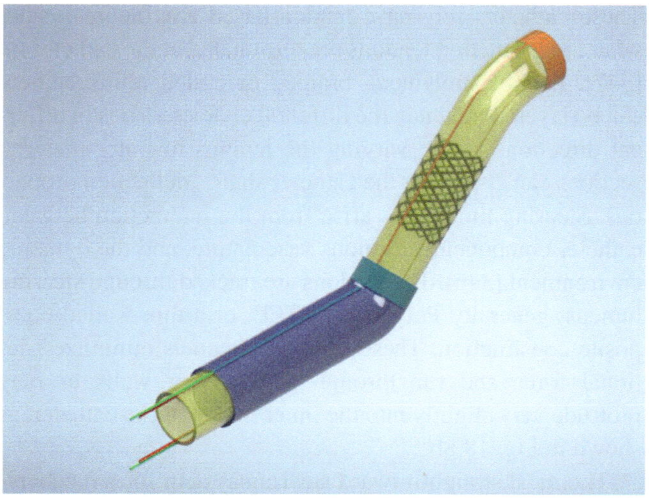

Fig. 18.9 Dual steering point catheter where both steering segments are in the same plane. Offsetting the steering cables by 90° allows multiplanar movement

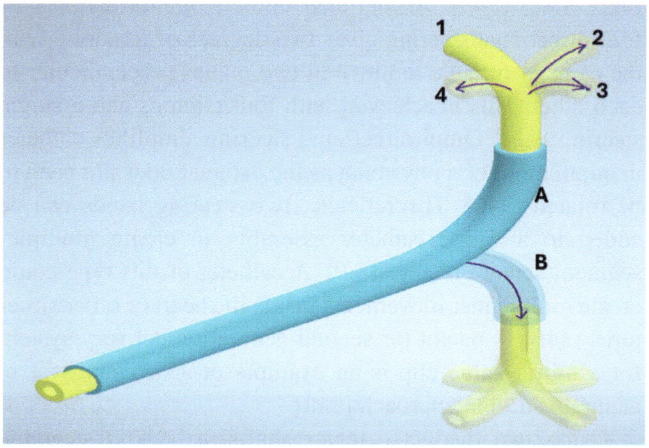

Fig. 18.10 Inner catheter steers in four directions (1–4). The outer catheter steers in two directions (A and B)

form. An inner steerable catheter with four deflection cables is used with the outer catheter (see Fig. 18.10). This system is used in the Sensei master-slave system developed for cardiac mapping and ablation procedures. Two catheters combine to create a system with a roughly toroidal workspace, defined by bending up to 270° [349]. The exact positioning of the catheter tip inside the heart remains challenging due to its dynamic and complex three-dimensional environment [346]. While fixed catheter shapes work in many catheter applications (radiology, angiography, etc.), in the heart, the lack of vessel wall support limits the ability to position catheter tips precisely [345]. Clinical trials have reported the beneficial effects of using steerable catheters in interventional cardiology [350–353]. Despite the challenges involved in their design, experience with steerable catheters has shown clinical advantages across different therapies and a relatively short learning curve [347, 351–354]. Steerable catheters that can facilitate a variety of complex shape tip curves may change conventional approaches toward more patient-specific and less invasive procedures [346].

Catheter Technology for Intra-Arterial Delivery of Chemotherapy

Chemotherapy is a drug that employs potent chemicals to kill fast-growing cells in the body. As a therapy, it focuses mainly on cancer treatment as cancer cells multiply much more quickly than most cells in the body. An accidental spill of mustard gas on troops in World War II led to the understanding that those men exposed to the mustard gas suffered from lower white blood cell counts. Building on that observation, Alfred Gilman and Louis Goodman at Yale experimented with mice bearing a transplanted lymphoid tumor who were then exposed to nitrogen mustard [355]. When they observed marked regressions in the animal trials, they convinced a colleague and thoracic surgeon, Gustaf Lindskog, to administer nitrogen mustard to a patient with non-Hodgkin's lymphoma and severe airway obstruction. Marked regression was observed, as described in Chap. 1 [356]. This marked the first use of chemotherapy. However, additional work, understanding, and development of additional drugs were required to make it an effective therapy.

In the 1940s, the newly discovered chemotherapy agents (nitrogen mustards) were administered intravenously [357]. It was understood that regional therapy would maximize the cytotoxic concentrations and minimize systemic side effects. In his paper, Calvin Klopp, a surgeon, outlined a novel technique for intra-arterial injection of chemotherapy agents to treat lung carcinoma [358]. Howard R. Bierman, an oncologist, outlined a technique for percutaneous catheterization of the aorta and celiac access through the brachial artery, acknowledged as the first report on the administration of chemotherapy through an artery [359]. At the beginning of the 1950s, single doses of chemotherapeutic agents were introduced directly into the hepatic artery [69]. The case for HAI (hepatic artery infusion therapy) was strengthened based on the work of Charles Breedis, a pathologist who objectively demonstrated that metastases in the liver are perfused almost exclusively from the hepatic artery [360]. Efforts to develop effective continuous intra-arterial infusion systems began in the 1960s. Technical challenges with developing effective continuous delivery systems meant that therapy was often limited to single injections or short-term delivery using external pumps. Serious risks with air embolism and other complications also had to be overcome before widespread use of HAI was possible. The 1970s saw the widespread use of an alternative drug, Floxuridine, which had a short half-life and very high first-pass metabolism in the liver after HAI. This drug became the standard for HAI therapy. This decade also saw the development of an implantable and refillable pump. The pump was developed by an engineer, Perry Blackshear Jr., and a surgeon, Henry Buchwald, who used it to infuse Floxuridine into the hepatic artery [361]. Silicone was introduced as a catheter material in this space in 1985 to reduce thrombosis.

Balloon-Assisted Techniques for Direct Cerebral Infusion

The challenge with direct infusion techniques is that they often suffer from poor local drug retention. Drugs inevitably enter systemic circulation due to inadequate tools/devices for optimizing delivery, leaky tumor vasculature, or changes in lymphatic drainage and interstitial pressure. In the context of brain cancer or metastasis to the brain, local drug delivery is particularly pertinent as the blood–brain barrier presents a challenge for drug transport. Despite extensive research, developing intracranial delivery systems for cancer treatment remains relentlessly challenging [362].

In 1994, a group led by Edward Oldfield, a neurosurgeon, published the first paper describing convection-enhanced delivery (CED) for the local delivery of drugs that were either limited by the BBB or too large to diffuse effectively [363]. CED is another promising catheter-based approach for local drug delivery to the central nervous system. CED employs the stereotactic placement of one or more catheters within an area of interest to facilitate the direct infusion of therapeutics. The catheters are connected to pumps that provide a continuous, positive-pressure micro-infusion of the desired agents to the target tissues [364]. Attempts have been made to improve the effectiveness of the techniques and the catheter approaches used to treat malignant brain tumors. An interesting paper by Riina [365] describes using a temporary occlusion balloon to occlude the basilar artery distal to the planned intra-arterial infusion site. The paper describes using a microcatheter positioned to give maximal infusion along the segment of the basilar artery where the pontine arteries arise to supply the pons and adjacent parts of the brain. The paper describes how a drug (bevacizumab) was infused through the microcatheter at 1 cc/min for 3 min with the balloon inflated. Then, the balloon was deflated for 2 min to allow blood flow to the posterior circulation. Reinfusion with the balloon inflated was then restarted. This cycle was repeated 12 times until the full 36 cc of drug solution was delivered. The proposed balloon-assisted superselective intra-arterial cerebral infusion (SIACI) of bevacizumab after blood–brain barrier disruption for malignant brainstem gliomas leans on the neurovascular catheter technology of the time (2010).

The balloon in Riina's publication was described as a Hyperglide but is a Hyperform 7 × 7 occlusion balloon (made by EV3 Neurovascular at the time and now Medtronic). This balloon catheter was used at that time as a component in coil placement procedures for the treatment of aneurysms to prevent hemorrhagic stroke. The other components mentioned, guide and microcatheters, were also used in hemorrhagic stroke therapy. It's interesting to note that developing sophisticated and trackable catheter systems for treating ischemic stroke over the last 14 years could provide even more advanced catheter tools for localized drug delivery in the brain. Balloon guide catheters, aspiration catheters, intermediate catheters, and more refined and trackable microcatheters are available today and have potentially significantly improved the ability of a clinician to navigate and access various areas of the neurovascular anatomy.

The Future of Transvascular Catheter Technology

Today's transvascular catheter technology offers a modular, adaptable platform tailored to new or emerging transcatheter therapies. This chapter has shown how the evolution of polymer material science, improved catheter manufacturing and reinforcement technologies, refined imaging technologies, and the specific requirements of the various therapies have all played a role in shaping the development of today's technology. Looking at the evolution of this space since the birth of interventional radiology with Dotter's work in 1964, it's clear that the desire to move from open surgery to less invasive approaches has driven this advancement. Today, we have catheter-based therapies for coronary arterial disease, ischemic stroke, small liver tumors, lower limb blockages, and a vast range of other clinical areas. This drive to create catheter-based therapies to replace remaining open surgical procedures will continue and be facilitated by further improvements in the base catheter technology. This capability platform is being augmented by the refinement of technologies to produce thinner catheter layers using solution-based coating methods rather than traditional extrusion techniques.

Thinner liner layers (inner layer of a composite catheter, see Fig. 18.11) coupled with softer tie-layer materials will produce thinner, more flexible, and more maneuverable catheters. This will facilitate the use of catheters in areas of the vasculature that cannot be navigated with today's technology (large parts of the cerebral vasculature). Some companies are investigating the use of ultra-low durometer polyurethane as tie layer materials. Also, fluoropolymer alternatives are being studied in the materials area as potential low-friction options that don't involve PFAS. Possible materials include copoly-

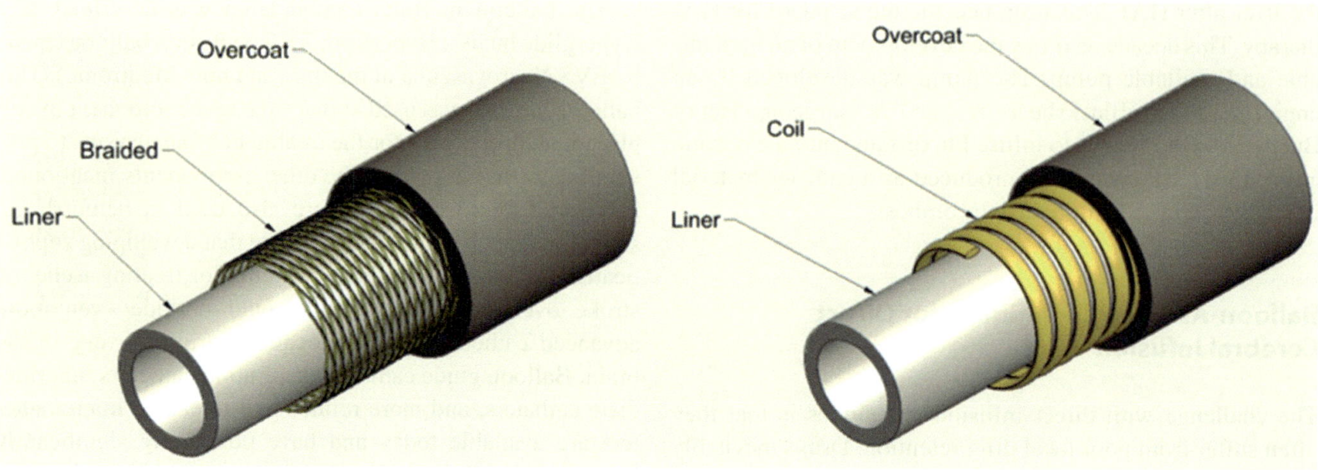

Fig. 18.11 **Left**: Braided and **Right**: Coiled composite catheter

mers of ethylene, siloxane, and several thermoplastic elastomers.

In terms of reinforcement, the use of stainless steel and increasingly nitinol-slotted hypo tubes in the distal sections of catheters are becoming more common for demanding applications right across the size range from microcatheters used for embolization to large-diameter structural heart delivery systems. Using a nitinol-slotted hypo-tube allows for improved torque ability of the catheter shaft while retaining pushability, trackability, and flexibility like other microcatheters [366]. For cardiac applications, it allows the design and fabrication of steerable delivery catheters that can be deflected using lower forces than traditionally fabricated designs based on a dense braid and coil reinforcement combination. This reduces the wall thickness profile. In electrophysiology applications, the ability of nitinol to straighten and recover after deflection in deflectable catheters is often critical to consistent and repeatable performance.

This trend toward nitinol will require developing simple and more robust joining and welding techniques to attach to other metals. As the properties of nitinol are generally only needed in the distal 100–150 mm of the composite catheter, joining it to a standard reinforcement skeleton of a conventional braid or coil will reduce the catheter cost point. Techniques for fabricating ever-thinner nitinol structures, such as thin film nitinol technology [367], will likely be used for thinner profile components rather than drawn nitinol tubing or components fabricated from nitinol sheets.

Traditionally, fluoroscopy has dominated imaging for transvascular catheter-based procedures. However, there are severe drawbacks to its use. Fluoroscopy exposes the catheter operator to significant doses of radiation. Heavy (lead-based) protective gear introduces other ergonomic risks for the catheter operator. Ideally, moving the physician out of the fluoroscopy field for all or most parts of the procedure would significantly reduce the radiation risk to the catheter operator. Much effort has gone into evaluating alternative imaging technologies and techniques for catheter-based transvascular therapies. Intravascular ultrasound (IVUS) and optical coherence tomography (OCT) have been developed and refined as diagnostic and guidance tools for interventional procedures over the past three decades. In the case of IVUS, the transducer is mounted within the catheter tip, and with OCT, the probe is also within the catheter. This means both technologies provide a view from the catheter perspective within the blood vessel. IVUS has a resolution of 100 μm with a high tissue penetration and the capability of assessing the entire structure of a coronary artery, including the external elastic membrane. OCT has a higher resolution of 10–20 μm to assess endoluminal structures but has limited tissue penetration compared to IVUS [368].

Intra-cardiac echocardiography (ICE) is like IVUS but is designed to image inside the heart using Doppler imaging. Compared to IVUS, it uses lower frequency transducers and allows the clinician to see structures and blood flow inside the heart. These lower-frequency transducers can have greater tissue penetration and imaging depth, permitting high-resolution two-dimensional imaging of the whole heart. It is a complement or an alternative to fluoroscopy for various interventional procedures in the electrophysiology and structural heart space. It offers advantages over transthoracic and transesophageal echo in terms of resolution and image quality due to the sensor's location within the heart structure rather than externally. As the sensing elements are miniaturized and catheters are downsized, they will likely grow in popularity. The critical difference between these imaging technologies is that they are catheter-based and can be very local to the specific procedure, so they offer possibilities that are not possible with traditional fluoroscopy.

Another notable development in imaging is piloting augmented or mixed reality (AR/MR) imaging. Centerline Biomedical is developing this technique, which allows simultaneous visualization of the surrounding physical environment overlaid with digital information. The clinician wears a digital head-mounted display with optical see-through lenses that project stereoscopic images called holograms. Preoperative tomographic imaging can generate anatomically correct and patient-specific 3D holograms of vascular structures [369]. The holograms can be projected onto the operative field in spatial registration with the patient's location and landmarks. When the surgeon looks directly at the operative field, the hologram of the subject's abdominal aorta, branch vessels, and relevant bony structures are visualized in the anatomically correct locations. This technology has potential in many areas and is an example of future technology that could transform imaging and, by extension, catheter-based therapies. The intravascular catheter must incorporate navigational sensing elements such as electromagnetic guidance. The electromagnetic navigation system attached to the surgical table generates a weak magnetic field around the patient. It allows the position and orientation of the sensors and, therefore, the catheter tip to be tracked. This technology or similar navigation and imaging-based technologies will transform catheter-based therapies over the next decade as they broaden the scope of what is possible with intra-vascular catheter technology. They will also facilitate the movement toward a wide use of robotic surgery-based approaches.

Robotic surgery is rapidly diffusing across a broad range of surgical procedures [370]. In 1998, the ZEUS robotic and Da Vinci surgical systems were introduced into the teleoperated surgery market. Rapid advancements have occurred in the intervening 27 years, and robotic systems have been widely used in medical fields such as neurological laparoscopy, radiosurgery, prosthetics, rehabilitation, orthopedics, and ophthalmology [371]. In orthopedic surgery, robotics and navigation techniques have been significantly adopted for hip and knee surgery. They are also increasingly adopted in elbow/shoulder, foot/ankle, spine, and arthroscopic surgeries.

The FDA has approved using several robotic navigation or CAS (computer-assisted surgery) platforms in the intravascular catheter space. Sensei X and the Magellan are among the robotic catheterization systems employed clinically. The Sensei system has been used for cardiac electrophysiology applications. Applying a constant force over a relatively long time is critical for consistent results in ablation procedures. It's easy to see how a robotic technique could work better in this clinical space. It has also been used in endovascular aneurysm repair. The focus of this procedure was potentially reducing procedure times and radiation exposure to the patient and operator [372].

Another commercial system is the Niobe robotic magnetic navigation system (Stereotaxis, St. Louis, MO, USA). This system uses two permanent magnets to produce a magnetic field to control the tip of the magnetic catheters/guidewires. This system has also been used in cardiac electrophysiological studies and coronary and peripheral arterial disease therapies [373]. The system has evolved, is smaller, more flexible, and faster today, and offers an alternative robotic approach for catheter-based procedures. Although still in development, the Amigo system (Catheter Precision) is a mechanically driven system developed to perform mapping and ablation for cardiac electrophysiology procedures. In catheter-based cardiac ablation procedures, the contact force between the cardiac tissue and the catheter tip is a significant factor for a good quality ablation. Current catheters, such as the 7 Fr TactiCath Quartz ablation catheter supplied by Abbott and the 7 Fr ThermoCool ablation catheter (Biosense Webster), incorporate force sensing technology into their design. The Abbott catheter employs Fiber Bragg Grating and incorporates force sensing technology to detect the force and the contact angle. The ThermoCool ablation catheter uses a magnetic transmitter to detect contact force at the tip.

While some examples of sensing are incorporated into catheters, most of today's catheters are similar to those developed 50 years ago. They have been refined through thinner walls and smaller diameters, and they predominantly use fluoropolymers, fine wire reinforcement, and thermoplastic elastomer outer layers. However, they are refined versions of the original technology platform. For robotics to be utilized entirely in the intra-vascular catheter space, sensing technology must be incorporated into catheters. Often, catheters incorporating sensing elements are referred to as smart catheters.

The EU providing Horizon funding for a pilot project for almost €11 million in the space of the next generation of smart catheters between 2018 and 2021. The stated objective of this POSITION II project was to bring innovation in the development and production of smart catheters by introducing open technology platforms for miniaturization, AD conversion at the tip, ultra-sound MEMS devices, and encapsulation. Open technology platforms will generate the production volume to enable sustainable innovation in this space. In the guidewire space, the pressure wire has revolutionized clinical practice in the coronary space and provided more subjective criteria for stent implantation.

The pressure wire has a pressure sensor at the distal tip. The wire is introduced into the coronary artery and tracked across the narrowed artery. The difference between the pressure measured in the artery beyond the narrowing is compared with that in the aorta (main blood vessel). The difference between the two can be expressed as the fractional flow reserve (FFR) ratio. This is measured at rest and after administration of a pharmaceutical agent to simulate the effects of exercise (increased blood flow). If the FFR ratio is >0.8, the narrowing is deemed insignificant and does not require treatment. If the ratio is <0.8, then there is evidence that coronary stenting would be beneficial. While the example relates to a guide wire rather than a catheter, it shows the incredible potential that the convergence of sensing technology into intra-vascular catheters represents.

As the critical technologies for sensors miniaturize, their value and potential will become more apparent in the intravascular catheter space. There is room for further improvement in micro-electro-mechanical systems (MEMS) and fiberoptic technologies for pressure measurement. Developing more sophisticated and smaller torque, force, and pressure sensors will allow haptic feedback into catheters. This will allow robotic surgery to progress more broadly in relation to catheter-based therapy. Electromagnetic navigational technologies are maturing, and again, as sensor technologies miniaturize and become more flexible, this will allow the development of ever smaller catheters that can be tracked further through more tortuous anatomy. These technological developments will be essential to enable robotic surgery systems for interventional catheters to develop a comprehensive sensing solution for what is today provided by the clinician's blend of experience and haptic feedback directly from the catheter.

While many challenges remain, and imaging, sensing, and robotic surgery technology need to evolve much further, it's clear that the catheter-based therapies of the future will involve more technically sophisticated catheters. These will likely be built with pressure, force, temperature, torque, and navigational sensing elements, enabling simpler and safer procedures for both patient and physician while continuously providing data to aid real-time clinical decision-making.

Conclusions

The purpose of this chapter was to provide an overview of the evolution of interventional or transvascular catheters from a technology and materials perspective. Understanding that technological evolution can open minds and inspire clinicians and designers to ask what's next in terms of transcatheter interventional therapy. Clearly, the technology has matured and become more refined through meeting the challenges of treating a variety of cardiovascular and vascular diseases. Hitherto, catheter-based technologies have offered novel physical solutions to cardiovascular diseases. This review aims to shift that paradigm toward pharmacological solutions. Perhaps those in catheter design and development space will be encouraged to develop catheters that enable such interventions.

While neurovascular catheter-based therapies are even more demanding due to the anatomical challenges and the accompanying risk of stroke, great technological strides have been made in that space in the last decade. With this improved clinical understanding of catheter design specific for the neurovascular space (i.e., triaxial microcatheter systems), the availability of new low-durometer polymers, and new reinforcement techniques, more maneuverable and effective catheter designs are now possible. It's also interesting to note the development of balloon guide catheters in the neurovascular space, which feature low profile and robust compliant occlusion balloons at the distal end of the sheath. These devices are used in mechanical thrombectomy and are associated with better safety and effectiveness outcomes for acute ischemic stroke, especially with stent retrievers.

Balloon-assisted techniques for direct cerebral infusion have the potential to leverage the significant technological refinements already achieved in the neurovascular catheter space. Arterial drug delivery in the cerebral vasculature will require drug delivery during concurrent blood flow reduction. Highly trackable, robust, customized microcatheters with distal-compliant balloon components will need to be developed for procedures that could last an hour in duration. These balloons will need to be capable of rapid inflation/deflation cycles without causing vascular trauma. The catheters themselves will need to be nonthrombogenic and elicit minimal tissue response. As the catheter technology supporting this clinical area develops and matures, future arterial drug delivery will likely require catheters that can be remotely or autonomously navigated.

Future innovations in the broad transvascular catheter therapy space are likely to be heavily influenced by innovations in complementary enabling technologies, as much or more so than by catheter-based technology itself. These include the miniaturization and incorporation of sensing elements in catheters, evolutions in catheter imaging technology, and the drive toward robotic surgery. While we can speculate on the exact nature of future innovation in the transvascular catheter space, we can be assured that it will be patient focused and continue to transform and refine clinical practices across a range of interventional therapies.

Returning to the specific area of arterial drug delivery, it's clear there is an enormous opportunity for advancing custom catheter technology to address the specific clinical needs of this area. The evolution and refinement of transvascular catheter technology, particularly in neurovascular space, has addressed many of the technical challenges in this area in terms of navigation, construction, and materials. It will be interesting to see how this specific area harnesses the developments and refinements in transvascular catheter technology into the future.

References

1. Marescaux J, Diana M. Inventing the future of surgery. World J Surg. 2015;39(3):615–22.
2. Tobis JM, Abudayyeh I. New devices and technology in interventional cardiology. J Cardiol. 2015;65(1):5–16.
3. Devanabanda AR, Tummala R, Galmer A, Grines C, Weinberg MD. Peripheral vascular interventional advances in 2017. J Interv Cardiol. 2018;31(5):553–61.
4. Zampi JD, Whiteside W. Innovative interventional catheterization techniques for congenital heart disease. Transl Pediatr. 2018;7(2):104.
5. Gülker J-E, Bansemir L, Klues HG, Bufe A. Chronic total coronary occlusion recanalization: current techniques and new devices. J Saudi Heart Assoc. 2017;29(2):110–5.
6. Rudin S, Bednarek DR, Hoffmann KR. Endovascular image-guided interventions (EIGIs). Med Phys. 2008;35(1):301–9.
7. Bonatti J. Minimally invasive cardiac surgery—from early steps to consolidation. Indian J Thorac Cardiovasc Surg. 2018;34(Suppl 2):84–5.
8. Baum RA, Baum S. Interventional radiology: a half century of innovation. Radiology. 2014;273(2S):S75–91.
9. Steinberg DH, Staubach S, Franke J, Sievert H. Defining structural heart disease in the adult patient: current scope, inherent challenges and future directions. Eur Heart J Suppl. 2010;12(Suppl_E):E2–9.
10. Sista AK, Moriarty JM. The future of catheter-directed therapy: data gaps, unmet needs, and future trials. Tech Vasc Interv Radiol. 2017;20(3):224–6.
11. Brenner M, Hoehn M, Teeter W, Stein D, Scalea T. Trading scalpels for sheaths: catheter-based treatment of vascular injury can be effectively performed by acute care surgeons trained in endovascular techniques. J Trauma Acute Care Surg. 2016;80(5):783–6.
12. de Baere T. The IR evolution in oncology: tools, treatments, and guidelines. Cardiovasc Interv Radiol. 2017;40:3–8.
13. Prabhakaran S, Ruff I, Bernstein RA. Acute stroke intervention: a systematic review. JAMA. 2015;313(14):1451–62.
14. Lakhan SE, Kaplan A, Laird C, Leiter Y. The interventionalism of medicine: interventional radiology, cardiology, and neuroradiology. Int Arch Med. 2009;2(1):27.
15. Hoerr NL, Osol A. Blakiston's new Gould medical dictionary: a modern comprehensive dictionary of the terms used in all branches of medicine and allied sciences. Blakiston Division, McGraw-Hill; 1956.
16. Goodman PC. The new light: discovery and introduction of the X-ray. AJR Am J Roentgenol. 1995;165(5):1041–5.
17. Bradley WG. History of medical imaging. Proc Am Philos Soc. 2008;152(3):349–61.
18. Teitelbaum GP, editor. A brief history of angiography and endovascular therapy, Seminars in anesthesia, perioperative medicine and pain. Elsevier; 2000.
19. Mueller RL, Sanborn TA. The history of interventional cardiology: cardiac catheterization, angioplasty, and related interventions. Am Heart J. 1995;129(1):146–72.
20. Zamora CA, Castillo M. Historical perspective of imaging contrast agents. Magn Reson Imaging Clin. 2017;25(4):685–96.
21. Stephenson LW, Rodengen JL. State of the heart: the practical guide to your heart and heart surgery. Write Stuff Syndicate; 1999.
22. Heiss H, Hurst JW. Werner Forssmann: a German problem with the Nobel prize. Clin Cardiol. 1992;15(7):547–9.
23. Meyer JA. Werner Forssmann and catheterization of the heart, 1929. Ann Thorac Surg. 1990;49(3):497–9.
24. Odman P. The radiopaque polythene catheter. Acta Radiol. 1959;52(1):52–64.
25. Mattelaer J, Billiet I. Catheters and sounds: the history of bladder catheterisation. Spinal Cord. 1995;33(8):429–33.
26. Brydson JA. Plastics materials. Newnes-Butterworths; 1975.
27. Grossman W. Grossman's cardiac catheterization, angiography, and intervention. Lippincott Williams & Wilkins; 2006.
28. Cournand A, Ranges HA. Catheterization of the right auricle in man. Proc Soc Exp Biol Med. 1941;46(3):462–6.
29. Braunwald E. The ten advances that have defined modern cardiology. Trends Cardiovasc Med. 2014;24(5):179–83.
30. Fishman AP. A century of pulmonary hemodynamics. Am J Respir Crit Care Med. 2004;170(2):109–13.
31. Narasimhan C, Balekundri V. Chapter 2: History of transcatheter interventions in adult cardiology. 2015. p. 21–33.
32. Cournand A, Riley RL, Breed ES, Baldwin ED, Richards DW, Lester MS, et al. Measurement of cardiac output in man using the technique of catheterization of the right auricle or ventricle. J Clin Invest. 1945;24(1):106–16.
33. Editorial. David Sheridan orbituary. Cath Lab Digest. Jun 2004.
34. Jeckel NC, inventor; Individual, assignee. US2494389A: Catheter: braided product and method for producing the same. USA, 1950.
35. Rodengen JL, Stefanova S. Bard: power of the past, force of the future. Write Stuff Enterprises, Incorporated; 2007.
36. Zimmermann B. Intravenous tubing for parenteral therapy. Science. 1945;101(2631):567–8.
37. Meyers L. Intravenous catheterization. AJN Am J Nurs. 1945;45(11):930–1.
38. Duffy BJ Jr. The clinical use of polyethylene tubing for intravenous therapy; a report on 72 cases. Ann Surg. 1949;130(5):929–36.
39. Massa DJ. A plastic needle. Anesthesiology. 1951;12(6):772–3.
40. Southorn PA, Narr BJ. The Massa or Rochester plastic needle. Mayo Clin Proc. 2008;83(10):1165–7.
41. Barr PO, Soila P. Introduction of soft cannula into artery by direct percutaneous puncture. Observations on technique and cannula materials. Angiology. 1960;11:168–72.
42. Martin JT. Plastic devices for intravascular therapy. Anesth Analg. 1965;44:25–9.
43. Sermon WL, inventor; Goodrich Corp, assignee. US Patent 2188396A: Method of preparing polyvinyl halide products patent US2188396A. 30 Jan 1940.
44. Zhao X, Courtney JM. Update on medical plasticised PVC. Smithers Rapra Publishing; 2009.
45. Chiellini F, Ferri M, Morelli A, Dipaola L, Latini G. Perspectives on alternatives to phthalate plasticized poly(vinyl chloride) in medical devices applications. Prog Polym Sci. 2013;38(7):1067–88.
46. Prowse CV, de Korte D, Hess JR, van der Meer PF. Commercially available blood storage containers. Vox Sang. 2014;106(1):1–13.
47. Rivera A, Strauss K, Van Zundert A, Mortier E. The history of peripheral intravenous catheters : how little plastic tubes revolutionized medicine. Acta Anaesthesiol Belg. 2005;56:271–82.
48. Rams JJ, Daicoff GR, Moulder PV. A simple method for central venous pressure measurements. Arch Surg. 1966;92(6):886.
49. Kempton JJ, Murray JM. Use of polyvinyl feeding-tube. Br Med J. 1958;1(5071):639.
50. Rubin RJ, Ness PM. What price progress? An update on vinyl plastic bags. Transfusion. 1989;29(4):358–61.
51. Testai E, Hartemann P, Rastogi SC, Bernauer U, Piersma A, De Jong W, et al. The safety of medical devices containing DEHP plasticized PVC or other plasticizers on neonates and other groups possibly at risk (2015 update). Regul Toxicol Pharmacol. 2016;76:209–10.
52. Lindgren E. Technique of abdominal aortography. Acta Radiol. 1953;39(3):205–18.
53. Peirce EC 2nd. Percutaneous femoral artery catheterization in man with special reference to aortography. Surg Gynecol Obstet. 1951;93(1):56–74.
54. Lindgren E. Another method of vertebral angiography. Acta Radiol. 1956;46(1–2):257–61.

55. Bloor BM, Wrenn FR Jr, Margolis G. An experimental evaluation of certain contrast media used for cerebral angiography; electroencephalographic and histopathological correlations. J Neurosurg. 1951;8(6):585–94.
56. Erwin P, Strickler JH, Rice CO. Use of polyethylene tubing in intravenous therapy for surgical patients. AMA Arch Surg. 1953;66(5):673–8.
57. Alexander E Jr, Small W, Campbell JB. A dependable method for constant intravenous therapy in infants using polyethylene tubing. Ann Surg. 1948;127(6):1212–6.
58. Greitz T. Sven-Ivar Seldinger. AJNR Am J Neuroradiol. 1999;20(6):1180–1.
59. Seldinger SI. Catheter replacement of the needle in percutaneous arteriography; a new technique. Acta Radiol. 1953;39(5):368–76.
60. Higgs ZCJ, Macafee DAL, Braithwaite BD, Maxwell-Armstrong CA. The Seldinger technique: 50 years on. Lancet. 2005;366(9494):1407–9.
61. Geddes LA, Geddes LNE. The catheter introducers. Mobium Press; 1993.
62. Rappaport AM, Graham RK, Kendrick WW. The use of siliconed polyethylene tubing in prolonged intravenous infusions. Can Med Assoc J. 1955;72(9):698–700.
63. Jaques LB, Fidlar E, Feldsted ET, Macdonald AG. Silicones and blood coagulation. Can Med Assoc J. 1946;55(1):26–31.
64. Margulies H, Barker NW. The coagulation time of blood in silicone tubes. Am J Med Sci. 1949;218(1):42–51.
65. Colas A, Curtis J. Silicone biomaterials: history and chemistry. Dow Corning Corporation; 2004. p. 80–6.
66. De Nicola RR. Permanent artificial, silicone, urethra. J Urol. 1950;63(1):168–72, illust.
67. Stewart RD, Sanislow CA. Silastic intravenous catheter. N Engl J Med. 1961;265(26):1283–5.
68. Luessenhop AJ, Velasquez AC. Observations on the tolerance of the intracranial arteries to catheterization. J Neurosurg. 1964;21:85–91.
69. Sullivan RD. Systemic and arterial infusion chemotherapy for metastatic liver cancer. Int J Radiat Oncol Biol Phys. 1976;1(9–10):973–6.
70. Feneley RC, Hopley IB, Wells PN. Urinary catheters: history, current status, adverse events and research agenda. J Med Eng Technol. 2015;39(8):459–70.
71. Peters JL. The history of central venous access. In: Central venous catheters. Wiley; 2009. p. 1–13.
72. Leveen HH, Barberio JR. Tissue reaction to plastics used in surgery with special reference to teflon. Ann Surg. 1949;129(1):74–84.
73. Starr A, Edwards ML. Mitral replacement: clinical experience with a ball-valve prosthesis. Ann Surg. 1961;154(4):726–40.
74. Bahnson HT, Spencer FC, Busse EF, Davis FW. Cusp replacement and coronary artery perfusion in open operations on the aortic valve. Ann Surg. 1960;152(3):494–503.
75. Bevegård S, Carlens E, Jonsson B, Karlöf I. A technique for transeptal left heart catheterization via the right external jugular vein. Thorax. 1960;15(4):299–302.
76. Nordenström B. Balloon catheters for percutaneous insertion into the vascular system. Acta Radiol. 1962;57(6):411–6.
77. Levy MJ, Lillehei CW. Percutaneous direct cardiac catheterization. A new method, with results in 122 patients. N Engl J Med. 1964;271:273–80.
78. McKee J, Shell J, Warren T, Campbell VP. Complications of I.V. therapy: vialon vs. teflon. J Infusion Nurs. 1990;13(4):259–60.
79. Lynn S, Moore B, Griffin C, Hayes D, Tanner D. Evaluating the performance of a configurable finite element model as a tool in composite catheter design. Proc Manuf. 2020;51:981–8.
80. Qin KR, Pittiruti M, Nataraja RM, Pacilli M. Long peripheral catheters and midline catheters: insights from a survey of vascular access specialists. J Vasc Access. 2021;22(6):905–10.
81. Chopra AM, Mehta M, Bismuth J, Shapiro M, Fishbein MC, Bridges AG, et al. Polymer coating embolism from intravascular medical devices—a clinical literature review. Cardiovasc Pathol. 2017;30:45–54.
82. Dudrick SJ, Wilmore DW, Vars HM, Rhoads JE. Long-term total parenteral nutrition with growth, development, and positive nitrogen balance. 1968. Nutr Hosp. 2001;16(6):287–92; discussion 6–7.
83. Dudrick SJ. History of vascular access. JPEN J Parenter Enteral Nutr. 2006;30(1 Suppl):S47–56.
84. Broviac JW, Cole JJ, Scribner BH. A silicone rubber atrial catheter for prolonged parenteral alimentation. Surg Gynecol Obstet. 1973;136(4):602–6.
85. Hickman RO, Buckner CD, Clift RA, Sanders JE, Stewart P, Thomas ED. A modified right atrial catheter for access to the venous system in marrow transplant recipients. Surg Gynecol Obstet. 1979;148(6):871–5.
86. Zerati AE, Wolosker N, de Luccia N, Puech-Leão P. Fully implantable venous catheters: history, implantation technique and complications. J Vasc Bras. 2017;16(2):128–39.
87. Galloway S, Bodenham A. Long-term central venous access. Br J Anaesth. 2004;92(5):722–34.
88. Raad I, Davis S, Becker M, Hohn D, Houston D, Umphrey J, et al. Low infection rate and long durability of nontunneled silastic catheters. A safe and cost-effective alternative for long-term venous access. Arch Intern Med. 1993;153(15):1791–6.
89. Horattas MC, Trupiano J, Hopkins S, Pasini D, Martino C, Murty A. Changing concepts in long-term central venous access: catheter selection and cost savings. Am J Infect Control. 2001;29(1):32–40.
90. Gallieni M, Pittiruti M, Biffi R. Vascular access in oncology patients. CA Cancer J Clin. 2008;58(6):323–46.
91. Temple HL, Steinberg I, Dotter CT. Angiocardiography utilizing photoroentgen apparatus with a rapid film changer. Am J Roentgenol Radium Ther. 1948;60(5):646–9.
92. Wallerich GW, inventor; V Muller and Company, assignee. Patent US 2212334: Catheter. 1940.
93. Odman P. Thoracic aortography by means of a radiopaque polythene catheter inserted percutaneously. Acta Radiol. 1956;45(2):117–24.
94. Fye WB. Coronary arteriography—it took a long time! Circulation. 1984;70(5):781–7.
95. Hoppe JO, Archer S. X-ray contrast media for cardiovascular angiography. Angiology. 1960;11(3):244–54.
96. Odman P. Percutaneous selective angiography of the main branches of the aorta. Acta Radiol. 1956;45(1):1–14.
97. Edholm P, Seldinger SI. Percutaneous catheterization of the renal artery. Acta Radiol. 1956;45(1):15–20.
98. Tillander H. Magnetic guidance of a catheter with articulated steel tip. Acta Radiol. 1951;35(1):62–4.
99. Radner S. Technical equipment for vasal catheterization. Acta Radiol. 1949;31(2):152–4.
100. Jonsson G, Broden B, Karnell J. Selective angiocardiography. Acta Radiol. 1949;32(5–6):486–97, illust.
101. Odman P. Percutaneous selective angiography of the coeliac artery. Acta Radiol Suppl. 1958;159:1–168.
102. Miller GM, Wylie EJ, Hinman F Jr. Renal complications from aortography. Surgery. 1954;35(6):885–96.
103. Tillander H. Selective angiography of the abdominal aorta with a guided catheter. Acta Radiol. 1956;45(1):21–6.
104. Kavanagh-Gray D. Cardiac catheterization. Can Med Assoc J. 1960;83(21):1095–100.
105. Lurie PR, Grajo MZ. Accidental cardiac puncture during right heart catheterization. Pediatrics. 1962;29(2):283–94.
106. Velat GJ, Lawson MF, Hoh BL, Mocco J. Novel application of an intermediate sized bridging catheter as an adjunct to aneurysm

coiling in patients with tortuous vasculature. Interv Neuroradiol. 2009;15(4):448–52.
107. Tornvall G. A modified catheter for percutaneous angiography. Acta Radiol. 1957;47(6):470–2.
108. Escher DJ, Shapiro JH, Rubinstein BM, Hurwitt ES, Schwartz SP. Perforation of the heart during cardiac catheterization and selective angiocardiography. Circulation. 1958;18(3):418–22.
109. Rodriguez-Alvarez A, Dorbecker N. Studies in angiocardiography: the problem of injection; presentation of a high-pressure automatic injecting machine to meet the needs of modern angiocardiography. Am Heart J. 1955;49(3):437–54.
110. Gidlund A. Development of apparatus and methods for roentgen studies in haemodynamics. Acta Radiol Suppl. 1956;130:7–70.
111. Blake HA, Inmon TW, Spencer FC. Emergency use of antegrade aortography in diagnosis of acute aortic rupture. Ann Surg. 1960;152(6):954–6.
112. Sloman G. Cine-aortography for the visualization of the aortic valve and coronary arteries. Proc R Soc Med. 1959;52(6):460–1.
113. Bruschke AV, Sheldon WC, Shirey EK, Proudfit WL. A half century of selective coronary arteriography. J Am Coll Cardiol. 2009;54(23):2139–44.
114. Monagan D, Williams DO. Journey into the heart: a tale of pioneering doctors and their race to transform cardiovascular medicine. Gotham Books; 2007.
115. Sones FM Jr, Shirey EK. Cine coronary arteriography. Mod Concepts Cardiovasc Dis. 1962;31:735–8.
116. Hale G, Jefferson K. Technique and interpretation of selective coronary arteriography in man. Br Heart J. 1963;25(5):644–54.
117. Sheldon WC. F. Mason Sones, Jr.—stormy petrel of cardiology. Clin Cardiol. 1994;17(7):405–7.
118. Favaloro RG. Saphenous vein autograft replacement of severe segmental coronary artery occlusion: operative technique. Ann Thorac Surg. 1968;5(4):334–9.
119. Ricketts HJ, Abrams HL. Percutaneous selective coronary cine arteriography. JAMA. 1962;181:620–4.
120. Ekberg O, Aspelin P, Baum S. Erik Boijsen, PhD. Radiology. 2018;286(1):365.
121. Amplatz K. Technics of coronary arteriography. Circulation. 1963;27(1):101–6.
122. Amplatz K, Formanek G, Stanger P, Wilson W. Mechanics of selective coronary artery catheterization via femoral approach. Radiology. 1967;89(6):1040–7.
123. Judkins MP. Selective coronary arteriography. I. A percutaneous transfemoral technic. Radiology. 1967;89(5):815–24.
124. Davis K, Kennedy JW, Kemp HG Jr, Judkins MP, Gosselin AJ, Killip T. Complications of coronary arteriography from the Collaborative Study of Coronary Artery Surgery (CASS). Circulation. 1979;59(6):1105–12.
125. Green GS, McKinnon CM, Rösch J, Judkins MP. Complications of selective percutaneous transfemoral coronary arteriography and their prevention. A review of 445 consecutive examinations. Circulation. 1972;45(3):552–7.
126. Bourassa MG, Lespérance J, Campeau L, Bois MA, Saltiel J. Selective coronary angiography using a percutaneous femoral technique. Can Med Assoc J. 1970;102(2):170–3.
127. Schoonmaker FW, King SB. Coronary arteriography by the single catheter percutaneous femoral technique. Circulation. 1974;50(4):735–40.
128. Windecker S, Meier B. X-ray coronary angiography. In: Lanzer P, Topol EJ, editors. Pan vascular medicine: integrated clinical management. Berlin: Springer; 2002. p. 602–35.
129. Dotter CT, Judkins MP, Frische LH. Safety guidespring for percutaneous cardiovascular catheterization. Am J Roentgenol Radium Ther Nucl Med. 1966;98(4):957–60.
130. Gensini GG. Positive torque control cardiac catheters. Circulation. 1965;32(6):932–5.
131. Stevens RC, inventor; Cordis Corp., assignee. Patent US 3485234: Tubular products and method of making same. USA, 1969.
132. Engbers GH, Dost L, Hennink WE, Aarts PA, Sixma JJ, Feijen J. An in vitro study of the adhesion of blood platelets onto vascular catheters. Part I. J Biomed Mater Res. 1987;21(5):613–27.
133. Duncan D. Strong and pliable, 50 years on. R & D Mag. 2009;51:27–9.
134. Haas JM, Peterson CR, Jones RC. Subintimal dissection of the coronary arteries. Circulation. 1968;38(4):678–83.
135. Wilner GD, Casarella WJ, Baier R, Fenoglio CM. Thrombogenicity of angiographic catheters. Circ Res. 1978;43(3):424–8.
136. Ayranci C. Predicting the elastic properties of two dimensionally braided tubular composite structures towards the design of braid-reinforced polymer medical catheters. 2010.
137. Carey J. Axial, flexural and torsional rigidities of two-dimensional braided fibre composite medical catheters. Ottawa: University of Ottawa; 2003.
138. Ledinsky R. Catheter design & achieving optimal performance. Medical Plastics News. 16 Aug 2017.
139. Roth R. Design considerations in small-diameter medical tubing. Medical Device and Diagnostic Industry. 2001.
140. Kucklick TR. Chapter 4: Bascics of catheter assembly. In: Kucklick TR, editor. The medical device R&D handbook. 2nd ed. Taylor & Francis; 2012. p. 85.
141. FDA. In: Center for Devices and Radiological Health, editor. Guidance document: Non-clinical engineering tests and recommended labeling for intravascular stents and associated delivery systems—guidance for industry and FDA staff. Washington, DC: FDA; 2010.
142. Laroya G. The design of interventional devices: an engineer's perspective. Cath Lab Digest; 2013.
143. Boijsen E, Judkins MP. A hook-tail "closed-end" catheter for percutaneous selective cardioangiography. Radiology. 1966;87(5):872–7.
144. Cowley MJ. Tribute to a legend in invasive/interventional cardiology Melvin P. Judkins, M.D (1922-85). Catheter Cardiovasc Interv. 2005;64(2):259–61.
145. Simmons CR, Tsao EC, Thompson JR. Angiographic approach to the difficult aortic arch: a new technique for transfemoral cerebral angiography in the aged. Am J Roentgenol Radium Ther Nucl Med. 1973;119(3):605–12.
146. Payne MM. Charles Theodore Dotter. The father of intervention. Tex Heart Inst J. 2001;28(1):28–38.
147. Murphy T, Soares G. The evolution of interventional radiology. Semin Interv Radiol. 2005;22:6–9.
148. Dotter CT. Cardiac catheterization and angiographic technics of the future. Background and current status of clinical catheter angiography. Cesk Radiol. 1965;19(4):217–36.
149. Rösch J. An interventional radiology odyssey: the story of my life and work. Springer International Publishing; 2016.
150. Dotter CT, Judkins MP. Transluminal treatment of arteriosclerotic obstruction. Circulation. 1964;30(5):654–70.
151. Rösch J, Keller FS, Kaufman JA. The birth, early years, and future of interventional radiology. J Vasc Interv Radiol. 2003;14(7):841–53.
152. Rösch J, Keller FS. Historical account: cardiovascular interventional radiology. In: Lanzer P, editor. Catheter-based cardiovascular interventions: a knowledge-based approach. Berlin: Springer; 2013. p. 15–26.
153. Kinney TB. Radiologic history exhibit. Charles T. Dotter: a pioneering interventional radiologist. Radiographics. 1996;16(3):697–707.
154. Dotter CT, Rösch J, Anderson JM, Antonovic R, Robinson M. Transluminal iliac artery dilatation: nonsurgical catheter treatment of atheromatous narrowing. JAMA. 1974;230(1):117–24.
155. Fogarty TJ, inventor; Edwards Labs, assignee. Patent US 3435826: Embolectomy catheter. 1969.

156. Ailawadi G, Nagji AS, Jones DR. The legends behind cardiothoracic surgical instruments. Ann Thorac Surg. 2010;89(5):1693–700.
157. Green RM, DeWeese JA, Rob CG. Arterial embolectomy before and after the Fogarty catheter. Surgery. 1975;77(1):24–33.
158. Krause RJ, Cranley JJ, Strasser ES, Hafner CD, Fogarty TJ. Further experience with a new embolectomy catheter. Surgery. 1966;59(1):81–7.
159. Zeitler E, Schoop W, Zahnow W. The treatment of occlusive arterial disease by transluminal catheter angioplasty. Radiology. 1971;99(1):19–26.
160. van Andel GJ. Percutaneous transluminal angioplasty: the Dotter procedure : a manual for the radiologist. Excerpta Medica; 1976.
161. Grüntzig A, Hopff H. Percutaneous recanalization after chronic arterial occlusion with a new dilator-catheter (modification of the Dotter technique) (author's transl). Dtsch Med Wochenschr. 1974;99(49):2502–10, 11.
162. Gaemperli O, Lüscher TF. Historical account: interventional cardiology. In: Lanzer P, editor. Catheter-based cardiovascular interventions: a knowledge-based approach. Berlin: Springer; 2013. p. 3–14.
163. King SB. The development of interventional cardiology. J Am Coll Cardiol. 1998;31(4 Suppl_2):64B–88B.
164. King SB. Angioplasty from bench to bedside to bench. Circulation. 1996;93(9):1621–9.
165. Grüntzig A. Die perkutane Rekanalisation chronischer arterieller Verschlüsse (Dotter-Prinzip) mit einem neuen doppellumigen Dilatationskatheter (The percutaneous recanalization of chronic arterial occlusions (Dotter principle) with a new double-lumen dilatation catheter). Fortschr Geb Rontgenstr Nuklearmed. 1976;124:80–6.
166. Gruntzig A, Gleichner H, inventors. US Patent US 4195637: Catheter arrangement, method of catheterization, and method of manufacturing a dilatation element. 1 Apr 1980.
167. Grüntzig A. Transluminal dilatation of coronary-artery stenosis. Lancet. 1978;311(8058):263.
168. Kelly ME, Taylor GJ, Moses HW, Mikell FL, Dove JT, Batchelder JE, et al. Comparative cost of myocardial revascularization: percutaneous transluminal angioplasty and coronary artery bypass surgery. J Am Coll Cardiol. 1985;5(1):16–20.
169. Roberts LJ, Wertman DJ, Mills S, Moore AJ, Heaston D. Transluminal angioplasty of the superior mesenteric artery: an alternative to surgical revascularization. Am J Roentgenol. 1983;141(5):1039–42.
170. Gruentzig AR. Percutaneous transluminal coronary angioplasty: six years' experience. Am Heart J. 1984;107(4):818–9.
171. Simpson JB, Baim DS, Robert EW, Harrison DC. A new catheter system for coronary angioplasty. Am J Cardiol. 1982;49(5):1216–22.
172. Simpson JB, Robert EW, inventors. Patent US 4323071: Vascular guiding catheter assembly and vascular dilating catheter assembly and a combination thereof and methods of making the same. 6 Apr 1982.
173. Simpson JB, Robert EW, inventors. Patent US 4411055: Vascular guiding catheter assembly and vascular dilating catheter assembly and a combination thereof and methods for making the same. 1983.
174. Colombo A, Reimers B. Coronary artery revascularization: percutaneous approach. In: Lanzer P, Topol EJ, editors. Pan vascular medicine: integrated clinical management. Berlin: Springer; 2002. p. 820–40.
175. Douglas JS, Gruentzig AR, King SB, Hollman J, Ischinger T, Meier B, et al. Percutaneous transluminal coronary angioplasty in patients with prior coronary bypass surgery. J Am Coll Cardiol. 1983;2(4):745–54.
176. Grech ED. ABC of interventional cardiology: percutaneous coronary intervention. I: history and development. BMJ. 2003;326(7398):1080–2.
177. Myler RK, Stertzer SH, Cumberland DC, Webb JG, Shaw RE. Coronary angioplasty: indications, contraindications, and limitations historical perspective and technological determinants. J Interv Cardiol. 1989;2(3):179–85.
178. Gruentzig A. Results from coronary angioplasty and implications for the future. Am Heart J. 1982;103(4, Part 2):779–83.
179. Detre K, Holubkov R, Kelsey S, Cowley M, Kent K, Williams D, et al. Percutaneous transluminal coronary angioplasty in 1985-1986 and 1977-1981. The National Heart, Lung, and Blood Institute registry. N Engl J Med. 1988;318(5):265–70.
180. Stack RS. New interventional technologies in cardiology. Mayo Clin Proc. 1989;64(7):867–70.
181. Newsome LT, Kutcher MA, Royster RL. Coronary artery stents: part I. Evolution of percutaneous coronary intervention. Anesth Analg. 2008;107(2):552–69.
182. Bhat TM, Afari ME, Garcia LA. Atherectomy in peripheral artery disease: a review. J Invasive Cardiol. 2017;29(4):135–44.
183. Akkus NI, Abdulbaki A, Jimenez E, Tandon N. Atherectomy devices: technology update. Med Devices (Auckl). 2015;8:1–10.
184. Topfer LA, Spry C, CADTH Horizon Scans. New technologies for the treatment of peripheral artery disease. In: CADTH issues in emerging health technologies. Ottawa, ON: Canadian Agency for Drugs and Technologies in Health; 2016. p. 1–19. You are permitted to reproduce this document for non-commercial purposes, provided it is not modified when reproduced and appropriate credit is given to CADTH.
185. Katsanos K, Spiliopoulos S, Reppas L, Karnabatidis D. Debulking atherectomy in the peripheral arteries: is there a role and what is the evidence? Cardiovasc Interv Radiol. 2017;40(7):964–77.
186. Iqbal J, Gunn J, Serruys PW. Coronary stents: historical development, current status and future directions. Br Med Bull. 2013;106:193–211.
187. Berger PB. The Cook Inc. Gianturco-Roubin flex-stent. J Interv Cardiol. 1996;9(2):145–52.
188. Kesselheim AS, Xu S, Avorn J. Clinicians' contributions to the development of coronary artery stents: a qualitative study of transformative device innovation. PLoS One. 2014;9(2):e88664.
189. Oesterle SN, Whitbourn R, Fitzgerald PJ, Yeung AC, Stertzer SH, Dake MD, et al. The stent decade: 1987 to 1997. Am Heart J. 1998;136(4):578–99.
190. Tan C, Schatz RA. The history of coronary stenting. Interv Cardiol Clin. 2016;5(3):271–80.
191. Sigwart U, Puel J, Mirkovitch V, Joffre F, Kappenberger L. Intravascular stents to prevent occlusion and re-stenosis after transluminal angioplasty. N Engl J Med. 1987;316(12):701–6.
192. Hoffmann R, Mintz GS, Dussaillant GR, Popma JJ, Pichard AD, Satler LF, et al. Patterns and mechanisms of in-stent restenosis. Circulation. 1996;94(6):1247–54.
193. Shrestha S, Patel J, Hollander G, Shani J. Coronary artery stents: from the beginning to the present. Consultant 360. 2019;60(6):1–13.
194. Kastrati A, Mehilli J, Dirschinger J, Dotzer F, Schühlen H, Neumann FJ, et al. Intracoronary stenting and angiographic results: strut thickness effect on restenosis outcome (ISAR-STEREO) trial. Circulation. 2001;103(23):2816–21.
195. Navarese E, Kowalewski M, Kandzari D, Lansky A, Gorny B, Koltowski L, et al. First-generation versus second-generation drug-eluting stents in current clinical practice: updated evidence from a comprehensive meta-analysis of randomised clinical trials comprising 31 379 patients. Open Heart. 2014;1:e000064.
196. Scheller B, Cremers B, Bienek S, Schnorr B, Clever Y, Speck U. Drug-coated balloons—history and peripheral vascular opportunities. Interv Cardiol Rev. 2010;5:70.

197. Windecker S, Kolh P, Alfonso F, Collet JP, Cremer J, Falk V, et al. 2014 ESC/EACTS guidelines on myocardial revascularization: the Task Force on Myocardial Revascularization of the European Society of Cardiology (ESC) and the European Association for Cardio-Thoracic Surgery (EACTS) developed with the special contribution of the European Association of Percutaneous Cardiovascular Interventions (EAPCI). Eur Heart J. 2014;35(37):2541–619.
198. Moukwa M. The development of polymer-based biomaterials since the 1920s. JOM. 1997;49(2):46–50.
199. Harrison JH. Synthetic materials as vascular prostheses. I. A comparative study in small vessels of nylon, dacron, orlon, ivalon sponge and teflon. Am J Surg. 1958;95(1):3–15.
200. Williams DF. On the mechanisms of biocompatibility. Biomaterials. 2008;29(20):2941–53.
201. Northup SJ. Safety evaluation of medical devices: US Food and Drug Administration and International Standards Organization Guidelines. Int J Toxicol. 1999;18(4):275–83.
202. Gensini GG. A new Teflon catheter for percutaneous catheterization and contrast material injection. Radiology. 1963;81(6):939–41.
203. Barr PO. Percutaneous puncture of the radial artery with a multi-purpose Teflon catheter for indwelling use. Acta Physiol Scand. 1961;51:343–7.
204. Dickson JFI, Hamer NAJ, Dow JW. Venoarterial pumping for relief of intractable cardiac failure in man. AMA Arch Surg. 1959;78(3):418–21.
205. McKissock W, Richardson A, L. W. Posterior communicating aneurysms: a controlled trial of conservative and surgical treatment of ruptured aneurysms of the internal carotid artery at or near the point of origin of the posterior communicating artery. Lancet. 1960;I:1203–6.
206. Reifschneider A. The new U.S. FDA regulations on biocompatibility and reprocessing for medical devices. 2018.
207. Ducheyne P, Healy K, Hutmacher DW, Grainger DW, Kirkpatrick CJ. Comprehensive biomaterials II. Elsevier Science; 2017.
208. Sall B. Regulation of medical devices. In: Madame curie bioscience database. Landes Bioscience; 2013.
209. Williams DF. There is no such thing as a biocompatible material. Biomaterials. 2014;35(38):10009–14.
210. Maitz M. Applications of synthetic polymers in clinical medicine. Biosurf Biotribol. 2015;1:161–76.
211. Molcho J, Karny HZ, Frei EH, Askenasy HM. Selective cerebral catheterization. IEEE Trans Biomed Eng. 1970;17(2):134–40.
212. Virtama P. A new closed-end catheter for angiography. Angiology. 1963;14(10):494–6.
213. Rossi P, Verdu CC. The floppy wire as an aid in arterial catheterization. Am J Roentgenol Radium Ther Nucl Med. 1966;97(2):511–8.
214. Schollenberger CS, inventor; Goodrich Corp., assignee. Patent US 2871218: Simulated vulcanizates of polyurethane elastomers. USA, 1959.
215. Gesner BD. Stabilization against chemical agents. New York: Wiley-Interscience; 1972.
216. Carson RA, Edwards A. Design and development of innovative medical devices using novel polyurethane elastomers. In: Polymers for the medical industry conference, London, UK; 1999. p. 1-5.
217. Rahimi A, Mashak A. Review on rubbers in medicine: natural, silicone and polyurethane rubbers. Plast Rubber Compos. 2013;42(6):223–30.
218. Ulrich H, Bonk HW. Emerging biomedical applications of polyurethane elastomers. J Cell Plast. 1983;19(2):83–8.
219. Bonk HW, Sardanopoli AA, Ulrich H, Sayigh AAR. Pellethane®: a new generation of polyurethane thermoplastic elastomers. J Elastoplast. 1971;3(3):157–86.
220. Szycher M, Poirier V. High performance tecoflex polyurethanes in biomedical applications. In: Lee SM, editor. Advances in biomaterials. Boca Raton: CRC Press; 1987.
221. Lamba NMK, Woodhouse KA, Cooper SL. Polyurethanes in biomedical applications. Taylor & Francis; 1997.
222. Szycher M. Biostability of polyurethane elastomers: a critical review. J Biomater Appl. 1988;3(2):297–402.
223. Szycher M. High performance biomaterials: a complete guide to medical and pharmceutical applications. Taylor & Francis; 1991.
224. Szycher M. Szycher's handbook of polyurethanes. 2nd ed. Taylor & Francis; 2012.
225. Mermel LA, Alang N. Adverse effects associated with ethanol catheter lock solutions: a systematic review. J Antimicrob Chemother. 2014;69(10):2611–9.
226. Tal MG, Ni N. Selecting optimal hemodialysis catheters: material, design, advanced features, and preferences. Tech Vasc Interv Radiol. 2008;11(3):186–91.
227. Kultys A, Rogulska M, Pikus S, Skrzypiec K. The synthesis and characterization of new thermoplastic poly(carbonate-urethane) elastomers derived from HDI and aliphatic–aromatic chain extenders. Eur Polym J. 2009;45(9):2629–43.
228. FDA. Penumbra 510K summary K 100826 2010. https://www.accessdata.fda.gov/cdrh_docs/pdf10/K100826.pdf.
229. Spiotta AM, Chaudry MI, Hui FK, Turner RD, Kellogg RT, Turk AS. Evolution of thrombectomy approaches and devices for acute stroke: a technical review. J Neurointerv Surg. 2015;7(1):2–7.
230. Jia Z-Y, Lee S-H, Kim Y, Choi J, Hwang S, Lee GY, et al. Optimal guiding catheter length for endovascular coiling of intracranial aneurysms in anterior circulation in era of flourishing distal access system. Neurointervention. 2017;12:91–9.
231. PolyOne. Healthcare NEU product selection guide. 2016. https://www.accessdata.fda.gov/cdrh_docs/pdf10/K100826.pdf.
232. Britton RC, Brown CH, Shirey EK. Intrahepatic veno-occlusive disease in cirrhosis with chronic ascites: diagnosis by hepatic phlebography and results of surgical treatment. Ann Surg. 1963;158(3):370.
233. Peckham GB, Chrysohou A, Aldridge HE, Wigle ED. Combined percutaneous retrograde aortic and transseptal left heart catheterization. Br Heart J. 1964;26(4):460–8.
234. Gray IR, Joshipura CS, Mackinnon J. Retrograde left ventricular cardioangiography in the diagnosis of mitral regurgitation. Br Heart J. 1963;25(2):145–52.
235. Feldman D. Polymer history. Des Monomers Polymers. 2008;11(1):1–15.
236. Page IB. Polyamides as engineering thermoplastic materials. Rapra Technology Limited; 2000.
237. Seymour RB, Porter RS. Manmade fibres: their origin and development. Dordrecht: Springer; 1993.
238. Jaganathan SK, Supriyanto E, Murugesan S, Balaji A, Asokan MK. Biomaterials in cardiovascular research: applications and clinical implications. Biomed Res Int. 2014;2014(1):459465.
239. Dang P, Marchioni R, Mason J, Werth M. Thermoplastic materials in oil and gas applications: 30 years experience with polyamide 11 from offshore production to onshore distribution. 2004. https://www.osti.gov/etdeweb/servlets/purl/21012070.
240. Flesher JR, editor. Pebax® polyether block amide—a new family of engineering thermoplastic elastomers. Dordrecht: Springer; 1986.
241. Rapra Technology Limited. TPE 2005: international conference: organised by Rapra Technology Ltd., Berlin, Germany, 14–15 Sept 2005. Rapra Technology; 2005.
242. Foy P, Jungblut C, Deleens G, inventors; ATO Chimie SA Arkema France SA, assignee. Patent US 4332920: Mouldable and extrudable polyether-ester-amide block copolymers. 1 Jun 1982.

243. Arsenault S. PEBAX® poly ether block amide copolymer a high performance TPE designed to meet the demands of tomorrow. In: 8th thermoplastic elastomers topical conference 2007. Akron, OH: Society of Plastic Engineers; 2007. p. 43–8.
244. Padsalgikar A. Plastics in medical devices for cardiovascular applications. 2017.
245. Kucklick TR. The medical device R&D handbook. 2nd ed. Taylor & Francis; 2012.
246. Lanzer P. Catheter-based cardiovascular interventions: a knowledge-based approach. Springer; 2013. p. 1–1046.
247. Formanek G, French RS, Amplatz K. Arterial thrombus formation during clinical percutaneous catheterization. Circulation. 1970;41(5):833–9.
248. Amplatz K. Catheter embolization. Radiology. 1968;91(2): 392–3.
249. Nejad MS, Klaper MA, Steggerda FR, Gianturco C. Clotting on the outer surfaces of vascular catheters. Radiology. 1968;91(2):248–50.
250. Kandarpa K. Peripheral vascular interventions. Lippincott Williams & Wilkins; 2008.
251. Fan YL. Hydrophilic lubricious coatings for medical applications. In: Gebelein CG, Cheng TC, Yang VC, editors. Cosmetic and pharmaceutical applications of polymers. Boston, MA: Springer; 1991. p. 311–9.
252. Amplatz K. A simple non-thrombogenic coating. Investig Radiol. 1971;6(4):280–9.
253. Durst S, Leslie J, Moore R, Amplatz K. A comparison of the thrombogenicity of commercially available catheters. Radiology. 1974;113(3):599–600.
254. Frech RS, Cramer R, Amplatz K, Nutini DM. A simple non-invasive technique to test non-thrombogenic surfaces. Am J Roentgenol. 1971;113(4):765–8.
255. Kikuchi Y, Graves VB, Strother CM, McDermott JC, Babel SG, Crummy AB. A new guidewire with kink-resistant core and low-friction coating. Cardiovasc Interv Radiol. 1989;12(2):107–9.
256. Nakagawa N, Yashiro N, Nakajima Y, Barnhart WH, Wakabayashi M. Hydrogel-coated glide catheter: experimental studies and initial clinical experience. AJR Am J Roentgenol. 1994;163(5):1227–9.
257. Back MR, White RA. Biomaterials: considerations for endovascular devices. In: White RA, Fogarty TJ, editors. Peripheral endovascular interventions. New York: Springer; 1999. p. 219–46.
258. Kenny S, McDermott E. Simulated testing in medical device design. Med Device Technol. 2006;17:22–5.
259. Wyman P. Hydrophilic coatings for biomedical applications in and ex vivo. In: Coatings for biomedical applications. Woodhead Publishing; 2012. p. 3–42.
260. Kiemeneij F, Fraser D, Slagboom T, Laarman G, van der Wieken R. Hydrophilic coating aids radial sheath withdrawal and reduces patient discomfort following transradial coronary intervention: a randomized double-blind comparison of coated and uncoated sheaths. Catheter Cardiovasc Interv. 2003;59(2):161–4.
261. Saito S, Tanaka S, Hiroe Y, Miyashita Y, Takahashi S, Satake S, et al. Usefulness of hydrophilic coating on arterial sheath introducer in transradial coronary intervention. Catheter Cardiovasc Interv. 2002;56(3):328–32.
262. Kallmes DF, McGraw JK, Evans AJ, Mathis JM, Hergenrother RW, Jensen ME, et al. Thrombogenicity of hydrophilic and non-hydrophilic microcatheters and guiding catheters. AJNR Am J Neuroradiol. 1997;18(7):1243–51.
263. Law KY. Definitions for hydrophilicity, hydrophobicity, and superhydrophobicity: getting the basics right. J Phys Chem Lett. 2014;5(4):686–8.
264. Mehta RI, Mehta RI. Hydrophilic polymer embolism: an update for physicians. Am J Med. 2017;130(7):e287–90.
265. Anthony LW. The evolution of low-profile endograft design: Are there tradeoffs being made for the improvements in these devices? 2011. https://evtoday.com/articles/2011-mar/the-evolution-of-low-profile-endograft-design.
266. Mahtta D, Elgendy IY, Bavry AA. From CoreValve to Evolut PRO: reviewing the journey of self-expanding transcatheter aortic valves. Cardiol Ther. 2017;6(2):183–92.
267. O'Neil C. So many polymers, so little time. 2010. p. 32.
268. Bigham KJ. Focus on polyimides. 2019.
269. Endrey AL, inventor; EIDP Inc., assignee. Patent US 3179630: Process for preparing polyimides by treating polyamide-acids with lower fatty monocarboxylic acid anhydrides. USA, 1965.
270. Thiruvasagam P, Venkatesan D. Synthesis and characterization of polyetherimides derived from AB monomers. J Macromol Sci A. 2009;46:419–24.
271. Brett S. Film-cast tubing specifications used in catheter-based medical devices medical product outsourcing. 2019. https://www.mpo-mag.com/contents/view_online-exclusives/2019-01-07/film-cast-tubing-specifications-used-in-catheter-based-medical-devices/.
272. Ranica A. A Serpentine Slip 'n Slide. 2014. https://www.mpo-mag.com/issues/2014-10-01/view_features/a-serpentine-slip-n-slide/.
273. Lynch TJ. Polyimide tubing: dispelling the myths. Med Device Technol. 2008;19(3):12–5.
274. Nordson Medical. Top 5 reasons to use film cast PTFE liner tubing for your next catheter design. 2017. p. 8. https://directory.qmed.com/.
275. Nordson Medical. Advantages of film-cast PTFE liner tubing. 2024. https://www.nordsonmedical.com/Components-and-Technologies/Medical-Tubing/PTFE-Tubing/Film-Cast-Liner-Tubing/.
276. Turk A, Manzoor MU, Nyberg EM, Turner RD, Chaudry I. Initial experience with distal guide catheter placement in the treatment of cerebrovascular disease: clinical safety and efficacy. J Neurointerv Surg. 2013;5(3):247–52.
277. Chaudhary N, Pandey AS, Thompson BG, Gandhi D, Ansari SA, Gemmete JJ. Utilization of the Neuron 6 French 0.053 inch inner luminal diameter guide catheter for treatment of cerebral vascular pathology: continued experience with ultra distal access into the cerebral vasculature. J Neurointerv Surg. 2012;4(4):301–6.
278. Topol EJ, Myler RK, Stertzer SH. Selection of dilatation hardware for PTCA—1985. Catheter Cardiovasc Diagn. 1985;11(6):629–37.
279. Van Tassel RA, Gobel FL, Rydell MA, Vlodaver Z, MacCarter DJ. A less traumatic catheter for coronary arteriography. Catheter Cardiovasc Diagn. 1985;11(2):187–99.
280. Grossman PM, Gurm HS, McNamara R, Lalonde T, Changezi H, Share D, et al. Percutaneous coronary intervention complications and guide catheter size: bigger is not better. JACC Cardiovasc Interv. 2009;2(7):636–44.
281. Ijichi T, Ikari Y. Transradial coronary angiography with virtual 1 French, sheathless 3 French catheter. Catheter Cardiovasc Interv. 2013;82(5):E676–7.
282. Kern MJ, Lim MJ, Sorajja P. The interventional cardiac catheterization handbook e-book. Elsevier Health Sciences; 2017.
283. Prashant UP. Current and emerging catheter technologies for percutaneous transluminal coronary angioplasty. Res Rep Clin Cardiol. 2014;5:213–26.
284. Brooksby IA, Swanton RH, Jenkins BS, Webb-Peploe MM. Long sheath technique for introduction of catheter tip manometer or endomyocardial bioptome into left or right heart. Br Heart J. 1974;36(9):908–12.
285. Desilets DT, Hoffman R. A new method of percutaneous catheterization. Radiology. 1965;85(1):147–8.
286. Grollman JH Jr. Editorial comment: The interventional vascular access sheath—the legacy of Donald T. Desilets, M.D. (1935–1996). Catheter Cardiovasc Diagn. 1997;40(1):84.

287. Desilets DT, Hoffman RB, Ruttenberg HD. A new method of percutaneous catheterization. Am J Roentgenol. 1966;97(2):519–22.
288. Cook M. From soda straw to Guiding Catheter Flexor Technology. 2017. PI-D20501-EN-F.
289. Hoffman RB, Grollman JH. Sequential progression from a large- to a small-diameter catheter during percutaneous arteriography. Radiology. 1974;113(2):479–80.
290. Cohen B. Cordis celebrates 50 years of transforming cardiovascular care. 2017. https://www.ptca.org/news/2009/0326_CORDIS.html.
291. Stevens RC, inventor; Cordis Corp., assignee. Patent US 4000739: Hemostasis cannula. 1977.
292. Barry WH, Levin DC, Green LH, Bettman MA, Mudge GH Jr, Phillips D. Left heart catheterization and angiography via the percutaneous femoral approach using an arterial sheath. Catheter Cardiovasc Diagn. 1979;5(4):401–9.
293. Hillis LD. Percutaneous left heart catheterization and coronary arteriography using a femoral artery sheath. Catheter Cardiovasc Diagn. 1979;5(4):393–9.
294. Schulte RR, inventor; Baxter International, assignee. Patent US V3618613: Antithrombotic intravascular catheter reinforced with nonkinking means. 1971.
295. Tate T, inventor; Medical Evaluation Devices and I, assignee. Patent US V3841308: Distally valved catheter device. 1974.
296. Kline WM, inventor; Medical Evaluation Devices and Instruments Corps, assignee. Patent US 4044765: Flexible tube for intravenous feeding. USA, 1977.
297. Kocak N, inventor; Bipore Inc., assignee. Patent US 4705511: Introducer sheath assembly. USA, 1987.
298. Teleflex. The history of the Arrow® Vascular Access Brand. 2024. https://www.teleflex.com/usa/en/product-areas/vascular-access/timeline/index#.
299. Fischell RE, inventor; Cathco Inc., assignee. Patent US 5180376: Non-buckling thin-walled sheath for the percutaneous insertion of intraluminal catheters. USPTO, 1993.
300. Parker FT, inventor. Patent CA 2075345: A flexible, kink-resistant, introducer sheath. Canada, 2003.
301. Schneider P. Endovascular skills: guidewire and catheter skills for endovascular surgery. CRC Press; 2019.
302. Moore WS. Moore's vascular and endovascular surgery e-book. Elsevier; 2018.
303. Lenhardt J, Michaels B. Think extrusion and beyond for optimal catheter design. 2014. https://www.mddionline.com/design-engineering/think-extrusion-and-beyond-for-optimal-catheter-design.
304. GmbH GJ. Jotec E-vita thoracic 3G stent graft system brochure. 2019.
305. Guglielmi G. History of endovascular endosaccular occlusion of brain aneurysms: 1965-1990. Interv Neuroradiol. 2007;13(3):217–24.
306. Bose A, Lockhart J, Barry D, Kuo SS. State-of-the-art and future perspective of devices for neuroendovascular treatment. In: Peschillo S, editor. Frontiers in neurosurgery neuroendovascular challenges, vol. 1. Bentham Science; 2015.
307. Guglielmi G. The beginning and the evolution of the endovascular treatment of intracranial aneurysms: from the first catheterization of brain arteries to the new stents. J Neurointerv Surg. 2009;1(1):53–5.
308. Debrun G, Lacour P, Caron JP, Hurth M, Comoy J, Keravel Y. Inflatable and released balloon technique experimentation in dog—application in man. Neuroradiology. 1975;9(5):267–71.
309. Hieshima GB, Grinnell VS, Mehringer CM. A detachable balloon for therapeutic transcatheter occlusions. Radiology. 1981;138(1):227–8.
310. Law M, Som PM, Naidich TP. Problem solving in neuroradiology e-book. Elsevier Health Sciences; 2011.
311. Engelson ET, inventor; Stryker European Operations Holdings LLC, assignee. Patent US 4739768: Catheter for guide-wire tracking. 1988.
312. Jiang B, Paff M, Colby GP, Coon AL, Lin LM. Cerebral aneurysm treatment: modern neurovascular techniques. Stroke Vasc Neurol. 2016;1(3):93–100.
313. Molyneux A. International subarachnoid aneurysm trial (ISAT) of neurosurgical clipping versus endovascular coiling in 2143 patients with ruptured intracranial aneurysms: a randomised trial. Lancet. 2002;360(9342):1267–74.
314. Spetzler RF, McDougall CG, Zabramski JM, Albuquerque FC, Hills NK, Russin JJ, et al. The Barrow ruptured aneurysm trial: 6-year results. J Neurosurg. 2015;123(3):609–17.
315. Dion JE, Duckwiler GR, Lylyk P, Viñuela F, Bentson J. Progressive suppleness pursil catheter: a new tool for superselective angiography and embolization. AJNR Am J Neuroradiol. 1989;10(5):1068–70.
316. Gore SM, Mueller M, Green N, Gold JG, Soltesz PP, inventors. Patent US 5733400: Intravascular catheter. 1998.
317. Engelson ET, Hergenrother R, Eder J, inventors; Target Therapeutics, assignee. Patent US 5531715: Lubricious catheters. USA, 1996.
318. Guglielmi G. History of the genesis of detachable coils: a review. J Neurosurg 2009;111(1):1–8, 1.
319. Lin LM, Colby GP, Huang J, Tamargo RJ, Coon AL. Ultra-distal large-bore intracranial access using the hyperflexible Navien distal intracranial catheter for the treatment of cerebrovascular pathologies: a technical note. J Neurointerv Surg. 2014;6(4):301–7.
320. Park MS, Stiefel MF, Fiorella D, Kelly M, McDougall CG, Albuquerque FC. Intracranial placement of a new, compliant guide catheter: technical note. Neurosurgery. 2008;63(3):E616–7; discussion E7.
321. Hui FK, et al., "Flexible tip guides and intermediate catheters: two center experience and a proposed taxonomy," J Neurointerv Surg, 2014;6(8):618–23. https://doi.org/10.1136/neurintsurg-2013-010892.
322. Raymond J, Guilbert F, Weill A, Georganos SA, Juravsky L, Lambert A, et al. Long-term angiographic recurrences after selective endovascular treatment of aneurysms with detachable coils. Stroke. 2003;34(6):1398–403.
323. Cohen ER, Meyers PM, Lavine SD, Higashida RT. Historical account of interventional neuroradiology. In: Lanzer P, editor. Textbook of catheter-based cardiovascular interventions: a knowledge-based approach. Cham: Springer International Publishing; 2018. p. 1863–76.
324. Alderazi YJ, Shastri D, Kass-Hout T, Prestigiacomo CJ, Gandhi CD. Flow diverters for intracranial aneurysms. Stroke Res Treat. 2014;2014:415653.
325. Arrese I, Sarabia R, Pintado R, Delgado-Rodriguez M. Flow-diverter devices for intracranial aneurysms: systematic review and meta-analysis. Neurosurgery. 2013;73(2):193–9; discussion 199–200.
326. Colby GP, Lin LM, Xu R, Beaty N, Bender MT, Jiang B, et al. Utilization of a novel, multi-durometer intracranial distal access catheter: nuances and experience in 110 consecutive cases of aneurysm flow diversion. Interv Neurol. 2017;6(1–2):90–104.
327. Hauck EF, Tawk RG, Karter NS, Binning MJ, Khalessi AA, Natarajan SK, et al. Use of the outreach distal access catheter as an intracranial platform facilitates coil embolization of select intracranial aneurysms: technical note. J Neurointerv Surg. 2011;3(2):172–6.
328. Spiotta AM, Hussain MS, Sivapatham T, Bain M, Gupta R, Moskowitz SI, et al. The versatile distal access catheter: the Cleveland clinic experience. Neurosurgery. 2011;68(6):1677–86; discussion 86.

329. Binning MJ, Yashar P, Orion D, Hauck EF, Levy EI, Hopkins LN, et al. Use of the outreach distal access catheter for microcatheter stabilization during intracranial arteriovenous malformation embolization. AJNR Am J Neuroradiol. 2012;33(9):E117–9.
330. Lee S, Gong TS, Lee YW, Kim HJ, Kweon CY. The benefits of Navien™ intracranial support catheter for endovascular treatment. J Cerebrovasc Endovasc Neurosurg. 2016;18(3):234–8.
331. Jankowitz B, Aghaebrahim A, Zirra A, Spataru O, Zaidi S, Jumaa M, et al. Manual aspiration thrombectomy: adjunctive endovascular recanalization technique in acute stroke interventions. Stroke. 2012;43(5):1408–11.
332. Driller J. Kinetics of magnetically guided catheters. IEEE Trans Magn. 1970;6(3):467–71.
333. Montgomery DB, Weggel RJ, Leupold MJ, Yodh SB, Wright RL. Superconducting magnet system for intravascular navigation. J Appl Phys. 1969;40(5):2129–32.
334. Lindsay BD. Perspectives on the development of a magnetic navigation system for remote control of electrophysiology catheters. Europace. 2006;8(4):231–2.
335. Fu Y, Liu H, Huang W, Wang S, Liang Z. Steerable catheters in minimally invasive vascular surgery. Int J Med Robot Comput Assist Surg. 2009;5(4):381–91.
336. Ernst S, Ouyang F, Linder C, Hertting K, Stahl F, Chun J, et al. Initial experience with remote catheter ablation using a novel magnetic navigation system: magnetic remote catheter ablation. Circulation. 2004;109(12):1472–5.
337. Pappone C, Vicedomini G, Manguso F, Gugliotta F, Mazzone P, Gulletta S, et al. Robotic magnetic navigation for atrial fibrillation ablation. J Am Coll Cardiol. 2006;47(7):1390–400.
338. Kiemeneij F, Patterson MS, Amoroso G, Laarman G, Slagboom T. Use of the Stereotaxis Niobe magnetic navigation system for percutaneous coronary intervention: results from 350 consecutive patients. Catheter Cardiovasc Interv. 2008;71(4):510–6.
339. Labelle JJ, Lucas RJ, Eisenstein B, Reed MD, Vaitkevicius VK, Wilson GS. Hepatic artery catheterization for chemotherapy. Arch Surg. 1968;96(4):683–92.
340. Takashima T, Yamamoto I, Mitani I, Shin M. Transfemoral superselective celiac angiography. Am J Roentgenol Radium Ther Nucl Med. 1970;110(4):813–7.
341. Grollman JH Jr, Hanafee W, MacAlpin R, Kattus A. Guided coronary arteriography and left ventriculography. Radiology. 1968;91(2):315–20.
342. Muller WF, inventor. US Patent: Spring guide manipulator. 1966.
343. Barchilon J, inventor. US Patent: Dirigible catheter. 1969.
344. Bentov IE, inventor. Patent US 3605725: Controlled motion devices. 1971.
345. Ali A, Plettenburg DH, Breedveld P. Steerable catheters in cardiology: classifying steerability and assessing future challenges. IEEE Trans Biomed Eng. 2016;63(4):679–93.
346. Ali A, Sakes A, Arkenbout EA, Henselmans P, van Starkenburg R, Szili-Torok T, et al. Catheter steering in interventional cardiology: mechanical analysis and novel solution. Proc Inst Mech Eng H. 2019;233(12):1207–18.
347. Rafii-Tari H, Payne CJ, Yang GZ. Current and emerging robot-assisted endovascular catheterization technologies: a review. Ann Biomed Eng. 2014;42(4):697–715.
348. Kabe AN, Thornton TN, Weiss AM, inventors. US Patent: Steerable assembly for surgical catheter patent US20140135685A1. 2014.
349. Kanagaratnam P, Koa-Wing M, Wallace DT, Goldenberg AS, Peters NS, Davies DW. Experience of robotic catheter ablation in humans using a novel remotely steerable catheter sheath. J Interv Card Electrophysiol. 2008;21(1):19–26.
350. Rajappan K, Baker V, Richmond L, Kistler PM, Thomas G, Redpath C, et al. A randomized trial to compare atrial fibrillation ablation using a steerable vs. a non-steerable sheath. Europace. 2009;11(5):571–5.
351. Piorkowski C, Sih H, Sommer P, Miller SP, Gaspar T, Teplitsky L, et al. First in human validation of impedance-based catheter tip-to-tissue contact assessment in the left atrium. J Cardiovasc Electrophysiol. 2009;20(12):1366–73.
352. Webb JG, Chandavimol M, Thompson CR, Ricci DR, Carere RG, Munt BI, et al. Percutaneous aortic valve implantation retrograde from the femoral artery. Circulation. 2006;113(6):842–50.
353. Arya A, Hindricks G, Sommer P, Huo Y, Bollmann A, Gaspar T, et al. Long-term results and the predictors of outcome of catheter ablation of atrial fibrillation using steerable sheath catheter navigation after single procedure in 674 patients. Europace. 2010;12(2):173–80.
354. Hascoet S, Fraisse A, Elbaz M. Successful percutaneous transcatheter patent foramen ovale closure through the right internal jugular vein using a steerable catheter. Catheter Cardiovasc Interv. 2013;82(4):E598–602.
355. DeVita VT Jr, Chu E. A history of cancer chemotherapy. Cancer Res. 2008;68(21):8643–53.
356. Goodman LS, Wintrobe MM, Dameshek W, Goodman MJ, Gilman A, Mclennan MT. Nitrogen mustard therapy: use of methyl-bis(beta-chloroethyl)amine hydrochloride and tris(beta-chloroethyl)amine hydrochloride for Hodgkin's disease, lymphosarcoma, leukemia and certain allied and miscellaneous disorders. JAMA J Am Med Assoc. 1946;132(3):126–32.
357. Rhoads CP. Nitrogen mustards in the treatment of neoplastic disease; official statement. JAMA J Am Med Assoc. 1946;131:656–8.
358. Klopp CT, Alford TC, Bateman J, Berry GN, Winship T. Fractionated intra-arterial cancer; chemotherapy with methyl bis amine hydrochloride; a preliminary report. Ann Surg. 1950;132(4):811–32.
359. Bierman HR, Byron RL Jr, Miller ER, Shimkin MB. Effects of intra-arterial administration of nitrogen mustard. Am J Med. 1950;8(4):535.
360. Anteby R, Kemeny NE, Kingham TP, D'Angelica MI, Wei AC, Balachandran VP, et al. Getting chemotherapy directly to the liver: the historical evolution of hepatic artery chemotherapy. J Am Coll Surg. 2021;232(3):332–8.
361. Buchwald H, Grage TB, Vassilopoulos PP, Rohde TD, Varco RL, Blackshear PJ. Intraarterial infusion chemotherapy for hepatic carcinoma using a totally implantable infusion pump. Cancer. 1980;45(5):866–9.
362. Chua CYX, Ho J, Demaria S, Ferrari M, Grattoni A. Emerging technologies for local cancer treatment. Adv Ther (Weinh). 2020;3(9):2000027.
363. Bobo RH, Laske DW, Akbasak A, Morrison PF, Dedrick RL, Oldfield EH. Convection-enhanced delivery of macromolecules in the brain. Proc Natl Acad Sci USA. 1994;91(6):2076–80.
364. D'Amico RS, Aghi MK, Vogelbaum MA, Bruce JN. Convection-enhanced drug delivery for glioblastoma: a review. J Neurooncol. 2021;151(3):415–27.
365. Riina HA, Knopman J, Greenfield JP, Fralin S, Gobin YP, Tsiouris AJ, et al. Balloon-assisted superselective intra-arterial cerebral infusion of bevacizumab for malignant brainstem glioma. A technical note. Interv Neuroradiol. 2010;16(1):71–6.
366. Dudeck O. Safety and efficacy of target vessel catheterization with the new steerable microcatheter Direxion compared with a standard microcatheter: a prospective, preclinical trial. Cardiovasc Interv Radiol. 2014;37(4):1041–6.
367. Shayan M, Chun Y. An overview of thin film nitinol endovascular devices. Acta Biomater. 2015;21:20–34.

368. Ono M, Kawashima H, Hara H, Gao C, Wang R, Kogame N, et al. Advances in IVUS/OCT and future clinical perspective of novel hybrid catheter system in coronary imaging. Front Cardiovasc Med. 2020;7:119.
369. West K, Al-Nimer S, Goel VR, Yanof JH, Hanlon AT, Weunski CJ, et al. Three-dimensional holographic guidance, navigation, and control (3D-GNC) for endograft positioning in porcine aorta: feasibility comparison with 2-dimensional X-ray fluoroscopy. J Endovasc Ther. 2021;28(5):796–803.
370. Sheetz KH, Claflin J, Dimick JB. Trends in the adoption of robotic surgery for common surgical procedures. JAMA Netw Open. 2020;3(1):e1918911.
371. Li T, Badre A, Alambeigi F, Tavakoli M. Robotic systems and navigation techniques in orthopedics: a historical review. Appl Sci. 2023;13(17):9768.
372. Riga C, Bicknell C, Cheshire N, Hamady M. Initial clinical application of a robotically steerable catheter system in endovascular aneurysm repair. J Endovasc Ther. 2009;16(2):149–53.
373. Gunduz S, Albadawi H, Oklu R. Robotic devices for minimally invasive endovascular interventions: a new dawn for interventional radiology. Adv Intell Syst. 2021;3(2):2000181.

19 Tools for Arterial Drug Delivery Research: The Case for Optical Measurements

John Lipiz and Shailendra Joshi

To measure is to know.

Lord Kelvin (1822–1911), Scottish Physicist and Engineer

Introduction

"I often say that when you can measure what you are speaking about and express it in numbers, you know something about it, but when you cannot measure it, when you cannot express it in numbers, your knowledge is of a meager and unsatisfactory kind." Lord Kelvin's often-used quotation about measurement is the bedrock of scientific advance [1]. Scientific advances are challenging, erratic, and often fail without accurate measurements. On the contrary, with reliable measurements, observations can be quantified, analyzed, and applied, and the applications refined and improved. Measurements of tissue drug concentrations in a sub-second time frame, without invading the tissue, are highly relevant to arterial drug delivery. While several techniques have tracked the blood–brain barrier (BBB) disruption in real time [2–6], very few pharmacokinetic studies have tracked arterial drug concentrations. Only a handful of studies by other investigators have looked at arterial pharmacokinetics using positron emission tomography [7, 8] and, more recently, with intravital microscopy [9]. Although the first-pass extraction of compounds was extensively investigated from the 1970s to the 1990s using radioisotopes to determine the brain uptake index (BUI) values of compounds [10–13], those studies were limited in scope. They did not always control injection parameters and were not designed to generate detailed pharmacokinetic profiles of arterial drug injections [14].

J. Lipiz
Columbia University, New York, NY, USA

S. Joshi (✉)
Department of Anesthesiology, Columbia University Irving Medical Center, New York, NY, USA
e-mail: sj121@cumc.columbia.edu

The pharmacokinetic advantages of arterial drug delivery are well described in the literature [15, 16]. The approach provides ubiquitous access to focal pathologies anywhere in the body. Delivering the drugs through the capillary networks significantly reduces the diffusion distance, a critical factor in drug delivery [17]. Thus, optimizing arterial drug delivery has enormous significance for focal diseases in many organs, especially for brain diseases where conventional approaches have failed [18]. Arterial drug delivery aims to achieve therapeutic drug concentrations with a fraction of the total body dose [19]. That goal has remained elusive over the past century. One can question the rationale of systemic drug delivery to the entire body weighing 60–80 kg for treating a small volume of pathological tissue, sometimes weighing a few grams. In the past two decades, cell targeting technologies have primarily focused on precision medicine, which relies on identifying specific cellular characteristics or pathological pathways. With this approach, systemic drugs have a localized effect on the pathological lesion. However, reaching the target site effectively in the central nervous system (CNS) remains challenging [20]. This is best illustrated by monoclonal antibodies, such as bevacizumab, that are effective in peripheral cancers but cannot cross the blood–brain barrier to treat brain cancers [21, 22]. Thus, despite the developments in precision medicine, there is a need to improve arterial drug delivery. There are many reasons why tissue targeting by arterial drug delivery has failed to gain clinical acceptance in treating neurological diseases. The failure could be due to potential risks, inconsistent benefits, or a lack of understanding of the underlying complexities of arterial delivery [16, 23]. The latter is the most important of the three as it could explain the other two failures.

S. Joshi (ed.), *Arterial Treatment of Neurological Diseases*, https://doi.org/10.1007/978-3-031-80173-0_19

An overview of the methods Used to Assess Arterial Drug Delivery

Traditional pharmacokinetic studies with intra-arterial (IA) drugs use chemical analysis of tissue samples, and do not usually focus on first-pass delivery through the target site [24–27]. These studies assess concentrations over several minutes. Perfusion studies with immediate (within 5–16 s) tissue harvest have been done with bolus injections [10, 11, 13, 28]. Such studies fail to provide time histories. A convenient approach is to use clearance of radioactive tracers to determine cerebral blood flow [29, 30]. Positron emission tomography (PET) and single photon-emission tomography (SPECT) studies can provide valuable human data, but they are resource- and time-intensive, and acquiring spatial data can take several minutes [7, 8]. Multifunction nanocarriers that can be tracked in real time by magnetic resonance, PET, SPECT, ultrasound, and optics are being developed for preclinical pharmacokinetic research [31]. Such carriers could help track delivery across the blood–brain barrier and investigate drug delivery protocols. One can also use anesthetic drugs. Assessing electroencephalographic (EEG) activity after intra-arterial injection of anesthetic drugs provides a surrogate of tissue concentrations and has been used to assess arterial drug kinetics [32–35]. Diffuse reflectance spectroscopy could be used to determine tissue concentrations for some cancer drugs with suitable absorption spectra, like mitoxantrone, doxorubicin, and daunorubicin [36–38]. Many dyes are available for pharmacokinetic research for labeling peptides, micelles, liposomes, and other nanoparticles [39]. Once again, however, it would be difficult to assess whether these labeling carriers would affect drug kinetics, specifically the delivery across the blood–brain barrier.

The Needs of Arterial Drug Delivery Research

Models of arterial drug delivery show that measurements of tissue drug concentrations have to be interpreted in context of regional blood flow. Collins and later Dedrick described the basic model of intra-arterial drug delivery in 1988, which is discussed in detail elsewhere in this book [16, 19]. However, the model ignores clinical complexities, such as injection characteristics, arterial anatomy, blood flow, and tissue and drug characteristics. Cooke et al. recently addressed some of these limitations [40]. Figure 19.1 shows

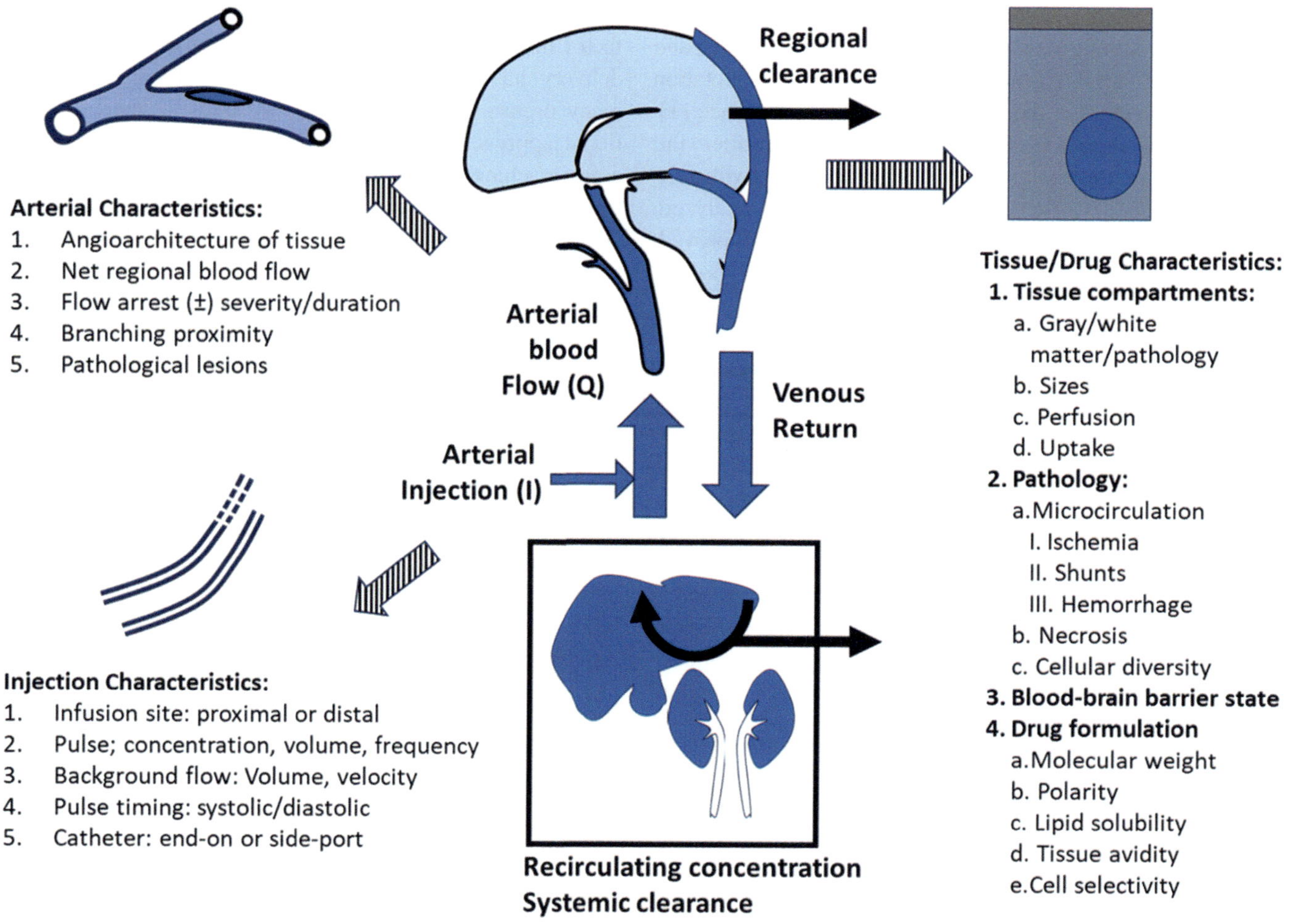

Fig. 19.1 The Dedrick model [16], shown in the center, largely ignores the characteristics of the injections, arteries, and perfused tissues that can affect arterial drug delivery

the complex nature of arterial injections. It is an erroneous oversimplification that, just by injecting drugs into arteries, the regional tissue concentration will be augmented in a sustained manner. Given the potential variables affecting arterial delivery, rigorous and cost-effective high-volume bench research will be needed to optimize and validate the approach. We are unaware of any model that comprehensively addresses arterial drug delivery.

The benefits of arterial drug delivery are due to the high concentrations that are transiently generated as the injected dose passes through the target site. Arterial delivery is most effective when the drug is better extracted and retained during the first pass through the tissue. However, cerebral circulation time in humans is about 3–5 s, and in small animals used for bench research, it is far less, <1 s [41]. Consequently, conventional tissue drug concentration measurements are challenging to apply. Arterial delivery requires precise bolus injections for consistent concentrations, making drug concentration measurements more challenging [14]. Steady-state infusion of drugs can be unreliable due to streaming [15, 42–44]. Drug concentrations generated by arterial injection are a complex function of blood flow, arterial anatomy, and injection parameters. Even for simple dilution, for example, 0.1 mL/s of drug bolus is injected into a tissue volume perfused with 1 mL/min of flow, generating different local concentrations than the same bolus injected with 4 mL/min of flow, due to differences in vascular dead space. An assessment of blood flow in the target tissue is therefore needed. *Thus, the ideal method for measurement of tissue drug concentrations for arterial drug delivery research would require tissue drug concentration measurements to be in a sub-second time frame, site-specific, tissue noninvasive, nondestructive, physiologically inert, repeatable, safe, cost-effective, and permit concurrent assessment of blood flow.*

Non-optical Techniques for Arterial Pharmacokinetic Research

Chemical Analysis

In-Situ Perfusion

The in-situ perfusion method often judges the net uptake of a compound by brain tissue [10–13]. In-situ perfusion experiments have traditionally been undertaken in rats, although the technique has been used in mice [45]. In classical experiments, hand infusion with driving pressure exceeding the systolic blood pressure was used such that the perfusate displaced the blood in the tissue. Hardebo emphasized the need to control the injection delivery precisely to interpret the BUI results correctly [14]. As shown in Fig. 19.2, a precise injection volume control system is needed. The tissue uptake could be assessed both by chemical and isotopic analysis.

Assessing Tissue Drug Uptake

If the concentration of the compound in the perfusate is C_{pf}, then the dose delivered is $C_{br} \times T$, where T is the time. If the amount of the drug taken up by the brain is Q_{br}, then:

$$K_{in} = Q_{br} / \left(C_{pf} \times T\right)$$

If the unidirectional influx factor (K_{in}) is known, then the unidirectional influx factor, permeability surface area (PSA) product can be determined from K_{in} and perfusion (F) by the Renkin–Crone equation:

$$\text{PSA product} = -F \ \ln \left(1 - K_{in} / F\right)$$

Limitation of in Situ Perfusion and Chemical Analysis

Chemical analysis with repeated tissue sampling has been undertaken in larger animals such as rabbits [24, 46]. Chemical analysis has several limitations compared to optical methods. These include:

- *Problems in tissue sampling*: There is enough experimental and clinical justification that arterial drug delivery is most effective when drugs are injected as boluses. Furthermore, modeling data suggest that the most significant benefit of arterial drug delivery is when the target site avidly retains the drug during the first pass through cerebral circulation [40]. In animals used for bench research, the cerebral transit time for a bolus injection is less than 1 s [41]. It is impossible to obtain reliable tissue samples in such a period. Chemical tissue analysis is a tissue-destructive approach. Although multiple tissue samples have been obtained in a single animal, the injury can confound drug delivery and will not permit site-specific measurements.
- *Need for arterial isolation*: Experimental animals' extra and intracranial arteries show considerable anatomical variations, also seen in human subjects [47, 48]. Figure 19.3 provides an example of the most common variations of the rabbit's common carotid artery [49]. Vendor-related variations in rats' cerebral circulation are also reported, which could affect perfusion-related experiments such as stroke or drug delivery [50]. Correct and complete isolation of the internal carotid artery (ICA) is necessary to investigate arterial drug delivery. Given the variable origin of the artery, it is desirable to test the isolation by retinal discoloration test. For the test, a small volume of saline (100–200 μL) injected into the isolated carotid artery results in blanching of the eye. The test is possible due to the origin of the ophthalmic artery, the first intracranial branch of the ICA [51]. The alternative to the test is angiography, which is usually not possible in most laboratories. One of the advantages of optical measurements, such as diffuse reflectance spectroscopy (DRS), is the effect of drug bolus injection on hemoglobin (Hb) concentrations due to dilution. A reproducible

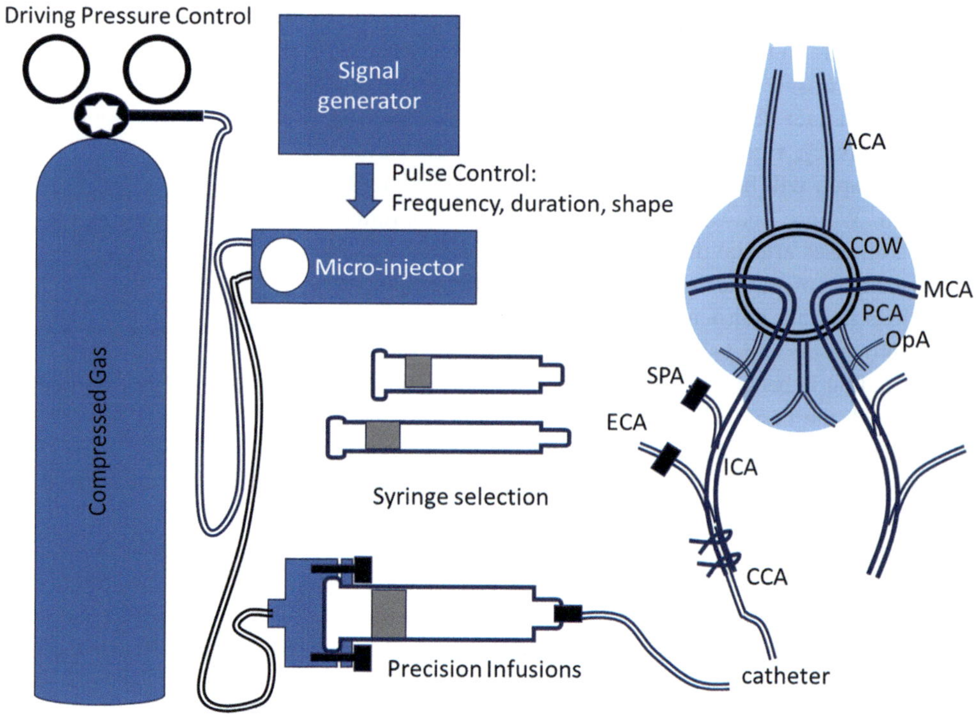

Fig. 19.2 Cerebral perfusion experiments in rats. *CCA* common carotid artery, *ECA* external carotid artery, *ICA* internal carotid artery, *COW* circle of Willis, *SPA* sphenopalatine artery, *OpA* ophthalmic artery, *ACA* anterior cerebral artery, *MCA* middle cerebral artery, *PCA* Posterior cerebral artery

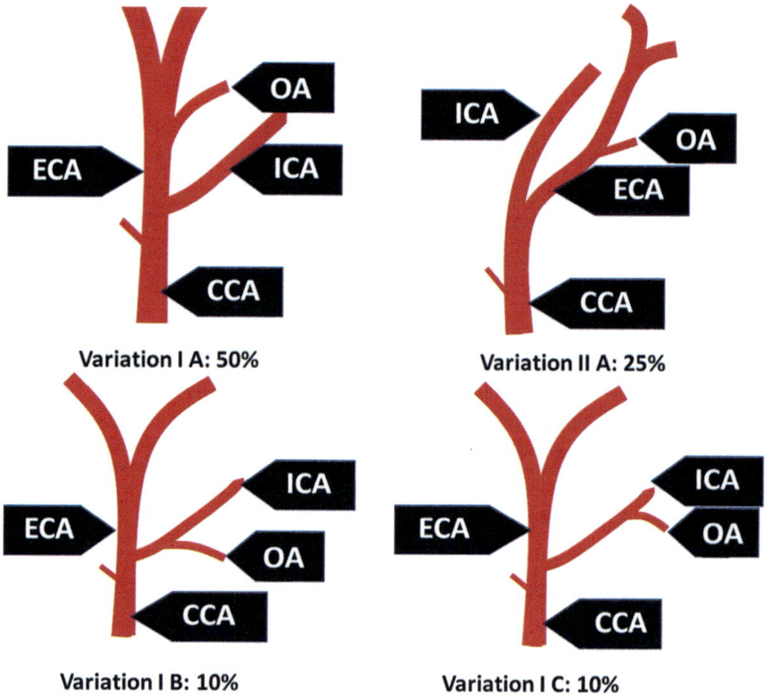

Fig. 19.3 The notable variations in rabbits' internal carotid artery origin. *CCA* common carotid artery, *ECA* external carotid artery, *ICA* Internal carotid artery, *OA* occipital artery

change in hemoglobin concentrations can also ensure consistent arterial injections.

- *Lack of spatial resolution*: Chemical analysis requires tissue homogenization, which results in the loss of spatial information [46, 52]. Furthermore, in a complex organ with widely different perfusion, lipid/water content, and transport characteristics, the concentrations within a tumor may be significantly different from gray or white matter. Optical sensing and imaging methods could provide spatial information that is lost with tissue homogenization for chemical analysis.
- *Chemical sample sources*: The limitation of chemical analysis is the resources and time expended to process samples.
  - *Tissue sampling*: Chemical analysis of tissue samples or the whole brain lacks spatial resolution and does not

give time history [10–13]. Given the test–retest variabilities, 6–10 tissue samples are needed for each time-point measurement. The limited samples obtained from an animal increase costs, cause time delays, and increase the number of animals required.

- *Microdialysis*: Microdialysis can be applied to determine tissue drug concentration if it can diffuse across a semipermeable membrane. The technique requires a steady-state infusion of a diffusible compound, such that in equilibrium, the returning dialysate reflects the drug's tissue concentration [53–55]. The technique can be applied to diffusible drugs, may not be applied to bolus drug delivery, is tissue-invasive, requires equilibrium time, is regional, and is site-specific. It can be used clinically and provides a time history. Recall, however, that bolus injection is far more clinically relevant than continuous infusion for IA drug delivery [56–58]. However, microdialysis may not be suitable for tracking arterial bolus delivery in the sub-second time frame or pulsed injections that will disturb the equilibrium state or limit effective drug diffusion.
- *Use of surrogates such as blood and CSF concentrations*: Due to difficulties in tissue sampling, surrogate measurements of drug concentration in blood and cerebrospinal fluid (CSF) have been used to investigate arterial drug delivery [59–62]. Drug concentration is the blood that could be used to estimate tissue concentration in an organ if the tissue (e.g., brain):blood partition coefficient at equilibrium is known [63, 64]. Similarly, CSF concentrations that assess arterial delivery require time to equilibrate with blood and tissues. Unlike the brain:blood partition coefficient, which is easily accessible, the brain:CSF partition data are not readily available. Zylber-Katz showed that the CSF methotrexate concentrations were directly related to the degree of osmotic blood–brain barrier disruption by intra-arterial mannitol [62].
- *Spatial localization with matrix-assisted laser desorption ionization (MALDI) imaging of tissue sections*: Spatial localization of drugs after arterial injection is necessary to assess the effectiveness of targeting strategies. MALDI preserves the tissue sample sections and does not require the labeling of drug molecules chemically or with isotopes. MALDI uses a matrix that extracts specific molecules. A laser beam line scans the matrix without damaging the tissue specimen, ionizing the molecules extracted by the matrix for mass spectroscopic analysis. The analysis has a resolution of 20–200 μm. The selection of different matrices allows different molecules to be quantified and spatially localized. These include lipids, proteins, and drug molecules [65]. MALDI could provide a valuable tool to investigate arterial drugs and carrier delivery in post-mortem tissue samples.

- *Lack of concurrent blood flow data*: Chemical and other drug concentration measurement methods do not provide blood flow data. In contrast, optical drug concentration measurements can easily be combined with optical blood flow measurement techniques. For example, laser Doppler, a widely used blood flow measurement method, can be combined with DRS. Regional blood flow is a significant determinant of both drug uptake and clearance. Quantifying drug delivery in the context of regional blood flow is a powerful tool to investigate the pharmacokinetics of arterial drug delivery.
- *Cost and time concerns*: Given the many systemic and regional parameters affecting arterial drug delivery, it is necessary to investigate it in cost-effective animal models. Chemical tissue analysis methods are fairly resource- and time-intensive. In contrast to optical and isotopic studies, chemical sample analysis is usually done in batches and can be considerably delayed.

Radioisotopic Methods

Several radioisotopic methods have been used to determine tissue drug concentration after intra-arterial injections. However, the limitations of the detection technology used, radiation hazards, and artifacts from drug metabolites versus unmetabolized drugs would be a concern. The sensitivity of radiation detection methods has improved, resulting in isotopic dose reduction. Isotopic whole-body pharmacokinetic studies with low radiation doses of stable isotopes have been proposed to quantify the uptake and distribution of drugs for oncologic applications. They could help future arterial drug delivery research [66].

These methods include:

- *Isotopes for brain uptake index (BUI) determination*: BUI is determined by the perfusion of the brain using radiolabeled reference and test compounds infused into the carotid artery at 200 μL in 0.5 s. Tissue is harvested 5–15 s after injection. The reference compound, usually ^{14}C-labeled butanol, is freely diffusible in the brain tissue. The test compounds are labeled with ^{3}H. As described by Jones et al. [28], BUI can be determined by:

$$\frac{{}^{3}\text{H brain} / {}^{14}\text{C brain}}{{}^{3}\text{H conc. injected} / {}^{14}\text{C concentration injected}}$$

BUI is the uptake of a drug relative to a standard compound. It can be expressed as a percentage of butanol uptake, which is considered to be 100% [28]. BUI represents the first-pass extraction of the drug and can be used to derive the PSA values [10–13, 64, 67, 68]. The main problem with BUI is that it does not generate time histories.

- *Quantitative autoradiographic imaging*: Quantitative autoradiography techniques use the injection of isotopes with serial blood samples. The target tissues are harvested at a fixed time. The tissue is serially sectioned and imaged. Radiolabeled sucrose, which is tissue impermeable, determines the intravascular volume. The method has been used to determine the K_{in} and PS of compounds delivered intravenously. Autoradiography was used to show maldistribution due to streaming after arterial drug delivery in rats and primates [42, 69]. Due to radiation risk, the method has not been widely applied in arterial drug delivery research. Optically labeling and imaging carrier-assisted drug delivery is more straightforward and safer and can provide cell-level details with confocal microscopy of tissue sections.
- *PET studies*: Tyler et al. used PET to compare intra-arterial and intravenous delivery of ^{14}C-labeled 1,3-bis (2-chloroethyl)-1-nitrosourea, also known as carmustine, (BCNU). PET can determine changes in tissue drug concentration over time in human subjects and PSA. However, it poses a radiation hazard, is cost-intensive, and is unsuitable for high-volume studies. PET imaging can measure tissue perfusion but has to be co-registered with anatomical imaging, such as CT, for spatial localization [8].
- *SPECT studies*: ^{99m}Tc imaging is widely used in SPECT studies. SPECT tracers have been used to track the delivery of nanoparticles. SPECT has been successfully used in human subjects for intra-arterial drug delivery. Consistent with simulations, SPECT investigation revealed no significant effect of streaming with infra-ophthalmic injections in human subjects [70].

MRI-Guided IA Delivery

MRI has several applications for arterial drug delivery research. MRI can help monitor the disruption of the blood–brain barrier to ensure effective drug delivery and enhance safety [71, 72]. Intra-arterial contrast injections with MRI have been used to select arteries for drug infusion and infusion rates necessary to optimize drug delivery [6]. MRI-assisted drug delivery is superior to delivery without MRI guidance [73]. MRI-detectable nanoparticle kinetics has been developed for preclinical pharmacokinetic research [74–77]. MRI-detectable stem cells could affect future stroke treatment [78]. Arterial delivery of stem cells requires careful monitoring of blood flow due to embolic risks posed by the stem cells [79, 80]. A potential use of this technology would be MRI guidance of stem cell therapy while carefully monitoring the blood flow for stroke and glioma treatments [81, 82].

Ultrasonic Tracers

Another emerging pharmacokinetic tool is ultrasound-detectable nanoparticles. Ultrasound can penetrate tissue and enable tracking of such nanoparticle delivery [83]. Ultrasound imaging permits depth interrogation in a sub-second time frame and does not pose operational hazards. However, in-vivo human ultrasound application is constrained by the skull, which restricts its application through specific insonation windows.

Electrocerebral Silence

EEG silence after arterial anesthetic drug injections: EEG silence with anesthetic drugs is well known and has been used to assess intra-arterial pharmacokinetics [32–35, 84]. Therefore, silence with intra-arterial anesthetic could be used to investigate the pharmacokinetics of IA administration. The duration of EEG silence or change could be used as a surrogate for real-time tissue drug concentrations. EEG silence has been used to investigate the relationship between arterial blood flow and the effect of intra-arterial anesthetic drugs [33]. However, such a method is limited to anesthetic drugs. This approach can only investigate a narrow dose range of anesthetic drugs as excessive doses could prolong local effects due to recirculation, and the duration can be confounded by tissue injury such as air or clot embolism.

Optical Techniques for Arterial Pharmacokinetic Research

The Advantages of Optical Methods

Maximizing the first-pass extraction of drugs is necessary to obtain the most benefit from arterial drug delivery. This requires optimizing injection and background flow parameters and developing drugs, carriers, peptides, micelles, liposomes, and nanoparticles that can be rapidly extracted and avidly retained during their first pass through the cerebral circulation. Given the vast array of potential carriers and experimental variables, extensive preclinical research is needed to advance models of arterial drug delivery. While isotopic measurements can inform and improve arterial drug delivery, they raise significant safety, scalability, and cost concerns. None of the currently available pharmacokinetic investigative methods fully meets the needs of arterial pharmacokinetic research. On the contrary, optical methods provide many tools to advance arterial pharmacokinetic research safely and efficiently. Optical methods can enormously impact arterial drug delivery research. Some of the interactions between light and tissues that enable optical measurements are shown in Fig. 19.4. This chapter shows how optical methods are being or can be applied to arterial

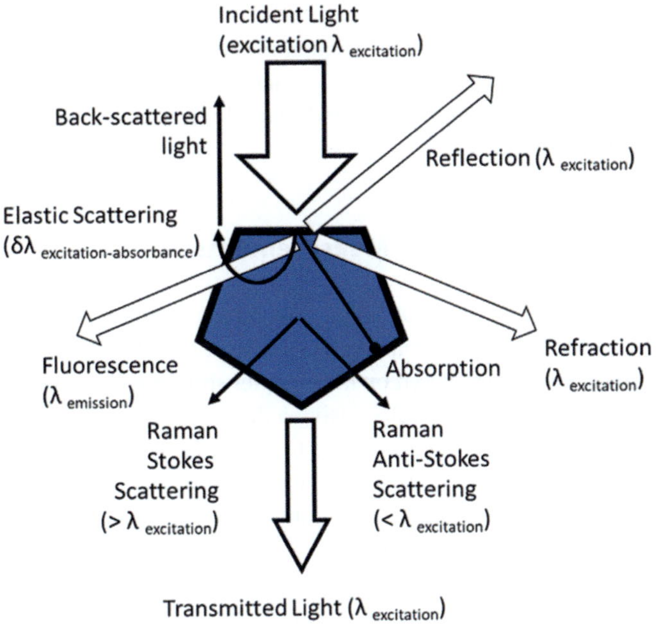

Fig. 19.4 The interaction of light with tissues

pharmacokinetic research. There could be other optical techniques to assess reliably relative or absolute tissue chromophore concentrations, which are not discussed here. Hopefully, this chapter will encourage the development of optical tools for arterial drug delivery research. The following are methods discussed here:

Intravital microscopy
- Laser Doppler flow measurements and imaging
- Diffuse reflectance spectroscopy [DRS]
- Tissue fluorescence and multispectral imaging (MSI)
- Hyperspectral imaging (HSI)
- Spatial frequency domain imaging (SFDI)
- Spectral optical coherence tomography
- Confocal microscopy

Intravital Microscopy

Technique

Intravital microscopy permits direct visualization of the vascular networks under a microscope. It provides a powerful tool to understand tissue-level blood flow changes and drug delivery. The basic technique consists of removing or thinning the skull, exposing the brain tissue, and directly observing an area of tissue beneath a glass window with appropriate illumination. The tissue is isolated in a chamber where local physiological conditions are kept stable or manipulated per experimental needs. The technique has been used extensively to investigate cerebral circulation [85]. Chronic windows have been used on brain tumor implants and peripherally implanted brain tumors. There are several applications of intravital microscopy relevant to arterial drug delivery:

- Detailed characterization and response of the vasculature to IA interventions
- Direct observation of vascular sizes, blood flow, and transit time through the circulation
- Uptake of tracers and drugs through the regional circulation
- Microspheres can enable regional blood flow measurements
- Optimizing arterial drug injections and drug release
- Drug delivery to pathological tissues

Chronic Cranial Window Technique

The overlying skin, skull, and dura matter limit the optical interrogation of the brain tissue. These impediments can be surgically removed to permit direct observation of tissue anatomy, pathology, and functioning. While some applications of acute windows are listed above, chronically implanted cranial windows also offer a powerful tool for investigating the effects of arterial drugs. Advances in optics instrumentation, microscopy, optogenetics, and genetic encoding for fluorescent proteins make chronic cranial windows a powerful investigative tool [86]. Chronic cranial windows broadly involve a breach of the cranial vault or thinning of the skull. When the skull is removed, it can be replaced by either glass slip, flexible polymer, or an optically assisting device such as a prism or cylindrical lens. The dura may be left intact or removed surgically. The space between the covering element and the brain can be filled with CSF, agarose, or silicone. The window can be removable to permit superfusion of the drugs and dyes and for implanting tumor cells or they may be permanently sealed. These windows vary in size from 1 to 10 mm. The interrogation depth depends on the optical techniques but could be as deep as 1400 μm with two-photon microscopy using glass windows. The window could be reinforced with methacrylate with or without the closure of the overlying skin. Chronic cranial windows can be used for several weeks. They may require re-thinning of the bone and pose a risk of infection, inflammation, astrocytosis, and alteration of neurological functions. However, their ability to provide information in-vivo on a microscopic scale over days or weeks to assess drug delivery and treatment response creates a powerful tool for arterial drug delivery research [86].

The Development of Optical Contrast Agents

A contrast agent, such as a dye, is a compound that selectively binds to a molecular target or cellular structure to differentiate it from the background when paired with a specific imaging method based on absorption, fluorescence, or both. For in-vivo use, the contrast agent should be nontoxic, photostable, have a high quantum yield, and have a broad Stoke shift (the separation of absorption and emission spectrum). A significant challenge in fluorescent signal processing is that the signal degrades due to the absorption and scattering of light and can be smeared by autofluorescence. In most tissues, hemoglobin and oxyhemoglobin (HbO) are the principal light absorbers in the visible range (400–700 nm), along with melanin, bilirubin, and cytochrome A3. However, modern imaging systems can operate well beyond the visual range. The in-vivo optical contrast agents have emission and absorption spectra in the visible to near-infrared (NIRS) range, from 400 to 1700 nm. There are three bands for optical measurements in the NIRS range: NIR-I (700–1100 nm), NIR-IIa (1300–1500) nm, and NIR-IIb (1500–1700 nm). The main advantages of longer wavelengths of light are greater tissue penetration and better signal-to-noise ratio due to less absorption, less scattering, and less autofluorescence. The wavelengths are beneficial in two-photon and multi-photon imaging that can image tissues to a depth of 3 mm [87].

Dyes for Visible and NIRS Imaging

Several classes of dyes are available in the visible and short NIR range. These include xanthene dyes, such as fluorescein and rhodamine. These dyes are safe and can easily be conjugated with a wide range of molecules to track their delivery. Fluorescein is approved for human use for tumor edge definition during surgery. The dye has a low quantum yield of 0.1 but a reasonable Stoke shift of 200 nm. It has been used in whole-animal pharmacokinetic studies [88]. *Cyanine* dyes are extensively used for research purposes. They are available in several discrete absorption bands. They have an intense, narrow absorption band with good quantum yield ranging from 0.32 to 0.69 and a Stoke shift of 140 nm. *Phthalocyanine and squaraine dyes* have an excellent quantum yield but a narrow Stoke shift (50–100 nm). These have poor aqueous solubility and tend to aggregate. Phthalocyanines are used for photodynamic therapy [39]. Cyanine dyes are commercially available and can track intra-arterial liposomes and micelles due to their lipid solubility. They can be conjugated with peptides for optical pharmacokinetic purposes. These dyes allow rapid postmortem assessment using tissue fluorescence and confocal microscopy [89–91].

Dyes in the NIR-II Range

Various tracers are being developed to exploit fluorescence with longer wavelengths. These include highly engineered inorganic fluorophores such as single-walled carbon nanotubes with or without polymer coating, quantum dots, rare earth-doped nanoparticles, several organic dyes, and genetically encoded NIR fluorescent proteins similar to green fluorescent protein (GFP) that are in the visible spectrum. These are designed to meet the needs of advanced microscopy techniques such as two-photon and multi-photon microscopy, light sheet microscopy and its variant forms, and super-resolution microscopy. These techniques allow considerable depth penetration and high-resolution imaging over more extended periods. Nanotubes have recently been used in mice to image cerebral vasculature through intact skulls. However, issues with their circulatory half-life, accumulation in the liver and spleen, and toxicological concerns need to be addressed [92].

Laser Doppler Flow Measurements

Technique: Continuous blood flow measurement is essential to understanding arterial drug delivery. Laser Doppler flow measurements are based on the Doppler shift of reflected light by moving red blood cells. Using a diffusing lens, a large tissue area can be imaged and used to determine tissue perfusion (Fig. 19.5) [93]. The main advantage of laser Doppler flowmetry is that the continuous flow data can be observed. For point measurements, small fibers 0.5–1 mm can be used. Laser Doppler measurements can be made with narrow bands of infrared (IR) light, such as around 800 nm [94]. Thus, laser Doppler flowmetry can be used with other optical devices [95].

Diffuse Reflectance (DRS) or Elastic Scattering Spectroscopy

Technique

DRS is a powerful tool for investigating the pharmacokinetics of arterial drugs. It provides tissue noninvasive drug concentration measurements in a sub-second time frame. It can sample to a depth of 3 mm and is thus ideally suited for high-volume small animal research. However, DRS is best used for drugs whose absorption spectra are distinct from hemoglobin (Hb) and oxyhemoglobin (HbO), two of the main chromogens in most tissues [36–38]. This limits the applicability of DRS for many drugs. Furthermore, the light absorption spectrum should be stable and not affected by in-vivo delivery. DRS can be used for many dyes conjugated to carriers and used to assess carrier kinetics. Even if DRS fails to provide absolute concentration measurements, it could be used to determine relative changes in tissue drug concentrations. One of the significant advantages of DRS in investigating drug delivery to the brain is the possibility of using a tracer to assess drug delivery as a function of the permeability of the blood–brain barrier [96–99].

DRS assesses the fraction of the backscattered light due to interaction with tissue components. DRS is based on the observation that concentrations of optically absorbing drugs can be measured in a small volume of tissue despite a wide range of scattering properties. When white light (450–850 nm) is applied to tissues at a specified distance ($\geq$0.5 cm), the spectrum of the backscattered light can determine the concentration of the chromophore. The DRS system typically uses afferent (400 μm) and efferent

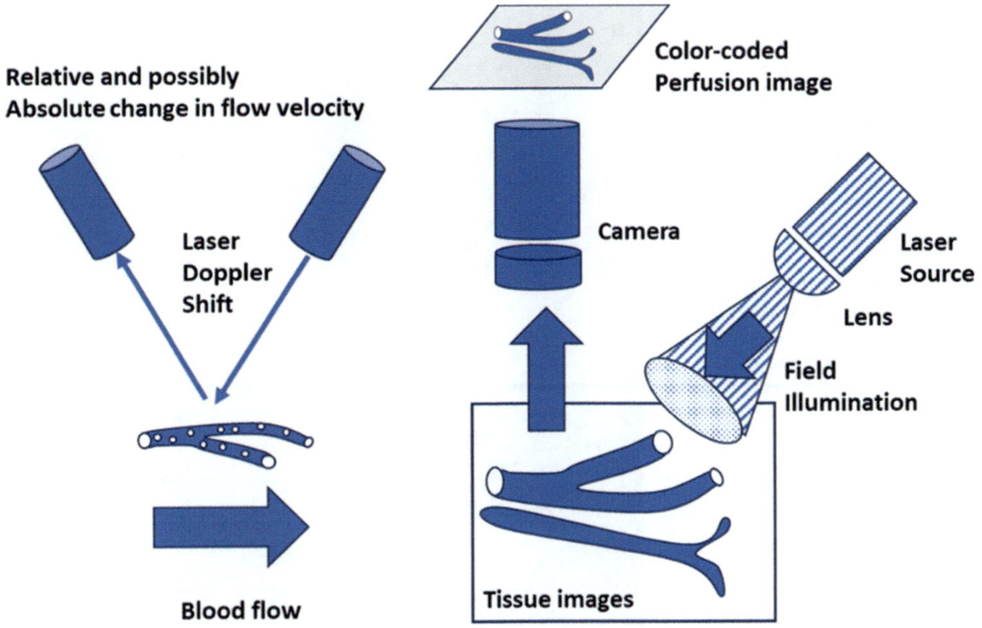

Fig. 19.5 Point and field measurements of perfusion with the laser Doppler technique

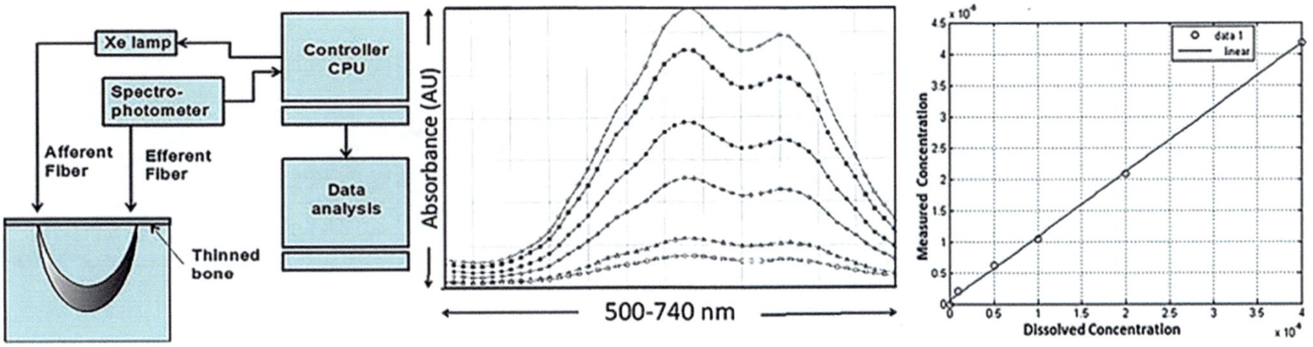

Fig. 19.6 **From left to the right**: DRS setup for arterial drug delivery to the brain, the spectrum of DiR dye, and the concentration of dye-labeled liposomes in a tissue phantom

(200 μm) optical fibers with a center-to-center separation of 2 mm. Both fibers have a numerical aperture of 0.22 and effectively sample tissue to a depth of up to 3 mm (Figs. 19.6 and 19.7). The method described by Reif et al. involves calibration of the probe-backscattered light tested against a white tissue phantom [100]. The system is then applied to the tissue to obtain baseline measurements followed by subsequent measurements of drug concentrations. For any given data point (I), the baseline measurement is subtracted from the observed value. The absorption coefficient ($\delta\mu_a$) is obtained as follows:

$$-\ln\left[I_{(t)} / I_{(0)}\right] = B + \delta\mu_a L(\mu_a)$$

where $I_{(t)}$ and $I_{(0)}$ are measurements at time t and baseline (t_0), respectively; $L(\mu_a)$ is the path length; B is the change due to scattering parameters between the two measurements. The baseline B is defined as

$$B = c_0(t) + c_1(t)\lambda + c_2(t)\lambda^2$$

where $c_0(t)$, $c_1(t)$, and $c_2(t)$ are baseline coefficients and λ is the wavelength. The pathlength (L) is determined by

$$L(\mu_a) = x_0 + x_1 \exp(-x_2\mu_a)$$

As shown above, the path length is wavelength-dependent and, over time, is a function of μ_a, where x_0, x_1, and x_2 are calibration constants determined in a light-scattering tissue phantom. As a tissue phantom, 1% intralipid can be used. It has a scattering coefficient of 10 cm^{-1} and an absorption coefficient of ~0.3 cm^{-1} at 700 nm, similar to tissue values. Furthermore, μ_a and $\delta\mu_a$ are

$$\mu_a = \left[\delta c_{HbO}(t) + c_{HbO}(t_0)\right]\varepsilon_{HbO}(\lambda) + \left[\delta c_{Hb}(t) + c_{Hb}(t_0)\right]\varepsilon_{Hb}(\lambda) + c_{\text{drug}}(t)\varepsilon_{\text{drug}}(\lambda)$$

$$\delta\mu_a = \delta c_{Hb}(t)\varepsilon_{Hb}(\lambda) + \delta c_{Hbo}(t)\varepsilon_{Hbo}(\lambda) + \delta c_{\text{drug}}(t)\varepsilon_{\text{drug}}(\lambda)$$

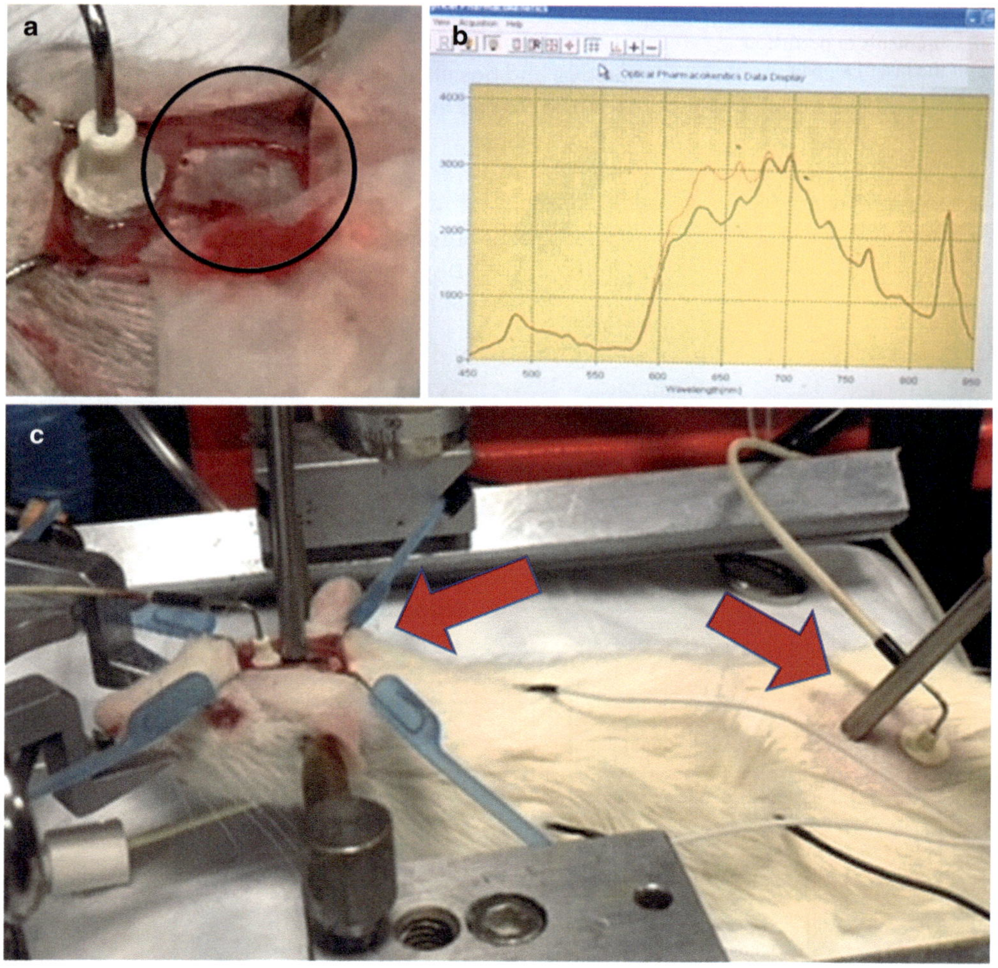

Fig. 19.7 DRS setup for brain drug delivery. (**a**) Laser Doppler probe measures cerebral blood flow, and the skull is thinned (circle). (**b**) Change in the spectrum of backscattered light after injection of an optically tagged carrier (Black) from baseline (red). (**c**) A steel-protected fiber-optic probe is placed on the skull and shaved skin (arrows) to measure regional blood flow and assess drug delivery

where $c_{Hb}(t)$, $c_{HbO}(t)$, and $c_{drug}(t)$ are concentrations of hemoglobin, oxyhemoglobin, and drug at time t, while $\varepsilon_{Hb}(\lambda)$, $\varepsilon_{HbO}(\lambda)$, and $\varepsilon_{drug}(\lambda)$ are the respective extinctions of Hb, HbO, and drug, respectively, the observed backscattered light spectrum is fitted to the individual light absorption data of Hb, HbO, and the drug(s) to determine the technique to assess brain tissue drug concentrations [100].

Technique to Assess Brain Tissue Drug Concentrations

To use DRS in rats and rabbits, the skull is shaved to transparency using a drill and sealed with bone wax. Fiber-optic DRS probes are placed over the shaved skull with a micromanipulator. A second DRS probe can be placed over the skin of the hind leg after carefully shaving the skin to assess systemic drug delivery. Baseline spectra are acquired before the drug is injected. During drug injection, data are acquired for every 300–500 ms for the first 2 min. This can capture the first-pass delivery and extraction of the drug. Subsequently, the data are acquired more slowly every 1 s for the following 300 observations. Finally, the data are acquired every 10 s for 300 measurements. Typically, 900 tissue drug measurements can be undertaken over an hour.

Limitations

DRS is a reliable tool with some limitations. It applies to drugs with a stable absorbance spectrum that is not affected by in-vivo delivery. The light absorbance should be separate from hemoglobin and oxyhemoglobin, which are strong absorbers in the visible spectral range. An additional practical problem is avoiding bleeding under the probe that can swamp the optical signal.

Arterial Drug Delivery Applications

1. *Delivery of native drugs*: The concentration of chemotherapy drugs like mitoxantrone and doxorubicin can directly be measured by the DRS method [36–38, 95]. DRS provides certain advantages over conventional chemical measurements:
   (a) DRS provides a rapid assessment of drug concentrations during the first pass through the tissues [100].
   (b) The DRS method can differentiate in-vivo tissue uptake and drug in the vascular compartment, comparing changes with a saline bolus injection.
   (c) Drug uptake can be assessed as a function of blood–brain permeability.

(d) Due to spectral shift due to binding with DNA, DRS may be able to provide the distribution of free and bound drugs [101].

(e) DRS can be supplemented with postmortem detailed imaging by other techniques such as hyperspectral imaging and confocal microscopy, which can be undertaken on tissue samples. It also permits the assessment of blood flow with laser Doppler measurements [102].

2. *Rapid screening method for carriers for arterial drug delivery*: Numerous carriers have been developed for delivering drugs to brain tumors and across the BBB. These include nanoparticles, peptides, transporter conjugates, liposomes, micelles, viral vectors, modified blood cells, and other nanoparticles [91, 95, 102, 103]. Labeling these entities with suitable dyes can permit the identification of suitable carriers for arterial delivery and test delivery protocols using the DRS method. Once the delivery effectiveness has been determined using dyes, drug cargo can replace the dye in the carrier.
3. *Monitoring BBB permeability*: DRS can be used to determine BBB permeability and the disruption method's effectiveness. Using the DRS, the opening of the BBB with intra-arterial mannitol was highly variable. Optically measured tracers like indocyanine green (ICG) can detect barrier disruption and improve drug delivery [97–99].

Fluorescence and Multispectral Imaging

Technique

Due to the presence of chromophores such as hemoglobin, myoglobin, bilirubin, melanin, cytochrome, and endogenous fluorescence of tissues due to collagen, elastin, lipids, proteins, and metabolites like nicotinamide adenine dinucleotide (NADH) and flavin adenine dinucleotide (FAD), direct quantitative fluorescence is more challenging than light absorption measurements. However, high-powered light-emitting diodes and low-cost fluorescence cameras enable the construction of devices that permit semiquantitative in-vivo measurements [104–106]. Fluorescent drugs and tracers enable gross assessment of drug distribution in postmortem specimens, while confocal microscopy can reveal cell-level uptake after tissue sectioning [91]. For pharmacokinetic studies, such measurements are best undertaken with non-toxic dyes with distinct absorption and emission peaks and high quantum yield that can map the uptake of distribution of drugs and carriers throughout the body [107]. Several anti-cancer drugs can be used for fluorescence quantification in the visual and near-infrared range; however, their quantum yield is relatively low compared to the dyes whose structure can be further optimized [108].

Figure 19.8 shows a simple, low-cost multispectral imaging system. Multispectral imaging (MSI) requires surgically exposed target tissue. In rats and rabbits, the skull has to be removed, and cranial windows with a suitable perfusion system might be needed to ensure physiological integrity. MSI systems must be ambient light-shielded; thus, it is often undertaken in dark room conditions where animal safety, physiological integrity, and immobility must be ensured. Fluorescence tomography using several light sources and detectors can generate more accurate localization of signals in small animals in vivo.

Limitations

MSI measurements in most animals require exposure to the target tissue. Clinically, MSI applies to eyes or exposed tissues, such as during neurosurgery. They are limited to compounds with suitably separated absorption and emission spectra. Fluorescent signals can be weak. Thus, light protection, rigorous standardization of experimental conditions, and calibration of the systems are needed. Tissue properties, endogenous fluorescence, absorbance, and quenching can affect precise MSI measurements. Quenching is the degradation of fluorescent signals with increasing exposure due to changes in tissue chemistry [109].

High-Speed Fluorescence Pharmacokinetics Studies

Arterial and intravenous pharmacokinetics require tissue concentration assessment at specified time points. This is usually a challenging process that is resource- and time-intensive. Dobosz et al. used near-infrared fluorescence to track the delivery of indocyanine green, OsteoSense 750, which targets bone, and Trastuzumab-Alexa750, which targets tumors. They could track their intravenous tail vein delivery and subsequent whole-body distribution in nude immunosuppressed mice using appropriate filter combinations for excitation and emission for the three compounds. Optical measurements were made through the eye and the whole body. Imaging was done using Perkin Elmer's Mastero imaging system. The pharmacokinetic data were acquired at 1 frame/s; the excitation lasted 200 ms while the animals remained anesthetized for 2 h. After their recovery, the images were acquired daily as needed. The experiments revealed that the half-life as determined by ocular measurements for ICG was 1.5 min due to its rapid clearance by the liver; OsteoSense 750's half-time was 3.8 min; and Trastuzumab-Alexa750's half-life was 2.5 days. The authors found that this was consistent with the reported results. More importantly, delayed imaging revealed OsteoSense 750 deposition in the long bones and spine. The experiment demonstrated the feasibility of obtaining systemic pharmacokinetic data by monitoring ocular fluorescence [88].

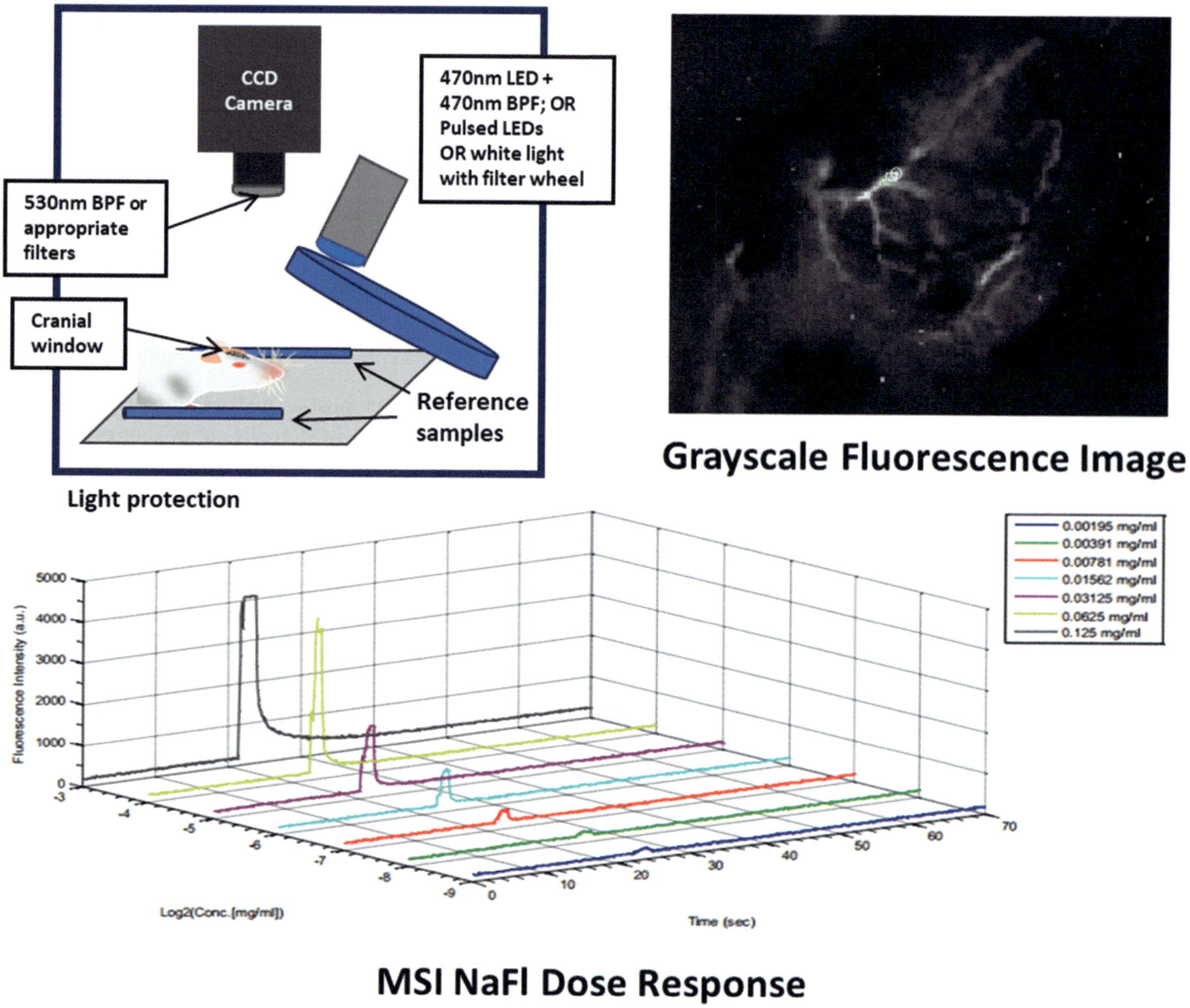

Fig. 19.8 In-vivo fluorescence imaging with arterial injections of sodium fluorescein

Arterial Drug Delivery Applications

- Rapid and repeated multispectral brain imaging is possible through cranial windows [110]
- Custom imaging devices are available for whole animal fluorescence imaging [88, 111]
- It can be used in-vivo and ex-vivo to assess carrier delivery [103, 112]
- Low-cost systems with laser diodes and fluorescence cameras can permit semiquantitative assessment of tissue fluorescence [105]
- It complements confocal microscopy to assess cell and cell-level effectiveness of carrier delivery [91]

Hyperspectral Imaging

Technique

Hyperspectral imaging (HSI) generates spectral information for each pixel of an image when illuminated with a broadband light source. The measurements can be remotely done. HSI creates a data cube consisting of planar (*X* and *Y* axis) and spectral information [113]. Illumination of tissues results in wavelength-specific scattering, absorbance, and fluorescence. While multispectral imaging uses fewer discrete wavelengths for illumination, hyperspectral imaging uses contiguous wavelengths [114]. Hyperspectral imaging can be in the ultraviolet

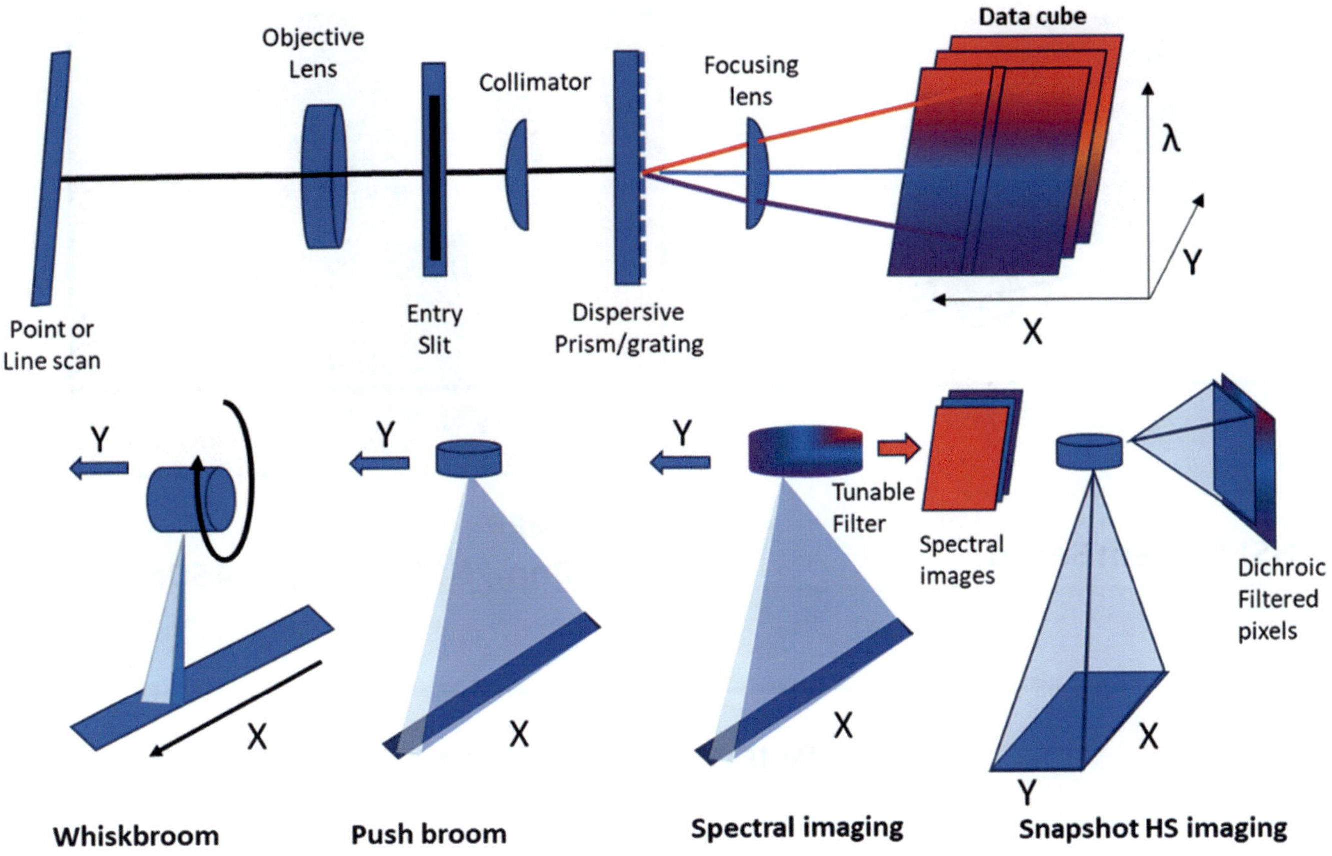

Fig. 19.9 Hyperspectral imaging (HSI). Top: Push broom HSI system. Below: Some HSI systems

(UV: 200–400 nm), visible (VIS: 400–780 nm), NIR (780–2500 nm), and mid-IR (2500–25,000 nm). The NIR range can be separated into IR-A (780–1400 nm), IR-B (1400–3000 nm), and IR-C (>3000 nm) [114]. Due to the light absorption properties of hemoglobin, 600–1100 nm is a suitable bandwidth for clinical imaging. Longer IR wavelengths are associated with thermal damage. Shorter wavelengths towards the UV range can result in phototoxic injuries.

The common types of HSI systems are shown in Fig. 19.9. The most common type of system used is the push broom system, which is highly efficient in capturing light but has longer scan times. They often use dispersive grating and are portable. Spectral imaging systems use a tunable filter that permits line scans at different wavelengths. The tunable filters can be liquid crystal tunable filters or acoustic-optical tunable filters. The former filters are slower; the latter are faster but bulkier. These are suited for microscopy imaging. Snapshot systems use pixels with dichroic filters that simultaneously acquire spatial and spectral data. These permit rapid imaging but are inefficient, have a low spectral and spatial resolution, and can be affected by the angle of imaging that alters the wavelength of incoming light.

Limitations

HSI enables noninvasive surface tissue imaging but requires surgical tissue exposure. Image processing takes time. Hyperspectral cameras are usually expensive. It generates vast amounts of data requiring sufficient computational capabilities.

Current Applications of HSI

- *Tumor detection*: Cervical, skin, colon, breast, head, and neck cancers have been identified using HSI with considerable specificity and sensitivity despite being a remote sensing modality [115]
- *Ophthalmology*: Detection of retinal and CNS diseases [116, 117]
- Peripheral vascular insufficiency and pharmacological responses by assessing skin Hb and HbO concentrations [118, 119]
- Assessment of shock [120]
- Rapid inspection of drug formulations during manufacturing [121]
- Clinical neurological applications of HSI:
  - Monitoring brain physiology [122]

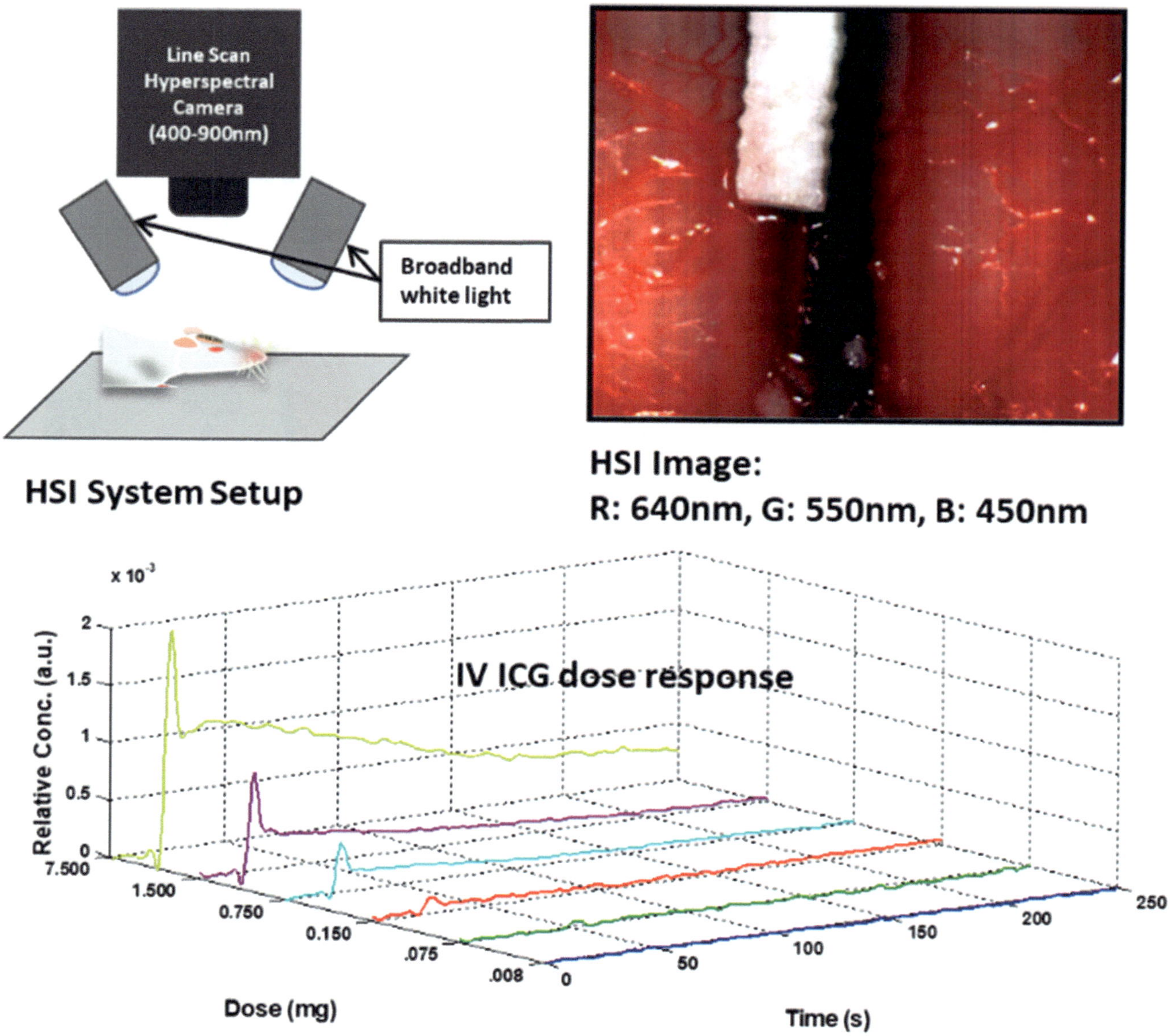

Fig. 19.10 HSI of rat brain showing ICG clearance data acquired every second in a small region of interest

- Tumor edge identification and tissue perfusion assessment [114]
- As a part of other optical devices such as SFDI [123]

Potential Arterial Drug Delivery Applications

- *Imaging drug and dye delivery by both by absorption and fluorescence measurements*: Figure 19.10 shows the clearance of IV indocyanine green after intravenous bolus injections. A line scan device could rapidly track the dye's bolus through the cerebral circulation by narrowing the region of interest.
- *Planar kinetics of drug delivery*: The ability to image drug and dye-tagged carrier delivery enables determining the regional kinetics of drugs in arteries, capillaries (tissues), and veins to build better computation models of regional drug delivery.
- Monitor the safety effects of arterial drugs by assessing tissue oxygenation and other spectral tissue injury changes.

Spatial Frequency Domain Imaging (SFDI)

Technique

SFDI permits real-time optical characterization of large tissue areas by assessing light transfer functions and determining wavelength-specific absorption and scattering using specific light illumination patterns (Fig. 19.11) [124]. Using sinusoidal illumination, large tissue areas

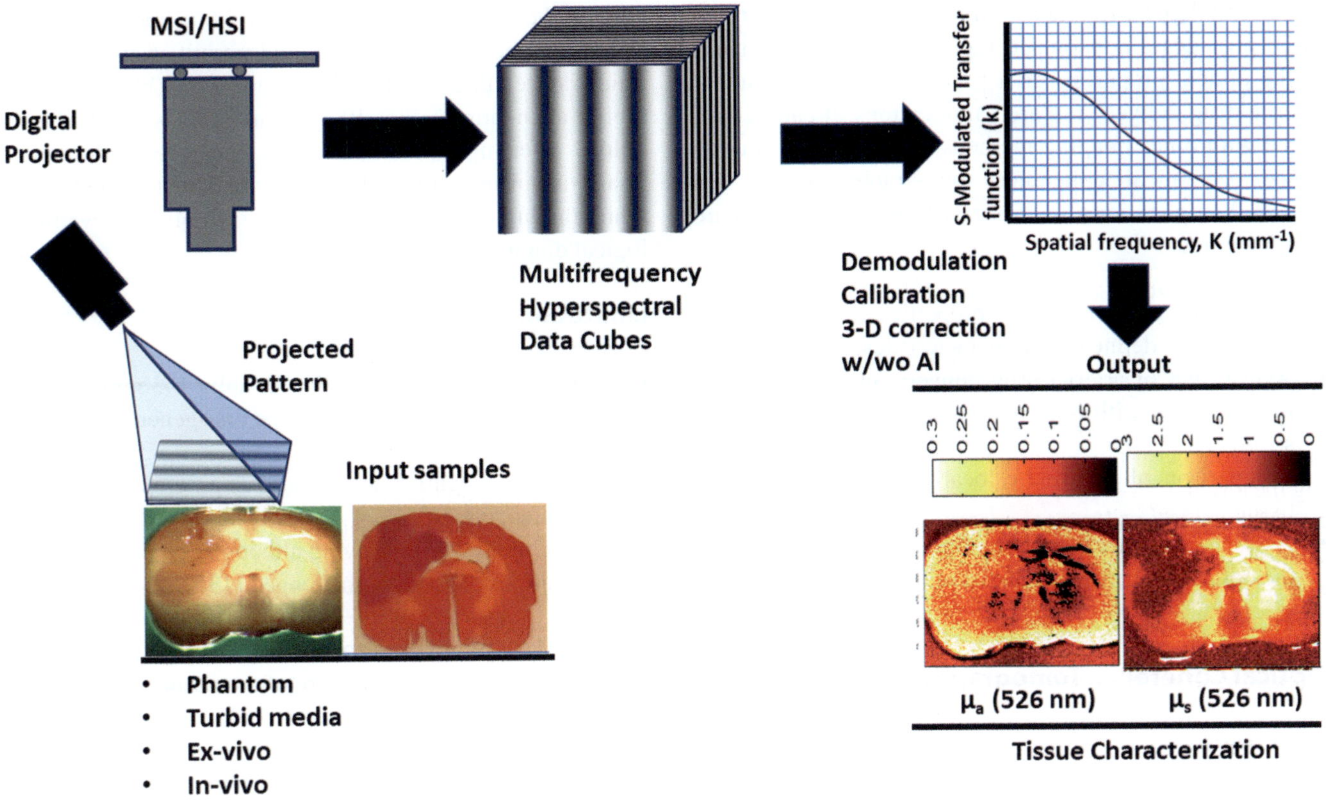

Fig. 19.11 Spatial frequency domain imaging method

several square centimeters across can be characterized in real time. Tissue characteristics such as oxygenation, drug and dye concentrations, pathological changes, and tumor margins can be determined without tissue contact. The SFDI method has evolved in the past decade. Recent advances involve improvements in three-dimensional (3-D) image correction and the use of artificial intelligence (AI) and machine learning to decrease the raw data requirement [125]. AI can reliably detect impaired tissue perfusion with snapshot imaging. Thus, SFDI imaging, combined with ICG fluorescence, now permits the characterization of large amounts of tissues, such as the intestines, during surgery [126]. Conversely, an ultra-miniature 3-mm SFDI system with dual-wavelength illumination that assesses chromophore, hemoglobin, and deoxyhemoglobin concentrations has been developed [127].

Limitation of SFDI for Arterial Drug Delivery

- Surgical exposure of tissues is needed.
- Unevenness of tissue surface can interfere with SFDI measurements.
- It is applicable to only certain drugs with suitable light absorbance characteristics.
- Most studies have hitherto focused on endogenous chromophores, and there needs to be more experience with drug or optically tagged carrier delivery [123].

Current Application of SFDI

SFDI enables real-time optical characterization of tissue properties covering areas several square centimeters. It is tissue noninvasive and can be undertaken remotely, avoiding contact with the target site. Effectively, SFDI enhances surgeons' color vision to enable them to assess tissue perfusion and oxygenation and aid tumor edge identification. SFDI's real-time ability to quantify light absorbance can enormously impact arterial drug delivery research. The applications of SFDI include:

- The quantification of chromophore concentration in real-time with SFDI can be used for:
  - Assessment of tissue perfusion and detection of ischemia [125, 128]
  - Assessment of the severity of burn injury [129]
  - Assessment of revascularization of graft [130]
  - Assessment of gut ischemia during surgery [126]
  - Assessment of cortical spreading depression [124]
  - Exceedingly dense time resolution of cerebral reperfusion after arrest [131]
  - Detection of and longitudinally follow the ischemic core in stroke models [132]
  - Tumor characterization and detection [124]
- In tissue phantoms, the remote SFDI measurements of chromophore concentrations correlate well with DRS measurements of tissue drug concentrations that correlate with diffuse reflectance spectroscopy [123].

Potential Applications for Arterial Drug Delivery

SFDI provides a noncontact, rapid assessment of changes in the optical properties on a tissue scale with significant arterial drug delivery research applications. It can be combined with other imaging methods, such as tissue fluorescence or optical coherence tomography (OCT). The potential applications to arterial drug delivery research could include:

- Characterization of baseline properties of tissue to assess perfusion or define tumor characteristics.
- Assessment of arterial drug delivery and regional pharmacokinetics with high temporal resolution on a tissue scale.
- Comparison of uptake by local pathology and healthy tissue.
- Assessment of treatment response based on changes in the optical properties of the tissue.

Optical Coherence Tomography

Technique

Optical coherence tomography is a form of interferometry that uses light interference between light returning from the interrogated tissue and that reflected by a mirror. Utilizing the interference pattern, OCT can create 3-D images of small volumes of tissues, typically with sampling depths of a few millimeters [133]. Such an imaging method has implications for small animal research. OCT technology was developed from techniques used to detect broken fiber-optic cables. It was first clinically applied to detect and investigate retinal disease. The original method, time-domain OCT, used a single wavelength of lasers. Since then, spectral OCT and swept spectral OCT have emerged (Fig. 19.12). The significant advances in the past decade using spectral OCT have decreased the scan time. This is important in fast-moving targets in the eye where movement artifacts degrade the images. One of the applications of the OCT is to track a bolus of saline or other contrast media and permit visualization of fluid transfer through the artery and veins (blood alone is highly attenuating) (Fig. 19.12). Innovations in OCT technology offer higher scan rates and image resolution. High image acquisition rates decrease movement-related noise, while the higher resolution could permit noninvasive histological diagnosis [134].

Limitation of OCT

- Surgical exposure of tissues.
- Limited depth of interrogation, usually 1–3 mm.
- Immobilization is needed with the first-generation devices using time-domain OCT.
- The clinical significance of deep angiography scans can be challenging [135].
- The technology is improving although certain OCT-based applications have been challenged [136].

Potential Applications for Arterial Drug Delivery

- Imaging the angioarchitecture of the tissue
- Determining optimum arterial bolus volume, such as saline bolus injection (Fig. 19.13)
- Pathology assessing and monitoring: rapid histological monitoring might be possible [137]

Photoacoustic Tomography

Technique

Photoacoustic tomography (PAT) or optoacoustic tomography is the cross-sectional or 3-D imaging of tissues using the photoacoustic phenomenon [138]. The photoacoustic phenomenon is the sound generation by absorbed light (Fig. 19.14). The availability of nanosecond pulsed lasers enables the safe and rapid heating of tissues (typically <0.01 °C), resulting in their expansion and subsequent generation of vibrations that an ultrasound array can detect

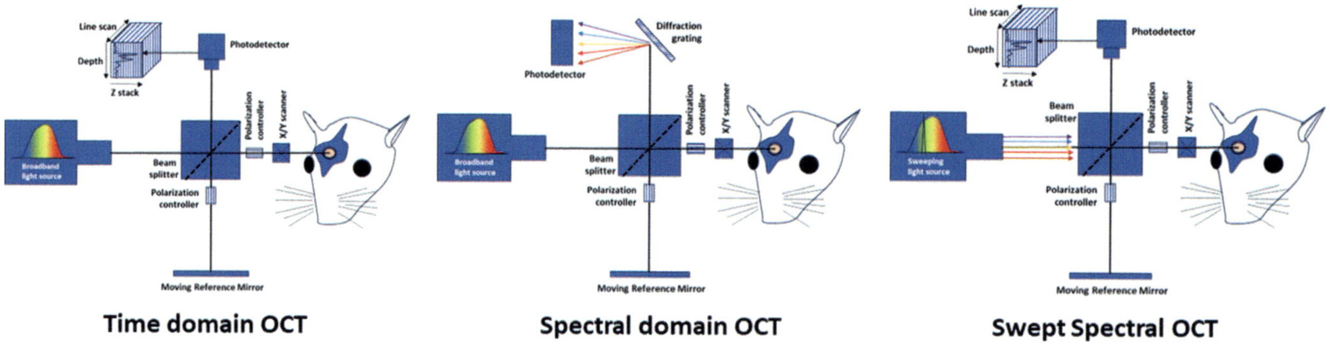

Fig. 19.12 A schematic representation of types of OCT

[139–141]. Depending on the wavelength of light, this method can image biological tissue to a depth of 3 cm. The images can provide anatomical, functional, and even cellular information. If used for functional imaging, the physiological changes and anatomical images are automatically overlaid as they both rely on receiving the ultrasound signals. Hitherto, most PAT research has been preclinical; however, human applications of PAT are rapidly advancing [142].

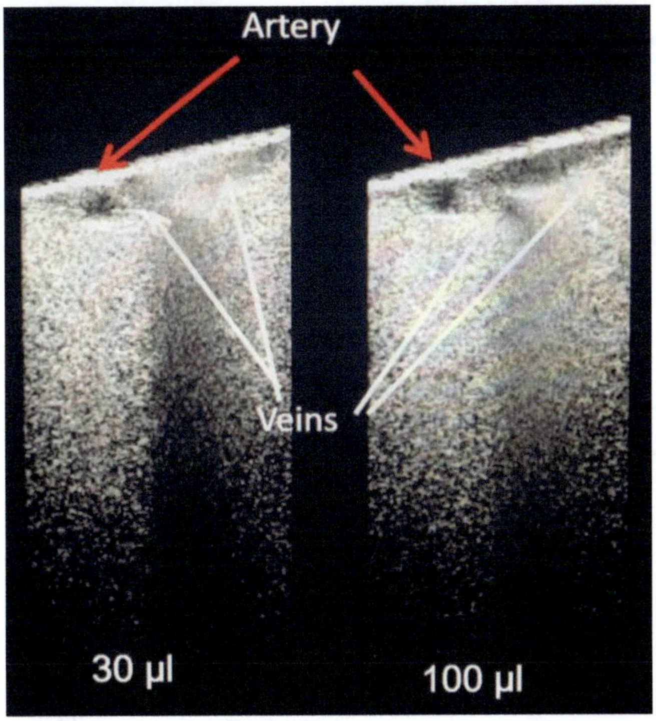

Fig. 19.13 Screenshot of OCT showing the effects of bolus volume on arterial drug delivery. A small bolus gradually transits through the capillary bed, while a large bolus rapidly flushes from the arterial to the venous side

Technological Concerns

We have yet to be aware of any application of PAT to arterial drug delivery research. However, this deep tissue imaging technology that generates anatomical data, such as vascular images, can track changes in fluorophore concentration at an extremely high rate (100–1000 Hz) and assess tissue perfusion, which could be invaluable to arterial drug delivery research. Although the field of PAT imaging is advancing rapidly, it will need the identification and testing of fluorophores, labeling of carriers, suitable lasers, and design of protocols based on instrument configuration for arterial delivery research. However, image reconstruction can be challenging, mainly when the tissues are heterogeneous and distant [143].

Limitations

PAT requires light absorption. The use of dyes restricts lasers in the visible and near-IR range. However, dyes are prone to photo-quenching and unsuitable for the 1000–1400 nm laser range. For such lasers, nanoparticles and nanorods are more suitable [144].

Potential Applications for Arterial Drug Delivery

PAT has many potential applications for arterial drug delivery research. These include:

- Imaging cerebral vasculature [145, 146]
- Imaging cerebral perfusion in health and disease [147, 148]
- Imaging brain tumors and chemotherapy response [148, 149]
- Imaging drug-carrier delivery labels with dyes and nanoparticles: Using ICG as the tracer, Taruttis et al. demonstrated the feasibility of cross-sectional imaging of multiple organs using a 64-detector array at 10 frames/s [150]. Data acquisition at such a frame rate is highly relevant to arterial drug delivery research.

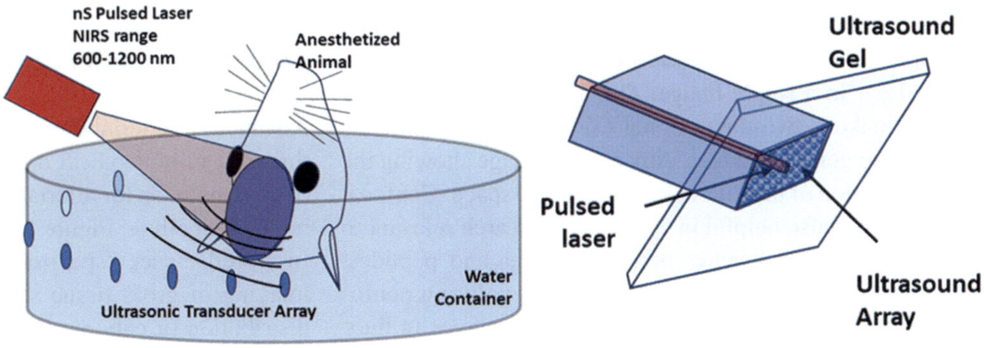

Fig. 19.14 Two approaches to PAT imaging: animals can be immersed in water (Left) to ensure conduction of ultrasonic waves. Right: Handheld compact ultrasonic transducer array with embedded laser delivery

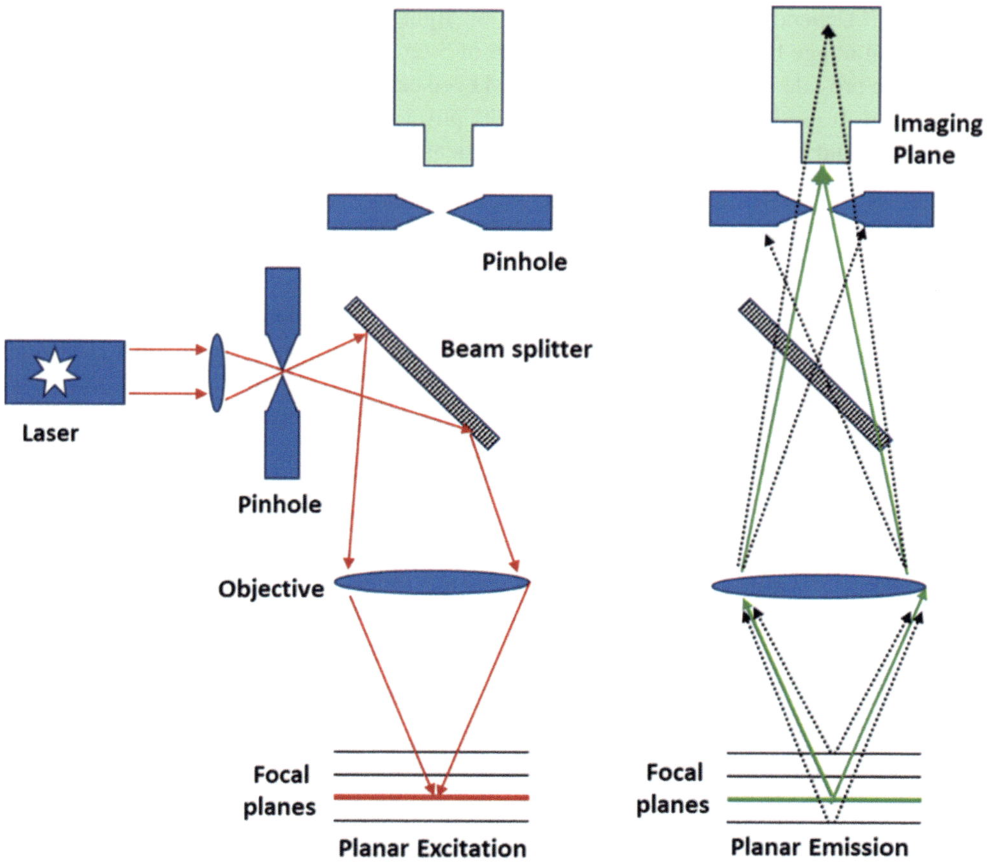

Fig. 19.15 Principle of confocal microscopy that uses pinholes to enable precise planar excitation and illumination

Confocal Microscopy

Confocal microscopy provides a compelling tool to assess arterial drug delivery in postmortem tissue samples. Delivery of naturally fluorescent drugs or peptides and nanoparticles that have been suitably labeled can be quantitatively determined at tissue and cell levels. Confocal microscopy is the forerunner of many advances in microscopic imaging methods that have emerged in the past two decades [151, 152]. The principle of confocal microscopy is to use pinhole images that capture light from a very narrow plane of excitation and emission (Fig. 19.15). Using fluorophore-specific excitation, the distribution of several fluorophores can be mapped out in a single image. The line scan image can be used to make a two-dimensional (*X*–*Y*) image that can be *z*-stacked to generate a three-dimensional image showing the precise location of the fluorophore in the 3-D space. Confocal microscopy is also helpful in cytological research relevant to the cellular uptake kinetics of nanoparticles and peptides. Quantitative measurement can be undertaken during confocal microscopy. They raise concerns about changes in fluorescence due to solubilizing, tissue uptake, pH effects, photobleaching, and quenching [153]. While some of these concerns can be addressed by comparing within tissue samples, such as tumor versus background uptake, their role in quantitative assessment should always be considered.

With low cost and versatile laser sources, extremely photon-sensitive cameras, powerful processors, and cheap memory storage. Laser-based microscopic methods have advanced immensely from postmortem imaging to in-vivo applications, in mainly two-photon microscopy that in rodent experiments can now probe depths of several hundred microns and detect both vascular and cellular changes over several weeks [154]. One can foresee the roles such technologies could play in advancing arterial drug delivery and monitoring the effects of such treatments.

Conclusions and Future Avenues

Advances in arterial drug delivery could benefit from breakthroughs in biomedical optics. The rationale for developing optical methods for arterial drug delivery research is exceedingly compelling. Figure 19.16 shows the application of diffuse reflectance spectroscopy (DRS) and postmortem imaging of gross tissue samples to track and map out the distribution of cationic liposomes using methods described in this chapter. The experiments required 1 h of animal preparation and another for drug delivery assessment. The analysis of data took another 30 min. Thus, 900 measurements and gross tissue analysis could be done in less than 3 h. Such experiments show how optics could permit rapid screening

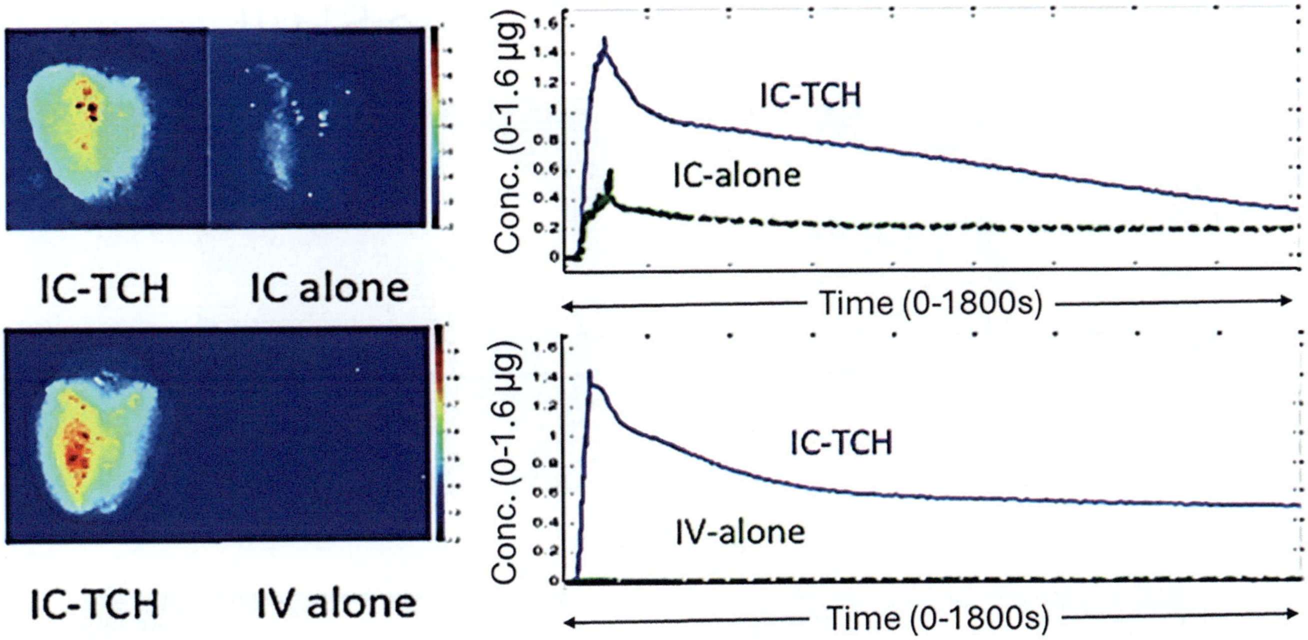

Fig. 19.16 The use of diffuse reflectance spectroscopy (DRS) and multispectral imaging (MSI) enables rapid assessment of carrier delivery to the brain tissue. Nine hundred measurements for each curve were completed in less than an hour. Conventional chemical or isotopic investigations into the arterial drugs kinetics will be challenging due to scientific, logistical, cost, safety, and manpower concerns

of arterial drug carriers and optimize drug delivery. No other imaging modality offers a sub-second assessment of tissue drug concentrations, which is tissue noninvasive, site-specific, or whole animal monitoring, poses no personal hazards, and is rapid and highly cost-effective. Nowhere is this more relevant than in the treatment of neurological diseases. Neurological diseases will continue to be a leading cause of morbidity and mortality in the foreseeable future. Timely and effective drug delivery will remain a major hurdle due to the restriction to drug delivery across the blood–brain barrier and the vulnerability of the brain to injury and the consequences thereof. Arterial drug delivery offers rapid, dependable, and effective access to treat focal neurological diseases. Current optical technologies have reached a point where dye-labeled compounds can be tracked in the whole bodies of small animals every second over several days. Translating these technologies to larger animals poses a significant challenge.

The next steps for better understanding the kinetics of arterial drug delivery include developing non-toxic dyes with higher quantum yields or far longer wavelengths that may permit the interrogation of deep tissues and research on larger animals. Methods such as photoacoustic imaging could permit noninvasive interrogation drug delivery through an intact skull. Through chronically implanted cranial windows, two-photon microscopy could track drug delivery at the cellular level in vivo. MRI could play a significant role in developing clinical applications of arterial drug delivery. MRI provides anatomical information, can assess blood flow and tissue oxygenation, and monitor tissue biochemical changes. It can guide catheters with ultrafast tracking, assess blood–brain barrier permeability, and enhance the safety of arterial injections. Iron oxide-loaded super-magnetic nanoparticles could be used to optimize arterial drug delivery. Hence, magnetic resonance (MR) technologies are bound to play a significant role in improving the safety and efficacy of arterial drug delivery in the path to clinical applications.

How could optical methods be used for arterial drug research in human subjects? Optical pharmacokinetic experiments could be done when the brain tissue is exposed during surgery. The second group of patients who could benefit from optical tissue interrogation are those with neurological injuries in whom the skull is removed, such as after a significant stroke, and in whom the brain tissue lies just beneath the skin to enable optical interrogation to monitor tissue viability of drug delivery. Finally, in the case of brain tumors, the skull could be replaced with a transparent cranial prosthesis (Fig. 19.17). The removal of the skull and its replacement with a transparent prosthesis can reduce light fluence, as shown in Fig. 19.16. Custom-printed acrylic skull prostheses are routinely used during neurosurgery. Skull phantoms have been used to test the performance of optical devices, but using skull implants could also enhance the clinical application of optical techniques [155]. If used after tumor resection, such prosthesis could help monitor tissue changes, function, and drug delivery. It is a humbling observation that most brain tumor recur-

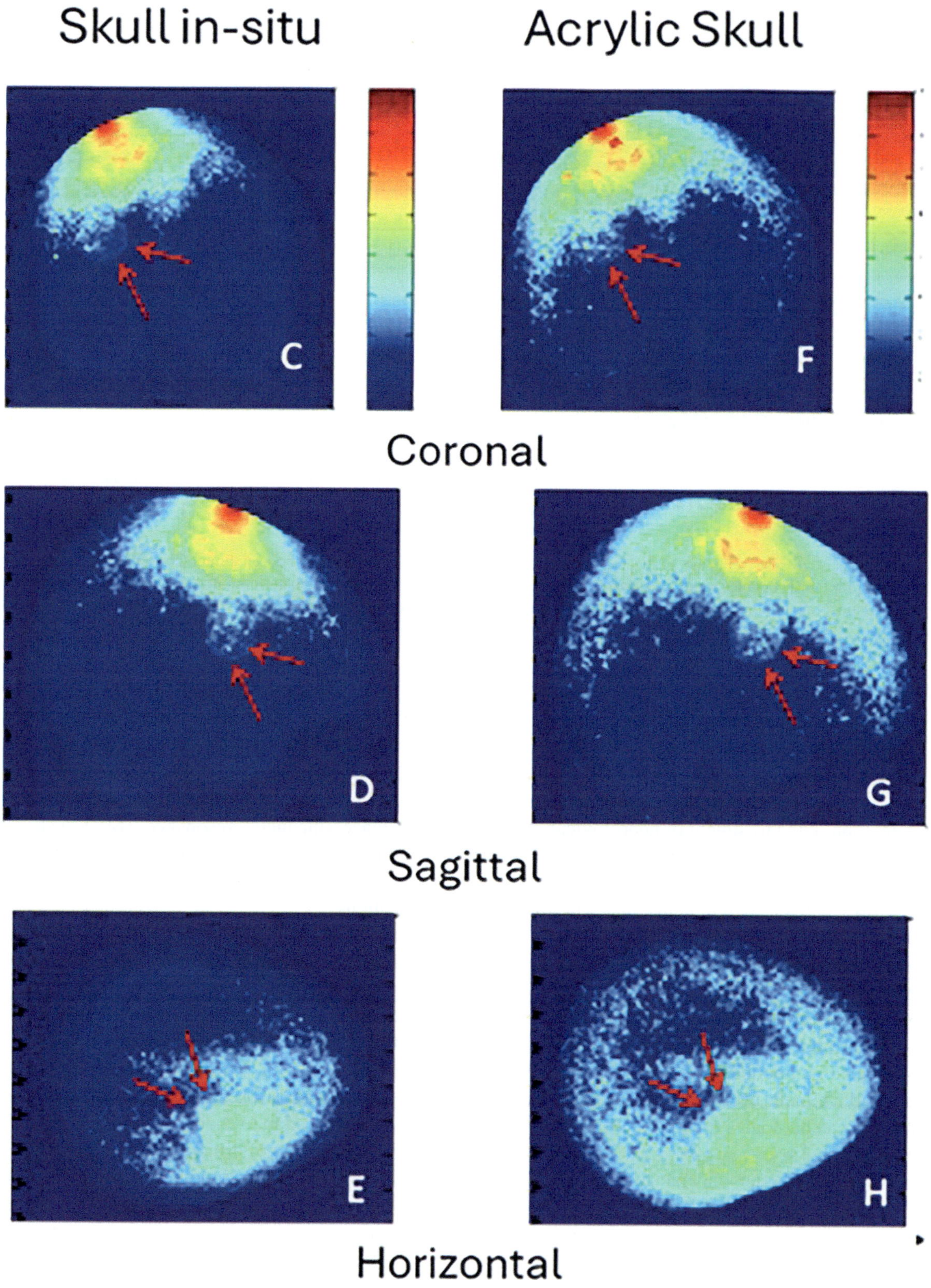

Fig. 19.17 Monte Carlo simulation of 780 nm light fluence (color bar) in brain tissue through an intact and an acrylic skull. An embedded tumor is shown with red arrows. Acrylic skull implants are clinically used and may permit long-term optical brain tissue monitoring after surgery (source: Rajinder Singh-Moon, PhD)

rences occur at the site of surgery. Thus, it is easy to foresee the profound impact optical technologies could play in the development of arterial drugs and their clinical applications.

References

1. Anonymous. In praise of Lord Kelvin. 2007 [updated 17 Dec 2007]. https://physicsworld.com/a/in-praise-of-lord-kelvin/.
2. Chen L, Liu J, Chu C, Han Z, Yadav N, Xu J, et al. Deuterium oxide as a contrast medium for real-time MRI-guided endovascular neurointervention. Theranostics. 2021;11(13):6240–50.
3. Chu C, Jablonska A, Gao Y, Lan X, Lesniak WG, Liang Y, et al. Hyperosmolar blood-brain barrier opening using intra-arterial injection of hyperosmotic mannitol in mice under real-time MRI guidance. Nat Protoc. 2022;17(1):76–94.
4. Chu C, Jablonska A, Lesniak WG, Thomas AM, Lan X, Linville RM, et al. Optimization of osmotic blood-brain barrier opening to enable intravital microscopy studies on drug delivery in mouse cortex. J Control Release. 2020;317:312–21.
5. Chu C, Liu G, Janowski M, Bulte JWM, Li S, Pearl M, et al. Real-time MRI guidance for reproducible hyperosmolar opening of the blood-brain barrier in mice. Front Neurol. 2018;9:921.
6. Janowski M, Walczak P, Pearl MS. Predicting and optimizing the territory of blood-brain barrier opening by superselective intra-arterial cerebral infusion under dynamic susceptibility contrast MRI guidance. J Cereb Blood Flow Metab. 2016;36(3):569–75.
7. Mitsuki S, Diksic M, Conway T, Yamamoto YL, Villemure JG, Feindel W. Pharmacokinetics of 11C-labelled BCNU and SarCNU in gliomas studied by PET. J Neurooncol. 1991;10(1):47–55.
8. Tyler JL, Yamamoto YL, Diksic M, Theron J, Villemure JG, Worthington C, et al. Pharmacokinetics of superselective intra-arterial and intravenous [11C]BCNU evaluated by PET. J Nucl Med. 1986;27(6):775–80.
9. Marcos-Contreras OA, Brenner JS, Kiseleva RY, Zuluaga-Ramirez V, Greineder CF, Villa CH, et al. Combining vascular targeting and the local first pass provides 100-fold higher uptake of ICAM-1-targeted vs untargeted nanocarriers in the inflamed brain. J Control Release. 2019;301:54–61.
10. Unger C, Eibl H, von Heyden HW, Kim DJ, Nagel GA. Aminoglutethimide. Penetration of the blood brain barrier. Investig New Drugs. 1986;4(3):237–40.
11. Van Uitert RL, Sage JI, Levy DE, Duffy TE. Comparison of radio-labeled butanol and iodoantipyrine as cerebral blood flow markers. Brain Res. 1981;222:365–72.
12. Winchell HS, Horst WD, Braun L, Oldendorf WH, Hattner R, Parker H. N-isopropyl-[123I] p-iodoamphetamine: single-pass brain uptake and washout; binding to brain synaptosomes; and localization in dog and monkey brain. J Nucl Med. 1980;21(10):947–52.
13. Unger C, Eibl H, Engel J, Nagel GA, Eisenbrand G. Brain uptake and CNS levels of 1-(2-chloroethyl)-1-nitroso-3-(2-hydroxyethyl) urea (HECNU). Investig New Drugs. 1987;5(4):361–4.
14. Hardebo JE, Nilsson B. Estimation of cerebral extraction of circulating compounds by the brain uptake index method: influence of circulation time, volume injection, and cerebral blood flow. Acta Physiol Scand. 1979;107(2):153–9.
15. Dedrick RL. Interspecies scaling of regional drug delivery. J Pharm Sci. 1986;75(11):1047–52.
16. Dedrick RL. Arterial drug infusion: pharmacokinetic problems and pitfalls. J Natl Cancer Inst. 1988;80(2):84–9.
17. Hammarlund-Udenaes M, Friden M, Syvanen S, Gupta A. On the rate and extent of drug delivery to the brain. Pharm Res. 2008;25(8):1737–50.
18. Ellis JA, Banu M, Hossain SS, Singh-Moon R, Lavine SD, Bruce JN, et al. Reassessing the role of intra-arterial drug delivery for glioblastoma multiforme treatment. J Drug Deliv. 2015;2015:405735.
19. Collins JM. Pharmacologic rationale for regional drug delivery. J Clin Oncol. 1984;2(5):498–504.
20. Pardridge WM. Drug transport across the blood-brain barrier. J Cereb Blood Flow Metab. 2012;32(11):1959–72.
21. Kovic B, Xie F. Economic evaluation of bevacizumab for the first-line treatment of newly diagnosed glioblastoma multiforme. J Clin Oncol. 2015;33(20):2296–302.
22. Riina HA, Burkhardt JK, Santillan A, Bassani L, Patsalides A, Boockvar JA. Short-term clinico-radiographic response to super-selective intra-arterial cerebral infusion of bevacizumab for the treatment of vestibular schwannomas in neurofibromatosis type 2. Interv Neuroradiol. 2012;18(2):127–32.
23. Bradbury MW, Patlak CS, Oldendorf WH. Analysis of brain uptake and loss or radiotracers after intracarotid injection. Am J Phys. 1975;229(4):1110–5.
24. Hassenbusch SJ, Anderson JH, Colvin OM. Predicted and actual BCNU concentrations in normal rabbit brain during intraarterial and intravenous infusions. J Neurooncol. 1996;30(1):7–18.
25. Hassenbusch SJ, Anderson JH, Whiting DM. Intra-arterial chemotherapy for brain tumors. Cleve Clin J Med. 1990;57(6):513–20.
26. Neuwelt EA, Barnett PA, Ramsey FL, Hellstrom I, Hellstrom KE, McCormick CI. Dexamethasone decreases the delivery of tumor-specific monoclonal antibody to both intracerebral and subcutaneous tumor xenografts. Neurosurgery. 1993;33(3):478–84; discussion 84.
27. Neuwelt EA, Diehl JT, Vu LH, Hill SA, Michael AJ, Frenkel EP. Monitoring of methotrexate delivery in patients with malignant brain tumors after osmotic blood-brain barrier disruption. Ann Intern Med. 1981;94(4 Pt 1):449–54.
28. Jones DR, Hall SD, Jackson EK, Branch RA, Wilkinson GR. Brain uptake of benzodiazepines: effects of lipophilicity and plasma protein binding. J Pharmacol Exp Ther. 1988;245(3):816–22.
29. Olesen J, Paulson OB, Lassen NA. Regional cerebral blood flow in man determined by the initial slope of the clearance of intra-arterially injected ^{133}Xe: theory of the method, normal values, error of measurement, correction for remaining radioactivity, relation to other flow parameters and response to $PaCO_2$ changes. Stroke. 1971;2:519–40.
30. Young WL, Prohovnik I, Schroeder T, Correll JW, Ostapkovich N. Intraoperative ^{133}Xe cerebral blood flow measurements by intravenous *versus* intracarotid methods. Anesthesiology. 1990;73:637–43.
31. Ding H, Wu F. Image guided biodistribution and pharmacokinetic studies of theranostics. Theranostics. 2012;2(11):1040–53.
32. Joshi S, Wang M, Etu J, Nishanian EV. Comparison of intracarotid anesthetics for EEG silence. J Neurosurg Anesthesiol. 2006;18(2):112–8.
33. Joshi S, Wang M, Etu JJ, Nishanian EV, Pile-Spellman J. Cerebral blood flow affects dose requirements of intracarotid propofol for electrocerebral silence. Anesthesiology. 2006;104(2):290–8; discussion 5A.
34. Joshi S, Wang M, Etu JJ, Pile-Spellman J. Bolus configuration affects dose requirements of intracarotid propofol for electroencephalographic silence. Anesth Analg. 2006;102(6):1816–22.
35. Wang M, Joshi S, Emerson RG. Comparison of intracarotid and intravenous propofol for electrocerebral silence in rabbits. Anesthesiology. 2003;99(4):904–10.
36. Bigio IJ, Mourant JR, Los G. Noninvasive, in-situ measurement of drug concentrations in tissue using optical spectroscopy. J Gravit Physiol. 1999;6(1):P173–5.
37. Mourant JR, Bigio IJ, Jack DA, Johnson TM, Miller HD. Measuring absorption coefficients in small volumes of highly scattering media: source-detector separations for which path lengths do not depend on scattering properties. Appl Opt. 1997;36(22):5655–61.

38. Mourant JR, Fuselier T, Boyer J, Johnson TM, Bigio IJ. Predictions and measurements of scattering and absorption over broad wavelength ranges in tissue phantoms. Appl Opt. 1997;36(4):949–57.
39. Escobedo JO, Rusin O, Lim S, Strongin RM. NIR dyes for bioimaging applications. Curr Opin Chem Biol. 2010;14(1):64–70.
40. Cooke JN, Ellis JA, Hossain S, Nguyen J, Bruce JN, Joshi S. Computational pharmacokinetic rationale for intra-arterial delivery to the brain. Drug Deliv Transl Res. 2016;6:622.
41. Thomas DL, Lythgoe MF, van der Weerd L, Ordidge RJ, Gadian DG. Regional variation of cerebral blood flow and arterial transit time in the normal and hypoperfused rat brain measured using continuous arterial spin labeling MRI. J Cereb Blood Flow Metab. 2006;26(2):274–82.
42. Blacklock JB, Wright DC, Dedrick RL, Blasberg RG, Lutz RJ, Doppman JL, et al. Drug streaming during intra-arterial chemotherapy. J Neurosurg. 1986;64:284–91.
43. Lutz RJ, Dedrick RL, Boretos JW, Oldfield EH, Blacklock JB, Doppman JL. Mixing studies during intracarotid artery infusions in an in vitro model. J Neurosurg. 1986;64(2):277–83.
44. Saris SC, Blasberg RG, Carson RE, deVroom HL, Lutz R, Dedrick RL, et al. Intravascular streaming during carotid artery infusions. Demonstration in humans and reduction using diastole-phased pulsatile administration. J Neurosurg. 1991;74(5):763–72.
45. Dagenais C, Rousselle C, Pollack GM, Scherrmann JM. Development of an in situ mouse brain perfusion model and its application to mdr1a P-glycoprotein-deficient mice. J Cereb Blood Flow Metab. 2000;20(2):381–6.
46. Hassenbusch SJ, Colvin OM, Anderson JH. Determination of nitrosourea compounds in brain tissue by gas chromatography and electron capture detection. J Pharm Sci. 1995;84(7):840–2.
47. Iqbal S. A comprehensive study of the anatomical variations of the circle of Willis in adult human brains. J Clin Diagn Res. 2013;7(11):2423–7.
48. Jones JD, Castanho P, Bazira P, Sanders K. Anatomical variations of the circle of Willis and their prevalence, with a focus on the posterior communicating artery: a literature review and meta-analysis. Clin Anat. 2021;34(7):978–90.
49. Lee JS, Hamilton MG, Zabramski JM. Variations in the anatomy of the rabbit cervical carotid artery. Stroke. 1994;25(2):501–3.
50. Oliff HS, Coyle P, Weber E. Rat strain and vendor differences in collateral anastomoses. J Cereb Blood Flow Metab. 1997;17(5):571–6.
51. Joshi S, Wang M, Hartl R. Retinal discoloration test. J Cereb Blood Flow Metab. 2004;24(3):305–8.
52. Joshi S, Wang M, Etu JJ, Suckow RF, Cooper TB, Feinmark SJ, et al. Transient cerebral hypoperfusion enhances intraarterial carmustine deposition into brain tissue. J Neurooncol. 2008;86(2):123–32.
53. Ding PT, Xu H, Zheng JM. Application of microdialysis in pharmacokinetic and drug metabolism studies. Yao Xue Xue Bao. 2002;37(4):316–20.
54. Elmquist WF, Sawchuk RJ. Application of microdialysis in pharmacokinetic studies. Pharm Res. 1997;14(3):267–88.
55. Wu Z, Wang D. Application of sites-microdialysis technology in pharmacokinetic studies. Zhongguo Zhong Yao Za Zhi. 2010;35(13):1765–8.
56. Cloughesy TF, Gobin YP, Black KL, Vinuela F, Taft F, Kadkhoda B, et al. Intra-arterial carboplatin chemotherapy for brain tumors: a dose escalation study based on cerebral blood flow. J Neurooncol. 1997;35(2):121–31.
57. Gobin YP, Cloughesy TF, Chow KL, Duckwiler GR, Sayre JW, Milanese K, et al. Intraarterial chemotherapy for brain tumors by using a spatial dose fractionation algorithm and pulsatile delivery. Radiology. 2001;218(3):724–32.
58. Gobin YP, Dunkel IJ, Marr BP, Brodie SE, Abramson DH. Intra-arterial chemotherapy for the management of retinoblastoma: four-year experience. Arch Ophthalmol. 2011;129(6):732–7.
59. Morikawa N, Mori T, Abe T, Kawashima H, Takeyama M, Hori S. Pharmacokinetics of cytosine arabinoside, methotrexate, nimustine and valproic acid in cerebrospinal fluid during cerebrospinal fluid perfusion chemotherapy. Biol Pharm Bull. 2000;23(6):784–7.
60. Morikawa N, Mori T, Kawashima H, Takeyama M, Abe T, Kobayashi H. Pharmacokinetics of nimustine, cytosine arabinoside, and methotrexate in cerebrospinal fluid during cerebrospinal fluid perfusion chemotherapy. Biol Pharm Bull. 2001;24(4):436–8.
61. Morikawa N, Mori T, Kawashima H, Takeyama M, Hori S. Methotrexate concentration in cerebrospinal fluid of the space created by tumor removal. Biol Pharm Bull. 2000;23(6):774–7.
62. Zylber-Katz E, Gomori JM, Schwartz A, Lossos A, Bokstein F, Siegal T. Pharmacokinetics of methotrexate in cerebrospinal fluid and serum after osmotic blood-brain barrier disruption in patients with brain lymphoma. Clin Pharmacol Ther. 2000;67(6):631–41.
63. Fischer H, Gottschlich R, Seelig A. Blood-brain barrier permeation: molecular parameters governing passive diffusion. J Membr Biol. 1998;165(3):201–11.
64. Lanevskij K, Japertas P, Didziapetris R, Petrauskas A. Ionization-specific prediction of blood-brain permeability. J Pharm Sci. 2009;98(1):122–34.
65. Aichler M, Walch A. MALDI imaging mass spectrometry: current frontiers and perspectives in pathology research and practice. Lab Investig. 2015;95(4):422–31.
66. Roosendaal J, Rosing H, Beijnen JH. Combining isotopic tracer techniques to increase efficiency of clinical pharmacokinetic trials in oncology. Drugs R D. 2020;20(2):147–54.
67. Charles AK, Chang YF, Myslinski NR. Blood-brain barrier transport of L-pipecolic acid in various rat brain regions. Neurochem Res. 1983;8(9):1087–96.
68. Shin WW, Fong WF, Pang SF, Wong PC. Limited blood-brain barrier transport of polyamines. J Neurochem. 1985;44(4):1056–9.
69. Saris SC, Wright DC, Oldfield EH, Blasberg RG. Intravascular streaming and variable delivery to brain following carotid artery infusions in the Sprague-Dawley rat. J Cereb Blood Flow Metab. 1988;8(1):116–20.
70. Agid R, Rubinstein R, Siegal T, Lester H, Bokstein F, Chisin R, et al. Does streaming affect the cerebral distribution of infraophthalmic intracarotid chemotherapy? AJNR Am J Neuroradiol. 2002;23(10):1732–5.
71. Mainprize T, Lipsman N, Huang Y, Meng Y, Bethune A, Ironside S, et al. Blood-brain barrier opening in primary brain tumors with non-invasive MR-guided focused ultrasound: a clinical safety and feasibility study. Sci Rep. 2019;9(1):321.
72. Park SH, Kim MJ, Jung HH, Chang WS, Choi HS, Rachmilevitch I, et al. Safety and feasibility of multiple blood-brain barrier disruptions for the treatment of glioblastoma in patients undergoing standard adjuvant chemotherapy. J Neurosurg. 2020;134(2):475–83.
73. Zawadzki M, Walecki J, Kostkiewicz B, Kostyra K, Pearl MS, Solaiyappan M, et al. Real-time MRI guidance for intra-arterial drug delivery in a patient with a brain tumor: technical note. BMJ Case Rep. 2019;12(1):e014469.
74. Neubauer AM, Sim H, Winter PM, Caruthers SD, Williams TA, Robertson JD, et al. Nanoparticle pharmacokinetic profiling in vivo using magnetic resonance imaging. Magn Reson Med. 2008;60(6):1353–61.
75. Nance E, Timbie K, Miller GW, Song J, Louttit C, Klibanov AL, et al. Non-invasive delivery of stealth, brain-penetrating nanoparticles across the blood-brain barrier using MRI-guided focused ultrasound. J Control Release. 2014;189:123–32.
76. Shen WB, Anastasiadis P, Nguyen B, Yarnell D, Yarowsky PJ, Frenkel V, et al. Magnetic enhancement of stem cell-targeted delivery into the brain following MR-guided focused ultrasound for opening the blood-brain barrier. Cell Transplant. 2017;26(7):1235–46.
77. Tomitaka A, Arami H, Raymond A, Yndart A, Kaushik A, Jayant RD, et al. Development of magneto-plasmonic nanoparticles

for multimodal image-guided therapy to the brain. Nanoscale. 2017;9(2):764–73.

78. Jasmin, de Souza GT, Louzada RA, Rosado-de-Castro PH, Mendez-Otero R, Campos de Carvalho AC. Tracking stem cells with superparamagnetic iron oxide nanoparticles: perspectives and considerations. Int J Nanomedicine. 2017;12:779–93.
79. Watanabe M, Yavagal DR. Intra-arterial delivery of mesenchymal stem cells. Brain Circ. 2016;2(3):114–7.
80. Yamaguchi S, Yoshida M, Horie N, Satoh K, Fukuda Y, Ishizaka S, et al. Stem cell therapy for acute/subacute ischemic stroke with a focus on intraarterial stem cell transplantation: from basic research to clinical trials. Bioengineering (Basel). 2022;10(1):33.
81. Chen SR, Chen MM, Ene C, Lang FF, Kan P. Perfusion-guided endovascular super-selective intra-arterial infusion for treatment of malignant brain tumors. J Neurointerv Surg. 2022;14(6):533–8.
82. Shichinohe H, Kawabori M, Iijima H, Teramoto T, Abumiya T, Nakayama N, et al. Research on advanced intervention using novel bone marrOW stem cell (RAINBOW): a study protocol for a phase I, open-label, uncontrolled, dose-response trial of autologous bone marrow stromal cell transplantation in patients with acute ischemic stroke. BMC Neurol. 2017;17(1):179.
83. Fu L, Ke HT. Nanomaterials incorporated ultrasound contrast agents for cancer theranostics. Cancer Biol Med. 2016;13(3):313–24.
84. Wang M, Joshi S. Electrocerebral silence after intracarotid propofol injection is a function of transit time. Anesth Analg. 2007;104(6):1498–503, table of contents.
85. Levasseur JE, Wei EP, Raper AJ, Kontos HA, Patterson JL. Detailed description of a cranial window technique for acute and chronic experiments. Stroke. 1975;6(3):308–17.
86. Cramer SW, Carter RE, Aronson JD, Kodandaramaiah SB, Ebner TJ, Chen CC. Through the looking glass: a review of cranial window technology for optical access to the brain. J Neurosci Methods. 2021;354:109100.
87. Liu P, Mu X, Zhang XD, Ming D. The near-infrared-II fluorophores and advanced microscopy technologies development and application in bioimaging. Bioconjug Chem. 2020;31(2):260–75.
88. Dobosz M, Strobel S, Stubenrauch KG, Osl F, Scheuer W. Noninvasive measurement of pharmacokinetics by near-infrared fluorescence imaging in the eye of mice. J Biomed Opt. 2014;19(1):16022.
89. Joshi S, Singh-Moon R, Wang M, Chaudhuri DB, Ellis JA, Bruce JN, et al. Cationic surface charge enhances early regional deposition of liposomes after intracarotid injection. J Neurooncol. 2014;120(3):489–97.
90. Joshi S, Cooke JR, Chan DK, Ellis JA, Hossain SS, Singh-Moon RP, et al. Liposome size and charge optimization for intraarterial delivery to gliomas. Drug Deliv Transl Res. 2016;6(3):225–33.
91. Joshi S, Cooke JRN, Ellis JA, Emala CW, Bruce JN. Targeting brain tumors by intra-arterial delivery of cell-penetrating peptides: a novel approach for primary and metastatic brain malignancy. J Neurooncol. 2017;135(3):497–506.
92. Ding F, Zhan Y, Lu X, Sun Y. Recent advances in near-infrared II fluorophores for multifunctional biomedical imaging. Chem Sci. 2018;9(19):4370–80.
93. Briers JD. Laser Doppler, speckle and related techniques for blood perfusion mapping and imaging. Physiol Meas. 2001;22(4):R35–66.
94. Stern MD, Lappe DL, Bowen PD, Chimosky JE, Holloway GA, Keiser HR, et al. Continuous measurement of tissue blood flow by laser-Doppler spectroscopy. Am J Phys Heart Circ Phys. 1977;232(4):H441–8.
95. Joshi S, Reif R, Wang M, Zhang J, Ergin A, Bruce JN, et al. Intra-arterial mitoxantrone delivery in rabbits: an optical pharmacokinetic study. Neurosurgery. 2011;69(3):706–12; discussion 12.
96. Joshi S, Ergin A, Wang M, Reif R, Zhang J, Bruce JN, et al. Inconsistent blood brain barrier disruption by intraarterial mannitol in rabbits: implications for chemotherapy. J Neurooncol. 2011;104:11.
97. Ergin A, Joshi S, Wang M, Bigio I, editors. Retention of indocyanine green as a potential marker for optical detection of blood brain barrier disruption. SPIE; 2011.
98. Ergin A, Wang M, Zhang J, Bigio I, Joshi S. Noninvasive in vivo optical assessment of blood brain barrier permeability and brain tissue drug deposition in rabbits. J Biomed Opt. 2012;17(5):057008.
99. Ergin A, Wang M, Zhang JY, Bruce JN, Fine RL, Bigio IJ, et al. The feasibility of real-time in vivo optical detection of blood-brain barrier disruption with indocyanine green. J Neurooncol. 2012;106(3):551–60.
100. Reif R, Wang M, Joshi S, A'Amar O, Bigio IJ. Optical method for real-time monitoring of drug concentrations facilitates the development of novel methods for drug delivery to brain tissue. J Biomed Opt. 2007;12(3):034036.
101. Dogra S, Awasthi P, Nair M, Barthwal R. Interaction of anticancer drug mitoxantrone with DNA hexamer sequence d-(CTCGAG)2 by absorption, fluorescence and circular dichroism spectroscopy. J Photochem Photobiol B. 2013;123:48–54.
102. Joshi S, Singh-Moon RP, Wang M, Chaudhuri DB, Holcomb M, Straubinger NL, et al. Transient cerebral hypoperfusion assisted intraarterial cationic liposome delivery to brain tissue. J Neurooncol. 2014;118(1):73–82.
103. Nguyen J, Cooke JR, Ellis JA, Deci M, Emala CW, Bruce JN, et al. Cationizable lipid micelles as vehicles for intraarterial glioma treatment. J Neurooncol. 2016;128(1):21–8.
104. Bouchard MB, Chen BR, Burgess SA, Hillman EM. Ultra-fast multispectral optical imaging of cortical oxygenation, blood flow, and intracellular calcium dynamics. Opt Express. 2009;17(18):15670–8.
105. Sun R, Bouchard M, Burgess S, Radosevich A, Hillman EMC, editors. A low-cost, portable system for high-speed multispectral optical imaging. Optical Society of America/BIOMED/DH; 2010.
106. Hillman EM. Optical brain imaging in vivo: techniques and applications from animal to man. J Biomed Opt. 2007;12(5):051402.
107. Etrych T, Janouskova O, Chytil P. Fluorescence imaging as a tool in preclinical evaluation of polymer-based nano-DDS systems intended for cancer treatment. Pharmaceutics. 2019;11(9):471.
108. Motlagh NS, Parvin P, Ghasemi F, Atyabi F. Fluorescence properties of several chemotherapy drugs: doxorubicin, paclitaxel and bleomycin. Biomed Opt Express. 2016;7(6):2400–6.
109. Anonymous. Quenching of fluorescence. In: Lakowicz JR, editor. Principles of fluorescence spectroscopy. Boston, MA: Springer; 2006. p. 277–330.
110. Kilic K, Desjardins M, Tang J, Thunemann M, Sunil S, Erdener SE, et al. Chronic cranial windows for long term multimodal neurovascular imaging in mice. Front Physiol. 2020;11:612678.
111. Vasquez KO, Casavant C, Peterson JD. Quantitative whole body biodistribution of fluorescent-labeled agents by non-invasive tomographic imaging. PLoS One. 2011;6(6):e20594.
112. Nguyen J, Hossain SS, Cooke JRN, Ellis JA, Deci MB, Emala CW, et al. Flow arrest intra-arterial delivery of small TAT-decorated and neutral micelles to gliomas. J Neurooncol. 2017;133:77.
113. Karim S, Qadir A, Farooq U, Shakir M, Laghari AA. Hyperspectral imaging: a review and trends towards medical imaging. Curr Med Imaging. 2022;19(5):417–27.
114. Wu Y, Xu Z, Yang W, Ning Z, Dong H. Review on the application of hyperspectral imaging technology of the exposed cortex in cerebral surgery. Front Bioeng Biotechnol. 2022;10:906728.
115. Zhang Y, Wu X, He L, Meng C, Du S, Bao J, et al. Applications of hyperspectral imaging in the detection and diagnosis of solid tumors. Transl Cancer Res. 2020;9(2):1265–77.
116. Lemmens S, Van Eijgen J, Van Keer K, Jacob J, Moylett S, De Groef L, et al. Hyperspectral imaging and the retina: worth the wave? Transl Vis Sci Technol. 2020;9(9):9.
117. Hadoux X, Hui F, Lim JKH, Masters CL, Pebay A, Chevalier S, et al. Non-invasive in vivo hyperspectral imaging of the retina for potential biomarker use in Alzheimer's disease. Nat Commun. 2019;10(1):4227.

118. Thiem DGE, Hans L, Blatt S, Romer P, Heimes D, Al-Nawas B, et al. Hyperspectral imaging to study dynamic skin perfusion after injection of articaine-4% with and without epinephrine-clinical implications on local vasoconstriction. J Clin Med. 2021;10(15):3411.
119. Kleiss SF, Ma KF, El Moumni M, Unlu C, Nijboer TS, Schuurmann RCL, et al. Detecting changes in tissue perfusion with hyperspectral imaging and thermal imaging following endovascular treatment for peripheral arterial disease. J Endovasc Ther. 2023;30(3):382–92.
120. Dietrich M, Ozdemir B, Gruneberg D, Petersen C, Studier-Fischer A, von der Forst M, et al. Hyperspectral imaging for the evaluation of microcirculatory tissue oxygenation and perfusion quality in haemorrhagic shock: a porcine study. Biomedicines. 2021;9(12):1829.
121. Al Ktash M, Stefanakis M, Boldrini B, Ostertag E, Brecht M. Characterization of pharmaceutical tablets using UV hyperspectral imaging as a rapid in-line analysis tool. Sensors (Basel). 2021;21(13):4436.
122. Giannoni L, Lange F, Tachtsidis I. Hyperspectral imaging solutions for brain tissue metabolic and hemodynamic monitoring: past, current and future developments. J Opt. 2018;20(4):044009.
123. Singh-Moon RP, Roblyer DM, Bigio IJ, Joshi S. Spatial mapping of drug delivery to brain tissue using hyperspectral spatial frequency-domain imaging. J Biomed Opt. 2014;19(9):96003.
124. Gioux S, Mazhar A, Cuccia DJ. Spatial frequency domain imaging in 2019: principles, applications, and perspectives. J Biomed Opt. 2019;24(7):1–18.
125. Chen MT, Durr NJ. Rapid tissue oxygenation mapping from snapshot structured-light images with adversarial deep learning. J Biomed Opt. 2020;25(11):112907.
126. Ségaud S, Baratelli L, Felli E, Bannone E, Cinelli L, Rita Rodríguez-Luna M, et al. Trident: a dual oxygenation and fluorescence imaging platform for real-time and quantitative surgical guidance. Front Photonics. 2022;3:1032776.
127. Crowley J, Gordon GSD. Ultra-miniature dual-wavelength spatial frequency domain imaging for micro-endoscopy. J Biomed Opt. 2024;29(2):026002.
128. Murphy GA, Singh-Moon RP, Mazhar A, Cuccia DJ, Rowe VL, Armstrong DG. Quantifying dermal microcirculatory changes of neuropathic and neuroischemic diabetic foot ulcers using spatial frequency domain imaging: a shade of things to come? BMJ Open Diabetes Res Care. 2020;8(2):e001815.
129. Ponticorvo A, Rowland R, Baldado M, Burmeister DM, Christy RJ, Bernal NP, et al. Evaluating clinical observation versus spatial frequency domain imaging (SFDI), laser speckle imaging (LSI) and thermal imaging for the assessment of burn depth. Burns. 2019;45(2):450–60.
130. Ren J, Ramirez GA, Proctor AR, Wu TT, Benoit DSW, Choe R. Spatial frequency domain imaging for the longitudinal monitoring of vascularization during mouse femoral graft healing. Biomed Opt Express. 2020;11(10):5442–55.
131. Wilson RH, Crouzet C, Torabzadeh M, Bazrafkan A, Farahabadi MH, Jamasian B, et al. High-speed spatial frequency domain imaging of rat cortex detects dynamic optical and physiological properties following cardiac arrest and resuscitation. Neurophotonics. 2017;4(4):045008.
132. Sunil S, Evren Erdener S, Cheng X, Kura S, Tang J, Jiang J, et al. Stroke core revealed by tissue scattering using spatial frequency domain imaging. Neuroimage Clin. 2021;29:102539.
133. Gabriele ML, Wollstein G, Ishikawa H, Kagemann L, Xu J, Folio LS, et al. Optical coherence tomography: history, current status, and laboratory work. Invest Ophthalmol Vis Sci. 2011;52(5):2425–36.
134. Bouma BE, de Boer JF, Huang D, Jang IK, Yonetsu T, Leggett CL, et al. Optical coherence tomography. Nat Rev Methods Primers. 2022;2:79.
135. Herbort CP Jr, Papasavvas I, Tugal-Tutkun I. Benefits and limitations of OCT-A in the diagnosis and follow-up of posterior intraocular inflammation in current clinical practice: a valuable tool or a deceiver? Diagnostics (Basel). 2022;12(10):2384.
136. Brezinski ME. Capabilities, limitations, and misconceptions of using OCT to assess vulnerable plaques. Nat Rev Cardiol. 2014;11(11):638.
137. Jung W, Boppart SA. Optical coherence tomography for rapid tissue screening and directed histological sectioning. Stud Health Technol Inform. 2013;185:109–28.
138. Gu Y, Sun Y, Wang X, Li H, Qiu J, Lu W. Application of photoacoustic computed tomography in biomedical imaging: a literature review. Bioeng Transl Med. 2023;8(2):e10419.
139. Beard P. Biomedical photoacoustic imaging. Interface Focus. 2011;1(4):602–31.
140. Xia J, Yao J, Wang LV. Photoacoustic tomography: principles and advances. Electromagn Waves (Camb). 2014;147:1–22.
141. Yang J, Choi S, Kim C. Practical review on photoacoustic computed tomography using curved ultrasound array transducer. Biomed Eng Lett. 2022;12(1):19–35.
142. Khan S, Vasudevan S. Biomedical instrumentation of photoacoustic imaging and quantitative sensing for clinical applications. Rev Sci Instrum. 2023;94(9):091502.
143. Choi W, Oh D, Kim C. Practical photoacoustic tomography: realistic limitations and technical solutions. J Appl Phys. 2020;127(23):230903.
144. Chen YS, Zhao Y, Yoon SJ, Gambhir SS, Emelianov S. Miniature gold nanorods for photoacoustic molecular imaging in the second near-infrared optical window. Nat Nanotechnol. 2019;14(5):465–72.
145. Novoselova MV, Abakumova TO, Khlebtsov BN, Zatsepin TS, Lazareva EN, Tuchin VV, et al. Optical clearing for photoacoustic lympho- and angiography beyond conventional depth limit in vivo. Photoacoustics. 2020;20:100186.
146. Wang X, Ku G, Wegiel MA, Bornhop DJ, Stoica G, Wang LV. Noninvasive photoacoustic angiography of animal brains in vivo with near-infrared light and an optical contrast agent. Opt Lett. 2004;29(7):730–2.
147. Menozzi L, Yang W, Feng W, Yao J. Sound out the impaired perfusion: photoacoustic imaging in preclinical ischemic stroke. Front Neurosci. 2022;16:1055552.
148. Qiu T, Lan Y, Gao W, Zhou M, Liu S, Huang W, et al. Photoacoustic imaging as a highly efficient and precise imaging strategy for the evaluation of brain diseases. Quant Imaging Med Surg. 2021;11(5):2169–86.
149. Wang D, Wu Y, Xia J. Review on photoacoustic imaging of the brain using nanoprobes. Neurophotonics. 2016;3(1):010901.
150. Taruttis A, Morscher S, Burton NC, Razansky D, Ntziachristos V. Fast multispectral optoacoustic tomography (MSOT) for dynamic imaging of pharmacokinetics and biodistribution in multiple organs. PLoS One. 2012;7(1):e30491.
151. Elliott AD. Confocal microscopy: principles and modern practices. Curr Protoc Cytom. 2020;92(1):e68.
152. Paddock SW. Principles and practices of laser scanning confocal microscopy. Mol Biotechnol. 2000;16(2):127–49.
153. Simonsen JB, Kromann EB. Pitfalls and opportunities in quantitative fluorescence-based nanomedicine studies—a commentary. J Control Release. 2021;335:660–7.
154. Yang Q, Vazquez AL, Cui XT. Long-term in vivo two-photon imaging of the neuroinflammatory response to intracortical implants and micro-vessel disruptions in awake mice. Biomaterials. 2021;276:121060.
155. Diep P, Pannem S, Sweer J, Lo J, Snyder M, Stueber G, et al. Three-dimensional printed optical phantoms with customized absorption and scattering properties. Biomed Opt Express. 2015;6(11):4212–20.

An Optical Approach to Intra-arterial Drug Development for Brain Tumor Treatment

20

Mei Wang, John Lipiz, and Shailendra Joshi

Falling down is not a failure. Failure comes when you stay where you have fallen.

Socrates (470–399 BCE), Greek Philosopher

Introduction

Although investigations into arterial drug delivery for treating brain tumors have been ongoing since the early 1950s, this approach remains essentially experimental [1–3]. To achieve the maximum benefit of arterial injections, the drugs must be absorbed and retained immediately after injection during their first pass through the tissue circulation [4]. Therefore, investigating the pharmacokinetics of arterial delivery requires a rapid assessment of tissue drug concentrations. In rodents, the most frequently used laboratory research model, the cerebral transit time is less than 1 s [5]. Physical tissue samples needed for chemical analysis cannot be obtained in such a short time frame. Although radioisotope-tagged drugs have been used to investigate arterial delivery, such studies are rare, costly, and less amenable to scaling [6, 7]. Optical methods to assess tissue drug concentrations can permit safe assessment in a sub-second time domain [8, 9]. This chapter describes the development of arterial carrier-drug conjugates for brain cancer treatment by optical means. It illustrates how optical methods, such as diffuse reflectance spectroscopy, multispectral imaging, and confocal microscopy, can investigate arterial drug kinetics and identify effective carriers. On the one hand, this chapter makes a case for neuroscience researchers to use optical methods to investigate arterial drug delivery. On the other hand, it urges optical engineers to develop novel tools that can sense and image arterial delivery and assess treatment responses. While the understanding of neurological diseases has vastly improved, their effective treatment has been hampered by ineffective drug delivery. Given the complexity of neurological diseases, their treatment requires effective, timely, and flexible drug delivery tailored to the evolving tissue needs, which arterial injections can achieve.

M. Wang
Columbia University, New York, NY, USA

Pain Medicine, Long Island Spine Rehabilitation Medicine, Great Neck, NY, USA

J. Lipiz
Columbia University, New York, NY, USA

S. Joshi (✉)
Department of Anesthesiology, Columbia University Irving Medical Center, New York, NY, USA
e-mail: sj121@cumc.columbia.edu

Evolution of Arterial Drug Delivery for Treating Neurological Diseases

Goyanes first invoked arterial drug delivery in 1908. As a pioneer in vascular surgery, Goyanes developed arteriotomy techniques in animals before successfully using them in human subjects to achieve regional anesthesia [10, 11]. This was an era when arteries had to be surgically exposed, metal needles provided vascular access, heparin was yet undiscovered, and understanding of blood coagulation was half a century away. Even at the time, as reviewed in Chap. 1, there was the desire to deliver drugs locally to the pathology to have a regional effect and increase the safety and effectiveness of treatments. It partly motivated Werner Forssmann to develop catheters in 1929 [12]. The first attempt to treat brain tumors by Klopp happened soon after the discovery of chemotherapy in the 1940s [1, 13]. The results were encouraging and temporarily effective. Over the next 30 years, considerable effort was put into optimizing drug delivery for

S. Joshi (ed.), *Arterial Treatment of Neurological Diseases*, https://doi.org/10.1007/978-3-031-80173-0_20

brain tumor treatment. Several conceptual models soon revealed arterial drug delivery's potential advantages and limitations [14–17]. Landmark studies at the National Institute of Health by Oldfeild and Dedrick [18–20], Stanely Rapport [21, 22], and Edward Neuwelt with osmotic blood-brain barrier disruption stood out [23–26]. Investigators looked into the treatment of other neurological diseases, such as cerebral vasospasm [27, 28] and acute stroke with intra-arterial thrombolysis [29–31]. However, like brain tumor treatment, the pharmacological effectiveness of arterial drugs for treating these neurological conditions did not make a compelling impact. In contrast, arterial drug delivery was accepted for treating certain cancers, such as retinoblastoma [32] and liver cancer [33–36]. One neurological application of arterial drugs that has withstood the test of time is the Wada test [20]. The injection of anesthetic drugs to localize brain functions was introduced in 1949 and is still used today [37, 38]. To some extent, the relative failure of arterial drug delivery in treating neurological diseases could reflect the complexity of the disease processes, the vulnerability of the host tissue to injury, or the failure of drug delivery—each one of these problems poses a daunting challenge.

Since the 1970s, much of the focus of drug delivery for cancer treatment has been the blood-brain barrier, which restricts the uptake of drugs [21, 22]. To increase transport across the BBB, several strategies were developed, such as osmotic disruption of the BBB [23–26], enhanced lipid solubility [39, 40], more glioma-specific alkylating agents such as nimustine or ACNU [41] and smaller molecules, such as temozolomide [42], focused ultrasound [43], neuro-targeting carrier systems such as transferrin receptor antibodies [44], neurotropic viruses [45], cationic albumin [46, 47], liposomes [48], micelles [49], gold nanoparticles [50], and cell-targeting peptides [51] In addition, other means of drug delivery, such as intranasal delivery [52], direct delivery by implanted catheters [53], intertumoral drug polymers [49, 54–57], hydrogels [58], wafers [59], and intrathecal delivery [60] were developed that bypassed the BBB. However, despite such an intense and wide search for a cure, the overall prognosis of glioblastomas - the most lethal brain cancer - has not improved significantly compared to other malignancies.

Perhaps the real challenge is posed by the glioblastomas is the morphological and cellular diversity of the tumor, such that the resistance cell strains evolve in response to treatment. Given the pathology's evolution, any rigid treatment regimen would likely fail. A similar evolution of pathology is also seen in stroke and reperfusion injury in a much shorter time frame. Thus, the ability to deliver drugs immediately, electively, and locally to the brain with minimum systemic exposure could provide the flexibility needed to deal with neurological diseases. Instantaneously achieving therapeutic concentrations with low total doses is a crucial advantage of arterial drug delivery. Achieving this objective could open new avenues for the treatment of neurological diseases. Optical sensing and imaging techniques that have rapidly evolved in the last two decades now offer means to monitor drug delivery and tissue parameters that could help to develop arterial treatments. Arterial drug delivery could be titrated to tissue response, creating a novel dynamic approach for treating neurological diseases. Furthermore, better arterial delivery methods could greatly enhance the neuro-targeting strategies developed for intravenous delivery.

Investigative Tools

Conventional Tissue Sampling

Conventional tissue samples with chemical analysis were used to investigate arterial drug delivery in preclinical studies [24, 26, 61, 62]. Uptake of drugs by the brain after arterial injections was reported during the determination of brain uptake index values [63–65]. However, these studies provided a single time point assessment, and the injection and sampling parameters were sometimes inconsistent [64–67]. Repeated brain tissue sampling was done in some instances, but obtaining time histories by tissue sampling is challenging due to injury [61, 68]. Therefore, cerebrospinal fluid (CSF), arterial, and venous blood concentrations have been used as surrogates [69–72]. When tissue sampling has been used to investigate arterial delivery, samples are usually obtained several minutes after arterial injections. Although such measurements have been used to compare drugs, they do not provide a means to investigate the sub-second first-pass pharmacokinetics of arterial drug injections through the cerebral circulation of experimental animals [5].

Radioactive Isotope Studies

Radioisotope studies such as positron emission tomography (PET) offer the advantage of continuous, site-specific tissue-noninvasive concentrations of radiolabeled drugs [6, 7, 73]. In the laboratory, autoradiographic methods can provide detailed spatial localization of the isotope [74]. Preclinical and clinical PET studies have revealed the benefits of arterial drug injections. In 1986, Tyler at McGill University compared the pharmacokinetics of intravenous and intra-arterial ^{11}C labeled BCNU using positron emission tomography in human subjects with biopsy-proven brain tumors. After a super-selective injection of 500 μCu of ^{11}C—BCNU, scans were obtained every 30 s for 5 min initially and less frequently over the next 45 min. They found that BCNU concentrations were 50× higher in the normal brain, and the drug or its metabolites were trapped in the tumor. Their clearance was significantly different from the contralateral healthy tissue. Although arterial injections increase peak tissue concentrations by 50× compared to intravenous injections, the drug is rapidly cleared after arterial injections, so the net benefit is only 2–3× intravenous delivery [6]. The limitations of PET investigations are problems in the preparation of isotopes, the relative lack of temporal and spatial resolution, the lack of concurrent blood flow data, the safety and regulatory concerns using isotopes, and the resource-intensive nature of PET studies that are challenging to scale. These PET limitations do not undermine the significance of this study, which provided human data and the ability to monitor the effects of the treatment. Isotopic autoradiographic studies investigated the relationship between the drug injection rate and the tracer distribution in primates. These studies confirmed the relationship between the drug injection and the distribution of the tracer. Higher arterial drug infusion rates avoided regional variations in tissue tracer concentrations due to streaming and achieved more homogeneous drug concentrations. Higher arterial drug infusion rates achieved more homogeneous drug concentrations [75].

One application of intra-arterial drug delivery is determining cerebral blood flow (CBF) by assessing the washout of ^{133}Xe, an extensively used technique at our center [76–80]. ^{133}Xe CBF measurements, in hindsight, provide a conceptual model of arterial drug delivery. They also illustrate the benefits and limitations of arterial drug delivery. For example, ^{133}Xe is a lipid-soluble isotope readily absorbed but poorly retained by gray and white matter. The decline in tissue concentrations is directly related to the tissue blood flow, and it follows a three-compartment model [79]. The three compartments represent washout from the gray matter (<80 s), the white matter (80–180 s), and other tissues (>180 s). A spike in isotope washout may be seen with arteriovenous fistula (<5 s) due to the rapid shunting of blood [81]. Short-acting drugs like adenosine that have an exceedingly transient effect on cerebral blood flow create an ultrafast compartment [82–84]. ^{133}Xe washouts revealed how the regional blood flow affects isotope retention. The area under the ^{133}Xe washout curve was significantly increased if the isotope perfuses the extracranial compartment with much lower blood flow than the brain. When ^{133}Xe is injected intravenously, its dose is five to ten times greater than the intra-arterial dose. These observations are broadly applicable to arterial drug delivery [79, 85].

EEG Silence by Intra-arterial Anesthetics

Intra-arterial injections of anesthetic drugs have been used to suppress neurological functions for over 70 years transiently [20]. Such injection produces transient reversible EEG silence [37]. The point of recovery of EEG activity can provide a real-time approximation of tissue concentrations of anesthetic drugs [86]. Assessing the duration of EEG silence relative to the dose of anesthetic drugs has been used to investigate the effect of blood flow on arterial drug delivery. EEG silence studies revealed that the duration of EEG silence after a dose of propofol was directly related to blood flow and was affected by bolus volume and concentrations (Fig. 20.1) [87–89]. Propofol, a white emulsion, can be contrasted with blood using intravital microscopy with a green light filter. It was found that the duration of EEG silence was directly related to the transit time of propofol bolus through the cerebral circulation [90]. The limitation of studies based on the duration of EEG silence is the assumption of a constant relationship between EEG silence threshold to the dose and the tissue anesthetic concentrations. Due to systemic accumulation of the drug, the dose-response of intra-arterial anesthetic can be altered with repeated challenges. Any embolic injury could also change the dose-response to the anesthetic drug. In addition, the pattern of EEG silence fur-

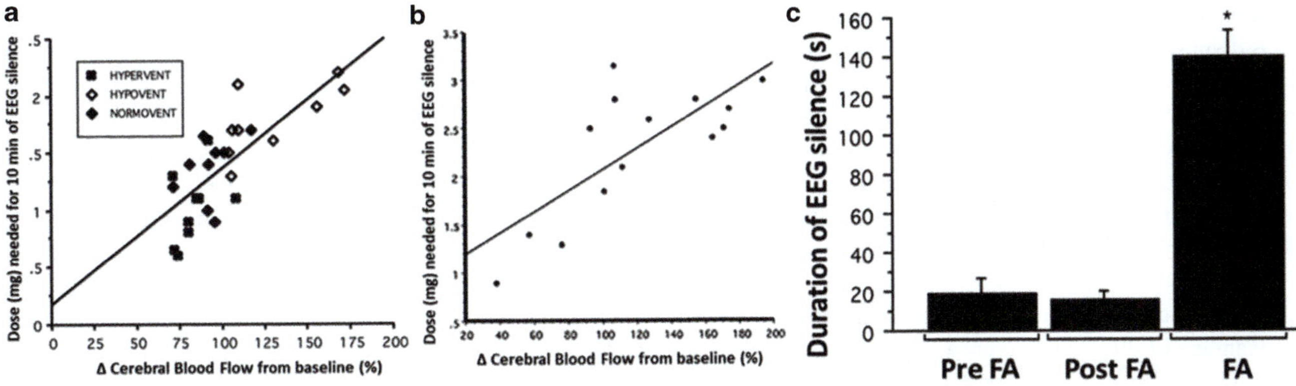

Fig. 20.1 Effect of changes in cerebral blood flow by alterations in ventilation (**a**) or intra-arterial injection of a vasodilator, verapamil 0.4 mg (**b**), directly affect the dose of anesthetic (propofol) needed to produce 10 min of EEG silence. (**c**) Also, injection of the anesthetic (propofol 3 mg) increased the duration of EEG silence by sevenfold during flow arrest (FA) compared to injection before and after the arrest

ther limits the application of this method mainly to propofol, which yields a more discernable pattern of EEG activity at the onset and the end of EEG silence [87].

Diffuse Reflectance Spectroscopy

The DRS Technique

Diffuse reflectance spectroscopy (DRS) or the optical pharmacokinetic method, analyzes tissue-backscattered light using afferent and efferent optical fibers. Halogen white light, between 450 and 850 nm, is transmitted by the afferent fiber. The backscattered light is transmitted to a spectrophotometer by the efferent fiber [91–94]. The analysis of the scattering-independent light absorption determines the concentration of a chromophore. This method can permit rapid (q 25–50 ms), site-specific, tissue-noninvasive determination of tissue chromophore concentration. DRS is helpful when the spectrum of the chromophore is relatively distinct from that of hemoglobin [8]. Ideally, DRS requires that the chromophore's spectrum remains stable and not affected by tissue pH or binding. The DRS method uses a simple fiber-optic spectroscopic system, can measure tissue concentrations in a sub-second time frame, and carries no exposure risks due to radiation, ultraviolet, or laser light. Thus, DRS is well-suited for arterial drug delivery research.

DRS is limited by the volume and depth of the tissue that can be interrogated. While multiple fibers can increase the area of tissue interrogation, the depth is limited to 3 mm. For brain tissue interrogation, the probe is placed on the carefully thinned skull. Meticulous care is needed to avoid bleeding under the probe by applying a thin layer of bone wax. The probe is calibrated to background white light and spectrum tested using a standardized tissue phantom. Light absorption at 2-nm wavelength increments is compared to baseline values before the injection of the chromophore. Typically, initial recordings are made at 3/s during arterial injections and more slowly as needed afterward. Raw spectrum is displayed on the screen, and changes in drug concentration can be detected by comparing them to the baseline, even during drug delivery. The data can be rapidly analyzed using MATLAB software within minutes of completing an experiment. Calibration curves are plotted across the anticipated measurement range using an intralipid or latex particle solution [8].

DRS with laser Doppler Flow Measurements

An advantage of diffuse reflectance spectroscopy is that it is compatible with laser Doppler flow measurements. Laser Doppler blood flow velocity measurements correlate with other flow measurement methods and can be used in the near-infrared range of 800 ± 10 nm [95–97]. Diffuse reflectance spectroscopy analyses change across the spectrum. Thus, it is immune to the narrow interference band by Doppler measurements if spectroscopic interference cannot be avoided by increasing the distance between the probes.

DRS in Conjunction with Postmortem Imaging of Drug Delivery

DRS is especially effective if the chromophore concentrations can also be assessed by quantitative fluorescence of postmortem samples. The multispectral imaging technique can enable rapid postmortem fluorescence imaging [98–103]. Under standardized imaging conditions, the tissue sample images are obtained along with reference samples using a photon-counting camera. Multispectral imaging provides a gross image of chromophore distribution. However, it assumes that the background optical properties of tissues are uniform across the image. Such an assumption raises concerns when imaging involves different types of tissues, such as brain tumors and the healthy brain. Brain tumors may differ in their optical characteristics and their hemoglobin content [104]. These limitations related to precise control of illumination of multispectral imaging can be overcome by confocal microscopy. Confocal imaging can reveal the chromophore's gross and cell-level distribution. The tissue fluorescence, such as through the eye, can be quantitatively assessed for pharmacokinetic purposes [9]. Another possible method to determine tissue drug concentrations in postmortem samples is spatial frequency domain imaging, which determines light absorption and scattering properties of tissue samples by modulated illumination [105].

Optical Approach to Intra-arterial Drug Development

An Overview of the Optical Approach

As suggested by Dedrick and Jenkins almost four decades ago, effective intra-arterial drug delivery requires three conditions [15–17]:

- Drugs are injected in states of reduced blood flow.
- The regional sites rapidly extract drugs.
- Drugs are rapidly cleared from systemic circulation.

Optical measurements can provide hundreds of site-specific measurements on a single animal without tissue extraction and chemical processing, both time- and resource-intensive. Dense pharmacokinetic data with hundreds of measurements can be acquired within minutes of completing the experiments. Simultaneously, it is possible to determine the blood flow with a laser Doppler device. A

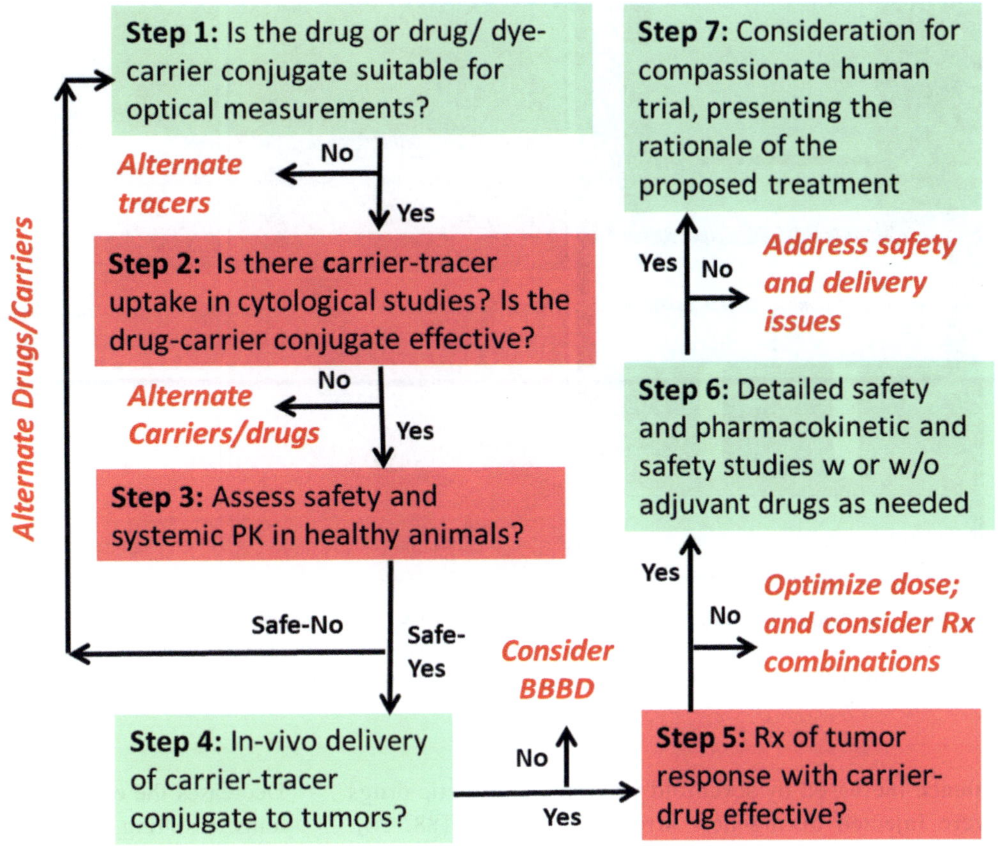

Fig. 20.2 A proposed optical pharmacokinetic approach to developing IA drugs for brain tumor treatment, bypassing chemical analysis. *BBBD* blood-brain barrier disruption

possible investigation strategy using optical measurements is shown in Fig. 20.2. The development process begins with **Step 1**, establishing the excitation and emission spectra of the drug or a dye, as in the case of a carrier. There are several anticancer drugs and dyes to choose from [94, 106–108]. Generally, carriers are large peptides and particles whose properties do not significantly alter when conjugated with the dyes. In vitro dissolved and measured concentrations are next tested in the tissue phantom to validate optical measurements [8, 94, 100, 103, 109, 110]. **Step 2**: Typical dyes for DRS are the lipid-soluble dialkyl-carbocyanine (Dir or DiD), cyanine (Cy 5, 5.5, 7, or 7.5) dyes, or Alexa fluor dyes, and can be used for labeling nanoparticles such as micelles and liposomes. Fluorescein isothiocyanate (FITC) labeling can be used for cytological studies to assess cell uptake of peptides using confocal microscopy [99]. **Step 3**: Once the drug, carrier dye, and drug conjugates have been tested in cytological studies, the safety and pharmacokinetics of the test compounds are established in healthy animals in survival and non-survival studies, respectively. In these experiments, probes can be put on the shaved skin and the brain to determine systemic and regional pharmacokinetics. **Step 4**: Testing drug delivery in pathological models in vivo with postmortem tissue sampling to establish the effectiveness of the carrier using drug/dye conjugates. **Step 5**: Once the effectiveness of the regional delivery method is established, treatment response can be assessed in a disease model. **Step 6**: Treatment protocols are further optimized by including adjuvant measures, such as systemic rescue, to enhance the safety and efficacy of arterial treatments. **Step 7**: If effective, the carrier-drug candidate can be a potential for compassionate human trials. Glioblastoma treatments could be investigated under the orphan drug program. Detailed pharmacokinetic and safety data is generally optional for such approval. However, it is prudent to provide additional pharmacokinetic and safety data for phase I human trials. Figure 20.3 shows the typical experimental setup for optical pharmacokinetic studies, as explained in Chap. 19.

Arterial Drug Injection During Hypoperfusion

Modeling data suggest that effective intra-arterial delivery requires rapid uptake and sustained retention of the drugs after the regional blood flow is decreased [4]. Compared to normal blood flow, the duration of EEG

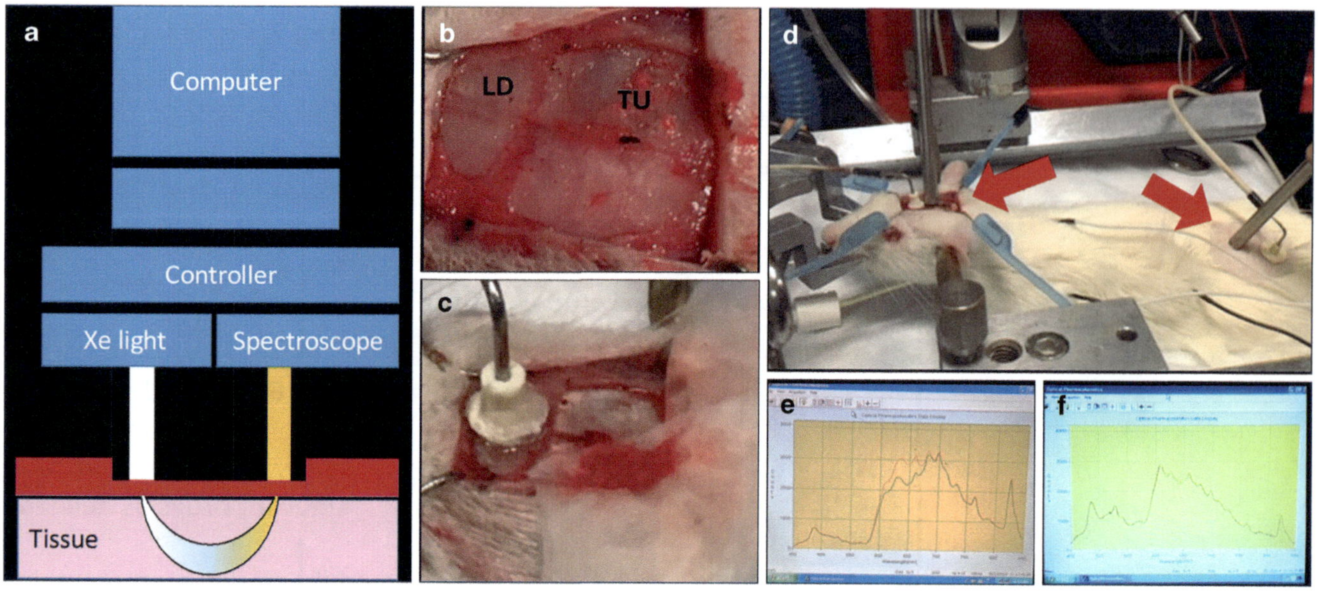

Fig. 20.3 (**a**) Setup for diffuse reflectance spectroscopy (DRS). (**b**) Superficially implanted brain tumor (Tu) can be seen through the skull. (**c, d**) The laser Doppler and the DRS probes are placed over the tumor and the skin (**arrows**). Spectrum was recorded from the tumor (**e**) and the skin (**f**) to determine concentrations of the dye-labeled carrier in the two tissues, along with laser Doppler (LD) blood flow measurements

silence increased by sevenfold when the anesthetic drugs were injected during flow arrest (Fig. 20.2c) [88, 90]. Subsequently, a direct comparison of intravenous, intra-arterial, and flow arrest (FA) intra-arterial delivery of BCNU was undertaken. It revealed that intra-arterial delivery of the drug increased sixfold with flow arrest compared to the arterial infusion (Fig. 20.4) [111]. Intravital microscopy revealed a distinct difference between flow arrest delivery and conventional arterial infusion. During FA, the bolus of BCNU completely displaced the blood intravascular dead space (Fig. 20.4). Subsequent studies with cationic liposomes also revealed a similar benefit of FA intra-arterial delivery on their regional deposition [102].

These results underscored the need to use flow arrest bolus drug delivery as an effective method of arterial drug delivery to the brain. Arterial injections during flow arrest offer several advantages over infusion. These include the following:

- Better control of the vascular distribution of the injected drug. Bolus injection is the method of contrast injection during angiography.
- Increases the arterial blood drug concentrations by minimizing dilution with blood.
- Increases transit time through the target circulation to permit drug diffusion.
- Decreases the exposure of drugs to blood cells and proteins, resulting in better tissue targeting by decreasing nonspecific opsonization.
- Decrease in blood flow decreases maldistribution due to streaming.
- Decreases shear stress on nanoparticles to increase the probability of adhesion to the endothelium.
- Lowers the distal perfusion pressure during flow arrest, potentially decreasing the pressure required to inject drug pulses. Decreased injection pressure could reduce the risk of vascular disruption in fragile pathological tissues. Hemorrhagic transformations have been reported with arterial drug delivery during the treatment of retinoblastomas and thrombolysis for stroke [85, 112].

Clinically, flow arrest is routinely used during vascular surgery, such as during clipping of brain aneurysms. During such surgeries, temporary clips are applied to transiently interrupt the flow to enable surgical dissection of the lesion. During interventional radiological procedures, flow arrest with high doses of intravenous adenosine has been clinically used to deliver embolic materials [113, 114]. Alternatively, balloon-occluding catheters can achieve a similar effect locally (Fig. 20.5) [115, 116]. In smaller animals carotid occlusion combined with bolus injections of adenosine, esmolol and cold saline produces reproducible and repeatable transient flow arrest to permit drug delivery [99, 101, 102, 111].

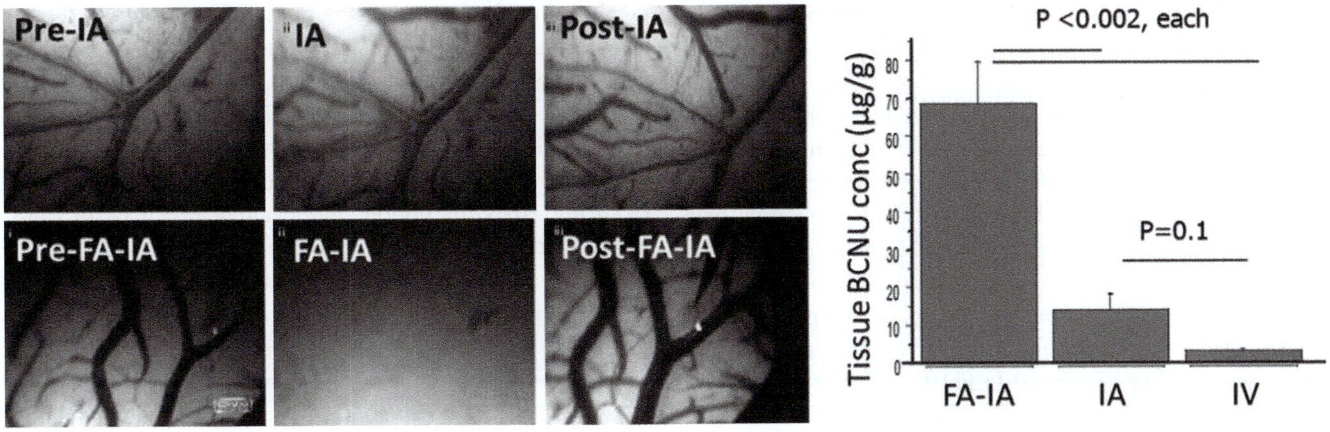

Fig. 20.4 Video microscopy of rabbit brain shows delivery of carmustine before, during, and after conventional intra-arterial infusion (**IA; top panel**) and similarly with flow arrest intra-arterial delivery (**FA-IA; bottom panel**). Compared to IA infusion, **FA-IA** increased carmustine deposition by 6×. During **FA-IA** injection, pure drug/carrier is delivered to the target site as blood is momentarily displaced from the vessels, and no vascular structures are visible

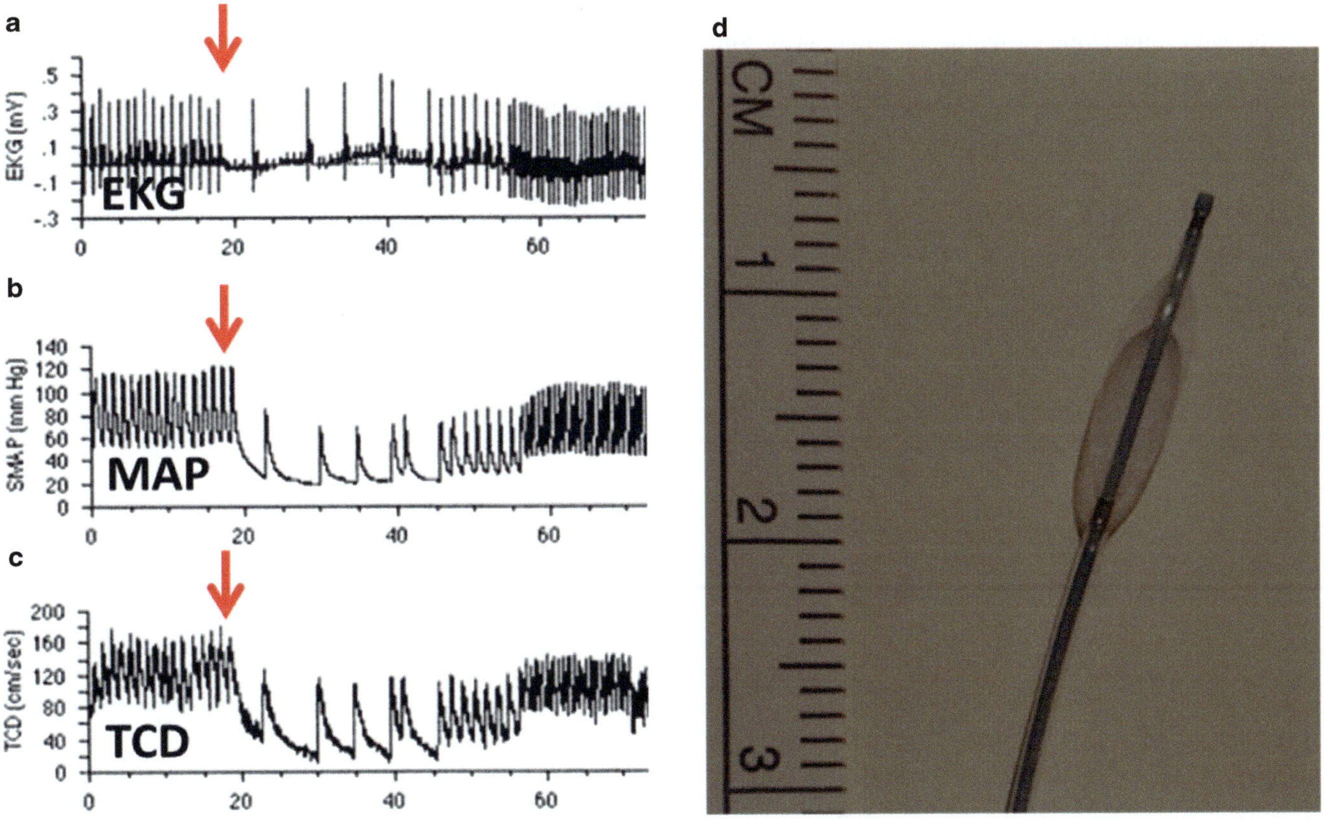

Fig. 20.5 Two clinical methods of FA-IA delivery: *First*, by systemic hypotension using IV adenosine (arrows), see Pile-Spellman et al. (1999). (**a–c**) are changes in EKG, mean arterial pressure (MAP), and transcranial Doppler (TCD) flow velocity during FA. *Second*, by a balloon-occluding catheter with distal port (**d**)

Optical Assessment of Blood-Brain Barrier Disruption

The blood-brain or blood-tumor barrier is a significant hurdle to effective drug delivery. Inconsistent disruption of the barrier can have a profound effect on drug delivery [72]. Rapidly assessing blood-brain barrier function can help understand and optimize drug delivery. Evans blue, indocyanine green, or fluorescein can test blood-brain barrier integrity [117–119]. Diffuse reflectance spectroscopy has been used to track tissue concentrations of dyes that can assess BBB permeability (Table 20.1) [110, 117–119]. The DRS method was used to track the concentrations of Evans blue after the disruption of the blood-brain barrier with intracarotid mannitol. A significant increase in Evans blue uptake by the brain tissue was evident. However, there were considerable differences across animals. Figure 20.6 shows that the DRS-determined ICG concentrations were considerably higher at the site of BBB disruption as determined by Evans blue staining. There was an enormous variability in BBB disruption with intracarotid mannitol injection [119]. Similar variability in BBB disruption with mannitol has been reported in human subjects [72]. In human subjects, the CSF concentrations of methotrexate are linearly related to the permeability of the BBB after mannitol. Given that the disruption of the BBB with mannitol varies between individuals and affects drug delivery, there is the need to achieve more consistent disruption or monitor BBB disruption using a compound that is rapidly cleared by the body, such as indocyanine green, or find carriers that can deliver drugs without requiring BBB disruption. Indocyanine green is an FDA-approved dye rapidly conjugated by the liver and excreted by the kidney. It has an elimination half-life of 3–4 min. Thus, it permits repeat assessment of BBB integrity. Using the DRS method, ICG can monitor BBB disruption in rabbits while assessing the mitoxantrone concentrations after arterial delivery [110]. Such an ability to determine drug concentrations about BBB permeability helps to understand and optimize arterial drug delivery when BBB disruption is required.

Tracking Arterial Drug Delivery with DRS

Mitoxantrone, an anticancer drug, has a peak absorption at 610 and 660 nm and peak emission at 685 nm. It is a non-cell cycle selective drug used for cancer treatments by intra-arterial injections. For brain tumor treatment, it was shown that effective FA-IA delivery required the disruption of the

Table 20.1 Dyes for assessing blood-brain barrier disruption

	Evan's blue	Indocyanine green	Fluorescein
Molecular formula	$C_{34}H_{28}N_6O_{14}S_5$	$C_{43}H_{47}N_2NaO_6S_2$	$C_{20}H_{12}O_5$
Molecular weight	873	775	376
Protein binding	68%	98%	53–83%
Peak absorption	620 nm	789 nm	460 nm
Peak emission	680 nm	814 nm	515 nm
Risk	Carcinogenic	Approved for human use	Approved for human use
Use	Plasma volume estimation Lymph flow	Angiography Liver blood flow Cardiac output Thermal therapy of cancer	Angiography Tumor edge identification

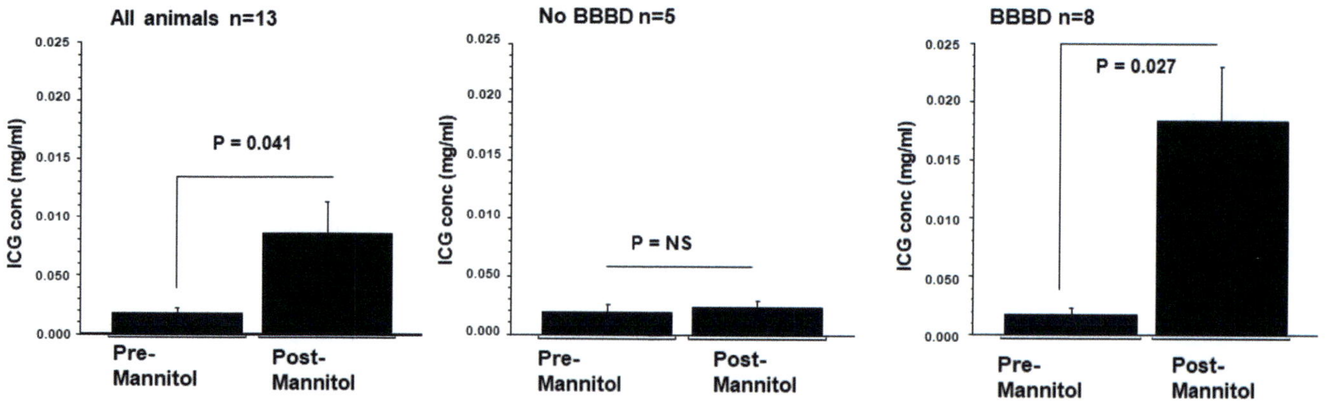

Fig. 20.6 DRS-determined brain tissue concentrations of indocyanine green in 13 rabbits before and after disruption of the BBB with mannitol in animals where there was no BBB disruption ($n = 5$) and in those where the BBB was disrupted ($n = 8$). Evans blue staining determined BBB disruption

BBB. However, due to the difficulty in disrupting the BBB with IA mannitol in the rabbit model, it is necessary to determine the degree of BBB disruption after mannitol treatment as that would determine the uptake of the mitoxantrone. Figure 20.7 shows the use of ICG as a guide to mitoxantrone delivery. The end concentration of mitoxantrone and the area under the concentration time curve after mannitol treatment were linearly related to ICG deposition, reflecting the extent of barrier opening. The optical approach can provide additional insight into drug delivery by permitting simultaneous assessment of BBB disruption and drug deposition [110].

Optimization of Liposomes for Arterial Delivery

Liposomal drug formulations have been proposed for drug delivery to the brain. Liposomal particles can be decorated with targeting molecules to enhance drug delivery to a specific site [121]. Liposomes can increase lipid solubility and penetrate the blood-brain barrier. In studies with 80-nm DiD 660 labeled liposomes, charge-neutral liposomes were ineffective in penetrating the BBB. The uptake of neutral liposomes required disruption of the BBB. The brain uptake was considerably greater with cationic liposomes than with charge-neutral or anionic liposomes (Fig. 20.8) [100]. Cationic liposomes did not require disrupting the blood-brain barrier. Larger liposomes (200 nm) were better retained than smaller ones [98, 101]. Cationic charge significantly improved liposomal deposition in the brain tissue. Limited survival data in these publications suggested that liposomal delivery was safe, and the particles were retained for several hours after a single injection. When tested in a tumor model, the liposomes deposited in the peritumor region compared to the center of the lesion [98]. Smaller micellar particles (20 nm) were assessed for greater tumor penetration because the capillary flow is impeded, and there is greater hydrostatic pressure in the core of tumors than in the periphery. Subsequent studies revealed that cationic micelles (20 nm) could penetrate the tumor core. Cationic micelles were superior on postmortem images but offered no additional advantage over the neutral micelles with the DRS measurements (Table 20.2). In addition, cat-ionizable micelles were tested. These particles increased their cationic charge in acidic pH and were better retained than the neutral ones. The smaller particles were more tumor selective, probably less dependent on charge. They were also deposited in the arteries, suggesting a secondary entrapment mechanism when delivered by the FA-IA injections [103, 120].

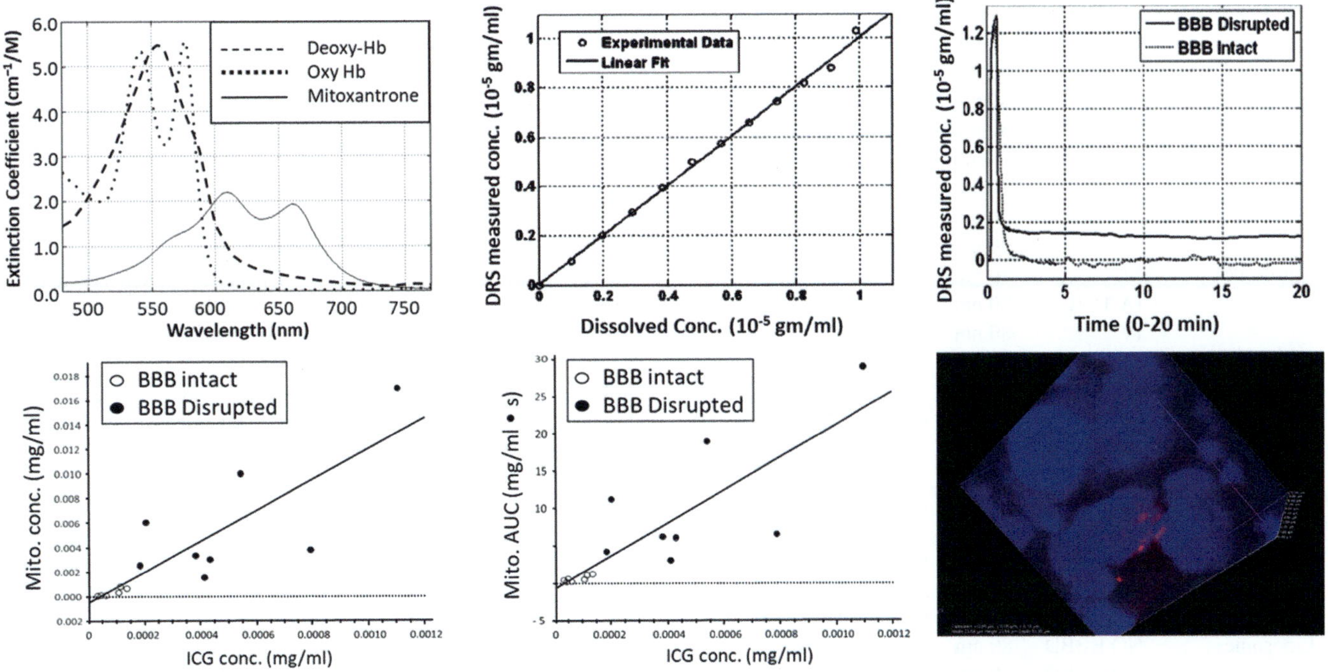

Fig. 20.7 Optical assessment of FA-IA mitoxantrone (Mito.) delivery: **Top panel**: Excitation spectrum of mitoxantrone, DRS measurements of mitoxantrone in a tissue phantom; preliminary data showing uptake of Mito. with and without blood-brain barrier. **Lower panel**: End concentration and the area under the concentration time curve (AUC) were directly related to ICG concentrations, reflecting the permeability of the BBB after disruption by hypertonic mannitol treatment. IA-FA mitoxantrone delivery was safe, and drug deposition in tumor implants was observed on confocal imaging. (Data from Reif 2008; Asegul 2010; Ellis 2016)

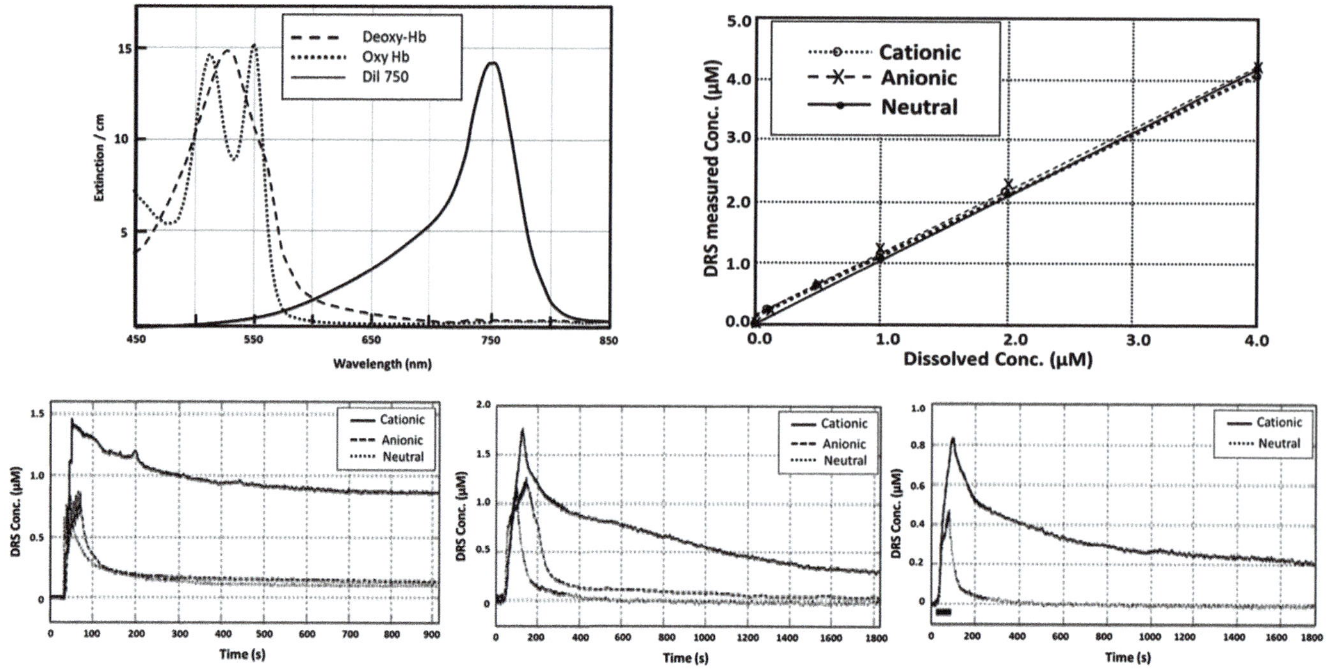

Fig. 20.8 DRS tracked delivery of labeled liposomes. The dye had a peak absorption at 750 nm. The dissolved and measured concentration of the dye in a tissue phantom linearly correlated with each for the three liposomes The uptake of cationic liposomes was assessed with three grades of BBB disruption using focused ultrasound. Left: high-intensity FUS disruption of the BBB; low-intensity disruption of BBB and no disruption. Under all three conditions, cationic liposomes (80 nm) were superior to other anionic and neutral liposomes

Table 20.2 Arterial delivery of liposomes and micelles during transient cerebral hypoperfusion (flow arrest)

Carrier type	Expt. conditions	Size	Charge (*n*)	Peak (μM)	AUC (μM s)	End conc. (μM)	Conclusion Reference
Liposomes	High-intensity FUS	80 nm	Cationic (6)	0.99 ± 0.43[a]	421 ± 249[a]	0.41 ± 0.1[a]	The cationic charge has a significantly greater uptake, and BBB disruption is unnecessary Joshi (2014) [100]
		80 nm	Neutral (6)	0.75 ± 0.44	146 ± 98	0.15 ± 0.08	
		80 nm	Anionic (6)	0.51 ± 0.2	71 ± 45	0.04 ± 0.05	
	Low-intensity FUS	80 nm	Cationic (5)	0.72 ± 0.07[a]	521 ± 143[a]	0.15 ± 0.09[a]	
		80 nm	Neutral (6)	0.4 ± 0.12	37 ± 49	0.0 ± 0.01	
		80 nm	Anionic (5)	0.4 ± 0.07	59 ± 25	0.01 ± 0.02	
	NO BBBD	80 nm	Cationic (8)	0.83 ± 0.3[a]	639 ± 271[a]	0.28 ± 0.12[a]	
		80 nm	Neutral (7)	0.27 ± 0.09[a]	71 ± 13	0.04 ± 0.02	
Liposomes	IA	80 nm	Cationic (5)	0.72 ± 0.28	297 ± 120	0.11 ± 0.06	IA-TCH delivery ≫ IA delivery and IA-TCH ≫ IV delivery Joshi (2014) [102]
	IA TCH	80 nm	Cationic (6)	1.32 ± 0.51[b]	1170 ± 502[b]	0.43 ± 0.17[b]	
	IV	80 nm	Cationic (5)	0.02 ± 0.01	9.1 ± 7.1	0.00 ± 0.01	
	IA-TCH	80 nm	Cationic (5)	1.59 ± 0.41[b]	928 ± 351[b]	0.43 ± 0.22[b]	
Liposomes	NO BBBD	80 nm	Anionic (5)	0.26 ± 0.12	48 ± 44	0.03 ± 0.03	Cationic surface charge enables regional liposomal deposition. No difference between 25% and 50% DOTAP Joshi (2015) [101]
	NO BBBD	80 nm	Cationic (5)	0.42 ± 0.07[a]	343 ± 36[a]	0.16 ± 0.03[a]	
	NO BBBD	80 nm	Neutral (5)	0.18 ± 0.04	56 ± 43	0.05 ± 0.03	
	NO BBBD	80 nm	5% DOTAP (6)	0.2 ± 0.07	39 ± 28	0.04 ± 0.03	
	NO BBBD	80 nm	25% DOTAP (6)	0.35 ± 0.08[b]	303 ± 110[b]	0.17 ± 0.06[b]	
	NO BBBD	80 nm	50% DOTAP (6)	0.42 ± 0.11[b]	326 ± 69[b]	0.15 ± 0.06[b]	
Liposomes	NO BBBD	80 nm	Cationic (7)	0.741 ± 0.339	162 ± 86[a]	0.135 ± 0.96[a]	Cationic surface and larger liposomes enhance regional delivery Joshi (2016) [98]
	NO BBBD	60 nm	Neutral (7)	0.581 ± 0.189	51 ± 10	0.043 ± 0.02	
	NO BBBD	200 nm	Cationic (7)	0.734 ± 0.357	233 ± 80[a]	0.216 ± 0.085[a,b]	
	NO BBBD	200 nm	Neutral (6)	0.477 ± 0.339	43 ± 20	0.02 ± 0.096	

(continued)

Table 20.2 (continued)

Carrier type	Expt. conditions	Size	Charge (*n*)	Peak (μM)	AUC (μM s)	End conc. (μM)	Conclusion Reference
pH-sensitive cationic micelles	NO BBBD No tumor	20 nm	Cationic (5)	2.2 ± 1.0	241 ± 71	0.34 ± 0.03[a]	Cat-ionizable micelle delivery to healthy and tumor tissue Nguyen (2016) [103]
		20 nm	Neutral (5)	1.3 ± 0.3	148 ± 71	0.17 ± 0.1[a]	
	No BBBD Tumor	20 nm	Cationic (5)	1.05 ± 0.7	258 ± 122	0.41 ± 0.23	
		20 nm	Neutral (5)	0.99 ± 0.67	146 ± 100	0.21 ± 0.21	
TAT-decorated micelles	NO BBBD High dose	20 nm	TAT-decorated (7)	2.44 ± 1.12	318 ± 175	0.32 ± 0.19	TAT-decorated micelles generate significantly higher concentrations Nguyen (2017) [120]
		20 nm	Neutral (7)	1.91 ± 0.87	293 ± 212	0.31 ± 0.2	
	NO BBBD Low dose	20 nm	TAT-decorated (7)	0.59 ± 0.23	115 ± 60	0.15 ± 0.13	
		20 nm	Neutral (7)	0.44 ± 0.11	37 ± 10	0.05 ± 0.02	

[a] Significant difference due to cationic charger
[b] Other significant differences

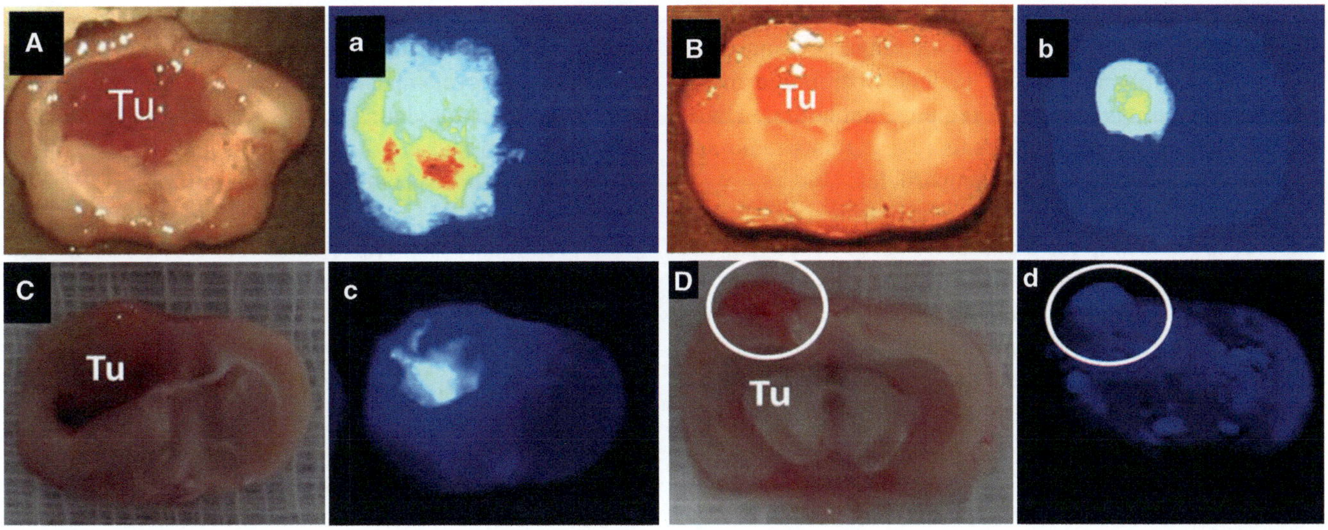

Fig. 20.9 Distribution of liposomes and micelles on postmortem fluorescence imaging: (**A**, **a**) 80-nm cationic liposomes had a peritumor distribution. (**B**, **b**) TAT was localized specifically to the tumors. (**C**, **c**) Tumor selectivity was also seen with cationic micelles and to some extent with neutral ones, (**D**, **d**) but the tumor uptake of neutral micelles was minimal

Cationic Peptides for Tumor-Selective Drug Delivery

Successful delivery of cationic liposomes to brain tissue raised the possibility of tumor-selective drug delivery with cationic peptides. In healthy cells, anionic lipids are located in the inner lipid surface of the cell membrane and endosomes. These lipids help to anchor the cationic proteins that play a vital role in cell function. However, these anionic phospholipids are redistributed to the external surface of the cell membrane of pre-apoptotic and malignant cells. When delivered by the FA-IA technique, these anionic lipids could provide tumor-specific targets for cationic drug carriers. The ability of FA-IA delivery to deliver high concentrations of cationic entities while minimizing or avoiding contact with blood proteins and prolonged capillary transit time could significantly enhance the capability of cationic peptides to target cancer cells [99].

Three converging lines of evidence support using cationic peptides to target malignant cells, in addition to evidence from cationic liposomes and micelles (Fig. 20.9). First, measuring cancer cells' surface potential reveals a greater negative charge [122–124]. Second, cationic nanoparticles have been developed to harvest circulating malignant cells from the peripheral blood. It has been reported that most cancer cells carry a significant negative surface charge that would permit such cell harvesting [122–125]. Finally, cationic peptides can penetrate the blood-brain barrier even after intravenous delivery [126, 127]. Thus, a compelling justification exists to evaluate the cationic peptides for targeting malignant cells by flow arrest delivery. The trans-activator of transcription (TAT) is a protein that contains 84–101 amino acids in the human immunodeficiency virus. TAT is one of the several cell-penetrating peptides that can translocate therapeutic entities across cell membranes. In the context of HIV, TAT greatly amplifies the transcription of the virus. The protein contains highly cationic peptide sequences that enable rapid virus translocation across the cell membranes. This 11-amino-acid chain (YGRKKRRQRRR) can cross the blood-brain barrier. Modeling data suggests that it penetrates the cell membranes within 100-200 ns [128]. In high concentrations likely to be achieved with IA-FA delivery, probably leads to the deposition of the peptide and its slow clearance thereafter results in penetrates the membrane and sutained deposition lasting hours after a single injection [129]. Cationic charge, particularly the GRKK sequence in TAT, enables it to localize on the nuclear membrane of the peptide [130]. TAT can deliver a wide range of compounds across cell membranes. These include hydrophilic molecules such as drugs, peptides, proteins, antibodies, DNA/RNA/siRNA/PNA, imaging agents (dyes/Q-dots/radio and MR ligands), liposomes, and nanoparticles.

Pharmacokinetic studies in tumor-bearing rats showed that TAT is retained in the brain tumor tissue with a half-life of 8 h [129]. In cytological studies uptake of TAT does not peak for several minutes. One possible explanation for sustained retention of TAT by implanted brain tumors could be that the peptide is trapped in the tumor when delivered in high concentrations by flow arrest delivery and the poor vascularity of the tumor delays its washout. The entrapped peptide could then slowly permeate the tumor cells. Prolonged retention of cationic liposomes was also observed in tumor-bearing rats [101]. Sustained tissue retention by brain tumors lasting hours after a single FA-IA injection could significantly affect the selection of drugs and carriers for specific clinical applications of FA-IA delivery. Thus, by targeting malignant and apoptotic cells, FA-IA delivery could offer novel treatments for cancers, stroke, and neurodegenerative diseases.

Cytological studies with TAT: Cytological studies with TAT showed a rapid uptake by L glioma cell lines. TAT uptake was evident with a variety of malignant cells, such as C6 (glioma), SKOV3 (ovarian cancer), MDA and 4T1 (breast cancer), and LLC (lung cancer) (Fig. 20.10). The dimer of TAT, when conjugated with melphalan, was more potent than the TAT conjugate.

Selection of drug cargo for cancer treatments: TAT was conjugated with doxorubicin and melphalan. Conjugation attenuated the toxicity of the native drugs; however, in both cases, it was greater than TAT alone.

There are several advantages of melphalan over doxorubicin for IA delivery. First, melphalan is a potent chemotherapeutic drug. It is clinically used for the intra-arterial treatment of retinoblastoma [131, 132]. Retinoblastoma is one of the clinically accepted intra-arterial treatments for cancers. Melphalan is an alkylating agent that acts on all cell cycle phases. Cell cycle selectivity can be an essential consideration in cancer chemotherapy. Doxorubicin acts in the G2/m phase of the cell cycle. A short drug exposure duration would spare cells that are not in the vulnerable phase of the growth cycle. When drugs are given intravenously, the therapeutic concentrations can be sustained for several hours or days. Therefore, cells in different stages of the cell cycle can be treated. However, with intra-arterial drug delivery, the drug concentration might not be sustained, so cell cycle-specific drugs might not be as effective. Like other alkylating agents, melphalan has a rapid onset of action and is not cell cycle selective. Thus, melphalan might be a better drug for intra-arterial cancer treatment.

In preliminary survival studies, FA-IA treatment with melphalan (Fig. 20.11), TAT-melphalan, and TAT-dimer melphalan using FA-IA delivery shows that melphalan demonstrated a trend toward improved survival of Fisher 344 rats with 9 L glioma implants. However, significant improvement in survival was noted with the other two treatments. The preliminary survival studies were undertaken in four groups of 9 L-Fisher 344 rats. They were primarily aimed to determine the feasibility and safety of FA-IA treatments, not to compare treatment outcomes. The treatment was undertaken 14 ± 2 days after tumor implantation. The animals were sacrificed after predetermined euthanasia criteria were reached. The survival data are presented in Fig. 20.10. Due to a lack of randomization, these results only establish the safety of all four interventions.

Current Limitations and Future Directions

The lack of pharmacokinetic justification for drug selection has often been blamed for the failure of arterial treatments. However, there is hardly any pharmacokinetic data to guide

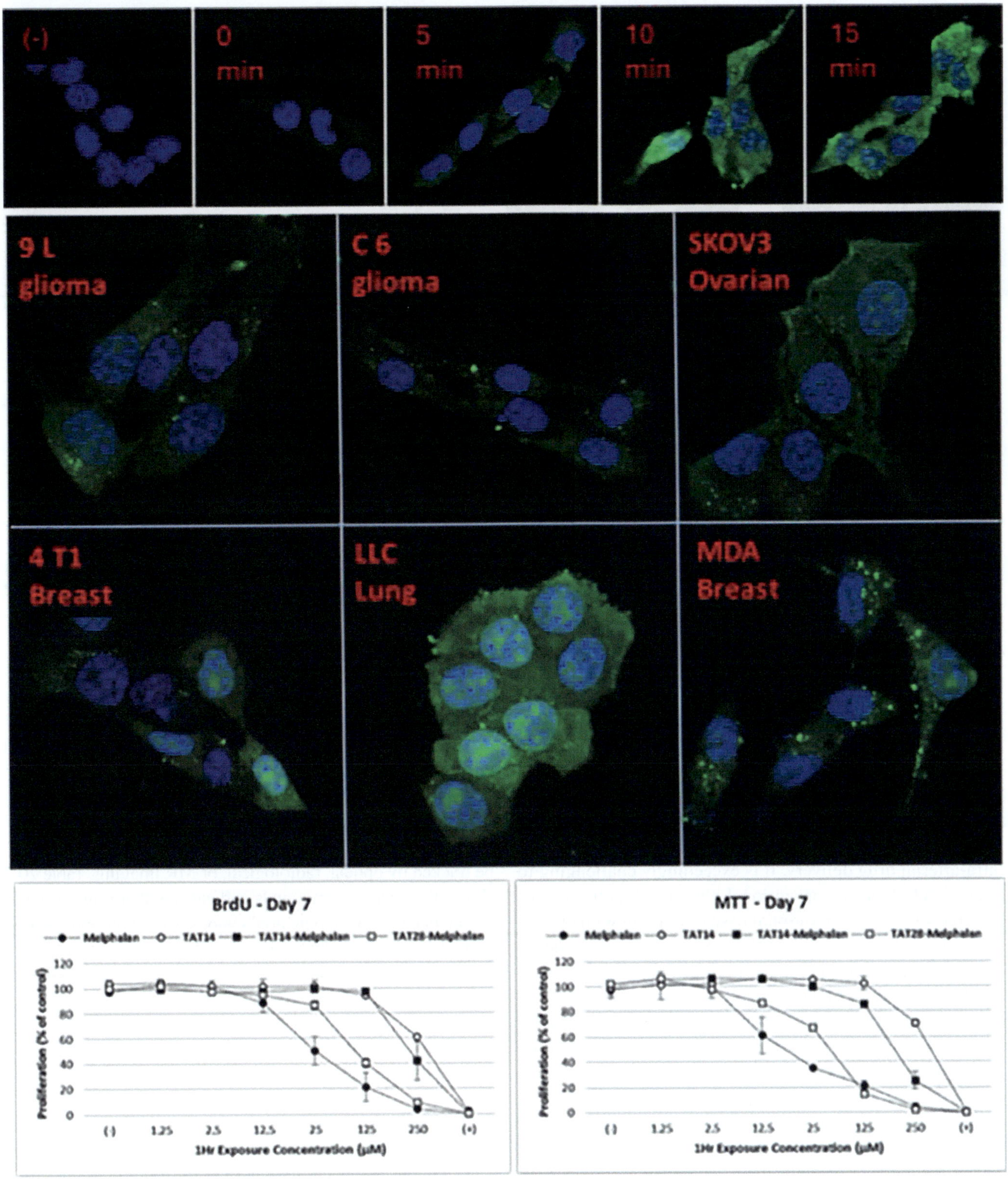

Fig. 20.10 Cytological studies show rapid uptake of TAT during 0–15 min of exposure (Top row). The middle two rows show that TAT is taken up by several cancer cell lines, and thus, TAT-conjugated drugs could be used to treat metastatic brain cancers. Conjugation of TAT (% cell viability compared to controls) shows an attenuation of melphalan toxicity after conjugation with TAT following a 1-h exposure over the next 7 days. Dimer of TAT was more cytotoxic than TAT-melphalan

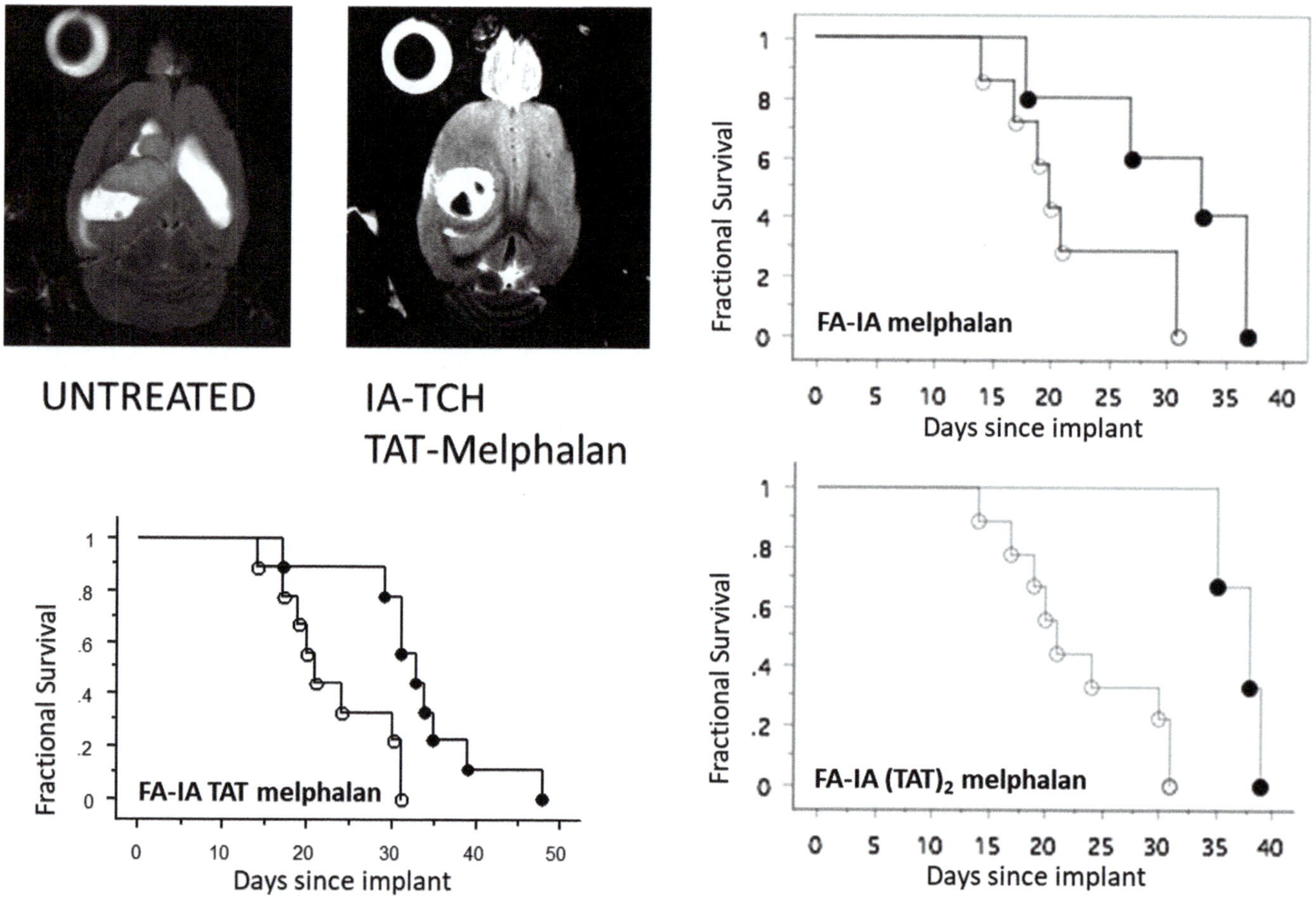

Fig. 20.11 Preliminary results of treatment of 9-L glioma implant in Fisher 344 rats. MRI imaging revealed circumscribed necrotic tumors with FA-IA TAT-melphalan. FA-IA melphalan increased survival from 22 ± 7 to 30 ± 8 days ($P = 0.07$); FA-IA TAT-melphalan increased survival from 23 ± 6 to 33 ± 8 days, $P = 0.01$; FA-IA delivery of TAT-dimer melphalan increased survival from 23 ± 6 to 37 ± 2 days ($P = 0.004$). TAT-chemotherapeutic drug conjugates probably represent the first drugs that were developed by optical methods specifically for intra-arterial delivery

intra-arterial drug delivery. It is exceedingly challenging to obtain such data by conventional pharmacokinetic means. Isotopic studies and traditional tissue sampling with chemical analysis have been undertaken, but they can raise safety concerns and are resource- and time-intensive.

The compelling impact of flow arrest intra-arterial drug delivery, which delivers the virtually pure drug to the target site, must be appreciated. Accessing the endothelium with a pure drug is a unique advantage of intra-arterial drug delivery. It greatly potentiates carrier-mediated targeted drug delivery while minimizing and avoiding contact with blood proteins or blood cells, unleashing the full potential of carrier-mediated or receptor-mediated transport. It is hard to predict where the technology for treating brain tumors will evolve. Regarding arterial drug delivery, it is likely that carrier-mediated drug delivery will play a significant role.

This chapter described the application of optical methods to investigate carriers for IA drug delivery. TAT is only one of the many cationic carriers available for drug delivery. An advantage of carrier-based delivery is that carriers could also be labeled with tracers to monitor drug delivery. These tracers can be tracked by optical, radiological, or MR imaging. Table 20.3 shows therapeutic compounds and carriers that might need to be screened for oncologic applications. Could an optics-based approach accelerate the screening of these compounds?

Four fundamental questions have to be addressed in developing carriers for arterial drug delivery:

- *What is the best carrier for a specific application?*
  - Is the carrier regionally and systemically safe? Allergic reactions to peptides could limit their use.
  - Can the carrier selectively target the pathology, such as malignant and apoptotic cells, by their negative surface charge, a specific ligand, or a transporter?
  - How long is the carrier retained after delivery?
- *What types of tracers can be attached to the carrier to monitor and optimize drug delivery?*
  - Which dye is suitable for preclinical research?
  - Can the carrier be tagged with iodinated or Gd contrast for radiological and MR imaging?
- *What drug cargo is best suited to treat the disease?*

  - What is the underlying complexity of the disease? Will it need a single-drug intervention for cancer treatment or a multidrug intervention for stroke?
  - What is the carrier's retention duration at the target site?
- Is the drug effective during the carrier's retention in the target tissue? *What is the nature of carrier-drug and carrier-tracer binding*?
  - Is the active drug released for the carrier?
  - Can the carrier also serve as a depot for sustained release?
  - Can tracer and drug be bound to the carrier to monitor drug delivery?

The development of TAT-chemotherapeutic conjugates was achieved purely by optical means [99]. There are eight pharmacokinetic curves in Fig. 20.8, each with 900 data points—just that panel alone has 7200 data points. It would be impossible to obtain tissue samples and even less likely to have the time and human resources needed to analyze those samples by chemical means. Table 20.3 lists some other cationic carriers that still need to be investigated using FA-IA delivery. In addition, hundreds of other cell-penetrating peptides and carriers may need to be investigated for intra-arterial delivery. It is only possible to undertake such research by optical means. An optics-based strategy is shown in Fig. 20.12. One could argue that the optical approach to arterial drug development will be simpler, quicker, safer, and more cost-effective than conventional pharmacokinetic means.

Table 20.3 Examples of carriers, drugs, and linkage methods show the need for a high-volume screening strategy

Cationic carrier	Cargo	Linker	Potency compared to parent drug	Reference
Cell-penetrating peptides	Doxorubicin, methotrexate	Maleimide sulfur carbon, H-bond	20× greater in vitro	[133, 134]
Protamine-albumin	Doxorubicin	Disulfide	6× greater in vitro; 2× greater in vivo	[135]
Cationic dextran	Doxorubicin, paclitaxel, methotrexate, mitoxantrone Gene delivery	Electrostatic interaction, hydrophobic interaction, amide and H-bond, disulfide	Same efficacy, 2.6× greater survivability	[55–57]
Cationic chitosan	Mitomycin C, doxorubicin, paclitaxel	Electrostatic interaction, hydrophobic interaction, amide and H-bond	2× greater in vivo 5–10× greater in vivo	[52, 136, 137]
Albumin	Doxorubicin, paclitaxel, methotrexate, camptothecin, carboplatin	H-bond, electrostatic interaction, peptide, ester	3× greater (in vitro) 2× greater in vivo	[138–143]
Chlorotoxin	Methotrexate, doxorubicin	Ester		[144]

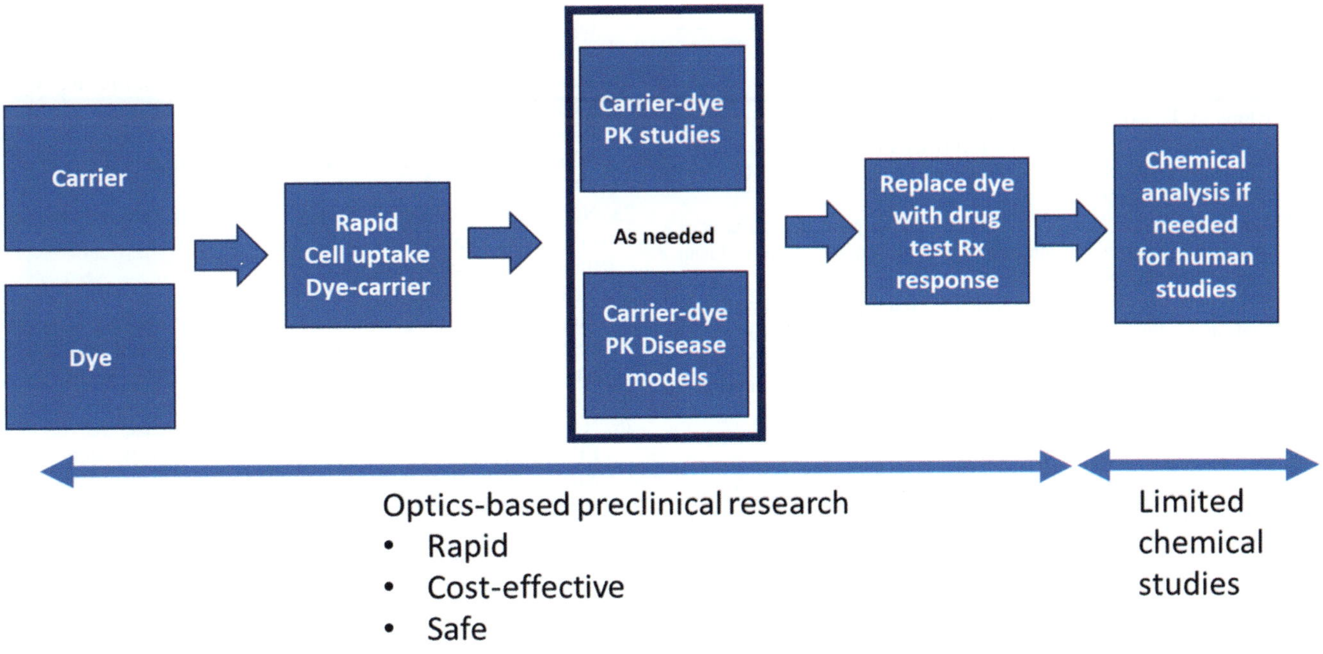

Fig. 20.12 Optics-based arterial drug development

Conclusions

The fundamental concept that drugs must be rapidly extracted during their first pass through the regional circulation for maximum benefits of arterial drug delivery cannot be overlooked. Conventional pharmacokinetic approaches do not permit rapid assessment of tissue drug concentrations in a sub-second time frame, which is needed to investigate first-pass drug delivery. However, optical sensing and imaging methods can rapidly assess tissue drug concentrations, particularly when the compounds have a light absorption spectrum distinct from oxy- and deoxyhemoglobin. It is likely that for maximum delivery, native drugs will require carriers that enable rapid uptake and retention by the target site. Such carriers will be especially needed for neurological applications where the BBB greatly restricts drug uptake. TAT carriers can rapidly penetrate the BBB and deliver diverse drug cargo. These carriers can be tagged with dyes that are tracked by optical means.

The unique feature of FA-IA drug delivery is the ability to deliver a nearly pure drug to the target site. Such a delivery method maximizes carrier-assisted drug delivery by minimizing contact with blood proteins and cells. Optical methods were used to develop the first carrier-drug conjugates for brain cancer treatment. However, TAT is one of the many cationic cell-penetrating peptides. Cell-penetrating peptides are one of the many carriers that can be used to improve arterial drug delivery. There is a vast library of carriers to explore. Once suitable carriers are identified, they could be conjugated with therapeutic compounds to develop novel treatments that have hitherto failed due to ineffective delivery. Thus, as in the case of TAT-melphalan development, highly cost-effective, site-specific, and safe optical methods already exist.

References

1. Klopp CT, Alford TC, Bateman J, Berry GN, Winship T. Fractionated intra-arterial cancer; chemotherapy with methyl bis amine hydrochloride; a preliminary report. Trans Meet Am Surg Assoc. 1950;68:490–511.
2. Huang R, Boltze J, Li S. Strategies for improved intra-arterial treatments targeting brain tumors: a systematic review. Front Oncol. 2020;10:1443.
3. Shikalov A, Koman I, Kogan NM. Targeted glioma therapy-clinical trials and future directions. Pharmaceutics. 2024;16(1):100.
4. Cooke JN, Ellis JA, Hossain S, Nguyen J, Bruce JN, Joshi S. Computational pharmacokinetic rationale for intra-arterial delivery to the brain. Drug Deliv Transl Res. 2016;6:622.
5. Thomas DL, Lythgoe MF, van der Weerd L, Ordidge RJ, Gadian DG. Regional variation of cerebral blood flow and arterial transit time in the normal and hypoperfused rat brain measured using continuous arterial spin labeling MRI. J Cereb Blood Flow Metab. 2006;26(2):274–82.
6. Tyler JL, Yamamoto YL, Diksic M, Theron J, Villemure JG, Worthington C, et al. Pharmacokinetics of superselective intra-arterial and intravenous [11C]BCNU evaluated by PET. J Nucl Med. 1986;27(6):775–80.
7. Mitsuki S, Diksic M, Conway T, Yamamoto YL, Villemure JG, Feindel W. Pharmacokinetics of 11C-labelled BCNU and SarCNU in gliomas studied by PET. J Neuro-Oncol. 1991;10(1):47–55.
8. Reif R, Wang M, Joshi S, A'Amar O, Bigio IJ. Optical method for real-time monitoring of drug concentrations facilitates the development of novel methods for drug delivery to brain tissue. J Biomed Opt. 2007;12(3):034036.
9. Dobosz M, Strobel S, Stubenrauch KG, Osl F, Scheuer W. Noninvasive measurement of pharmacokinetics by near-infrared fluorescence imaging in the eye of mice. J Biomed Opt. 2014;19(1):16022.
10. Criado E, Giron F. Jose Goyanes Capdevila, unsung pioneer of vascular surgery. Ann Vasc Surg. 2006;20(3):422–5.
11. Die-Goyanes A, Die-Trill J. Jose Goyanes. Surgeon and humanist. Cir Esp. 2008;83(1):8–11.
12. Afshar A, Steensma DP, Kyle RA. Werner Forssmann: a Pioneer of interventional cardiology and auto-experimentation. Mayo Clin Proc. 2018;93(9):e97–8.
13. Klopp CT, Smith DF, Alford TC. Palliation achieved in carcinoma of the head and neck with intra-arterial chemotherapy. Am J Surg. 1961;102:830–4.
14. Eckman WW, Patlak CS, Fenstermacher JD. A critical evaluation of the principles governing the advantages of intra-arterial infusions. J Pharmacokinet Biopharm. 1974;2(3):257–85.
15. Collins JM. Pharmacologic rationale for regional drug delivery. J Clin Oncol. 1984;2(5):498–504.
16. Dedrick RL. Interspecies scaling of regional drug delivery. J Pharm Sci. 1986;75(11):1047–52.
17. Dedrick RL. Arterial drug infusion: pharmacokinetic problems and pitfalls. J Natl Cancer Inst. 1988;80(2):84–9.
18. Dedrick RL, Oldfield EH, Collins JM. Arterial drug infusion with extracorporeal removal. I. Theoretic basis with particular reference to the brain. Cancer Treat Rep. 1984;68(2):373–80.
19. Oldfield EH, Dedrick RL, Chatterji DC, Yeager RL, Girton ME, Kornblith PL, et al. Arterial drug infusion with extracorporeal removal. II. Internal carotid carmustine in the rhesus monkey. Cancer Treat Rep. 1985;69(3):293–303.
20. Oldfield EH, Dedrick RL, Yeager RL, Clark WC, DeVroom HL, Chatterji DC, et al. Reduced systemic drug exposure by combining intra-arterial chemotherapy with hemoperfusion of regional venous drainage. J Neurosurg. 1985;63(5):726–32.
21. Rapoport SI, Hori M, Klatzo I. Reversible osmotic opening of the blood-brain barrier. Science. 1971;173(4001):1026–8.
22. Rapoport SI, Hori M, Klatzo I. Testing of a hypothesis for osmotic opening of the blood-brain barrier. Am J Phys. 1972;223(2):323–31.
23. Neuwelt EA. Reversible osmotic blood-brain barrier disruption in humans: implications for the chemotherapy of malignant brain tumors. Neurosurgery. 1980;7(2):204.
24. Neuwelt EA, Barnett PA, Ramsey FL, Hellstrom I, Hellstrom KE, McCormick CI. Dexamethasone decreases the delivery of tumor-specific monoclonal antibody to both intracerebral and subcutaneous tumor xenografts. Neurosurgery. 1993;33(3):478–84; discussion 84.
25. Neuwelt EA, Diehl JT, Vu LH, Hill SA, Michael AJ, Frenkel EP. Monitoring of methotrexate delivery in patients with malignant brain tumors after osmotic blood-brain barrier disruption. Ann Intern Med. 1981;94(4 pt 1):449–54.
26. Neuwelt EA, Pagel M, Barnett P, Glassberg M, Frenkel EP. Pharmacology and toxicity of intracarotid adriamycin admin-

istration following osmotic blood-brain barrier modification. Cancer Res. 1981;41(11 Pt 1):4466–70.
27. Rahimi SY, Brown JH, Macomson SD, Jensen MA, Alleyne CH Jr. Evolution of the treatment of cerebral vasospasm. Neurosurg Focus. 2006;20(6):E4.
28. Kaku Y, Yonekawa Y, Tsukahara T, Kazekawa K. Superselective intra-arterial infusion of papaverine for the treatment of cerebral vasospasm after subarachnoid hemorrhage. J Neurosurg. 1992;77(6):842–7.
29. del Zoppo GJ, Ferbert A, Otis S, Bruckmann H, Hacke W, Zyroff J, et al. Local intra-arterial fibrinolytic therapy in acute carotid territory stroke. A pilot study. Stroke. 1988;19(3):307–13.
30. Abou-Chebl A. Intra-arterial therapy for acute ischemic stroke. Neurotherapeutics. 2011;8(3):400–13.
31. Lewandowski CA, Frankel M, Tomsick TA, Broderick J, Frey J, Clark W, et al. Combined intravenous and intra-arterial r-TPA versus intra-arterial therapy of acute ischemic stroke: emergency management of stroke (EMS) bridging trial. Stroke. 1999;30(12):2598–605.
32. Kocharian G, Gobin YP, Kharas N, Knopman J, Francis JH, Abramson DH. Advancements in super-selective catheterization and drug selection for intra-arterial chemotherapy for retinoblastoma: a 15-year evolution. J Neurointerv Surg. 2024;16(4):398–404.
33. Napier KJ, Lidsky ME, James OG, Wildman-Tobriner B. Hepatic arterial infusion pumps: what the radiologist needs to know. Radiographics. 2021;41(3):895–908.
34. Kim JH, Kim YH, Nam HC, Kim CW, Yoo JS, Han JW, et al. Consistent efficacy of hepatic artery infusion chemotherapy irrespective of PD-L1 positivity in unresectable hepatocellular carcinoma. Oncol Lett. 2024;28(2):388.
35. Lin YS, Li S, Yang X, Guo RP, Huang YH, Bai KH, et al. First-line hepatic arterial infusion chemotherapy plus lenvatinib and PD-(L)1 inhibitors versus systemic chemotherapy alone or with PD-(L)1 inhibitors in unresectable intrahepatic cholangiocarcinoma. J Cancer Res Clin Oncol. 2024;150(6):309.
36. Wang QF, Li ZW, Zhou HF, Zhu KZ, Wang YJ, Wang YQ, et al. Predicting the prognosis of hepatic arterial infusion chemotherapy in hepatocellular carcinoma. World J Gastrointest Oncol. 2024;16(6):2380–93.
37. Wada J. A new method for the determination of the side of cerebral dominance. A preliminary report of intracarotid injection of sodium amytal in man. Igaku to Seibutsugaki. 1949;14:221–2.
38. Conradi N, Rosenberg F, Knake S, Biermann L, Haag A, Gorny I, et al. Wada test results contribute to the prediction of change in verbal learning and verbal memory function after temporal lobe epilepsy surgery. Sci Rep. 2021;11(1):10979.
39. Greig NH, Daly EM, Sweeney DJ, Rapoport SI. Pharmacokinetics of chlorambucil-tertiary butyl ester, a lipophilic chlorambucil derivative that achieves and maintains high concentrations in brain. Cancer Chemother Pharmacol. 1990;25(5):320–5.
40. Greig NH, Genka S, Daly EM, Sweeney DJ, Rapoport SI. Physicochemical and pharmacokinetic parameters of seven lipophilic chlorambucil esters designed for brain penetration. Cancer Chemother Pharmacol. 1990;25(5):311–9.
41. Saito R, Kanamori M, Sonoda Y, Yamashita Y, Nagamatsu K, Murata T, et al. Phase I trial of convection-enhanced delivery of nimustine hydrochloride (ACNU) for brainstem recurrent glioma. Neurooncol Adv. 2020;2(1):vdaa033.
42. Stevens MF, Hickman JA, Langdon SP, Chubb D, Vickers L, Stone R, et al. Antitumor activity and pharmacokinetics in mice of 8-carbamoyl-3-methyl-imidazo[5,1-d]-1,2,3,5-tetrazin-4(3H)-one (CCRG 81045; M & B 39831), a novel drug with potential as an alternative to dacarbazine. Cancer Res. 1987;47(22):5846–52.
43. Chien CY, Xu L, Yuan J, Fadera S, Stark AH, Athiraman U, et al. Quality assurance for focused ultrasound-induced blood-brain barrier opening procedure using passive acoustic detection. EBioMedicine. 2024;102:105066.
44. Candelaria PV, Leoh LS, Penichet ML, Daniels-Wells TR. Antibodies targeting the transferrin receptor 1 (TfR1) as direct anti-cancer agents. Front Immunol. 2021;12:607692.
45. Haddad AF, Young JS, Aghi MK. Using viral vectors to deliver local immunotherapy to glioblastoma. Neurosurg Focus. 2021;50(2):E4.
46. Li X, Oh JS, Lee Y, Lee EC, Yang M, Kwon N, et al. Albumin-binding photosensitizer capable of targeting glioma via the SPARC pathway. Biomater Res. 2023;27(1):23.
47. Lu W, Sun Q, Wan J, She Z, Jiang XG. Cationic albumin-conjugated pegylated nanoparticles allow gene delivery into brain tumors via intravenous administration. Cancer Res. 2006;66(24):11878–87.
48. Raju R, Abuwatfa WH, Pitt WG, Husseini GA. Liposomes for the treatment of brain cancer-a review. Pharmaceuticals (Basel). 2023;16(8):1056.
49. Morshed RA, Cheng Y, Auffinger B, Wegscheid ML, Lesniak MS. The potential of polymeric micelles in the context of glioblastoma therapy. Front Pharmacol. 2013;4:157.
50. Norouzi M. Gold nanoparticles in glioma theranostics. Pharmacol Res. 2020;156:104753.
51. Kim J, Potez M, She C, Huang P, Wu Q, Bao S, et al. Glioblastoma stem cell targeting peptide isolated through phage display binds cadherin 2. Stem Cells. 2023;41(8):762–74.
52. Casettari L, Illum L. Chitosan in nasal delivery systems for therapeutic drugs. J Control Release. 2014;190C:189–200.
53. Spinazzi EF, Argenziano MG, Upadhyayula PS, Banu MA, Neira JA, Higgins DMO, et al. Chronic convection-enhanced delivery of topotecan for patients with recurrent glioblastoma: a first-in-patient, single-centre, single-arm, phase 1b trial. Lancet Oncol. 2022;23(11):1409–18.
54. Liu CA, Liu WH, Ma HI, Chen YH, Hueng DY, Tsai WC, et al. Interstitial control-released polymer carrying a targeting small-molecule drug reduces PD-L1 and MGMT expression in recurrent high-grade gliomas with TMZ resistance. Cancers (Basel). 2022;14(4):1051.
55. Hao H, Ma Q, Huang C, He F, Yao P. Preparation, characterization, and in vivo evaluation of doxorubicin loaded BSA nanoparticles with folic acid modified dextran surface. Int J Pharm. 2013;444(1–2):77–84.
56. Nakamura J, Nakajima N, Matsumura K, Hyon SH. Water-soluble taxol conjugates with dextran and targets tumor cells by folic acid immobilization. Anticancer Res. 2010;30(3):903–9.
57. Song Y, Lou B, Zhao P, Lin C. Multifunctional disulfide-based cationic dextran conjugates for intravenous gene delivery targeting ovarian cancer cells. Mol Pharm. 2014;11(7):2250–61.
58. Wanjale MV, Sunil Jaikumar V, Sivakumar KC, Ann Paul R, James J, Kumar GSV. Supramolecular hydrogel based post-surgical implant system for hydrophobic drug delivery against glioma recurrence. Int J Nanomedicine. 2022;17:2203–24.
59. Bettag C, Hussein A, Sachkova A, Bock HC, Mielke D, Rohde V, et al. Implantation of Carmustine wafers after resection of malignant glioma with and without opening of the ventricular system. J Neurooncol. 2021;153(3):519–25.
60. Witham TF, Fukui MB, Meltzer CC, Burns R, Kondziolka D, Bozik ME. Survival of patients with high grade glioma treated with intrathecal thiotriethylenephosphoramide for ependymal or leptomeningeal gliomatosis. Cancer. 1999;86(7):1347–53.

61. Hassenbusch SJ, Anderson JH, Whiting DM. Intra-arterial chemotherapy for brain tumors. Cleve Clin J Med. 1990;57(6):513–20.
62. Hassenbusch SJ, Colvin OM, Anderson JH. Determination of nitrosourea compounds in brain tissue by gas chromatography and electron capture detection. J Pharm Sci. 1995;84(7):840–2.
63. Shin WW, Fong WF, Pang SF, Wong PC. Limited blood-brain barrier transport of polyamines. J Neurochem. 1985;44(4):1056–9.
64. Jones DR, Hall SD, Jackson EK, Branch RA, Wilkinson GR. Brain uptake of benzodiazepines: effects of lipophilicity and plasma protein binding. J Pharmacol Exp Ther. 1988;245(3):816–22.
65. Bradbury MW, Patlak CS, Oldendorf WH. Analysis of brain uptake and loss or radiotracers after intracarotid injection. Am J Phys. 1975;229(4):1110–5.
66. Winchell HS, Horst WD, Braun L, Oldendorf WH, Hattner R, Parker H. N-isopropyl-[123I] p-iodoamphetamine: single-pass brain uptake and washout; binding to brain synaptosomes; and localization in dog and monkey brain. J Nucl Med. 1980;21(10):947–52.
67. Hardebo JE, Nilsson B. Estimation of cerebral extraction of circulating compounds by the brain uptake index method: influence of circulation time, volume injection, and cerebral blood flow. Acta Physiol Scand. 1979;107(2):153–9.
68. Hassenbusch SJ, Anderson JH, Colvin OM. Predicted and actual BCNU concentrations in normal rabbit brain during intraarterial and intravenous infusions. J Neuro-Oncol. 1996;30(1):7–18.
69. Unger C, Eibl H, Engel J, Nagel GA, Eisenbrand G. Brain uptake and CNS levels of 1-(2-chloroethyl)-1-nitroso-3-(2-hydroxyethyl) urea (HECNU). Investig New Drugs. 1987;5(4):361–4.
70. Unger C, Eibl H, von Heyden HW, Kim DJ, Nagel GA. Aminoglutethimide. Penetration of the blood brain barrier. Investig New Drugs. 1986;4(3):237–40.
71. Morikawa N, Mori T, Abe T, Ghoda M, Takeyama M, Hori S. Pharmacokinetics of methotrexate in plasma and cerebrospinal fluid. Ann Pharmacother. 1997;31(10):1153–6.
72. Zylber-Katz E, Gomori JM, Schwartz A, Lossos A, Bokstein F, Siegal T. Pharmacokinetics of methotrexate in cerebrospinal fluid and serum after osmotic blood-brain barrier disruption in patients with brain lymphoma. Clin Pharmacol Ther. 2000;67(6):631–41.
73. Saris SC, Blasberg RG, Carson RE, deVroom HL, Lutz R, Dedrick RL, et al. Intravascular streaming during carotid artery infusions. Demonstration in humans and reduction using diastole-phased pulsatile administration. J Neurosurg. 1991;74(5):763–72.
74. Saris SC, Wright DC, Oldfield EH, Blasberg RG. Intravascular streaming and variable delivery to brain following carotid artery infusions in the Sprague-Dawley rat. J Cereb Blood Flow Metab. 1988;8(1):116–20.
75. Blacklock JB, Wright DC, Dedrick RL, Blasberg RG, Lutz RJ, Doppman JL, et al. Drug streaming during intra-arterial chemotherapy. J Neurosurg. 1986;64:284–91.
76. Lassen NA, Palvolgyi R. Cerebral steal during hypercapnia and the inverse reaction during hypocapnia observed by the ^{133}Xenon technique in man (Abstract). Scand J Lab Clin Invest Suppl. 1968;102:XIII-D.
77. Olesen J, Paulson OB, Lassen NA. Regional cerebral blood flow in man determined by the initial slope of the clearance of intra-arterially injected ^{133}Xe: theory of the method, normal values, error of measurement, correction for remaining radioactivity, relation to other flow parameters and response to $PaCO_2$ changes. Stroke. 1971;2:519–40.
78. Young WL, Prohovnik I, Ornstein E, Lucas LR, Wang TST, Correll JW, et al. Rapid monitoring of intraoperative cerebral blood flow using ^{133}Xe. J Cereb Blood Flow Metab. 1988;8(5):691–6.
79. Young WL, Prohovnik I, Schroeder T, Correll JW, Ostapkovich N. Intraoperative ^{133}Xe cerebral blood flow measurements by intravenous *versus* intracarotid methods. Anesthesiology. 1990;73:637–43.
80. Young WL, Solomon RA, Prohovnik I, Ornstein E, Weinstein J, Stein BM. ^{133}Xe blood flow monitoring during arteriovenous malformation resection: a case of intraoperative hyperperfusion with subsequent brain swelling. Neurosurgery. 1988;22(4):765–9.
81. Young WL, Pile-Spellman J, Prohovnik I, Kader A, Stein BM. Evidence for adaptive autoregulatory displacement in hypotensive cortical territories adjacent to arteriovenous malformations. Columbia University AVM Study Project. Neurosurgery. 1994;34(4):601–10; discussion 10–11.
82. Joshi S, Young WL, Pile-Spellman J, Duong DH, Vang MC, Hacein-Bey L, et al. The feasibility of intracarotid adenosine for the manipulation of human cerebrovascular resistance. Anesth Analg. 1998;87(6):1291–8.
83. Joshi S, Duong H, Mangla S, Wang M, Libow AD, Popilskis SJ, et al. In nonhuman primates intracarotid adenosine, but not sodium nitroprusside, increases cerebral blood flow. Anesth Analg. 2002;94(2):393–9, table of contents.
84. Joshi S, Mangla S, Wang M, Sciacca RR, Young WL. Intra-arterial 133Xe measurements suggest a dose-dependent increase in cerebral blood flow during intracarotid infusion of adenosine in nonhuman primates. J Neurosurg Anesthesiol. 2002;14(2):108–13.
85. Jenkins R, Lemire C, Altamirano-Lamarque F, Orbach DB, Vanderveen D, Shah AS, et al. Complications of intra-arterial chemotherapy (IAC) for retinoblastoma: an updated, comprehensive review. American Academy of Ophthalmology; 2023 [updated 24 Aug 2023]. https://www.aao.org/education/disease-review/complications-of-intra-arterial-chemotherapy-iac-r.
86. Wang M, Joshi S, Emerson RG. Comparison of intracarotid and intravenous propofol for electrocerebral silence in rabbits. Anesthesiology. 2003;99(4):904–10.
87. Joshi S, Wang M, Etu J, Nishanian EV. Comparison of intracarotid anesthetics for EEG silence. J Neurosurg Anesthesiol. 2006;18(2):112–8.
88. Joshi S, Wang M, Etu JJ, Nishanian EV, Pile-Spellman J. Cerebral blood flow affects dose requirements of intracarotid propofol for electrocerebral silence. Anesthesiology. 2006;104(2):290–8, discussion 5A.
89. Joshi S, Wang M, Etu JJ, Pile-Spellman J. Bolus configuration affects dose requirements of intracarotid propofol for electroencephalographic silence. Anesth Analg. 2006;102(6):1816–22.
90. Wang M, Joshi S. Electrocerebral silence after intracarotid propofol injection is a function of transit time. Anesth Analg. 2007;104(6):1498–503, table of contents.
91. Mourant JR, Bigio IJ, Boyer J, Conn RL, Johnson T, Shimada T. Spectroscopic diagnosis of bladder cancer with elastic light scattering. Lasers Surg Med. 1995;17(4):350–7.
92. Mourant JR, Bigio IJ, Jack DA, Johnson TM, Miller HD. Measuring absorption coefficients in small volumes of highly scattering media: source-detector separations for which path lengths do not depend on scattering properties. Appl Opt. 1997;36(22):5655–61.
93. Mourant JR, Fuselier T, Boyer J, Johnson TM, Bigio IJ. Predictions and measurements of scattering and absorption over broad wavelength ranges in tissue phantoms. Appl Opt. 1997;36(4):949–57.
94. Bigio IJ, Mourant JR, Los G. Noninvasive, in-situ measurement of drug concentrations in tissue using optical spectroscopy. J Gravit Physiol. 1999;6(1):P173–5.
95. Eyre JA, Essex TJ, Flecknell PA, Bartholomew PH, Sinclair JI. A comparison of measurements of cerebral blood flow in the rabbit using laser Doppler spectroscopy and radionuclide labelled microspheres. Clin Phys Physiol Meas. 1988;9(1):65–74.
96. Skarphedinsson JO, Harding H, Thoren P. Repeated measurements of cerebral blood flow in rats. Comparisons between the hydrogen clearance method and laser Doppler flowmetry. Acta Physiol Scand. 1988;134(1):133–42.

97. Odor TM, Pitt Ford TR, McDonald F. Effect of wavelength and bandwidth on the clinical reliability of laser Doppler recordings. Endod Dent Traumatol. 1996;12(1):9–15.
98. Joshi S, Cooke JR, Chan DK, Ellis JA, Hossain SS, Singh-Moon RP, et al. Liposome size and charge optimization for intraarterial delivery to gliomas. Drug Deliv Transl Res. 2016;6(3):225–33.
99. Joshi S, Cooke JRN, Ellis JA, Emala CW, Bruce JN. Targeting brain tumors by intra-arterial delivery of cell-penetrating peptides: a novel approach for primary and metastatic brain malignancy. J Neurooncol. 2017;135(3):497–506.
100. Joshi S, Singh-Moon R, Wang M, Chaudhuri DB, Ellis JA, Bruce JN, et al. Cationic surface charge enhances early regional deposition of liposomes after intracarotid injection. J Neurooncol. 2014;120(3):489–97.
101. Joshi S, Singh-Moon RP, Ellis JA, Chaudhuri DB, Wang M, Reif R, et al. Cerebral hypoperfusion-assisted intra-arterial deposition of liposomes in normal and glioma-bearing rats. Neurosurgery. 2015;76(1):92–100.
102. Joshi S, Singh-Moon RP, Wang M, Chaudhuri DB, Holcomb M, Straubinger NL, et al. Transient cerebral hypoperfusion assisted intraarterial cationic liposome delivery to brain tissue. J Neurooncol. 2014;118(1):73–82.
103. Nguyen J, Cooke JR, Ellis JA, Deci M, Emala CW, Bruce JN, et al. Cationizable lipid micelles as vehicles for intraarterial glioma treatment. J Neurooncol. 2016;128(1):21–8.
104. Simonsen JB, Kromann EB. Pitfalls and opportunities in quantitative fluorescence-based nanomedicine studies—a commentary. J Control Release. 2021;335:660–7.
105. Singh-Moon RP, Roblyer DM, Bigio IJ, Joshi S. Spatial mapping of drug delivery to brain tissue using hyperspectral spatial frequency-domain imaging. J Biomed Opt. 2014;19(9):96003.
106. Motlagh NS, Parvin P, Ghasemi F, Atyabi F. Fluorescence properties of several chemotherapy drugs: doxorubicin, paclitaxel and bleomycin. Biomed Opt Express. 2016;7(6):2400–6.
107. Escobedo JO, Rusin O, Lim S, Strongin RM. NIR dyes for bioimaging applications. Curr Opin Chem Biol. 2010;14(1):64–70.
108. Liu P, Mu X, Zhang XD, Ming D. The near-infrared-II fluorophores and advanced microscopy technologies development and application in bioimaging. Bioconjug Chem. 2020;31(2):260–75.
109. Joshi S, Reif R, Wang M, Zhang J, Ergin A, Bruce JN, et al. Intra-arterial mitoxantrone delivery in rabbits: an optical pharmacokinetic study. Neurosurgery. 2011;69(3):706–12; discussion 12.
110. Ergin A, Wang M, Zhang J, Bigio I, Joshi S. Noninvasive in vivo optical assessment of blood brain barrier permeability and brain tissue drug deposition in rabbits. J Biomed Opt. 2012;17(5):057008.
111. Joshi S, Wang M, Etu JJ, Suckow RF, Cooper TB, Feinmark SJ, et al. Transient cerebral hypoperfusion enhances intraarterial carmustine deposition into brain tissue. J Neuro-Oncol. 2008;86(2):123–32.
112. Spronk E, Sykes G, Falcione S, Munsterman D, Joy T, Kamtchum-Tatuene J, et al. Hemorrhagic transformation in ischemic stroke and the role of inflammation. Front Neurol. 2021;12:661955.
113. Pile-Spellman J, Young WL, Joshi S, Duong H, Vang MC, Hartmann A, et al. Adenosine-induced cardiac pause for endovascular embolization of cerebral arteriovenous malformations: technical case report. Neurosurgery. 1999;44(4):881–6; discussion 6–7.
114. Hashimoto T, Young WL, Aagaard BD, Joshi S, Ostapkovich ND, Pile-Spellman J. Adenosine-induced ventricular asystole to induce transient profound systemic hypotension in patients undergoing endovascular therapy: dose-response characteristics [in process citation]. Anesthesiology. 2000;93(4):998–1001.
115. Riina HA, Burkhardt JK, Santillan A, Bassani L, Patsalides A, Boockvar JA. Short-term clinico-radiographic response to superselective intra-arterial cerebral infusion of bevacizumab for the treatment of vestibular schwannomas in Neurofibromatosis type 2. Interv Neuroradiol. 2012;18(2):127–32.
116. Riina HA, Fraser JF, Fralin S, Knopman J, Scheff RJ, Boockvar JA. Superselective intraarterial cerebral infusion of bevacizumab: a revival of interventional neuro-oncology for malignant glioma. J Exp Ther Oncol. 2009;8(2):145–50.
117. Ergin A, Joshi S, Wang M, Bigio I, editors. Retention of indocyanine green as a potential marker for optical detection of blood brain barrier disruption. SPIE; 2011.
118. Ergin A, Wang M, Zhang JY, Bruce JN, Fine RL, Bigio IJ, et al. The feasibility of real-time in vivo optical detection of blood-brain barrier disruption with indocyanine green. J Neuro-Oncol. 2012;106(3):551–60.
119. Joshi S, Ergin A, Wang M, Reif R, Zhang J, Bruce JN, et al. Inconsistent blood brain barrier disruption by intraarterial mannitol in rabbits: implications for chemotherapy. J Neurooncol. 2011;104:11.
120. Nguyen J, Hossain SS, Cooke JRN, Ellis JA, Deci MB, Emala CW, et al. Flow arrest intra-arterial delivery of small TAT-decorated and neutral micelles to gliomas. J Neurooncol. 2017;133:77.
121. Sharma US, Sharma A, Chau RI, Straubinger RM. Liposome-mediated therapy of intracranial brain tumors in a rat model. Pharm Res. 1997;14(8):992–8.
122. Dobrzynska I, Skrzydlewska E, Figaszewski ZA. Changes in electric properties of human breast cancer cells. J Membr Biol. 2013;246(2):161–6.
123. Dobrzynska I, Szachowicz-Petelska B, Darewicz B, Figaszewski ZA. Characterization of human bladder cell membrane during cancer transformation. J Membr Biol. 2015;248(2):301–7.
124. Dobrzynska I, Szachowicz-Petelska B, Sulkowski S, Figaszewski Z. Changes in electric charge and phospholipids composition in human colorectal cancer cells. Mol Cell Biochem. 2005;276(1–2):113–9.
125. Chen B, Le W, Wang Y, Li Z, Wang D, Ren L, et al. Targeting negative surface charges of cancer cells by multifunctional nanoprobes. Theranostics. 2016;6(11):1887–98.
126. Sarkar G, Curran GL, Sarkaria JN, Lowe VJ, Jenkins RB. Peptide carrier-mediated non-covalent delivery of unmodified cisplatin, methotrexate and other agents via intravenous route to the brain. PLoS One. 2014;9(5):e97655.
127. Drin G, Cottin S, Blanc E, Rees AR, Temsamani J. Studies on the internalization mechanism of cationic cell-penetrating peptides. J Biol Chem. 2003;278(33):31192–201.
128. Herce HD, Garcia AE. Molecular dynamics simulations suggest a mechanism for translocation of the HIV-1 TAT peptide across lipid membranes. Proc Natl Acad Sci U S A. 2007;104(52):20805–10.
129. Cooke J, Joshi S. Optical Pharmacokinetics of Intraarterial Delivery of Cy5 labeled Cell Penetrating Peptide- TAT to 9 L Brain Tumors. J Neurosurg Anesth. 2019;31(4):462.
130. Kurnaeva MA, Zalevsky AO, Arifulin EA, Lisitsyna OM, Tvorogova AV, Shubina MY, et al. Molecular coevolution of nuclear and nucleolar localization signals inside basic domain of HIV-1 Tat. bioRxiv. 2021:2021.04.20.440437.
131. Jones RB. Clinical pharmacology of melphalan and its implications for clinical resistance to anticancer agents. Cancer Treat Res. 2002;112:305–22.
132. Pekacka A. The role of intraarterial chemotherapy in the management of retinoblastoma. J Ophthalmol. 2020;2020:3638410.
133. Regberg J, Srimanee A, Langel U. Applications of cell-penetrating peptides for tumor targeting and future cancer therapies. Pharmaceuticals (Basel). 2012;5(9):991–1007.
134. Shi NQ, Gao W, Xiang B, Qi XR. Enhancing cellular uptake of activable cell-penetrating peptide-doxorubicin conjugate by enzymatic cleavage. Int J Nanomedicine. 2012;7:1613–21.

135. Guo QQ, Wang HY, Zhao YX, Wang HX, Zeng F, Hua HY, et al. Cell-penetrating albumin conjugates for enhanced doxorubicin delivery. Polym Chem UK. 2013;4(17):4584–7.
136. Yang Y, Wang S, Wang Y, Wang X, Wang Q, Chen M. Advances in self-assembled chitosan nanomaterials for drug delivery. Biotechnol Adv. 2014;32:1301.
137. Bilensoy E, Sarisozen C, Esendagli G, Dogan AL, Aktas Y, Sen M, et al. Intravesical cationic nanoparticles of chitosan and polycaprolactone for the delivery of Mitomycin C to bladder tumors. Int J Pharm. 2009;371(1–2):170–6.
138. Schmid B, Chung DE, Warnecke A, Fichtner I, Kratz F. Albumin-binding prodrugs of camptothecin and doxorubicin with an Ala-Leu-Ala-Leu-linker that are cleaved by cathepsin B: synthesis and antitumor efficacy. Bioconjug Chem. 2007;18(3):702–16.
139. Chung DE, Kratz F. Development of a novel albumin-binding prodrug that is cleaved by urokinase-type-plasminogen activator (uPA). Bioorg Med Chem Lett. 2006;16(19):5157–63.
140. Warnecke A, Fichtner I, Sass G, Kratz F. Synthesis, cleavage profile, and antitumor efficacy of an albumin-binding prodrug of methotrexate that is cleaved by plasmin and cathepsin B. Arch Pharm. 2007;340(8):389–95.
141. Agudelo D, Bourassa P, Bruneau J, Berube G, Asselin E, Tajmir-Riahi HA. Probing the binding sites of antibiotic drugs doxorubicin and N-(trifluoroacetyl) doxorubicin with human and bovine serum albumins. PLoS One. 2012;7(8):e43814.
142. Abbasi S, Paul A, Shao W, Prakash S. Cationic albumin nanoparticles for enhanced drug delivery to treat breast cancer: preparation and in vitro assessment. J Drug Deliv. 2012;2012:686108.
143. Bolling C, Graefe T, Lubbing C, Jankevicius F, Uktveris S, Cesas A, et al. Phase II study of MTX-HSA in combination with cisplatin as first line treatment in patients with advanced or metastatic transitional cell carcinoma. Invest New Drug. 2006;24(6):521–7.
144. Sun C, Veiseh O, Gunn J, Fang C, Hansen S, Lee D, et al. In vivo MRI detection of gliomas by chlorotoxin-conjugated superparamagnetic nanoprobes. Small. 2008;4(3):372–9.

Robotics in Neurointervention

21

Amir M. Molaie, Naoki Kaneko, Satoshi Tateshima, and Charles Beaman

Machines were devised not to do a man out of a job, but to take the heavy labor from man's back and place it on the broad back of the machine.

Henry Ford (1863–1947), American Engineer and Futurist

Introduction

Neurointervention refers to the endovascular treatment of vascular disorders affecting the brain and spine. The field has witnessed remarkable growth in recent years, expanding to treat an ever-broadening list of neurovascular diseases. Recently published trials have broadened the eligibility criteria for thrombectomy in stroke [1–3], while ongoing device innovations have revolutionized catheter-based treatment for complex aneurysms [4]. Even in disease processes previously thought amenable only to open surgical treatment, such as subdural hematomas, endovascular approaches are now being explored and show favorable potential [5, 6].

As the volume of these procedures escalates, optimizing practice patterns in all aspects of care becomes increasingly crucial, from technical issues such as operator safety and tool precision to patient care individually and across communities. Particularly in the treatment of acute ischemic stroke, where endovascular thrombectomy is now the standard of care, ensuring access to this lifesaving therapy is a principal goal. Earlier time to treatment is known to be associated with better outcomes [7], and even delays of 15 min can increase the risk of poor outcomes [8]. However, in the USA, only 20% of the population lives within 15 min of a thrombectomy-capable center, and only 30% are within 30 min [9]. The implementation of telestroke has decreased door-to-needle times and rates of death and dependency and is a step in the right direction [10, 11]. Applying this concept to thrombectomy may be the next frontier in decreasing the time needed for endovascular treatment.

Physician safety is also an important consideration. The occupational hazards of working as an interventionalist have been known for many years; however, there is alarming data to suggest these risks are more significant than once thought. A nationwide cohort of radiologic technologists revealed an increased risk of brain cancer, breast cancer, and skin cancer (both melanoma and nonmelanoma) among technologists who worked in fluoroscopy [12, 13]. Furthermore, in a cohort of interventionalists with brain tumors, a disproportionately high number had left-sided lesions [14, 15]. Another study revealed a higher burden of subclinical atherosclerosis, measured by carotid intima-media thickness on ultrasound, in high radiation-exposed workers, further noting a correlation between left-sided carotid intima-media thickness and higher "radiation risk" scores [16]. Compared to controls, interventional cardiologists also had a higher risk of developing radiation-induced cataracts [17]. Even a single procedure alone has been shown to cause measurable changes in DNA damage response markers in the circulating lymphocytes of operators [18]. Aside from radiation-related hazards, operators also suffer from higher rates of orthopedic injuries due to long hours donning lead aprons in suboptimal ergonomic conditions [19]. Lastly, in the era of COVID-19, it is relevant to consider the risks of microbial transmission to staff operating near afflicted patients if future pandemics arise. As the hours in the angiosuite continue to grow, measures will need to be taken to alleviate some of these risks to ensure the long-

A. M. Molaie
Department of Neurology, David Geffen School of Medicine at UCLA, Los Angeles, CA, USA
e-mail: Amolaie@mednet.ucla.edu

N. Kaneko · S. Tateshima · C. Beaman (✉)
Division of Interventional Neuroradiology, David Geffen School of Medicine at UCLA, Los Angeles, CA, USA
e-mail: Nkaneko@mednet.ucla.edu; Stateshima@mednet.ucla.edu

S. Joshi (ed.), *Arterial Treatment of Neurological Diseases*, https://doi.org/10.1007/978-3-031-80173-0_21

term health of physicians, technologists, nurses, and staff. The integration of robotic technology stands to offer a promising solution to address these concerns.

This chapter aims to provide a comprehensive overview of the latest breakthroughs in robotic neurointerventional procedures. From robot-assisted catheter navigation systems to automated imaging analysis, we will explore cutting-edge technologies reshaping how we approach the treatment of neurovascular pathologies. Moreover, we will delve into the potential implications of these advancements on patient care, clinical outcomes, and the future of neurointervention.

Robotics in Surgery

When discussing medical robots, it has been proposed to categorize them into varying levels of autonomy to allow for precise regulatory, ethical, and legal discussions. One model classifies robots into six categories, ranging from no autonomy (*Level 0*) to full automation (*Level 5*) [20]. The technology we discuss below belongs to *Level 0*, which describes directly manipulated robots and telerobotic functions. *Level 1* invokes some robotic assistance, while the operator retains continuous control (e.g., *virtual fixtures*). At *Level 2*, task automation takes place (e.g., *suturing*). *Level 3* and *4* systems are progressively more independent, with robots in the latter expected to make medical decisions under the supervision of a physician, while at *Level 5*, no humans are needed. More practically, surgical robotic systems can be divided into three categories: active, semiautonomous, or surgeon-driven [21, 22]. *Surgeon-driven* systems lack preprogramming and constitute the majority of medical robots, which are under the complete control of the operator. *Semi-active* systems take automation one step further and utilize some preprogramming, whereas *active* systems are fully preprogrammed and work autonomously.

Brief History

Robotic technologies were first employed in modern surgical practice in the late 1980s. The first robotic procedures are credited to orthopedic surgeons in Canada who used their "Arthrobot" to aid in positioning limbs [23] and a neurosurgeon in the USA who used the PUMA 560 robotic system to position the biopsy cannula precisely [24]. These were followed in short succession by using similar systems in other domains, such as the PROBOT in transurethral resection of the prostate [25]. Ultimately, the US military foresaw an opportunity to develop telesystems to improve battlefield care, and supporting collaboration between researchers at Stanford and NASA sparked an acceleration in surgical robotic development. Through this partnership, the AESOP (*Automated Endoscopic System for Optimal Positioning*) telemanipulator platform was developed, allowing control of a traditional laparoscope via foot pedal and later voice command [21]. This was then modified to the better known ZEUS robotic system, which was approved by the FDA in 2001. Contemporaneously, the da Vinci platform was developed and FDA-approved in 2000 and has since dominated the surgical field, with the number of procedures performed worldwide surpassing 10 million in 2021 [26]. The advantages touted by advocates of the da Vinci system include augmented surgical dexterity, superior high-definition vision, and obvious ergonomic benefits [27]. The technology to manipulate surgical devices precisely through narrow ports is relevant to neurointervention applications, but it is not currently being effectively utilized.

Vascular Interventional Robotic Systems

When envisioning robotic applications to neurovascular care, one can consider the exploration of two frontiers: (1) the transformation of neurovascular devices to robotic platforms or (2) the creation of robotic systems that control conventional endovascular devices. Regarding the former, the primary obstacle in creating robotic or self-navigating catheters for neurointervention is the miniaturization of robotic devices that navigate through the narrow and tortuous neurovasculature. During conventional catheter angiography, a guidewire is manually shaped and oriented to a desired direction to guide a catheter to the desired location. Once suitably shaped, the guidewire is torqued at the proximal end to engage the target. Indeed, steering the catheter tip around sharp turns or into geometrically complex spaces, such as aneurysms, can be laborious, particularly when navigating in distal territories [28]. Creating steerable devices is an active area of research [29, 30]. However, miniaturizing these devices to the submillimeter scale is challenging using standard actuation mechanisms that pull mechanical wires or use embedded rigid magnets [28, 31, 32]. Some groups have defied this conventional approach. For example, Gopesh et al. constructed a steerable tip microcatheter using hydraulically actuated hyperelastic polymers at the distal ends [28]. Furthermore, several innovators have capitalized on magnetic technologies to rethink robotic devices [32, 33], which we will discuss below. However, considering the obstacles in shrinking robotic fabrication schemes, the industry has generally focused on developing robotic platforms that can manipulate conventional guidewires and catheters under remote control.

As we delve into the mechanics of these modern-day robotic systems, it is helpful to first consider the conceptual task at hand. An endovascular robotic system must integrate mechanisms for sensing, tool clamping, and actuation (*the production of rotary or linear motion*). These actions are driven by a separate user interface that controls the system [34]. As such, a typical setup is two-pronged, combining a remote cockpit containing the control panel (*leader device*) with a patient-side robotic arm that physically manipulates the catheters and wires using linear and rotational drive motors (*follower device*) [35]. The cockpit is radiation-shielded, equipped with multiple display monitors and a control device connected to the bedside robot wirelessly or through an electronic cable (Fig. 21.1). Having explored the fundamental conceptual framework of endovascular robotic systems, we now focus on the specific components that make these systems function. We examine the actuation mechanisms essential to understanding how these robotic systems translate human commands into mechanical actions.

Actuation Mechanisms

Understanding the details of the patient- and operator-side processes is essential for an in-depth review. In conventional catheter angiography, the surgeon uses delicate maneuvers to advance, retract, and twist the wire or catheter between the forefinger and thumb. Similarly, a robotic actuation system must have the ability to clamp, translate, and rotate tools to produce both axial and rotatory motion. To date, three driver mechanisms are primarily employed to achieve *axial* motion: friction roller-based motion, clamp-based sliding motion, or magnetic navigation (Fig. 21.1). The generation of *rotary* motion typically involves friction wheels or a rotating clamp.

For axial motion, a *friction roller-based* mechanism implements a friction roller by pressing the wire against another roller or a capstan, propelling it forward and backward. In contrast, a *clamp-based* mechanism uses a holder

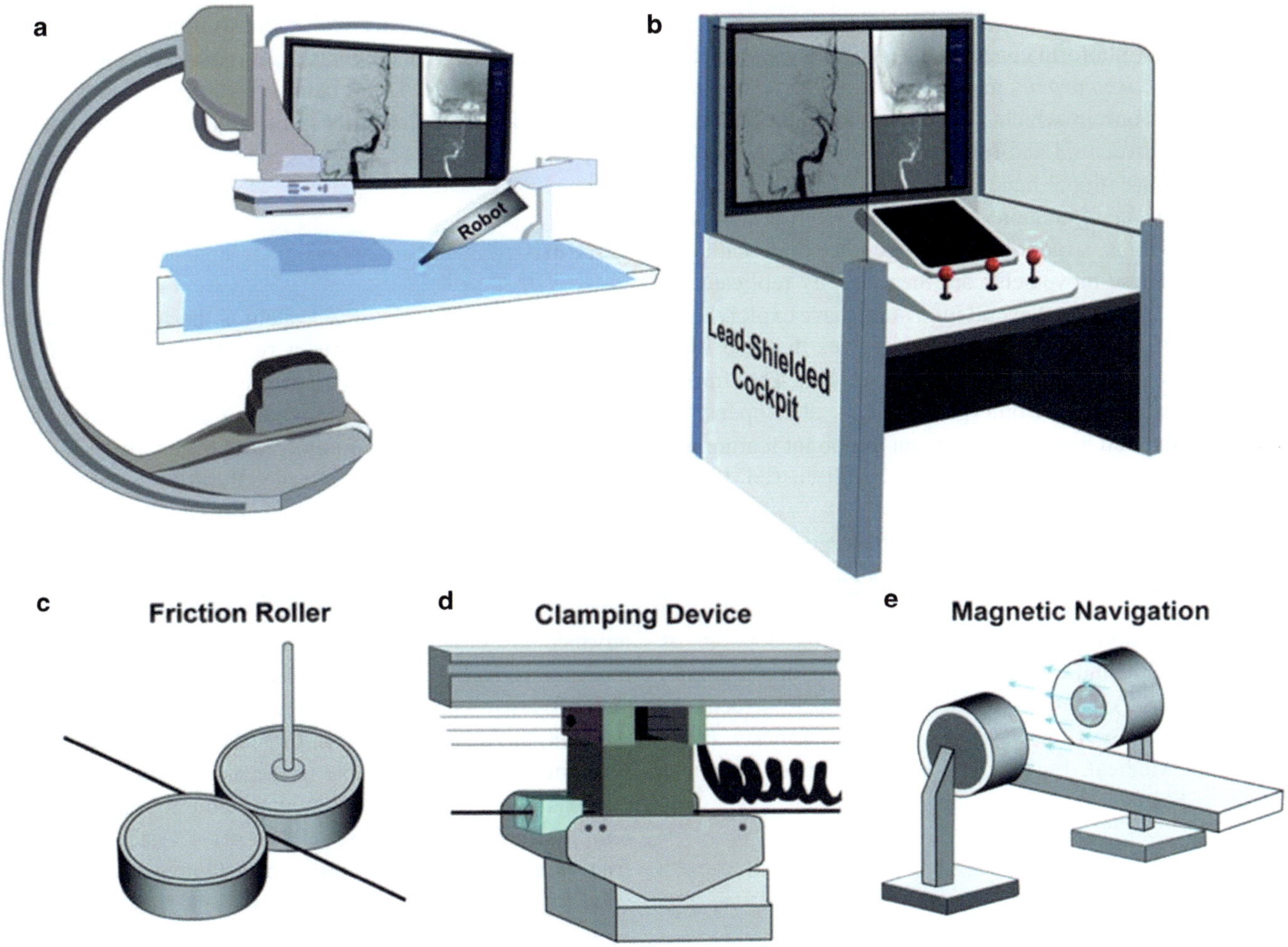

Fig. 21.1 Robotic system overview and common actuation mechanisms. (**a**) Patient-side robot with articulating arm. (**b**) Lead-shielded cockpit with monitors and controls. (**c**) Friction roller drive mechanism. (**d**) Clamping device mechanism. (**e**) Magnetic navigation system. (*Reprinted with permission from Beaman et al.* [35]. *Copyright American Journal of Neuroradiology*)

module to grasp the wire and a linear actuator to drive the wire linearly along a slider rail. After each stroke, the slider rail returns to the home position, allowing for continued translation. A clamp holding the wire can be positioned on a rotating wheel to achieve wire rotation, typically driven by gears and belts. Alternatively, two friction wheels can clinch a wire and act analogously to two fingers, moving up and down in opposite directions to rotate the wire. Each of these mechanisms has advantages and disadvantages; for example, friction roller-based drivers are prone to slippage between the friction wheel and the catheter or guidewire, and sliding drivers risk damaging tools with the force of clamping. Some authors have invented workarounds, such as a hybrid translation mechanism utilizing a friction roller and sliding components [36] or grouping multiple friction wheels to avoid slippage [37].

Controller Platforms

Two controller platform concepts have been devised for tool manipulation: *isomorphic* and *non-isomorphic*. An *isomorphic* setup is one in which the control and output devices have similar structural and functional designs. The operator simulates conventional hand movements and natural catheter/guidewire manipulation techniques upon the control device, which is structurally homogenous to a catheter/guidewire. These movements are then directly replicated in the patient-side device. Several innovators have explored this approach [38, 39] and have created devices that use force feedback to produce flexible clamping [40]. The further development of these isomorphic designs also opens the door for improved haptic feedback, an important feature that limits current technology and will be discussed further below.

Non-isomorphic designs represent the majority of control systems in use today. Here, there is a distinct difference between the structure and form of the control interface and the bedside robotic platform. For example, the cockpits of the CorPath 200 and CorPath GRX systems (Corindus, Inc., Waltham, USA) contain joysticks and touch screens to manipulate tools. Other systems like the Liberty robot (Microbot Medical, Inc., MA, USA) implement handheld remote controls.

Early Robotic Systems

The first type of robot described in endovascular literature dates back to the early 2000s. Drawing from surgeons' experience applying telemanipulation to surgical instruments, innovators in endovascular therapy developed a prototype non-isomorphic telesystem to drive and manipulate catheters using rollers controlled by a distant joystick [41]. Several years later, the Sensei robotic navigation system (Hansen Medical, Inc., CA, USA) was unveiled as one of the first commercially available robots. The system was FDA-approved in 2007 and initially designed to facilitate catheter positioning in cardiac ablations [42]. It used an electromechanical tendon-driven mechanism to steer the tip of its custom guide catheter. The rigidity of this system raised concerns for complication risks, leading to the development of its next-generation system, Magellan (Hansen Medical, Inc., CA, USA) [43]. The Magellan robotic system used a similar steering mechanism in the distal coaxial tip of custom-made 6Fr, 9Fr, and 10Fr robotic catheters [44]. It was FDA-approved in 2012 for peripheral vascular interventions and has since been used clinically in thousands of peripheral cases, including carotid artery stenting [45]. However, the exceptionally high cost of acquiring the system and using proprietary catheters limited its use. The Amigo remote catheter system (Catheter Precision, Inc., NJ, USA) is another electromechanical robot similar to Sensei and Magellan but is guided by a handheld remote control. It was FDA-approved in 2012 for cardiac electrophysiology procedures, but its use is generally limited by its cumbersome size [43].

CorPath

Currently, the CorPath GRX system is the most widespread robotic system. It comprises a remote, radiation-shielded workstation and a table-side robotic unit [46]. The cockpit has a touch screen control console, three joysticks, and a high-definition display monitor, which can display up to eight images from live or reference fluoroscopy and patient vital signs. The system tracks the proximal movement of devices, showing their linear movements on the touch screen with 0.1-mm resolution. Using either forward/backward or rotational adjustments of the joystick, the operator can advance or retract the guidewire in 1-mm increments or torque it as desired. The operator can also shift from the joysticks to arrows on the touch screen console to perform steps requiring high precision for millimetric control. The cockpit is connected through a cable to the patient-side unit, which consists of an articulating robotic arm, the robotic drive system, and a single-use cassette. The drive system combines friction and rotary wheels for catheter/guidewire movement (Fig. 21.2).

Magnetic Navigation

The technology for *magnetically guided* devices has existed for decades [48]. The Niobe magnetic navigation system

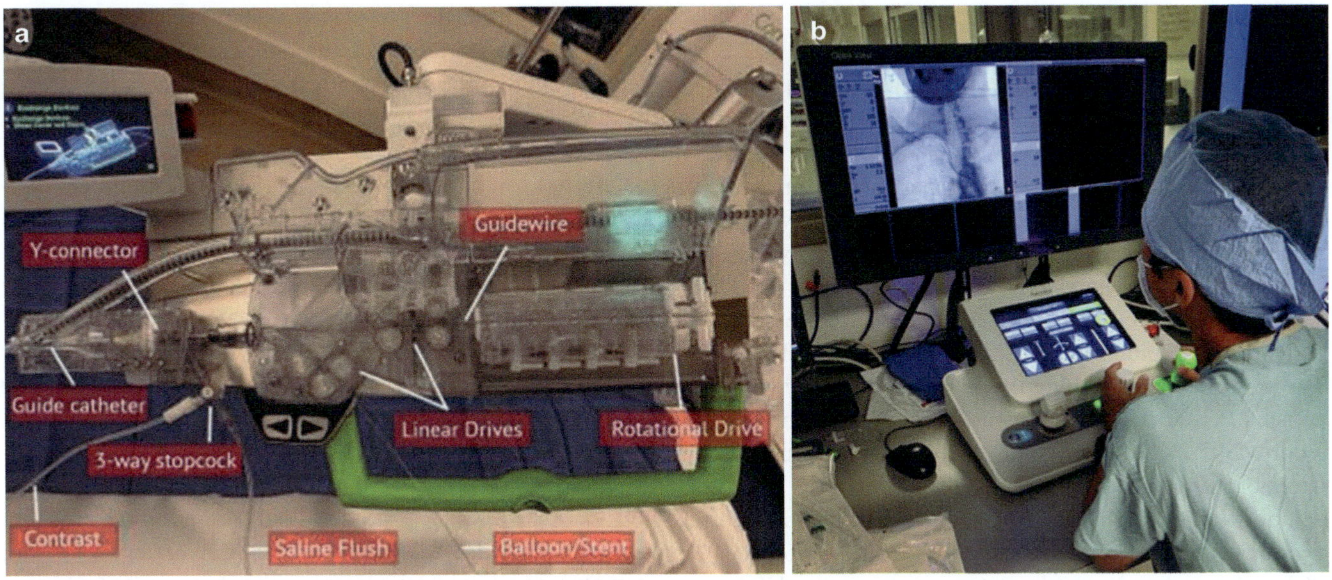

Fig. 21.2 The CorPath GRX robotic platform. (**a**) The patient-side unit comprises an articulating robotic arm, a robotic drive system, and a single-use cassette. (*Reprinted with permission from Narsinh et al.* [47]. *Copyright SAGE Publications*). (**b**) The cockpit with a touch screen control console, three joysticks, and a high-definition display monitor. (*Reprinted with permission from Beaman et al.* [35]. *Copyright American Journal of Neuroradiology*)

(Stereotaxis, St. Louis, USA) was an early robotic system introduced in 2002 for cardiac radiofrequency ablation [47]. Here, patients were situated between magnets that generated a magnetic field to navigate a catheter remotely with three magnets embedded in the distal segment. However, these magnet-tipped guidewires were bulky and immobile, and the large magnets that flanked the patient limited C-arm angulation [49]. Since then, magnetic technology has significantly advanced: Kim et al. recently described a novel robotic system comprising a magnetically steerable, flexible ferromagnetic guidewire, a robotic arm equipped with an actuating magnet for steering the guidewire, and a series of motorized linear drives to facilitate the advancement and retraction of the guidewire/microcatheter [31]. The team employed their system for aneurysm coil embolization and thrombectomy in a neurovascular model. Further, it demonstrated the system's steering and navigational capabilities using a porcine brachial artery tortuosity model. The authors' magnetic guidewire was based on their previous work on *ferromagnetic soft materials*, wherein magnetizable microparticles are uniformly dispersed in soft polymeric matrices, acting as distributed actuation sources, allowing for miniaturization to submillimeter scales [33]—effectively remedying the difficulties mentioned above of robotic miniaturization. A Zurich-based company, Nanoflex Robotics (Zurich, CHE), recently developed a robotic system designed explicitly for neurointervention that utilizes a compact, mobile magnetic field generator to precisely navigate guidewires and catheters through tortuous vascular anatomy [50]. As a proof of concept, surgeons at the Mayo Clinic in Arizona recently used the Nanoflex remote magnetic navigation system to perform a mechanical thrombectomy on a phantom vascular model in Zurich, Switzerland [51]. The company recently announced upcoming plans for first-in-human trials.

Pancaldi et al. also recently reexamined magnetic actuation, developing magnetically steerable ultra-flexible flow-driven microscopic probes [32]. In this model, magnetic forces exert torque on the distal head of the device, which interacts with the flow so that the chosen trajectory is taken. Microprobes potentially allow for catheterization of deeper and more distal vessels previously inaccessible to traditional catheterization. One step further, Xie and colleagues developed magnetic soft microrobots that deliver and release thrombolytic drugs via magneto-collective control [52]. Similarly, one could imagine using micro- or nanorobotic drug delivery systems [53] to transport neuroprotective agents to stroke targets [54] or even for other indications in neurointervention, such as embolization with particles, liquid embolic, or glue. The Missouri-based company *Euphrates Vascular* (St. Louis, MO, USA) recently started an in-human early feasibility clinical trial testing iron oxide-based magnetic microbeads in helping guide tissue plasminogen activator (t-PA) in reaching more distal occlusions [55]. We delve further into the possibilities of magnet-based microrobotics in later sections. Though promising, the disadvantage of magnetic systems generally includes the necessity to employ specialized tools and machinery incompatible with today's standard equipment.

Clinical Use

Cardiologists and peripheral vascular interventionalists laid the groundwork for the clinical execution of robot-assisted procedures. Beginning in 2006, Beyar et al. proved the safety and feasibility of percutaneous coronary intervention (PCI) using an experimental robotic model (the Remote Navigation System, RNS, NaviCath, Haifa, Israel), which served as the basis for the development of the CorPath robot [56]. The CorPath 200 system was utilized in a small case series of patients undergoing PCI [57]. In 2013, the PRECISE study was published, establishing the safety and efficacy of robot-assisted PCI in a large multicenter cohort [58]. The authors reported 95.2% lower radiation exposure for the primary operator than traditional methods. The RAPID trial followed, demonstrating safety and efficacy in peripheral arterial revascularization [59]. CorPath GRX is FDA-approved for PCI and peripheral vascular interventions in the USA and many countries abroad.

Interestingly, the use of magnetism in neuroendovascular therapy dates back to the 1960s, when a magnetic catheter was used to catheterize the middle cerebral artery from a percutaneous puncture of the carotid artery in the neck of a patient, just 5 years after the first superselective catheterization of intracranial vessels took place [60, 61]. Later studies using this technology unfolded in the early 2000s when Dabus et al. employed magnetic navigation to treat six intracranial aneurysms, three vessel sacrifices, and one extracranial AVM [62]. Subsequently, robotically driven intracranial procedures were not reported until the late 2010s.

Vuong and colleagues reported using the Magellan robotic catheter system in 15 months between 2015 and 2016 in 23 patients in diagnostic cerebral angiograms (DCAs) and intracranial interventions. However, they did not specify the interventions [63]. Lu et al. reported successful DCAs in 15 patients with their experimental system (VIR-2) in China in 2016 [64]. A single DCA was then performed successfully by Yuhua Jiang et al. in 2018 using their experimental "Robot of Endovascular Treatment (RobEnt)," designed in collaboration with the Beijing Institute of Technology [65].

CorPath was tested for neurovascular use by Britz et al. in an in vitro aneurysm flow model for stent-assisted coiling and to deliver Onyx liquid embolic (ev3, Irvine, Calif) in swine models [46, 66]. In 2020, Sajja and colleagues described their experience using CorPath GRX for seven DCAs and three carotid stent procedures [67]. Though all cases were successful without complications, conversion to manual angiography occurred in three diagnostic cases due to bovine arch anatomy. Nogueira et al. published a case series of robotically assisted carotid angioplasty and stenting in four cases of severe carotid stenosis with the CorPath GRX, reporting 100% technical success. However, stent navigation and deployment were not done robotically due to incompatibility with the system [68]. Weinberg and colleagues also performed six trans-radial robot-assisted carotid artery stenting procedures with technical success [69]. Desai et al. described their experience using CorPath for DCAs and the first reported Onyx embolization of a dural arteriovenous fistula fed by the occipital artery [70]. Tateshima and colleagues performed the first robotic spinal angiography in 2021 [71] and, the following year, reported robotic embolization of extracranial vessels in a patient with COVID-19 and acute epistaxis [72]. Costa et al. reported DCAs in 37 patients, 3 extracranial carotid stents, and 1 transverse sinus stenting with CorPath [73]. Pereira et al. described the first clinical use of robotics in intracranial aneurysm treatment, successfully treating a wide-necked, >10 mm saccular sidewall basilar artery aneurysm with stent-assisted coiling using the CorPath GRX [74]. Since then, the authors' group in Toronto, Canada, has expanded their experience treating complex intracranial aneurysms with robot-assisted intravascular devices and flow diversion [75]. Chivot et al. reported using CorPath GRX to deploy flow diverter stents in ten patients [76]. More recently, Beaman and collaborators among 3 separate University of California institutions published a series of 113 robotically assisted DCAs with CorPath GRX, of which 88 (77.9%) were completed without unplanned manual conversion [77]. Femoral access was used in 98 (86.7%) cases, 14 (12.4%) cases obtained access through the radial approach, and 1 (0.9%) case was conducted with the ulnar approach. The primary reasons for unplanned manual conversion were attributed to challenging anatomy (10.6%), technical difficulties with the bedside robotic cassette (3.5%), "hubbing out" of the robot due to inadequate working length (3.5%), and rarely mechanical failure, either of the console (0.9%) or robotic arm (1.8%).

Most recently, Mendes Pereira and colleagues published the results of an international, multicenter, single-arm, prospective study of CorPath GRX-assisted aneurysm or stent-assisted coiling. The study enrolled 117 participants from 10 clinical locations in 6 different countries. The group demonstrated technical success in 110 of 117 (94%) procedures, with 7 requiring manual conversion. Seventy-one of 110 (64.5%) subjects had complete obliteration of the aneurysm by follow-up. In terms of safety outcomes, two patients suffered intraprocedural aneurysm rupture, and two patients suffered strokes [78]. At this time, CorPath GRX has earned CE marking for neurovascular procedures but is not FDA-approved for this indication in the USA.

Endovascular thrombectomy (EVT) has yet to be clinically attempted using robotics. However, preclinical in vitro studies suggest technical success may be comparable to conventional methods. Kaneko and colleagues performed robotic M1 branch mechanical thrombectomies using CorPath GRX to deploy the EmboTrap stent retriever (CERENOVUS, Johnson & Johnson Medical Devices,

Irvine, California, USA) [79]. The authors demonstrated a 100% technical success rate among seven procedures and no statistically significant difference in first-pass recanalization (28.6% vs. 42.9%, $p = 0.557$). In addition to technical feasibility, they showed a substantial reduction in radiation exposure to the operators (robotic 0.02 μSv vs. manual 0.22 μSv, $p < 0.0001$). The main limitation identified in this study's analysis of the current robotic model was a substantial increase in procedural time compared to manual thrombectomy. Other limitations included microwire and catheter size incompatibility, limited working length, and inability to load an aspiration catheter with the microcatheter simultaneously. In a later section, we expound on these constraints posed by the most recent CorPath GRX system. As more preclinical data emerges and devices, procedures, and processes are optimized for mechanical thrombectomy to be clinically conceived using robots, the first robot-assisted EVT will transpire in the near future.

Automation

When looking toward the future, increasing automation in robotic systems will likely be vital to improving precision and decreasing procedure time. Endovascular systems hitherto are almost entirely surgeon-driven, but automation capabilities are beginning to appear. For example, in the upgrade from CorPath 200 to GRX, optional automation modes were added to the platform's guidance software, including "rotate on retract," "active device fixation," "wiggle," "spin," "dotter," and "constant speed" [35, 80]. "Rotate on retract" automatically rotates the guidewire when retracting to facilitate vessel selection and was demonstrated to decrease wiring time in a porcine model [81]. "Active device fixation" was devised to prevent unanticipated guidewire movement when the microcatheter is engaged, allowing for more precise control of the relative device positions as they move [66]. Pereira and colleagues found this application particularly useful for carefully advancing the microcatheter over the wire when entering the aneurysm sac during coiling procedures [82]. Down the line, increasing automation will become part and parcel of robotic procedures. Guided by advances in artificial intelligence, robotic systems may offer data-driven abilities to perform safe and precise automated maneuvers.

Artificial Intelligence and Machine Learning in Neuroimaging

The term *artificial intelligence* (AI) was first coined in 1956 by John McCarthy, 6 years after Alan Turing introduced the idea of intelligent machines. Today, AI describes the capacity of a machine to simulate human intelligence and learn, problem-solve, and make decisions. Incorporation of AI into everyday life has been gradual; however, integrating these applications into routine practice has become imminent with the groundbreaking release of ChatGPT and related software. From AI-led diagnoses to improved therapeutic decision-making, the possibilities are vast. However, it is helpful to take a step back to review the current uses and the recent data surrounding AI. We will start with a general overview of the concepts to understand when describing "AI," which refers to a collection of technologies, including machine learning, deep learning, computer vision, natural language processing, and physical robots [83].

Machine learning (ML) is a broad subset of AI that involves building algorithms that allow machines to learn from data and make predictions or decisions without being explicitly programmed. Algorithms in ML are trained on a dataset to discern patterns and relationships within the data. They subsequently apply this learned knowledge to new, unseen data to make predictions or take action. A typical basic application of traditional ML in medicine is *precision medicine*, which involves using patient data and treatment context to predict which treatment protocols are most likely to be successful for an individual patient [84].

Neural networks (NN) are ML algorithms consisting of layers of interconnected "nodes," i.e., neurons, which take inputs from the previous layer to produce an output passed on. Deep learning (DL) involves more complex neural networks with multiple layers of interconnected nodes that can process vast amounts of data and recognize patterns, allowing them to learn, make independent decisions, and perform advanced tasks such as image recognition (Fig. 21.3). A *convolutional neural network* (CNN) is a deep learning neural network commonly used for imaging discrimination tasks. In CNN, "feature maps" are automatically generated (*without human intervention*), which function as filters and identify visual patterns within the data, memorizing patterns with the highest frequency. The CNN model comprises convolution layers, pooling layers, and normalization layers, and after producing a final output, it is compared with the actual output to calculate the model's accuracy. The model is then optimized by reweighting inputs until the best performance is achieved (Fig. 21.3b). These techniques in AI have expanded rapidly over the past decade and have led to dozens of efforts to improve the diagnosis, treatment, and clinical optimization of neurovascular disease [22].

AI in Stroke

For cerebrovascular diagnosis, AI and deep learning have already been incorporated into many academic centers, particularly for large vessel occlusion (LVO) detection in the setting of ischemic stroke or detection of stroke size.

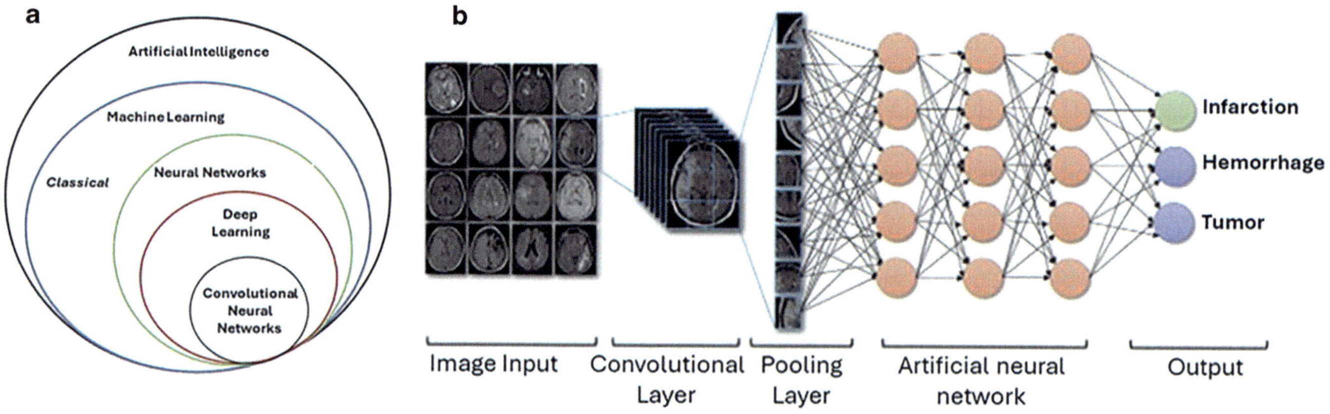

Fig. 21.3 (**a**) Subsets of artificial intelligence: *machine learning* broadly involves *classical* and *neural network*-based algorithms. *Deep learning* involves complex neural networks, and *convolutional neural networks* are specific DL algorithms employed in imaging software. (**b**) Sequential processing steps in a convolutional neural network: The convolutional layer extracts local features and produces feature maps highlighting important patterns and spatial relationships in the image. The pooling layer decreases the spatial dimensions of the data to extract the most robust components. The pooled feature maps then pass through neural networks consisting of multiple layers of interconnected neurons called neurons to produce the final output. (*Reprinted with permission from Zaharchuk et al.* [85]. *Copyright American Journal of Neuroradiology*)

Automated, timely, and accurate LVO detection has the potential to significantly impact patient care by streamlining hospital workflow in emergent stroke settings. Several AI-based diagnostic aids have come to the market in recent years: Viz.ai (San Francisco, California, USA) is an increasingly utilized program that employs CNNs, and multiple recent studies have confirmed its accuracy and sensitivity in detecting LVO [86–89]. Recent retrospective analyses also demonstrated decreased door-to-neuroendovascular team notification times and faster transfer times from peripheral to thrombectomy-capable centers using Viz AI [90–92]. Similarly, RapidAI technology (iSchemaView, Inc.) is a mobile application that can detect proximal LVOs and has demonstrated decreased door-to-recanalization times and associations with lower post-procedure NIHSS [88]. A study by the Neuroendovascular group at the Barrow Neurologic Institute found that the specificity and positive predictive value of detecting an M1 occlusion are 100% if RapidAI results are combined with gaze deviation and a hyperdense sign [92].

Another area showing promise in the stroke literature is using ML-based approaches to forecast final infarct size using acute stroke scans. A systematic review of the heterogenous studies published to date summarized 13 studies that used conventional ML models and 25 that used DL techniques, deriving data from CT perfusion source data or various MRI sequences [90]. Pooling 11 studies in a meta-analysis, the authors concluded that ML algorithms showed moderate performance, with an overall prediction performance dice similarity coefficient score of 0.50 (*ranging from 0 to 1*). DL-based models outperformed conventional ML-based programs.

These advances have demonstrated improved clinical outcomes with the subsequent widespread adoption of these technologies in stroke diagnosis and treatment decision support. However, it will be pertinent in the coming years to approach the implementation of these technologies with diligence. A recent review investigated the methodologies used to develop and validate current AI-based clinical decision support systems and found significant variability in methods and reporting parameters [91]. For example, the authors report inconsistent technical robustness of algorithms. This criterion is typically achieved by splitting data into training, validation, and test sets to optimize a model. Many of the reviewed articles did not use test sets or properly separate datasets, suggesting further validation is likely required to assess the clinical applicability of the tested systems.

AI in Aneurysm Treatment

Intracranial aneurysm detection and rupture risk assessment have been extensively examined over the past few years, primarily employing CNNs. A systematic review and meta-analysis of 20 studies reported impressive accuracy, with a sensitivity of CNN models in detecting >98% of aneurysms >3 mm in size and roughly 75% for aneurysms less than 3 mm [93]. Two more recent systematic reviews and meta-analyses echoed the high-performance accuracy reported in the literature. However, again, caution was expressed in interpreting these studies, noting that most studies employed retrospective, single-center, case-control designs using relatively small samples, limiting generalizability and providing an overall low level of evidence [94, 95].

Regarding risk detection, early work used neural networks to predict anterior communicating aneurysm rupture risk with almost 95% accuracy [96]. More recently, three classical ML models [random forest (RF), linear support vector machine (SVM), and radial basis function kernel SVM] were shown to identify high-risk aneurysm features and accurately distinguish ruptured from unruptured aneurysms [97]. Zhu et al. demonstrated that SVM, RF, and NN outperformed the logistic regression and PHASES scores in assessing aneurysm stability [98]. Interestingly, studies have also shown accurate prediction models for vasospasm and delayed cerebral ischemia in the setting of ruptured subarachnoid hemorrhage: Again, NN [99, 100] and other ML methods (SVM, random forests, and multilayer perceptron) [101] outperformed logistic regression models. To investigate complications after the intervention of arteriovenous malformations, Asadi et al. employed a neural network model that exhibited superior accuracy for predicting mortality compared to a standard regression analysis model, 97.5% vs. 43% [102].

These advancements in neuroimaging offer a glimpse into the potential applications of AI-powered imaging to enhance neurointerventional practices. Merging these technologies with robotics at the bedside unveils the possibility of a future with optimized and possibly autonomous diagnostic and therapeutic neurovascular management approaches.

Technological Advances

Though AI and robotic systems have advanced exponentially over the past decade, their use in neurointervention remains in infancy. To continue the growth of this field, attention will need to be directed toward device optimization, telesystem development, and rigorous expansion and testing of AI algorithms.

Device Optimization

Various obstacles related to devices need to be addressed to enhance the comfort of using robotic technology and safely expand its application to neurovascular interventions. The lack of haptic feedback is a frequently cited concern. Interventionalists depend heavily on tactile perception to aid in selecting vessels and gauge the potential energy within a microsystem to prevent sudden, unexpected wire or catheter advancements. For this to be implemented in robots, the system must be able to (1) sense the force felt by the catheter or between the tool and vessel wall and (2) transmit this force back to the operator-side control station. A miniaturized sensor is typically implanted into the distal tip to measure the force between the catheter and the vessel wall. In the cardiac electrophysiology literature, devices such as the TactiCath Catheter (Endosense SA, Geneva, Switzerland) have integrated force sensors into 7Fr radiofrequency-ablation catheters [103]. Force sensing has been studied most often using an implementation of strain gauges [38, 101]. However, these sensors are unfortunately limited in neurovascular cases by their size. Guo et al. described a fiberoptic pressure sensor (OPP-M40, Opsens, Quebec City, QC, Canada) with a diameter of only 0.25 mm, which also implements a warning function that alerts the operator when the contact force of the catheter tip is more significant than a predefined safety threshold [104]. Recently, force detection based on fiber Bragg grating (FBG) sensors has shown promise, with device diameters generally smaller than 0.25 mm [105]. Interestingly, model-based force-prediction methods have also attracted attention: here, force is calculated and estimated by integrating sensor boundary conditions, imaging, and vascular anatomy [106]. The next challenge is translating the force the sensors detect into haptic perception. As alluded to above, groups have developed *isomorphic* robotic prototypes whose control modules simulate the natural handling of catheters, allowing force feedback received from distal force sensors to be felt intuitively and tactilely [39]. Other experiments to create haptic perception have included vision-based feedback [107] and magnetorheological fluid-based systems [108]. The difficulty with applying haptics to operators in *non-isomorphic* control panels is the counterintuitive methods of tool manipulation that go against conventional catheterization practices [109].

However, it is essential to note that many believe this parameter may not be crucial to address, as alternative modes of sensory input and feedback may avoid relying so heavily on haptics in the future. In this regard, we can look to surgical colleagues in fields such as urology who have fully integrated robots into their practice. Here, it has been described that haptic feedback surrogates in the form of visual cues, such as local tissue deformation or shadows, adequately compensate for this loss of sensory force feedback [110]. Similarly, it is conceivable that interventionalists may increasingly focus on visually observing microcatheter or microwire behavior, using a heightened awareness of tool deflection during procedures. In line with this, Pereira and colleagues reported visual feedback was sufficient in their series of robot-assisted aneurysm treatments, compensating with surveillance of microcatheter kickback or "snaking" of coils [82]. The authors add that senior neurointerventionalists routinely rely on these visual cues when supervising trainees during cases. While performing robot-assisted spinal angiography, Dr. Satoshi Tateshima described a novel "wire-aid guidance" technique to confirm the successful catheterization of a segmental artery, relying solely on visual aids [71]. In this strategy, when the operator believes the segmental artery has been engaged, a soft microguidewire is pushed through the microcatheter. If the guidewire runs in a straight path, this is confirmed; however, if the tip of the guidewire is deflected up or down and seen to run along the wall of the aorta, this suggests the artery has not been hooked into. This approach also obviates the need for repeated contrast puffs by a bedside supporting operator, increasing ease and decreasing overall contrast load.

Dr. Pereira, who has performed over 70 robotic neurointerventional procedures, also points out that the combination of visual input and available alarms on robotic systems (which may indicate excess resistance, for instance) can substitute for haptic feedback. He illustrates that in this way, complex mechanical parameters, such as slack in a microcatheter/microwire system, can be precisely controlled to ensure one-to-one manipulation (i.e., *with each joystick movement, the device moves as expected*) [111]. Likewise, Dr. Tjoumakaris, another expert with significant robotic experience, has touted the stability of the robotic system, even when led through tortuous anatomy [112]. For example, when the microguidewire is securely locked in place using software automation, introducing intracranial devices becomes seamless, facilitated by the stable and anchored microguidewire.

Added procedural time is one limitation that may be difficult to overcome with the current robot systems, as the extra time required to set up the robotic arm and load devices is largely unavoidable. One can imagine that treating a sizeable aneurysm with many coils, for example, may be cumbersome. However, it is likely that as robotic technology enhances, the improved efficiency and precision during active procedural time will make up this difference. It has also been postulated that once the learning curve is attained, less experienced manual operators may be faster with robotic assistance. Interestingly, when considering telestroke treatment—where time is most pertinent—these procedural delays may be less consequential: Using geospatial analysis models, Beaman et al. demonstrated that the conversion of tPA-capable centers into telerobotic EVT centers significantly decreased median travel time for patients and suggested that the substantial time saved for patients living far from current thrombectomy-capable centers rendered minor procedural delays tolerable, as long as procedural success was comparable to conventional manual methods [113]. An in vitro EVT study by Kaneko et al. [76] using a flow model revealed that the mean total procedural time for a robotic thrombectomy was 892 s, significantly longer than the 357 s required for manual thrombectomy. The delay was due to the time needed for the guiding catheter from the aorta to the cervical ICA, the intracranial guidance of a microcatheter, the mechanical thrombectomy by the stent retriever, and the time needed to set devices into the robot's cassette. Although the robotic procedure took longer than the manual, it is essential to note that the difference was less than 10 min. As suggested, this delay in procedural time with a robotic system may be acceptable, particularly in cases where stroke patients are located at a distance from a stroke center capable of performing mechanical thrombectomy. The evolution of robotic designs and increased efficiency may help bridge this time gap in the future, adding to the overall viability of robotics in neurovascular treatments.

A notable design improvement that warrants consideration revolves around the constraint posed by limited working length, which remains a significant barrier to the extension of robotics to many neurovascular procedures. The CorPath system, for instance, has a 20-cm travel distance; therefore, manual navigation of distal access catheters to the neck is required to allow forward and backward navigation of intracranial devices. In the series by Beaman et al., inadequate working length led to unplanned manual conversion in 3.5% of cases [77]. Importantly, this is an idiosyncratic issue related to current robot designs, which can be adjusted in future renditions to incorporate a working length of ideally 40 cm or greater. The authors also noted in their series that the CorPath robotic arm was occasionally too short, offering their recommendation to lengthen it in future iterations to increase the range of motion. In this same vein, developing future generations of robotic systems specifically designed to accept and manipulate neuroendovascular tools will be imperative. For example, as CorPath was initially intended for coronary intervention, the robot only accepts smaller 0.014-in. or 0.018-in. wires, rendering commonly used 0.035- and 0.038-in. wires incompatible. Furthermore, only 5–7Fr catheters are suitable, precluding the use of larger guiding or balloon-guide catheters. Equally pertinent will be to ensure the ability to accommodate triaxial systems in future renditions to allow the utilization of intermediate catheters in distal intracranial procedures. An aspiration catheter and microcatheter cannot simultaneously be loaded into the cassette.

Certain procedures in the neurointerventionalists' arsenal also come with unique challenges that must be considered. For instance, in embolizing extracranial tumors or dural arteriovenous fistulas, operators often need repeated superselective angiograms with continuously updated roadmaps. Therefore, using the robot for such procedures necessitates frequent bedside wire unloading for contrast injections. To this end, developing new tools designed specifically for robot use may be necessary. Magnetically steerable microcatheters, such as the Nanoflex mentioned above, may alleviate these concerns, as the ability to steer the microcatheter could remove the reliance on microwires and allow angiograms to be intermittently obtained through the microcatheter with a pump without repeated wire unloading. Furthermore, as advancements are made with steerable devices, automation is also set to play an increasingly significant role. In 2022, Abah et al. presented their research on semiautonomous catheters, utilizing preoperative CT scans of carotid vasculature to optimize catheter design parameters [114]. By employing series-elastic actuation methods, the catheter tip was shown to respond autonomously to forces, enabling active steering and branch selection in mock vasculature.

Lastly, the integration of interventional angiography systems and robotic control is crucial. Manipulating catheters and guidewires is only a part of neurointerventional procedures; interpretation of superselective intermittent angiograms with constant readjustment of the table height or the flat-panel detector plays a significant role in the procedure. To minimize the delay in procedure time or provide a seamless procedure remotely, neurointerventionalists must have complete control of the catheter-guidewire combination and the other functions equipped in neurointervention suites.

Each of these technological advancements and adjustments will represent significant strides in enhancing the capabilities of our current devices. However, when we peer further into the future, a new realm in robotic devices may emerge: the domain of micro- and nanorobotics, which may harbor revolutionary concepts for precise and autonomous minimally invasive and interventional surgery.

Micro- and Nanorobots

Over the last decade, significant research has been conducted into the development and biomedical applications of biodegradable robots at the micro- and nanoscale [115]. Using untethered microrobots in the neurovascular field offers the potential for drug delivery and navigation to distal vasculature in the narrowest capillaries with high precision [116]. As aforementioned, given the difference in physical properties of micro and macro environments, simple miniaturization of traditional robotic designs becomes unfeasible, necessitating new sensing, navigation, actuation, and fabrication mechanisms [117]. Generally, microrobots are chemically powered, harvesting energy from the local environment or drawing their power from external stimuli, primarily from magnetic, optical, acoustic, or electric fields [118]. For example, the underlying propelling principle of chemically driven microrobots often revolves around the asymmetric distribution of redox reaction products [119]. As bubbles leak from the robot, momentum generates motion. Furthermore, when constituent materials are magnetic, propulsion can be achieved by applying magnetic fields [120]. Several excellent reviews have addressed the vast array of mechanisms of micro-/nanomotors and the progression of breakthroughs that have built the foundation of the current state of microrobotic therapeutics [115–119].

In microsurgery, advances in untethered tools such as nanodrillers, microgrippers, and microbullets promise to deliver uniquely precise operative capabilities [116]. A notable example of this can be seen in the development of thermochemically actuated microgrippers able to capture live fibroblast cells, an advancement with implications in precision biopsies [121]. In terms of applications to neurointervention, multiple modalities have been explored to address thrombolysis. Wan and colleagues built self-driven nanomotors encapsulated by platelet membrane on the outer layer of a platinum-loaded porous nanostructure loaded with urokinase and heparin [122]. The platelet membrane allows for targeting of the thrombus, while the platinum provides near-infrared light-driven motion capability. However, the focus of microscale robotics has also been concentrated on drug delivery systems in tumor treatment. Zhang et al., for example, reported the delivery of biohybrid neutrophil-based microrobots ("neurobots") to a malignant glioma in vivo [123]. The system was developed by phagocytosis of *E. coli* membrane-enveloped, drug-loaded magnetic nanogels by neutrophils, with controlled movement in the setting of a rotating magnetic field and the ability to cross the blood-brain barrier through positive chemotactic motion along the gradient of inflammatory factors.

Innovations in magnetically actuated technology such as this have been pivotal in microrobot development. Magnetic fields are ideal for use in micro-/nanosystems, as they obviate the need for alterations in chemical compositions, like in chemical activation, and do not require high-intensity lasers for activation, such as in light activation [124]. As aforementioned, biomimetic magnetic microrobots were developed for targeted thrombolytic therapy [52]. Inspired by magnetotactic bacteria, Xie and colleagues used magneto-collective control to navigate and propel the devices via iron oxide nanoparticle chains inside biocompatible microgel shells. Bakenecker et al. steered a helical magnetic microrobot through a phantom of a human cerebral aneurysm with high accuracy using a magnetic particle imaging (MPI) scanner [125]. Hosney and colleagues subsequently described using a helical microrobot to drill through gelatin thrombi with a magnetic-based robotic system [126]. Servant et al. demonstrated in vivo actuation and navigation of a *swarm* of artificial bacterial flagella in the peritoneal cavity of an anesthetized mouse using rotating magnetic fields [127]. Employing microrobotic magnetic particle swarms in this way has attracted attention lately, inspired by the collective behaviors present in nature (e.g., schools of fish), which allow for increased efficiency and task performance [128]. Related to the neurovascular space, actuation of thrombin-coated magnetic particle swarms was recently used to selectively embolize in vivo porcine kidneys, a demonstration with implications in embolization of cerebral pathologies [128]. Jin and colleagues subsequently demonstrated a tethered approach for aneurysm embolization in an ex vivo model using a swarm of microspheres composed of a pH-responsive self-healing hydrogel matrix, magnetic nanoparticles, and imaging dopants [129]. These are delivered with a catheter to the aneurysm neck, and by subsequently applying an external magnetic field, the swarming microrobots are concentrated into the aneurysm sac. An acidic buffer solution is then injected through the catheter to activate the self-healing behavior of microgels, welding the matrix together. In due course, the coming years will likely witness the addition of autonomy to these microsystems. Yang et al. applied deep learning algorithms to micro-/nanorobots in this endeavor, demonstrating the potential for autonomous navigation of magnetic nanoparticle swarms in unstructured environments [130].

These breakthroughs hold tremendous potential for revolutionizing the field of robotics in the context of targeted drug delivery and intravascular procedures. Indeed, an in-human clinical trial has recently commenced testing the Pulse NanoMED™ system developed by Euphrates Vascular in improving reperfusion in acute ischemic stroke [55]. This technology, analogous to the concepts described above, comprises intravenously delivered magnetic microbeads manipulated by an externally rotating magnet to assemble and act as "stirring rods" to direct blood flow and thrombolytic particles toward the clot. In this early feasibility study, the magnetic system is being tested first in patients who have residual distal, medium vessel occlusions that remain after mechanical thrombectomy is performed and in whom t-PA was administered. Though the routine application of such nanotechnologies in human settings remains somewhat distant, it is promising that forward-thinking groups will translate these advancements to in vivo models and human clinical trials in the coming years.

Telesystems

In a field where "time is brain," probably the most transformative implication of robotic technology is the application of tele-thrombectomy to acute ischemic stroke patients in remote regions. The feasibility of remote PCI with the operator 20 miles away from patients was demonstrated in 2019 [131]. Robotic cardiac telestenting was subsequently tested transcontinentally (*from Boston to San Francisco, >3000 miles*) in an ex vivo model over both wired and fifth-generation (5G) wireless networks. Compared to trans-regional telestenting (*from Boston to New York, ~200 miles*), there were minor latency differences, graded as "imperceptible," and procedure times and performance did not differ between the groups [132]. When deliberately adding signal latencies to telestenting procedures in ex vivo and in vivo animal models, Madder et al. reported a delay threshold for perceptible operator latency of >250 ms, higher than typical network connection systems [133]. These findings are consistent with the telesurgical literature, which demonstrated that delays below 300 ms did not significantly affect task performance [134, 135]. Though encouraging, the impact of other network parameters remains to be investigated, such as bandwidth (*which refers to the maximum amount of data that can be transmitted*), jitter (*variations in network delay*), and data security concerns.

With the initiation of remote procedures, the distribution of responsibilities among the interventional team will be markedly changed. Most notably, the bedside team (*often technologists*) may need to take on the role of table and biplane adjustment, rotating hemostatic valve manipulation, flushing, and exchanging or loading devices. As previously suggested, a potential avenue for future robotic systems is to construct integrated hardware and software systems to simultaneously control many factors, including patient table movement, biplane adjustment, and contrast injection, to streamline procedures and enhance efficiency. Interestingly, robot-assisted femoral vascular cannulation has been explored to obtain access using a system specifically designed for this task [136]. The robot uses ultrasound imaging to scan for an optimal puncture site and insert the needle. Successful access in silicone tissue phantom and in vivo porcine models was demonstrated by a single operator with no medical experience. The authors foresee a path toward full automation of the catheterization process and the Seldinger technique using more advanced imaging models and machine learning. Brattain et al. also prototyped a handheld AI-enabled device, AI-GUIDE (artificial intelligence-guided ultrasound interventional device), for use in femoral vein puncture [137]. The system locates the femoral vein, performs needle insertion, and assists with guidewire insertion. It was likewise tested successfully on tissue phantom and porcine models by operators with minimal experience.

However, until these advances are further matured, interventional teams and technicians must be trained on their expanded roles and procedures, ideally optimized to minimize wire and device exchanges. Interestingly, though using robotic systems does follow a steep learning curve, in a retrospective series by Abbas et al., it took only about five procedures to achieve high team efficiency during carotid artery stenting [138]. However, EVT cases will likely require more experience before overcoming the learning curve. Indeed, developing standard operating procedures to follow in the case of emergent manual conversion is an important task. In this context, analogies have been drawn to aviation, where emergencies are rare, but preparation is deliberately made with repeated simulations. Similarly, simulation-based training for emergent thrombectomy, particularly in lower-volume centers, will require stringent quality improvement programs.

Ethical and Medicolegal Concerns

In addition to the technological and systems-level challenges that must be overcome in robotic intervention, ethical considerations must also be addressed [139]. First and foremost, on the physician side, obtaining informed consent from patients after full disclosure regarding the preliminary nature of the current technology and updated supporting evidence will be critical. Neurointerventionalists must also take steps to confront the altered physician-patient dynamics inherent in performing remote procedures. This may include conducting immediate pre- and postoperative tele-calls to improve the doctor-patient relationship and minimize the risk of decreased empathy in this setting.

Furthermore, despite the estimated benefit of bringing remote procedures to rural areas, the reality remains that the cost may be prohibitive for community hospitals to implement these technologies. For example, a single cassette port for CorPath GRX costs $600, with the entire system costing $480,000–650,000 [44]. Certain companies are, therefore, testing cheaper one-time-use alternatives: the Liberty robot, developed by *Microbot*, is a fully disposable robot to eliminate expensive capital equipment. In May 2023, the company announced its 100th preclinical catheterization, reporting a 95% success rate in reaching predetermined vascular targets, though intracranial vessels were not mentioned [140, 141]. Avoiding a future where only large academic centers can access unattainably expensive robotic equipment will be imperative.

Lastly, having a remote operator brings potential ethical and medicolegal concerns related to the diffusion of responsibility. Namely, ownership of the procedure and professional liability in the case of adverse events will be complex issues given the range of participants involved in each case (e.g., remote operators, local physicians, hardware manufacturers, and software programmers). All stakeholders must cultivate active collaboration at each step of this care delivery chain, overseen by the FDA and related governing bodies. One plausible approach could resemble telestroke, wherein remote providers are granted hospital privileges to offer procedural services.

A Preview of AI Assisted Neurointerventions

Present AI programs have shown promising results in diagnosis and prognosis in stroke and aneurysm management. However, future studies will need to focus on the feasibility and applicability of these AI algorithms [142]. Akay et al. elegantly offered four recommendations to promote this: (1) rigorous adherence to best practices in model development, (2) strict reporting requirements, (3) prioritization of research that offers clinical applicability and real-life implementation plans, and (4) emphasis on the availability of large, diverse, and thoroughly annotated datasets to produce high-quality training and validation data [143].

Future innovations will involve merging AI with robotic systems, bringing machine learning-led automation to the forefront of management. For example, the Clotild Smart Guidewire System (Sensome, Massy, France) is a recently developed guidewire equipped with a 2-mm microsensor near the distal end that performs impedance data upon contact with a thrombus [144]. The sensor provides higher impedance measurements for red blood cell-rich clots and lower impedance measurements for fibrin-rich clots, offering the ability to distinguish between the two and allowing for thrombus length estimation. To achieve this, the developers trained a machine learning algorithm using a database of known clot compositions, enabling it to predict the composition of a clot. The device is currently being tested in an in-human single-arm, multicenter study of M1 occlusions. Other types of virtual simulation aids are also being investigated. Stent sizing can be challenging in flow diversion due to stent foreshortening. Software such as AneuGuide™ (ArteryFlow Technology, Hangzhou, China) [145] and Sim&Size (Sim&Cure, Grabels, France) [146] perform virtual sizing before stent deployment using preoperative three-dimensional rotational angiography acquisition. Multiple retrospective reviews of flow diversion for aneurysm treatment demonstrated that using the Sim&Size software led to shorter stent use and decreased procedural time, with fewer corrective interventions [146] and fewer aneurysms requiring multiple stents [147]. AI algorithms can also be used to address the challenges of microcatheter shaping in aneurysm treatment: Liu and colleagues described a software that formulates optimal microcatheter pathways after inputting location, size, and 3D structure of the aneurysm, in addition to the axis of the parent artery and microcatheter information [148]. Computer-assisted microcatheter shaping was used in a randomized controlled trial, demonstrating higher rates of first-trial success, successful microcatheter placement within 5 min, and microcatheter stability compared to manual shaping methods [149]. Taking simulations one step further, training AI algorithms to suggest techniques with the highest probability of success may be possible. These tools ultimately have the potential to aid in choosing the most efficacious, efficient, and cost-effective treatment modalities.

Conclusions

Robotics in neurointervention holds considerable promise in improving neurovascular care. The next step toward integrating robotics into the field requires the development of neurovascular-specific technologies that ensure reliable and efficient procedures. This entails focusing on adequate working length, minimal tool exchanges, optimized steerability, and haptic feedback. Additionally, it is crucial to establish reliable remote networks to support the implementation of robotic systems. Subsequent trials should be conducted to demonstrate the safety, efficacy, and equivalence of outcomes compared to conventional manual techniques. Lastly, prioritizing comprehensive training for operators and support staff and extending these technologies to remote centers remain essential.

In the realm of AI, once the feasibility and applicability of algorithms have been demonstrated, one can envision broad technical support in both diagnostic and therapeutic arenas. The neuroendovascular field thrives on collaboration and regularly emerging new tools and techniques. AI has the potential to facilitate this collaboration at the bedside in real time. For instance, imagine encountering a patient during a preoperative clinic visit where an AI program founded on extensive datasets of similar aneurysms offers insights into treatment modalities based on aneurysm characteristics. Similarly, intraoperatively, as an interventionalist prepares for thrombectomy, an AI algorithm provides valuable feedback on the technique that may be most effective upfront.

Once AI evolves to the point of reliable decision-making, these algorithms can then be used to guide a robot to execute the required treatment. In this manner, combining robotics and AI, one can envision a future of neurovascular intervention that looks much like an airplane cockpit: the interventionalist in place of a pilot, overseeing a primarily automated system built to optimize therapeutic decisions and management while enhancing occupational safety and increasing access to care.

And these changes will likely happen fast. Based on the rapid evolution of the technologies over the past decade and the growing interest in neurointerventional devices by researchers and industry partners alike, it can be expected that in just a short time, significant advances will take place in this arena. Physician-scientist visionaries and biotechnology companies are advancing rapidly to tailor robotics to the neurointervention suite; development of such devices would be adopted and studied briskly, motivated by the potential impact remote procedures can have on globalizing care. In parallel, introducing microrobotics to optimize drug delivery will refine our therapeutic options. Finally, adding AI with exponentially more robust computational capabilities will make neurointervention safer, more efficient, efficacious, and accessible. The next two to three decades will surely bring about an evolution and expansion of the field that may be as drastic of a change as 2024 may look to those practicing neurointervention in 2004. For robotics and automation in neurovascular care, this is only the beginning.

References

1. Yoshimura S, Sakai N, Yamagami H, Uchida K, Beppu M, Toyoda K, et al. Endovascular therapy for acute stroke with a large ischemic region. N Engl J Med. 2022;386(14):1303–13.
2. Huo X, Ma G, Tong X, Zhang X, Pan Y, Nguyen TN, et al. Trial of endovascular therapy for acute ischemic stroke with large infarct. N Engl J Med. 2023;388(14):1272–83.
3. Sarraj A, Hassan AE, Abraham MG, Ortega-Gutierrez S, Kasner SE, Hussain MS, et al. Trial of endovascular thrombectomy for large ischemic strokes. N Engl J Med. 2023;388(14):1259–71.
4. Lauzier DC, Huguenard AL, Srienc AI, Cler SJ, Osbun JW, Chatterjee AR, et al. A review of technological innovations leading to modern endovascular brain aneurysm treatment. Front Neurol. 2023;14:1156887.
5. Rudy RF, Catapano JS, Jadhav AP, Albuquerque FC, Ducruet AF. Middle meningeal artery embolization to treat chronic subdural hematoma. Stroke Vasc Interv Neurol. 2023;3(1):e000490.
6. Levitt MR, Hirsch JA, Chen M. Middle meningeal artery embolization for chronic subdural hematoma: an effective treatment with a bright future. J Neurointerv Surg. 2024;16(4):329–30.
7. Saver JL, Goyal M, van der Lugt A, Menon BK, Majoie CB, Dippel DW, et al. Time to treatment with endovascular thrombectomy and outcomes from ischemic stroke: a meta-analysis. JAMA. 2016;316(12):1279–88.
8. He AH, Churilov L, Mitchell PJ, Dowling RJ, Yan B. Every 15-min delay in recanalization by intra-arterial therapy in acute ischemic stroke increases risk of poor outcome. Int J Stroke. 2015;10(7):1062–7.
9. Sarraj A, Savitz S, Pujara D, Kamal H, Carroll K, Shaker F, et al. Endovascular thrombectomy for acute ischemic strokes. Stroke. 2020;51(4):1207–17.
10. Audebert HJ, Schultes K, Tietz V, Heuschmann PU, Bogdahn U, Haberl RL, Schenkel J. Long-term effects of specialized stroke care with telemedicine support in community hospitals on behalf of the Telemedical Project for Integrative Stroke Care (TEMPiS). Stroke. 2009;40(3):902–8.
11. Müller-Barna P, Hubert GJ, Boy S, Bogdahn U, Wiedmann S, Heuschmann PU, Audebert HJ. TeleStroke units serving as a model of care in rural areas. Stroke. 2014;45(9):2739–44.
12. Rajaraman P, Doody MM, Yu CL, Preston DL, Miller JS, Sigurdson AJ, et al. Cancer risks in U.S. radiologic technologists working with fluoroscopically guided interventional procedures, 1994–2008. AJR Am J Roentgenol. 2016;206(5):1101–8; quiz 9.
13. Yoshinaga S, Hauptmann M, Sigurdson AJ, Doody MM, Freedman DM, Alexander BH, et al. Nonmelanoma skin cancer in relation to ionizing radiation exposure among U.S. radiologic technologists. Int J Cancer. 2005;115(5):828–34.
14. Roguin A, Goldstein J, Bar O. Brain tumours among interventional cardiologists: a cause for alarm? Report of four new cases from two cities and a review of the literature. EuroIntervention. 2012;7(9):1081–6.
15. Roguin A, Goldstein J, Bar O, Goldstein JA. Brain and neck tumors among physicians performing interventional procedures. Am J Cardiol. 2013;111(9):1368–72.
16. Andreassi MG, Piccaluga E, Gargani L, Sabatino L, Borghini A, Faita F, et al. Subclinical carotid atherosclerosis and early vascular aging from long-term low-dose ionizing radiation exposure: a genetic, telomere, and vascular ultrasound study in cardiac catheterization laboratory staff. JACC Cardiovasc Interv. 2015;8(4):616–27.
17. Elmaraezy A, Ebraheem Morra M, Tarek Mohammed A, Al-Habaa A, Elgebaly A, Abdelmotaleb Ghazy A, et al. Risk of cataract among interventional cardiologists and catheterization lab staff: a systematic review and meta-analysis. Catheter Cardiovasc Interv. 2017;90(1):1–9.
18. El-Sayed T, Patel AS, Cho JS, Kelly JA, Ludwinski FE, Saha P, et al. Radiation-induced DNA damage in operators performing endovascular aortic repair. Circulation. 2017;136(25):2406–16.
19. Goldstein JA, Balter S, Cowley M, Hodgson J, Klein LW. Occupational hazards of interventional cardiologists: prevalence of orthopedic health problems in contemporary practice. Catheter Cardiovasc Interv. 2004;63(4):407–11.

20. Yang GZ, Cambias J, Cleary K, Daimler E, Drake J, Dupont PE, et al. Medical robotics—regulatory, ethical, and legal considerations for increasing levels of autonomy. Sci Robot. 2017;2(4):eaam8638.
21. Lane T. A short history of robotic surgery. Ann R Coll Surg Engl. 2018;100(6_Suppl):5–7.
22. Bravo J, Wali AR, Hirshman BR, Gopesh T, Steinberg JA, Yan B, et al. Robotics and artificial intelligence in endovascular neurosurgery. Cureus. 2022;14(3):e23662.
23. Mohammad S. Robotic surgery. J Oral Biol Craniofac Res. 2013;3(1):2.
24. Kwoh YS, Hou J, Jonckheere EA, Hayati S. A robot with improved absolute positioning accuracy for CT guided stereotactic brain surgery. IEEE Trans Biomed Eng. 1988;35(2):153–60.
25. Harris SJ, Arambula-Cosio F, Mei Q, Hibberd RD, Davies BL, Wickham JE, et al. The Probot—an active robot for prostate resection. Proc Inst Mech Eng H. 1997;211(4):317–25.
26. Intuitive reaches 10 million procedures performed using da Vinci Surgical Systems [press release]. 12/14/2021. 2021.
27. Schwaibold H, Wiesend F, Bach C. The age of robotic surgery—is laparoscopy dead? Arab J Urol. 2018;16(3):262–9.
28. Gopesh T, Wen JH, Santiago-Dieppa D, Yan B, Pannell JS, Khalessi A, et al. Soft robotic steerable microcatheter for the endovascular treatment of cerebral disorders. Sci Robot. 2021;6(57):eabf0601.
29. Killer-Oberpfalzer M, Chapot R, Orion D, Barr JD, Cabiri O, Berenstein A. Clinical experience with the Bendit steerable microcatheter: a new paradigm for endovascular treatment. J Neurointerv Surg. 2023;15:771–5.
30. Berenstein A, Cabiri O, Broussalis E, Hufnagl C, Killer-Oberpfalzer M. New concept in neurovascular navigation: technical description and preclinical experience with the Bendit 17 and Bendit 21 microcatheters in a rabbit aneurysm model. J Neurointerv Surg. 2023;15(2):172–5.
31. Kim Y, Genevriere E, Harker P, Choe J, Balicki M, Regenhardt RW, et al. Telerobotic neurovascular interventions with magnetic manipulation. Sci Robot. 2022;7(65):eabg9907.
32. Pancaldi L, Dirix P, Fanelli A, Lima AM, Stergiopulos N, Mosimann PJ, et al. Flow driven robotic navigation of microengineered endovascular probes. Nat Commun. 2020;11(1):6356.
33. Kim Y, Parada GA, Liu S, Zhao X. Ferromagnetic soft continuum robots. Sci Robot. 2019;4(33):eaax7329.
34. Duan W, Akinyemi T, Du W, Ma J, Chen X, Wang F, et al. Technical and clinical progress on robot-assisted endovascular interventions: a review. Micromachines (Basel). 2023;14(1):197.
35. Beaman CB, Kaneko N, Meyers PM, Tateshima S. A review of robotic interventional neuroradiology. Am J Neuroradiol. 2021;42(5):808–14.
36. Shen H, Wang C, Xie L, Zhou S, Gu L, Xie H. A novel remote-controlled robotic system for cerebrovascular intervention. Int J Med Robot. 2018;14(6):e1943.
37. Choi J, Park S, Kim YH, Moon Y, Choi J. A vascular intervention assist device using bi-motional roller cartridge structure and clinical evaluation. Biosensors (Basel). 2021;11(9):329.
38. Thakur Y, Bax JS, Holdsworth DW, Drangova M. Design and performance evaluation of a remote catheter navigation system. IEEE Trans Biomed Eng. 2009;56(7):1901–8.
39. Payne CJ, Rafii-Tari H, Yang G-Z. A force feedback system for endovascular catheterisation. In: 2012 IEEE/RSJ International Conference on Intelligent Robots and Systems; 2012. p. 1298–304.
40. Yu H, Wang H, Chang J, Niu J, Wang F, Yan Y, et al. A novel vascular intervention surgical robot based on force feedback and flexible clamping. Appl Sci. 2021;11(2):611.
41. Negoro M, Tanimoto M, Arai F, Fukuda T, Fukasaku K, Takahashi I, Miyachi S. An intelligent catheter system robotic controlled catheter system. Interv Neuroradiol. 2001;7(Suppl 1):111–3.
42. Cruddas L, Martin G, Riga C. Robotic endovascular surgery: current and future practice. Semin Vasc Surg. 2021;34(4):233–40.
43. Cercenelli L, Bortolani B, Marcelli E. CathROB: a highly compact and versatile remote catheter navigation system. Appl Bionics Biomech. 2017;2017:2712453.
44. Najafi G, Kreiser K, Abdelaziz M, Hamady MS. Current state of robotics in interventional radiology. Cardiovasc Intervent Radiol. 2023;46(5):549–61.
45. Lumsden AB, Bismuth J. Current status of endovascular catheter robotics. J Cardiovasc Surg. 2018;59(3):310–6.
46. Britz GW, Tomas J, Lumsden A. Feasibility of robotic-assisted neurovascular interventions: initial experience in flow model and porcine model. Neurosurgery. 2020;86(2):309–14.
47. Narsinh KH, Paez R, Mueller K, Caton MT, Baker A, Higashida RT, et al. Robotics for neuroendovascular intervention: background and primer. Neuroradiol J. 2022;35(1):25–35.
48. Tillander H. Magnetic guidance of a catheter with articulated steel tip. Acta Radiol. 1951;35(1):62–4.
49. Krings T, Finney J, Niggemann P, Reinacher P, Lück N, Drexler A, et al. Magnetic versus manual guidewire manipulation in neuroradiology: in vitro results. Neuroradiology. 2006;48(6):394–401.
50. Swiss robotic endovascular navigation platform secures over USD12m in funding support [press release]. 9/2/2023. 2023.
51. Nelson BJ, Bendok BR, Turcotte EL, Batjer HH. Remote magnetic navigation enables precision telesurgery. Sci Robot. 2024;9(87):eado3187.
52. Xie M, Zhang W, Fan C, Wu C, Feng Q, Wu J, et al. Bioinspired soft microrobots with precise magneto-collective control for microvascular thrombolysis. Adv Mater. 2020;32(26):e2000366.
53. Wang Z, Xu Z, Zhu B, Zhang Y, Lin J, Wu Y, Wu D. Design, fabrication and application of magnetically actuated micro/nanorobots: a review. Nanotechnology. 2022;33(15):152001.
54. Lin X, Li N, Tang H. Recent advances in nanomaterials for diagnosis, treatments, and neurorestoration in ischemic stroke. Front Cell Neurosci. 2022;16:885190.
55. Sen S. PERFUSION AIS—Pulse endovascular ReperFUSION for acute ischemic stroke: an early feasibility clinical study. 2023. https://classic.clinicaltrials.gov/ct2/show/NCT06052969. [2024].
56. Beyar R, Gruberg L, Deleanu D, Roguin A, Almagor Y, Cohen S, et al. Remote-control percutaneous coronary interventions: concept, validation, and first-in-humans pilot clinical trial. J Am Coll Cardiol. 2006;47(2):296–300.
57. Granada JF, Delgado JA, Uribe MP, Fernandez A, Blanco G, Leon MB, Weisz G. First-in-human evaluation of a novel robotic-assisted coronary angioplasty system. J Am Coll Cardiol Intv. 2011;4(4):460–5.
58. Weisz G, Metzger DC, Caputo RP, Delgado JA, Marshall JJ, Vetrovec GW, et al. Safety and feasibility of robotic percutaneous coronary intervention: PRECISE (Percutaneous Robotically-Enhanced Coronary Intervention) Study. J Am Coll Cardiol. 2013;61(15):1596–600.
59. Mahmud E, Schmid F, Kalmar P, Deutschmann H, Hafner F, Rief P, Brodmann M. Feasibility and safety of robotic peripheral vascular interventions: results of the RAPID trial. JACC Cardiovasc Interv. 2016;9(19):2058–64.
60. Guglielmi G. The beginning and the evolution of the endovascular treatment of intracranial aneurysms: from the first catheterization of brain arteries to the new stents. J Neurointerv Surg. 2009;1(1):53–5.
61. Hilal SK, Michelsen WJ, Driller J. POD catheter: a means for small vessel exploration. J Appl Phys. 2003;40(3):1046.
62. Dabus G, Gerstle RJ, Cross DT 3rd, Derdeyn CP, Moran CJ. Neuroendovascular magnetic navigation: clinical experience in ten patients. Neuroradiology. 2007;49(4):351–5.

63. Vuong SM, Carroll CP, Tackla RD, Jeong WJ, Ringer AJ. Application of emerging technologies to improve access to ischemic stroke care. Neurosurg Focus. 2017;42(4):E8.
64. Lu WS, Xu WY, Pan F, Liu D, Tian ZM, Zeng Y. Clinical application of a vascular interventional robot in cerebral angiography. Int J Med Robot. 2016;12(1):132–6.
65. Jiang Y, Liu K, Li Y. Initial clinical trial of robot of endovascular treatment with force feedback and cooperating of catheter and guidewire. Appl Bionics Biomech. 2018;2018:9735979.
66. Britz GW, Panesar SS, Falb P, Tomas J, Desai V, Lumsden A. Neuroendovascular-specific engineering modifications to the CorPath GRX Robotic System. J Neurosurg. 2020;133(6):1830–6.
67. Sajja KC, Sweid A, Saiegh FA, Chalouhi N, Avery MB, Schmidt RF, et al. Endovascular robotic: feasibility and proof of principle for diagnostic cerebral angiography and carotid artery stenting. J Neurointerv Surg. 2020;12(4):345–9.
68. Nogueira RG, Sachdeva R, Al-Bayati AR, Mohammaden MH, Frankel MR, Haussen DC. Robotic assisted carotid artery stenting for the treatment of symptomatic carotid disease: technical feasibility and preliminary results. J Neurointerv Surg. 2020;12(4):341–4.
69. Weinberg JH, Sweid A, Sajja K, Gooch MR, Herial N, Tjoumakaris S, et al. Comparison of robotic-assisted carotid stenting and manual carotid stenting through the transradial approach. J Neurosurg. 2020;135(1):21–8.
70. Desai VR, Lee JJ, Sample T, Kleiman NS, Lumsden A, Britz GW. First in man pilot feasibility study in extracranial carotid robotic-assisted endovascular intervention. Neurosurgery. 2021;88(3):506–14.
71. Tateshima S, Saber H, Colby GP, Enzmann D, Duckwiler G. Robotic assistant spinal angiography: a case report and technical considerations. BMJ Case Rep. 2021;14(3):1–3.
72. Saber H, Beaman C, Tateshima S. Complete robotic intervention for acute epistaxis in a patient with COVID-19 pneumonia: technical considerations and device selection tips. J Neurointerv Surg. 2022;14(5):500–2.
73. Costa M, Tataryn Z, Alobaid A, Pierre C, Basamh M, Somji M, et al. Robotically-assisted neuro-endovascular procedures: single-center experience and a review of the literature. Interv Neuroradiol. 2023;29(2):201–10.
74. Mendes Pereira V, Cancelliere NM, Nicholson P, Radovanovic I, Drake KE, Sungur JM, et al. First-in-human, robotic-assisted neuroendovascular intervention. J Neurointerv Surg. 2020;12(4):338–40.
75. Pereira VM, Cancelliere N, Liu E, Marotta T, Spears J. P-018 treatment of complex intracranial aneurysms using new robotic-assisted techniques: flow diverter and intrasaccular device experience. J Neurointerv Surg. 2022;14(Suppl 1):A59–60.
76. Chivot C, Bouzerar R, Peltier J, Lefranc M, Yzet T. Robotically assisted deployment of flow diverter stents for the treatment of cerebral and cervical aneurysms. J Neurointerv Surg. 2023;16:412.
77. Beaman C, Gautam A, Peterson C, Kaneko N, Ponce L, Saber H, et al. Robotic diagnostic cerebral angiography: a multicenter experience of 113 patients. J Neurointerv Surg. 2024;16:726–30.
78. Mendes Pereira V, Rice H, De Villiers L, Sourour N, Clarencon F, Spears J, et al. Evaluation of effectiveness and safety of the CorPath GRX robotic system in endovascular embolization procedures of cerebral aneurysms. J Neurointerv Surg. 2024;16(4):405–11.
79. Kaneko N, Beaman C, Imahori T, Takayanagi A, Saber H, Tateshima S. In vitro comparison of manual and robotic endovascular thrombectomy for acute ischemic stroke. Interv Neuroradiol. 2023;2023:15910199231206315.
80. Al Nooryani A, Aboushokka W. Rotate-on-retract procedural automation for robotic-assisted percutaneous coronary intervention: first clinical experience. Case Rep Cardiol. 2018;2018:6086034.
81. Madder R, Lombardi W, Parikh M, Kandzari D, Grantham JA, Rao S. TCT-539 impact of a novel advanced robotic wiring algorithm on time to wire a coronary artery bifurcation in a porcine model. J Am Coll Cardiol. 2017;70(18_Suppl):B223.
82. Mendes Pereira V, Nicholson P, Cancelliere NM, Liu XYE, Agid R, Radovanovic I, Krings T. Feasibility of robot-assisted neuroendovascular procedures. J Neurosurg. 2022;136(4):992–1004.
83. Kaul V, Enslin S, Gross SA. History of artificial intelligence in medicine. Gastrointest Endosc. 2020;92(4):807–12.
84. Davenport T, Kalakota R. The potential for artificial intelligence in healthcare. Future Healthc J. 2019;6(2):94–8.
85. Zaharchuk G, Gong E, Wintermark M, Rubin D, Langlotz CP. Deep learning in neuroradiology. AJNR Am J Neuroradiol. 2018;39(10):1776–84.
86. Shlobin NA, Baig AA, Waqas M, Patel TR, Dossani RH, Wilson M, et al. Artificial intelligence for large-vessel occlusion stroke: a systematic review. World Neurosurg. 2022;159:207–20.e1.
87. Yahav-Dovrat A, Saban M, Merhav G, Lankri I, Abergel E, Eran A, et al. Evaluation of artificial intelligence-powered identification of large-vessel occlusions in a comprehensive stroke center. AJNR Am J Neuroradiol. 2021;42(2):247–54.
88. Karamchandani RR, Helms AM, Satyanarayana S, Yang H, Clemente JD, Defilipp G, et al. Automated detection of intracranial large vessel occlusions using Viz.AI software: experience in a large, integrated stroke network. Brain Behav. 2023;13(1):e2808.
89. Matsoukas S, Morey J, Lock G, Chada D, Shigematsu T, Marayati NF, et al. AI software detection of large vessel occlusion stroke on CT angiography: a real-world prospective diagnostic test accuracy study. J Neurointerv Surg. 2023;15(1):52–6.
90. Hassan AE, Ringheanu VM, Rabah RR, Preston L, Tekle WG, Qureshi AI. Early experience utilizing artificial intelligence shows significant reduction in transfer times and length of stay in a hub and spoke model. Interv Neuroradiol. 2020;26(5):615–22.
91. Morey JR, Zhang X, Yaeger KA, Fiano E, Marayati NF, Kellner CP, et al. Real-world experience with artificial intelligence-based triage in transferred large vessel occlusion stroke patients. Cerebrovasc Dis. 2021;50(4):450–5.
92. Matsoukas S, Stein LK, Fifi JT. Artificial intelligence-assisted software significantly decreases all workflow metrics for large vessel occlusion transfer patients, within a large spoke and hub system. Cerebrovasc Dis Extra. 2023;13(1):41–6.
93. Abdollahifard S, Farrokhi A, Kheshti F, Jalali M, Mowla A. Application of convolutional network models in detection of intracranial aneurysms: a systematic review and meta-analysis. Interv Neuroradiol. 2023;29(6):738–47.
94. Gu F, Wu X, Wu W, Wang Z, Yang X, Chen Z, et al. Performance of deep learning in the detection of intracranial aneurysm: a systematic review and meta-analysis. Eur J Radiol. 2022;155:110457.
95. Din M, Agarwal S, Grzeda M, Wood DA, Modat M, Booth TC. Detection of cerebral aneurysms using artificial intelligence: a systematic review and meta-analysis. J Neurointerv Surg. 2023;15(3):262–71.
96. Liu J, Chen Y, Lan L, Lin B, Chen W, Wang M, et al. Prediction of rupture risk in anterior communicating artery aneurysms with a feed-forward artificial neural network. Eur Radiol. 2018;28(8):3268–75.
97. Silva MA, Patel J, Kavouridis V, Gallerani T, Beers A, Chang K, et al. Machine learning models can detect aneurysm rupture and identify clinical features associated with rupture. World Neurosurg. 2019;131:e46–51.
98. Zhu W, Li W, Tian Z, Zhang Y, Wang K, Zhang Y, et al. Stability assessment of intracranial aneurysms using machine learning based on clinical and morphological features. Transl Stroke Res. 2020;11(6):1287–95.
99. Dumont TM, Rughani AI, Tranmer BI. Prediction of symptomatic cerebral vasospasm after aneurysmal subarachnoid hemorrhage

with an artificial neural network: feasibility and comparison with logistic regression models. World Neurosurg. 2011;75(1):57–63; discussion 25–8.
100. de Jong G, Aquarius R, Sanaan B, Bartels R, Grotenhuis JA, Henssen D, Boogaarts HD. Prediction models in aneurysmal subarachnoid hemorrhage: forecasting clinical outcome with artificial intelligence. Neurosurgery. 2021;88(5):E427–34.
101. Ramos LA, van der Steen WE, Sales Barros R, Majoie C, van den Berg R, Verbaan D, et al. Machine learning improves prediction of delayed cerebral ischemia in patients with subarachnoid hemorrhage. J Neurointerv Surg. 2019;11(5):497–502.
102. Asadi H, Kok HK, Looby S, Brennan P, O'Hare A, Thornton J. Outcomes and complications after endovascular treatment of brain arteriovenous malformations: a prognostication attempt using artificial intelligence. World Neurosurg. 2016;96:562–9.e1.
103. Reddy VY, Shah D, Kautzner J, Schmidt B, Saoudi N, Herrera C, et al. The relationship between contact force and clinical outcome during radiofrequency catheter ablation of atrial fibrillation in the TOCCATA study. Heart Rhythm. 2012;9(11):1789–95.
104. Guo J, Jin X, Guo S. Study of the operational safety of a vascular interventional surgical robotic system. Micromachines (Basel). 2018;9(3):119.
105. He C, Wang S, Zuo S. A linear stepping endovascular intervention robot with variable stiffness and force sensing. Int J Comput Assist Radiol Surg. 2018;13(5):671–82.
106. Hasanzadeh S, Janabi-Sharifi F. Model-based force estimation for intracardiac catheters. IEEE/ASME Trans Mech. 2016;21:154–62.
107. Dagnino G, Liu J, Abdelaziz MEMK, Chi W, Riga CV, Yang G-Z. Haptic feedback and dynamic active constraints for robot-assisted endovascular catheterization. In: 2018 IEEE/RSJ International Conference on Intelligent Robots and Systems (IROS); 2018. p. 1770–5.
108. Guo S, Song Y, Yin X, Zhang L, Tamiya T, Hirata H, Ishihara H. A novel robot-assisted endovascular catheterization system with haptic force feedback. IEEE Trans Robot. 2019;35(3):685–96.
109. Shen H, Wang C, Xie L, Zhou S, Gu L, Xie H. A novel robotic system for vascular intervention: principles, performances, and applications. Int J Comput Assist Radiol Surg. 2019;14(4):671–83.
110. Reiley CE, Akinbiyi T, Burschka D, Chang DC, Okamura AM, Yuh DD. Effects of visual force feedback on robot-assisted surgical task performance. J Thorac Cardiovasc Surg. 2008;135(1):196–202.
111. Mendes-Pereira V. AI in robotics in the neurointerventional field. Master and Fellow; 2023.
112. Tjoumakaris S. Robotics in neurovascular surgery. Seattle Science Foundation; 2023.
113. Beaman C, Holodinsky JK, Goyal M, Tateshima S, Hill MD, Saver JL, Kamal N. Modeling optimal patient transport in a stroke network capable of remote telerobotic endovascular therapy. Interv Neuroradiol. 2024;30(4):506–16.
114. Abah C, Lawson J, Simaan N, Chitale R. O-017 towards self-steering microcatheters for neurointervention. J Neurointerv Surg. 2022;14(Suppl 1):A11–A2.
115. Li J, Yu J. Biodegradable microrobots and their biomedical applications: a review. Nanomaterials (Basel). 2023;13(10):1590.
116. Li J, Esteban-Fernández de Ávila B, Gao W, Zhang L, Wang J. Micro/nanorobots for biomedicine: delivery, surgery, sensing, and detoxification. Sci Robot. 2017;2(4):eaam6431.
117. Zhang D, Gorochowski TE, Marucci L, Lee HT, Gil B, Li B, et al. Advanced medical micro-robotics for early diagnosis and therapeutic interventions. Front Robot AI. 2022;9:1086043.
118. Jiang J, Yang Z, Ferreira A, Zhang L. Control and autonomy of microrobots: recent Progress and perspective. Adv Intell Syst. 2022;4(5):2100279.
119. Guo Y, Jing D, Liu S, Yuan Q. Construction of intelligent moving micro/nanomotors and their applications in biosensing and disease treatment. Theranostics. 2023;13(9):2993–3020.
120. Kadiri VM, Bussi C, Holle AW, Son K, Kwon H, Schütz G, et al. Biocompatible magnetic micro- and nanodevices: fabrication of FePt nanopropellers and cell transfection. Adv Mater. 2020;32(25):e2001114.
121. Leong TG, Randall CL, Benson BR, Bassik N, Stern GM, Gracias DH. Tetherless thermobiochemically actuated microgrippers. Proc Natl Acad Sci USA. 2009;106(3):703–8.
122. Wan M, Wang Q, Wang R, Wu R, Li T, Fang D, et al. Platelet-derived porous nanomotor for thrombus therapy. Sci Adv. 2020;6(22):eaaz9014.
123. Zhang H, Li Z, Gao C, Fan X, Pang Y, Li T, et al. Dual-responsive biohybrid neutrobots for active target delivery. Sci Robot. 2021;6(52):eaaz9519.
124. Liu F, Liu X, Huang Q, Arai T. Recent progress of magnetically actuated DNA micro/nanorobots. Cyborg Bionic Syst. 2022;2022:9758460.
125. Bakenecker AC, von Gladiss A, Schwenke H, Behrends A, Friedrich T, Lüdtke-Buzug K, et al. Navigation of a magnetic micro-robot through a cerebral aneurysm phantom with magnetic particle imaging. Sci Rep. 2021;11(1):14082.
126. Hosney A, Abdalla J, Amin IS, Hamdi N, Khalil ISM, editors. In vitro validation of clearing clogged vessels using microrobots. In: 2016 6th IEEE International Conference on Biomedical Robotics and Biomechatronics (BioRob); 2016. p. 26–9.
127. Servant A, Qiu F, Mazza M, Kostarelos K, Nelson BJ. Controlled in vivo swimming of a swarm of bacteria-like microrobotic flagella. Adv Mater. 2015;27(19):2981–8.
128. Law J, Wang X, Luo M, Xin L, Du X, Dou W, et al. Microrobotic swarms for selective embolization. Sci Adv. 2022;8(29):eabm5752.
129. Jin D, Wang Q, Chan KF, Xia N, Yang H, Wang Q, et al. Swarming self-adhesive microgels enabled aneurysm on-demand embolization in physiological blood flow. Sci Adv. 2023;9(19):eadf9278.
130. Yang L, Jiang J, Gao X, Wang Q, Dou Q, Zhang L. Autonomous environment-adaptive microrobot swarm navigation enabled by deep learning-based real-time distribution planning. Nat Mach Intell. 2022;4(5):480–93.
131. Patel TM, Shah SC, Pancholy SB. Long distance tele-robotic-assisted percutaneous coronary intervention: a report of first-in-human experience. EClinicalMedicine. 2019;14:53–8.
132. Madder RD, VanOosterhout S, Parker J, Sconzert K, Li Y, Kottenstette N, et al. Robotic telestenting performance in transcontinental and regional pre-clinical models. Catheter Cardiovasc Interv. 2021;97(3):E327–32.
133. Madder RD, VanOosterhout S, Mulder A, Bush J, Martin S, Rash AJ, et al. Network latency and long-distance robotic telestenting: exploring the potential impact of network delays on telestenting performance. Catheter Cardiovasc Interv. 2020;95(5):914–9.
134. Rayman R, Croome K, Galbraith N, McClure R, Morady R, Peterson S, et al. Long-distance robotic telesurgery: a feasibility study for care in remote environments. Int J Med Robot. 2006;2(3):216–24.
135. Xu S, Perez M, Yang K, Perrenot C, Felblinger J, Hubert J. Determination of the latency effects on surgical performance and the acceptable latency levels in telesurgery using the dV-Trainer(®) simulator. Surg Endosc. 2014;28(9):2569–76.
136. Zevallos N, Harber E, Abhimanyu PK, Gu Y, Sladick K, et al. Toward robotically automated femoral vascular access. In: 2021 International Symposium on Medical Robotics (ISMR); 2021. p. 17–9.
137. Brattain LJ, Pierce TT, Gjesteby LA, Johnson MR, DeLosa ND, Werblin JS, et al. AI-enabled, ultrasound-guided handheld robotic device for femoral vascular access. Biosensors (Basel). 2021;11(12):522.
138. Abbas R, Al Saiegh F, El Naamani K, Chen CJ, Velagapudi L, Sioutas GS, et al. Robot-assisted carotid artery stenting: out-

comes, safety, and operational learning curve. Neurosurg Focus. 2022;52(1):E17.
139. Saver J. Episode 1: informed patient consent and other pressing ethical issues in robot-assisted neurointervention. 2022. https://neuronewsinternational.com/episode-1-informed-patient-consent-and-other-pressing-ethical-issues-in-robot-assisted-neurointervention/.
140. Microbot Medical's LIBERTY® Robotic System Surpasses 100th Catheterization [press release]. 5/3/2023. 2023.
141. Moschovaki-Zeiger O, Arkoudis NA, Spiliopoulos S. Safety and feasibility study of a novel robotic system in an in vivo porcine vascular model. CVIR Endovasc. 2024;7(1):14.
142. Bravata DM, Ranta A. Artificial intelligence in clinical decisions support for stroke: balancing opportunity with caution. Stroke. 2023;54(6):1517–8.
143. Akay EMZ, Hilbert A, Carlisle BG, Madai VI, Mutke MA, Frey D. Artificial intelligence for clinical decision support in acute ischemic stroke: a systematic review. Stroke. 2023;54(6):1505–16.
144. Sensome begins human trial for its AI-powered stroke guidewire [press release].
145. Tong X, Shan Y, Leng X, Chen J, Fiehler J, Siddiqui AH, et al. Predicting flow diverter sizing using the AneuGuide(TM) software: a validation study. J Neurointerv Surg. 2023;15(1):57–62.
146. Piergallini L, Cagnazzo F, Conte G, Dargazanli C, Derraz I, Lefevre PH, et al. Virtual simulation with Sim&Size software for Pipeline Flex Embolization: evaluation of the technical and clinical impact. J Neurointerv Surg. 2020;12(10):968–73.
147. Mantilla D, Ferreira-Prada CA, Galvis M, Vargas O, Valenzuela-Santos C, Canci P, et al. Clinical impact of Sim & Size(®) simulation software in the treatment of patients with cerebral aneurysms with flow-diverter Pipeline stents. Interv Neuroradiol. 2023;29(1):47–55.
148. Liu C, Shen Y, Wu X, Qian K, Hu X, Yang H. Artificial intelligence-assisted microcatheter shaping for intracranial aneurysm coiling: a preliminary study. Ann Vasc Surg. 2022;85:228–36.
149. Yang H, Ni W, Xu L, Geng J, He X, Ba H, et al. Computer-assisted microcatheter shaping for intracranial aneurysm embolization: evaluation of safety and efficacy in a multicenter randomized controlled trial. J Neurointerv Surg. 2023;16:177.

Implications of Artificial Intelligence for Arterial Drug Delivery and Beyond

22

Zhenrui Liao, Vidur Joshi, and Shailendra Joshi

A computer would deserve to be called intelligent if it could deceive a human into believing it was human.

Alan Turing (1912–1954), Computer Scientist and Mathematician

Introduction

Artificial intelligence (AI) has become a ubiquitous buzzword in the twenty-first century, permeating discussions across diverse domains. In the current era of big data and high throughput, AI stands poised to reshape the landscape of medicine and healthcare. Although our ability to generate, aggregate, and process massive data has exploded, our capacity to decipher this wealth of information, discern meaningful patterns from noise, and avoid interpretive fallacies and pitfalls remains the bottleneck in our ability to use this proliferation of data to optimize care and improve patient outcomes. Artificial intelligence offers new possibilities that may revolutionize all aspects of healthcare, from the laboratory to the procedural suite. However, it also poses new and unique technical and ethical challenges that we must confront in the domains of privacy, data security, and inaccurate or biased decision-making.

The concept of automating feats that previously required human thought and labor has antecedents dating back to antiquity. The ancient Greeks, for instance, built the Antikythera mechanism to automate the prediction of eclipses [1–3]. Simpler single-application computing devices were used in many places and historical periods. The first documented general-purpose computer was Charles Babbage's analytical engine, a machine that was flexible enough in theory to perform any computation. This engine, which Babbage designed but never built, sparked the curiosity of early programmer Ada Lovelace, who pondered whether a machine could ever be said to "think" or "reason." A century later, Alan Turing independently posed the question "Can machines think?" in his 1950 paper "Computing Machinery and Intelligence," in which he also introduced the famous test that now bears his eponym. In this work, Turing presciently considered the possibility that a machine could be programmed to learn to pass this test on its own, based on inputs and feedback, much like a human child learns, even outlining a rudimentary genetic algorithm for doing so.

The AI field in the twentieth century was characterized by boom-and-bust cycles of widespread public excitement and investment (fueled by sensational claims of being on the brink of achieving human-level cognition), followed by yearslong "winters" of interest and research funding once the promised breakthroughs failed to materialize. Although the basic concepts of modern AI were established in the mid-to-late twentieth century, advancements in computing power, memory storage capacity, and data available for training have led to an explosion of progress in the field in the twenty-first century, primarily driven by the "unreasonable effectiveness" of neural networks at solving a wide array of problems [4]. Beginning in the 2000s, deep neural networks and improved hardware for linear algebraic operations ushered in a new AI wave based on machine learning that successfully delivered on many of the promises of humanlike performance in historically challenging tasks such as image recognition, speech processing, complex gameplay, and, recently,

Z. Liao (✉)
Columbia University, New York, NY, USA
e-mail: zl2359@cumc.columbia.edu

V. Joshi
Steven's Institute of Technology, Hoboken, NJ, USA

S. Joshi
Department of Anesthesiology, Columbia University Irving Medical Center, New York, NY, USA
e-mail: sj121@cumc.columbia.edu

S. Joshi (ed.), *Arterial Treatment of Neurological Diseases*, https://doi.org/10.1007/978-3-031-80173-0_22

natural language and image generation. In the past 20 years, AI has transformed from a field of speculation and science fiction into one offering practical algorithms to solve useful problems intractable to conventional methods. Nonetheless, given this history, it is essential to be cautious of overstating the capabilities of existing AI and distinguish genuine advances from overhyped claims.

This chapter discusses the potential benefits of AI in arterial drug delivery. This broad topic spans preclinical research, clinical data interpretation, treatment planning, and procedural guidance, with significant implications in medical ethics. These issues serve as a microcosm of the larger questions raised by AI's integration into healthcare. We present several illustrative examples and specific applications to provide a glimpse of how AI could revolutionize arterial drug delivery. Throughout this chapter, we aim to explicitly connect the specific cases we examine with the broader healthcare issues they represent, where possible. While this chapter does not cover every possible AI application in medicine, it does aim to introduce the topic at a level that's digestible for medical providers across disciplines, offering a framework to navigate the intersection of AI and healthcare.

We understand that most readers of this chapter may not have the time or expertise for in-depth study of the mathematical and implementational details of specific AI models; to keep the information provided here practical and clinically relevant, we refer readers interested in a deeper dive to excellent reviews by Bishop [5]; Hastie et al. [6]; Russell and Norvig [7]; and Sutton and Barto [8]. However, we do note two frequent and related but counterproductive reactions to this lack of expertise among clinicians: (1) resignation to the belief that there is no way for them to evaluate or contribute to conversations about AI constructively and (2) uncritical acceptance of claims made about AI or embrace of the mysticism surrounding AI. We will endeavor to show that both of these reactions are unnecessary; in the same way that clinicians routinely evaluate the evidence for a test or a drug without knowing each protein interaction or amino acid residue, the clinician can also learn to critically evaluate the advantages and disadvantages of specific models in different applications, including those not discussed here, without being an AI expert. An essential skill for doing so is *abstraction*: the ability to formulate imperfect, high-level mental models that enable us to connect pieces of knowledge and make predictions. By abstracting specific details and complexities, clinicians can engage with the subject at a level that aligns with their expertise, allowing conversations about AI in healthcare to become more bilateral. This is likely a skill most readers already have extensive experience exercising in domains adjacent to medicine and physiology; one goal of this chapter is to provide some appropriate abstractions for thinking about AI.

By the end of this chapter, the reader will become familiar with some of the most commonly used terms in AI and come to a high-level understanding of a typical AI workflow for different situations. We will discuss existing and possible applications of AI in drug development and delivery, clinical data analysis, and other aspects of healthcare. Undoubtedly, there will be essential applications that we will not have a chance to discuss or may not yet exist as of this writing. We hope the reader will come away equipped to recognize possible applications of AI in their research or practice and recognize what features of a clinical problem predict the impact of AI on the issue in the near term. Finally, the reader should pay particular attention to limitations shared by almost all existing AI systems, such as the availability of training data, bias present in the training set, the problem of discriminating correlation from causation, interpretability, and others, as well as the ethical responsibilities borne by human actors in its deployment and use.

AI Primer for Clinicians

Despite the term's ubiquity, there is no universally accepted definition of what constitutes "artificial intelligence." Russell and Norvig (2021) characterize AI through parallels to human capabilities such as perception, reasoning, prediction, and interaction with the environment, including other agents in it [7, 9]. *For this work, we will loosely define artificial intelligence as the attempt to recreate some aspect of human cognition in a computer* (Fig. 22.1).

In almost all cases, the science fiction-influenced vision of AI as an autonomous agent capable of independently collecting data and making decisions conveys the wrong mental model for thinking about AI systems as they exist today. Philosophers of AI have traditionally distinguished "strong" AI with a humanlike general capability of interacting with the world, as opposed to "weak" AI fulfilling a narrow self-contained function. Weak AI also falls on a spectrum, from narrow models only capable of answering a single question (e.g., is there a mass in this radiograph) to specialized systems capable of a limited degree of autonomy (such as a hypothetical "AI radiologist" capable of generating reports from any imaging modality). All AI that currently exists is weak. Almost all current systems to which the term "AI" is applied in medicine and other domains are extremely narrow machine learning systems dedicated to singular tasks. In a later section of this chapter, *AI Agents in Healthcare*, we discuss a future in which "stronger" automated systems may have an expanded role more consistent with the popular perception of "artificial intelligence."

The field of AI encompasses many overlapping subfields, which lack a singular systematic classification. Subfields may be classified based on the type of data used (e.g., computer vision, natural language processing), the methodology used (probabilistic vs. deterministic, neural networks), or a particular practical or engineering goal (e.g., speech recognition, robotics). These classifications are not mutually exclu-

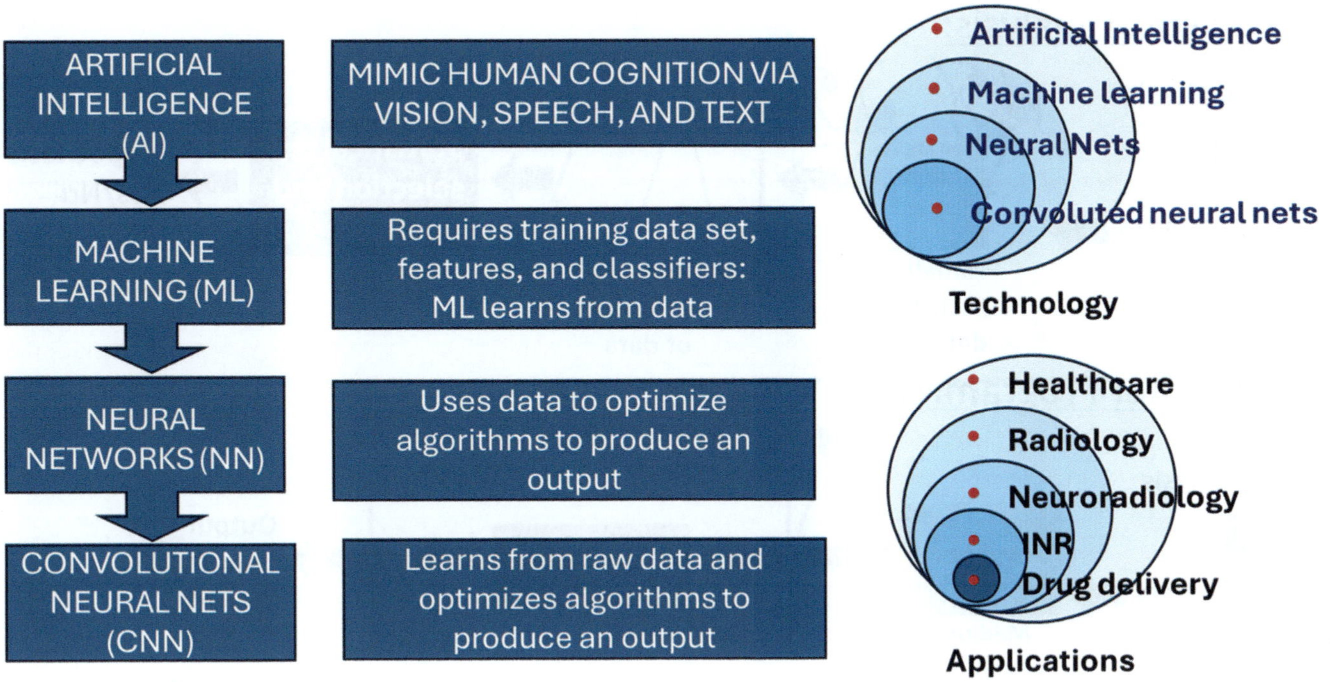

Fig. 22.1 Conceptual hierarchy of common AI-related terms, with examples. Artificial intelligence refers to the goal of computationally reproducing some element of human cognition. Machine learning, a subset of AI, refers to the approach of accomplishing that goal by training with data. Neural networks represent one highly successful class of machine learning algorithms. Convolutional neural networks (CNNs) are one type of neural network particularly suited to processing image-type data. Potential applications of AI from healthcare to drug delivery

sive—some of the same approaches have been highly successful in multiple domains.

Machine learning (ML) uses *data* to iteratively train a system to perceive, reason, predict, or interact with its environment. It is important to note that ML and AI are not synonymous—AI refers to the overarching goal of replicating human faculties in a computer. In contrast, ML refers to the specific approach of learning patterns from data in an automated manner to accomplish this goal. Non-ML approaches, such as search algorithms and symbolic reasoning, occupied a significant role in the history of AI and, in some domains, have remained essential or experienced a resurgence. Nonetheless, as medicine is a data-driven field, a large proportion of the questions of interest in the domain of drug development and drug delivery can be reframed as machine learning questions; hence, the bulk of this chapter will be devoted to discussing techniques that broadly fall under the ML umbrella, though we will also briefly mention non-ML approaches to AI.

Virtually all problems for which AI has been proposed as a solution involve producing some output given some input. The input may be an explicit data point from which the answer to a specific question is desired, but it may also be the state of a system or an environment to which the AI must respond dynamically. Under the conventional programming paradigm (Fig. 22.2), a human programmer provides a set of specific, step-by-step instructions to a computer to transform a particular input into a desired output. Specific input and output types lend themselves particularly well to this paradigm. For example, calculations involving multistep repeated arithmetic operations on numerical inputs to return a numerical output would be extremely tedious for a human to perform by hand. Yet, they are relatively easy to encode in computer-readable language and execute on computer hardware. On the other hand, it isn't easy to imagine how one would write step-by-step instructions for specific tasks that are trivial for a human to perform, such as viewing the pixels of an image and determining whether it contains a bird. The **model** or **algorithm** is the black box that transforms the input into the output; the knowledge the model uses to perform this transformation is encoded in its **parameters**. In machine learning, these parameters are shaped through a **training** process, wherein the model learns from many inputs or input-output pairs. Subsequently, the system's performance is evaluated on previously unseen ("held-out") test data to verify its performance before being deployed in a real-world application (Fig. 22.2).

Machine learning can further be divided into subfields based on the inputs and the problem to be solved. Problems that takes the form: "From a piece of data (e.g., a chest radiograph), predict a label (e.g., cancer vs. not cancer)" or a numerical value (e.g., lesion volume) fall under the purview of *supervised learning*. Problems that take the form of "From a large dataset (e.g., genomic data from a large population), discover the patterns within it (e.g., genetic subgroups, directions of variation in the data)" fall under the purview of *unsupervised learning*. Problems in the form of "Given a set of observations from the world, decide or take an action that

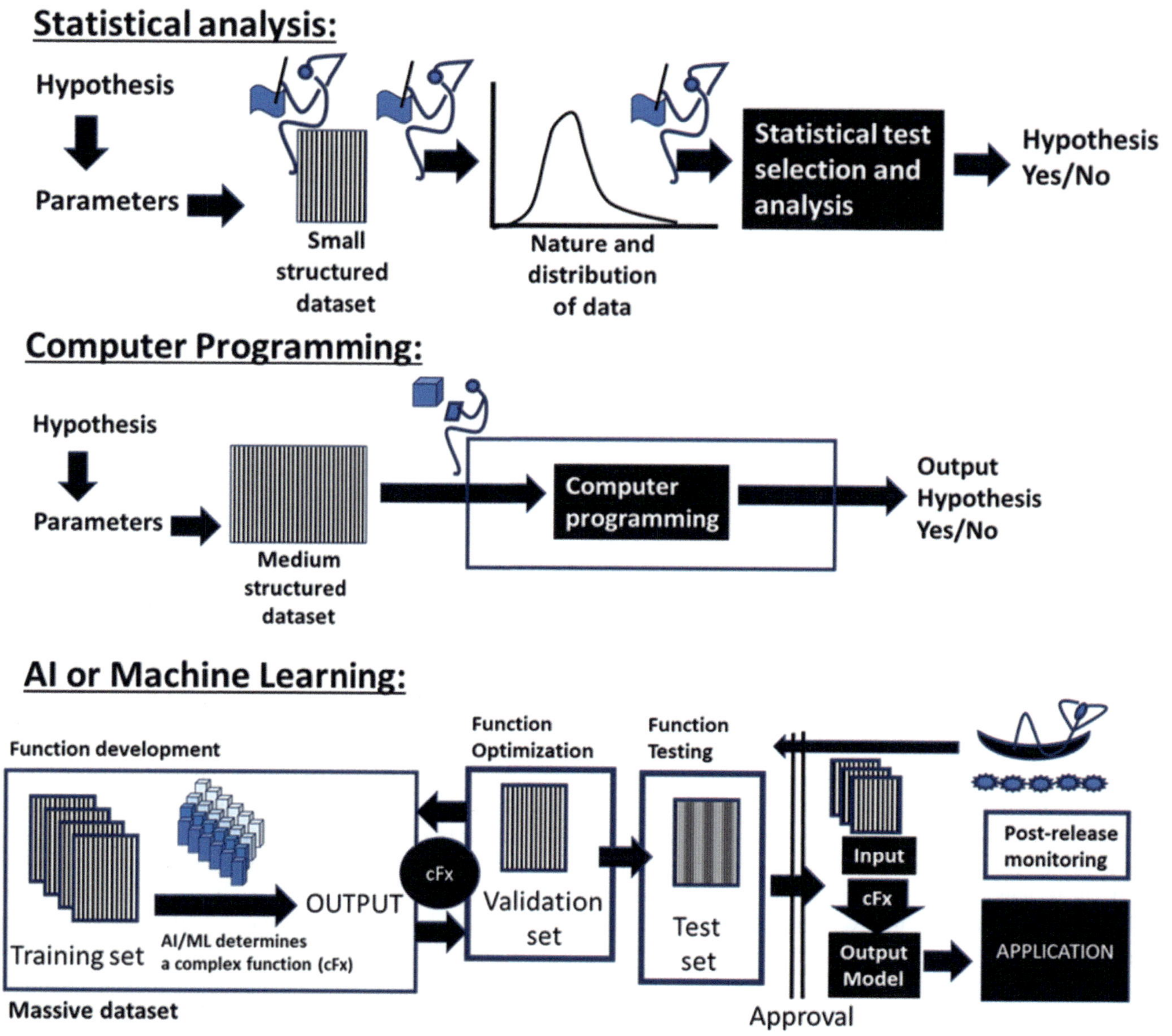

Fig. 22.2 Distinct paradigms for computationally producing a desired output given specified inputs. These paradigms are not necessarily mutually exclusive. Top: Under the frequentist statistical analysis paradigm, hypotheses are expressed in terms of a null distribution and a critical value. The probability of the data under the null distribution is calculated, and the null hypothesis is rejected or not rejected. Middle: Under the explicit computer programming paradigm, a human programmer explicitly conceives and writes down a procedure to go from the input to the desired output and precisely expresses that procedure using computer code. Bottom: Under the machine learning paradigm, the algorithm is programmed to learn input-output functions from data using optimization, but the desired function is not programmed explicitly. The learned model is evaluated based on held-out (validation and test) data

will change the state of the world, then collecting a new set of observations and repeating the learning process" are *reinforcement learning* problems.

Under the **supervised learning** paradigm, the input-output transformation does not have to be programmed manually but rather is *learned* from many examples, similar to how a child might learn to recognize unfamiliar animals by being given pictures of the animals in different environments, paired with verbal cues from a teacher about the identity of the animal in each picture. Any data encoded as a list of numbers are valid inputs, for example, laboratory values, radiographic images, pathology slides, or combinations of the above. The training set consists of many input samples, each with a list of *features*, such as pixels in an image or laboratory values. The outputs may either be *categorical* (yes/no or a choice from a list) or *continuous* (a decimal number). Supervised learning models subsume some tools from classical statistics, such as logistic regression and linear regression, and models specific to the machine learning field, such as neural networks (Figs. 22.2 and 22.3). They are trained on input-output *pairs* where the output is a "ground truth," i.e., the desired answer obtained some other way.

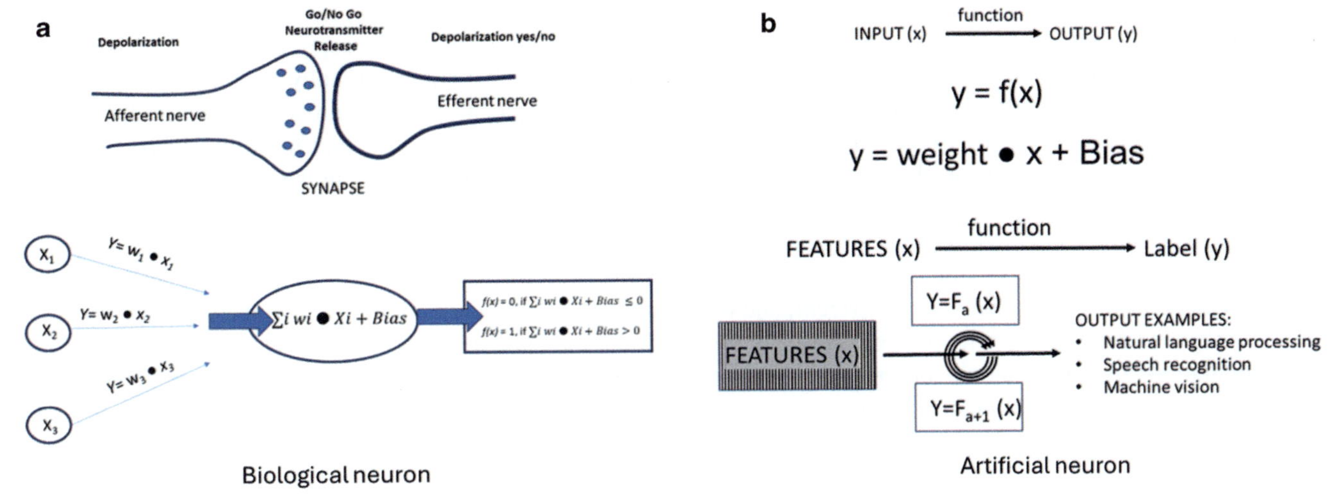

Fig. 22.3 Biological and artificial neurons. (**a**) Simplified biological neuron. Top: Inputs arrive at the neuron at synapses in the form of presynaptic neurotransmitter release and association with postsynaptic receptors, which may cause postsynaptic depolarization or hyperpolarization. Bottom: The activity at the neuronal cell body can be modeled as a weighted sum of the received inputs passed through a nonlinearity. (**b**) Single artificial neuron. Input features are multiplied by a weight vector, with or without a bias term, and transformed via a nonlinearity into an output

Machine learning models typically require thousands or millions of examples, unlike human children, who can learn new object classes with few examples. How enough data is obtained is a recurring issue when applying AI to new domains. Usually, the training data is collected and annotated by hand, which is labor-intensive and expensive. Some pre-annotated public datasets exist for everyday tasks, such as recognizing handwritten digits or common objects. However, specialized applications still require manual data curation and annotation, which is usually the rate-limiting step of model training. A model may behave unpredictably if encountering data in the real world that differs from its training set; for example, facial recognition models trained primarily on white faces have difficulty accurately recognizing faces of color. We discuss the problem of biases in the training set further in the section on *AI Ethics*.

Supervised learning answers questions such as the following:

- Given chemical properties, what is a drug's PO/IV/arterial bioavailability likely to be?
- Given an X-ray, is a fracture present?
- Given a brain MRI, what is the volume of the ventricles?
- Given patient characteristics, what is the patient's risk of disease X?

The **unsupervised learning** paradigm differs from the supervised learning paradigm in that there is no ground-truth label to be predicted; instead, the goal is to understand the *structure* within the data. As with supervised learning, any data encoded numerically can be used for this purpose. These models typically explore input data to identify patterns. They do not rely on extensive manual ground-truth labeling to generate a training set. Extending the previous analogy, unsupervised learning is akin to a child noticing without any explicit instruction that there are natural groups or "clusters" among animals based on observable characteristics—e.g., scaled animals that swim, feathered animals that fly, warm-blooded animals with fur, and so on. Although the learner may not have specific external names ("labels") for these groups, it can answer questions such as which group a new observation is most similar to. More complex structure in data can also be learned using unsupervised learning, often based on notions of how "similar" or "different" (or in other words, "close" or "far") points in the dataset are from each other and what "shape" the data takes. Commonly used data visualization and interpretation methods such as K-means clusters, principal component analysis, t-SNE, and manifold learning all fall under the unsupervised learning umbrella. An important limitation is that the output of these methods may be sensitive to noise in the original dataset or the specific preprocessing that is applied to the data.

Unsupervised learning answers questions such as the following:

- Given a population genetic dataset, what cluster structure is present, if any?
- Given an EEG dataset, what combinations of leads represent the directions of the highest variance?
- How can trends in a 50,000-dimensional point cloud be visualized in two or three dimensions?

One particularly successful class of algorithms is the previously mentioned artificial neural networks (ANNs), often referred to as *neural networks* (Fig. 22.3). Neurons inspired the creation of neural networks. However, they differ from biological neural networks in many essential ways, and the extent to which analogies from artificial neural networks provide insight into biological cognition remains a hotly debated question. In a simplified model, a single biological neuron receives synaptic *inputs* from many upstream neurons, each modulated by a distinct synaptic *weight*, and nonlinearly integrates these inputs with intrinsic biases or local neuromodulation to produce an *output* firing pattern (Fig. 22.3a). A single artificial neuron works very similarly to this simplified model: it receives a set of input features, to which it applies a weighted sum followed by a nonlinear mathematical function, producing an output (Fig. 22.3b). Although a single artificial neuron alone can solve some simple tasks, *networks* in which many such neurons are connected in multiple layers are far more powerful. The successes for which neural networks have been celebrated have been driven by "deep" networks, i.e., networks consisting of many neurons in many such layers (Fig. 22.4). Theoretical work suggests that deeper networks are more expressive and can learn more complex input-output relationships. There are, however, significant differences between biological and artificial neural networks. Artificial neurons used in practice are significantly simpler than biological neurons and typically do not model the complex 3D morphology, binary (spike/no spike) output, or neuromodulatory inputs of biological neurons. Weight is also a significant abstraction of the complexity of the biological synapse, which distills the complexities of vesicles, receptors, and other synaptic proteins into a single number. Finally, although highly effective, the backpropagation algorithm with which artificial neural networks are trained is distinct from the Hebbian rule [10] associated with biological neural networks and generally not considered biologically plausible.

Even though AI models may make very accurate predictions, it is difficult for humans to comprehend how the model arrived at these predictions, even with complete information about the input and model parameters. This problem, sometimes referred to as the "black box" problem, particularly plagues deep neural networks, which complicates understanding what went wrong when performance is poor and raises the possibility that the AI may be reasoning in incorrect or undesirable ways, such as drawing prohibited inferences from patient demographic characteristics. Compounding this problem, this undesired behavior may be nonobvious or masked by apparently good "bottom-line" performance. Therefore, AI interpretability is one of AI's most critical unresolved problems for drug development. As AI systems become more complex and more relied upon for impactful decisions, transparency and explainability become paramount. Explaining internal models comprehensibly allows researchers and clinicians to understand the reasoning behind AI-generated predictions and independently verify their accuracy. This interpretability is critical for building trust in AI applications within the medical community and setting the terms of collaboration between AI systems and human experts.

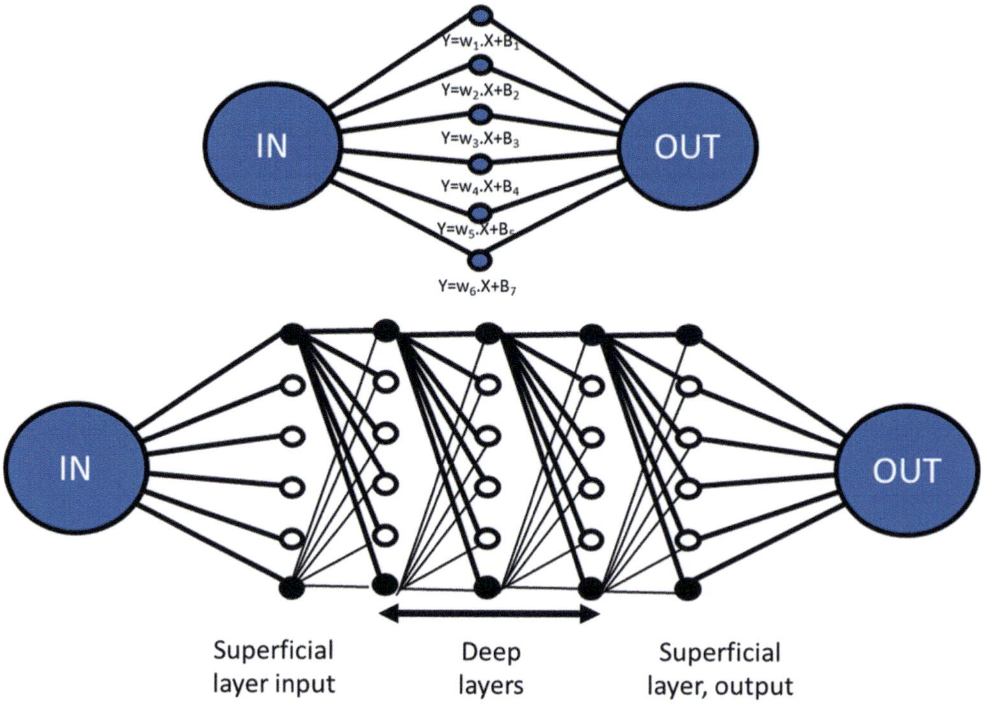

Fig. 22.4 Artificial neural network schematic. Many artificial neurons as shown in Fig. 22.3 are chained together in successive layers: each circle represents an artificial neuron, and each line represents one weight ("synapse"). Layers that are not the input or output are referred to as hidden layers. The "depth" of a neural network refers to the number of hidden layers: a "shallow" network may have only one hidden layer (top), whereas a deep network may have many hidden layers (bottom). Deep networks have been highly successful in learning complex input-output functions that are difficult to program explicitly

Table 22.1 Recognizable characteristics of problems on which AI-driven progress is likely vs. characteristics of problems that will likely be challenging for AI in the near to medium term

Amenable to AI	Challenging for AI
Human experts can solve the problem with high accuracy and inter-rater agreement, even if • Solving the problem is expensive, time-consuming, and/or subject to human factors • Experts may have difficulty explicitly articulating or programming in a computer exactly what process they go through to produce the solution	Human experts often disagree on the solution, even without practical constraints such as limited time
Limited solution space: The solution can be expressed as categorical choices (yes/no or choice from a predetermined list), numbers or lists of numbers, or natural language text following a predictable formula	Solutions are open-ended or freeform: sequence of actions in a procedure, freeform natural language
Objective, evidence-based performance readouts and feedback are available to assess a solution in real time	Few readouts available for real-time objective/evidence-based feedback
Human experts can verify AI solutions somehow (or overrule them if necessary)	AI-generated solutions cannot easily be evaluated or overruled by human experts
Extensive, high-dimensional training data available	Limited or low-dimensional training data

Finally, it is essential to recognize that AI solutions are not required or desirable for every problem. Although barriers to application have been lowered by the widespread availability of public datasets and pretrained models as well as user-friendly software packages such as Torch and TensorFlow, bringing AI to bear on many tasks still requires significant upfront investment in development, data collection, curation, and testing. The return on this investment is scalability: well-trained models can be scaled up simply by purchasing more computing power, which is much more cost-efficient in many cases than scaling up human effort. However, the gain from this investment is not necessarily worth the opportunity cost in all cases: for example, if a conventional algorithm already performs well, if it is relatively easy to solve the problem manually, or if the scale of the problem is small. As we have discussed, unlike explicitly programmed algorithms, the behavior of AI models may not be wholly interpretable or predictable on new inputs; AI solutions are not yet sufficiently mature for deployment in high-stakes settings where consistency in performance is obligatory. We summarize characteristics of problems that are likely amenable to AI progress in the near to medium term, compared to attributes of problems where AI currently still falls short, in Table 22.1.

AI for Preclinical Research and Drug Development

AI has already emerged as a transformative force in preclinical research, with drug development a particularly promising arena. The main impacts of AI on preclinical research fall into two interrelated categories: (1) the automated generation of high-quality testable hypotheses and (2) the extraction of patterns from large datasets. In the realm of drug discovery, AI is already making significant strides on both fronts.

Historically, identifying good drug candidates from the overwhelming array of possible chemical and structural permutations has been the most expensive and time-consuming step of the drug development pipeline. Because in vitro and in vivo screening are costly, identifying compounds that are better investments with a higher chance of passing these early stages could markedly reduce the cost of and accelerate drug development [11, 12]. Research is active in the area of in silico screening of pharmaceutical compounds, predicting their pharmacokinetic properties based on chemical structure and properties and in vitro data, optimizing the experimental design to a minimum number of necessary animal studies, scaling animal models to human studies, and finally optimizing human doses and predicting and minimizing side effects [13–17].

Short of discovering entirely new drugs, structural modifications to existing drugs can reduce side effects, enhance efficacy, improve absorption, and optimize pharmacokinetic and pharmacodynamic properties [15]. While the potential impact of modifying existing drugs is smaller than the possibility of discovering new drugs, this space remains far too vast to explore by brute force. Thus far, screening such modifications requires a combination of human intuition and expensive high-throughput assays. AI may be able to propose changes with a higher likelihood of success, reducing the number of assays that need to be performed and possibly increasing the likelihood and accelerating the rate at which these favorable modifications are discovered [18, 19]. Relevant to arterial drug development, AI can predict a wide range of drug responses [20–26].

Drug-protein interactions are another promising avenue for AI-driven progress. The ability to predict structure-activity relationships, i.e., how a drug will interact with target and off-target receptors and proteins, would be transformational for drug development, predicting drug efficacy and side effects. Traditionally, predicting these interactions required a laborious combination of structural biology, in vitro assays, and a certain degree of "guess-and-check." Human intervention and expertise remain essential in refining and interpreting the results. Some creativity is required to generate reasonable hypotheses; each hypothesis can be verified or falsified experimentally, although doing so for many hypotheses by brute force is prohibitively expensive. AI has already been used to develop pK and pD models to predict potential complications and therapeutic effects [15, 16]. However, automated structural prediction has recently advanced dramatically with DeepMind's AlphaFold, a neural network-based supervised learning model for predicting protein 3D structure from its amino acid sequence [27]. Although this problem is not identical to the drug interaction problem, it shares essential similarities: both are considered intractable by brute force; hypotheses may be verified or falsified experimentally; humans have made progress on subproblems corresponding to individual proteins or drug-protein pairs in the past, but the space of subproblems is vast out of proportion to the number of researchers working on them. Encouragingly, AlphaFold revolutionized the field of protein structure prediction, with accuracies far higher than any preceding system. The ability to predict protein structures enables researchers to identify potential drug targets with greater precision, with research ongoing into how to leverage this breakthrough to design ligands.

In the long term, AI's potential in drug development extends to creating molecules de novo to manipulate biological pathways. This ambitious goal involves leveraging AI to design molecules from scratch, tailoring them to modulate specific biological processes in desired ways, and exploring structural variants to optimize biophysical parameters. Moreover, the long-term vision includes incorporating feedback mechanisms, allowing AI systems to learn and adapt from multiple sources, such as experimental results and human feedback. This adaptability enhances the system's efficacy and responsiveness to dynamic changes in the drug development landscape.

AI for Arterial Drug Delivery

Most drugs that pass preclinical or early-stage human trials eventually fail at the clinical trial stage. The reasons for this high proportion of failure are multifactorial and include problems with drug metabolism, challenges in achieving therapeutic concentrations, and unexpected toxicity. While some of these drugs have the potential to overcome these obstacles with appropriate adjustments to delivery and pharmacologic parameters, a large number of drug candidates have been abandoned after a failure at this stage as clinical trials are costly to conduct and are often industry-funded, which may be averse to "throwing good money after bad" given the uncertain return and the opportunity cost to the pursuit of other promising candidates. A validated, automated method for predicting the effect of varying dosing parameters and the delivery route on efficacy, safety, and side effects could make further investigation of many of these failed drugs viable [21, 28–32].

Arterial delivery is a promising route for many reasons discussed elsewhere in this book, notably due to the ability to avoid hepatic first-pass metabolism and precisely target desired organs or tissues. There is a critical lack of data describing the pharmacokinetics of arterial drug delivery for most drugs, as the IV route remains the overwhelming standard in pharmacological studies. A limited number of animal and tissue sampling studies measure tissue drug concentrations after IA injection, and most do not track tissue drug concentration over time after injection. Many variables include injection characteristics, vascular anatomy, regional blood flow, tissue-specific drug properties, regional uptake metabolism, and clearances [33]. It would be prohibitively expensive to repeat all of the trials that yielded this information for conventional intravenous delivery again for arterial delivery for every drug of interest, especially as many are likely to show no advantage to IA delivery. However, a supervised learning approach could be used to predict drug properties under arterial delivery, which could help identify those with advantageous properties meriting further investigation; these properties could then be validated experimentally in this much smaller set of drugs before human trials [19].

In the previous section, we discussed the use of AI in predicting treatment responses [20–26]. However, as discussed in this book, hundreds of carrier molecules and their cargos still need to be investigated for arterial drug delivery. Over a thousand neuroprotective compounds that failed with intravenous delivery might benefit from arterial delivery [34]. For over 30 years, it has been recognized that unless the regional extraction of the drug is maximized, the benefits of arterial delivery will be limited. The availability of a new carrier system with efficient regional uptake and a broad range of drugs could benefit from AI-assisted carrier-drug selection for arterial injections (Fig. 22.5).

In neuro-oncology, delivering drugs across the blood-brain barrier has been a topic of great interest for the last decade. However, the BBB is not the only hurdle to effective drug delivery: the disintegration of the vascular network, hydrodynamic changes in the capillary bed such as the increase in hydrostatic pressure at the core of a tumor, clonal diversity of cancer cells, etc. could all contribute to therapeutic failure. However, it seems that with AI drug delivery, cationic carriers could penetrate the BBB and retain it for a long time in the tissues. One application of AI is designing and evaluating carriers for specific target sites. Such an approach will significantly help improve carrier-assisted arterial drug delivery [35, 36].

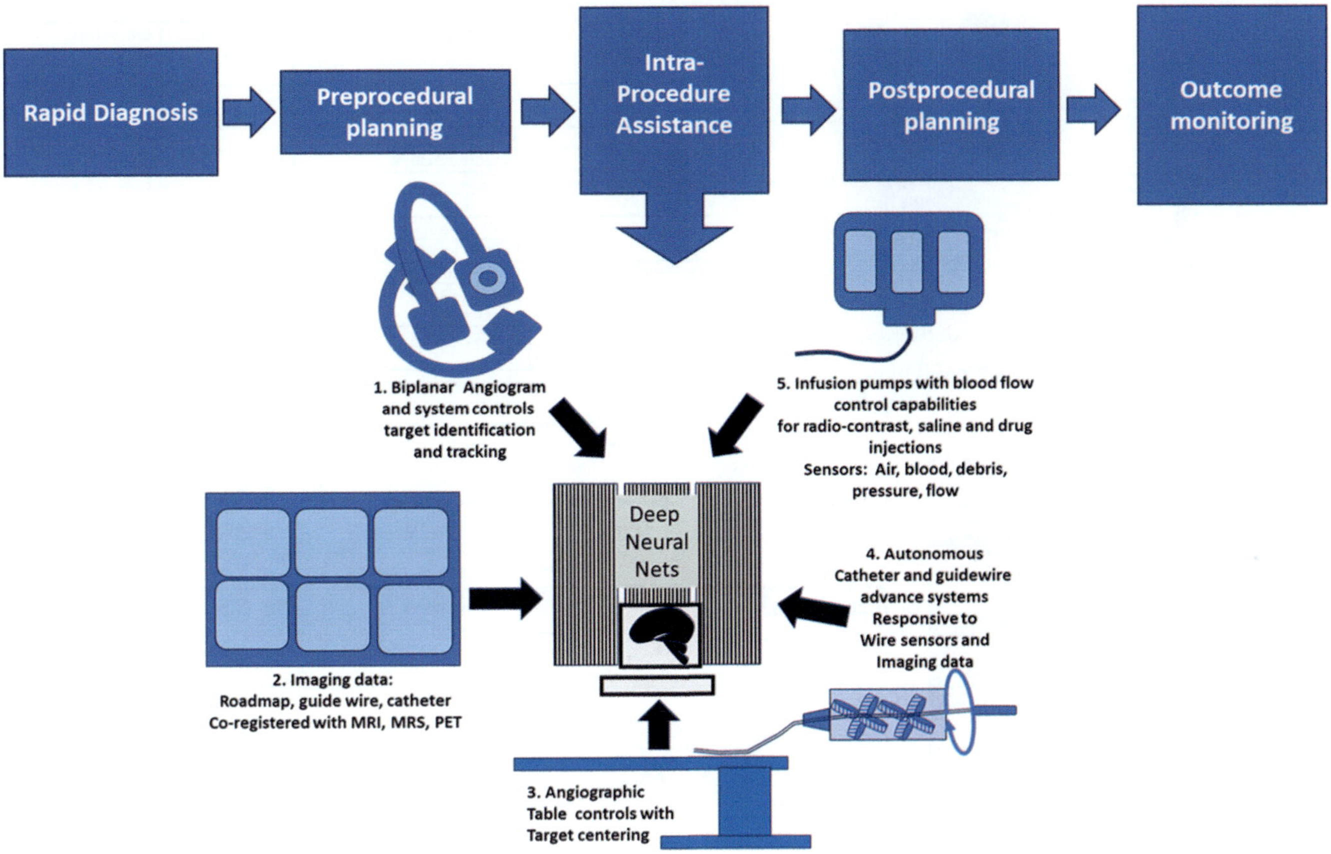

Fig. 22.5 The possible role of AI in arterial drug delivery

How to obtain data of sufficient volume, quality, and richness to train any models of the pharmacologic parameters of a drug under arterial delivery remains an open question. Chapters 19 and 20 elaborate on how optical methods can be applied to investigate arterial drug delivery: A combination of optical techniques can rapidly screen carriers tagged with dyes by elastic scatter spectroscopy and postmortem fluorescence imaging. Most of these early studies use relatively simple regional pharmacokinetic analysis, generating hemodynamic, regional blood flow, and carrier kinetics data. It is possible to track real-time changes in pathogenic pathways of neural injury using tissue imaging by optical means (Fig. 22.6). The data can be acquired several times a second for sensing, fluorescence, and reflectance imaging. Other optical imaging methods, such as photoacoustic and optical coherence tomography, can acquire data with similarly high temporal resolution. At the same time, hyperspectral imaging can acquire dense data in a slightly longer time frame. Unsupervised and supervised learning models could maximize the usefulness of these data by clarifying the regional pharmacokinetics of carriers as it relates to injection, regional physiological conditions, carrier characteristics, and systemic parameters.

Chapter 23 describes the current simple approach to clinical neuroscience research. Given the structural complexity of the host tissue, the multitude of potential injury pathways, and the functional impact of injuries, a simple linear cause-effect approach is unlikely to succeed. What might be needed is to monitor the multiple pathways of neurological injuries by optical or magnetic resonance imaging methods. These will generate vast amounts of data. Neurological diseases and their treatment result in a "problem mess." The large volume of data such investigations will generate will require supervised and unsupervised learning models.

The potential impacts of AI on arterial drug delivery are vast and multifaceted (Table 22.2). From short-term applications in basic research and drug discovery to medium-term prospects in predicting interactions and optimizing arterial delivery and, finally, the long-term vision of de novo molecule design and interpretability, AI stands as a catalyst for innovation in drug development. As researchers continue to navigate the dynamic landscape of AI applications, a thoughtful integration of these technologies holds the promise of revolutionizing the field, ultimately leading to more targeted, efficient, and personalized approaches to arterial drug delivery and healthcare at large.

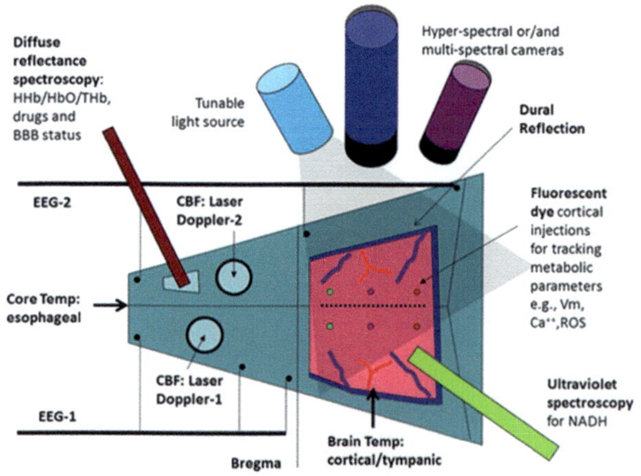

Measured parameter	Optical probe	Excitation max (nm)	Emission max (nm)
Micro-vascular O2	Oxyphor G3	635	810
NADH	auto-florescence	350	465
ROS (O2-)	Dihydroethidium	518	605
pH sensitive dye	BCECF	470	535
K+	SKC 463		
Voltage (Vm)	JPW series	650	>720
Ca++	Fura 2	330/360	510
Neutrophil activation	CFCE labeled neutrophils	491	518
platelet activation	carboxy-fluorescein labeled platelets	488	525
cell viability/ apoptosis	cytoGLO	488	530

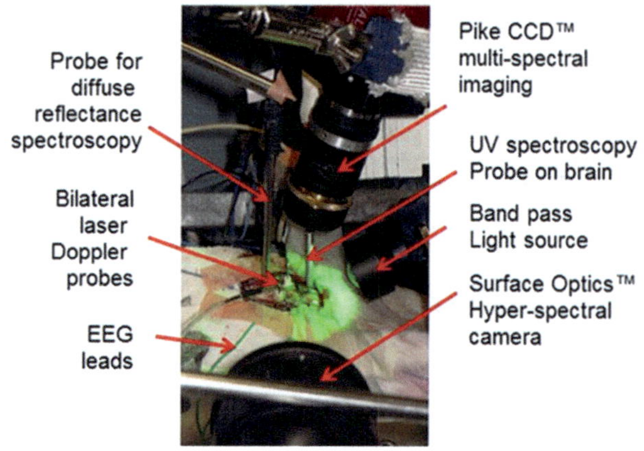

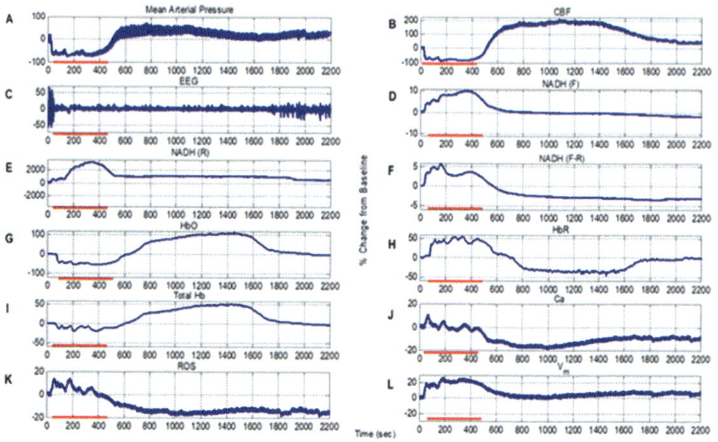

Fig. 22.6 Dense imaging and time-sequenced data are generated while investigating cerebral neurological reperfusion injuries in preclinical research in a rabbit model. A similar approach could be used to investigate therapeutic interventions. Typically, such experiments sample tissue several times a second and last several hours, generating gigabytes of data

Table 22.2 Potential applications of AI to clinical pharmacokinetics

Applications of AI in clinical pharmacokinetics	References
Drug development	[37, 38]
Integrating EHR with drug databases to ensure safer drug delivery	[39–41]
Determining accurate drug doses for a given patient	[15, 42–46]
Developing pharmacokinetic models	[15–17, 42, 47]
Predicting unknown adverse drug reactions	[48–54]
Pharmacogenetic variability	[17–19]
Predicting drug interactions with other drugs or food intake	[55–60]
Designing efficient clinical trials	[61–64]
Predicting treatment response, such as brain tumors and stroke	[65–67]

AI for Diagnostic and Interventional Radiology

Image analysis, comprising diagnostic scans, images acquired during interventional radiology procedures, and cell and tissue images from pathology, is currently at the frontier of AI in medicine [68–72]. Computer vision, which seeks to automate the extraction of information from images and videos, has been predated by modern AI for decades. However, deep neural networks have revolutionized the field within the past 20 years. Neuroscience has always enjoyed a symbiotic relationship with computer vision; deep convolutional networks, the current most successful computer vision architecture, are inspired by the architecture of the mammalian visual system [73]. The best deep networks perform comparably to or better than humans on general-purpose object recognition benchmarks [74–76]. This domain presents many opportunities for AI-driven progress, establishing guidelines for AI image analysis [77], collating information from multiple sources [78, 79], accurately assessing treatment response [80], integration and registration, and treatment guidance [81]. While the rollout of AI in some of these areas is already underway, research into expanding the utility of these tools in procedural fields such as interventional neuroradiology (INR) is ongoing, as time delays and the unavailability of human skills could impact procedure outcomes [82–86]. In radiology, AI-assisted reads of routine imaging are already in active use or being tested at many hospitals. However, a human radiologist still validates and confirms the report before signing it. Similarly, in pathology, studies have demonstrated that AI can outperform human pathologists in detecting cancer in stained tissue slides. This early success has generated considerable excitement, but it is also crucial to acknowledge the limitations of these technologies, which are often overlooked in media reports.

Many image analysis tasks naturally lend themselves to AI based on the criteria outlined at the beginning of this chapter: they involve large, high-dimensional datasets; humans can perform them reliably with training and effort; AI reads can be verified by a human radiologist or pathologist. AI may be able to detect subtle changes or correlates in these datasets that the human eye cannot pick up on. In addition, AI may reduce the impact of human factors such as distraction, exhaustion, understaffing, and individual variation in skill or training on clinical outcomes. Conversely, AI may introduce new sources of error that human clinicians must remain vigilant against—in some cases. Otherwise, well-trained AI models may give results far outside what any human interpreter would consider reasonable. This may be the case when the input is unusual in some way that has not been encountered in the training set; it is possible to design adversarial inputs to "trick" computer vision algorithms into giving an absurd result. How to guarantee fault tolerance in such systems remains an open question. AI may also introduce unconscious bias while conveying a false sense of objectivity; we discuss this problem further in the section *AI Ethics*.

Diagnostic imaging produces large datasets that remain bottlenecked by the rate at which human radiologists can accurately interpret and report them. Brain MRI image analysis is an area of rapid technology development [68–72]. Computer vision algorithms can reliably diagnose pulmonary lesions with 92% positive predictive value, sometimes surpassing the performance of human radiologists [87]. AI has yet to reach similar capabilities in neuroradiology but is advancing rapidly. Neurological applications of AI/ML include diagnosing and classifying brain tumors [71, 88–92], neurodegenerative diseases [73, 93, 94], stroke [95–98], and intracranial hemorrhage [99]. Connectomics, in combination with white matter imaging, diffusion imaging, and fMRI, could provide novel insights into the functional impact of neurological injuries [100–104]. Machine learning algorithms have also been used in fMRI studies to map task-specific neural functions in different regions of the brain, as well as assess changes in functional connectivity in disorders such as autism [103], attention deficit hyperactivity disorder [105], and psychiatric illnesses [106]. ML may also assist in EEG signal processing [93, 107]. ML has also been used to assess treatment response, such as response to steroid treatment for multiple sclerosis as judged by MRI [108, 109]. Given the complexity of neurological diseases and the potentially devastating impact of not urgently treating them, AI could play a significant role in patient and drug selection for arterial treatments. AI offers data analysis that is beyond human capabilities. Figure 22.2 shows the three approaches to handling a dataset with increasing complexity.

Research into the intraprocedural use of AI for real-time image analysis, registration, and procedural guidance is also ongoing [86]. In neurosurgery, surgical planning and navigation with preoperative volumetric imaging combined with computer vision has been used for decades, with companies such as BrainLab and Medtronic already providing widely used products. In interventional neuroradiology, a system for real-time image analysis integrated with other data streams could assist with catheter and guidewire selection and navigation. Such a system could reduce the duration of procedures and procedural complications. In addition, realistic procedural simulations with real-time feedback could be very valuable in medical education and patient communication. As with the other applications we have discussed, a lack of standardized data poses a barrier to training any such system, and patient privacy considerations may make collecting a sufficiently large dataset difficult. AI in procedures poses unique risks of patient harm from errors in real-time image analysis that are acted upon by the proceduralist without independent verification. At a minimum, the raw images on which the analysis is performed should also be available to the proceduralist in real time. However, once AI can detect imaging subtleties that are not readily perceptible by humans, the "black box" problem could become more pronounced, emphasizing the need for interpretable AI.

Several recent publications that have received attention in the popular press have claimed that an AI model performs better than a human physician [87] on various image diagnostic tasks. An important caveat to these claims is that these comparisons occur under highly artificial conditions, which differ markedly from practical conditions in several important ways. AI models are typically highly specialized, providing binary yes/no answers to specific single diagnoses for which they are extensively trained on datasets of millions of images. Many of the skills of the human radiologist or pathologist, including the capacity to reason about uncertainty, breadth of knowledge, and diagnostic repertoire, remain very challenging for AI systems to replicate. Human diagnosticians cannot just consider and distinguish multiple differential diagnoses; they can also

Table 22.3 Pros and cons of artificial intelligence

Advantages	Disadvantages
Instantaneous, ubiquitous access, indefatigable	Significant developmental cost
Lack of observer bias	Lack of reliable datasets to learn from
INR involves rapid assessment of image-based information that is mostly digital in nature	Technology in evolution provides insufficient data for reliable AI/ML applications
Rapid preprocedural analysis	Unexplainablilty due to algorithmic propriety or incomprehensible complexity
Improve procedural performance	Narrow margin for errors
Customize interventions	Potential concealed bias in training data
Al can enhance safety	Lack of creative innovation
Al can assist in related research: preclinical and clinical outcome assessment	ML has resulted in serious errors. In some instances, predictive capacity less than human intelligence

recognize incidental findings that were not part of the instruction set for the AI model. This ability extends beyond mere diagnosis; human diagnosticians can transfer knowledge, e.g., recognizing patterns in one type of cancer to aid in diagnosing another, and are capable of learning intentionally and in a structured way from multiple sources rather than relying solely on brute force from datasets of millions of images. Moreover, humans can function under nonideal conditions such as degraded or artifact-laden studies, a trait not easily replicated by AI. Similarly, image recognition models claimed to outperform humans on general-purpose object recognition in a controlled setting have been found to underperform in real-world conditions with noise and uncertainty. Table 22.3 lists the pros and cons of AI that need to be considered during clinical applications [110, 111].

Ethical Considerations of AI in Medicine

The deployment of AI in healthcare raises critical ethical considerations which merit careful consideration. The role of AI in patient care remains limited to narrow domains and early trials. Nonetheless, some ethical issues have emerged, and others are easily foreseeable as these technologies evolve and gain a more significant role. While, in this chapter, we have strived to emphasize the limits of AI as it currently exists and the importance of not exaggerating its capabilities, we believe there is also a pressing need to preemptively establish professional frameworks and guidelines for thinking about the ethics of technologies still on the horizon, to avoid a scenario in which problematic technologies are deployed in an ad hoc manner, in a regulatory environment unprepared for their implications or to provide necessary oversight.

Classically, medical ethics rests on the pillars of beneficence, non-maleficence, autonomy, and justice. Issues with existing and future AI technologies in medicine touch on all these pillars. In this section, we discuss some of these issues under a rough categorization, although we acknowledge that many touch on more than one simultaneously and could arguably be categorized differently; the precise categorization is less important than the issues themselves.

Beneficence

At the heart of medical practice is the principle of beneficence: medicine's goal is to benefit patients. AI has the potential to revolutionize healthcare, offering more accurate and rapid diagnoses, personalized treatment plans, and reductions in the cost of care. However, a formidable challenge arises in the form of financial incentives favoring cost-effective AI solutions, even if outcomes are equivalent or slightly inferior. The principle of beneficence urges us to limit the deployment of AI solutions to cases where there is some active benefit to patients rather than solely to the hospital's or practice's finances. Balancing technological progress with genuine patient welfare is crucial, considering AI implementation's multifaceted direct and opportunity costs.

Non-maleficence

The principle of non-maleficence ("do no harm") refers to the obligation to avoid harm to patients. The rapid integration of AI into healthcare introduces new avenues for potential harm, including diagnostic errors, inappropriate treatment plans, and procedural errors. Determining responsibility in cases of AI-related medical errors raises critical ethical and legal questions. For example, will hospitals deflect liability by attributing errors to machines, potentially reducing patient legal protections? So far, these questions have only been tested to a limited degree in the courts. Additionally, the intersection of AI bias and social inequality may harm vulnerable populations, warranting a careful examination of these dynamics; we discuss this issue further in the *Justice* subsection.

Autonomy

Autonomy refers to the right of patients to make informed decisions about their bodies and health. In the future, when AI takes a more prominent role in healthcare, questions arise about patient autonomy in decision-making. For example, can patients decline AI involvement in their care, or will the degree of human physician involvement break along the lines of income and insurance status, as many aspects of care currently do? Will AI exacerbate our current two-tier healthcare system? This issue intensifies as AI assumes a more active role in delivering care than solely analyzing data. Patients must have the autonomy to choose human physicians over AI, request human interpretation of clinical data, and decline AI-assisted interventions, mainly when such assistants are still experimental. However, as specific tasks become routine for AI, human operators may become deskilled in those areas, paradoxically increasing risks associated with human-provided care.

Justice

The ethical principle of justice encompasses fairness, equity, and the distribution of benefits and burdens. AI bias poses a significant challenge, as certain technologies may work less effectively in diverse populations, potentially exacerbating existing disparities. The prospect of a two-tier healthcare system, where affluent patients can access human physicians while low-income patients rely on AI, raises concerns about equitable healthcare access. This scenario parallels existing experiments in legal defense, where those unable to afford lawyers turn to AI chatbots.

Furthermore, the impact of AI on healthcare workers, particularly nonphysician team members, warrants attention. As AI assumes responsibilities previously held by human workers, questions about fair compensation, humane work hours, and the potential redundancy of certain roles arise. Ensuring the just treatment of healthcare workers involves guaranteeing opportunities for retraining, modified roles, or early retirement for those affected by technological shifts. The cost-effectiveness of AI deployment must be scrutinized, with any cost savings used to uphold ethical standards in workforce management.

In conclusion, the ethical considerations surrounding AI in medicine are intricate and multifaceted. As we navigate the integration of AI into healthcare, a proactive and vigilant approach is imperative. Upholding the principles of beneficence, non-maleficence, autonomy, and justice in the context of AI requires ongoing dialog, ethical guidelines, and a commitment to prioritizing patient well-being over financial gains. By addressing these ethical challenges comprehensively, we can ensure that AI in medicine remains a force for positive transformation, enhancing patient care while maintaining the fundamental tenets of medical ethics.

Future Directions: Large Language Models, AI Agents, and Medicine

Thus far, we have discussed relatively "narrow" realizations of AI in solving specific problems using data. This type of AI is already in use in many areas of healthcare, from preclinical research to drug development to image analysis. In this section, we will discuss recent advances in the AI field that have not yet gained wide traction in medicine but have the potential to introduce AI "agents" with some level of autonomy into healthcare. An "agent" is an autonomous entity capable of perceiving the world, making decisions, and acting toward a specific goal. AI agents are typically thought of as operating in real time: each action taken can change the world somehow, which the agent must then perceive and respond to continuously. How to train agents to maximize their objectives in dynamic environments, from games to social interactions to robotics, is the central goal of reinforcement learning.

Reinforcement learning has been an extremely successful paradigm for system control in various fields including navigation in space, aerial, aquatic, and terrestrial environments. It will likely play a role in any future automated procedural tasks in medicine. Arterial drug delivery will require exceedingly safe placement of catheters and interventional neuroradiology techniques (Fig. 22.5). A significant advantage of arterial drug delivery is that underlying core techniques are not organ-specific. AI-guided catheter placement is in development [112]. Automation in catheter navigation could significantly address the workforce's unavailability due to time constraints or geographical location.

Another recent innovation within the field of neural networks has been the transformer architecture, on which large language models (LLMs) such as ChatGPT are based. These models, trained in a self-supervised manner on vast amounts of data, are designed to generate humanlike text based on input prompts and represent the most successful natural language production models. On a basic level, these models are trained to predict text completion: given a sentence with a missing word, the model must produce plausible hypotheses for what the missing word might be. Although this idea seems simple, it is extremely potent when combined with an attention-based model architecture that allows the learning of long-term dependencies. The same architecture can be used to learn and generate patterns in sequential data, such as EEG. Notoriously, these models suffer from the "hallucination" problem. As plausibility is the goal during training rather than truth, LLMs may generate language output that is grammatically correct and coherent on the surface but factually incorrect, posing obvious challenges for healthcare contexts.

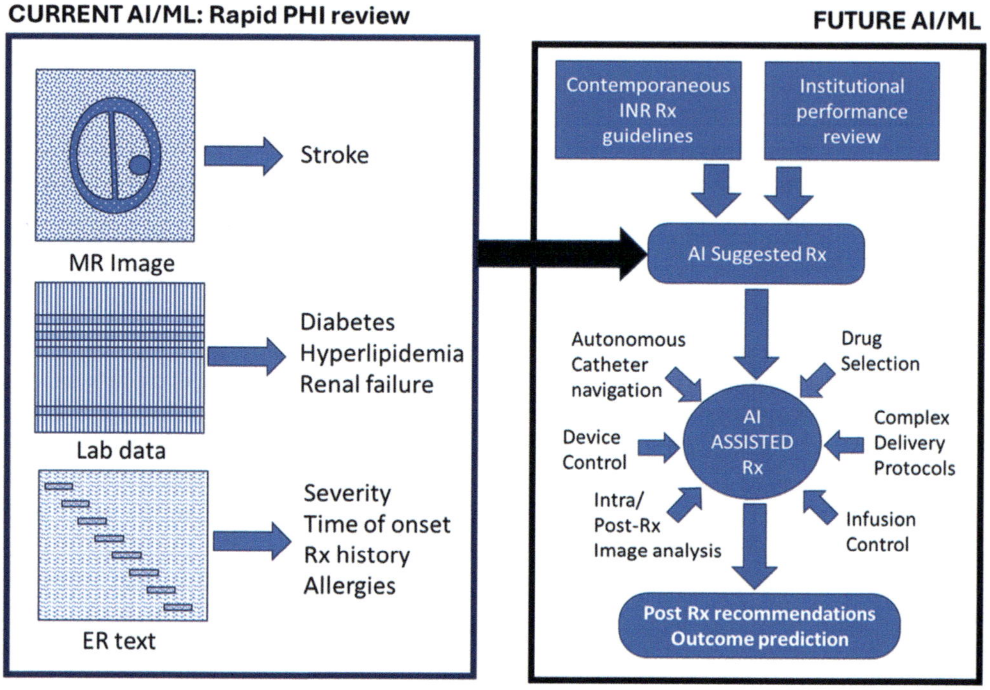

Fig. 22.7 Current and future uses of AI in healthcare. Left: Machine learning algorithms are currently being tested for clinical image analysis, interpretation of laboratory data, and pertinent data extraction from EMR natural language text. Right: Possible future applications of AI in healthcare. More advanced and reliable algorithms may be entrusted with the integration of multisource clinical data, suggesting diagnoses and plans and guiding procedures

While LLMs and AI agents are not officially integrated into healthcare systems, extensive research is underway to explore their potential applications. One area of focus is the automation of routine tasks, such as documentation and appointment reminders, offering a streamlined approach to patient communication. Additionally, these AI agents could play a role in answering basic patient queries and providing information and support on time; several large companies have already rolled out LLM-based virtual assistants or customer service agents. However, introducing even simple tasks involving direct and unsupervised patient interaction by AI raises significant ethical and liability concerns. The potential for misinformation, misinterpretation, or the generation of inaccurate recommendations underscores the importance of maintaining a human oversight role in healthcare interactions, using the "standard of care" principle that although currently accepted practice may be imperfect, any changes must be shown to be non-inferior before being widely deployed to prevent unintentional harm. As healthcare decisions carry profound consequences, ensuring accountability and minimizing the risk of errors become paramount considerations.

Conclusion

In the long term, the scope of AI involvement in healthcare will undoubtedly expand to more complex tasks (Fig. 22.7). Could an AI, for instance, collect a patient's history and perform a physical examination independently? Could AI directly guide medical or surgical intervention? The prospect of AI formulating medical plans and independently executing them, either with minimal human oversight or with only periodic review, raises both technical and ethical questions.

The integration of AI agents in medicine is not without challenges. The reliability, interpretability, and ethical implications of AI-generated recommendations in the intricate realm of drug delivery demand careful consideration. Moreover, questions surrounding liability for AI-driven decisions and the potential for unforeseen consequences underscore the need for a cautious and phased approach to implementation. It is essential to balance excitement about technological advancements with a thoughtful acknowledgment of the limitations and ethical dimensions inherent in using AI in healthcare. The evolving role of AI should reflect not just the promise of technological innovation but also the imperative to establish clear ethical guidelines and safeguards to ensure patient safety and quality of care. The promises and perils of AI come at a time when arterial drug delivery is being reassessed. Arterial drugs and their delivery, which have hitherto been largely ignored, are a promising avenue of pharmaceutical research. AI could significantly hasten arterial carrier and drug development, arterial pharmacokinetic research, and their clinical translation to offer novel treatments for neurological diseases.

References

1. Freeth T. Eclipse prediction on the ancient Greek astronomical calculating machine known as the Antikythera mechanism. PLoS One. 2014;9(7):e103275.
2. Freeth T, Higgon D, Dacanalis A, MacDonald L, Georgakopoulou M, Wojcik A. A model of the cosmos in the ancient Greek Antikythera mechanism. Sci Rep. 2021;11(1):5821.

3. Iavazzo C, Gkegke XE, Iavazzo PE, Gkegkes ID. Evolution of robots throughout history from Hephaestus to Da Vinci robot. Acta Med Hist Adriat. 2014;12(2):247–58.
4. Sejnowski TJ. The unreasonable effectiveness of deep learning in artificial intelligence. Proc Natl Acad Sci USA. 2020;117(48):30033–8.
5. Bishop CM. Pattern recognition and machine learning. New York: Springer; 2006.
6. Hastie T, Tibshirani R, Friedman JH. The elements of statistical learning: data mining, inference, and prediction. New York: Springer; 2009.
7. Russell S, Norvig P. Artificial intelligence: a modern approach. New Jersey: Pearson; 2021. 1166 p
8. Sutton RS, Barto AG. Reinforcement learning. In: An introduction (adaptive computation and machine learning series). 2nd ed. Cambridge, MA: Bradford Books; 2018. 552 p.
9. Garg PK. Chapter 1: Overview of artificial intelligence. In: Sharma L, Garg PK, editors. Artificial intelligence technologies, applications, and challenges. Boca Raton: CRC Press, Taylor & Francis Group; 2022. p. 3–18.
10. Keysers C, Gazzola V. Hebbian learning and predictive mirror neurons for actions, sensations and emotions. Philos Trans R Soc Lond Ser B Biol Sci. 2014;369(1644):20130175.
11. Raza A, Chohan TA, Buabeid M, Arafa EA, Chohan TA, Fatima B, et al. Deep learning in drug discovery: a futuristic modality to materialize the large datasets for cheminformatics. J Biomol Struct Dyn. 2023;41(18):9177–92.
12. Srivathsa AV, Sadashivappa NM, Hegde AK, Radha S, Mahesh AR, Ammunje DN, et al. A review on artificial intelligence approaches and rational approaches in drug discovery. Curr Pharm Des. 2023;29(15):1180–92.
13. Johnson M, Patel M, Phipps A, van der Schaar M, Boulton D, Gibbs M. The potential and pitfalls of artificial intelligence in clinical pharmacology. CPT Pharmacometrics Syst Pharmacol. 2023;12(3):279–84.
14. Chaturvedula A, Calad-Thomson S, Liu C, Sale M, Gattu N, Goyal N. Artificial intelligence and pharmacometrics: time to embrace, capitalize, and advance? CPT Pharmacometrics Syst Pharmacol. 2019;8(7):440–3.
15. Obrezanova O. Artificial intelligence for compound pharmacokinetics prediction. Curr Opin Struct Biol. 2023;79:102546.
16. Chou WC, Chen Q, Yuan L, Cheng YH, He C, Monteiro-Riviere NA, et al. An artificial intelligence-assisted physiologically-based pharmacokinetic model to predict nanoparticle delivery to tumors in mice. J Control Release. 2023;361:53–63.
17. Lin Z, Chou WC. Machine learning and artificial intelligence in toxicological sciences. Toxicol Sci. 2022;189(1):7–19.
18. Vora LK, Gholap AD, Jetha K, Thakur RRS, Solanki HK, Chavda VP. Artificial intelligence in pharmaceutical technology and drug delivery design. Pharmaceutics. 2023;15(7):1916.
19. Oliveira AL. Biotechnology, big data and artificial intelligence. Biotechnol J. 2019;14(8):e1800613.
20. Hakeem H, Feng W, Chen Z, Choong J, Brodie MJ, Fong SL, et al. Development and validation of a deep learning model for predicting treatment response in patients with newly diagnosed epilepsy. JAMA Neurol. 2022;79(10):986–96.
21. Gao M, Igata H, Takeuchi A, Sato K, Ikegaya Y. Machine learning-based prediction of adverse drug effects: an example of seizure-inducing compounds. J Pharmacol Sci. 2017;133(2):70–8.
22. Stephenson N, Shane E, Chase J, Rowland J, Ries D, Justice N, et al. Survey of machine learning techniques in drug discovery. Curr Drug Metab. 2019;20(3):185–93.
23. Eagleman SL, Drover DR. Calculations of consciousness: electroencephalography analyses to determine anesthetic depth. Curr Opin Anaesthesiol. 2018;31(4):431–8.
24. Pascucci M, Royer G, Adamek J, Asmar MA, Aristizabal D, Blanche L, et al. AI-based mobile application to fight antibiotic resistance. Nat Commun. 2021;12(1):1173.
25. Wahl RL, Chareonthaitawee P, Clarke B, Drzezga A, Lindenberg L, Rahmim A, et al. Mars shot for nuclear medicine, molecular imaging, and molecularly targeted radiopharmaceutical therapy. J Nucl Med. 2021;62(1):6–14.
26. Wei H, Wang Y, Zhang Y, Du S, Shen J, Li X, et al. Outcomes and risk factors of perforating and non-perforating middle cerebral artery infarctions after intravenous thrombolysis. J Thromb Thrombolysis. 2022;53(3):722–30.
27. Jumper J, Evans R, Pritzel A, Green T, Figurnov M, Ronneberger O, et al. Highly accurate protein structure prediction with AlphaFold. Nature. 2021;596(7873):583–9.
28. Gao M, Sato M, Ikegaya Y. Machine learning-based prediction of seizure-inducing action as an adverse drug effect. Yakugaku Zasshi. 2018;138(6):809–13.
29. Komorowski M, Celi LA, Badawi O, Gordon AC, Faisal AA. The artificial intelligence clinician learns optimal treatment strategies for sepsis in intensive care. Nat Med. 2018;24(11):1716–20.
30. Naushad SM, Kutala VK. Artificial neural network and bioavailability of the immunosuppression drug. Curr Opin Organ Transplant. 2020;25(4):435–41.
31. Chen WM, Yu YH, Chen M, Shia BC, Wu SY. Statin use during concurrent chemoradiotherapy with improved survival outcomes in esophageal squamous cell carcinoma: a propensity score-matched nationwide cohort study. J Thorac Oncol. 2023;18(8):1082–93.
32. Huang YC, Cheng YC, Jhou MJ, Chen M, Lu CJ. Integrated machine learning decision tree model for risk evaluation in patients with non-valvular atrial fibrillation when taking different doses of dabigatran. Int J Environ Res Public Health. 2023;20(3):2359.
33. Dedrick RL. Interspecies scaling of regional drug delivery. J Pharm Sci. 1986;75(11):1047–52.
34. Editorial. Neuroprotection: the end of an era? Lancet. 2006;368(9547):1548.
35. de Oliveira ECL, da Costa KS, Taube PS, Lima AH, Junior CSS. Biological membrane-penetrating peptides: computational prediction and applications. Front Cell Infect Microbiol. 2022;12:838259.
36. Guixer B, Arroyo X, Belda I, Sabido E, Teixido M, Giralt E. Chemically synthesized peptide libraries as a new source of BBB shuttles. Use of mass spectrometry for peptide identification. J Pept Sci. 2016;22(9):577–91.
37. Moingeon P. Applications of artificial intelligence to new drug development. Ann Pharm Fr. 2021;79(5):566–71.
38. Hasan MR, Alsaiari AA, Fakhurji BZ, Molla MHR, Asseri AH, Sumon MAA, et al. Application of mathematical modeling and computational tools in the modern drug design and development process. Molecules. 2022;27(13):4169.
39. Al Kuwaiti A, Nazer K, Al-Reedy A, Al-Shehri S, Al-Muhanna A, Subbarayalu AV, et al. A review of the role of artificial intelligence in healthcare. J Pers Med. 2023;13(6):951.
40. Willyard C, Can AI. Fix medical records? Nature. 2019;576(7787):S59–62.
41. Gaspar F, Lutters M, Beeler PE, Lang PO, Burnand B, Rinaldi F, et al. Automatic detection of adverse drug events in geriatric care: study proposal. JMIR Res Protoc. 2022;11(11):e40456.
42. He Y, Peng S, Chen M, Yang Z, Chen Y. A transformer-based prediction method for depth of anesthesia during target-controlled infusion of propofol and remifentanil. IEEE Trans Neural Syst Rehabil Eng. 2023;31:3363–74.
43. Lee HC, Ryu HG, Chung EJ, Jung CW. Prediction of bispectral index during target-controlled infusion of propofol and remifentanil: a deep learning approach. Anesthesiology. 2018;128(3):492–501.

44. Miyaguchi N, Takeuchi K, Kashima H, Morita M, Morimatsu H. Predicting anesthetic infusion events using machine learning. Sci Rep. 2021;11(1):23648.
45. Ribba B, Dudal S, Lave T, Peck RW. Model-informed artificial intelligence: reinforcement learning for precision dosing. Clin Pharmacol Ther. 2020;107(4):853–7.
46. Nair R, Mohan DD, Setlur S, Govindaraju V, Ramanathan M. Generative models for age, race/ethnicity, and disease state dependence of physiological determinants of drug dosing. J Pharmacokinet Pharmacodyn. 2023;50(2):111–22.
47. Chou WC, Lin Z. Machine learning and artificial intelligence in physiologically based pharmacokinetic modeling. Toxicol Sci. 2023;191(1):1–14.
48. Edrees H, Song W, Syrowatka A, Simona A, Amato MG, Bates DW. Intelligent telehealth in pharmacovigilance: a future perspective. Drug Saf. 2022;45(5):449–58.
49. Primorac D, Bach-Rojecky L, Vadunec D, Juginovic A, Zunic K, Matisic V, et al. Pharmacogenomics at the center of precision medicine: challenges and perspective in an era of Big Data. Pharmacogenomics. 2020;21(2):141–56.
50. Riva N, Ibarra M, Parra-Guillen ZP, Galvan ME, Perez E, Trezeguet Renatti G, et al. Population pharmacokinetics of sublingually administered tacrolimus in infants and young children with liver transplantation. Br J Clin Pharmacol. 2023;89(3):1115–26.
51. Molokhia M, Majeed A. Current and future perspectives on the management of polypharmacy. BMC Fam Pract. 2017;18(1):70.
52. Basile AO, Yahi A, Tatonetti NP. Artificial intelligence for drug toxicity and safety. Trends Pharmacol Sci. 2019;40(9):624–35.
53. Ball R, Dal Pan G. "Artificial intelligence" for pharmacovigilance: ready for prime time? Drug Saf. 2022;45(5):429–38.
54. Zhao Y, Yu Y, Wang H, Li Y, Deng Y, Jiang G, et al. Machine learning in causal inference: application in pharmacovigilance. Drug Saf. 2022;45(5):459–76.
55. Mumtaz H, Saqib M, Jabeen S, Muneeb M, Mughal W, Sohail H, et al. Exploring alternative approaches to precision medicine through genomics and artificial intelligence—a systematic review. Front Med (Lausanne). 2023;10:1227168.
56. Del Fiol G, Rocha BH, Kuperman GJ, Bates DW, Nohama P. Comparison of two knowledge bases on the detection of drug-drug interactions. In: Proc AMIA Symp; 2000. p. 171–5.
57. Del Fiol G, Rocha BH, Nohama P. Design, implementation and evaluation of a clinical decision support system to prevent adverse drug events. Stud Health Technol Inform. 2000;77:740–4.
58. Wongpoowarak W, Wongpoowarak P. Unified algorithm for real-time detection of drug interaction and drug allergy. Comput Methods Prog Biomed. 2002;68(1):63–72.
59. Teramoto R, Kato T. Transfer learning for cytochrome P450 isozyme selectivity prediction. J Bioinforma Comput Biol. 2011;9(4):521–40.
60. Chalasani SH, Syed J, Ramesh M, Patil V, Pramod Kumar TM. Artificial intelligence in the field of pharmacy practice: a literature review. Explor Res Clin Soc Pharm. 2023;12:100346.
61. Taylor M, Liu X, Denniston A, Esteva A, Ko J, Daneshjou R, et al. Raising the bar for randomized trials involving artificial intelligence: the SPIRIT-artificial intelligence and CONSORT—artificial intelligence guidelines. J Invest Dermatol. 2021;141(9):2109–11.
62. Kolluri S, Lin J, Liu R, Zhang Y, Zhang W. Machine learning and artificial intelligence in pharmaceutical research and development: a review. AAPS J. 2022;24(1):19.
63. Liu C, Liu H, Ta C, Roger J, Butler A, Lee J, et al. Evaluation of Criteria2Query: towards augmented intelligence for cohort identification. Stud Health Technol Inform. 2022;290:297–300.
64. Aliper A, Kudrin R, Polykovskiy D, Kamya P, Tutubalina E, Chen S, et al. Prediction of clinical trials outcomes based on target choice and clinical trial design with multi-modal artificial intelligence. Clin Pharmacol Ther. 2023;114(5):972–80.
65. Clarke LP, Velthuizen RP, Clark M, Gaviria J, Hall L, Goldgof D, et al. MRI measurement of brain tumor response: comparison of visual metric and automatic segmentation. Magn Reson Imaging. 1998;16(3):271–9.
66. Hu X, Wong KK, Young GS, Guo L, Wong ST. Support vector machine multiparametric MRI identification of pseudoprogression from tumor recurrence in patients with resected glioblastoma. J Magn Reson Imaging. 2011;33(2):296–305.
67. Boers AMM, Jansen IGH, Brown S, Lingsma HF, Beenen LFM, Devlin TG, et al. Mediation of the relationship between endovascular therapy and functional outcome by follow-up infarct volume in patients with acute ischemic stroke. JAMA Neurol. 2019;76(2):194–202.
68. Asif S, Zhao M, Chen X, Zhu Y. BMRI-NET: a deep stacked ensemble model for multi-class brain tumor classification from MRI images. Interdiscip Sci. 2023;15(3):499–514.
69. Bailleul J, Ruan S, Constans JM. Statistical shape model-based segmentation of brain MRI images. Annu Int Conf IEEE Eng Med Biol Soc. 2007;2007:5255–8.
70. Papadomanolakis TN, Sergaki ES, Polydorou AA, Krasoudakis AG, Makris-Tsalikis GN, Polydorou AA, et al. Tumor diagnosis against other brain diseases using T2 MRI brain images and CNN binary classifier and DWT. Brain Sci. 2023;13(2):348.
71. Ranjbarzadeh R, Caputo A, Tirkolaee EB, Jafarzadeh Ghoushchi S, Bendechache M. Brain tumor segmentation of MRI images: a comprehensive review on the application of artificial intelligence tools. Comput Biol Med. 2023;152:106405.
72. Sheejakumari V, Sankara GB. MRI brain images healthy and pathological tissues classification with the aid of improved particle swarm optimization and neural network. Comput Math Methods Med. 2015;2015:807826.
73. Surianarayanan C, Lawrence JJ, Chelliah PR, Prakash E, Hewage C. Convergence of artificial intelligence and neuroscience towards the diagnosis of neurological disorders—a scoping review. Sensors (Basel). 2023;23(6):3062.
74. He K, Zhang X, Ren S, Sun J, editors. Delving deep into rectifiers: Surpassing human-level performance on imagenet classification. In: Proceedings of the IEEE International Conference on Computer Vision. 2015.
75. Vasudevan V, Caine B, Gontijo Lopes R, Fridovich-Keil S, Roelofs R. When does dough become a bagel? Analyzing the remaining mistakes on imagenet. Adv Neural Inf Proces Syst. 2022;35:6720–34.
76. Dehghani M, Djolonga J, Mustafa B, Padlewski P, Heek J, Gilmer J, et al. Scaling vision transformers to 22 billion parameters. In: Andreas K, Emma B, Kyunghyun C, Barbara E, Sivan S, Jonathan S, editors. Proceedings of the 40th International Conference on Machine Learning, Proceedings of Machine Learning Research. PMLR; 2023. p. 7480–512.
77. Aggarwal K, Manso Jimeno M, Ravi KS, Gonzalez G, Geethanath S. Developing and deploying deep learning models in brain magnetic resonance imaging: a review. NMR Biomed. 2023;36:e5014.
78. de Godoy LL, Chawla S, Brem S, Mohan S. Taming glioblastoma in "real time": integrating multimodal advanced neuroimaging/AI tools towards creating a robust and therapy agnostic model for response assessment in neuro-oncology. Clin Cancer Res. 2023;29(14):2588–92.
79. Raghavendra U, Acharya UR, Adeli H. Artificial intelligence techniques for automated diagnosis of neurological disorders. Eur Neurol. 2019;82(1–3):41–64.
80. Henssen D, Meijer F, Verburg FA, Smits M. Challenges and opportunities for advanced neuroimaging of glioblastoma. Br J Radiol. 2023;96(1141):20211232.

81. Pedersen M, Verspoor K, Jenkinson M, Law M, Abbott DF, Jackson GD. Artificial intelligence for clinical decision support in neurology. Brain Commun. 2020;2(2):fcaa096.
82. Boeken T, Feydy J, Lecler A, Soyer P, Feydy A, Barat M, et al. Artificial intelligence in diagnostic and interventional radiology: where are we now? Diagn Interv Imaging. 2023;104(1):1–5.
83. Gurgitano M, Angileri SA, Roda GM, Liguori A, Pandolfi M, Ierardi AM, et al. Interventional radiology ex-machina: impact of artificial intelligence on practice. Radiol Med. 2021;126(7):998–1006.
84. Iezzi R, Goldberg SN, Merlino B, Posa A, Valentini V, Manfredi R. Artificial intelligence in interventional radiology: a literature review and future perspectives. J Oncol. 2019;2019:6153041.
85. Murugiah K, Chen L, Castro-Dominguez Y, Khera R, Krumholz HM. Scope of practice of US interventional cardiologists from an analysis of Medicare billing data. Am J Cardiol. 2021;160:40–5.
86. Seah J, Boeken T, Sapoval M, Goh GS. Prime time for artificial intelligence in interventional radiology. Cardiovasc Intervent Radiol. 2022;45(3):283–9.
87. Horry M, Chakraborty S, Pradhan B, Paul M, Gomes D, Ul-Haq A, et al. Deep mining generation of lung cancer malignancy models from chest X-ray images. Sensors (Basel). 2021;21(19):6655.
88. Ce M, Irmici G, Foschini C, Danesini GM, Falsitta LV, Serio ML, et al. Artificial intelligence in brain tumor imaging: a step toward personalized medicine. Curr Oncol. 2023;30(3):2673–701.
89. Kocher M, Ruge MI, Galldiks N, Lohmann P. Applications of radiomics and machine learning for radiotherapy of malignant brain tumors. Strahlenther Onkol. 2020;196(10):856–67.
90. Zhu M, Li S, Kuang Y, Hill VB, Heimberger AB, Zhai L, et al. Artificial intelligence in the radiomic analysis of glioblastomas: a review, taxonomy, and perspective. Front Oncol. 2022;12:924245.
91. Vollmuth P, Foltyn M, Huang RY, Galldiks N, Petersen J, Isensee F, et al. Artificial intelligence (AI)-based decision support improves reproducibility of tumor response assessment in neuro-oncology: an international multi-reader study. Neuro-Oncology. 2023;25(3):533–43.
92. Sakly H, Said M, Seekins J, Guetari R, Kraiem N, Marzougui M. Brain tumor radiogenomic classification of O(6)-methylguanine-DNA methyltransferase promoter methylation in malignant gliomas-based transfer learning. Cancer Control. 2023;30:10732748231169149.
93. Vinny PW, Vishnu VY, Padma Srivastava MV. Artificial intelligence shaping the future of neurology practice. Med J Armed Forces India. 2021;77(3):276–82.
94. Sharma S, Borski C, Hanson J, Garcia MA, Link CD, Hoeffer C, et al. Identifying an optimal neuroinflammation treatment using a nanoligomer discovery engine. ACS Chem Neurosci. 2022;13(23):3247–56.
95. Corrias G, Mazzotta A, Melis M, Cademartiri F, Yang Q, Suri JS, et al. Emerging role of artificial intelligence in stroke imaging. Expert Rev Neurother. 2021;21(7):745–54.
96. Bivard A, Churilov L, Parsons M. Artificial intelligence for decision support in acute stroke—current roles and potential. Nat Rev Neurol. 2020;16(10):575–85.
97. Bivard A, Levi C, Lin L, Cheng X, Aviv R, Spratt NJ, et al. Assessing the relative value of CT perfusion compared to non-contrast CT and CT angiography in prognosticating reperfusion-eligible acute ischemic stroke patients. Front Neurol. 2021;12:736768.
98. Zhu G, Jiang B, Chen H, Tong E, Xie Y, Faizy TD, et al. Artificial intelligence and stroke imaging: a west coast perspective. Neuroimaging Clin N Am. 2020;30(4):479–92.
99. Sun J, Zheng X, Gao Q, Wang X, Qiao Y, Li J. Computed tomography images under artificial intelligence algorithms on the treatment evaluation of intracerebral hemorrhage with minimally invasive aspiration. Comput Math Methods Med. 2022;2022:6204089.
100. Ali R, Li H, Dillman JR, Altaye M, Wang H, Parikh NA, et al. A self-training deep neural network for early prediction of cognitive deficits in very preterm infants using brain functional connectome data. Pediatr Radiol. 2022;52(11):2227–40.
101. Peng SJ, Chen YW, Hung A, Wang KW, Tsai JZ. Connectome-based predictive modeling for functional recovery of acute ischemic stroke. Neuroimage Clin. 2023;38:103369.
102. Stocco A, Sibert C, Steine-Hanson Z, Koh N, Laird JE, Lebiere CJ, et al. Analysis of the human connectome data supports the notion of a "Common Model of Cognition" for human and human-like intelligence across domains. NeuroImage. 2021;235:118035.
103. Yang S, Jin D, Liu J, He Y. Identification of Young high-functioning autism individuals based on functional connectome using graph isomorphism network: a pilot study. Brain Sci. 2022;12(7):883.
104. Rabinowitch I. What would a synthetic connectome look like? Phys Life Rev. 2020;33:1–15.
105. Chen T, Tachmazidis I, Batsakis S, Adamou M, Papadakis E, Antoniou G. Diagnosing attention-deficit hyperactivity disorder (ADHD) using artificial intelligence: a clinical study in the UK. Front Psych. 2023;14:1164433.
106. Torous J, Bucci S, Bell IH, Kessing LV, Faurholt-Jepsen M, Whelan P, et al. The growing field of digital psychiatry: current evidence and the future of apps, social media, chatbots, and virtual reality. World Psychiatry. 2021;20(3):318–35.
107. Davey Z, Gupta PB, Li DR, Nayak RU, Govindarajan P. Rapid response EEG: current state and future directions. Curr Neurol Neurosci Rep. 2022;22(12):839–46.
108. Jakimovski D, Silva D, Niels B, Dwyer MG, Weinstock-Guttman B, Benedict RH, et al. Therapy effect on AI-derived thalamic atrophy using clinical routine MRI protocol: a longitudinal, multicenter, propensity-matched multiple sclerosis study. Mult Scler Relat Disord. 2023;74:104708.
109. Roca P, Attye A, Colas L, Tucholka A, Rubini P, Cackowski S, et al. Artificial intelligence to predict clinical disability in patients with multiple sclerosis using FLAIR MRI. Diagn Interv Imaging. 2020;101(12):795–802.
110. Geirhos R, Temme CRM, Rauber J, Schütt HH, Bethge M, Wichmann FA. Generalisation in humans and deep neural networks. In: Bengio S, Wallach H, Larochelle H, Grauman K, Cesa-Bianchi N, Garnett R, editors. ; 2018.
111. Ollikka N, Abbas A, Perin A, Kilpeläinen M, Deny S. Humans beat deep networks at recognizing objects in unusual poses, given enough time. arXiv preprint arXiv:240203973. 2024.
112. Ghosh R, Wong K, Zhang YJ, Britz GW, Wong STC. Automated catheter segmentation and tip detection in cerebral angiography with topology-aware geometric deep learning. J Neurointerv Surg. 2023;16:290.

Arterial Drug Delivery in the Future: Addressing Complex Problems as Acute Ischemic Stroke

23

Shailendra Joshi and Alexander Ramos

Logic will get you from A to B; imagination will get you everywhere.

Albert Einstein (1879–1955), Theoretical Physicist

A Future Case Report

March 2101: During the 10-sol Martian mission, a 52-year-old crewmember with a low genetic predisposition to vascular and malignant diseases, who was fully compliant with the mandatory health monitoring protocols received a cautionary medical alert and had to report immediately to the Planetary Medical Center. Wearable personal sensors and those in the vehicle had reported a lack of a stress-triggered increase in heart rate and blood pressure, concurrent with the abnormal pupillary and skin photogalvanic responses, during flight. An unexplained transient loss of attention resulted in critical flight deviation. The thought-controlled flight helmet that monitored the EEG activity reported two abnormal focal spikes in the dominant temporal lobe during these lapses in attention. Postflight radiomic scans at the Planetary Medical Base revealed partial occlusion of the distal lenticular-striate arteries with atherosclerotic lesions in the middle cerebral artery. The lesions resulted in a minor asymptomatic embolic stroke. There was no encroachment of the arterial lumen beyond the partially occluded vessel. There was no hypoperfusion in the surrounding vascular territory. Motor functions that are sometimes impaired with such stroke were preserved in his case. Due to the unresolved endothelial injury, there was a high probability of recurrence. The concerns excluded the astronaut from independent activities until the vascular injury was resolved. He was prescribed an anti-inflammatory platelet aggregation-inhibiting drug. On the third day of his return, sometime during the last 3 h, when he was resting in his bay, he became aphasic and developed a right-sided weakness. He was diagnosed with a left embolic middle cerebral artery stroke. The automated MERCI (Medical Evaluation and Rectification of Critical Incidents) report faulted the initial management and subsequent monitoring of the subject after he arrived at the Planetary Medical Center, which failed to prevent the stroke.

S. Joshi (✉)
Department of Anesthesiology, Columbia University Irving Medical Center, New York, NY, USA
e-mail: sj121@cumc.columbia.edu

A. Ramos
Columbia University, New York, NY, USA

Introduction

Looking over the time horizon in science comes with obvious risks [1]. Predicting the impact of science, even with modern informatic analysis, can be challenging. On a longer time scale, a distant vision can set goals that seem unachievable in the begining but may drive technology development in the future. Some distant visions proove to be inherently unachievable, like Bhaskar's perpetual motion machine from the twelfth century [2]. Others, like Wan Hu's mythical journey to the moon using rockets in the sixteenth century, have succeeded beyond the human imagination of the time [3]. However, relevant to this case history, we can predict that by 2101 neurological diseases will be diagnosed very early in their evolution [4]. The higher levels of human functionality, better predictive models, and wearable sensors constantly monitoring performance, and health parameters will generate massive amounts of medical information. Medical imaging will be capable of detecting and characterizing pathology in very early stages. Thus, it is foreseeable that therapeutic interventions will be undertaken when the pathological tissue volume is relatively small [5–7]. How will we deal with brain

S. Joshi (ed.), *Arterial Treatment of Neurological Diseases*, https://doi.org/10.1007/978-3-031-80173-0_23

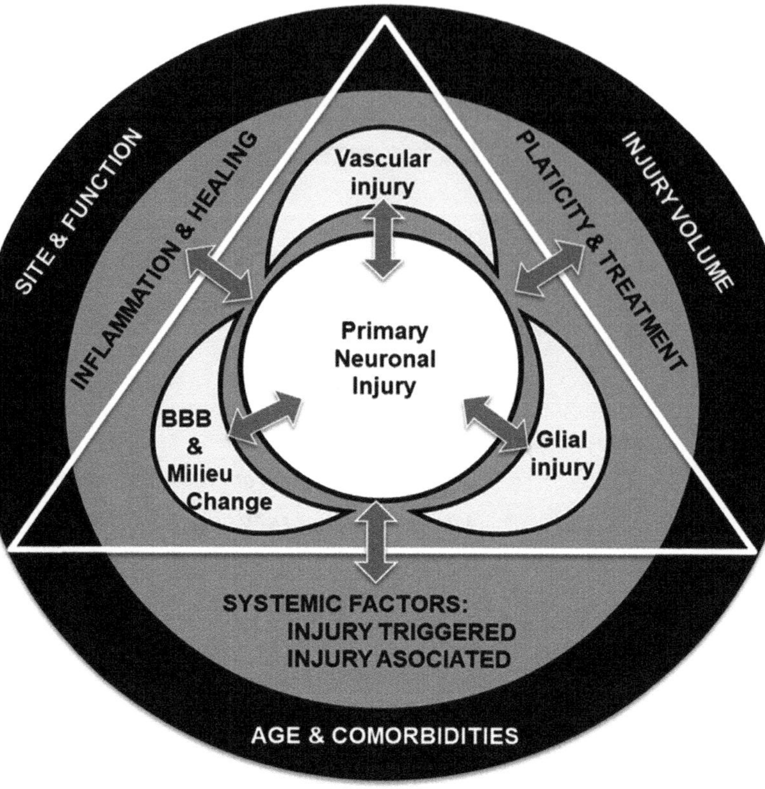

Fig. 23.1 The net outcome of neurological injuries is determined by several pathogenic pathways. A holistic approach based on complex problem-solving might help identify more effective treatments

tumors, stroke, and neurodegenerative diseases at their very inception when the pathology is limited to a few hundred or a thousand cells? Knowing well that if we do not intervene, the outcome will be disastrous in weeks and months ahead.

In recent years, much of the endovascular success in treating stroke has been due to mechanical thrombectomy, which contrasts with the general failure of treating stroke with neuroprotective drugs [8]. It is similar to the medical treatment of brain tumors, where survival, particularly in the elderly, has not significantly improved in the last four decades [9]. Likewise, for degenerative diseases such as Parkinson's, symptomatic treatments have advanced, but the pathology cannot be reversed [10, 11]. These failures of neuropharmacology, such as in stroke, have been attributed to deficiencies in preclinical research that led to the STAIR guidelines [12–14]. Over a decade since the STAIR guidelines were established, drugs have failed in clinical trials despite compliance with the guidelines [13, 15, 16]. The question arises as to whether the failure could be due to broader problems in translational neuroscience research. The failure contrasts with the significant advances that are being made in mapping neurological anatomy and function at virtually cellular levels [17, 18]. Although our understanding of neurological injuries has increased immensely, the ability to halt and reverse neurological injuries remains elusive. Given the complexity of neurological injuries and the numerous factors that could affect their outcome (Fig. 23.1), the question arises whether the failure of translational neuropharmacology represents a failure of approach. Has the oversimplification of the problem led to this failure? If so, do we need a new approach?

This chapter examines the role of arterial interventions in understanding and treating neurological diseases in the future on the conceptual and practical levels. On the conceptual level, using stroke as a prototype disease looks at the complexity of neurological diseases that affect the outcome. Given the complexity of the underlying injury mechanism, it questions if the direct cause-effect assessment approach is the correct means to assess the evolution or treatment of neurological injuries. Second, on the practical level, the chapter offers an approach with multiparameter tissue injury monitoring to look at the effect of treatments on those parameters rather than the net injury outcome. To solve the problem piecemeal with optical monitoring and arterial drug delivery to arrive at a probabilistically rather than a binary outcome. To constantly learn and improve the nature and timing of interventions to turn a "wicked problem" into a set of "simple" ones which can be reliably solved.

Applying Complex Problem-Solving to Translational Neuroscience Research

Translational Neuroscience Poses Complex Problems

Despite the immense complexity of neurological diseases, the contemporary approach in neuroscience research usually seeks to disrupt a "specific pathogenic mechanism" within the complex and ill-understood web of pathogenic interactions. The inherent complexity of clinical and pathological variables makes treatment selection challenging [19]. In clinical trials and laboratory investigations, the effect of the experimental treatment is usually determined by comparing treated vs. untreated groups. While positive findings are widely publicized and pursued, negative findings are usually ignored and discarded, as in other research endeavors [20–22]. The latter could be as valuable as the former [23]. In a longer time frame, neuroprotective research seems to be driven by the interests and capabilities of individual groups, and moving from one intervention to the next without impacting the outcome [13]. In the clinical realm, even when the results are encouraging, the extent to which an intervention is successful is often unclear, as many outcome parameters are used to assess treatments [24, 25]. The confusion is mirrored in bench research that uses various animal models. These models have subtle differences across laboratories. They often lack dose-response studies, have negligible pharmacokinetic data, and use different injury parameters observed at varying time points [26, 27]. The assumptions in bench and clinical research often go unchallenged [28]. Causality is frequently attributed to associations without distinction [29]. There is an overprojection of the significance of the results, often biased favorably toward the funding source [30]. With such an approach, a random, fragmented solution to complex problems can lead to erroneous positive conclusions and false negative results. Given the complexity and dynamic nature of neurological injuries, such an approach prevents any reliable causal correlation between studies or integrating their results meaningfully. As is the case for neurodegenerative diseases and aging, the pathogenic pathways may have an even more compicated course [31, 32]. Tracking pathological events in real time and assessing their interactions is hence necessary. The current research approach does not usually permit such an assessment. Therefore, there is a need to look at the problem from a different perspective.

Acknowledging Complexity

Complex problem-solving is traditionally applied to psychology and sociology, where goals are hard to define, the inputs are unpredictable, there is a nonlinear relationship between those inputs, and the output is poorly defined [33]. Complex problems are encountered frequently in human resources training, political negotiations, day-to-day personal decisions, cognition, and even while investigating neural connectivity [34, 35]. Applying this approach to clinical neuroscience research is provocative, although system biology and computational neurosciences are examples that pose complex problems as well. However, the dominant application of complex problem-solving seems to be related to human behavior. One could see the similarities between collective human behavior and the population of cells in the nervous system that are diverse, sometimes individually unique, where the relationships between pathogenic mechanisms are often ill-defined, the system has redundancy and is self-correcting and heals to a variable extent, and the outcome of studies is variably assessed from histology to functionality, and survival at various time points, often arriving at different results. Figure 23.1 shows that several pathways of neuronal injuries interact to affect the outcome, creating a web of interactions that determines the result.

The complex problem-solving field arose when it was realized that computationally based universal problem-solver programs would not address specific problems when the input variables are poorly characterized and defined, the relationships between the variables are unpredictable, the system changes with interventions, and there are nebulous and ill-defined goals. Complex problems contrast sharply with well-defined problems, such as puzzles. For example, "Correct the equation IV = III + III by moving one match stick." Here, the solution is well-defined: VI = III + III. That is not the case when dealing with complex problems with many variables that provide poorly characterized inputs [33].

Complex problems are characterized by the following:

- *Complexity* due to the large number of variables involved.
- *Connectivity or the nature* of mutual dependency of variables.
- *Dynamic nature of the problem as it* evolves over time and in response to interventions.
- *Intransparency*, ill-defined nature of variables.
- *Polytely* or multiple conflicting goals at different levels of analysis.

Complexity of Clinical Neuroscience Problems

It is easy to see that translation neuroscience problems share many of the above characteristics. We could create equivalent scenarios to illustrate how complex problem solving could apply to translational research. *A well-defined problem* in translational neuroscience, akin to the matchstick problem, would be "Whether intra-arterial verapamil causes angiographic vasodilation in healthy human subjects?" Here, the intervention, conditions, and experimental outcome are relatively well-defined, and the hypothesis can be reliably tested by measuring pre- and posttreatment angiographic diameters. In contrast, consider the question, "Does intra-arterial verapamil improve survival in patients with vasospasm after subarachnoid hemorrhage?". In the context of survival, the question immediately brings into play several patient-related factors: the definition of vasospasm, the severity of vasospasm, the severity of the hemorrhage, the dose and duration of verapamil treatment, the management of complications, and so on [36]. Complexity, connectivity, dynamism, ill-transparency, and even polytely come into play. Even when the outcome seems to be binary survival or no survival, the time points of assessment and the survival quality might confuse the intervention's clinical value. Furthermore studies also report significant complications that are at times subjectively defined by the investigators. Collectively, making it difficult to assess the net benefits of treatments. Comparing the outcome of treatment vs. non-treatment groups is further challenging when there are several pathogenic mechanisms and the treatment affects only part of the problem, an inherent risk of oversimplification [37].

Complex problem-solving requires a holistic approach with diverse multilevel, intuitive, and logical problem analyses. It can generate multiple hypotheses. It requires formulating, applying, and assessing several solutions. The aim is to downgrade the problem, improve understanding, and arrive at the best possible options rather than a definite solution. Complex problem-solving iteratively addresses the central hypothesis by fragmenting it into solvable questions by the best available means from several different perspectives. The experiments lead to new information and refinement of the central hypothesis. The solutions may not be perfect, but there is a better understanding of the conditions under which a specific solution will likely work. Figure 23.2 shows several possible factors that affect the outcome of cerebral vasospasm. Cerebral vasospasm, which appeared to be a simple vascular phenomenon, may have a far more complex etiology with hitherto unknown pathogenic mechanisms. Understanding factors other than vasospasm could affect the impact of intra-arterial verapamil treatment or the design of future experiments that may require additional parameters of remote brain functions such as electroencephalographic monitoring or MRI assessment, not just angiographic response. Similarly, Fig. 23.3 shows the potential factors that could affect the outcome of glioma treatment, but only some of them, as shown in red, assume statistical significance [38–41]. Figures 23.1, 23.2, and 23.3 suggest clinical neuroscience research is not a simple linear cause-effect relationship. Given the unknown nature of factors, the indeterminate pattern of interactions, and several ways of assessing outcomes, the simple linear cause-effect relationship is unlikely to succeed, and a complex problem-solving approach is needed to evaluate treatments.

Structure of Complex Problems

A problem classification that could be applied clinically could divide clinical neuroscience problems into **well-structured and poorly structured problems**.

Well-Structured Problems

Well-structured problems have a definable solution or a predictable conclusion. They can be puzzles, problems, or simple messes. Unstructured problems are principally complex messes. The following are some possible examples of well-structured problems analogous to neuroscience research.

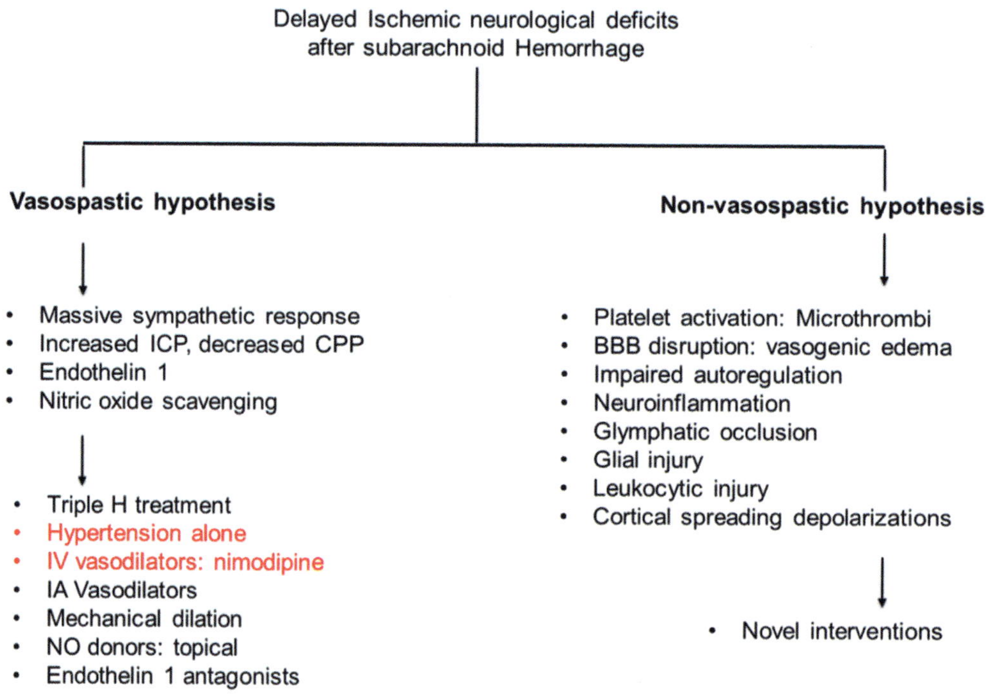

Fig. 23.2 Cerebral vasospasm after aneurysmal sub-arachnoid hemorrhage (SAH). For years, it was thought to be a simple pathological narrowing of arteries, but recent evidence suggests that the pathology is far more complicated

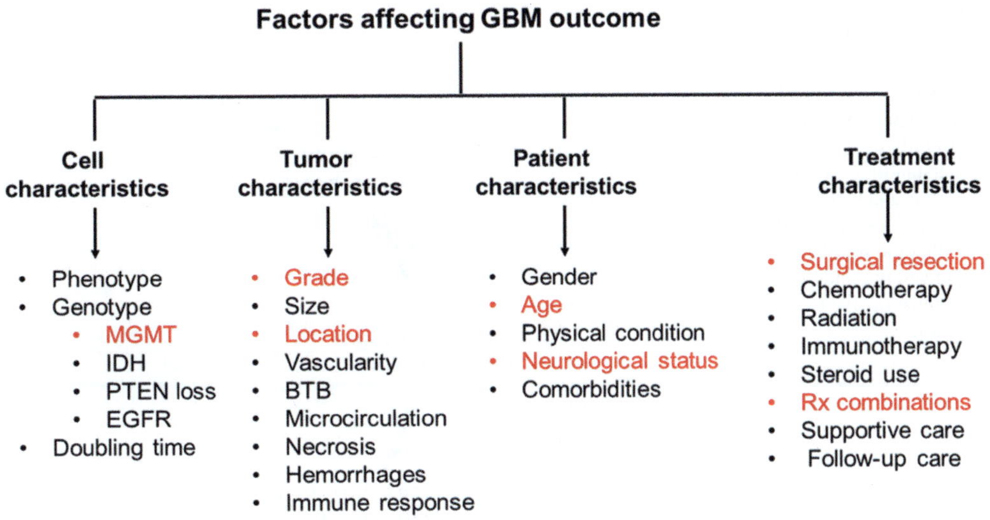

Fig. 23.3 Factors affecting the outcome of glioblastoma multiforme, a virulent and lethal brain cancer whose survival has minimally improved in the last six decades. Factors shown in red are generally considered to be statistically significant

- A well-structured *puzzle* has a single known solution. The classic puzzle definition cannot be directly applied to research, as research addresses unsolved problems. However, the clinical equivalent of a puzzle can be an experiment that arrives at highly consistent results, such as the effect of hypothermia on brain metabolism. Brain metabolism predictably decreases by about 6% for every degree fall in core temperature [42]. Therefore, in a healthy subject, we can reasonably predict the effect of a 5 °C decrease in core temperature on brain metabolism as judged by jugular venous sampling/PET imaging. So, if with hypothermia, the anticipated reduction in metabolism is not evident, one is certain some other factors (persistent seizures, drugs, or failure to cool effectively) might be involved.
- A well-structured *problem* has an unknown solution—for example, does intra-arterial milrinone rapidly increase angiographic diameters in healthy human subjects? Here, the question, is the experimental intervention that is narrow and well-defined. The hypothesis can be adequately tested with available clinical tools such as angiography and biological variables such as, age and gender have minimal effect, yet the solution/result is unknown.

Poorly Structured Problems

These can be as follows:

- *A poorly structured, complicated mess* has two or more subproblems that predictably interact—for example, the effect of hypothermia on the outcome of arterial occlusion. Here, we know that the neuroprotective effects of hypothermia will interact with time-dependent injury due to arterial occlusion. For example, while 3 min of arterial occlusion during hypothermia with a 34 °C core temperature reduction is safe, the outcome of 30 min of arterial occlusion despite moderate hypothermia becomes uncertain. Although both the effects of temperature on brain metabolism and the effect of brain metabolism on the resulting injury can be predicted in the short term, the relationship becomes more complex and unpredictable as time passes.
- *A poorly structured complex mess* is when the underlying problems are poorly defined and ill-understood, interact nonlinearly, evolve, are subjectively assessed, or are unknown. Experimental neuronal injuries, create a poorly structured complex mess where only some confounding factors are understood and can be experimentally addressed. Even if we rigorously standardize experimental conditions, many variables that cannot be fully characterized will affect the outcome of the injury. An example would be intra-arterial thrombolysis. Here, the outcome is affected by the time, site, and severity of the stroke, the effectiveness of treatment, and potential complications, such as hemorrhagic conversion.
- *A wicked mess* is a complex problem that defies a solution. Many neurodegenerative diseases that are exceedingly ill-understood and have no known treatment, can probably be considered wicked. The underlying factors, interactions between factors, and even assessment parameters are unknown, but what is likely is that these diseases are patterned after the neural injury and healing matrix shown in Fig. 23.1. Another example is predicting outcomes of treatment in elderly patients with previous stroke who may have preexisting deficits, preconditioning events, very poor functional reserve, lack of neuroplasticity, vascular comorbidities, residual effects of prior stroke, nutritional factors, and concurrent treatments. While imaging may provide some insight into the problem, assessing therapeutic intervention poses a challenge. Predicting outcomes and response to treatments reliably in these situations creates a wicked problem mess.

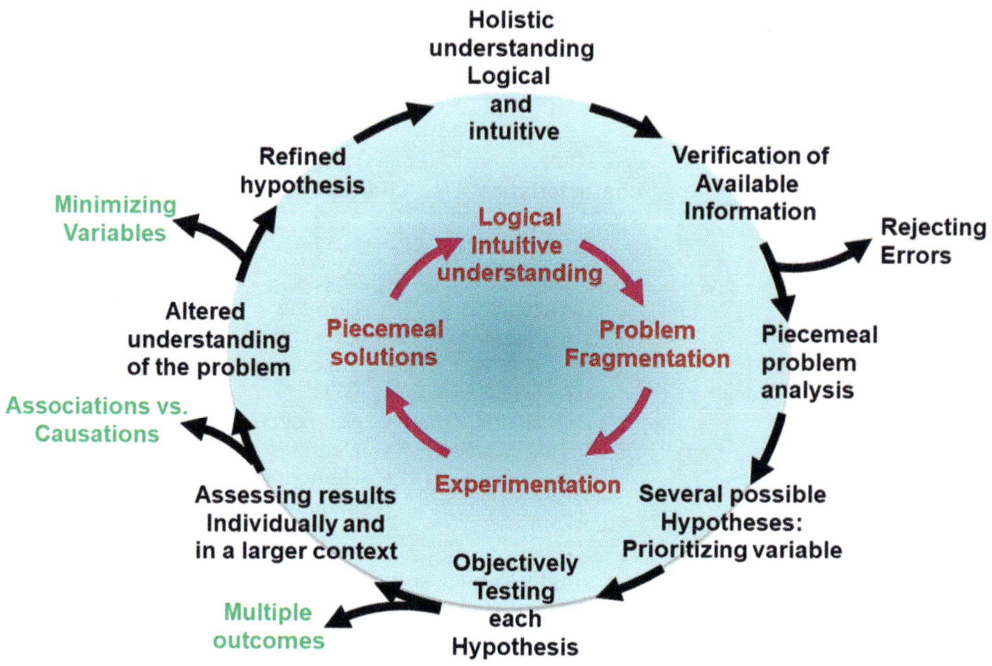

Fig. 23.4 Solving complex problems is a dynamic process that involves holistic assessment, piecemeal experimentation, and a constantly evolving understanding. This dynamic nature is a key characteristic of the process, reflecting the fact that the problem is not static and the understanding of it must evolve to render it solvable

Approach to Complex Problem-Solving

At the outset, complex problem-solving requires a deep understanding of the problem based on logic and intuition to establish priorities. It also requires building and testing several hypotheses, applying multiple tools and approaches to solve the problem, and constantly evaluating and reassessing the problem based on evolving information (Fig. 23.4) [34]. Solving a complex problem requires persistence, even without apparent progress. Complex problem-solving is, at times, open-ended. It may not arrive at a definite solution, but a better understanding of the problems can render unsolvable problems solvable.

The generic approach to complex problem-solving involves the following:

- A deep understanding of the nature of the problem.
- Defining the problem.
- Gathering reliable information.
- Decomposing the problem logically.
- Formulating solutions.
- Applying solution.
- Evaluating outcome.
- Reassessing the approach.

The deeper understanding needed for complex problem-solving has to be logical as well as intuitive. Generating background information is critical to understanding the problems. The possible sources of information for neuroscience research come with advantages and limitations (Fig. 23.5). Assessing the best available information free of bias and errors is necessary for complex problem solutions. There are several possible solutions to complex problem-solving, each with some constraints. The process is judged by progress in understanding rather than the conclusive results. The solutions assessed could support or reject a hypothesis. However, both positive and negative results are relevant as they enlarge the understanding of the problem and help seek better solutions. Thus, in solving complex problems, the negative results are as important as the positive ones. Solving a complex problem is a dynamic and iterative process wherein the hypothesis constantly changes as novel information is generated. The outcome of solving a complex mess problem can be a definite solution or arriving at an acceptable understanding, or the problem may remain unsolvable, awaiting the development of technologies that can test the underlying hypotheses.

Though unrelated to medicine, a common complex problem which illustrates complex problem solving process is predicting the weather. For centuries, the weather was predicted by looking at the skies. Those predictions were local and often erroneous. However, it became possible to measure barometric pressures in the seventeenth century. A combination of temperature, humidity, and pressure led to the development of weather stations in the eighteenth century. These weather stations could locally forecast the weather a few hours ahead. The emergence of the telegraph in the nineteenth century made it possible to network weather stations to predict the weather over land. However, there was a lack of understanding of the atmospheric jet stream and oceanic factors. The development of weather balloons, radar, satellites, and Doppler technology in the twentieth century helped provide the missing data. In this century, supercomputers process the massive amount of weather data from worldwide sources. Based on this, various models predict the weather

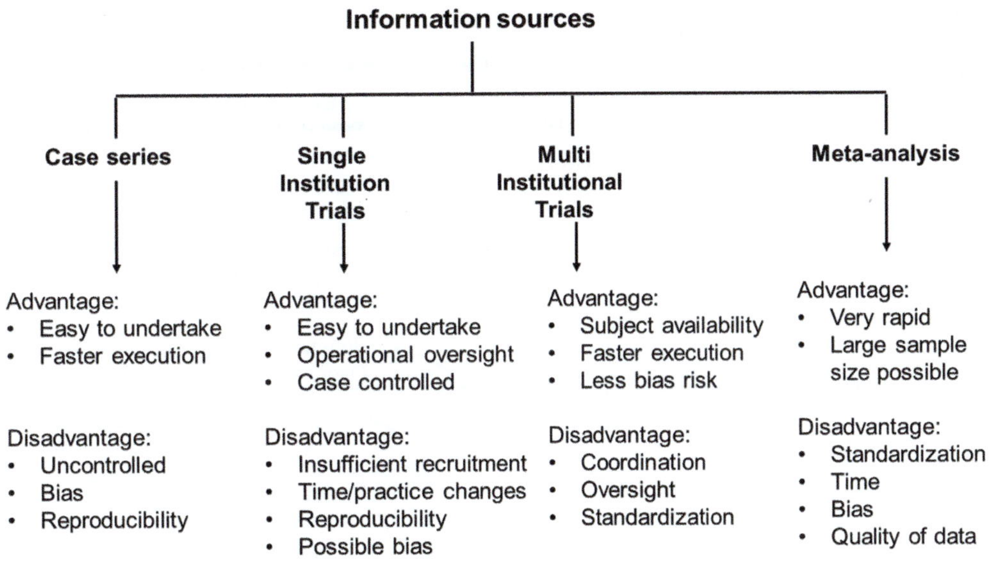

Fig. 23.5 Usual sources of clinical information available for understanding clinical neuroscience problems

outcome several days ahead. These models usually arrive at somewhat different results. It is up to the observer to decide which result to select based on their experience. As new technologies, parameters, and data emerge, the models evolve to correct and refine themselves, which makes weather forecasting more reliable.

Applying Complex Problem-Solving to Acute Ischemic Stroke

Acute Ischemic Stroke as a Complex Problem:

As illustrated in Fig. 23.1 and explained above, several factors affect the stroke outcome, creating a wicked problem mess. In the case of simple clinical problems such as the dose-response of an anesthetic drug in healthy volunteers, it is relatively easy to establish a cause-effect relationship and reliably test any relationship between the two. Here, the experimental variables are limited, the baseline and the final conditions are well-defined, and accessory tools to establish causation, such as EEG effects or blood and brain anesthetic concentrations, are feasible and reliable. Thus, a cause-effect relationship is easy to assess, but finding one in a complex situation, such as an acute ischemic stroke, is exceedingly challenging (Fig. 23.6).

Acute ischemic stroke represents a neurological disease that presents as a "wicked problem mess." The underlying pathological pathways in stroke evolve, and they interact to create a complex web of injurious events (Fig. 23.7) [43]. The cascade of pathogenic events becomes increasingly complex over time. These events result first in the attenuation of neural functions, subsequently the cessation of function, reversible metabolic injury, injury progression, and ultimately irreversible injury. The rapidity with which neurological injuries occur often makes it impossible to contain initial neuronal injury, as is underscored by the adage, "Time is brain." Although the restoration of perfusion has widened the intervention window, the consequences of delayed intervention are challenging to contain and reverse [44, 45]. Applying a complex problem-solving approach to preclinical research could help understand the pathogenic pathways, the evolution of the pathogenic mechanism, and their interactions. Hitherto, most preclinical research in acute stroke generally treats the neural injury as a black box. While the STAIR guidelines have significantly addressed many limitations of preclinical research, much has changed in technology since then [46]. The four technological advances relevant to neuroscience research are: (1) Advances in optical sensing and imaging that can potentially map cell-level anatomy and functions. (2) Advances in drug delivery and novel therapeutic agents. (3) Advances in artificial intelligence. capable of processing vast volumes of data with minimal bias. (4) Advances, magnetic resonance imaging and spectroscopy, that could help with clinical translation.

Currently, most preclinical research treats neurological injuries as a black box but there is increasing recognition to pry the box open [47, 48]. While the STAIR guidelines (Table 23.1) improve the clinical relevance of preclinical stroke models, they do not provide critical insight into whether the intervention alters the injury pathway. STAIR does not assure that the drug reaches the pathological site and whether it did so promptly. There are many reports of effective neuroprotective interventions if given before ischemia although they fail after ischemia occurs. This either reflects a failure of drug delivery or their ineffectiveness with delayed treatment. To understand and advance the treatment of stroke one needs to monitor the pathogenic mechanism ensure drug delivery. We make the case that *optical imaging* and sensing methods could help monitor several injury

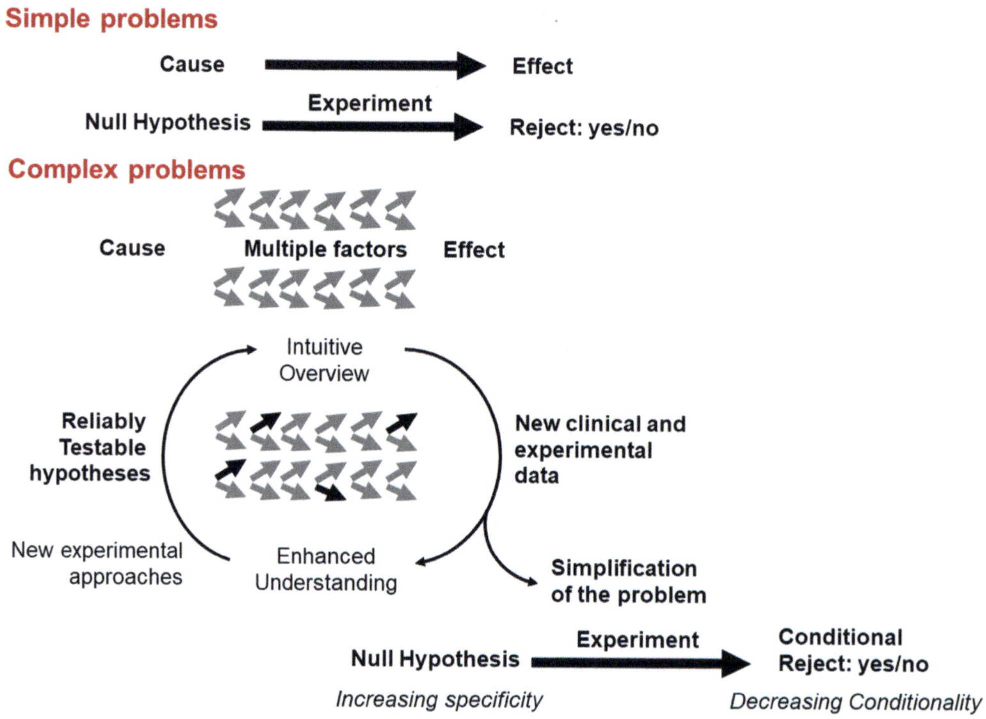

Fig. 23.6 Simple vs. complex problem-solving approaches

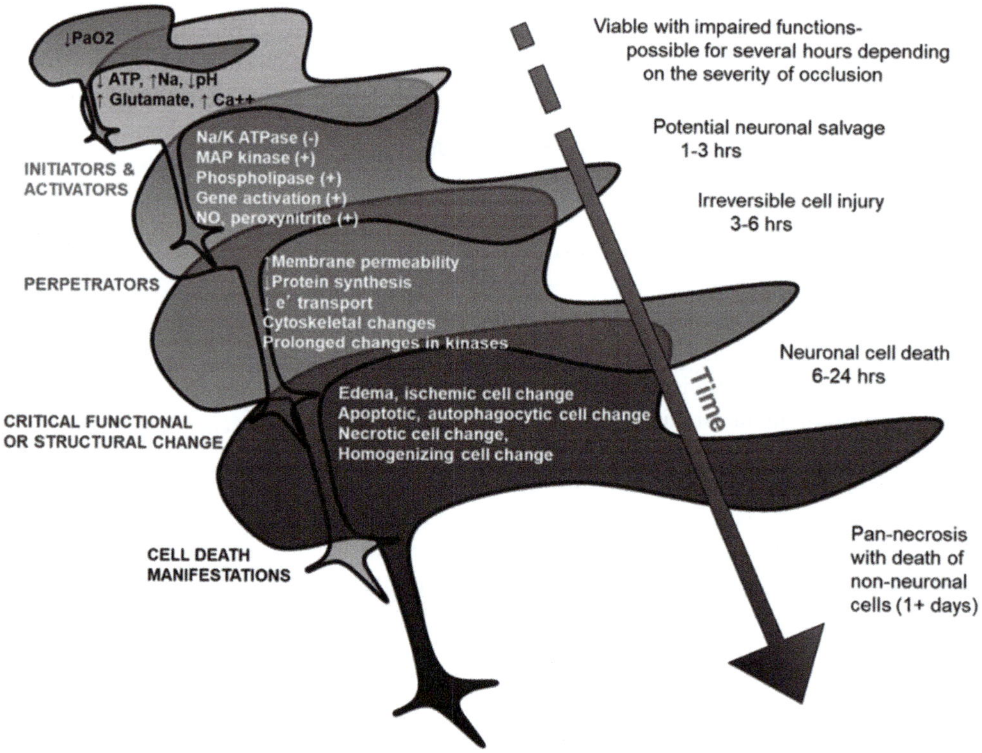

Fig. 23.7 Pathways of ischemic neurological injuries cross-talk with each other and evolve, making it progressively challenging to assess treatments

parameters in bench research. The three objectives of tracking multiple pathogenic mechanisms are (1) to establish their role, (2) to see how they evolve and interact with each other, and (3) to establish a hierarchical pattern that could guide clinical interventions [49]. Hence, we suggest advancing optical technologies in bench research to monitor stroke pathogenesis, drug delivery and treatment response.

Mapping Injury Pathways in Stroke by Optical Methods

Figure 23.7 provides some of the paths of ischemic stroke that increase over time and interact nonlinearly. Any treatment of stroke aimed at a specific mechanism may have a time-dependent effect. If these pathogenic pathways could be tracked, it would be possible to optimize treatments. Due to the complexity of neurological injuries, comparing the real-time evolution of injury pathways with and without experimental interventions will generate novel insights into the pathogenic pathways and how they interact [49]. The availability of various chemical-sensitive dyes can help track concentrations of ischemic markers using multispectral imaging (Table 23.2) [50, 51]. These can be combined with ultraviolet and diffuse reflectance spectroscopies and laser Doppler flow measurements [52–54]. Electroencephalographic recordings and evoked responses can monitor functional brain activity.

Table 23.1 Stroke therapy academic industry roundtable (STAIR) guidelines

STAIR original recommendations	Added recommendations
Initial rodent, then gyrencephalic models	Sample size justification
Permanent, later transient occlusion	Inclusion and exclusion criteria
Adequate dose response data	Randomization
Well characterized model	Allocation concealed or justification
Specified time line of intervention	Accounting for loss of animals
Adequate blinding	Blinded outcome assessment
Physiological monitoring data	Reporting conflicts of interest
Histological outcome	
Functional outcome	
Long term survival	

Figure 23.8 shows this multimodality approach to tracking ischemic injury parameters in intubated anesthetized rabbits and how optical methods can be supplemented with microdialysis and systemic hemodynamic monitoring. Figures 23.9 and 23.10 show how injury parameters can be tracked to map the evolution of ischemic injury. In Fig. 23.9, the ischemia is transient, lasting 60 s, and observed over the next 15 min. Such a brief period of ischemia provides an example of entirely reversible changes during cerebral ischemia. All changes are normalized to baseline values. Currently, the only reliable means of preventing ischemic neurological injury is instituting hypothermia before or sometimes shortly after the ischemic challenge. Hypothermia provides a positive control for neuroprotective compounds. Preliminary investigations using the model revealed that ischemic changes did not correlate with arterial occlusion but were evident only with the onset of hypotension that possibly prevented collateral blood flow. Changes during ischemia and reperfusion hyperemia affect blood flow, oxy- and deoxyhemoglobin, and NADH concentration. Transient changes in Ca^{2+}, reactive oxygen species, and voltage channels were seen and reversed over time. However, it was also

Table 23.2 Ischemic injury parameters that can be quantified by optical means

Parameter	Rationale for monitoring	Optical method	Optical tracer	μ_a (nm)	μ_e (nm)	Positive challenge	Negative challenge	Cross-validation method
Endogenous optical tracers								
Oxy-Hb	Tissue O_2 availability	DRS	NA	NA	NA	100% O_2	N_2 inhalation	MSI/tissue HbO_2
Reduced-Hb	Ischemia severity	DRS	NA	NA	NA	N_2 inhalation	100% O_2	MSI/tissue Hb
NADH	Mitochondrial electron transport	UV-S	NA	350 nm	465 nm	N_2 inhalation	100% O_2	MSI/NADH imaging
Microinjected biosensors								
Voltage change	Neuronal functions	MSI	JPW, (RH-1691, AH 414)	650 nm	>750 nm	Evoked response	IV anesthesia bolus	EEG activity on stimulation
pH sensitive	pH sensitive Ca influx	MSI	BCECF	470 nm	535 nm	3 min hypoventilation	3 min hyperventilation	MD/pH dialsylate
Ca^{2+}	Injury evolution	MSI	Fura-2	330/360 nm	510 nm	Evoked response	Deep anesthesia	EEG/evoked response
Reactive O_2 species[a]	Lipid peroxidation	MSI	Dihydro-ethidium	518 nm	605 nm	Ischemia	NC 186	MD/glutamate
Optical tracer labeled cells/tracers injected systemically								
Platelet[a] activation	Secondary vascular injury	MSI	Carboy-fluorescein labeling	491 nm	518 nm	CF-labeled platelet injection	INS 50589 (platelet inhibitor)	Histology
Neutrophil activation[a]	Inflammatory damage	MSI	Carboy-fluorescein labeling	488 nm	525 nm	CF-labeled interferon activated	LXA4 (activation inhibitor)	Histology

DRS diffuse reflectance spectroscopy, *UV-S* ultra-violet spectroscopy, *MSI* multispectral imaging, *MD* micro-dialysis, *Hb* hemoglobin, alternate dyes in brackets

[a] Positive challenge may not be needed, as sustained ischemia (filament occlusion) will needed and ischemic and non-ischemic hemispheres could be compared

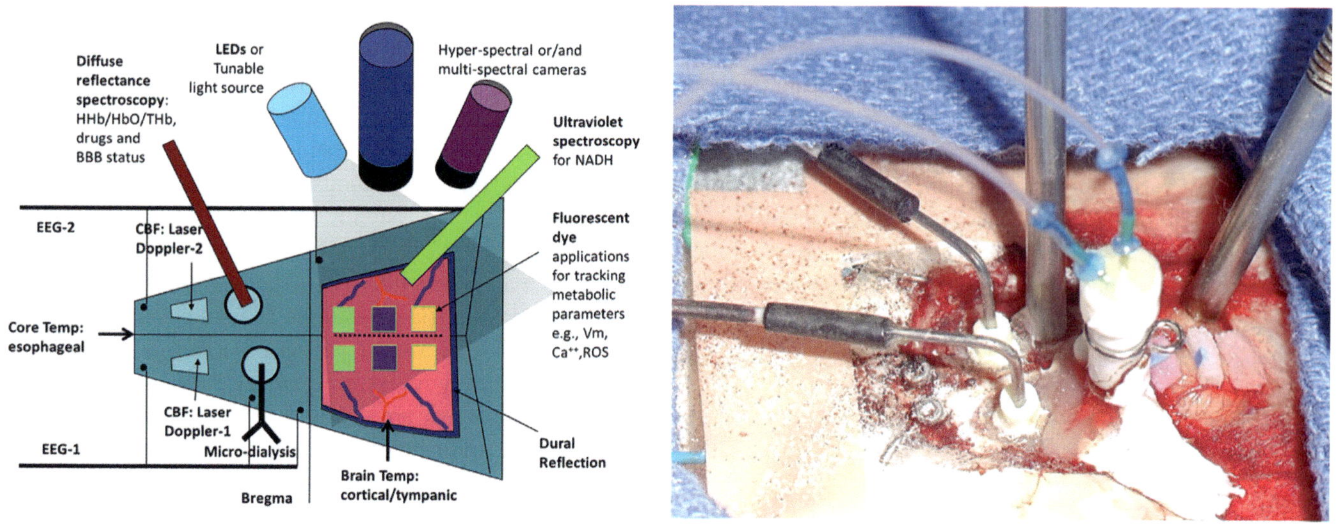

Fig. 23.8 Multimodality monitoring of ischemic injury parameters to establish the evolution of injuries and interactions between the pathogenic pathways

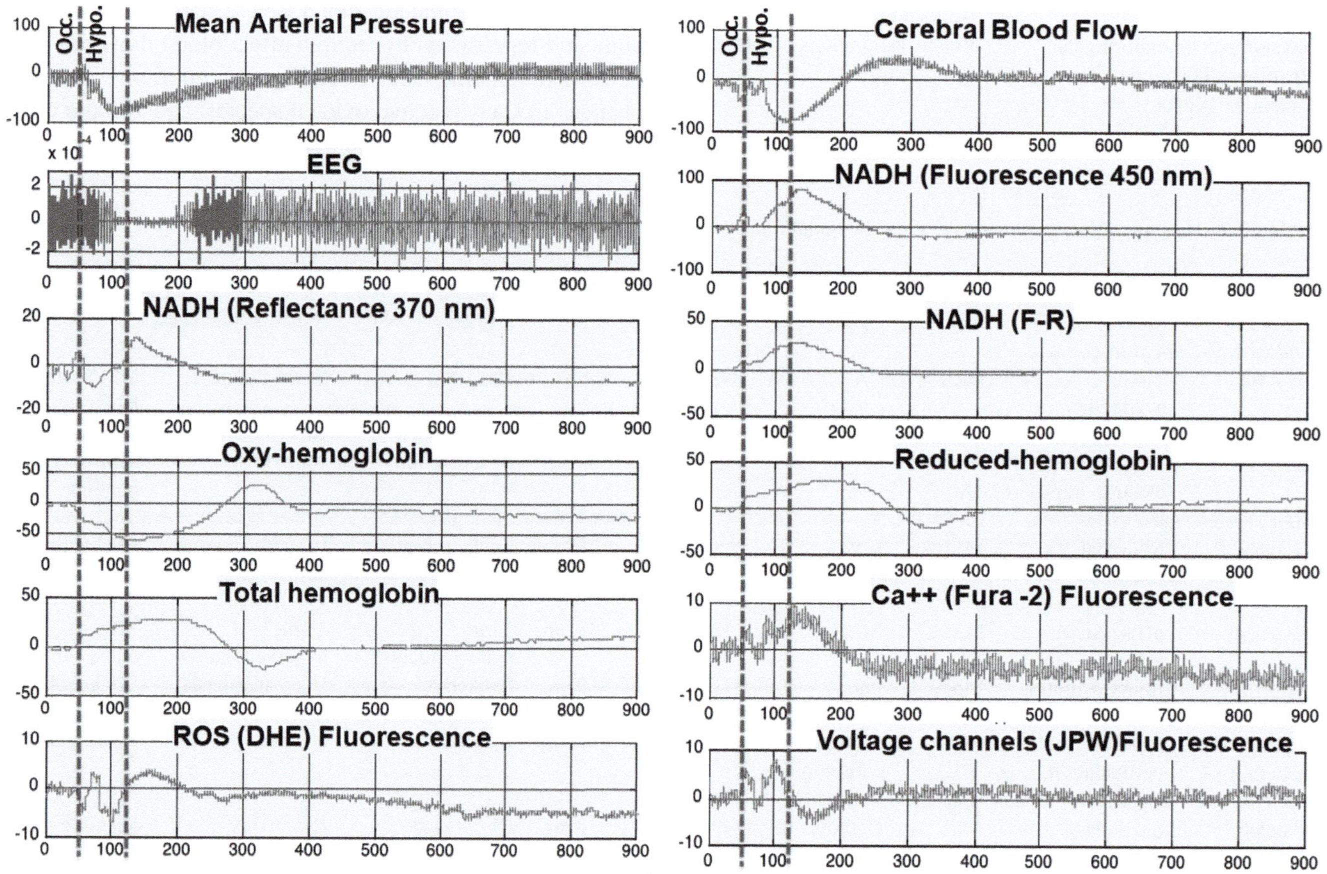

Fig. 23.9 An example of reversible changes in optically monitored parameters with 60 s of bilateral carotid occlusion (Occ.) and hypotension (Hypo.) tracked over 15 min

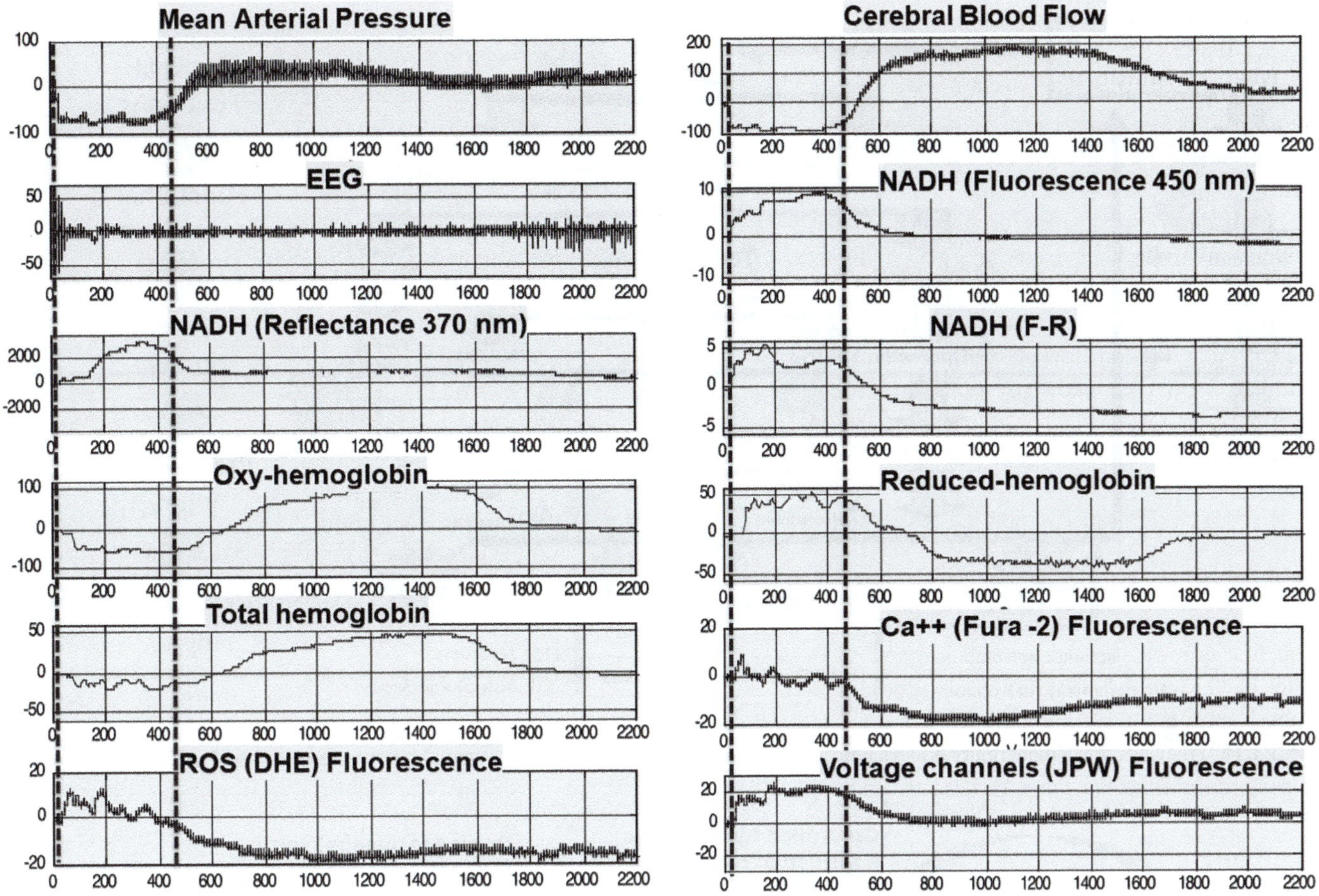

Fig. 23.10 An example of changes in optically monitored parameters with 8 min of bilateral carotid occlusion and systemic hypotension (O/H), tracked over the next 30 min after reperfusion (RP)

observed that when the same challenge of occlusion hypotension was extended to 8 min (Fig. 23.10), some parameters, including EEG activity, did not recover over the next 30 min. Profound hyperperfusion was seen during reperfusion, with an initial rise in NADH florescence during ischemia and a rapid recovery. Voltage-sensitive dye (JPW) was infused topically. It showed no recovery correlating with a suppressed EEG activity with prolonged arterial occlusion, in contrast to the prompt recovery seen with 60-s occlusion hypotension challenge. Results of these preliminary experiments show that multiparameter tissue monitoring is feasible in preclinical research and could help understand stroke evolution and therapeutic impact.

Pitfall and Potential Applications of Optical Monitoring of Cortical Integrity and Functions

Monitoring cortical functions with the permeabilization of tissue-sensitive fluorescent dyes poses several theoretical and technical problems. Some are shared between low- and high-resolution optical and radiological imaging [56, 69]. The optical concerns include effective permeabilization of the tissue by the dye, change in tissue behavior due to the dye permeabilization, selective excitation of the dye, loss of fluorescence due to quenching, changes in light absorption due to changes in hemoglobin concentrations, and interference due to autofluorescence and other fluorophores. However, these problems can be overcome by using programmed excitation by tunable filters, adequate shielding of the probes, corrections of hemoglobin concentrations assessed independently, and optimum selection of test dyes and their combinations. The ability to track potential neuronal injury parameters in real time could have many applications, such as investigating ischemic neurological injury through graded challenges, investigating reperfusion injuries, assessing neurotoxicities such as with anesthetics or chemotherapeutic drugs, investigating the effectiveness and optimum use of neuroprotective drugs, and evaluating the effectiveness of stroke treatment. Figures 23.11 and 23.12 show the multiple sites for potential intervention in ischemic stroke. Many of these interventions have yet to be tested with intra-arterial delivery [49].

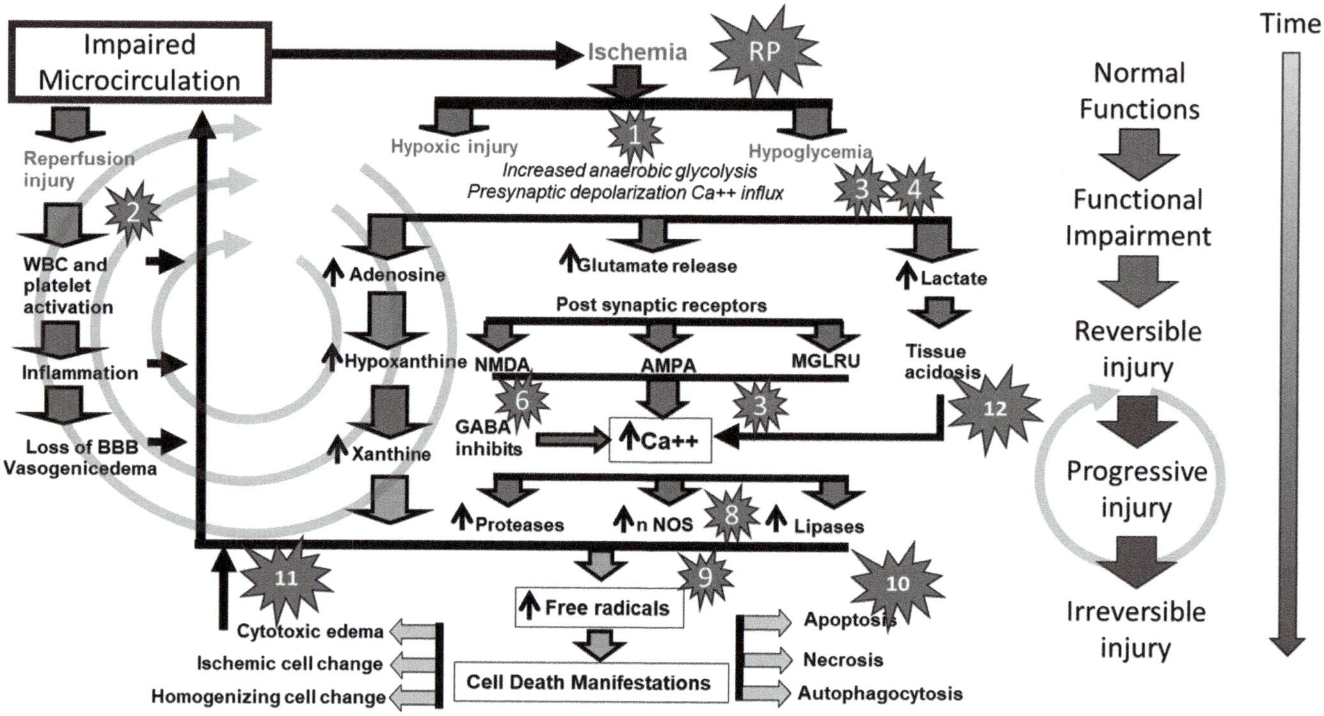

Fig. 23.11 Pathways of neuronal injury are dynamic and cross talk with each other. The potential interventions are listed in Table 23.3

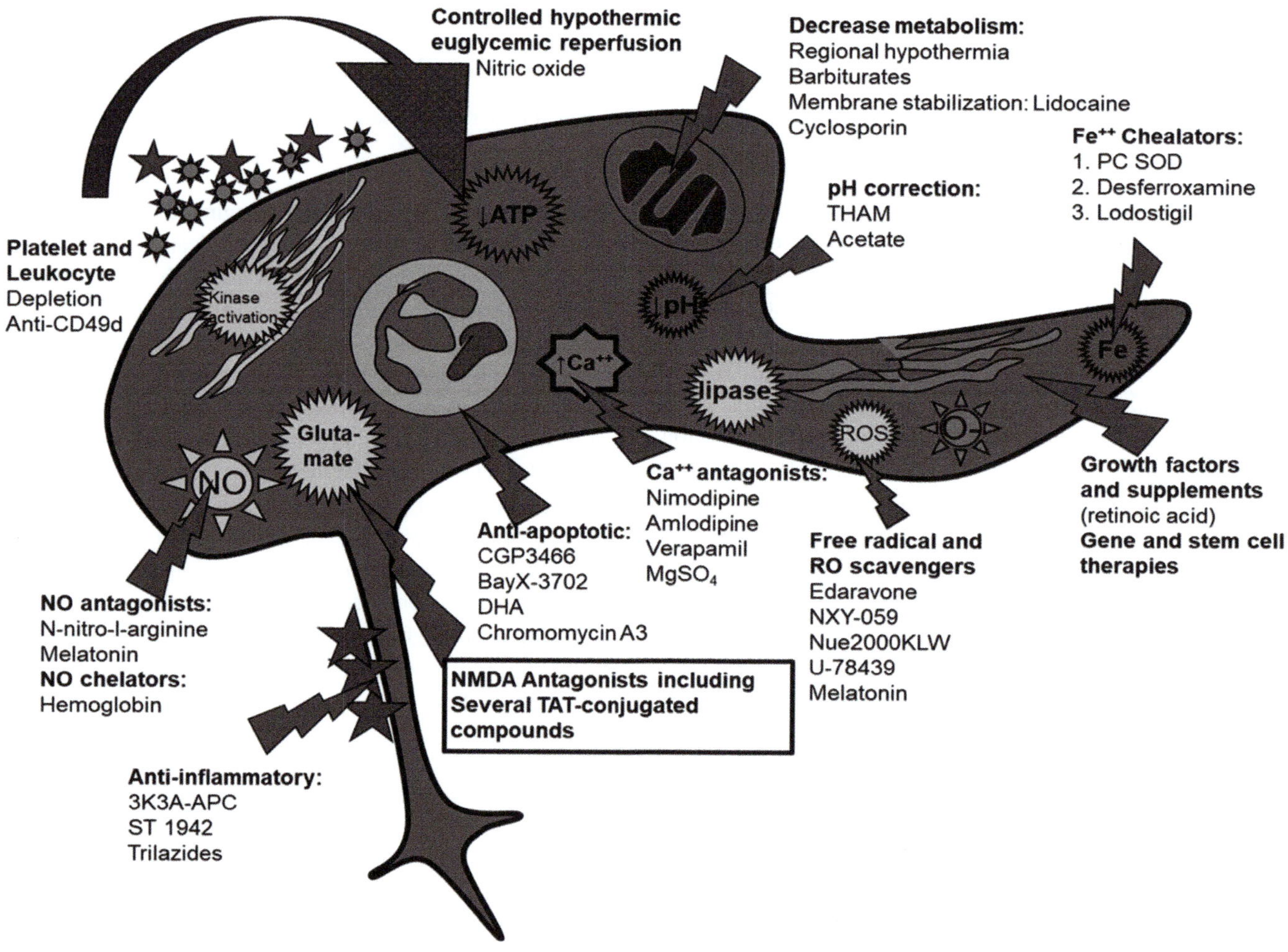

Fig. 23.12 Many possible interventions for stroke and reperfusion injuries, with most yet to be optimized for arterial delivery

Table 23.3 List and justifications of potential arterial interventions

Drug (mechanism)	Outcome of clinical stroke studies: main side effect of IV Rx	The rationale for IA delivery
RP: Reperfusion mechanical or thrombolytic Rx	*The significant impact of early reperfusion has been established, and the treatment window is being expanded*	*Mechanical or intra-arterial thrombolysis creates the opportunity for intra-arterial interventions and reperfusion triggers for subsequent injury cascades* [55]
1. *Hypothermia* (decreased neuronal excitability and metabolism)	Optimum results from moderate hypothermia, approx. 34 °C; severe hypothermia ↓ coagulation, ↑ infection, and ↑ arrhythmias	Cold low-viscosity fluids (e.g., blood with low hematocrit) can ↓ local brain temperature and control reoxygenation, while ↓ WBC and platelet content can ↓ inflammatory response [56]
2. *Enlimomab* (anti-ICAM antibody)	Worsened outcome: ↑ fever/infection/ inflammation [57]	Specific local binding with the endothelial cell surface receptor. CD-31 could substantially ↓increase the dose with IA bolus delivery and flow manipulation
3. *Nimodipine* (voltage-gated Ca^{2+} ch. blocker)	No benefit on meta-analysis of human data; ↑mortality with early rapid IV Rx; ↑ IV dose, ↓BP and worsened outcome	Prompt onset of action is desirable because maximum benefit is seen if given <20 min in animal stroke models; however, rapid IV dosing worsens prognosis. Highly effective after SAH [58]
4. *BMS-204352* (K^+ ch. opener)	Lack of efficacy via. the IV route: well tolerated	Concentrations by IA delivery may be greater than those achieved by the IV route [59]
5. *Gavestinel* (glycine antagonist)	Lack of efficacy ↓ hallucinations compared to other NMDA antagonists	Selective delivery to ischemic tissue, ↑ concentrations, and ↑ therapeutic effects. Ineffective IV [60]
6. *Clomethiazole* (GABA agonist)	Lack of efficacy, particularly with large strokes: ↑ sedation	Selective delivery to ischemic tissue combined with ↓the total dose may ↓sedation. Ineffective IV [61]
7. *Tirilazad* (free radical scavenger)	Increased mortality: ↑ systemic effects of steroids a major concern	↓Total dose may ↓systemic effects yet achieve effective tissue concentrations. Ineffective IV [62]
8. *Lubeluzole* (prevents glutamate increase. And ↓ses NO-mediated injury)	Lack of efficacy: ↑ QT prolongation/ transient arrhythmias	Selective delivery to ischemic tissue combined with ↓the total dose may ↓ cardiac side effects. IV safe and ↓ mortality [63]
9. *NXY-059* (free radical scavenger)	Lack of efficacy: limited BBB penetration: polar compound, poor lipid solubility	Better analogs are being developed, and more lipid-soluble analogs might be suited for IA delivery. Intravenous NXY-059 is ineffective [64]
10. *Trafermin* (fibroblast growth factor)	Lack of efficacy: hypotension, leukocytosis, best results with low doses [65]	Brain-selective liposomal delivery with sustained release is possible
11. *Mannitol* (hyperosmotic dehydration)	Lack of efficacy; IV mannitol can increase mortality in acute stroke [66]	With intact BBB, IA mannitol will ↓ cytotoxic edema and improve microcirculation and, if needed, ↑ drug delivery [67]
12. *Tham* (Tris hydroxymethyl amino methane)	Some benefits of pH correction in preclinical studies [68]	Correction of intracellular acidosis will ↓ ionized Ca^{2+} concentrations

Arterial Drug Delivery

Many methods of targeted drug delivery are being developed. Given that the most successful stroke intervention hitherto has been thrombectomy, arterial drug delivery is the most relevant approach to intervene in acute ischemic stroke because the catheter for drug delivery can be readily deployed. The ability of arterial delivery to instantaneously achieve therapeutic concentrations and to do so at a fraction of systemic dose is highly relevant to both research and clinical treatments. On the one hand, it provides the tool to investigate pathological pathways, and on the other, it enables multiple therapeutic interventions while minimizing the risk of systemic interactions [70].

The advantages of arterial drug delivery include the following:

- It provides relatively safe and easy access to the target site.
- The procedures are not physiologically stressful and pose minimal risk.
- The core techniques of arterial delivery can be applied across organs and diseases.
- The drugs can instantly achieve therapeutic concentrations.
- With improved methods of first-pass drug extraction, significant dose reductions may be possible.
- Multiple drugs may be delivered to the target site.
- To counter the systemic side effects, drugs could be neutralized by an antidote or removed by extracorporeal extractions.
- Can deliver a variety of therapeutic cargo, including drugs, genes, and stem cells.
- In the context of stroke, the catheter for drug delivery is already in situ after the clot is extracted, as the injury is initiated, and the perfusion is reestablished. The case for arterial interventions is exceedingly compelling.

The main benefit of arterial drug delivery is that it could permit the use of multiple drugs as independent pulses. In the case of stroke, when multiple pathways of ischemic injuries interact, arterial treatment could allow dynamic interventions based on evolving tissue needs. The arterial approach can also permit regional cooling and modulate blood flow physically and pharmacologically. Modulating blood flow can optimize drug delivery and mitigate ischemic and hyperperfusion injuries.

Feasibility of Selective Targeting Ischemic and Apoptotic Neurons

In healthy cells, anionic lipids such as phosphatidylserine (PtdSer) are present in the inner membrane layer and anchor key signaling mechanisms [71]. Stressed, malignant, and apoptotic cells demonstrate the migration of PtdSer onto the cell surface [72]. This translocation is affected by caspases, reacting oxygen species, or increased intracellular Ca^{2+}. The translocation of PtdSer from the inner to the outer leaflet of the cell membrane plays a crucial role in recognizing apoptotic cells by phagocytes and modulating the immune response. Phagocytic cells have transmembrane receptors that directly bind to PtdSer, brain-specific angiogenic inhibitor-1, and stablin-1. Several proteins also bind to PtdSer, which include Protein S, Gas 6, C1q, and MFG-E8. PtdSer could be used to target stressed, apoptotic cells and malignant cells [73].

Anionic PtdSer targeting in vivo and in vitro can be achieved by cationic peptides. The translocation of human immunodeficiency virus-derived cell-penetrating peptide, trans-activator of transcription (TAT): HIV-derived protein TAT consists of 81–101 amino acids. TAT has a cell-penetrating peptide (TAT-CPP) sequence comprising 11 to 13 amino acids (YGRKKRRQRRR to GRKKRRQRRRPPQ) and is highly cationic. Unlike the entire TAT molecule, the TAT-CPP does not require binding to heparan sulfate to penetrate the cells. Furthermore, the arginine and lysine-rich, GRKK amino acid sequence, enables TAT to target the nuclear membrane [74, 75]. The internalization of TAT-CPP is exceedingly rapid within 100–200 ns in computational models [76]. CPPs can penetrate the cell membrane without disrupting its integrity. CPPs can cross the cell membrane by energy-dependent and energy-independent mechanisms. TAT can deliver a wide range of cargos across the cell membrane [77]. The former include endocytosis through micropinocytosis, caveolin-mediated or clathrin-mediated. The energy-independent mechanism includes direct penetration. TAT primarily enters the cells at high concentrations by directly penetrating the cell membrane. Several cationic peptides other than TAT can penetrate the cell membrane and be used for targeted drug delivery. They could have neurooncological and stroke applications [78].

TAT can carry large drug cargo and nanoparticles across the cell membrane. Like the apoptotic cells, cancer cells also show transmigration of anionic lipids of the outer leaflet of the cell membranes. In these cells and animals with implanted brain tumors, there is a rapid uptake of TAT after intra-arterial delivery [79]. Whole animal experiments show relatedly poor uptake of TAT in healthy brain tissue even after optimized arterial delivery. Preliminary reports with conjugates of TAT and a chemotherapeutic drug, melphalan, show a substantial reduction of doses with improved survival after intra-arterial delivery (Chap. 20). Figure 23.13 shows the comparative uptake of FITC-labeled TAT after intravenous and intra-arterial delivery. The figure illustrates the potential benefits of arterial delivery of TAT conjugates and nanoparticles to brain tumors [80]. The apoptotic cells, like tumors with overexpression of PtdSer on their out leaflets, could similarly benefit targeting by TAT-conjugated peptides [72].

Several neuroprotective peptides have been conjugated with TAT. Table 23.4 reports their neuroprotective benefits in cell studies, brain slices, and stroke models after topical or intravenous delivery. However, we found no reports of TAT or TAT-conjugated arterial drug delivery for stroke/reperfusion injury. Arterial drug delivery by delivering a pure drug to the target site has the potential to overcome fundamental limitations of systemic cationic peptides, namely, immunological reactions and nontarget site uptake.

Rationalization of Stroke Treatments

The anatomic and cytological complexity of the neural tissue, the functional specificity of each region of the brain, the need for a stable milieu for cells to function, the tight linkage between regional blood flow and neural activity, the high tissue metabolic rate, the lack of energy reserves, the presence of the blood-brain barrier, the regional susceptibility to ischemic injury, and the diversity of injury pathways that cross-talk with each other and become increasingly complex as time elapses are some of the many challenges that are faced with stroke treatment. The one-size-fits-all approach to stroke treatment is unlikely to improve neurological outcomes. Detection, characterization, and prediction of stroke's clinical course and treatment will become increasingly individualized as diagnostic and treatment modalities evolve. With increasing human life expectancy worldwide, the burden of acute ischemic stroke on healthcare systems and costs will escalate. Furthermore, there will be an expectation of qualitative, not just quantitative improvement.

Time-Based Stroke Interventions

Pathogenic pathways in stroke evolve rapidly, and as time passes, the complexity of interventions increases with a declining likelihood of a favorable outcome. As shown in Table 23.2, there is an optimum therapeutic window for stroke interventions. In the last decade, a flurry of reports has demonstrated the effectiveness of mechanical clot-extracting devices. There is also an effort to set up endovascular treatment units equipped with MR and CT capabilities close to the emergency and operating rooms. Mobile stroke units

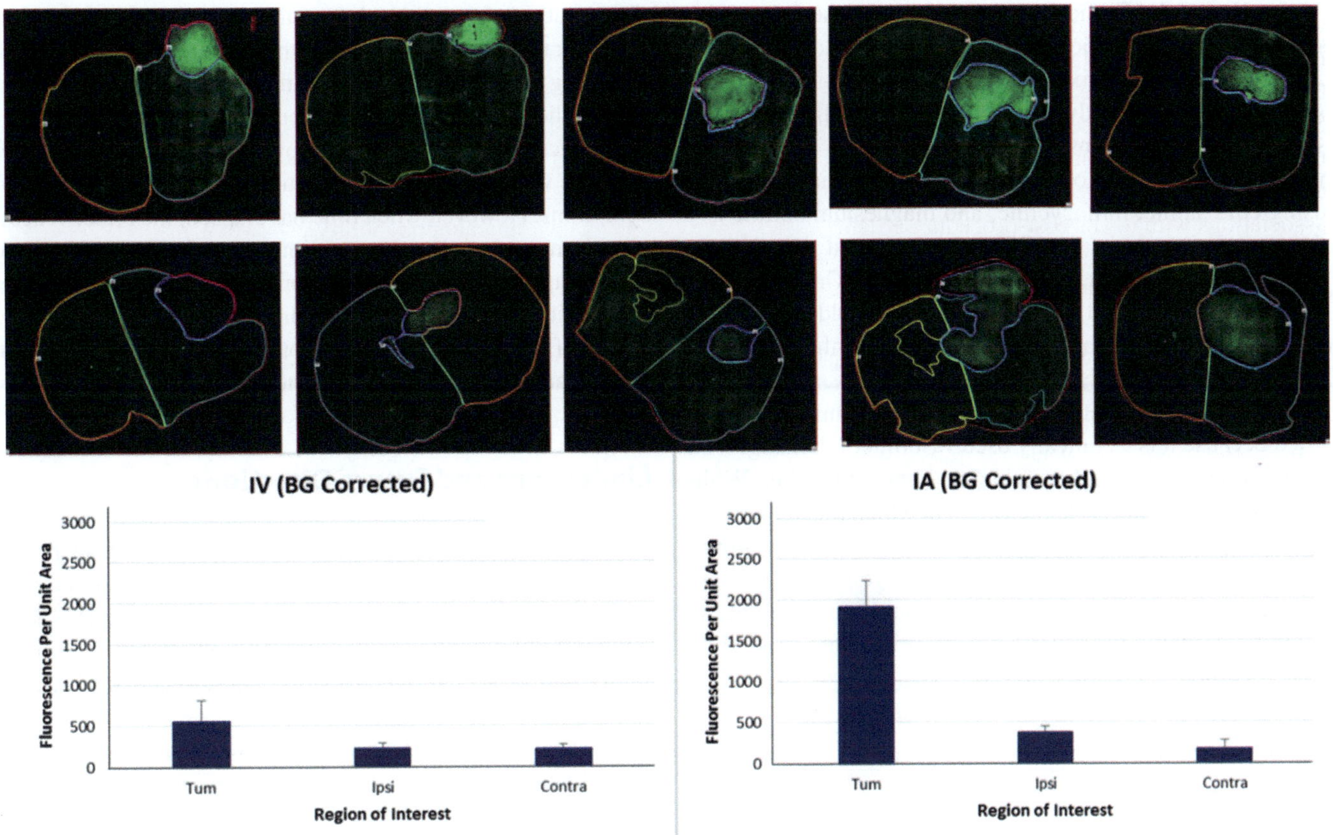

Fig. 23.13 Intra-arterial (IA) delivery of FITC-labeled TAT that targets anionic lipids of the cell membrane, delivered to tumor-bearing rats by IA (top row) and intravenous (IV; bottom row) injections. Measurements were made in three regions—tumor, ipsilateral, and contralateral brain—using confocal microscopy. With IV injection, the tumor FITC-TAT uptake was 2.5× the ipsilateral and contralateral brain tissue. With IA injection, tumor uptake was 11× the contralateral and 5× the remaining ipsilateral tissue. IA delivery of TAT-conjugated compounds could target anionic lipids on the cell surface of malignant and apoptotic cells

Table 23.4 TAT-conjugated neuroprotective compounds in development with potential intra-arterial applications

Apoptotic pathway	TAT conjugate	Therapeutic window	Model	References
Glutamate—NMDR-GluN2B				
Neuronal and BBB protection: GluN2B-Ca^{2+}-PSD95-nNOS/MMP9	TAT-NR2B9C	1–3 h IV	MCAO, rats	[81, 82]
Death associated protein kinase and	TAT-Glu2B$^{CT1292-1304}$	0–60 min	MCAO, mice	[83]
P53 interaction: GluN2B-CAPK1-p53	TAT-P53DM	6 h	MCAO, mice	[84]
Nuclear translocation of PTEN: GluN2B-PTEN	TAT-K-13	6 h	MCAO, rats	[85]
Pannexin-1 Channel: GluN2B-SFK-Panx1	TAT-Panx1$_{305-318}$	0 or 1 h after	Anoxia, acute hippocampal slices of rats and mice	[86]
Secondary messenger				
Neuronal differentiation, survival and function by ankyrin repeat-rich membrane spanning (ARMS) substrate proteolysis: Calpain	TAT-Kidins220	N/A	Cultured neurons MOA: preservation of ERK1/2 and CERB	[87]
	TAT-STEP	0 and 6 h	Cultured neurons and MCAO occlusion STEP KO mice	[88]
	TAT-mGluR1	Pretreatment	Post-SAH	[89]

capable of diagnosing stroke and shortening the treatment time have been shown to improve outcomes. Early intravenous thrombolysis within 3–4.5 h after the onset of symptoms and subsequent mechanical extraction within 6 h are generally recommended. The treatment window can be extended based on imaging data. Yet, neuroprotective strategies are seldom routinely used in the ICU setting after thrombectomy.

A National Clinical Trials website search using stroke + neuroprotection as search terms yields 91 hits in 2024. Of these, only six studies involved intra-arterial interventions. One trial study involved regional cooling with cold saline arterial infusions. Two trials evaluated intra-arterial verapamil. The fourth one evaluated intra-arterial treatments using cold saline, minocycline, and magnesium sulfate as a dose escalation study. The fifth trial evaluated an unproven neuroprotective agent, 3-*n*-butylphthalide. The sixth trial evaluated intra-arterial magnesium sulfate. Cold saline could be helpful after recanalization by decreasing the brain temperature and viscosity, restoring tissue pH, and perhaps washing the accumulated metabolites. Verapamil can be justified because it is a clinically used vasodilator that augments cerebral blood flow and is a calcium channel blocker. While there is some dispute as to the extent to which $MgSO_4$ crosses the blood-brain barrier, it is a Ca^{2+} and NMDA antagonist that could benefit acute stroke. Minocycline is an anti-inflammatory and immunomodulator that has been effective in stroke models. While these efforts are laudable and clinically justified, they also highlight the lack of preclinical studies to select drugs, their doses, and the timing to be fully effective in a rapidly evolving situation.

The Route to Clinical Translation

After the failure of NXY059, which was developed in compliance with the STAIR guidelines, the guidelines had to be ammended [13]. The basic idea was to obtain effective, reproducible, and unbiased results. However, no matter how reliable preclinical research is, it is only possible to replicate some aspects of clinical injury in the laboratory. Many factors that operate in the clinical realm, such as variability in age, comorbidities, concurrent treatment, and precise onset time, cannot be reproduced in laboratory research. The STAIR guidelines are a faithful attempt to standardize factors in complex problems. However, several factors that determine the outcome remain unknown. The alternate approach to preclinical and clinical stroke research might be to apply optical methods to pry open the black box of neuropathology and identify specific treatments based on observed injury parameters. The experimental approach for investigating neuroprotection using multimodality tissue monitoring is shown in Fig. 23.8, while Table 23.5 shows the advances in MRI imaging that are available for clinical translation. A detailed characterization of injury could lead to specific interventions by arterial drug delivery for a given patient at a specific time point.

A patient-specific approach to stroke treatment is already emerging in determining when to intervene after embolic stroke based on MRI data rather than simply relying on the time since the onset of symptoms. Several new stroke injury parameters are being developed that could better characterize the evolution of the injury. At the same time, carriers and drugs that seek to treat these specific pathological pathways are also emerging (Table 23.4). Currently, the emphasis of stroke treatment relies on establishing reperfusion. Data suggest that mechanical clot extraction and flow augmentation are highly effective when the treatment is initiated soon after the onset of symptoms. However, when time has elapsed, the effectiveness of treatment declines. At that time, reperfusion itself could trigger apoptosis. There is a compelling case for treating reperfusion injuries with arterial drugs at that time. The availability of carrier-linked antiapoptotic compounds (Table 23.4) could lead to novel treatment when reperfusion is delayed.

Limitations and Future Directions

Translational neuroscience poses many challenging problems, mainly due to the characteristics of the host organ, the brain. An organ that is uniquely vulnerable to injury yet is inherently smart with redundancy and a diversity of compensatory and protective mechanisms. These mechanisms, like autoregulation, blood-brain barrier, excessive blood flow, neuroplasticity, and adaptability, can conceal pathology, sometimes to the detriment of survival. It is enormously challenging to halt, recover, and heal from injury when failure occurs. Since antiquity, neuronal injuries have been classified as in the Egyptian papyri, "Something I can treat, something I am content with, and something that cannot be treated" [119]. Such an approach needs to change in the future. This chapter proposes uses of the emerging advances in optics, drug delivery, AI, and MR imaging that could offer a path to do so (Table 23.5).

Although we present preliminary data, it suggests the possible role of optical imaging and arterial drug delivery in understanding the evolution and treatment of acute ischemic stroke. While there are challenges in using optical approaches, the advances in the field are so rapid that a wide array of techniques will be available to enable optical pharmacokinetics and monitor drug effects. Arterial drug delivery is most effective when the drugs are rapidly extracted and retained during their first pass through the cerebral circulation. Improving arterial drug delivery requires tracking tissue concentrations in a sub-second time domain. The instantaneous delivery of drugs selectively to pathological sites with minimal systemic overflow creates the possibility of multidrug arterial interventions. Stroke, malignancies, and neurodegenerative diseases provide a common cell surface target, PtdSer. Targeting PtdSer with intra-arterial cationic cell-penetrating peptides/nanoparticles may deliver therapeutics selectively to the target cells. Assessing the effectiveness and safety of pharmacological interventions on neuronal activity also requires monitoring in a millisecond time domain. In theory, with rapid assessment of injury parameters could permit the selection of drug treatments based on evolving injury. Optical technologies provide

Table 23.5 Optical and magnetic resonance imaging/spectroscopic tools to investigate stroke pathology

Injury mechanism	Optical monitoring	MR monitoring	Intra-arterial treatment
Microvascular anatomy	Laser Doppler speckled imaging [90], ICG angiography [91], PAT angiography [92]	Contrast and non-contrast MR angiography [93, 94]	Thrombolysis Mechanical clot retrieval
Tissue perfusion	Microsphere transit time [95]	Perfusion MRI [96]	Intra-arterial vasodilators
Tissue oxygenation	Near-infrared spectroscopy [97–99]	BOLD [100], $^{31}P/^{1}H$ MRS [101, 102]	Local perfusion cold low-viscosity fluorocarbons or WBCs and platelet-depleted blood
Tissue acidosis	pH-sensitive dyes [103]	^{1}H MRS [102]	IA THAM, reperfusion
Impaired electron transport	NAD+/NADH ratio: UV spectroscopy [104] Cytochrome A3 [107]	$^{31}P/^{1}H$ MRS [106]	Cold perfusion; IA anesthetics
Ca^{2+} imaging	Calcium sensitive dyes [109]	Ca responsive MRI probes [108]	Ca^{2+} antagonists
Neuronal activity	Near-infrared spectroscopy [109] Functional PAT [110]	FMRI [111]	IA anesthetics
Cytotoxic brain edema	PAT [112] diffuse reflectance spectroscopy (DRS) [113]	Diffusion-weighted imaging MRI [114]	IA mannitol
Free radical damage	Free radical sensitive dyes [115]	Overhauser-enhanced MRI [116]	IA ROS scavengers
Apoptosis	DRS [117]	Phosphatidylserine externalization and MRI tracer tags [118]	Early: Ca and NMDA antagonists Late: Antiapoptotic drugs and peptide conjugates

ICG indocyanine green, *BOLD* blood oxygen level-dependent, *NAD+* nicotinamide adenine dinucleotide, *MRS* magnetic reflectance spectroscopy, *FMRI* functional magnetic resonance imaging, *PAT* photoacoustic imaging, *DRS* diffuse reflectance spectroscopy, *ROS* reactive oxygen species, *NMDA* *N*-methyl-D-aspartate

the only possible safe and cost-effective means to interrogate tissue in a time-dense manner. Thus, it is easy to foresee ongoing advances in biomedical optics, experimental neuroscience techniques, and arterial pharmacology converge to create new avenues for translational neuroscience research.

In terms of assessing outcomes, we suggest using a complex problem-solving approach. Complex problems are an unpredictable aggregation of several subproblems. The subproblems are ill-understood and unpredictable, interact nonlinearly, evolve, are subjectively assessed, and could be unknown. Such a description can be applied to neurological diseases like stroke, vasospasm, head injury, neurodegenerative diseases, and brain tumors. In most neurological diseases, the pathogenic pathways that affect cellular injury, tissue perfusion, inflammation, repair, and neural functions evolve and interact unpredictably to create a problem mess. The mess makes it difficult to determine the impact of any treatment. Optical and magentic resonance imaging alongwith arterial drug delivery could offer new treatments for acute ischemic stroke and the other hitherto challenging neurological diseases.

Conclusion

The description of a medical event on Mars seventy-five years in the future was to expand the time frame for technological development. As technology advances, neurological diseases will often be diagnosed before clinical symptoms are evident. There will also be a greater need to preserve and restore functionality with minimal lifestyle disruption. When the neuropathology is limited to such a small scale, drugs must be delivered locally as per tissue needs. Although many drug delivery methods are being developed, arterial drug delivery provides the most reliable means of delivering multiple drugs to the target site to achieve therapeutic concentrations immediately. The complex nature of neurological injuries, with many underlying mechanisms, has prevented the effective containment and reversal of neurological pathologies. The mechanisms are often ill-understood and nonlinear, interact with each other, and evolve to create a complex problem mess. Solving such problem messes requires a fundamentally different approach. The current model is usually based on comparing isolated treatments of a specific pathogenic component. This chapter offered an alternative approach to investigating neuroprotective drugs after acute ischemic stroke—an area where huge investments were made to develop treatments but to no avail. Optically tracking neuronal injury parameters and tissue changes could help understand and treat neurological injuries with intra-arterial drugs for their eventual clinical translation in the MR environment.

References

1. Min C, Bu Y, Sun J. Predicting scientific breakthroughs based on knowledge structure variations. Technol Forecast Soc Change. 2021;164:120502.
2. Tsaousis D. Perpetual motion machine. J Eng Sci Technol Rev. 2008;1:53–7.
3. Anonymous. A pictorial history of rockets. https://www.grc.nasa.gov/www/k-12/rocket/BottleRocket/13thru16.htm.

4. Wang DZ, Schwamm LH, Qian T, Dai Q. Decoding the brain through research—the future of brain health. BMJ. 2020;371:m3735.
5. Siuly S, Zhang Y. Medical big data: medical data diagnosis through medical data analysis. Data Sci Eng. 2016;1(2):54–64.
6. Chandrabhatla AS, Kuo EA, Sokolowski JD, Kellogg RT, Park M, Mastorakos P. Artificial intelligence and machine learning in the diagnosis and management of stroke: a narrative review of United States Food and Drug Administration—approved technologies. J Clin Med. 2023;12(11):3755.
7. Manera V, Rovini E, Wais P. Editorial: Early detection of neurodegenerative disorders using behavioral markers and new technologies: new methods and perspectives. Front Aging Neurosci. 2023;15:1149886.
8. Raha O, Hall C, Malik A, D'Anna L, Lobotesis K, Kwan J, et al. Advances in mechanical thrombectomy for acute ischaemic stroke. BMJ Med. 2023;2(1):e000407.
9. Liu J, Li C, Wang Y, Ji P, Guo S, Zhai Y, et al. Prognostic and predictive factors in elderly patients with glioblastoma: a single-center retrospective study. Front Aging Neurosci. 2021;13:777962.
10. Murakami H, Shiraishi T, Umehara T, Omoto S, Iguchi Y. Recent advances in drug therapy for Parkinson's disease. Intern Med. 2023;62(1):33–42.
11. Obeso JA, Monje MHG, Matarazzo M. Major advances in Parkinson's disease over the past two decades and future research directions. Lancet Neurol. 2022;21(12):1076–9.
12. Gladstone DJ, Black SE, Hakim AM, Heart, Stroke Foundation of Ontario Centre of Excellence in Stroke Recovery. Toward wisdom from failure: lessons from neuroprotective stroke trials and new therapeutic directions. Stroke. 2002;33(8):2123–36.
13. Editorial. Neuroprotection: the end of an era? Lancet. 2006;368(9547):1548.
14. STAIR. Recommendations for standards regarding preclinical neuroprotective and restorative drug development. Stroke. 1999;30(12):2752–8.
15. Lapchak PA, Zhang JH, Noble-Haeusslein LJ. RIGOR guidelines: escalating STAIR and STEPS for effective translational research. Transl Stroke Res. 2013;4(3):279–85.
16. Thomas A, Detilleux J, Flecknell P, Sandersen C. Impact of Stroke Therapy Academic Industry Roundtable (STAIR) guidelines on peri-anesthesia care for rat models of stroke: a meta-analysis comparing the years 2005 and 2015. PLoS One. 2017;12(1):e0170243.
17. Wintermark M, Colen R, Whitlow CT, Zaharchuk G. The vast potential and bright future of neuroimaging. Br J Radiol. 2018;91(1087):20170505.
18. Vazquez-Guardado A, Yang Y, Bandodkar AJ, Rogers JA. Recent advances in neurotechnologies with broad potential for neuroscience research. Nat Neurosci. 2020;23(12):1522–36.
19. Goyal M, Ospel JM, Kappelhof M, Ganesh A. Challenges of outcome prediction for acute stroke treatment decisions. Stroke. 2021;52(5):1921–8.
20. Fanelli D. Negative results are disappearing from most disciplines and countries. Scientometrics. 2012;90:891–904.
21. Littner Y, Mimouni FB, Dollberg S, Mandel D. Negative results and impact factor: a lesson from neonatology. Arch Pediatr Adolesc Med. 2005;159(11):1036–7.
22. DeVito NJ, Goldacre B. Catalogue of bias: publication bias. BMJ Evid Based Med. 2019;24(2):53–4.
23. Mlinaric A, Horvat M, Supak SV. Dealing with the positive publication bias: why you should really publish your negative results. Biochem Med (Zagreb). 2017;27(3):030201.
24. He S, Wu S, Zeng Q, Zhang S, Lin S, Zhang C, et al. Assessment of methodological quality and outcome measures of acute stroke randomized controlled trials in China in recent 15 years. J Evid Based Med. 2012;5(3):174–82.
25. Duncan PW, Jorgensen HS, Wade DT. Outcome measures in acute stroke trials: a systematic review and some recommendations to improve practice. Stroke. 2000;31(6):1429–38.
26. Li Y, Zhang J. Animal models of stroke. Animal Model Exp Med. 2021;4(3):204–19.
27. Kaiser EE, West FD. Large animal ischemic stroke models: replicating human stroke pathophysiology. Neural Regen Res. 2020;15(8):1377–87.
28. Thiagarajan T. 3 Assumptions that could topple neuroscience. 2019. https://sapienlabs.org/lab-talk/3-assumptions-that-could-topple-neuroscience/.
29. Barack DL, Miller EK, Moore CI, Packer AM, Pessoa L, Ross LN, et al. A call for more clarity around causality in neuroscience. Trends Neurosci. 2022;45(9):654–5.
30. Fabbri A, Lai A, Grundy Q, Bero LA. The influence of industry sponsorship on the research agenda: a scoping review. Am J Public Health. 2018;108(11):e9–e16.
31. Jellinger KA. Interaction between pathogenic proteins in neurodegenerative disorders. J Cell Mol Med. 2012;16(6):1166–83.
32. Gupta MK, Jayaram S, Madugundu AK, Chavan S, Advani J, Pandey A, et al. Chromosome-centric human proteome project: deciphering proteins associated with glioma and neurodegenerative disorders on chromosome 12. J Proteome Res. 2014;13(7):3178–90.
33. Dorner D, Funke J. Complex problem solving: what it is and what it is not. Front Psychol. 2017;8:1153.
34. Fischer A, Neubert JC. The multiple faces of complex problems: a model of problem solving competency and its implications for training and assessment. J Dyn Decis Making. 2016;1(6):1–13.
35. Alchihabi A, Ekmekci O, Kivilcim BB, Newman SD, Yarman Vural FT. Analyzing complex problem solving by dynamic brain networks. Front Neuroinform. 2021;15:670052.
36. Dodd WS, Laurent D, Dumont AS, Hasan DM, Jabbour PM, Starke RM, et al. Pathophysiology of delayed cerebral ischemia after subarachnoid hemorrhage: a review. J Am Heart Assoc. 2021;10(15):e021845.
37. Funke J, Fischer A, Holt DV. When less is less: solving multiple simple problems is not complex problem solving—a comment on Greiff et al. (2015). J Intell. 2017;5(1):5.
38. Jia Z, Li X, Yan Y, Shen X, Wang J, Yang H, et al. Exploring the relationship between age and prognosis in glioma: rethinking current age stratification. BMC Neurol. 2022;22(1):350.
39. Aiyappa-Maudsley R, Chalmers AJ, Parsons JL. Factors affecting the radiation response in glioblastoma. Neurooncol Adv. 2022;4(1):vdac156.
40. Davis ME. Glioblastoma: overview of disease and treatment. Clin J Oncol Nurs. 2016;20(5 Suppl):S2–8.
41. Abedi AA, Grunnet K, Christensen IJ, Michaelsen SR, Muhic A, Moller S, et al. A prognostic model for glioblastoma patients treated with standard therapy based on a prospective cohort of consecutive non-selected patients from a single institution. Front Oncol. 2021;11:597587.
42. Steen PA, Newberg L, Milde JH, Michenfelder JD. Hypothermia and barbiturates: individual and combined effects on canine cerebral oxygen consumption. Anesthesiology. 1983;58(6):527–32.
43. Lipton P. Ischemic cell death in brain neurons. Physiol Rev. 1999;79(4):1431–568.
44. Jiang Y, Liu Z, Liao Y, Sun S, Dai Y, Tang Y. Ischemic stroke: from pathological mechanisms to neuroprotective strategies. Front Neurol. 2022;13:1013083.
45. Zhang TL, Zhang ZW, Lin W, Lin XR, Lin KX, Fang MC, et al. Reperfusion after hypoxia-ischemia exacerbates brain injury with compensatory activation of the anti-ferroptosis system: based on a novel rat model. Neural Regen Res. 2023;18(10):2229–36.
46. Fisher M, Feuerstein G, Howells DW, Hurn PD, Kent TA, Savitz SI, et al. Update of the stroke therapy academic industry roundtable preclinical recommendations. Stroke. 2009;40(6):2244–50.
47. Loussert-Fonta C, Stoppini L, Neuenschwander Y, Righini O, Prim D, Schmidt C, et al. Opening the black box of traumatic brain injury: a holistic approach combining human 3D neural tis-

sue and an in vitro traumatic brain injury induction device. Front Neurosci. 2023;17:1189615.
48. She HQ, Sun YF, Chen L, Xiao QX, Luo BY, Zhou HS, et al. Current analysis of hypoxic-ischemic encephalopathy research issues and future treatment modalities. Front Neurosci. 2023;17:1136500.
49. Joshi S, Agarwal S. The proposed role of optical sensing in translational stroke research. Ann N Y Acad Sci. 2010;1199:149–57.
50. Bouchard MB, Chen BR, Burgess SA, Hillman EM. Ultrafast multispectral optical imaging of cortical oxygenation, blood flow, and intracellular calcium dynamics. Opt Express. 2009;17(18):15670–8.
51. Sun R, Bouchard MB, Burgess SA, Radosevich AJ, Hillman EMC. A low-cost, portable system for high-speed multispectral optical imaging. In: Biomedical optics and 3-D imaging. Miami, FL: Optica Publishing Group; 2010.
52. Mayevsky A, Rogatsky GG. Mitochondrial function in vivo evaluated by NADH fluorescence: from animal models to human studies. Am J Physiol Cell Physiol. 2007;292(2):C615–40.
53. Bigio IJ, Mourant JR. Ultraviolet and visible spectroscopies for tissue diagnostics: fluorescence spectroscopy and elastic-scattering spectroscopy. Phys Med Biol. 1997;42(5):803–14.
54. Humeau A, Steenbergen W, Nilsson H, Stromberg T. Laser Doppler perfusion monitoring and imaging: novel approaches. Med Biol Eng Comput. 2007;45(5):421–35.
55. Bageac DV, Gershon BS, De Leacy RA. The evolution of devices and techniques in endovascular stroke therapy. Brisbane, Australia: Exon Publications; 2021. https://www.ncbi.nlm.nih.gov/books/NBK572010/.
56. Wu D, Chen J, Hussain M, Wu L, Shi J, Wu C, et al. Selective intra-arterial brain cooling improves long-term outcomes in a non-human primate model of embolic stroke: efficacy depending on reperfusion status. J Cereb Blood Flow Metab. 2020;40(7):1415–26.
57. Furuya K, Takeda H, Azhar S, McCarron RM, Chen Y, Ruetzler CA, et al. Examination of several potential mechanisms for the negative outcome in a clinical stroke trial of enlimomab, a murine anti-human intercellular adhesion molecule-1 antibody: a bedside-to-bench study. Stroke. 2001;32(11):2665–74.
58. Vossen LV, Weiss M, Albanna W, Conzen-Dilger C, Schulze-Steinen H, Rossmann T, et al. Intra-arterial nimodipine for the treatment of refractory delayed cerebral ischemia after aneurysmal subarachnoid hemorrhage. J NeuroIntery Surg. 2024;2024:jnis-2023-021151.
59. Krishna R, Shah VR, Srinivas N. Pharmacokinetics and dose proportionality of BMS-204352 after intraarterial administration to rats. Biopharm Drug Dispos. 2002;23(6):233–7.
60. Sacco RL, DeRosa JT, Haley EC Jr, Levin B, Ordronneau P, Phillips SJ, et al. Glycine antagonist in neuroprotection for patients with acute stroke: GAIN Americas: a randomized controlled trial. JAMA. 2001;285(13):1719–28.
61. Lyden P, Shuaib A, Ng K, Levin K, Atkinson RP, Rajput A, et al. Clomethiazole Acute Stroke Study in ischemic stroke (CLASS-I): final results. Stroke. 2002;33(1):122–8.
62. STIPASSafety study of tirilazad mesylate in patients with acute ischemic stroke (STIPAS). Stroke. 1994;25(2):418–23.
63. Diener HC, Hacke W, Hennerici M, Rådberg J, Hantson L, De Keyser J. Lubeluzole in acute ischemic stroke. A double-blind, placebo-controlled phase II trial. Lubeluzole International Study Group. Stroke. 1996;27(1):76–81.
64. Diener HC, Lees KR, Lyden P, Grotta J, Davalos A, Davis SM, et al. NXY-059 for the treatment of acute stroke: pooled analysis of the SAINT I and II Trials. Stroke. 2008;39(6):1751–8.
65. Bogousslavsky J, Victor SJ, Salinas EO, Pallay A, Donnan GA, Fieschi C, et al. Fiblast (Trafermin) in acute stroke: results of the European-Australian phase II/III safety and efficacy trial. Cerebrovasc Dis. 2002;14(3–4):239–51.
66. Papagianni M, Tziomalos K, Kostaki S, Angelopoulou SM, Christou K, Bouziana SD, et al. Treatment with mannitol is associated with increased risk for in-hospital mortality in patients with acute ischemic stroke and cerebral edema. Am J Cardiovasc Drugs. 2018;18(5):397–403.
67. Chu C, Jablonska A, Gao Y, Lan X, Lesniak WG, Liang Y, et al. Hyperosmolar blood-brain barrier opening using intra-arterial injection of hyperosmotic mannitol in mice under real-time MRI guidance. Nat Protoc. 2022;17(1):76–94.
68. Nagao S, Kitaoka T, Fujita K, Kuyama H, Ohkawa M. Effect of tris-(hydroxymethyl)-aminomethane on experimental focal cerebral ischemia. Exp Brain Res. 1996;111(1):51–6.
69. Bon P, Cognet L. On some current challenges in high-resolution optical bioimaging. ACS Photon. 2022;9(8):2538–46.
70. Joshi S, Meyers PM, Ornstein E. Intracarotid delivery of drugs: the potential and the pitfalls. Anesthesiology. 2008;109(3):543–64.
71. Lemke G. Biology of the TAM receptors. Cold Spring Harb Perspect Biol. 2013;5(11):a009076.
72. Lemke G. Phosphatidylserine is the signal for TAM receptors and their ligands. Trends Biochem Sci. 2017;42(9):738–48.
73. Barth ND, Marwick JA, Vendrell M, Rossi AG, Dransfield I. The "phagocytic synapse" and clearance of apoptotic cells. Front Immunol. 2017;8:1708.
74. Kurnaeva MA, Zalevsky AO, Arifulin EA, Lisitsyna OM, Tvorogova AV, Shubina MY, et al. Molecular coevolution of nuclear and nucleolar localization signals inside basic domain of HIV-1 Tat. bioRxiv. 2021; https://doi.org/10.1101/2021.04.20.440437.
75. Herve F, Ghinea N, Scherrmann JM. CNS delivery via adsorptive transcytosis. AAPS J. 2008;10(3):455–72.
76. Herce HD, Garcia AE. Molecular dynamics simulations suggest a mechanism for translocation of the HIV-1 TAT peptide across lipid membranes. Proc Natl Acad Sci U S A. 2007;104(52):20805–10.
77. Rizzuti M, Nizzardo M, Zanetta C, Ramirez A, Corti S. Therapeutic applications of the cell-penetrating HIV-1 Tat peptide. Drug Discov Today. 2015;20(1):76–85.
78. Rusiecka I, Gągało I, Kocić I. Cell-penetrating peptides improve pharmacokinetics and pharmacodynamics of anticancer drugs. Tissue Barrier. 2022;10(1):1965418.
79. Joshi S, Cooke JRN, Ellis JA, Emala CW, Bruce JN. Targeting brain tumors by intra-arterial delivery of cell-penetrating peptides: a novel approach for primary and metastatic brain malignancy. J Neurooncol. 2017;135(3):497–506.
80. Nguyen J, Hossain SS, Cooke JRN, Ellis JA, Deci MB, Emala CW, et al. Flow arrest intra-arterial delivery of small TAT-decorated and neutral micelles to gliomas. J Neurooncol. 2017;133(1):77–85.
81. Sun HS, Doucette TA, Liu Y, Fang Y, Teves L, Aarts M, et al. Effectiveness of PSD95 inhibitors in permanent and transient focal ischemia in the rat. Stroke. 2008;39(9):2544–53.
82. Xu Y, Xu L, Xu C, Zhao M, Xu T, Xia L, et al. PSD-95 inhibitor Tat-NR2B9c (NA-1) protects the integrity of the blood-brain barrier after transient middle artery occlusion in rats by downregulating matrix metalloprotease-9 and upregulating endothelial nitric oxide synthase. Brain Res Bull. 2024;206:110836.
83. Tu W, Xu X, Peng L, Zhong X, Zhang W, Soundarapandian MM, et al. DAPK1 interaction with NMDA receptor NR2B subunits mediates brain damage in stroke. Cell. 2010;140(2):222–34.
84. Wang X, Pei L, Yan H, Wang Z, Wei N, Wang S, et al. Intervention of death-associated protein kinase 1-p53 interaction exerts the therapeutic effects against stroke. Stroke. 2014;45(10):3089–91.
85. Zhang S, Taghibiglou C, Girling K, Dong Z, Lin SZ, Lee W, et al. Critical role of increased PTEN nuclear translocation in excitotoxic and ischemic neuronal injuries. J Neurosci. 2013;33(18):7997–8008.
86. Weilinger NL, Tang PL, Thompson RJ. Anoxia-induced NMDA receptor activation opens pannexin channels via Src family kinases. J Neurosci. 2012;32(36):12579–88.

87. Gamir-Morralla A, Lopez-Menendez C, Ayuso-Dolado S, Tejeda GS, Montaner J, Rosell A, et al. Development of a neuroprotective peptide that preserves survival pathways by preventing Kidins220/ARMS calpain processing induced by excitotoxicity. Cell Death Dis. 2015;6(10):e1939.
88. Deb I, Manhas N, Poddar R, Rajagopal S, Allan AM, Lombroso PJ, et al. Neuroprotective role of a brain-enriched tyrosine phosphatase, STEP, in focal cerebral ischemia. J Neurosci. 2013;33(45):17814–26.
89. Wang W, Han P, Xie R, Yang M, Zhang C, Mi Q, et al. TAT-mGluR1 attenuation of neuronal apoptosis through prevention of MGluR1alpha truncation after experimental subarachnoid hemorrhage. ACS Chem Neurosci. 2019;10(1):746–56.
90. Guven G, Dijkstra A, Kuijper TM, Trommel N, van Baar ME, Topeli A, et al. Comparison of laser speckle contrast imaging with laser Doppler perfusion imaging for tissue perfusion measurement. Microcirculation. 2023;30(1):e12795.
91. Teng CW, Huang V, Arguelles GR, Zhou C, Cho SS, Harmsen S, et al. Applications of indocyanine green in brain tumor surgery: review of clinical evidence and emerging technologies. Neurosurg Focus. 2021;50(1):E4.
92. Qiu T, Lan Y, Gao W, Zhou M, Liu S, Huang W, et al. Photoacoustic imaging as a highly efficient and precise imaging strategy for the evaluation of brain diseases. Quant Imaging Med Surg. 2021;11(5):2169–86.
93. Navot B, Hecht EM, Lim RP, Edelman RR, Koktzoglou I. MR angiography series: fundamentals of non-contrast-enhanced MR angiography. Radiographics. 2021;41(5):E157–E8.
94. Hartung MP, Grist TM, Francois CJ. Magnetic resonance angiography: current status and future directions. J Cardiovasc Magn Reson. 2011;13(1):19.
95. De Visscher G, Haseldonckx M, Flameng W. Fluorescent microsphere technique to measure cerebral blood flow in the rat. Nat Protoc. 2006;1(4):2162–70.
96. Jahng GH, Li KL, Ostergaard L, Calamante F. Perfusion magnetic resonance imaging: a comprehensive update on principles and techniques. Korean J Radiol. 2014;15(5):554–77.
97. Yu Y, Zhang K, Zhang L, Zong H, Meng L, Han R. Cerebral near-infrared spectroscopy (NIRS) for perioperative monitoring of brain oxygenation in children and adults. Cochrane Database Syst Rev. 2018;1(1):CD010947.
98. van Bel F, Mintzer JP. Monitoring cerebral oxygenation of the immature brain: a neuroprotective strategy? Pediatr Res. 2018;84(2):159–64.
99. van Bel F, Mintzer JP. Correction: Monitoring cerebral oxygenation of the immature brain: a neuroprotective strategy? Pediatr Res. 2018;84(5):786.
100. Christen T, Bouzat P, Pannetier N, Coquery N, Moisan A, Lemasson B, et al. Tissue oxygen saturation mapping with magnetic resonance imaging. J Cereb Blood Flow Metab. 2014;34(9):1550–7.
101. Rietzler A, Steiger R, Mangesius S, Walchhofer LM, Gothe RM, Schocke M, et al. Energy metabolism measured by 31P magnetic resonance spectroscopy in the healthy human brain. J Neuroradiol. 2022;49(5):370–9.
102. Felber SR, Aichner FT, Sauter R, Gerstenbrand F. Combined magnetic resonance imaging and proton magnetic resonance spectroscopy of patients with acute stroke. Stroke. 1992;23(8):1106–10.
103. Swanson WB, Durdan M, Eberle M, Woodbury S, Mauser A, Gregory J, et al. A library of Rhodamine6G-based pH-sensitive fluorescent probes with versatile in vivo and in vitro applications. RSC Chem Biol. 2022;3(6):748–64.
104. Ince C, Coremans JMCC, Bruining HA. In vivo NADH fluorescence. In: Erdmann W, Bruley DF, editors. Oxygen transport to tissue XIV. Boston, MA: Springer US; 1992. p. 277–96.
105. Kariman K, Jobsis FF, Saltzman HA. Cytochrome a,a3 reoxidation. Early indicator of metabolic recovery from hemorrhagic shock in rats. J Clin Invest. 1983;72(1):180–91.
106. Skupienski R, Do KQ, Xin L. In vivo 31P magnetic resonance spectroscopy study of mouse cerebral NAD content and redox state during neurodevelopment. Sci Rep. 2020;10(1):15623.
107. Ma H, Harris S, Rahmani R, Lacefield CO, Zhao M, Daniel AG, et al. Wide-field in vivo neocortical calcium dye imaging using a convection-enhanced loading technique combined with simultaneous multiwavelength imaging of voltage-sensitive dyes and hemodynamic signals. Neurophotonics. 2014;1(1):015003.
108. Savic T, Gambino G, Bokharaie VS, Noori HR, Logothetis NK, Angelovski G. Early detection and monitoring of cerebral ischemia using calcium-responsive MRI probes. Proc Natl Acad Sci USA. 2019;116(41):20666–71.
109. Yucel MA, Selb JJ, Huppert TJ, Franceschini MA, Boas DA. Functional near infrared spectroscopy: enabling routine functional brain imaging. Curr Opin Biomed Eng. 2017;4:78–86.
110. Na S, Russin JJ, Lin L, Yuan X, Hu P, Jann KB, et al. Massively parallel functional photoacoustic computed tomography of the human brain. Nat Biomed Eng. 2022;6(5):584–92.
111. Heeger DJ, Ress D. What does fMRI tell us about neuronal activity? Nat Rev Neurosci. 2002;3(2):142–51.
112. Xu Z, Zhu Q, Wang LV. In vivo photoacoustic tomography of mouse cerebral edema induced by cold injury. J Biomed Opt. 2011;16(6):066020.
113. Rodriguez JG, Sisson C, Hendricks C, Pattillo C, McWaters M, Hardjasudarma M, et al., editors. Feasibility of using diffuse reflectance spectroscopy for the quantification of brain edema. Saratov Fall Meeting 2000: Optical Technologies in Biophysics and Medicine II; 2001.
114. Ito J, Marmarou A, Barzó P, Fatouros P, Corwin F. Characterization of edema by diffusion-weighted imaging in experimental traumatic brain injury. J Neurosurg. 1996;84(1):97–103.
115. Wardman P. Fluorescent and luminescent probes for measurement of oxidative and nitrosative species in cells and tissues: progress, pitfalls, and prospects. Free Radic Biol Med. 2007;43(7):995–1022.
116. Waddington DEJ, Sarracanie M, Salameh N, Herisson F, Ayata C, Rosen MS. An overhauser-enhanced-MRI platform for dynamic free radical imaging in vivo. NMR Biomed. 2018;31(5):e3896.
117. Kucuksayan E, Sircan-Kucuksayan A. Real-time detection of doxorubicin-induced apoptosis in breast cancer cells using the back reflection spectroscopy. Eastern J Med. 2021;26:128–34.
118. Jiang X, McKinley ET, Xie J, Li H, Xu J, Gore JC. In vivo magnetic resonance imaging of treatment-induced apoptosis. Sci Rep. 2019;9(1):9540.
119. Sanchez GM, Burridge AL. Decision making in head injury management in the Edwin Smith Papyrus. Neurosurg Focus. 2007;23(1):E5.

Index

S. Joshi (ed.), *Arterial Treatment of Neurological Diseases*, https://doi.org/10.1007/978-3-031-80173-0

Y

Z

GPSR Compliance

The European Union's (EU) General Product Safety Regulation (GPSR) is a set of rules that requires consumer products to be safe and our obligations to ensure this.

If you have any concerns about our products, you can contact us on ProductSafety@springernature.com

In case Publisher is established outside the EU, the EU authorized representative is:

Springer Nature Customer Service Center GmbH
Europaplatz 3
69115 Heidelberg, Germany

Batch number: 08452568

Printed by Printforce, the Netherlands